World Scientific Handbook of Global Health Economics and Public Policy

❸ Health System Characteristics and Performance

World Scientific Series in Global Health Economics and Public Policy

ISSN: 2010-2089

Published:

Vol. 1 Accountability and Responsibility in Health Care:
Issues in Addressing an Emerging Global Challenge
edited by Bruce Rosen, Avi Israeli and Stephen Shortell

Vol. 2 The Economics of Social Capital and Health:
A Conceptual and Empirical Roadmap
edited by Sherman Folland and Lorenzo Rocco

Vol. 3 World Scientific Handbook of Global Health Economics and Public Policy
edited by Richard M Scheffler

World Scientific Series in Global Health Economics and Public Policy – Vol. 3

World Scientific Handbook of Global Health Economics and Public Policy

❸ Health System Characteristics and Performance

Edited by

Richard M. Scheffler

University of California, Berkeley, USA

World Scientific

NEW JERSEY • LONDON • SINGAPORE • BEIJING • SHANGHAI • HONG KONG • TAIPEI • CHENNAI • TOKYO

Published by

World Scientific Publishing Co. Pte. Ltd.
5 Toh Tuck Link, Singapore 596224
USA office: 27 Warren Street, Suite 401-402, Hackensack, NJ 07601
UK office: 57 Shelton Street, Covent Garden, London WC2H 9HE

Library of Congress Cataloging-in-Publication Data
Names: Scheffler, Richard M., editor.
Title: World Scientific handbook of global health economics and public policy /
[edited by] Richard M. Scheffler.
Other titles: Handbook of global health economics and public policy
Description: New Jersey : World Scientific, 2016. | Includes bibliographical references and index.
Identifiers: LCCN 2015040481| ISBN 9789814612319 (set : alk. paper) |
ISBN 9789814612340 (v. 1 : alk. paper) | ISBN 9789814612357 (v. 2 : alk. paper) |
ISBN 9789814612364 (v. 3 : alk. paper)
Subjects: | MESH: Economics, Medical. | Delivery of Health Care. | Global Health. |
Health Policy. | Quality of Health Care. | Social Determinants of Health.
Classification: LCC RA410.5 | NLM W 74.1 | DDC 338.4/73621--dc23
LC record available at http://lccn.loc.gov/2015040481

British Library Cataloguing-in-Publication Data
A catalogue record for this book is available from the British Library.

In-house Editors: Herbert Moses/Li Hongyan

Typeset by Stallion Press
Email: enquiries@stallionpress.com

Printed in Singapore

Acknowledgment

Jessica Foster was my editorial assistant and partner. She helped me in every way possible. I am very grateful to her. Kati Phillips made the handbook happen. She handled all the details and coordinated all the moving parts without missing a beat. Finally, I would like to thank Zvi Ruder. He worked hard over a long period of time to convince me that the handbook could be done. He was so right.

—Dr. Richard M. Scheffler

Contents

Acknowledgment v

About the Editor ix

List of Contributors xi

Introduction to Volume 3 xix
Richard M. Scheffler

Hospital Quality and Performance Around the Globe 1
Barbara McPake

Global Human Resources for Health 55
Joanne Spetz, Michelle Tellez, and Brent Fulton

Impact and Costs of Pharmaceuticals and Biotechnology 107
Panos Kanavos

Technological Innovation in Health Care: A Global Perspective 189
Sheila Smith

Primary Care: Effectiveness and Costs 231
Tor Iversen

Health Systems Performance 269
Peter Berman

Pay for Performance in Health Systems: Theory, Evidence and Case Studies 295
Jed Friedman and Richard M Scheffler

Medical Tourism 333
Johanna Hanefeld, Richard Smith, and Thinakorn Noree

Public–Private Partnerships 351
Pedro Pita Barros and Rui Sousa Monteiro

Translational Health Economics 405
Wolf Rogowski, Jürgen John, and Maarten IJzerman

Index 441

About the Editor

Richard M. Scheffler is Distinguished Professor of Health Economics and Public Policy at the School of Public Health and the Goldman School of Public Policy at the University of California, Berkeley and holds the endowed Chair in Healthcare Markets and Consumer Welfare. In 2003 Dr. Scheffler served as the elected president of the International Health Economics Association. He has been a visiting professor at a number of universities including the London School of Economics, Charles University in Prague, at the Department of Economics at the University of Pompeu Fabra in Barcelona and at Carlos III University of Madrid, Spain. Dr. Scheffler has been a visiting scholar at the World Bank, the Rockefeller Foundation in Bellagio, and the Institute of Medicine at the National Academy of Sciences. He has been a consultant for the World Bank, the WHO, and the OECD. Professor Scheffler has been a Fulbright Scholar at Pontifica Universidad Catolica de Chile in Santiago, Chile, and at Charles University, Prague, Czech Republic. He was also awarded the Chair of Excellence Award at the Carlos III University of Madrid in 2013. In 2015 Dr. Scheffler was awarded the Gold Medal for Charles University in Prague for his longstanding and continued support of international scientific and educational collaboration. He earned his PhD in economics with honors at New York University.

List of Contributors

(Author bios are listed as per the Chapter order)

Barbara McPake is a health economist specializing in health policy and health systems research. She has 25 years of experience in these areas based in three UK university departments. She is currently Director, Institute for International Health and Development, Queen Margaret University, Edinburgh and one of two Research Directors of 'REBUILD' a UK Department for International Development funded Research Programme Consortium on health systems development. She was formerly (2001–2006) Programme Director, Health Systems Development Knowledge Programme. She has extensive research degree supervision and other postgraduate teaching experience and extensive international experience in health systems research and policy analysis and advice to UN agencies and low- and middle-income country governments.

Joanne Spetz is a Professor at the Institute for Health Policy Studies and Associate Director for Research at the Healthforce Center at the University of California, San Francisco. She is a Professor in the Department of Family and Community Medicine and the School of Nursing, and the Director of the UCSF Health Workforce Research Center on Long-Term Care. She has conducted research on health care labor markets, education, and practice for more than 20 years. Dr Spetz has been the Principal Investigator of national and state surveys of registered nurses and nursing schools, and led research on the quality of hospital nursing care, organization of the hospital industry, impact of health information technology, effect of medical marijuana policy on youth substance use, and quality of patient care. Dr Spetz was a member of the Institute of Medicine Standing Committee on Credentialing Research in Nursing and was a consultant to the Institute of Medicine Committee on the Future of Nursing. She is an Honorary Fellow of the American Academy of Nursing.

Michelle Téllez is Associate Professor of Nursing and Health Science at the College of Science at the California State University, East Bay. She has been a visiting Professor at the School of Nursing at the University of Sao Paulo, Brazil. Dr Téllez was a Betty Irene Moore Fellow at the University of California, San Francisco. She has conducted research in the labor supply of nurses in California. She is presently working on a project for the University Hospital of Sao Paulo (Brazil) evaluating how nurses use health information technology.

Brent Fulton is an Assistant Adjunct Professor of Health Economics and Public Policy, Division of Health Policy and Management, School of Public Health at University of California, Berkeley. He is the Associate Director of the Nicholas C Petris Center on Health Care Markets and Consumer Welfare and the Global Center for Health Economics and Policy Research. His current research areas include health reform, health insurance markets (rate review regulation, risk adjustment and reinsurance), the healthcare workforce (task shifting and pay for performance in the US and globally), mental health (attention-deficit/hyperactivity disorder treatments and disparities), and oral health care (disparities). Brent received his doctorate in public policy analysis from the Pardee RAND Graduate School and his MBA from The Anderson School at UCLA.

Panos Kanavos is Associate Professor in International Health Policy in the Department of Social Policy, London School of Economics and Political Science (LSE), Programme Director of the Medical Technology Research Group and Deputy Director at LSE Health. He has previously been Harkness Fellow in Health Care Policy in the Department of Ambulatory Care and Prevention, Harvard Medical School, and has held visiting appointments at the University of Lausanne, the University of Basel, the London School of Hygiene and Tropical Medicine and the University of Delaware. An economist by training, he currently coordinates the Programme in International Health Policy at LSE. He has acted as an advisor to a number of international governmental and nongovernmental organizations, including the European Commission, the European Parliament, the World Bank, the World Health Organization, the Organization for Economic Co-operation and Development, the American Association for Retired Persons, and Ministries of Health of over 28 transition and developing countries.

Panos' research interests include comparative health policy and healthcare reform, pharmaceutical economics and policy from a developed and developing country perspective, quality and access in healthcare, and socio-economic determinants of health.

Sheila Smith is a Senior Economist with the Office of the Actuary at the Centers for Medicare and Medicaid Services (CMS). She is the principle economist responsible for the development of the Factors Contributions to Growth (FCG) Model (with Mark Freeland). This model was recommended by the 2010–2011 Medicare Technical Panel for use in long-term projections of Medicare spending, and currently plays a key role in determining projections of Medicare spending in the annual reports of the Medicare Boards of Trustees to Congress on the financial status of the Medicare program. She also led the original process of development of the CMS National Health Expenditures (NHE) 10-Year Projections Model. Her current research addresses issues of long-term structural change in international markets for health care, and interaction effects between technological change and demographic change for long-term growth in health spending.

Prior to joining CMS in 1998, Ms Smith was the senior health economist for the Cost Information Service of Standard and Poors'/DRI (now Global Insights). She holds an MA in Economics from the University of Virginia.

Tor Iversen is an economist with specialization in health economics. He was one of the initiators of the Health Economics Research Program at the University of Oslo (HERO) and from 2006 research director for HERO. He has had research stays at the University of York, England and the University of California, Berkeley. Iversen's primary interest is the impact of market conditions and economic instruments in the health sector. Projects under work include the interaction between primary health care and specialist health services, economic incentives in long-term care, relationships between social capital and health and comparisons of treatment outcomes and costs across regions and countries. Internationally, he has cooperation with universities and researchers in Europe, the US and China. Iversen is Associate Editor of Health Economics, member of the editorial team of Nordic Journal of Health Economics and member of the editorial board of the International Journal of Health Economics and Management.

Peter Berman is a health economist with 40 years of experience in research, policy analysis and development, and training and education in global health. He is currently Professor of the Practice of Global Health Systems and Economics at Harvard T. H. Chan School of Public Health. Professor Berman is also Faculty Director of the Harvard DrPH and Coordinator of Harvard Chan's India Health Partnership. He is Visiting Professor at the Public Health Foundation of India, New Delhi and advisor to the China National Health Development Research Center for health care financing and health accounts. His current research focuses on health financing, system reform, and primary care development in Ethiopia, India, and Malaysia.

From 2004–2011, Professor Berman worked with World Bank as Lead Economist. He worked in the HNP anchor department and was Practice Leader for the World Bank's Health Systems Global Expert Team from 2008 to 2011. From

2004–2008, he was based in the World Bank's New Delhi office as Lead Economist for Health, Nutrition, and Population in India.

Jed Friedman is a senior economist in the Poverty and Inequality Unit of the Development Research Group at the World Bank. His research interests include the measurement of poverty dynamics and the interactions between poverty and health. Jed holds a BA in Philosophy from Stanford University and a PhD in Economics from the University of Michigan. Before joining the World Bank in 2003, Jed worked at the RAND Corporation. His previous work has appeared in the *Review of Economics and Statistics*, the *Journal of Development Economics*, and the *American Journal of Public Health*, among other outlets. Jed is currently the principal investigator for impact evaluations on: the effectiveness of malaria control programs in India, Nigeria, and Zambia; national health financing reforms in Kyrgyzstan, Zambia, and Zimbabwe; and conditional cash transfers in the Philippines.

Richard M. Scheffler is Distinguished Professor of Health Economics and Public Policy at the School of Public Health and the Goldman School of Public Policy at the University of California, Berkeley and holds the endowed Chair in Healthcare Markets and Consumer Welfare. In 2003 Dr. Scheffler served as the elected president of the International Health Economics Association. He has been a visiting professor at a number of universities including the London School of Economics, Charles University in Prague, at the Department of Economics at the University of Pompeu Fabra in Barcelona and at Carlos III University of Madrid, Spain. Dr. Scheffler has been a visiting scholar at the World Bank, the Rockefeller Foundation in Bellagio, and the Institute of Medicine at the National Academy of Sciences. He has been a consultant for the World Bank, the WHO, and the OECD. Professor Scheffler has been a Fulbright Scholar at Pontifica Universidad Catolica de Chile in Santiago, Chile, and at Charles University, Prague, Czech Republic. He was also awarded the Chair of Excellence Award at the Carlos III University of Madrid in 2013. In 2015 Dr. Scheffler was awarded the Gold Medal for Charles University in Prague for his longstanding and continued support of international scientific and educational collaboration. He earned his PhD in economics with honors at New York University.

Johanna Hanefeld is Lecturer in Health Systems Economics in the department of Global Health and Development focusing on trade and health, health systems, governance, and quantitative and qualitative policy analysis mainly in low- and middle-income countries. Together with Professor Richard Smith and colleagues at the University of York, UK she recently completed a large research project examining the impact of medical tourism on the UK NHS. She is co-editor of the forthcoming *Edward Elgar Handbook on Medical Tourism and Patient Mobility*.

Richard Smith is Professor of Health System Economics and Dean of the Faculty of Public Health and Policy at the London School of Hygiene & Tropical Medicine. Following undergraduate and postgraduate studies in economics at the University of York, Richard worked in Sydney, Cambridge, Bristol, Melbourne and Norwich, before joining the School in 2007. Richard has held various other appointments, including honorary posts at the Universities of Hong Kong and East Anglia, Associate Fellow at The Royal Institute of International Affairs, and editorial roles for journals including Health Economics, the Journal of Public Health and Globalization and Health. He has also acted as an expert advisor for a number of international bodies, including the World Health Organization, World Trade Organization, World Economic Forum and OECD, as well as several national government departments.

Richard's research has covered a number of areas of health economics, in recent years focusing upon developing the methods for macro-economic analysis of health, the economics of globalization and health, and aspects of trade in health goods, services, people and ideas. Richard has received over £30 million in grant income, published five books, more than 100 journal papers, and dozens of other works.

Thinakorn Noree is a researcher at the International Health Policy Program of the Ministry of — Thailand. He worked as general practitioner and hospital director in rural Thailand for 12 years before moving to the Thai Ministry of Public Health in 2005. His research focuses on human resources for health. He received his PhD from the London School of Hygiene and Tropical Medicine with a thesis focused on the impact of medical tourism on the domestic economy and private health system: A case study of Thailand.

Pedro Pita Barros is Professor of Economics at Universidade Nova de Lisboa. He is also a member of the Expert Panel on Effective Ways of Investing in Health at the European Commission and a research fellow at the Centre for Economic Policy Research (London). Pedro's research focuses on health economics and on regulation and competition policy, covering different topics including: health expenditure determinants, waiting lists, bargaining in health care, competition policy in Portugal and in the European Union, among others. His research has appeared in many academic journals, and he has contributed to several books on health economics. Recent publications include the *Handbook of Health Economics Vol II* (co-edited with Mark Pauly and Tom McGuire) and *Health Economics — An IO*

Perspective (co-authored with Xavier Martinez-Giralt). He has served as Member of the Board of the Portuguese Energy Regulator (2005/2006), on the Governmental Commission for the Financial Sustainability of the National Health Service (2006/2007) and on the National Council of Financial Supervisors (2014/2015). He has consulted for both private and public entities, in Portugal and at the European level, in the areas of health economics, competition policy and economic regulation.

Rui Sousa Monteiro joined the World Bank as Senior Public-Private Partnerships Specialist in 2010, after having been for more than 10 years PPP advisor to the Treasury Secretary and representative of the Finance Minister of Portugal in steering committees and tender boards for several major rail, tram, highway and health PPP projects and public tenders, including six PPP-hospital contracts (four of them including the provision of clinical services) and several highways and high-speed rail lines. Furthermore, he sat on (re)negotiation committees and provided training and support for PPP contract managers and the Court of Auditors. Prior to his Ministry of Finance activities, he did applied research on fiscal matters and on large public projects (urban renewal, public infrastructure). In the international field, Rui has an extensive experience in bilateral cooperation with many governments in Europe, Africa, Asia and the Americas, including field missions for institutional diagnosis regarding infrastructure procurement reform and PPP project development. He has been an active member of several PPP networks. As an economist, he puts strong emphasis on the use of incentive contracts and competitive schemes.

Wolf Rogowski is a health economist at the Helmholtz Center Munich, Institute of Health Economics and Health Care Management in Germany. Since August 2009, he heads the institute's research unit "Translational Health Economics". He holds a PhD from Ludwig-Maximilians Universität in Munich and has held visiting fellowships at the Centre of Health Economics at the University of York, the Hastings Center in Garrison, New York and the Harvard School of Public Health. Wolf explores the process of translational medicine from a health economics perspective. This includes: the application of cost-effectiveness and value of information analysis to new health technologies; the empirical and theoretical assessment of methods and procedures applied in decision making; and the development of instruments for decision support. He has a particular interest in the intersection of ethics and economics in medical innovation. Wolf serves as a member of the European Society for Human Genetics' Professional and Public Policy Committee and the scientific advisory board of the *Journal of Community* Genetics. He teaches health economics, health systems analysis and health care business planning at the Ludwig Maximilians University, Munich, Germany.

Jürgen John is an economist with more than 30 years of experience in research, teaching and consulting in the area of health economics. Until his retirement, he was head of the research unit for health systems analysis and deputy director of the Institute of Health Economics and Health Care Management at the German National Center for Environmental Health, Munich. He received his MA from the University of Heidelberg and his PhD from the Ludwig Maximilian University Munich.

Jürgen's research interests include economics of obesity, equity in health and health care, economics of prevention, and methods of economic evaluation in health care. He teaches health economics and methods of health services and health care evaluation research at the Ludwig Maximilian University Munich and universities of applied sciences in Germany and Austria.

Maarten IJzerman is full professor and head of the department of Health Technology & Services Research (HTSR) of the University of Twente. He has received an MSc in Biomedical Health Science from the Medical School at the University of Nijmegen in 1993 and a PhD at the MIRA institute for biomedical engineering and technical medicine in 1997. He is a board registered clinical epidemiologist. He has worked as research fellow at the Vrije Universiteit Medical Centre, dept. Rehabilitation Medicine. In March 2000 he became scientific director of Roessingh Research and Development. Between 2007 and 2012, he was the Program Director Health Sciences, with tracks in Health Technology Assessment and Health Services & Management. He has more than 130 peer-reviewed articles in the intersection of engineering, medicine and outcomes research. Known for his interest in translational research and technology development, most of his work is on applying and developing outcomes research methods to early stages of development. Maarten has an adjunct position as clinical professor of PM&R at Case Western Reserve University. Since February 2013, he is project leader at CRP-Santé in Luxemburg responsible for initiating and developing a center for health economics and personalized medicine.

Introduction to Volume 3: Health System Characteristics and Performance

Richard M. Scheffler
Distinguished Professor of Health Economics and Public Policy
Director of the Global Center for Health Economics and Policy Research
University of California, Berkeley

Chapter 1 in this volume, *Hospital Quality and Performance Around the Globe*, looks at the issues of hospital quality and performance globally. There is vast evidence that shows that there is a huge variation between cost and quality around the globe, and little reliable empirical evidence of why this is the case. This chapter carefully examines new empirical evidence and economic indicators. Specifically, it addresses the issue of the performance of hospitals in LMICs and the factors that improved quality and performance. Chapter 2 explains why human resources are a key factor in the performance of health care systems. The shortages of health care workers globally, and especially in LMICs, is a major problem. Chapter 2, *Global Human Resources for Health*, lays out an economic framework of supply and demand and the factors that impact them. It then looks on the role of the public, private sector, and donor organizations in planning to eliminate the shortage of human resources and its misdistribution.

Pharmaceutical expenditures around the globe range from one-third to one-sixth of the health care spending in OECD and emerging countries, which is the second largest part of health budgets after salaries. Pharmaceutical markets are complicated and have a multiple stakeholders, oligopolistic structure, as well as imperfect information and agency problems, which lead to inefficiencies in the cost of and access to drugs. Chapter 3, *Impact and Costs of Pharmaceuticals and Biotechnology*, looks at the role of governments and insurers and their role in the pharmaceutical market. The chapter demonstrates a mix of public and private policies that can be used to limit the increase in pharmaceutical prices and expenditures. Like pharmaceuticals, technology is understood to be a major input in the improvement of health and has a major impact on global spending on health. Chapter 4, *Technological Innovation in Health Care: A Global Perspective*, describes the relationship between health policy, medical innovation, and health care spending from a global perspective. Recent impact of medical technology on health spending across a broad range of countries and time periods has been declining. A causal link is difficult to explicitly demonstrate, but it does show that it has important implications on health care spending and coverage.

A key ingredient in all health care systems is the organization and payment of primary care. Chapter 5, *Primary Care: Effectiveness and Costs*, looks at two constructs of the financing of primary care — one in countries that have a low density of physicians. In this framework, the payment system does not greatly influence the volume of health services provided to each patient. In another framework with a high density of primary care physicians, it asserts that fee-for-service is a better measure to encourage a more service-oriented practice style than capitation. Empirical examples are given to assess this policy.

Chapters 6–7 deal with the issues of health system performance and methods to improve it. Chapter 6, *Health Systems Performance*, discusses the conceptual and empirical issues and developments in examining the health systems performance. It addresses the key issue of what determines performance in health systems and differences in performance between and within countries. The authors look at key elements impacting performance as well as the role of consumers and providers. Chapter 7, *Pay for Performance in Health Systems: Theory, Evidence, and Case Studies*, examines the expanded use of the pay for performance (P4P) payment system. Pay for performance is the fastest growing new payment system being used throughout the globe. It is used to increase efficiency and quality of health care systems. They are generally designed with the following elements in mind: measurement, performance, form of reward, and the basis of the reward (financial and non-financial). P4P systems are quite prevalent in OECD countries, as detailed in this chapter, though the evidence on their impact is still emerging. The chapter also looks at selected low-income countries where P4P is used to strengthen the health care system.

Chapters 8–10 begins by looking at the rising trend of medical tourism, where patients travel long distances to receive medical care. Chapter 8, *Medical Tourism*, looks at the issue of medical tourism, specific patterns, and the rise of south-to-south medical tourism, along with the mechanism that is causing it. The authors point out that there are no regulations or accepted standards, and the data that examines the impact on health outcomes is extremely limited. The authors use

Thailand and the UK as case examples of countries with large amounts of medical tourism. Chapter 9 goes on to discuss limited resources in the health care sector, particularly for the building of new facilities. This has led hospitals, as well as other parts of the health care delivery system, to turn to the use of public–private partnerships. Many of these partnerships are controversial and have risks and challenges. These are carefully explained in Chapter 9, *Public–Private Partnerships*, which details the use of optimal incentives and the transfer of risk from the public sector to the private sector. It lays out specific policies and programs to improve the functioning and use of public–private partnerships in health care. The volume concludes with Chapter 10 on Translational Medicine (*Translational Health Economics*). Translational Medicine is a new field in health economics, which uses theoretical concepts and empirical methods to bridge the gap between the decision to fund and use a health technology in clinical practice and the decision to invest in its development. It seeks to analyze how to value medical technology and its eventual use in the health care sector. It confronts the issue of uncertainty, motivation and cooperation, in institutions that seek to implement new technologies. The integrated approach to Translational Medicine provides a linkage between the health care business perspective and the translation of new technologies in the health care system.

Hospital Quality and Performance Around the Globe

Barbara McPake
Nossal Institute for Global Health
University of Melbourne School of Population and Global Health

The issues of hospital quality and performance have always received significant attention, at least in part because hospitals absorb large shares of health sector resources. Yet there is wide variation in quality and performance across hospitals globally, with concerns about shortfalls expressed in public and political debates in most countries of the world. Ensuring high quality and good performance is challenging even in the best resourced systems and is a considerably difficult task for the least well-resourced ones. This chapter examines hospital quality and performance through an empirical and economic lens. It addresses levels of hospital quality and performance in low- and middle-income countries; the factors that influence the hospital quality and performance; and strategies to improve hospital quality and performance and their practical applications.

Keywords: Hospital Quality; Performance; Efficiency; Equity; Access Reform.

Introduction

The boundaries of what constitutes a hospital are poorly defined. The World Health Organization (WHO) defines hospitals as '*health care institutions that have an organized medical and other professional staff, and inpatient facilities, and deliver medical, nursing and related services 24 hours per day, 7 days per week*'.[1] Within most health systems, the hospital is often at one end of a spectrum of health service providing institutions that can reach from small to large, community-based to centralized, low- to high-technology, or general to specialized care. Looking globally

[1] http://www.who.int/topics/hospitals/en/

across health systems, institutions known as hospitals span a large part of that spectrum and are therefore a highly heterogenous collection of institutions, with shifting boundaries between hospitals and other types of health care-providing institutions, such as health centers or long-term care facilities for the elderly. Nor can hospitals be clearly defined as covering the activities only within their physical boundaries, as extension to provision of off-site services becomes more common and the idea of 'hospitals without walls' has been advanced (McKee and Healy, 2002).

Medical practice and, in consequence, the role and nature of this collection of institutions, are subject to constant change responding to changes in populations, patterns of disease, opportunities for medical interventions, and public and political expectations (Healy and McKee, 2002). Some changes appear to be long-term trends over large parts of the globe. Technology is enabling less invasive intervention and allowing for better supported primary care and home-based convalescence, and necessary lengths of hospital stays are shortening. In Western European countries, numbers of hospital beds have been declining, and numbers of hospitals themselves have been declining even faster as hospital functions become increasingly specialized and are thought to require greater concentration and centralization to be delivered effectively (although Ahgren (2008) makes the case that this belief is based on remarkably little research evidence).

Changes in populations, patterns of disease, opportunities for medical interventions, and public and political expectations vary from country to country. For example, while population aging is occurring globally, one source of global demographic data lists 88 countries as having more than 30% of their population under the age of 15[2]; Niger is reported to have 52% of its population under the age of 15. The epidemiological transition is occurring globally, but many countries are still characterized by a burden of disease dominated by infectious conditions (Lozano *et al.*., 2012). The economic benefits of applying new medical technologies, and thus the likelihood of adoption, depend on the relative costs of those technologies versus the labor or other inputs to health service provision that they substitute; the cost-effectiveness levels required for inclusion in publicly financed service packages; and their affordability to users of private systems. All these factors weigh in favor of a slower pace of change in lower-income economies than higher. Hospitals and the political systems within which they operate also resist change for a number of reasons (Farrington-Douglas and Brooks, 2007), implying that the extent to which change occurs is in part dependent on the ability of those systems to adapt to providing secure health and medical benefits for their populations through reform. Nevertheless, the pressures and rationale for change have much in common across the world given the common directions of population, epidemiological, and technological change.

---

[2] http://kff.org/global-indicator/population-under-age-15/.

The issues of hospital quality and performance have always received significant attention, at least in part because hospitals absorb large shares of health sector resources. McKee and Healy (2002) indicate that they absorb about 50% of health care budgets in Western European countries and 70% or more in Eastern European ones. Hanson *et al.* (2002) report evidence from the early 1990s that in Sub-Saharan African countries, levels may be similar to those suggested in Eastern Europe, with two hospitals alone in Malawi consuming 40% of the public health budget; four in Zimbabwe consuming 45%; and three in Zambia consuming 30%. More recently, Oxfam (2014) has described a single hospital project in Lesotho as consuming 51% of the public health budget, although that appears to be a special case.

The importance of ensuring that such large volumes of resource are well used is clear. This chapter focuses on hospital quality and performance, where the word 'quality' is used to mean high standards of service delivery for the services made available, and the word 'performance' is used to reflect the many dimensions of efficiency, including the appropriateness of the mix of available services and the extent to which the resources used to provide those services are adequate and used without waste. Ambiguities remain in both of these definitions, but these broad concepts will be further explored and defined in the following sections.

There is wide variation in quality and performance across hospitals globally, with concerns about shortfalls expressed in public and political debates in most countries of the world. Ensuring high quality and good performance challenges even the best resourced systems and is a considerably difficult task for the least well-resourced ones.

Focusing on low- and middle-income countries, acknowledged to be poorly served by the existing literature (McKee and Healy, 2002), this chapter will explore the challenges involved by first of all sampling available studies that have attempted to measure hospital quality and performance and considering what they are able to contribute to an understanding of the two concepts at the global level (Section "Levels of Hospital Quality and Performance in Low- and Middle-Income Countries"). This is divided into two sections on quality and performance, respectively, which consider the different ways of defining and framing the concepts and providing examples of studies that have used alternative frameworks, and their conclusions. Section "What Factors Have Been Identified as Influencing Hospital Quality and Performance?" provides a review of the evidence regarding the factors that influence hospital quality and performance, considering evidence for the roles of scale and scope, market conditions, and the public or private ownership status of hospitals. Section "Strategies for Improving Hospital Quality and Performance" considers opportunities to intervene to improve quality and performance, including quality improvement programs at the micro-level as well as sectoral interventions including regulatory approaches and system reform. Section "Conclusions" concludes with the public policy implications of the evidence reviewed, and the most important evidence gaps that form the research priority agenda.

Levels of Hospital Quality and Performance in Low- and Middle-Income Countries

Quality

• *Quality concepts*

There are many definitions of hospital quality, but the most widely referenced starting point for consideration is the work of Avedis Donabedian, whose landmark 1966 publication on this subject first described the three elements of structure, process and outcome. *Structure* concerns the characteristics of the providers of care, including organizational characteristics; *Process* concerns the caregiving transaction between the provider and the patient, including both its interpersonal characteristics and its technical characteristics, such as conformity with evidence-based protocols; *Outcomes* are the changes resulting from health care, in terms of improved health, health knowledge or health-related behavior's, and in terms of patient satisfaction. There have been many uses, applications and modifications of Donabedian's framework (for example, Qu *et al.*, 2010; Carayon *et al.*, 2006), some recognizing the need to better understand the linkages between structure, process, and outcome; others the need to consider a wider range of inputs to the process, such as patient characteristics and the health facility's environment; and yet others a more comprehensive view of outputs, including for example institutional outputs for the organization and its employees. The model has nevertheless proved remarkably resilient to half a century of health services research.

Other conceptual models used to evaluate hospital quality have largely originated in business and have been adapted. For example, Vakani *et al.* (2009) apply a European Federation of Quality Management (EFQM) scale, normally applied to business organizations, to a Pakistani teaching hospital in response to pressures of increasing competition in the higher education market.

Minvielle *et al.* (2008) delineate four models of organizational performance derived from business: (1) The rational goal model (focused on achieving objectives); (2) the open system model (focused on the organization's interactions with its environment); (3) the internal process model (focused on specific organizational processes); and (4) the human relations model (focused on enabling staff to fulfill potential and hence make a greater contribution to the organization). They review the applicability of these models to French hospitals, recognizing that each provides a somewhat one-sided view of organizational performance and that not all components of the models are mutually compatible: They can't simply be merged. For example, flexibility and openness to change are valued in the human relations and open system models, while control and stability are valued in the rational goal and internal process models. Although the authors found a degree of convergence in relation to the values underlying the hospital performance measurement across three stakeholder groups (physicians, caregivers and administrative staff), this work provides grounds for caution in interpreting the rest of the literature, both with respect to differing measures of quality and to strategies for quality improvement. First, what constitutes quality is contestable: Many models, including the Donabedian Model, take a single (even if multi-dimensional) perspective which cannot accommodate the conflicts unearthed by Minvielle *et al.* (2008). Second, evaluations of quality improvement strategies may share models of both measurement and change; in other words, they may not measure the quality dimensions that their quality improvement strategy has also ignored. These limitations qualify most of the findings reported below, which are overwhelmingly uncritically adopting of a single perspective.

- *Measures of quality applied*

The most common approach adopted to the measurement of quality is the criterion-based audit. In this approach, a set of procedures is identified as expected in good practice, and a measurement strategy is developed to establish whether these procedures were undertaken in the case under examination. The expected procedures are sometimes established by carefully considered methods, such as the convening of expert panel meetings (for example, Graham *et al.*, 2000); the use of the Delphi Technique to resolve differences of opinion between experts (for example, Lodewijckx *et al.*, 2013; Sun *et al.*, 2011); the use of established standards published by recognized bodies such as the WHO (for example, Duke *et al.*, 2006; Ibrahim, 2010; Lind *et al.*, 2011; Sidik *et al.*, 2013); the consideration of local protocols (for example, Hongoro *et al.*, 2005; Kidanto *et al.*, 2012) and/or other literature review (Graham *et al.*, 2000); or the use of experts in the review process itself (for example, Nolan *et al.*, 2001). In other cases, the process for establishing criteria is unstated (for example, English *et al.*, 2004; Harzallah *et al.*, 2004), with it perhaps implicit that the reviewers were experts themselves. The criterion-based audit approach has been used to measure quality for a wide range of hospital conditions and processes, including hospital tuberculosis care (Hongoro *et al.*, 2005), diabetes care (Harzallah *et al.*, 2004); obstetric care (Graham *et al.*, 2000; Tunçalp *et al.*, 2013); pediatric care (Duke *et al.*, 2006); brain injury care (Alexander *et al.*, 2009), and many others.

Another common approach is to analyze administrative data with the objective of reaching conclusions about the quality of hospital services. Data that are reported routinely from hospitals, such as mortality rates, readmissions, length of stay, number of operations postponed, and other measures, have obvious relevance to quality, but caution is needed in using them directly as quality measures because of the influence of case mix and environment. Bottle *et al.* (2013) consider the extent to which international comparisons of hospital quality can be derived from such data. Comparing five European countries and the US, it was concluded that even after risk adjustments, it was not possible to attribute differences in outcomes to quality of care, but rather that the data could be used to initiate dialogue around explanations. Onwudike *et al.* (2001), however, suggest that the higher mortality rates in trauma care in a Lagos teaching hospital (relative to similar hospitals in the UK and US), after controlling for injury severity, could be attributed to quality differences; and Shahraz *et al.* (2012) use risk-adjusted mortality and length of stay data to compare a hospital in Iran to those in the US.

Other studies have used patient opinion surveys as their measure of care quality. The rationale for a focus on patient views ranges from a recognition of the market pressures under which hospitals often operate, leading to an interest in understanding the client's perspective, to a need to balance professional and expert views with lay views that may reflect different values as well as a different perspective. Most studies take the validity of patient views of quality as a starting point. For example, one study in Malawi (Kumbani *et al.*, 2012) considered women using perinatal care at a district hospital to be uncritical of the care they received, other than its interpersonal aspects. Pai and Chary (2010) review the range of efforts of this type from a global perspective, comparing the dimensions about which patients have been consulted and the approaches used to decide on those. They identified 47 studies from 25 countries that met inclusion criteria; 23 of the studies had used the SERVQUAL instrument as the basis of their approach, an instrument that originates in the work of Parasuraman (1985; 1988; 1990; 1991). The SERVQUAL tool has 5 dimensions (responsiveness, assurance, reliability, empathy, and tangibility) and 22 components for measuring expectations and perceptions of health care. Aghamolaei *et al.* (2014) report one recent use of the approach in an Iranian hospital. Because the tool has been used in multiple locations, the authors were able to conclude that the hospital performed well relative to those of other studies in Malaysia and Singapore, while they were also able to identify where differences between perceptions and expectations were greatest (in this case in the area of responsiveness). The studies included in Pai and Chary's analysis that used approaches other than SERVQUAL also used instruments to assess multiple dimensions of quality (between 2 and 14).

Still other studies have focused on the views of professional staff. Rabbani *et al.* (2009) surveyed the 54 faculty members of a large private university hospital in Karachi, capturing their views of hospital quality using an instrument developed by Shortell (2001) for use in the US and focused on the extent to which the hospital implements quality of care measures. The instrument has seven dimensions (leadership, information and analysis, human resource utilization, strategic quality planning, quality management, quality results, and customer satisfaction) and 58 items, although the study team included only the first three dimensions. More common for studies that have surveyed staff perceptions is to compare these with patient perceptions (Olusina *et al.*, 2002; Zhao *et al.*, 2008; You *et al.*, 2013), highlighting areas of difference. For example, Olusina *et al.* (2002) found both staff and patients rated most highly the element of quality related to staff-patient relationships in a Nigerian hospital although patients were least satisfied with meals and 'staff talking in belittling manners,' while the physical environment was least satisfactory to staff. Similarly, Zhao *et al.* (2008) found that while evaluations indicated agreement over a high quality of nursing care in a Chinese hospital, there were significant differences in the relative scores of different elements. You *et al.* (2013) conducted large surveys of 9,688 nurses and 5,786 patients in 191 Chinese hospitals, sufficient to identify factors influencing care perceptions, such as the importance of staff-patient ratios for staff perceptions, and of more qualified nursing staff for patient perceptions. Other studies have focused more specifically on the nature of staff and patient interaction (Olusina *et al.*, 2003), on how that interaction is influenced by culture (Nguyen *et al.*, 2007), and organizational culture (Rabbani, 2009) in Nigeria, Vietnam, and Pakistan, respectively.

Kaplan and Norton (1996) developed the concept of a 'balanced scorecard' to emphasize the importance of presenting a multi-dimensional picture of quality in any organization; this thinking has been increasingly applied in hospitals and health care in high-income countries, and has more recently been extended to low- and middle-income countries. This approach is consistent with Donabedian's multi-dimensional conception of quality, as well as other multi-dimensional quality constructs, such as those of the US Institute of Medicine (2001) or that of the Joint Commission on Accreditation of Healthcare (Lloyd, 2004). Castaneda Mendez *et al.* (1998) identified the opportunity to apply the balanced scorecard approach in health care, suggesting that health care organizations need to think in multiple dimensions about the value they create, in a similar way to business organizations, and suggest translating Kaplan and Norton's four dimensions to those of (1) 'patient-value added'; (2) 'employee-value added'; (3) 'business-value added (learning perspective)' and (4) 'business-value added (financial perspective)'. Rabbani *et al.* (2007) review the applicability of these ideas to health care organizations in low-income countries, concluding that committed leadership, cultural readiness, quality information systems, viable strategic plans and 'optimum resources' are the pre-requisites. Rabbani *et al.* (2010) report on the design of an approach and Rabbani *et al.* (2011) proceed with the pilot testing of the applicability of the approach in a Pakistani hospital, finding significant constraints to implementation which may have been predicted by the pre-requisites identified in Rabbani *et al.* (2007). For example, staff shortfalls, absence of incentives and cultural resistance were among the reasons some units in the hospital resisted participation. Nevertheless, Chen *et al.* (2006) had earlier applied the balanced scorecard approach to Chinese hospitals in a comparative exercise with Japanese hospitals, finding the approach effective both in measuring the contribution made by the hospitals to the countries' health systems and in identifying specific problems and opportunities for improvement. El-Jardali *et al.* (2011) report successful use of the approach in hospitals in the Lebanon but report similar constraints to those reported by Rabbani *et al.* (2011). Beyond measuring aspects of quality, the balanced scorecard is also used as an approach for quality improvement and is further discussed as such in Section "Strategies for Improving Hospital Quality and Performance".

Other elements of performance

- *Efficiency*

A general definition of efficiency is the use of resources to achieve the maximum effectiveness in achieving an objective. Economists distinguish between different levels at which efficiency can be obtained. In any given production process, it might be possible to achieve a higher level of output with the set of inputs used; or to use fewer inputs to achieve the same level of output. This concept is known as *technical efficiency*. Even if a production process is technically efficient, it may be possible to use a different combination of inputs or a different technology to produce the same level of output at a lower opportunity cost (the value of that resource in an alternative use): For example, a machine with low opportunity costs may be able to replace several workers with high opportunity costs. Achieving the highest output for a given opportunity cost or achieving the same output for a lower opportunity cost is known as *economic efficiency*. At a third level, the outputs being produced may not be those most highly valued by those they are being produced for. *Allocative efficiency* requires that resources be used to produce the mix of goods or outputs for which consumers or society have the highest value, or from which they receive the greatest benefit. Finally, a production process might meet all the above conditions but could achieve a better ratio of inputs to outputs if it were operated at different scale, most commonly because of *economies of scale* allow lower levels of resource input per unit of output as the volume of production increases. Achieving the minimum resource use per unit of output, then, additionally requires *scale efficiency*. Efficiency in the general sense is only obtained when all sets of conditions have been met.

Measurement of each level of efficiency is attempted by economic evaluations such as cost-effectiveness and cost–utility analyses. Few of these have been applied to hospital production processes at the general level, although there is a substantial body of work applying this approach to specific hospital treatments: For example, there are studies considering the cost-effectiveness of alternative malaria (e.g., Mori *et al.*, 2014: Tanzania) and pneumonia (e.g., Wessels *et al.*, 1998: South Africa) pharmaceutical therapies for hospitalized cases; of alternative chemotherapy approaches (e.g., Keat and Ghani, 2013: Malaysia); of alternative hospital treatments of fractures (e.g., Gosselin *et al.*, 2009: Cambodia; Opondo *et al.*, 2013: Kenya) and so on. None of these studies are capable of evaluating the performance of a hospital in general, nor are they intended for that purpose. Nevertheless, they exemplify the level of detail that would be required with respect to every hospital function before a full efficiency analysis of a hospital could be considered complete and hence explain the difficulty of achieving such an objective.

Despite the difficulties, a few studies have attempted cost-effectiveness analysis at the level of the whole hospital (McCord and Chowdhury, 2003 in Bangladesh; Gosselin *et al.*, 2006 in Sierra Leone; and Gosselin and Heitto, 2008 in Cambodia). While these fall short of comprehensively evaluating the efficiency of each hospital process, they provide an overall estimate of the rate at which expenditure is translated into outputs (in the cited cases, measured in terms of disability-adjusted life years (DALYs) using an approach developed by McCord and Chowdhury (2003)), which can be compared with other health sector investments. Both studies suggest that the efficiency of the use of resources in the hospital sector (at least in relation to surgical interventions, the dominant activity in both hospitals studied) is higher than the authors consider is generally thought.

More achievable is a comparison of cost per standardized hospital activity, for example, per inpatient day or admission, or per outpatient visit. This has been attempted by a number of studies, some of which have given careful attention to the question of the comparability of the units compared and adjusted accordingly.

When large numbers of hospitals are being compared, their costs can be estimated from administrative data reporting some measure of their global resource use, such as their allocation from a public health budget; their total billings; or their reported total expenditures (Hung and Chang, 2008; Wong *et al.*, 2011). This approach for estimating costs is rarely used in low- and middle-income countries (the two studies cited are from high-income Taiwan and Hong Kong) because administrative data are unreliable and relatively difficult to obtain for the whole population of hospitals in most of these countries. A more detailed understanding of one or a few hospital cost structures can be obtained from hospital costing exercises which use a combination of *'step-down' costing* (working from total expenditure reports and allocating reported totals down to departments, sub-departments and then to service level by using estimates of the relevant proportions) and *'bottom–up' costing* (working from observations or records of resource use at the service level and aggregating to that resource use to wards, departments, and upwards to hospital level) to provide this detail (for example, Flessa, 1998; Guinness *et al.*, 2002; Audibert *et al.*, 2007). A variant of these approaches, known as *activity-based costing*, uses a cost center that pools similar hospital processes together, regardless of the administrative department they fall under (Yereli, 2009). Costs might be allocated to activities by observing or estimating from records the use of resources by each activity (Yereli, 2009), or by modeling a standard process (Riewpaiboon *et al.*, 2011).

The relatively poor quality of administrative data in most low- and middle-income settings and the substantial research resources needed to develop detailed costing studies that can improve on such data have made the large-scale analysis of hospital costs in such settings difficult and rare. Adam *et al.* (2014) aim to establish a method by which better quality costing data can be used to compare larger numbers of hospitals in low- and middle-income settings by identifying the sources of ward-level cost variability in 41 hospitals in China, and using the results to predict ward-level costs, finding that costs were strongly predicted by the number of staff and bed days in inpatient wards. The authors emphasize that this result is not of great interest in itself, but its implication for the feasibility of estimating ward-level costs from routinely reported administrative data could be important. The study's replication in a wider range of settings would clarify whether this might be possible in settings which might exhibit a greater degree of heterogeneity in some respects than China.

The comparison of cost and input levels with hospital activity levels is developed in the approach of data envelopment analysis (DEA). DEA is a frontier technique. Hospitals are positioned in a two-(or more) dimensional space with each dimension a type of input, such as beds or health staff. A frontier is identified by which a given level of output or vector of outputs is produced using lowest observed combinations of inputs; any hospital which uses more of both (or all) inputs to produce the same (or smaller) output is considered inefficient and its degree of inefficiency is measured by its distance from the frontier. The frontier is a curve along which different types of inputs are substituted: more beds for less staff, for example. The approach has been widely used. Table 1 provides examples of studies that have applied the technique in low- and middle-income countries.

Table 1. Selected DEA studies 1997–2014

References	Location	No. of hospitals	% of hospitals deemed efficient	Average technical efficiency score (CRS where both CRS and VRS estimated)
Ersoy *et al.* (1997)	Turkey	573	9.4%	
Sahin and Ozcan (2000)	Turkey	682	55%	
Kirigia *et al.* (2002)	Kenya	54	74%	0.956
Osei *et al.* (2005)	Ghana	17	53%	0.61
Renner *et al.* (2005)	Sierra Leone	37	40.5%	0.78
Zere *et al.* (2006)	Namibia	30		0.627–0.743 1997–2001
Hajialiafzali *et al.* (2007)	Iran	53	51	0.904
Masiye (2007)	Zambia	30	40%	0.67
Kirigia *et al.* (2008)	Angola	28	39% (2000) 43% (2001) 36% (2002)	0.662 0.658 0.675
Puenpatom and Rosenman (2008)	Thailand	19–48	23.9% (2000) 14.1% (2001) 37.0% (2002)	0.819–0.860
Ketabi (2011)	Iran	23	53%	0.97
Tlotlego *et al.* (2010)	Botswana	21	23.8% (2006) 23.8% (2007) 38.1% (2008)	
Gai *et al.* (2010)	China	3391		
Özgen and Sahin (2010)	Turkey	830 dialysis facilities	3%	0.503
Pham (2011)	Vietnam	101		0.65–0.76
Shahhoseini *et al.* (2011)	Iran	12	58%	0.875
Sulku (2011)	Turkey	751 (2001) 769 (2006)	Change rather than levels reported	
Gok and Sezen (2013)	Turkey	348	46%	0.76
Jat and Sebastian (2013)	India (Madhya Pradesh)	40	50%	0.90
Kiadaliri *et al.* (2013)	Iran			0.846 (pooled estimate)
Kirigia and Asbu (2013)	Eritrea	19	47%	0.903
Keith and Prior (2014)	Mexico	2105	1.76%	0.256
Li *et al.* (2014)	China (Beijing)	12	Reports changes rather than levels	

Source: Author.

Table 1 also shows a series of estimates of levels of efficiency in the last column; the distance from the estimated efficiency level and the value 1 (maximum efficiency) is interpreted as the proportion of additional output that hospitals could produce with the same level of input, or that inputs could be reduced with the same level of output, if all hospitals operated efficiently. Most studies also report the proportion of hospitals operating on versus inside the estimated efficiency frontier. The fourth column of Table 1 reports the proportion of hospitals estimated to be efficient by this analysis.

The attribution of efficiency according to a hospitals' position in relation to the frontier is problematic. Hospitals' performance measures may place them away from the frontier, where they're deemed inefficient in relation to other hospitals, for a number of reasons apart from inefficient operation. The measurement takes no account of the differences in the environment of different hospitals which may make service delivery more difficult in some areas — for example, some hospitals operate in a conflict-affected area, a factor affecting several of the countries in Table 1. Hospitals may also deal with a more complex case load. Additionally, there is no measure of the value or quality of the output. High levels of 'output' may reflect excessive use of procedures in circumstances in which they are of low or no value to the patient. Or, those whose performance is deemed 'efficient' by the technique may be operating with insufficient resources, rendering the services they provide low quality. The latter issue particularly affects low-income countries where such operating conditions are common. Most of the studies do not sufficiently recognize this problem and operate on the assumption that hospitals away from the frontier could and should operate on it. Some attempt to control for case mix; some recognize the problem of disparate quality levels by excluding quality from the definition of efficiency; and a further group identify a list of factors that might affect the results, suggesting that the results offer a starting point for an analysis of such factors. The last approach is the only one that recognizes the need for qualitative understanding of the context of results before applying the terms 'efficient' and 'inefficient' with useful meaning.

Kiadaliri *et al.* (2013) report a meta-analysis of frontier studies of hospital efficiency in Iran, noting also the limited adjustment for case mix and quality of care. Comparing 29 such studies, they conclude that inclusion of larger numbers of variables and greater heterogeneity of hospital types results in higher estimates of technical efficiency.

However, Gok and Sezen (2013) focus on the relationship between efficiency, as measured by the frontier approach, and quality, as measured by a routine Turkish Ministry of Health data set suggested to capture 'structural quality' (as defined above), and a patient satisfaction survey. The results indicate that hospital size has a negative effect on patient satisfaction, and structural quality has a positive effect on patient satisfaction, but that higher levels of efficiency weaken the relationship between structural quality and patient satisfaction. One interpretation of this is that efficiency, as measured, is indeed obtained at the expense of quality of care. This is confirmed in small hospitals, where there is a negative relationship between efficiency and patient satisfaction; but not in large ones, where there is positive correlation between efficiency and patient satisfaction. The last result, the authors suggest, is consistent with the total quality management approach that considers efficiency and quality to be jointly produced.

What is much better recognized across the set of studies is that the technical efficiency measure estimated is restricted to technical efficiency according to the definitions set out above. The approach places no relative values on the different outputs on the frontier, usually including outpatient visits, admissions and/or bed days and variously surgeries or other specific activities. DEA results can be decomposed to separately consider the issues of technical efficiency and scale efficiency, addressing the determinants of hospital performance. The determinants of hospital performance and quality are addressed in Section "What factors have been identified as influencing hospital quality and performance" later in the chapter.

A few studies have used DEA to measure productivity change rather than absolute productivity levels; others have estimated both (as shown in Table 1). These have mostly been undertaken in order to estimate the effect of policy change.

The results of DEA indicate the relative efficiency of hospitals to each other within a geographical area, so it is not possible to compare the results of different studies without reanalysis of the primary data. Direct comparison of the data in Table 1 is therefore not recommended. There is little correlation between the proportion of hospitals deemed efficient and the overall level of efficiency, even although both are relative measures, indicating that the shapes of the distributions of results generated by this analysis vary across studies — in some cases, a small proportion of hospitals locate a significant distance from the frontier, with many on the frontier; in others, a large proportion locate close to the frontier.

- *Accessibility and equity*

Hospitals might also be compared with respect to the extent to which their services are accessible or they contribute to the equity of the health system. This is arguably a system rather than institutional responsibility: one hospital may serve one section of the population while another serves a different one, potentially producing overall universal access and equity at the system level. Nevertheless, elements of hospital institutional policy or behavior may positively or negatively affect the access of a given population and equity across the population.

There are a number of frameworks that both define access and consider the factors that affect it, which can be adapted to conceptualize access to an individual hospital. The most useful of these frameworks for this purpose focus on factors that operate at the micro-level in shaping individuals' ability to use health services, rather than those that focus on larger sectoral, systemic, and environmental factors (such as the well-known model of Aday and Anderson, 1974), which give most attention to issues outside the hospital's sphere of control. One such model is that of Penchansky and Thomas (1981), in which five dimensions of access are deemed to determine the 'fit' between a patient's needs and the response of the health system (or hospital). The five dimensions of access are delineated:

1. *Availability* (volume and type of supply, matched to volume and need);
2. *Accessibility* (location of supply, matched to patients' location and ability to travel);
3. *Accommodation* (such as clinic hours and waiting times fitting patients' needs);
4. *Affordability* (patients' financial capacities and insurance coverage relative to hospital charges); and
5. *Acceptability* (services provided are in a form and of a standard that patients find acceptable).

There are few studies that consider issues of equity and access at the hospital level, but a large number that consider the question in relation to specific hospital services such as maternal care and AIDS treatment.

Availability and *accessibility* are strongly inter-related: One cannot apply without the other, in that all conceived-of services are available somewhere to some group of patients, and can only be considered available to those patients if also accessible. Both have rarely been explicitly evaluated as a component of access, perhaps because it is self-evident that without availability and accessibility, there can be no access. Those studies that have explicitly addressed availability have recognized that availability is not a sufficient condition and considered the extent to which increasing availability improves access. For example, Prata *et al.* (2013) consider the extent to which increased provision of comprehensive abortion care reduced cases of incomplete abortion in the Tigray Region of Ethiopia, recognizing that abortion services are subject to a complex set of requirements of 'fit' in the five dimensions of the Penchansky and Thomas Framework. They find a significant decrease in incomplete abortion cases, implying that availability alone had a strong influence on access. Gao and Barclay (2010) find significant gaps in the availability of emergency obstetric care services in the Shanxi Province of China, affecting access. Similarly, studies of accessibility focus on how variable accessibility (measured by distance or travel time) effects utilization, or outcomes from episodes of ill health. A recent example is the study reported by Manongi *et al.* (2014), from which it was concluded that for every hour of additional travel time to a hospital, deaths associated with failing to access the hospital increased by 21.4%.

The main issue identified as an access constraint in relation to *accommodation* is that of delay in receipt of care after arrival at a hospital. Two studies from Nigeria identify this as an important barrier to achieving access to effective care, with implications for outcomes (Ifesanya and Ifesanya, 2012) and patient satisfaction (Oluwadiya *et al.*, 2010).

By far the most frequently studied element of the Penchansky and Thomas framework in low- and middle-income countries is *affordability*. The issue of the financial accessibility of health care generally has been a major source of contention and, although most of the attention has not been directed at hospital charges or the implications of insurance coverage for hospital utilization and access, there are still a considerable number of studies that address this. Mostert *et al.* (2014) find that cancer outcomes for children in Kenya are negatively affected by not being covered by the National Hospital Insurance Fund, while Yawson *et al.* (2012) find that those covered by the National Health Insurance Scheme in Ghana receive excess medications. Health equity funds, externally funded exemption systems established in Cambodia, and Community Health Insurance in the district of Gudalur in Tamil Nadu (Devadasan *et al.*, 2009) have been shown to improve access to hospital care for the poor (Noirhomme *et al.*, 2007). However, few of the financial factors affecting affordability and therefore access that have been addressed in these studies are the policies of individual hospitals, although further discussion of hospital user fees policies follows in Section "Strategies for Improving Hospital Quality and Performance".

Acceptability has been extensively studied through the approach of patient satisfaction surveys, a literature that has been discussed above as one of the components of quality.

A number of studies consider and compare different elements of access to hospital care. Samad *et al.* (2013), for example, seek to identify the major constraints to accessing surgical care in Karachi, Pakistan and find the most important constraint to be lack of knowledge about treatment options — something not considered by Penchansky and Thomas but to which low rates of utilization of health services in general are widely attributed in low- and middle-income countries. Next most important, however, were accommodation issues (waiting times for surgery after consultation), affordability issues, and accessibility issues. For Gao *et al.* (2010), the most important barrier was affordability, followed by acceptability (perceptions of poor quality) and accessibility (transport problems) in the Shanxi Province of China. Levesque *et al.* (2007) point to the heightened importance of affordability issues in those urban areas of Kerala less well served by the public sector, where people are more reliant on the private sector.

Studies of the *equity* implications of hospital performance are rare — most of the relevant focus is on access. Equity has been addressed from the perspective of evaluating whether specific population groups are appropriately represented in the hospital attending population: For example, Shrestha *et al.* (2012) conclude that women and girls are under-represented among those seeking hospital care for eye problems in Nepal, and Wilunda *et al.* (2013) find that those accessing emergency obstetric care in Ethiopia were highly disproportionately representative of the richest wealth quintile, which was attributed to differential access to transport. Niens *et al.* (2014), however, failed to find a significant difference across socio-economic quintiles in benefits from hospital-based cancer treatment (although the non-significant difference was in the expected direction).

Equity has also been addressed from the perspective of the distribution of hospital resources and patient's out-of-pocket payments. McPake *et al.* (2007) show that where hospitals engage in two-tier charging strategies, the separation of services into higher-priced and higher-quality, and lower-priced and lower-quality segments (for example, where 'private' wards are separated from the main wards of a public hospital) the hospital's incentives may favor cross-subsidization in either direction (from high-priced to low-priced or from low-priced to high-priced). McPake *et al.* (2011) suggest that the situation in Maputo Central Hospital in Mozambique favored those using the high-priced services of the Special Clinic. Turning to equity issues in India, Roy and Howard (2007) show that out-of-pocket payments for hospital care do not decline with the ability to pay in India. They attribute the problem to the absence of risk pooling arrangements for the poorer population.

What Factors have been Identified as Influencing Hospital Quality and Performance?

Size and scope

Economies of scale mean that costs per unit of activity decline as a hospital increases in size — for example, because it is able to make more intensive use of capital equipment. Economies of scope imply that costs per unit of activity decline as a hospital's range of service provision extends — for example, because of continuity of care opportunities between outpatient and inpatient services, or because outpatient and inpatient providers can share a laboratory service. Diseconomies of scale and scope may also be encountered, for example, because large scale or scope increase the complexity of activities, which become increasingly difficult to manage.

These considerations have inspired much research focused on the optimum scale and scope of hospital activity, now generally addressed using the DEA approach described in the previous section. Efficiency scores can be computed by the DEA approach under the assumptions of constant or variable returns to scale. Under the assumption of constant returns to scale (CRS), the efficient ratio of inputs to outputs is constant irrespective of scale; under variable returns to scale (VRS) it is allowed to vary, increasing the technical efficiency estimate by the extent to which scale is estimated to have affected the ratio. Hence, efficiency estimates calculated by the constant returns to scale measure are always lower than those calculated by the variable returns to scale measure and the ratio between the two scales provides an estimate of the extent to which scale explains a higher ratio of inputs to outputs. This scale efficiency index (equated to the ratio of CRS to VRS estimates) therefore varies between 0 and 1, with 1 indicating constant returns to scale, and values less than 1 indicating increasing or decreasing returns to scale. Only some studies report whether the scale efficiency measure is associated with operating in an area of increasing or decreasing returns to scale, something that cannot be determined by the scale efficiency index itself.

Among the studies in Table 1, the most complete analysis of scale effects is found in the analysis of Zambian hospitals by Masiye (2007). Masiye provides a table showing the nature of scale returns (increasing, constant or decreasing) and a measure of scale itself (hospital bed numbers), as reproduced in Table 2. The table supports the intuition that increasing returns to scale predominate among smaller hospitals while decreasing returns to scale predominate in larger ones, although there are exceptions. It is notable, however, that decreasing returns to scale are universal among the six hospitals with more than 500 beds, a hospital scale quite common in Africa. While the same analysis is not undertaken by Kirigia and Asbu (2013), hospital size (bed numbers) and the nature of scale returns are both provided for a subset of six Ethiopian hospitals in different tables. For that subset, four hospitals larger than 100 beds all exhibit decreasing returns to scale while two smaller than 100 beds exhibit increasing returns to scale. Otherwise, it is not possible to judge the implications for optimal hospital size from the DEA studies, which would appear a missed opportunity. Weaver and Deolalikar (2004) use a different methodology to assess returns to scale among public hospitals in Vietnam. Their analysis suggests that cost functions differed significantly across hospital categories (central, provincial, and district), with central hospitals exhibiting approximately constant returns to scale, provincial hospitals exhibiting significant decreasing returns to scale, and modest economies of scale for district hospitals.

Table 2. Scale efficiency scores and returns-to-scale characteristics of Zambian hospitals

Hospitals	No. of beds and cots	Scale effeciency score	Type of scale inefficiency
Kalomo	52	0.49	IRS
Kamuchanga	60	0.78	DRS
Gwembe	68	0.19	IRS
Nyimba	73	0.65	IRS
St. Theresa's Mission	93	0.97	DRS
Sinozam	93	0.89	IRS
Kabwe Mine	101	0.77	IRS
Thomson District	115	0.96	IRS
Lumezi	117	1.00	No scale inefficiency
Konkola Mine Hospital	125	1.00	No scale inefficiency
Kalulushi Mine	132	0.66	IRS
Minga Mission	133	0.95	IRS
Lundazi District	138	0.45	IRS
Zimba Mission	141	0.60	IRS
Mazabuka	142	1.00	No scale inefficiency
Petauke	142	0.98	DRS
Nchanga South	171	0.96	DRS
Mwami Mission	187	0.89	IRS
Choma General	218	0.99	IRS
Arthur Davison	250	0.78	DRS
Nchanga North	293	0.96	DRS
Monze Mission Hospital	322	0.98	IRS
St. Francis	455	0.95	DRS
Wusakile Hospital	478	1.00	No scale inefficiency
Livingstone	501	0.58	DRS
Kabwe	515	0.36	DRS
Chipata General	536	0.75	DRS
Chikankata	540	0.98	DRS
Kitwe Central	645	0.88	DRS
Ndola Central	948	0.56	DRS

Source: Masiye (2007).

Even was the answer more definitive, there are a number of other considerations before implications for 'right sizing' hospitals could be identified. As discussed in the previous section, hospital supply needs to be matched geographically with need or demand, and this matching may not be consistent with ensuring that all hospitals are operating at the point of scale efficiency. Furthermore, the recognition that the outputs used in these analyses are, at best, approximate measures of productivity as discussed above, implies that it is wise to consider further evidence about the potential confounding influences of factors such as case complexity, quality of care, and environmental constraints. The current literature does not allow such further consideration.

Market structure and characteristics

Standard economic approaches suggest that the performance of an economic entity is shaped by its position in the market. The 'structure–conduct–performance' model assumes that market structure (number of sellers in the market) determines conduct (such as price, what things are produced and in what quantities and qualities), which in turn determines performance (efficiency). There is a substantial body of work that critiques and offers alternatives to the standard approach (McPake *et al.*, 2013).

This section considers the evidence that the market disciplines hospitals to varying degrees according to the level of competition, with predictable implications for the quality and performance of hospitals. There are considerable difficulties in reaching clear conclusions in relation to this question. Defining and measuring competition and the boundaries of the market are problematic. Conceptually, the market for a good or a service is made of the providers of a given good or service together with the providers of its substitutes. Economists have traditionally defined product markets in terms of prices: a service belongs to a given product market if the cross-price elasticity is high and positive, or in other words, if it is clear that consumers substitute one for the other on the basis of comparing price (Griffiths and Wall, 2001). Typically, this is described in terms of the degree of concentration, measured either in 'n-firm concentration ratios' (which describe the sum of the market shares of the n — usually 3 or 5 — largest firms in the market, with higher values reflecting more concentrated, less competitive, markets), or summarized in a Hirschman–Herfindahl Index (the sum of the squared market shares of all the firms in the market, taking the value 1 if there is a monopoly and tending to 0 in a highly competitive market) (Nakamba *et al.*, 2002).

The specificity with which the product is defined will have an important effect on the market definition. For example, the market for alcoholic drinks will be populated by more firms than the market for a more narrowly defined product such as beer. Product definitions are therefore critical in thinking through issues of market structure (Griffiths and Wall, 2001). This raises particular difficulties in defining appropriate product groups for hospitals, since they produce a heterogeneous mix of services. It might be argued that the tertiary services provided by a national referral hospital have a single supplier for an entire national market. However, from another perspective, the service mix of such facilities might include a considerable element of primary care provision, also offered at lower levels of the system, equally allowing the conclusion that there is a high degree of competition for those services. Hence, different services provided by a single facility may face different levels of competition.

Defining the geographic boundary within which competition is measured is also problematic. Even in principle, this is difficult to conceptualize, as each consumer may consider a unique set of options from which to obtain hospital services, among which they select dependent on their home location, routine travel patterns, access to transport and the means to pay transport costs. Empirical approaches include using administrative boundaries such as towns or districts, whose boundaries are delineated for other purposes (for example, Mills *et al.*, 2001 uses administrative districts as the geographic boundary of the markets analyzed in Bangladesh), defining competition faced by a specific facility as all other providers within a given radius of that facility (for example, Bennett, 1997 uses the number of hospitals with 2 and 5 kilometer radii in Bangkok); and analyzing actual patterns of patient flow, such that the geographic boundary captures a given percentage of users (for example, Chang *et al.* (2011) describes a hospital's market in the US as a geographical area defined by the postal codes capturing 75% of the hospital's patients).

Data limitations in low- and middle-income countries have limited the extent to which the impact of hospital markets on outcomes or efficiency have been evaluated in these settings, with the studies cited above of Bennett (1997) and Mills *et al.* (2001) providing rare examples. Torun *et al.* (2013) analyzed the level of competition among hospitals in Turkey, concluding that competition had a positive effect on hospital efficiency but not on quality. Nakamba *et al.* (2002) describe the markets of two urban Zambian areas, demonstrating the data-related difficulties. Detailed analysis was required, for example, to estimate prices of accessing the hospitals for a small subset of conditions that might warrant hospitalization: Analysis that would not be feasible for a sufficiently large number of hospitals to reliably estimate effects on any outcome measure. Moreover, the price analysis exercise demonstrated that hospitals used price discrimination strategies to segment the market by ability to pay, implying that a given set of services in a given hospital could incur different levels of charge. Hence, it would be necessary to specify markets not only for specific sets of services, but also by population group, and the set of 16 hospitals operating in the two urban areas in question would not be sufficient to draw strong conclusions at these levels of disaggregation.

While in other markets, greater levels of competition are expected to increase efficiency by driving out of business hospitals that do not offer consumers the best combinations of price and quality, it has been observed in some hospital markets that the opposite can be the case. Consumers may be insensitive to price if covered by insurance, but responsive to quality signals that may mislead or only partially reflect a full understanding of the quality of care provided. Under these conditions, hospitals may respond to competitive pressure by inefficiently increasing quality signals with price inflationary implications. This has been suggested as an explanation of hospital behavior in the US (Dranove and White, 1994; Thomson, 1994) and also in Bangkok and Bangladesh (Bennett, 1997; Amin, 2001).

Gaynor and Town (2011) review the literature in high-income countries, where data permit analysis across large numbers of hospitals. The review suggests that the literature is heavily dominated by US studies at national or state levels, but finds in addition, a number of European studies. Studies of hospital markets under administered prices mainly find negative association between market concentration and quality, usually proxied by mortality rates, in some cases suggesting quite large impacts on hospital mortality rates predicted by market concentration. Gaynor and Town suggest that what may be happening is that hospitals in more concentrated markets exert lower effort while hospitals in more competitive environments are under more pressure to perform. Studies of behavior under market determined prices provide much more mixed assessments of the relationship between market concentration and quality. The review highlights the importance of the institutional features of the market in shaping the ways that market forces operate, and the effects of higher and lower levels of concentration.

While the discussion to this point considers payment mechanism an exogenously determined institutional factor, Maceira and Poblete (2003) provide empirical evidence in Argentina of the relationship between market structure and payment mechanism, recognizing that insurance agencies' ability to set prices varies with the degree of concentration of the provision market, while hospitals' control over prices negotiated in contracts with hospital doctors also varies with market concentration. In two districts in Argentina, the study finds patterns of risk distribution present in the mix of contracts in operation between payer, hospital, and doctor consistent with these hypotheses.

Public and private ownership characteristics

Hospitals owned by public versus private institutions, and characterized as for-profit versus not-for-profit might also be expected to prioritize differently among objectives of quality, volume, affordability, and profit. A number of studies have sought to measure differences in performance between hospitals with different ownership and objective characteristics.

For example, studies in Bangladesh (Andaleeb, 2000), Turkey (Taner and Antony, 2006), and South Africa (Coetzee *et al.*., 2013) have attempted to compare the quality levels of public and private hospitals. Both Andaleeb (2000) and Taner and Antony (2006) adapted the SERVQUAL framework discussed previously to establish patients' quality perceptions and found that private hospitals were considered superior by patients. The superior elements in Bangladesh were responsiveness, communication, and discipline dimensions, with communication replacing empathy in the SERVQUAL adaptation and discipline added to capture elements related to absenteeism, order in the hospital environment, and facility maintenance, all of which are deemed important in the Bangladesh context. In Turkey, doctors, nurses, and supportive services were judged superior in private hospitals. By focusing exclusively on patient perspectives, both studies do not address professionally or technically judged quality, or the question of whether private hospitals focus exclusively on those factors that signal quality to patients.

Coetzee *et al.* (2013) evaluated nurses' perception of quality of care in public and private hospitals in South Africa. Coetzee *et al.* used the RN4CAST survey which is also concerned with the practice environment and job satisfaction of nurses. The section focused on quality of care includes questions on nurses' perceptions of quality, patient safety issues and the occurrence of adverse incidents. Coetzee *et al.* report that these questions have been demonstrated to be significantly correlated with independent data on patient outcomes. The study reports that 11.8% of private hospital nurses compared to 21.0% of public hospital nurses would definitely or probably not recommend the hospital to family and friends if they needed hospital care; 18.1% of private hospital nurses and 24.5% of public hospital nurses report ward quality to be fair or poor; 33.5% of private hospital nurses and 62.9% of public hospital nurses considered that they were not confident that management would resolve patients' problems; and that 3.4% of private hospital nurses and 8.9% of public hospital nurses report a poor or failing safety grade. All differences but those in the ward quality score were significant at the 1% level. While this study uses a validated measure of quality, it sampled from 55 private hospitals that were presumably operating at smaller scale to the 7 public national referral hospitals with which they were compared, which may not produce the same results as if hospitals of similar size were compared. Nevertheless, in Africa, public hospitals tend to be larger than private ones and a more comparable sample of hospitals may not have been feasible.

Mathiyazhgan (2006) compared the efficiency of public and private hospitals in India using frontier approaches, similar to and including a DEA method that has been described in detail previously in this chapter, but capturing data on costs and quality levels in more detail than has typically been feasible in the studies discussed, and controlling for case mix using a Diagnostic Related Group (DRG) approach. The hospitals in both public and private groups exhibited wide variation in their efficiency levels, but overall, private hospitals were evaluated as more technically efficient than their public counterparts, and this difference was statistically significant at the 1% level. The hospital quality index constructed did not help to explain differences in efficiency, implying that low cost-to-output ratios could not systematically be explained by quality differences.

Liu *et al.* (2009) and Dilip (2010) consider the equity implications of a changing public–private mix of hospitals in China, and in the state of Kerala, India, respectively. In both contexts, demand for hospital care is increasing, the supply of public hospital care has failed to match this increase, and private for-profit hospitals are playing an increasing role in the market. The focus of Liu *et al.* is on patients' out-of-pocket expenditures, which was high (according to a cited study, an average admission at a Ministry of Health hospital was estimated at nearly 90% of per capita annual GDP in 2006), and the incidence of catastrophic payments for health care[3] was regressive, meaning they reduced in probability with higher income (Wagstaff and Lindelow, 2005). Liu *et al.* find that the effect of increasing market penetration of private for-profit hospitals serves to reduce the average expenditures for both outpatient and inpatient services in public general hospitals, especially for pharmaceuticals. While the Chinese case is unusual in that public hospitals were considered to operate as if profit-driven, and their regulatory environment encouraged that (Eggleston and Yip, 2004), the underlying explanation that the competition stimulated by private for-profit hospitals could exert downward pressure on public hospital pricing might apply in other contexts.

The relationships between the market penetration of private hospitals, prices, and patterns of utilization in Kerala were judged to have shifted between three surveys analyzed by Dilip (2010) between 1986 and 2004, with changing implications for the equity of utilization patterns and the incidence of associated financial burdens. Equity, considered from the two perspectives of utilization and financial burden, are likely to trade off to some extent: The more that poorer population groups succeed in achieving access to private hospitals, the greater their share of the financial burden of hospital fees is likely to be. Dilip finds that between 1995/1996 and 2004, the rich–poor divide in the consumption of inpatient treatment from private hospitals declined. Private hospitals' pricing strategies evolved to offer different pricing options to those populations. However, the burden of out-of-pocket expenditure among the poor was higher.

[3]Catastrophic payments are defined here as exceeding 10% of the household's own per capita income.

As with the estimation of the effect of increasing competition on hospital quality and performance, the number of studies evaluating the relative quality and performance of public and private hospitals in low- and middle-income countries is limited to a handful, exemplified by those described above. Eggleston *et al.* (2008) review the much larger number of studies of the implications of ownership type in the US, which supply inconsistent answers regarding the relative qualities of public, private for-profit, and private not-for-profit hospitals. The studies reviewed mostly find no difference in adverse events (most studies used mortality data, a few used other types of adverse events) between for-profit and not-for-profit hospitals but tend to find that government hospitals have either higher or similar rates of adverse events than not-for-profit hospitals. Eggleston *et al.* find that the inconsistency in results arises from the use of different data sources, the time period examined, and the region covered. Overall, studies that consider the whole of the US tend to find lower quality among for-profits than not-for-profits.

Strategies for Improving Hospital Quality and Performance

Given the many concerns about hospital quality and performance that arise from the studies addressed in the preceding sections, and from other sources, significant innovation and effort has been applied to finding approaches to improve outcomes. This section considers these approaches by the level of the system at which they operate, which can be at the level of the individual hospital, groups of hospitals, or the sector as a whole, and can address financing levels or mechanisms, management or regulation, or aim to reform the structure of the sector or its institutions.

Increased investment

Little attention has been given to the returns to increasing investment in hospitals, despite insufficient finances appearing as a frequent explanation of poor performance. Most interventions discussed in this section rely on investment and each considers the evidence that the specific investments involved generate returns. A number of studies document a much simpler route to improved outcomes through investing in infrastructure, equipment, training or information systems — all of these being health system elements that are clearly required as part of an effective hospital system but which may or may not in any individual application, yield returns. Such approaches are voluminous and seldom considered worthy of research or publication and they inevitably exhibit a wide range of impacts on hospital performance and rates of return on the investment.

In the instability of conditions in a lot of low- and middle-income countries, there are particular risks that investments' returns will be curtailed. For example

Ande *et al.* (1997) document the impact of re-equipping an operating theatre, labor suite and laboratory; repairing a blood bank and standby generator; restocking essential drugs and consumables; and updating staff training on provision of obstetric care in a district hospital in Nigeria. They documented an increase in the utilization of the hospital for complicated obstetric cases, which was not sustained perhaps because of increased political, social and economic unrest in the area, or perhaps because of the opening of a new hospital. Oyesola *et al.* (1997) report similar results (improved quality and utilization of the hospital for complicated obstetric cases but a failure to sustain the gains) from a more modest investment in another Nigerian state. A similar intervention in a teaching hospital in a third Nigerian state generated improvements in quality of care but was introduced alongside effective fee increases, resulting in large decreases in utilization of the service (Ifenne *et al.*, 1997). The two studies demonstrate the complexity of achieving sustainable returns to investments in hospital services in fragile environments, and the risks that such investments carry. Increased investment is likely to be a necessary but not sufficient condition for achieving improved health outcomes from hospital care in such settings.

Management initiatives at the hospital or hospital group level

There is a complex terrain of quality improvement approaches and labeling. The US Department of Health and Human Services describes the five models in Box 1. While there are multiple labels and packages of measures, most can be identified as a variant of the approaches in Box 1.

In what follows, we divide the approaches found in the literature applied to low- and middle-income countries into the two more generic types of approach:

(1) Those that derive definitions of quality through their process, like the Care Model and the Lean Model. These derive quality definitions from the patient (consumer), as in the case of the Lean Model, or from the interactions between patients and providers, through which providers' expert views can also influence the definition, as in the Care Model.
(2) Those that define a planning and management process and use indicators deemed to be measures of quality by implementers or evaluators of the intervention (as in the Model for Improvement, FADE, and Six Sigma).

The low- and middle-income country literature contains few examples of the first type of model from our classification of approaches. Most of the examples identified in this section use expert views as the reference point for determining quality, whether these are internal to a research or change team, or sourced from

Box 1. Introduction to quality improvement (QI) models

There are a variety of QI models currently in use and five are highlighted here. Two of the models highlighted, the *Care Model* and the *Lean Model*, provide a framework to improve patient care. The other three models, Model for Improvement, FADE, and Six Sigma, focus on processes that monitor the results of measures:

1. **Care Model:** There are six fundamental aspects of care identified in the Care Model, which creates a system that promotes high-quality disease and prevention management. It does this by supporting productive interactions between patients, who take an active part in their care, and providers, who have the necessary resources and expertise.
2. **Lean Model:** This model defines value by what a customer (i.e., patient) wants. It maps how the value flows to the customer and ensures the competency of the process by making it cost effective and time efficient.
3. **Model for Improvement:** In order to set the aim or organizational goal, establish measures, and select changes, this model focuses on three questions: What are we trying to accomplish? How will we know that a change is an improvement? And, what changes can we make that will result in improvement? It incorporates Plan–Do–Study–Act (PDSA) cycles to test changes on a small scale.
4. **FADE:** There are four broad steps to the FADE QI model:
   - ***Focus***: Define the process to be improved
   - ***Analyze***: Collect and analyze data
   - ***Develop***: Develop action plans for improvement
   - ***Execute***: Implement the action plans, and
   - ***Evaluate***: Measure and monitor the system to ensure success
5. **Six Sigma:** Six Sigma is a measurement-based strategy for process improvement and problem reduction. It is completed through the application of the QI project and accomplished with the use of two Six Sigma models: (1) DMAIC (define, measure, analyze, improve, control), which is designed to examine existing processes, and (2) DMADV (define, measure, analyze, design, verify) which is used to develop new processes.

Notes: Experts are beginning to combine the Six Sigma and Lean models into the one term, Lean Six Sigma. This is because they both require a focus on analyzing processes, and use mapping as a means to achieve improvement.

Sources: US Department of Health and Human Services, Health Resources and Services Administration at: http://www.hrsa.gov/quality/toolbox/methodology/qualityimprovement/part3.html.

external authorities such as WHO. For example, Nausheen *et al.* (2013) used guidelines from the American College of Obstetricians and Gynecologists to improve antibiotic use in obstetric care; Latham *et al.* (2012) referenced WHO guidelines in implementing a process of improving patient identification within Malawian hospitals; while Srofenyoh *et al.* (2012) describe an external change team from a US university leading a process of deriving guidelines from published evidence and encouraging their implementation; and Hunyinbo *et al.* (2008) describe a criterionbased audit whereby the change team applied their own expert knowledge to a review of patient records and led a process of feedback and change in response. Others who have used externally validated guideline approaches to benchmarking quality levels include Berman *et al.* (2014) for a range of hospital services in Lesotho; Du *et al.* (2014) for the introduction of clinical pathways in cardiology in China; Cong *et al.* (2012) for improving quality in pressure ulcer prevention in China; Mohammadi *et al.* (2007) for non-clinical aspects of patient care in Tehran; and Ovretveit and Al Serouri (2006) for a range of patient care areas in Yemen.

An exception to the externally driven quality standard setting processes of these studies is exemplified by the study of Mbovane *et al.* (2007) who used a quality circle approach to enable hospital nurses to define quality improvements needed. This study did not evaluate the effectiveness of the intervention, only its acceptability and feasibility, but concluded that the approach was well accepted by those involved.

Those that have used the balanced scorecard approach, not only as a quality measurement approach as discussed earlier, but also as a mechanism for driving quality improvement, have mainly at least considered an element of patient perspective in the quality standard setting process, as the balanced scorecard approach recommends. Rohsiswatmo *et al.* (2014) included patient satisfaction in their balanced scorecard approach to improving prevention and control of blood stream infection in Indonesia and it was among those measures of quality that they succeeded in improving. However, there is some evidence of reluctance to give patient and staff views the weight the balanced scorecard suggests. For example, Rabbani *et al.* (2011), seeking to understand the constraints to the implementation of the balanced scorecard in a Pakistani hospital found that staff and faculty perceived employee and patient satisfaction indicators to be *'non-clinical in nature and therefore not of direct concern'* (p. 6). Mvula-Mwenda (2009) concluded that in Zambia: *'it is imperative for management at UTH to internalize that patients have a role to play in determining what is quality health care services and treatment.'* (p. 142). Meanwhile, in the Lebanon El-Jardali *et al.* (2011) study, the authors assessed the measure of patient satisfaction applied unreliable and infeasible, mainly because of the difficulty of the survey methods required to collect it.

The effects of quality improvement programs have been mixed, with studies such as those of Berman *et al.* (2014), Srofenyoh *et al.* (2012), and Hunyinbo *et al.*

(2008) measuring significant impacts while others such as those of Du *et al.* (2014) and Latham *et al.* (2012) judging their impact limited. Both the studies of Rabbani *et al.* (2011) and Ovretveit and Al Serouri (2006) distinguished between the extent of implementation and the effectiveness of implementation, both commenting on implementation difficulties. Quality improvement is constrained by resource limitations: It is difficult to apply Western models of quality improvement when there are absolute shortages of basic resources like staff and essential medicines, for example (Agyeman-Duah *et al.*, 2014). It is also constrained by hierarchical perspectives that may explain the scarcity of approaches that give weight to staff and patient perspectives. These perspectives are exemplified by the quotes from Rabbani *et al.* (2011) and Mvula-Mwenda (2009) above and the conclusion of Latham *et al.* (2012) that staff simply considered the aspect of quality in question — in this case, reducing the risk of misidentifying patients — unimportant. Ranasinghe *et al.* (2014) also found that an absence of leadership support constituted a barrier to successful quality improvement in hospitals in China.

Sectoral intervention

While individual hospitals may aim to improve their own standards, there are also a number of mechanisms used by hospitals and other health sector agents to improve hospital performance and quality across the sector or large sections of it. The mechanisms reviewed in this section are regulation mechanisms, including statutory certification; accreditation programs defined as systems of voluntary certification; and system-level supports to the operations of individual provider institutions, such as systems of supervision.

- *Regulation*

Regulation has been defined as the government or state exerting control over activities of individuals and firms (Roemer, 1993). McPake *et al.* (2013) classify the major areas of health care regulation as either regulation of *quantity* (for example, limiting the number of providers or the volume of specific types of services that can be provided) or regulation of *quality* (for example, regulation of minimum standards or input levels).

An example of quantity regulation is the Certificate of Need laws that are prevalent in the United States and require state agencies to approve the entry of new hospitals, the expansion or modernization of hospitals, and the provision of services, aiming to ensure that provision matches need and to control supplier-induced demand and its consequences for health care cost inflation (McPake *et al.*, 2013). While similar regulations are scarce in low- and middle-income countries, health technology assessment (HTA) plays a role in controlling what technologies can be made available by hospitals in what volumes, whether in public or private sectors. Thailand has a well-developed system managed by the Health Intervention and Technology Assessment Program (HITAP), applying national standards and methodological guidelines for technology assessment. HITAP evaluations determine the reimbursement lists for pharmaceuticals. Public health plans have also based their resource allocation decisions on HITAP analyses, and the assessment of high-cost medical devices (costing more than US$3.3 million in 2009) is mandatory before market authorization (Teerawattananon *et al.*, 2009). Although less developed, HTA is beginning to be used for similar purposes in China (Chen *et al.*, 2009); it is used within the national health insurance program in the Philippines (De Rosas-Valera, 2009); and it has some at least informal application in most Asia-Pacific countries (Sivalal, 2009). Kriza *et al.* (2014) report very limited use in Sub-Saharan Africa.

Quality regulation exists in a basic form almost everywhere. For example, it is present in minimum standard setting for hospital designation, usually based on the presence of specific facilities and staffing cadres, with the staffing cadres defined by regulated educational requirements (McPake *et al.*, 2013). The approach of accreditation — which might classify as regulation according to the definition above, as mechanisms of control are exerted to require hospitals to participate in accreditation programs — is discussed in the next section. Its more usual status as a voluntary activity would exclude it from this definition of regulation. Another approach to quality regulation is to strengthen legal frameworks that penalize negligence in hospital services. In India, the Consumer Protection Act of 1986 attempted to strengthen the rights of consumers and their ability to seek redress through the courts in cases of medical malpractice. Bhat (1996) reviews experience under this legislation but concludes that such measures are not in themselves sufficient to significantly impact poor quality of care in the private sector. Bhat cites the evidence that 71% of cases filed in the state of Gujarat were decided in favor of the defendant, complainants faced considerable difficulty in getting experts to support their cases, and half of outstanding cases at the time of the review were 'pending.' Kessler *et al.* (2006) conclude that the effect of such provisions in the UK and US is to promote 'defensive medicine' involving both unnecessary intervention to protect against an allegation of neglect; and the avoidance of involvement in care delivery in risky circumstances.

- *Accreditation*

Systems of accreditation have been defined as 'external quality assessment' based on written standards (Montagu, 2003). For the purpose of this chapter, we further qualify the definition as those entered voluntarily to distinguish from the types of standard setting and certification addressed in the preceding section. Montagu (2003) further describes accreditation as having the following components: (1) A base in written and published standards; (2) review conducted by professional peers; (3) administered by an independent body and (4) aimed at encouragement of organizational development.

Shaw (2003) describes the rapid growth of accreditation systems, especially in Europe, but makes the point that the evidence base on this topic is very weak, specifically in relation to the coverage of accreditation programs (meaning, what proportion of national hospital markets are covered); the consistency, compatibility, and validity of programs as a basis for comparing hospitals internationally; and the costs and benefits of programs to hospitals. Accreditation programs may quickly increase compliance, although that may not be sustained; the relationship between compliance and quality judged otherwise has not been well established.

Consistent with this, a randomized controlled trial in Kwa Zulu Natal (Salmon *et al.*, 2003) found that compliance with Council for Health Services Accreditation of Southern Africa (COHSASA) standards improved 38 percentage points, from 38% to 76%, in intervention hospitals, while increasing only 1 percentage point, from 37% to 38%, in control hospitals. However, the research team failed to see evidence of improved quality in their separate observations. More recently, Linegar *et al.* (2012) have evaluated the effects of the accreditation program in a hospital in Bloemfontein, finding that its effect of improving quality has provided a conducive environment into which to introduce new services.

Also based largely on the experience of South Africa, Montagu (2003) concludes that it is feasible for an accreditation program in a middle-income country to raise standards of care in incremental stages and also increase equity because smaller facilities serving marginalized populations can be included. However, he argues that subsidy is important in achieving this, as there are economies of scale in the process that disadvantage this type of facility, and facilities that serve marginalized populations are often not market-oriented so lack strong incentives to participate.

Besides the South African experience, the experience of Lebanon has been reasonably well documented (Ammar *et al.*, 2013; El-Jardali *et al.*, 2012; Ammar *et al.*, 2007). Ammar *et al.* (2007) describe the introduction of the accreditation program in Lebanon. Its prior system of hospital grading based on availability of facilities that created incentives to purchase excessive sophisticated equipment; over-provide associated services and inflate hospital cost was replaced by one aiming to create incentives for quality improvement by focusing on external evaluation of patient and staff safety, output and outcome data reporting, infection control measures, and patient advocacy. El-Jardali *et al.* (2012) focus on the process of integrating patient safety standards into the system, finding that few hospitals had effectively integrated patient safety standards into their practice and that a significant investment in training and education would be required to shift culture in this respect. Ammar *et al.* (2013) find that the results of the accreditation exercise do not provide a fair basis for reimbursement because proxy measures of case mix are not sufficiently accurate. This implies that some redesign of the Lebanese system is needed.

Few studies of accreditation and limited accreditation programs seem to exist in low-income countries. Bateganya (2009) suggests that there is strong support and scope to introduce such a program in Uganda, but that support is needed to ease resource and technical capacity deficits. Nandraj *et al.* (2001) make the same argument for India (also middle income).

- *System-level support to health provider institutions*

Although the importance of supportive management systems across the health system is frequently alluded to and its absence often considered the explanation of problems and failed programs (for example, Hofman and Mohammed, 2014; Mselle *et al.*, 2013; Ray *et al.*, 2013; Asp *et al.*, 2011), there is little formal evidence to support these judgments. Some studies show that health workers are better able to achieve reduced stress or achieve better work–life balance in the context of supportive management systems (for example, Zhang *et al.*, 2014; Farhadi *et al.*, 2013; Nantsupawat *et al.*, 2011), and other studies show that intensive support to specific staff functions can achieve improved staff performance (for example, Masika *et al.*, 2006; Khan *et al.*, 2011). However, the literature fails to support an evidence-based understanding of the forms and elements of management and support systems that influence hospital performance and quality at any level of the health system.

Financial reform

Hospitals may be paid directly by patients who use their services, out-of-pocket; by a branch of government, financed through taxation revenues; or by insurance agencies, who in turn may receive payments from those buying insurance against health and health-related cost risks and from government agencies subsidizing those policies. Each payer may negotiate the basis of payment. Payment options include fee-for-service, by which each service element is charged separately; prospective payment, by which an episode of care is charged at a maximum or total price; capitation, by which a hospital charges to provide services to a defined population, irrespective of their pattern of demand for care; or, the hospital may receive a budget to cover the costs of providing care to a less well-defined population, with variable constraints on how it can be spent. For example a 'global' budget can be spent as the budget holder deems appropriate with minimal constraints, or a line item budget may be spent only according to ceilings for each 'item' such as staff or medicines. Given the evident differences in the incentives, risk distribution, and constraints associated with these different institutional arrangements and payment mechanisms, it is likely that hospital performance is influenced by the mix prevailing, and therefore that intervention may focus on improving performance by altering these arrangements.

The implications of alternative payment arrangements may differ according to the characteristics of hospitals, too. Section "Public and Private Ownership Characteristics" discussed the evidence that the public or private ownership characteristics of a hospital may influence its performance: In some cases, it was recognized that the impact was mediated by the influence of payment mechanism. Section "Market Structure and Characteristics" suggested that the payment system itself, as a negotiation over the distribution of risk between the payer and the service provider, is influenced by the structure of the market and the economic power balance between the two.

This section considers the evidence concerning the relationship between payment mechanism and hospital performance. The available research varies in the extent to which it considers the complexities discussed in the previous paragraph. There is a body of work about user fees and out-of-pocket payments; and the replacement of budgeted arrangements with purchasing arrangements using a range of payment mechanisms within the public sector or between public payers and hospitals in both sectors; otherwise the literature is patchy, and inconclusive about the opportunities of improving hospital performance through restructuring payment methods.

User fees and out-of-pocket payments

Most focus on user fees has been on their impact on access and equity. Studies conducted across a range of time periods and settings confirm that other things being equal, the introduction or increase of user fees deters hospital use (for example, Dao *et al.*, 2008; Stekelenburg *et al.*, 2004; Malama *et al.*, 2002; Nordberg *et al.*, 1996) and constitute a significant financial burden for poor households (Vuong *et al.*, 2014; Onwujekwe *et al.*, 2013; Dao *et al.*, 2008; Kadir *et al.*, 2000; Chisadza *et al.*, 1995), and were even associated with non-payers being detained in hospitals in Burundi (Kippenberg *et al.*, 2007). Although exemption systems aim to counter these problems, they work poorly at targeting those in need (for example, Meng, 2002) and have mixed effects in supporting access (Weaver, 1995) or reducing the financial burdens associated with seeking hospital care (Chisadza *et al.*, 1995). These findings are similar to those that relate to seeking health care at other levels of the health system.

User fees at the hospital level have sometimes been designed with the aim of supporting referral structures that often work poorly in low- and middle-income countries. By structuring fees so that hospital services are more expensive; or are reduced for those patients who have been referred from lower levels of the system, policy architects have often hoped to encourage patients to use under-utilized primary care systems (Hongoro *et al.*, 1988; Weaver, 1995; Nordberg *et al.*, 1996). These objectives have often been frustrated. Hongoro *et al.* (1988) found a poor understanding of the difference between levels of care and a failure to observe fee waivers for referred patients at the hospital level. Nordberg *et al.* (1996) found the referral process ineffective, failing to refer patients appropriately, and patients deterred from following referral instructions by fees. Weaver (1995) found that the system would be effective in the case of inpatients but not outpatients.

Given the constraint that fees place on the demand for hospital services, their justification is largely based on their ability to support the supply of services by improving quality and rationalizing use of services, thereby allowing resources to be focused on higher priority services. Few studies have documented these benefits from the introduction or increasing of fees at hospital level. Although utilization can be shown to be supported by quality improvement counterbalancing the effect of fees, the resulting change in the distribution of users has been shown to be inequitable in a case study in India (Rao and Peters, 2007). Eggleston and Yip (2004) show that the relative price levels of different services are critical for the rationalization of service provision. Fee structures that are intended to motivate rational choice of services on the part of the service user may instead motivate irrational supply of services on the part of service providers in the presence of significant provider moral hazard, as in China in the early 2000s.

- *Purchasing for public service provision*

The concept of purchasing discussed here is that of negotiating a contract for services on behalf of the general public with the strategic intent of securing gains in efficiency, quality or other dimensions of performance. This incorporates a number of models, including the 'purchaser–provider split' as a reorganization of a whole health system, contracting out by a public funder, and pay-for-performance approaches, although the intention is to discuss evidence related to larger sectoral programs in this section rather than small projects.

Turkey, Kygyzstan, Zambia, and Senegal, are among low- and middle-income countries that have applied a purchaser–provider split arrangement across their entire hospital systems. The arrangements involved in Turkey and Kyrgyzstan are described but not evaluated by Tatar *et al.* (2011) and Ibraimova *et al.* (2011), respectively. Gueye and Kopp (2009) describe the process of implementation and its early results in Senegal. Fifteen contracts were signed in early 2006 and evaluated in July 2007 with the evaluation results determining a performance subsidy to be allocated in 2008. The contracts were judged to have had a positive impact on performance. A second phase of contracts was being negotiated at the time the authors were writing.

Hanson *et al.* (2002) describe the earlier experience of Zambia (initiated in 1992), which was later reversed. The 1992 reforms created a purchasing authority, called the Central Board of Health, and 22 Hospital Boards at second and third referral level hospitals. The relationship between the two was governed by contracts, setting out services the hospital committed to provide for its catchment population. Hospitals were also expected to sell services directly to patients at cost recovery prices that fell outside the negotiated package of services. The reforms coincided with a period of economic recession in which health sector expenditures contracted. While elements of the reforms appeared to improve service provision, for example the ability to contract locally with certain categories of staff rather than employing them through the Public Service Commission, positive performance trends were not observed overall and the hospitals responded most actively to the opportunity to gain additional revenue through marketing services deemed outside the package. Such responsiveness to market opportunities has been observed in other countries in which public hospitals have been freed to generate revenue from the market (see Section "Structural Reform").

More limited contracting for public sector services has been evaluated as delivering benefits in terms of hospital performance. For example, Igwegbe *et al.* (2012) find that a contract with a University Teaching Hospital in Nigeria resulted in a progressive reduction in maternal mortality (which was not statistically significant), a progressive increase in the number of live births, and a reduction in the delay between patient presentation at the hospital and intervention.

Contracting of private hospitals to provide services to the general public has been undertaken in a number of countries. Ssengooba *et al.* (2012) describe the experience of seven hospitals in Uganda in intervention and control arms of a national experiment to contract with private-not-for-profit hospitals: An experiment their analysis revealed to be poorly designed and implemented and not to have achieved its intended outcomes. McPake and Hongoro (1995) earlier reviewed a contract between the Zimbabwean government and a mining hospital, concluding that it succeeded in providing services of higher quality and equivalent cost to those of public hospitals but failed to control costs overall, implying that the contract absorbed a disproportionate share of public expenditure.

Heberholz and Supakankunti (2015) describe the experience of Thailand and the Philippines. In Thailand, public authorities contract with 98 private and 2313 network hospitals (who are contracted by other providers) to contribute to service provision for the general population under the Universal Health Coverage scheme. The contracts mainly use capitation rates, supplemented by additional payments for meeting targets. In the Philippines, the contracting is tied to an accreditation process of a type discussed above. To join the program, hospitals submit Performance Commitments which form the basis of a contract and are reimbursed on a fee-for-service basis. In neither country has the process been smooth, or is there clear evidence of hospital performance gains through the approach but the authors argue that longer experience in high-income countries suggest that the relationships between contracting parties may improve over time and form the basis of greater success.

Structural reform

The final type of reform to be considered in this chapter is that of changing the governance arrangements of public hospitals. The direction of reform over the past 20 years has been to increase the operational autonomy of hospitals that were traditionally directly managed by national Ministries of Health, Health Service Divisions, or their regional counterparts. Hanson *et al.* (2002) point out that this involves an element of decentralization or more local control of operations, and usually also an element of greater exposure to market forces. Among the increased freedoms is usually the option of generating revenue in addition to public funds by directly selling services to patients, or employers or other organizations buying services on behalf of patients.

Harding and Preker (2003) propose a typology of governance arrangements for public hospitals as in Figure 1. A public hospital directly managed by government is termed a 'budgetary unit.' The hospital arrangements can be characterized

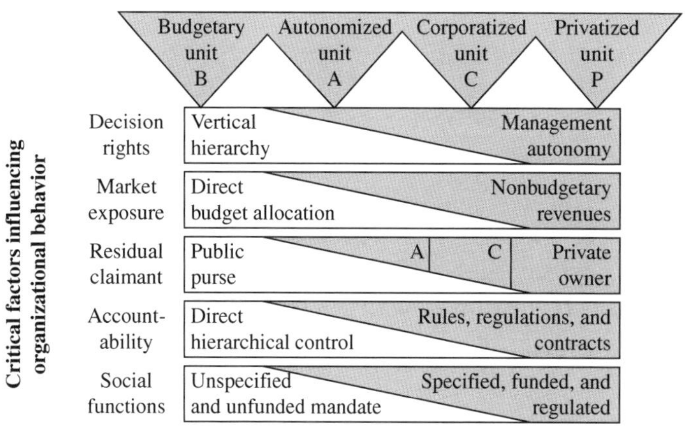

Figure 1. Typology of governance arrangements for public hospitals

Source: Harding and Preker (2003).

as those of autonomized units, corporatized units, or privatized units — this characterization is based on the level of management autonomy, reliance on non-budgetary revenues, and the emergence of residual claimants on any financial surplus leveraged by increases in hospital operations. The characterization also shifts as accountability shifts from operating through a system of direct hierarchical control to operating through rules, regulations and contracts, and as the mandate to deliver social functions (i.e., services for public benefit rather than private profit) shifts from unspecified and unfunded to specified, funded and regulated. In practice, the arrangements characterizing reformed hospitals may mix levels of each of the dimensions in ways other than suggested by the figure, and the last dimension is least clearly related to the others, but the framework provides a useful typology and set of dimensions with which arrangements in different countries can be compared.

The empirical literature evaluating case studies of hospital reform discusses cases in a wide range of low- and middle-income countries, including Vietnam (London, 2013); Colombia (Castaño and Mills, 2012); Senegal (Gueye and Kopp, 2009); Pakistan (Abdullah and Shaw, 2007); Iran (Jafari *et al.*, 2011); Tunisia (Achouri and Jarawan, 2003); Indonesia (Lieberman and Alkatiri, 2003); Uganda and Zambia (Hanson *et al.*, 2002); India (Sharma and Hotchkiss, 2001); and Kenya (Collins, 1999).

There are considerable difficulties in evaluating the impact of this reform, often embedded in other reforms and seldom under implementation against a background of stability in relation to economy or governance. Those hospitals that have been included in reforms that increase their autonomy are not randomly selected, so controls are not available. Few studies are even able to call on baseline data. Reforms are complex and have multiple components.

There has been mixed evaluation of the experience of hospital reform, with some cases presented as successes (for example Collins, 1999), and others identifying specific problems, especially in relation to quality of care and equity (Govindaraj and Chawla, 1996), even on the basis of rather partial analysis.

Many of the case studies conclude that the level of autonomy implemented is significantly less than that implied by the rhetoric of the policy or its formal design. For example, Achouri and Jarawan (2003) and Jafari *et al.* (2011) both conclude that the post-reform hospitals differ little from the budgetary units of the Harding and Preker (2003) framework; and Abdullah and Shaw (2007) describe the steps taken by provincial government officials to frustrate the processes that were intended to decentralize authority.

However, even where only minimal new authority was judged to have been delegated, the clear response in most cases was the use of that authority to increase revenue generation from fees: Both general fees and separated 'private' service provision within the public hospital. For example, even in the Pakistani case, which Abdullah and Shaw (2007) concluded had barely shifted the level of the hospitals' autonomy, the creation of an "Institution-Based (Private) Practice" was noted to have generated significant revenues in one of the hospitals under study. In the case of Kenyatta National Hospital — which, considered as an early success, may have contributed to the impetus for similar reforms elsewhere — documented the increase of recurrent income from fees from 1% pre-reform to 10% post-reform *excluding private wing revenue*. Similar response to any degree of greater autonomy has been documented in Zambia and Indonesia (McPake and Hanson, 2004); Vietnam (London, 2013); and India (Sharma and Hotchkiss, 2001) among others.

Otherwise, assessments of the effects on performance aspects such as quality, efficiency, volume of services provided and budgetary management are highly varied across the case studies. This probably reflects differences in performance in very different contexts, institutional arrangements and reforms to those arrangements, and very diverse research methodologies.

Conclusions

Hospitals have been experiencing challenging times. They are at the forefront of the conflict between the technically possible and resource limits. This is premised in part on the possibilities opened up by new technologies to intervene in our health at all stages of the lifecycle, in part on the success of health care and other advances that have extended life expectancy and produced ageing societies, and in part on the failures that have allowed chronic non-communicable diseases to become endemic. The achievement of high quality and good performance must occur in this difficult context. In low- and middle-income countries, it must occur typically with the additional constraint of severe resource limits relative to demand and expectations of services.

This chapter has reviewed a large number of concepts of hospital quality and performance and a range of research with a bearing on the factors producing them in low- and middle-income contexts. It is far from exhaustive in either the range of issues addressed, the approaches taken to address them, or the published research. All aspects of quality and performance are complex and difficult to measure and they mostly are contingent on the perspective taken, which is not always identified or acknowledged.

While not attempting to be comprehensive, the review of available literature has suggested a great unevenness in the coverage of different topics.

For example, there is now quite a significant body of work using DEA to measure hospital efficiency and to judge the effectiveness of policies in improving hospital efficiency. Despite the limitations of the approach, it seems conducive to available data opportunities in a large number of settings and generates interesting if less than conclusive analyses about the profile of inputs, activities, and outputs of hospitals in different settings. It specifically generates evidence in relation to scale effects, which could be useful for public policy if further analyzed in the context of patterns of demand and need to produce an understanding of what hospital scale of operation is consistent with efficiency. Given the extent to which the approach has been developed and refined, with increasing applications in low- and middle-income countries, and given that it may be a more reliable guide to efficiency change than to overall levels of efficiency, it could be used more extensively to evaluate the efficiency impacts of interventions at hospital or sectoral levels than it has been to date.

In contrast, there is very little understanding of the nature of hospital markets in low- and middle-income countries, and these are consequently poorly understood. Clearly, there is an incompatibility between typical data availability and the capacity to undertake market analysis, with few national institutions generating routine data about prices, service volumes and patient characteristics that would be required to undertake such analyses. In many low- and middle-income countries, hospital markets appear more monopolistic than in high-income countries, implying that particular types of regulation may be needed to moderate their efficiency toward better quality and performance. However, this is insufficiently understood to generate such policy implications.

In general, the surveys of evidence in relation to the range of intervention approaches that had attracted published research suggested inconsistent results from the application of similar interventions. This is not an unusual conclusion from wide ranging reviews of policy-related research. The search for policies that are universally successful wherever applied is usually a fruitless one. What becomes clear in such exercises is that the effects of policies depend on the context into which they are applied, on the micro-detail of the policy design and its fit with that context, and on the nature of the policy as implemented, which can differ significantly to how it was designed, especially where a policy poses particular implementation challenges. Hospitals are politically important institutions and researchers are not immune from the pressures that it creates. London (2013) notes that researchers have been restricted in their access to data related to the impacts of hospital autonomy in Vietnam, and that the literature in general is politicized, some of it authored by people with clear stakes in the success of reform; others with clear ideological antagonism. While this is a particular problem for high profile and market liberalizing measures like hospital autonomy, it can also be a factor in evaluation of less clearly political questions.

Considering the evidence about the quite prevalent attempts to introduce quality improvement programs premised on a criterion-based audit approach highlights these issues and the need. At least three studies reported significant performance benefits from these quality improvement attempts (Berman *et al.*, 2014; Srofenyoh *et al.*, 2012; Hunyinbo *et al.* 2008); at least two reported less success (Du *et al.*, 2014; Latham *et al.*, 2012); while two explicitly considered the difficulties constraining the extent of implementation of the program as designed (Rabbani *et al.*, 2011; Ovretveit and Al Serouri, 2006). Further analysis of the seven cases might provide a better comparative understanding of the conducive and unconducive contextual characteristics; the detailed differences in program design that might account for the different results, or the random factors that influenced implementation at the time and place that it was attempted and reshaped the program into a different intervention. The published accounts generally cannot support this type of analysis. It is left to those interested to explore the opportunities that such programs might present, to seek to understand better how to go about it from published literature and any other sources of evidence about past experience they are able to access, to experiment and learn from experience in context, and to hope to avoid adverse random implementation constraints. It is not clear that simply more research would obviate these measures.

On the other hand, a much clearer picture emerges in relation to more patient-centric approaches to hospital quality improvement: they are much more rarely attempted in low- and middle-income countries, and where attempted, they seem to encounter strong cultural resistance in settings as different as Pakistan and Zambia. This has quite clear implications for the need to specifically address likely cultural resistance in attempts to introduce such programs — which may also be required in high-income countries. Similarly, the limited experience with accreditation approaches in low- and middle-income countries might reflect the relatively intensive institutional capacity demands of such approaches, and suggest that the need for investment in specific kinds of institutions needs to precede attempts to introduce accreditation.

As suggested earlier, limits to specific types of data availability seem to explain the dearth of published research in a number of important areas in low- and middle-income countries, relative to high-income countries. It is seldom the case that major data collection efforts are premised entirely on research purposes, but rather that data sets are a by product of management and accounting processes that tend to accompany more complex institutional arrangements. Much US research is premised on the availability of billing records that allow for estimation of resource flows, which are more difficult to estimate everywhere that health services are provided without charge and without billing. Reforms that have introduced purchasing as the financing mechanism, even within public systems that are free at the point of use to the patient, are increasing the extent to which such data are being created, and research has followed. For example, Gaynor and Town (2011) were able to include several European studies in their review of the importance of market structure for hospital performance. As institutional arrangements become more complex in larger numbers of low- and middle-income countries, research opportunities are likely to open up to better understand a number of factors shaping hospital quality and performance.

Comparative analysis will remain challenging even in the context of the availability of better data. The analysis of Bottle *et al.* (2013), attempting to compare quality across data rich settings still concluded that differences in variable definitions, measurement processes and institutional contexts left results inconclusive and most useful as a basis for further qualitative inquiry. This provides a helpful cautionary note in relation to appropriate ambition for research agendas in hospital quality and performance. We can greatly improve the availability of data and evidence for decision-making, but decisions and strategies will still require judgment based on a broader understanding of context and unmeasured and unmeasurable considerations about fit between interventions and context and constraints to implementation.

References

Abdullah MT, Shaw J. 2007. A review of the experience of hospital autonomy in Pakistan. *International Journal of Health Planning and Management* 22: 45–62.

Achouri H, Jarawan E. 2003. Autonomous Structures — with Incomplete Autonomy: Unusual hospital reform in Tunisia, Chapter 13. In: In Preker AS, Harding A. (eds.). Innovations in Health Service Delivery: The Corporatization of Hospitals. Washington DC: The World Bank.

Adam T, Evans DB, Ying B, Murray CJL. 2014. Variability in costs across hospital wards. A study of Chinese hospitals. *PLOS One* 9(5): e97874. doi:101371/journal.pone.0097874.

Aghamolaei T, Eftekhaari TE, Rafati S, Kahnouji K, Ahangari S, Shahrzad ME, Kahnouji A, Hoseini SH. 2014. Service quality assessment of a referral hospital in Southern Iran with SERVQUAL technique: Patients' perspective. *BMC Health Services Research* 14: 322.

Agyeman-Duah JNA, Theurer A, Munthali C, Alide N, Neuhann F. (2014). Understanding the barriers to setting up a healthcare quality improvement process in resource-limited settings: A situational analysis at the medical department of Kamuzu Central Hospital in Lilongwe, Malawi. *BMC Health Services Research* 14: 1.

Ahgren B. 2008. Is it better to be big? The reconfiguration of 21st century hospitals: Responses to a hospital merger in Sweden. *Health Policy* 87: 92–99.

Alexander T, Fuller G, Hargovan P, Clarke DL, Muckart DJ, Thomson SR. 2009. An audit of the quality of care of traumatic brain injury at a busy regional hospital in South Africa. *South African Journal of Surgery* 47(4): 120–126.

Ammar W, Wakim R, Hajj I. 2007. Accreditation of hospitals in Lebanon: A challenging experience. *La Revue de Santé de la Méditerranée orientale* 13(1): 138–149.

Ammar W, Khalife J, El-Jardali F, Romanos J, Harb H, Hamadeh G, Dimassi H. 2013. Hospital accreditation, reimbursement and case mix: Links and insights for contractual systems. *BMC Health Services Research* 13: 505.

Andaleeb SS. 2000. Public and private hospitals in Bangladesh: Service quality and predictors of hospital choice. *Health Policy and Planning* 15(1): 95–102.

Ande, B, Chiwuzie J, Akpala W, Oronsaye A, Okojie O, Okolocha C, Omorogbe S, Onoguwe B, Oikeh E. 1997. Improving obstetric care at the district hospital, Ekpoma, Nigeria. *International Journal of Gynecology and Obstetrics* 59: S47–S53.

Asp G, Sandberg J, Ezechi O, Petterson KO. 2011. Challenges of immediate newborn care in maternity units in Lagos, Nigeria: An observational study. *Journal of Obstetrics and Gynaecology* 31(7): 612–616.

Audibert M, Mathonnat J, Pareil D, Kabamba R. 2007. Analysis of hospital costs as a basis for pricing services in Mali. *International Journal of Health Planning and Management* 22: 205–224.

Bateganya M, Hagopian A, Tavrow P, Luboga S, Barnhart S. 2009. Incentives and barriers to implement national hospital standards in Uganda. *International Journal for Quality in Health Care* 21(6): 421–426.

Bennett S. 1997. The nature of competition among private hospitals in Bangkok. In *Private Health Providers in Developing Countries*. Bennett S, McPake B, Mills A. (eds.). Zed Press: London.

Berman J, Nkabane EL, Malope S, Machai S, Jack B, Bicknell W. 2014. Developing a hospital quality improvement initiative in Lesotho. *International Journal of Health Care Quality Assurance* 27(1): 15–24.

Bhat R. 1996. Regulating the private health care sector: The case of the Indian Consumer Protection Act. *Health Policy and Planning* 1(3): 265–279.

Bottle A, Middleton S, Kalkman CJ, Livingston EH, Aylin P. 2013. Global comparators project: International comparison of hospital outcomes using administrative data. *Health Services Research* 2081–2100.

Carayon P, Schoofs Hundt A, Karsh BT, Gurses AP, Alvarado GJ, Smith M, Flatley-Brennan P. 2006. Work system design for patient safety: The SEIPS model. *Quality and Safety in Health Care* 15(Suppl 1): I50–i58.

Castañeda-Mendez K, Mangan K, Lavery AM. 1998. The role and application of the balanced scorecard in healthcare quality management. *Journal for Healthcare Quality* 20(1): 10–13.

Castano R, Mills A. 2012. The consequences of hospital autonomization in Colombia: A transaction cost economics analysis. *Health Policy and Planning* 28: 157–164.

Chang DC, Nguyen LL, Chrouser LL, Freischlag JA, Colombani PM, Abdullah F. 2011. Cost of inpatient care and its association with hospital competition. *Journal of the American College of Surgeons* 212(1): 12–19.

Chen Y, Banta D, Tang Z. 2009. Health technology assessment development in China. *International Journal of Technology Assessment in Health Care* 25(Supplement 1): 202–209.

Chen X, Yamauchi K, Kato K, Nishimura A, Ito K. 2006. Using the balanced scorecard to measure Chinese and Japanese hospital performance. *International Journal of Health Care Quality Assurance* 19(4): 339–350.

Chisadza E, Maponga CC, Nazerali H. 1995. User fees and drug pricing prolicies: A study at Harare Central Hospital, Zimbabwe. *Health Policy and Planning* 10(3): 319–326.

Coetzee SK, Klopper HC, Ellis SM, Aiken LH. 2013. A tale of two systems — nurses practice environment, well being, perceived quality of care and patient safety in private and public hospitals in South Africa: A questionnaire survey. *International Journal of Nursing Studies* 50: 162–173.

Collins D, Njeru G, Meme J, Newbrander W. 1999. Hospital autonomy: The experience of Kenyatta National Hospital. *International Journal of Health Planning and Management* 14: 129–153.

Cong L, Yu J, Liu Y. 2012. Implementing a continuous quality improvement program for reducing pressure prevalence in a teaching hospital in China. *Journal of Wound Ostomy Continence Nursing* 39(5): 509–513.

Dao HT, Waters H, Le QV. 2008. User fees and health service utilization in Vietnam: How to protect the poor? *Public Health* 122: 1069–1078.

De Rosas-Valera M. 2009. Health technology assessment in the Philippines. *International Journal of Technology assessment in Health Care* 25(Supplement 1): 231–213.

Devadasan N, Criel B, Van Damme W, Manoharan S, Sankara Sarma P, Van der Stuyft P. 2009. Community health insurance in Gudalur, India, increases access to hospital care. *Health Policy and Planning* 25: 145–154.

Dilip TR. 2010. Utilization of inpatient care from private hospitals: Trends emerging from Kerala, India. *Health Policy and Planning* 25: 437–446.

Donabedian A. 1966. Evaluating the quality of medical care. *The Milbank Quarterly* 83(4): 691–729.

Dranove D, White WD. 1994. Recent theory and evidence on competition in hospital markets. *Journal of Economic Management and Strategy* 3: 169–209.

Du X, *et al.* 2014. Hospital quality improvement initiative for Patients with acute coronary syndromes in China: A cluster randomized, controlled trial. *Circulation Cardiovascular Quality Outcomes* 7: 217–226.

Duke T, Keshishiyan E, Kuttumuratova A, Ostergren M, Ryumina I, Stasii E, Weber MW, Tamburlini G. 2006. Quality of hospital care for children in Kazakhstan, Republic of Moldova, and Russia: Systematic observational assessment. *The Lancet* 367: 919–925.

Eggleston K, Yip W. 2004. Hospital competition under regulated prices: Application to urban health sector reforms in China. *International Journal of Health Care Finance and Economics* 4: 343–368.

Eggleston K, Shen Y-C, Lau J, Schmid CH, Chan J. 2008. Hospital ownership and quality of care: What explains the different results in the literature? *Health Economics* 17: 1345–1362.

El-Jardali F, Saleh S, Ataya N, Jamal D. 2011. Design, implementation and scaling up of the balanced scorecard for hospitals in Lebanon: Policy coherence and application lessons for low and middle income countries. *Health Policy* 103: 305–314.

El-Jardali, Jaafar M, Jamal D, Rabbaa S. 2012. Integrating patient safety standards in to the accreditation program: A qualitative study to assess the readiness of Lebanese hospitals to implement into routine practice. *Journal of Patient Satisfaction* 8: 97–103.

English M, Esamai F, Wasunna A, Were F, Ogutu B, Wamae A, Snow RW, Peshu N. 2004. Assessment of inpatient paediatric care in first referral level hospitals in 13 districts in Kenya. *The Lancet* 363: 1948–1953.

Ersoy K, Kavuncubasi S, Ozcan YA, Harris JM. 1997. Technical efficiencies of Turkish hospitals: DEA approach. *Journal of Medical Systems* 21(2): 67–74.

Farhadi P, Sharifian R, Feili A, Shokrpour N. 2013. The effects of supervisors' supportive role, job stress, and work–family conflicts on the nurses' attitudes. *The Health Care Manager* 32(2): 107–122.

Farrington-Douglas J, Brooks R. 2007. *The Future Hospital: The Politics of Change*, London: Institute for Public Policy Research.

Flessa S. 1998. The costs of hospital services: A case study of Evangelical Lutheran church hospitals in Tanzania. *Health Policy and Planning* 13(4): 397–407.

Gai R, Zhou C, Xu L, Zhu M, Wang X, Li S, Zheng W, Song P, Yang X, Fang L, Zhen Y, Tang W. 2010. Health resource allocation and productive efficiency of Chinese county hospitals: Data from 1993 to 2005. *BioScience Trends* 4(5): 218–224.

Gao Y, Barclay L. 2010. Availability and quality of emergency obstetric care in Shanxi Province, China. *International Journal of Gynecology and Obstetrics* 110: 181–185.

Gao Y, Barclay L, Kildea, S, Hao, M, Belton, S. 2010. Barriers to increasing hospital birth rates in rural Shanxi Province, China. *Reproductive Health Matters* 18(36): 35–45.

Gaynor, M, Town RJ. 2011. Competition in health care markets, *Working Paper* 17208, National Bureau of Economic Research, Cambridge MA.

Gok MS Sezen B. 2013. Analyzing the ambiguous relationship between efficiency, quality and patient satisfaction in healthcare services: The case of public hospitals in Turkey. *Health Policy* 111: 290–300.

Gosselin RA, Thind A, Bellardinelli A. 2006. Cost/DALY averted in a small hospital in Sierra Leone: What is the relative contribution of different services? *World Journal of Surgery* 30: 505–511.

Gosselin RA. Heitto, M. 2008. Cost-effectiveness of a district trauma hospital in Battambang, Cambodia. *World Journal of Surgery* 32: 2450–2453.

Gosselin RA, Hietto M, Zirkle L. 2009. Cost-effectiveness of replacing skeletal traction by interlocked intramedullary nailing for femoral shaft fractures in a provincial trauma hospital in Cambodia. *International Orthopaedics* 33: 1445–1448.

Govindaraj R, Chawla M. 1996. Recent experiences with hospital autonomy in developing countries, What can we learn?, Data for Decision Making Project, Harvard School of Public Health.

Graham W, Wagaarachchi P, Penney G, McCaw-Binns A, Yeboah Antwi K, Hall MH. 2000. Criteria for clinical audit of the quality of hospital-based obstetric care in developing countries. *Bulletin of the World Health Organization* 78(5): 614–620.

Griffiths A, Wall S. 2001. *Applied Economics*, 9th Edition, Pearson Education.

Gueye MA, Kopp JE. 2009. [Hospital performance contract: The Senegalese experience] (article in French). *Sante Publique* 21(1): 77–87.

Guinness L, Arthur G, Bhatt SM, Achiya G, Kariuki S. Gilks CF. 2002. Costs of hospital care for HIV-positive and HIV-negative patients at Kenyatta National Hospital, Nairobi, Kenya. *AIDS* 16: 901–908.

Hajialiafzali H, Moss JR. Mahmood MA. 2007. Efficiency measurement for hospitals owned by the Iranian Social Security Organisation. *Journal of Medical Systems* 31: 166–172.

Hanson K, Atuyambe L, Kamwanga J, McPake B, Mungule O, Ssengooba F. 2002. Towards improving hospital performance in Uganda and Zambia: Reflections and opportunities for autonomy. *Health Policy* 61: 73–94.

Harding A, Preker AS. 2003. A conceptual framework for the organizational reforms of hospitals Chapter 1. In Preker AS, Harding A. (eds.). *Innovations in Health Service Delivery: The Corporatization of Hospitals*. Washington DC: The World Bank.

Harzallah F, Alberti H, Kanoun F, Elhouch F, Slimane H. 2004. Quality of care of patients with type 2 diabetes in a Tunisian university hospital. *Diabetes Metabolism* 30: 523–526.

Healy J, McKee M. 2002. The evolution of hospital systems Chapter 2. In: Healy J, McKee M. (eds.). *Hospitals in a Changing Europe*, European Observatory on Health Care Systems Series, Buckingham and Philadelphia: Open University Press.

Heberholz C, Supakankunti S. 2015. Contracting private hospitals: Experiences from southeast and east Asia. *Health Policy* (epub ahead of print).

Hofman JJ, Mohammed H. 2014. Experiences with facility-based maternal death reviews in northern Nigeria. *International Journal of Gynecology and Obstetrics* 126: 111–114.

Hongoro C, McPake B, Vickerman P. 2005. Measuring the quality of hospital tuberculosis services: A prospective study in four Zimbabwe hospitals. *International Journal for Quality in Health Care* 17(4): 287–292.

Hongoro C, Musonza TG, Macq J, Anozie A. 1988. A qualitative assessment of the referral system at district level in Zimbabwe: Implications on efficiency and effective delivery of health services. *Central African Journal of Medicine* 44(4): 93–97.

Hung J-H, Chang L. 2008. Has cost containment after the National Health Insurance system been successful? Determinants of Taiwan hospital costs. *Health Policy* 85: 321–335.

Hunyinbo KI, Fawole AO, Sotiloye OS, Otolorin EO. 2008. Evaulation of criteria-based audit at improving quality of obstetric care in a developing country hospital. *African Journal of Reproductive Health* 12(3): 59–70.

Ibrahim S. 2010. Quality of care assessment and adherence to the international guidelines considering dialysis, water treatment, and protection against transmission of infections in university hospital-based dialysis units in Cairo, Egypt. *Hemodialysis International* 14: 61–67.

Ibraimova A, Akkazieva B, Ibraimov A, Manzhieva E, Rechel B. 2011. *Kyrgyzstan: Health System Review*, Health Systems in Transition, 13, 3, European Observatory on Health Systems and Policies, Copenhagen: World Health Organization.

Ifenne D, Essien E, Golji N, Sabitu K, Alti-Mu-azu M, Musa A, Adidu V, Mukaddas M. 1997. Improving the quality of obstetric care at the teaching hospital, Zaria, Nigeria. *International Journal of Gynecology and Obstetrics* 59(Suppl. 2): S37–S46.

Igwegbe AO, Eleje GU, Ugboaja JO, Ofiaeli RO. 2012. Improving maternal mortality at a university teaching hospital in Nnewi, Nigeria. *International Journal of Gynecology and Obstetrics* 116: 197–200.

Jafari M, Rashidian A, Abolhasani F, Mohammad K, Yazdani S, Parkerton P, Yunesian M, Akbari F, Arab M. 2011. Space or no space for managing public hospitals; a qualitative study of hospital autonomy in Iran. *International Journal of Health Planning and Management* 26: e121–e137.

Jat TR, Sebastian MS. 2013. Technical efficiency of public district hospitals in Madhya Pradesh, India: A data envelopment analysis. *Global Health Action* 6: 21742.

Kadir MM, Khan A, Sadrudding S, Luby SP. 2000. Out-of-pocket expenses borne by the user of obstetric services at government hospitals in Karachi, Pakistan. *Journal of the Pakistan Medical Association* 50(12): 412–415.

Kaplan RS, Norton DP. 1996. *The Balanced Scorecard: Translating Strategy into Action.* Boston, MA: Harvard Business School Press.

Keat CH, Ghani NA. 2013. Cost-effectiveness analysis of Granisetron-based versus standard antiemetic regimens in low-emetogenic chemotherapy: A hospital based perspective from Malaysia. *Asian Pacific Journal of Cancer Prevention* 14(12): 7701–7706.

Keith J, Prior D. 2014. Scale and scope economies in Mexican private medical units. *Salud Publica de México* 56: 348–354.

Kessler DP, Summerton N, Graham JR. 2006. Effects of the medical liability system in Australia, the UK and the USA. *The Lancet* 368(9531): 240–246.

Ketabi S. 2011. Efficiency measurement of cardiac care units of Isfahan hospitals in Iran. *Journal of Medical Systems* 35: 143–150.

Khan MS, Suwannapong N, Howteerakul N, Pacheum O, Rajatanun T. 2011. Improvement of district hospital service system to increase treatment adherence among tuberculosis patients in Pakistan. *Southeast Asian Journal of Tropical Medicine and Public Health* 42(3): 664–673.

Kiadaliri AA, Jafari M, Gerdtham U-G. 2013. Frontier based techniques in measuring hospital efficiency in Iran: A systematic review and meta-regression analysis. *BMC Health Services Research* 13: 312.

Kidanto HL, Wangwe P, Kilewo CD, Nystrom L, Lindmark G. 2012. Improved quality of management of eclampsia patients through criteria based autdit at Muhimbili National Hospital, Dar es Salaam, Tanzani. Bridging the quality. *BMC Pregnancy and Childbirth* 12: 134.

Kippenberg J, Sahokwasama JB, Amon JJ. 2007. Detention of insolvent patients in Burundian hospitals. *Health Policy and Planning* 23: 14–23.

Kirigia JM, Emrouznejad A, Sambo LG. 2002. Measurement of technical efficiency of public hospitals in Kenya: Using data envelopment analysis. *Journal of Medical Systems* 26(1): 39–45.

Kirigia JM, Emrouznehad A, Cassoma B, Asbu EZ, Barry S. 2008. A performance assessment method for hospitals: The case of municipal hospitals in Angola. *Journal of Medical Systems* 32: 509–519.

Kirigia JM, Asbu EZ. 2013. Technical and scale efficiency of public community hospitals in Eritrea: An exploratory study. *Health Economics Review* 3: 6.

Kriza C, Hanass-Hancock J, Ankrah Odame E, Deghaye N, Aman R, Wahlster P, Marin M, Gebe N, Akhwale W, Wachsmuth I, Kolominsky-Rabas PL. 2014. A systematic review of health technology assessment tools in Sub-Saharan Africa: Methodological issues and implications. *Health Research Policy and Systems* 12: 66.

Kumbani LC, Chirwa E, Malata A, Odland JO, Bjune G. 2012. Do Malawian women critically assess the quality of care? A qualitative study on women's perceptions of perinatal care at a district hospital in Malawi. *Reproductive Health* 9: 30.

Latham T, Malomboza O, Nyirenda L, Ashford P, Emmanuel J, M'Baya B, Bates I. 2012. Quality in practice: Implementation of hospital guidelines for patient identification in Malawi. *International Journal for Quality in Health Care* 24(6): 626–633.

Levesque JF, Haddad S, Narayana D, Fournier P. (2007). Insular pathways to health care in the city: A multilevel analysis of access to hospital care in urban Kerala, India. *Tropical Medicine and International Health* 12(7): 802–814.

Li H, Dong S, Liu T. 2014. Relative efficiency and productivity: A preliminary exploration of public hospitals in Beijing, China. *BMC Health Services Research* 14: 158.

Lieberman SS, Alkatiri A. 2003. Autonomization in Indonesia: The wrong path to reduce hospital expenditures in: In Preker AS, Harding A. (eds.). Innovations in Health Service Delivery: The corporatization of hospitals, Washington DC: The World Bank.

Lind A, Edward A, Bonhoure P, Mustafa L, Hansen P, Burnham G, Peters DH. 2011. Quality of outpatient hospital care for children under 5 years in Afghanistan. *International Journal for Quality in Health Care* 23(2): 108–116.

Linegar A, Whittaker S, van Zyl G. 2012. Academic hospital accreditation strengthens postgraduate training programmes: Case study from Universitas Academic Hospital. *South African Medical Journal* 102: 146–148.

Liu GG, Li L, Hou X, Xu J, Hyslop D. 2009. The role of for-profit hospitals in medical expenditures: Evidence from aggregate data in China. *China Economic Review* 20: 625–633.

Lloyd RC. 2004. *Quality Health Care: A guide to Developing and Using Indicators*, Burlington, MA: Jones and Bartlett Learning.

Lodewijckx C, Sermeus W, Panella M, Deneckere S, Leigheb F, Troosters T, Boto PA, Mendes RV, Decramer M, Vanhaecht K. 2013. Quality indicators for in-hospital management of exacerbation of chronic obstructive pulmonary disease: Results of an international Delphi study. *Journal of Advanced Nursing* 69(2): 348–362.

London JD. 2013. The promises and perils of hospital autonomy, Reform by degree in Viet Nam. *Social Science and Medicine* 96: 232–240.

Lozano R. *et al.* 2012. Global and regional mortality from 235 causes of death for 20 age groups in 1990 and 2010: A systematic analysis for the Global Burden of Disease Study 2010. *The Lancet* 380: 2095–2128.

McCord C, Chowdhury Q. 2003. A cost effective small hospital in Bangladesh: What it can mean for emergency obstetric care. *International Journal of Gynaecology and Obstetrics* 81: 83–92.

Maceira D, Poblete C. 2003. Estructura de Mercado y mecanismos de pago en salud: Experiencias en la provincial de Mendoza, Argentina, 1989–1999. *Desarrollo Económico* 43(171): 443–468.

McKee M, Healy J. 2002. The significance of hospitals: An introduction. Chapter 1 in: Healy J, McKee M. (eds.) *Hospitals in a Changing Europe*, European Observatory on Health Care Systems Series, Buckingham and Philadelphia: Open University Press.

McPake B, Hongoro C. 1995. Contracting out of clinical services in Zimbabwe. *Social Science and Medicine* 41(1): 13–24.

McPake B, Hanson K. 2004. Implementation of hospital reform policies: Lessons of experience. Available at: http://webcache.googleusercontent.com/search?q=cache:ZiNGGecS7YEJ:www1.worldbank.org/publicsector/decentralization/Feb2004Course/Background%2520materials/McPake.doc+&cd=1&hl=en&ct=clnk&gl=au.

McPake B, Hanson K, Adam C. 2007. Two-tier charging strategies in public hospitals: Implications for intra-hospital resource allocation and equity of access to hospital services. *Journal of Health Economics* 26: 447–462.

McPake B, Hongoro C, Russo G. 2011. Two-tier charging in Maputo Central Hospital: Costs, revenues and effects on equity of access to hospital services. *BMC Health Services Research* 11: 143.

McPake B, Normand C, Smith S. 2013. Health Economics: An international perspective. 3rd Edition, London and New York: Routledge Kegan Paul.

Malama C, Chen Q, de Vogli R, Birbeck GL. 2002. User fees impact access to healthcare for female in rural Zambia. *Journal of Tropical Pediatrics* 48: 371–372.

Manongi R, Mtei F, Mtove G, Nadjm B, Muro F, Alegan V, Noor AM, Todd J, Reyburn H. 2014. Inpatient child mortality by travel time to hospital in a rural area of Tanzania. *Tropical Medicine and International Health* 19(5): 555–562.

Masika, PM, Semarundu WJ, Urassa R, Mosha J, Chandramohan D, Gosling RD. 2006. Over-diagnosis of malaria is not a lost cause. *Malaria Journal* 5: I20.

Masiye F. 2007. Investigating health system performance: An application of data envelopment analysis to Zambian hospitals. *BMC Health Services Research* 7: 58.

Mathiyazhgan MK. 2006. Cost efficiency of public and private hospitals: Evidence from Karnataka state in India, Institute of South Asian Studies, *Working Paper*, 8.

Mbovane MM, Mavundla TR, Roos JH. 2007. Professional nurses' perception of the implementation of quality circle programme in a public hospital in the Eastern Cape province. *Curationis* 30(1): 62–70.

Meng Q, Sun Q, Hearst N. 2002. Hospital charge exmptions for the poor in Shandong, China. *Health Policy and Planning* 17(Supplement 1): 56–63.

Mills A, Amin M, Hanson K. 2001. Understanding competition among private hospitals in Bangladesh. International Health Economics Association Conference, New York.

Minvielle E, Sicotte C, Champagne F, Contandripoulos A-P, Jeantet M, Préaubert N, Bourdil A, Richard C. 2008. Hospital performance: Competing or shared values? *Health Policy* 87: 8–19.

Mohammadi SM, Mohammadi SF, Hedges JR, Zohrabi M, Ameli O. 2007. Introduction of a quality improvement program in a children's hospital in Tehran: Design, implementation, evaluation and lessons learned. *International Journal of Quality in Health Care* 19(4): 237–243.

Montagu D. 2003. Accreditation and other external quality assessment systems for health-care, Health Systems Resource Centre: London.

Mori AT, Ngalesoni F, Norheim OF, Robberstad B. 2014. Cost-effectiveness of dihydroartemisinin-piperaquine compared with artemether-lumefantrine for treating uncomplicated malaria in children at a district hospital in Tanzania. *Malaria Journal* 13: 363.

Mostert S, Njuguna F, van de Ven PM, Olbara G, Kemps LJPA, Musimbi J, Strother RM, Aluoch LM, Skiles J, Buziba NG, Sitaresmi MN, Vreeman RC, Kaspers GJL. 2014. Influence of health insurance access and hospital retention policies on childhood cancer treatment in Kenya. *Pediatric Blood Cancer* 61: 913–918.

Mselle LT, Moland KM, Mvungi A, Evjen-Olsen B, Kohi TW. 2013. Why give birth in health facility? Users' and providers' accounts of poor quality of birth care in Tanzania. *BMC Health Services Research* 13: 174.

Mvula-Mwenda J. 2009. Total quality management and health services administration: The case of Zambia's University Teaching Hospital in Kaoma Mwenda K. and Ikombo Muuka, G. *The Challenge of Change in Africa's Higher Education in the 21st Century*, Cambria Press.

Nakamba P, Hanson K, McPake B. 2002. Markets for hospital services in Zambia. *International Journal of Health Planning and Management* 17: 229–247.

Nandraj S, Khot A, Menon S, Brugha R. 2001. A stakeholder approach towards hospital accredition in India. *Health Policy and Planning* 16(Supplement 2): 70–79.

Nantsupawat A, Srisuphan, W, Kunaviktikul W, Wichaikhum OA, Aungsuroch Y, Aiken LH. 2011. Impact of nurse work environment and staffing on hospital nurse and quality of care in Thailand. *Journal of Nursing Scholarship* 43(4): 426–432.

Nausheen S, Hammad R, Khan A. 2013. Rational use of antibiotics — a quality improvement initiative in hospital setting. *Journal of the Pakistan Medical Association* 63: 60.

Nguyen MH, Gammeltoft T, Rasch V. 2007. Situation analysis of quality of abortion care in the main maternity hospital in Hai Phong, Viet Nam. *Reproductive Health Matters* 15(29): 172–182.

Niens LM, Nyarko KM, Zelle SG, Jehu-Appiah C, Rutten FH. 2014. Equity in Ghanaian breast cancer treatment outcomes — a modelling study in Komfo Anokye Teaching Hospital. *The Breast Journal* 20(1): 100–102.

Noirhomme M, Meessen B, Griffiths F, Ir P, Jacobs B, Thor R, Criel B, van Damme W. 2007. Improving access to hospital care for the poor: Comparative analysis of four health equity funds in Cambodia. *Health Policy and Planning* 22: 246–262.

Nolan T, Angos P, Cunha AJLA, Muhe L, Qazi S, Simoes EAF, Tamburlini G, Wbere M, Pierce NF. 2001. Quality of hospital care for seriously ill children in less-developed countries. *The Lancet* 357: 106–110.

Nordberg E, Holmberg S, Kiugu S. 1996. Exploring the interface between first and second level of care: Referrals in rural Africa. *Tropical Medicine and International Health* 1(1): 107–111.

Olusina AK, Ohaeri JU, Olatawura MO. 2002. Patient and staff satisfaction with the quality of in-patient psychiatric care in a Nigerian general hospital. *Society for Psychiatry and Psychiatric Epidemiology* 37: 283–288.

Olusina AK, Ohaeri JU, Olatawura MO. 2003. The quality of interactions between staff and psychiatric inpatients in a Nigerian General Hospital. *Psychopathology* 36(5): 269–275.

Oluwadiya K, Olatoke SA, Ariba AJ, OMotosho OA, Olakulehin OA. 2010. Patients satisfaction with emergency care and priorities for change in a university teaching hospital in Nigeria. *International Emergency Nursing* 18: 203–209.

Onwujekwe O, Uguru N, Etiaba E, Chikezie I, Uzochukwu B, Adjagba A. 2013. The economic burden of malaria on households and the health system in Enugu State Southeast Nigeria. *PLOS One* 9(11): e78362.

Opondo E, Wanzala P, Makokha. 2013. Cost effectiveness of using surgery versus skeletal traction in management of femoral shaft fractures at Thika level 5 hospital, Kenya. *Pan African Medical Journal* 15: 42.

Onwudike M, Olaloye OA, Orth M, Olusola OA, Oni MD. 2001. Teaching hospital perspective on the quality of trauma care in Lagos, Nigeria. *World Journal of Surgery* 25: 112–115.

Osei D, d'Almeida S, George MO, Kirigia JM, Mensah AO, Kainyu LH. 2005. Technical efficiency of public district hospitals and health centres in Ghana: A pilot study. *Cost Effectiveness and Resource Allocation* 3: 9.

Ovretveit J. Al Serouri A. 2006. Hospital quality management system in a low income Arabic country: An evaluation. *International Journal of Health Care Quality Assurance* 19(6): 516–532.

Oxfam. 2014. A Dangerous Diversion: Will the IFC's Flagship Health PPP Bankrupt Lesotho's Ministry of Health, Oxfam Briefing Note, 7 April.

Oyesola R, Shehu D, Ikeh AT, Maru I. 1997. Improving emergency obstetric care at a state referral hospital, Kebbi State, Nigeria. *International Journal of Gynecology and Obstetrics* 59: S75–S81.

Özgen H, Sahin I. 2010. Measurement of efficiency of the dialysis sector in Turkey using data envelopment analysis. *Health Policy* 95: 185–193.

Pai YP, Chary ST. 2010. Dimensions of hospital services quality: A critical review. *International Journal of Health Care Quality Assurance* 26(4): 308–341.

Parasuraman A, Zeithaml VA, Berry LL. 1985. A conceptual model of service quality and its implications for future research. *Journal of Marketing* 49: 41–50.

Parasuraman A, Zeithaml VA. Berry LL. 1988. SERVQUAL: A multiple item scale for measuring consumer perceptions of service quality. *Journal of Retailing* 64(1): 12–40.

Parasuraman A, Berry LL, Zeithaml VA. 1990. *An Empirical Test of the Extended Gaps Model of Service Quality, Working Paper No.* 90-122, Marketing Science Institute, Cambridge.

Parasuraman A, Berry LL, Zeithaml VA. 1991. Refinement and reassessment of the SERVQUAL scale. *Journal of Retailing* 67(4): 420–450.

Penchansky R, Thomas JW. 1981. The concept of access: Definition and relationship to consumer satisfaction. *Medical Care* 19(2): 127–140.

Pham TL. 2011. Efficiency and productivity of hospitals in Vietnam. *Journal of Health Organization and Management* 25(2): 195–213.

Prata N, Bell S, Gessessew A. 2013. Comprehensive abortion care: Evidence of improvements in hospital-level indicators in Tigray, Ethiopia. *BMJ Open* 3.

Puenpatom RA, Rosenman R. 2008. Efficiency of Thai provincial public hospitals during the introduction of universal health coverage using capitation. *Health Care Management Science* 11: 319–338.

Qu H, Shewchuk RM, Chen Y, Scott Richards J. 2010. Evaluating the quality of acute rehabilitation care for patients with spinal cord injury: An extended Donabedian model. *Quality Management Health Care* 19(1): 47–61.

Rabbani F, Jafri SMW, Abbas F, Pappas G, Brommels M, Tomson G. 2007. Reviewing the application of the balanced scorecard with implications for low-income health settings. *Journal for Healthcare Quality* 29(5): 21–34.

Rabbani F, Jafri SMW, Abbas F, Shah M, Azam SI, Shaikh BT, Brommels M, Tomson G. 2010. Designing a balanced scorecard for a tertiary care hospital in Pakistan: A modified Delphi group exercise. *International Journal of Health Planning and Management* 25: 74–90.

Rabbani F, Lalji SNH, Abbas F, Jafri SMW, Razzak JA, Nabi N, Janan F, Ajmal A, Petzold M, Brommels M, Tomson G. 2011. Understanding the context of balanced scorecard implementation: A hospital-based case study in Pakistan. *Implementation Science* 6: 31.

Ranasinghe I, Rong Y, Du X, Wang Y, Gao R, Patel A, Wu Y, Iedema R, Hao Z, Hu D, Turnbull F. 2014. System barriers to the evidence based care of acute coronary syndrome patients in China. Qualitative Analysis. *Circulatory and Cardiovascular Quality Outcomes* 7: 209–216.

Rao KD, Peters DH. 2007. Quality improvement and its impact on the use and equality of outpatient health services in India. *Health Economics* 16: 799–813.

Ray S, Madzimbamuto FD, Ramagola-Masire D, Phillips R, Mogobe KD, Haverkamp M, Mokatedi M, Motana, M. 2013. Review of causes of maternal deaths in Botswana in 2010. *South African Medical Journal* 103(8): 537–542.

Renner A, Kirigia JM, Zere EA, Barry SP, Kirigia DG, Kamara C, Muthuri LHK. 2005. Technical efficiency of peripheral health units in Pujehun district of Sierra Leone: A DEA application. *BMC Health Services Research* 5: 77.

Rohsiswatmo R, Rafika S, Marsubrin PMT. 2014. Prevention and control of lood stream infection using the balanced scorecard approach. *Acta Medica Indonesiana* 46(3): 209–216.

Riewpaiboon A, Kumluang S. The Pharmacy Cost Study Group. 2011. Cost analysis of reimbursement-rate setting of hospital pharmaceutical services in Thailand. *International Journal of Pharmacy Practice* 19: 333–341.

Roemer MI. 1993. *National Health Systems of the World, II.* Oxford: Oxford University Press.

Roy K, Howard DH. 2007. Equity in out-of-pocket payments for hospital care: Evidence from India. *Health Policy* 80: 297–307.

Sahin I, Ozcan YA. 2000. Public sector hospital efficiency for provincial markets in Turkey. *Journal of Medical Systems* 24(6): 307–330.

Salmon JW, Heavens J, Lombard C, Tavrow P. 2003. The impact of accreditation on the quality of hospital care: KwaZulu-Natal Province, Republic of South Africa, University Research Co. LC, Bethesda MD.

Samad L, Jawed F, Sajun SZ, Arshad MH, Baig-Ansari N. 2013. Barriers to accessing surgical care: A cross-sectional survey conducted at a tertiary care hospital in Karachi, Pakistan. *World Journal of Surgery* 37: 2313–2321.

Shahhoseini R, Tofighi S, Jaafaripooyan E, Safiaryan R. 2011. Efficiency measurement in developing countries: Application of data envelopment analysis for Iranian hospitals. *Health Services Management Research* 24: 75–80.

Shahraz S, Barzanjeh A, Bahari A, Nadery Y, Farzadfar F, Beyranvsand MR, Stason WB. 2012. The completeness of medical records to assess quality of hospital care: The case of acute myocardial infarction in a district-level general hospital in Iran. *Archives of Iranian Medicine* 15(10): 592–595.

Sharma S, Hotchkiss DR. 2001. Developing financial autonomy in public hospitals in India: Rajasthan's model. *Health Policy* 55: 1–18.

Shaw CD. 2003. Evaluating accreditation. *International Journal for Quality in Health Care* 15(6): 455–456.

Shrestha MK, Chan H, Gurung R. 2012. Gender equity in eye health of Nepal: A hospital based study. *Nepal Journal of Opthamology* 4(2): 277–281.

Sidik NA, Lazuardi L, Agung FH, Pritasari K, Roespandi H, Setiawan T, Pawitro U, Nurhamzah W, Weber MW. 2013. The Indonesian Paediatric Hospital Assessment Group, Assessment of the quality of hospital care for children in Indonesia. *Tropical Medicine and International Health* 18(4): 407–415.

Sivalal S. 2009. Health technology assessment in the Asia Pacific Region. *International Journal of Technology Assessment in Health Care* 25(Supplement 1): 196–201.

Srofenyoh E, Ivester T, Engmann C, Olufolabi A, Bookman L, Owen M. 2012. Advancing obstetric and neonatal care in a regional hospital in Ghana via continuous quality improvement. *International Journal of Gynecology and Obstetrics* 116: 17–21.

Ssengooba F, McPake B, Palmer N. 2012. Why performance-based contracting failed in Uganda — An "open-box" evaluation of a complex health system intervention. *Social Science and Medicine* 75: 377–383.

Stekelenburg J, Kyanamina S, Mukelabai M, Wolffers I, van Roosmalen J. 2004. Waiting too long: Low use of maternal health services in Kalabo, Zambia. *Tropical Medicine and International Health* 9(3): 390–398.

Sulku SN. 2011. The health sector reforms and the efficiency of public hospitals in Turkey: Provincial markets. *European Journal of Public Health* 22(5): 634–638.

Sun H, Liu M, Hou S. 2011. Quality indicators for acute myocardial infarction care in China. *International Journal of Quality in Health Care* 23: 365–374.

Taner T, Antony J. 2006. Comparing public and private hospital care service quality in Turkey. *Leadership in Health Services* 19(2): i–x.

Tatar M, Mollahalilogly, Sahin B, Aydin S, Maresso A, Hernández-Quevedo C. 2011. Turkey: *Health System Review*, Health Systems in Transition, 13, 6, European Observatory on Health Systems and Policies, Copenhagen: World Health Organization.

Teerawattananon Y, Tantivess S, Yothasamut J, Kingkaew P, Chaisiri K. 2009. Historical development of health technology assessment in Thailand. *International Journal of Technology Assessment in Health Care* 25(Supplement 1): 241–252.

Thomson RB. 1994. Competition among hospitals in the United States. *Health Policy* 27: 205–231.

Tlotlego N, Nonvignon J, Sambo LG, Asbu EZ, Kirigia JM. 2010. Assessment of productivity of hospitals in Botswana: A DEA application. *International Archives of Medicine* 3: 27.

Torun N, Celik Y, Younis MZ. 2013. Competition among Turkish hospitals and its effect on hospital efficiency and service quality. *Journal of Health Care Finance* 40(2): 42–58.

Tunçalp O, Hindin MJ, Adu-Bonsaffoh K, Adanu RM. 2013. Assessment of maternal near-miss and quality of care in a hospital-based study in Accra, Ghana. *International Journal of Gynecology and Obstetrics* 123: 58–63.

Vakani F, Fatmi Z, Naqvi K. 2009. Three-level quality assessment of a dental hospital using EFQM. *International Journal of Health Care Quality Assurance* 24(8): 582–591.

Vuong DA, Flessa S, Marschall P, Thai Ha S, Luong KN, Busse R. 2014. Determining the impacts of hospital cost-sharing on the uninsured near-poor households in Vietnam. *International Journal for Equity in Health* 13: 40.

Wagstaff A, Lindelow M. 2005. Can insurance increase financial risk? The curious case of health insurance in China. *Journal of Health Economics* 27(4): 990–1005.

Weaver M. 1995. User fees and patient behaviour: Evidence from Niamey National Hospital. *Health Policy and Planning* 10(4): 350–361.

Weaver M, Deolalikar A. 2004. Economies of scale and scope in Vietnamese hospitals. *Social Science and Medicine* 59: 199–208.

Wessels F, Anderson AN, Ebrahim O. 1998. Cost-effectiveness of ceftriaxone in the treatment of community-acquired pneumonia in adult hospital patients: A pharmaco-economic study based on a meta-analysis. *South African Medical Journal* 88(3): 251–255.

Wilunda C, Putoto G, Manenti F, Castiglioni M, Azzimonti G, Edessa W, Atzori A, Merialdi M, Betrán AP, Vogel J, Criel B. 2013. Measuring equity in utilization of emergency obstetric care at Wolisso Hospital in Oromiya, Ethiopia: A cross sectional study. *International Journal for Equity in Health* 12: 27.

Wong EL, Cheung AWL, Leung MCM, Yam CHK, Chan FWK, Wong FYY, Yeoh E-K 2011. Unplanned readmission rates, length of hospital stay, mortality, and medical costs of ten common medical conditions: A retrospective analysis of Hong Kong hospital data. *BMC Health Services Research* 11: 149.

Yawson AE, Biritwum RB, Nimo PK. 2012. Efffects of consumer and provider moral hazard at a municipal hospital outpatient deparment on Ghana's national health insurance scheme. *Ghana Medical Journal* 46(4): 200–210.

Yereli AN. 2009. Activity-based costing and its application in a Turkish University Hospital. *AORN Journal* 89(3): 573–589.

You L, Aiken LJ, Sloane DM, Liu K, He G, Hu Y, Jiang X, Li X, Li X, Liu H, Shang S, Kutney-Lee A, Sermeus W. 2013. Hospital nursing, care quality, and patient satisfaction: Cross-sectional surveys of nurses and patients in hospitals in China and Europe. *International Journal of Nursing Studies* 50: 154–161.

Zere E, Mbeeli T, Shangula K, Nadlhate C, Mutirua K, Tjivambi B, Kapenambili W. 2006. Technical efficiency of district hospitals: Evidence from Namibia using Data Envelopment Analysis. *Cost Effectiveness and Resource Allocation* 4: 5.

Zhang L, You L, Liu K, Zheng J, Fang J, Lu M, Lu A, Ma W, Wang J, Want S, Wu X, Zhu X, Xiu-qing B. 2014. The association of Chinese hospital work environment with nurse burnout, job satisfaction, and intention to leave. *Nursing Outlook* 62: 128–137.

Zhao SJ, Akkadechanunt T, Xue XL. 2008. Quality nursing care as perceived by nurses and patients in a Chinese hospital. *Journal of Clinical Nursing* 18: 1722–1728.

Global Human Resources for Health

Joanne Spetz
University of California, San Francisco

Michelle Tellez
California State University, East Bay

Brent Fulton
University of California, Berkeley

Human resources for health (HRH) play a central role in the delivery of health care services. Global health policymakers need to understand the key factors that impact HRH, because shortages adversely impact population health and surpluses inefficiently consume a country's resources. This chapter describes key issues surrounding the global health workforce and HRH planning. It begins by describing the HRH workforce and the supply of HRH workers across countries by income level. An economic framework of supply and demand is presented, along with the factors that affect the demand for and supply of HRH. The chapter then delves into the challenge of ensuring that HRH are well distributed across and within countries, including the issue of international migration. Next, it discusses the roles of the public sector, private sector, and donor organizations in HRH planning. Although, there has been significant progress over recent decades in the development of HRH severe shortages and maldistribution remain. Moreover, the future workforce will need to be designed to meet the care needs of an aging population that will become increasingly burdened by chronic conditions and mental health disorders. These trends require proactive HRH planning by global health policymakers.

Keywords: Human Resources; Health Workforce; Labor Supply; Labor Demand; Labor Productivity; Wages.

Introduction

In *Working Together for Health* (2006), the World Health Organization (WHO) analyzed the problem of human resources for health and proposed that a central focus of international health policy should be “to get the right workers with the right skills in the right place doing the right things” (WHO, 2006). Human resources that provide health care services — also called the health workforce — are essential to all health care systems (Campbell *et al.*, 2013). The provision of health care services is inherently labor-intensive, and a lack of adequately trained workers is a primary cause of poor access to services. As noted by the WHO in 2011, “Today, over 1 billion people worldwide lack access to quality health care services — in large part because of a huge shortage, imbalanced skill mix, and uneven geographical distribution of professionally qualified health workers such as doctors, nurses and midwives” (WHO, 2011b). The WHO estimated that there was a shortage of approximately 2.4 million health care workers (WHO, 2011b). The accessibility of the health workforce to those who need care, the capacity of the health workforce to treat all patients with dignity, and the quality of the skills possessed by the health workforce are key to determining whether human resources for health are adequate to meet health care needs (Campbell *et al.*, 2013).

The number of people working as health care service providers is only one important dimension of human resources for health (Dal Poz *et al.*, 2007). Health care service providers include professionals such as physicians and nurses, other workers who provide health care services such as associate nurses and laboratory technicians, and community-based health workers. In addition to these workers, there are managerial and administrative staff that operate key components of a country’s health system, including accountants, clerical workers, ambulance drivers, and facilities maintenance staff. In 2004, the WHO estimated that there were about 500 managers and support staff for every 1,000 health services providers (Dal Poz *et al.*, 2007).

Many countries are reforming their health care systems to decrease health care spending in order to balance their budgets in the wake of the financial and economic crises of 2007 (OECD, 2013). Total health spending declined between 2009 and 2011 in 11 of 34 member countries of the Organisation for Economic Co-Operation and Development (OECD) (OECD, 2013). The health workforce is a focus of some nations’ efforts to increase efficiency and reduce health spending, largely because human resource spending accounts for a significant share of total health spending in every country. For example, in the United States about half of all health spending is for the wages and benefits of those who work in the health sector (US Bureau of Economic Analysis (BEA), 2011). Health workforce spending accounted for more than 90% of total health spending in Ghana in 2006 (Hernández *et al.*, 2009). In some countries, efficiency improvements might come from greater numbers of health workers engaged in basic public health and prevention, while in other countries the reorganization of traditional health care workforce roles may be more important to controlling costs and improving health (OECD, 2013).

Ensuring that health care systems have enough workers to provide the services necessary to improve or at least maintain the health of the population is an essential goal for global health policymakers. Given that the global market for health care services is directly linked to the global market of human resources for health (HRH), it is critical to understand the key factors that impact HRH. This chapter describes key issues surrounding the global health workforce and HRH planning. It begins by describing the HRH workforce and the supply of HRH workers across countries by income level. An economic framework of supply and demand is presented, along with the factors that affect the demand for and supply of HRH. The chapter then delves into the challenge of ensuring that HRH are well distributed across and within countries, including the issue of international migration. Next, it discusses the roles of the public sector, private sector, and donor organizations in HRH planning. Finally, this chapter assesses pertinent policy issues and recommends proactive HRH planning by global health policymakers.

Supply of Human Resources for Health by Country Income Levels

Human resources for health (HRH) are defined as including "those that provide health services such as doctors, nurses etc. and those that support the health services such as hospital managers, ambulance drivers etc." (WHO, 2014). The *Handbook on Monitoring and Evaluation of Human Resources for Health* suggests that training, occupation, and place of worker are critical elements for defining the health workforce and classifying distinct occupations (WHO, 2009). The health care workforce includes the well-known professions of medicine, nursing, pharmacy, and dentistry, which are tightly linked to the provision of health care services. There are also myriad other occupations that directly deliver health care services, such as medical officers, clinical officers, and a wide variety of technicians, therapists, and assistants. Community health workers, who are trained to provide basic health services and work in the communities in which they reside, are an important part of the health workforce in many countries. Many other occupations are associated with the provision of health care services, although they do not deliver health services directly, such as social work and counseling, environmental protection, and occupational health and safety (WHO, 2009).

Employment of HRH varies substantially across countries. Figure 1 presents the number of health services providers per 1,000 population by WHO Region. The African region has the lowest density of providers, averaging 1.9 per 1,000. There is notable variation within Africa, with a greater supply of providers in northern Africa. For example, a WHO analysis of the country-level supply of doctors, nurses, and midwives in Africa, relative to a need of 2.28 of these workers per

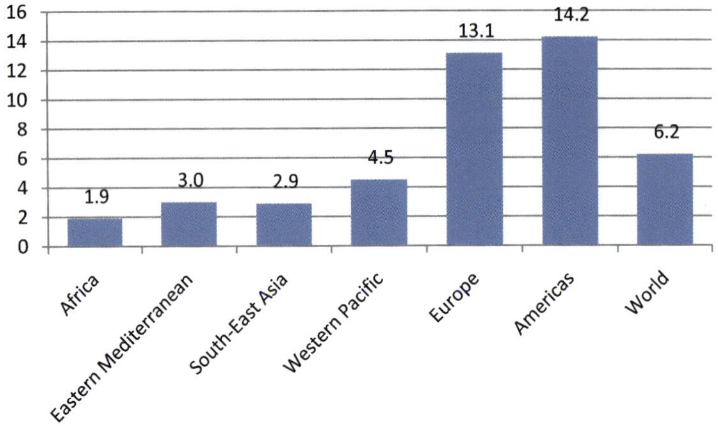

Figure 1. Density of health services providers per 1,000 population, by WHO region

Notes: Health services providers include all clinically-trained personnel, such as physicians, nurses, pharmacists, laboratory technicians, and public health workers.
Source: WHO (2006).

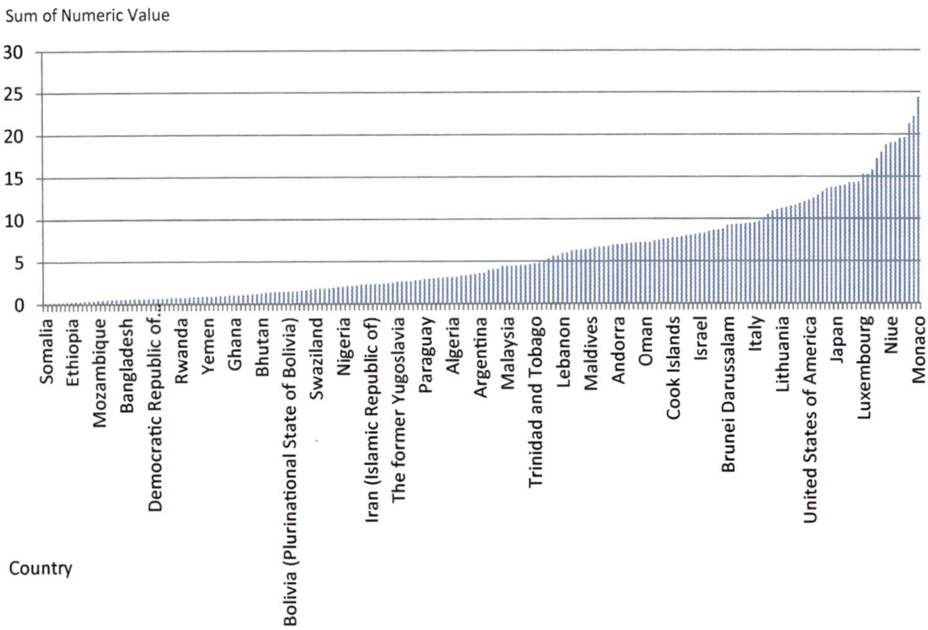

Figure 2. Density of physicians, nurses, and midwives per 10,000 population

Source: WHO (2013).

1,000 population, found that 36 of 46 countries had critical shortages that did not meet this threshold (WHO, 2006). In contrast, there is an average of 14.2 health services providers per 1,000 in the Americas, and 13.1 per 1,000 in Europe. Five countries in the Americas have shortages of doctors, nurses, and midwives, while no European country has a shortage (WHO, 2006).

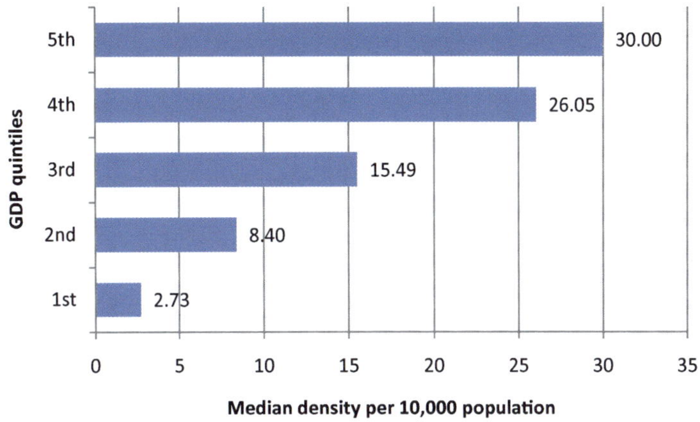

Figure 3. Median density of skilled health professionals per 10,000 population, with countries grouped by quintiles of gross domestic product (GDP) per capita (adjusted for purchasing power parity)

Source: Campbell *et al.* (2013).

Figure 2 presents data on the density of physicians, nurses, and midwives per 10,000 population for all countries that report to the WHO Global Health Observatory. Many health workers are not physicians, nurses, and midwives, and thus the county-level density of these professions is much lower than for all health workers. There is notable variation in country-level densities of health workers.

The availability of health workers is associated with national income levels, as seen in Figure 3. The average number of skilled health workers per 10,000 population for countries in the top quintile of GDP per capita is 30. This is more than 10 times greater than the density for countries in the lowest quintile of GDP: 2.73. The relationship between GDP per capita and workforce density is fairly consistent, with a few exceptions (Chen *et al.*, 2004). Equatorial Guinea has a relatively low density of health workers despite their somewhat high level of GDP per capita, while Gabon's health worker density is also lower than would be expected given their GDP. In contrast, Tajikistan has a relatively high density of health workers despite having a low level of GDP per capita. The factors underlying the income–workforce relationship differ across national income levels.

Low-income countries

Low-income countries are resource-limited and therefore often experience a shortage of HRH. It can be challenging to document the degree to which low-income countries face shortages because the lack of resources contributes to the lack of data. A review of the literature on the workforce among low- and middle-income countries (LMICs) found comprehensive data were only available for six countries and no data were available for 23 of the 57 countries considered by the WHO to be in a health workforce crisis (Hoyler *et al.*, 2014). The Harvard Global Surgery Workforce Initiative and the WHO Global Surgical Workforce Database are working to address this need for the surgical occupations by surveying Ministries of Health and surgical professional organizations around the world (Hoyler *et al.*, 2014).

Most low-income countries have difficulty generating enough supply of HRH with the competencies necessary to fulfill the needs of their communities. In the United States, there is an average of 230 medical doctors per 100,000 people, while in Sub-Saharan Africa, the ratio is 100 health care workers (all categories) per 100,000 population (WHO, 2011b). There are 168 medical schools in Africa but only about 10,000 graduates complete the programs each year. Of those who graduate, 22% migrate outside of Africa (WHO, 2011b).

Low availability of health workers contributes to the burden of disease in low-income countries. Most of these countries have high rates of communicable diseases and adverse health conditions associated with nutritional deficiencies, but there is a lack of health care workers to address these basic health care needs. Sub-Saharan Africa, e.g., has only 3% of the world's health workforce, but about 25% of the world's disease burden (Kasper and Bajunirwe, 2012). The challenges these countries face in meeting basic health care needs contributes to a lack of other important services such as mental and behavioral health care (McBain *et al.*, 2012).

Middle-income countries

Countries with middle-income levels typically have different health care needs than low-income countries. Many of these countries, such as the Pacific Island countries and territories, have reduced the burden of communicable diseases through basic public health measures, but are experiencing rising rates of chronic illness (Yamamoto *et al.*, 2012). Cancer is one of the major non-communicable diseases posing a threat to the health of residents of middle-income countries. In countries such as China, India, and Russia, people are adopting the diets and lifestyles of high-income countries such as the United States (Goss *et al.*, 2014). In addition, environmental contamination has been a consequence of rapid economic development in countries such as China, leading to increasing rates of cancer and asthma (Goss *et al.*, 2014).

Half of the world's population lives in Brazil, Russia, India, China, and South Africa, also known as the BRICS countries. The governments of all of the BRICS countries have committed to providing universal health coverage (UHC) for their populations (Marten *et al.*, 2014), although progress toward UHC has been varied due to differences in public spending, workforce supply, stewardship of public health systems, management of changing disease burdens, and addressing the social determinants of health (Figure 4).

	Brazil	Russia	India	China	South Africa
Life expectancy (years, 2011)[8]	73	70	65	73	53
Maternal mortality ratio (per 100 000 livebirths, 2010)[9]	56	34	200	37	300
Under-5 mortality rate (per 1000 livebirths, 2012)[10]	14·4	10·3	56·3	14	44·6
Prevalence of HIV in adults aged 15–49 years (%, year)[11,12]	0·3% (2011)	0·8–1·4% (2011)	0·3% (2009)	<0·1% (2011)	17·3%(2011)
Physicians density (per 1000 population, year)[13]	1·76 (2009)	4·3 (2006)	0·65 (2009)	1·46 (2010)	0·76 (2011)
Probability of dying between ages 30 and 70 years from any of cardiovascular disease, cancer, diabetes, or chronic respiratory disease (%, 2008)[14]	20%	32%	27%	21%	27%

BRICS=Brazil, Russia, India, China, and South Africa.

Table 1: Comparison of key indicators across BRICS countries

Figure 4. Physician density and health characteristics of the BRICS countries

Source: Marten *et al.* (2014).

Many emerging economies are working to increase their supply of HRH and improve their skills. Most middle-income countries are facing challenges associated with inequitable rural–urban distribution of health workers, income inequality, and aging populations (Goss *et al.*, 2014). Changes in the prevalence of chronic illnesses and non-communicable diseases in middle-income countries demand different skills from the health workforce and thus additional training is required (Yamamoto *et al.*, 2012). Some of these countries are using technology to extend health workforce education, such as e-learning tools that allow educational content to be delivered through the internet (Frehywot *et al.*, 2013). These tools are most commonly used for physician training, and preliminary research suggests that they can successfully and efficiently enhance knowledge (Frehywot *et al.*, 2013).

- *Country case study: Brazil*

In 1980, Brazil established a new constitution that declared that health care is a right of all citizens (Buchan *et al.*, 2011). In 1988, the government decentralized the health care system, realizing that it was not meeting the needs of the diverse and dispersed population, and in 1998, it created the centralized Unified Health System (SUS). The SUS is a government-run health system that offers health care services to 75% of Brazil's 250 million population, accounting for half of the country's health care spending (Buchan *et al.*, 2011).

Each of the clinics of the SUS is comprised of teams. Each team has one physician, one nurse and several community health workers who provide care for 2,000 to 3,500 families (Dayrit *et al.*, 2011). The community health workers are expected to live in the communities served by the SUS clinic. Each state of Brazil has engaged in numerous coordinated efforts to develop the HRH required for the SUS. There has been active collaboration with trade unions as well as professional and educational organizations (Buchan *et al.*, 2011). Despite these efforts, however, recent research has found that in some rural communities a large share of health care teams are incomplete. For example, in a small town in the state of Rio de Janeiro, 87.5% of the health care teams lacked physicians (dos Reis Moreira and O'Dwyer, 2013).

An ongoing challenge for the SUS is bridging the gap between the education received in academic settings and the needs of the population in practice. The national Pro-Saude (Pro-Health) program is seeking to address this problem by improving the selection, recruitment, training, and assessment of HRH (Andre *et al.*, 2013). There also have been some efforts to decentralize the financing and management of HRH from the federal level to the state level (Pierantoni and Garcia, 2011). However, some local health departments lack resources to adequately monitor and develop HRH. Nearly one-quarter of health departments lack an HRH unit, and more than one-third do not have an HRH information system (Pierantoni and Garcia, 2011).

- *Country case study: China*

China's rapid economic development has been accompanied by expansions of its public health care system. The government is the main source of health care for China's 1.3 billion people (Glass *et al.*, 2013). Unlike most countries, China has more doctors than nurses (Anand *et al.*, 2008), and several analyses have determined that the supply of physicians is adequate (Wang *et al.*, 2013). However, there are comparatively few nurses in China, with a doctor-to-nurse ratio of 0.9 to 1.0 in 2010 (Wang *et al.*, 2013). There is also a shortage of mental health service providers such as psychiatrists, social workers, and clinical psychologists, although in 2012 China adopted a new Mental Health Law to address the needs of its population (Li *et al.*, 2014).

China has a large population of residents in rural areas, and urban–rural disparities in doctor and nurse density account for about a third of overall intra-country health inequality (Anand *et al.*, 2008). Public health service efforts have been viewed as the key strategy to address the needs of rural populations (Hu and Chen, 2014). According to the *China Statistical Yearbooks Database* (CSYD) the number of HRH in rural areas' health centers increased from 1.16 per 1,000 to 1.32 per 1,000 from 2005 to 2011, although an analysis of rural health care needs suggests that the ratio should be 1.54 to 1,000 (Hu and Chen, 2014). In rural areas, the "township–village health centers" play a central role in the provision of health services. In many areas, these centers have been privatized in an effort to improve the delivery of health care, however some research suggests that privatization has been associated with reductions in the number of permanent staff in township–village health centers, possibly due to reductions in salary and caseload (Huang *et al.*, 2013).

Another important challenge for China is the rapid aging of its population, in part due to the policy that each couple has only one child (adopted in 1979).

One-third of the Chinese population is projected to be over 65 years of age by 2015 (Glass *et al.*, 2013). Traditionally, younger generations are responsible for caring for aging parents and grandparents, but with fewer children and grandchildren, the burden of such arrangements has increased dramatically. In addition, there is a high rate of migration of young people from rural to urban areas. Together, these trends have created a crisis of long-term care. There are very few long-term care facilities and those that exist are expensive (Glass *et al.*, 2013). In the near term, China will have to address the care needs of the aging population, perhaps by introducing new cadres of workers.

High-income countries

Countries with high-income levels usually have comparatively high health status and high supplies of health workers. However, they often face disparities in the distribution of workers across urban and rural areas, shortages of some types of workers, and the need to constrain health care costs (Spetz, 2012). Health care spending as a percentage of GDP is approximately 17% in the United States, 10% in the United Kingdom and Sweden, and 12% in France and Germany (Propper and Venables, 2013). Although health care spending in these countries has slowed in recent years, the supply of physicians has risen since 2000 (OECD, 2013).

The mix of health workers varies across high-income countries. In many OECD countries, the supply of specialist physicians exceeds that of generalists (OECD, 2013), although some countries have faced an outflow of specialists. For example, there has been a net outflow of thoracic, vascular, and cardiac surgeons in France (Laskar *et al.*, 2013; Berger and Mace, 2012). Nurses greatly outnumber physicians in most high-income countries, although some countries have ongoing concerns about shortages of nurses (OECD, 2013). The employment of nurses with advanced training is growing in some countries. For example, primary health care nursing in European countries is being used as a strategy to respond to the increase in demand for health care services while controlling costs (Martin *et al.*, 2013). Some countries have relatively high supplies of midwives, such as Iceland, Sweden, and Australia, while others rely more heavily on obstetricians for maternal care (OECD, 2013).

Some high-income countries have benefitted from an inflow of health workers from other countries (Aluttis *et al.*, 2014). The migration of nurses from low-income countries to high-income countries has received considerable attention by policymakers (Khaliq *et al.*, 2008). However, there also has been migration of physicians to high-income countries. For example, the Irish Health Service has had increasing difficulty retaining physicians, and thus the recruitment of foreign doctors rose substantially between 2000 and 2010 (Murphy, 2014). Many high-income countries have increased the numbers of health professionals they educate to increase their locally-educated supply and address concerns about shortages (OECD, 2013).

A Simple Economic Model of Labor Supply and Demand

Health worker employment levels result from the interaction between demand and supply (Spetz, 2011). Demand is a function of the need for health services, the money available to finance those services, and the organizational structure of the health care delivery system. In general, when the wage for workers is high, health care employers demand fewer of them because the population will demand fewer. This is illustrated in Figure 6. The line labeled "demand" slopes downward because at lower wages, more nurses are demanded than at higher wages. The supply of workers results from the number of people qualified to work and the individual choices they make regarding whether to work and how much. In general, as the wage paid to workers rises, their employment rises — both because those currently working choose to work more hours and because more people choose to work in the health sector versus other sectors. This is indicated in Figure 6 by the line labeled "supply."

If there is a greater demand for workers than supply, a shortage will exist. Economic theory predicts that when there is a shortage of workers, compensation will rise because employers will compete to recruit workers by offering higher wages and improvements to working conditions and employment benefits. In Figure 5, this is indicated by the lower horizontal line, because demand is greater than supply.

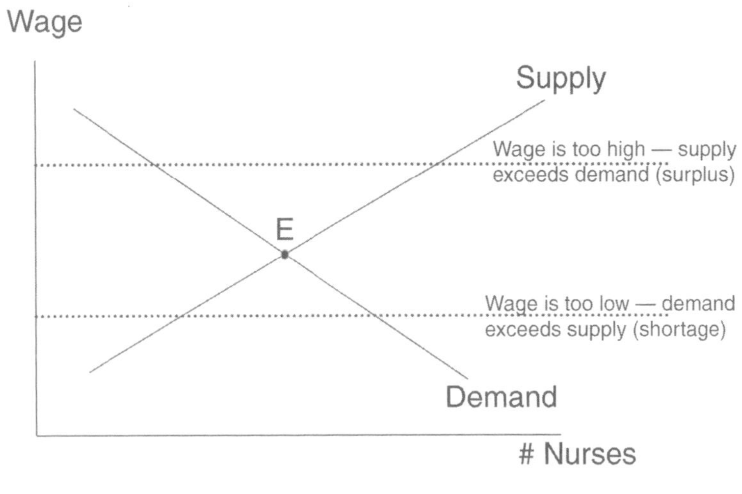

Figure 5. The basic economic model of a health worker labor market

The growth in compensation will lead to greater supply because employment is more lucrative and also will reduce demand, because employers will not be able to afford as many workers (Spetz, 2012). The net effect is a rebalancing of the labor market and an end to the shortage, leading the labor market to the point where the supply and demand lines cross, which is called the equilibrium point and is labeled "E". If there were more workers than jobs, as indicated by the higher horizontal line in Figure 5, then wages would drop to reach the equilibrium point.

However, there are many cases in which the normal economic model does not function as described above, particularly in the short term within the health care sector (Scheffler *et al.*, 2012; Vujicic, 2014). First, wages and other forms of compensation may not adjust rapidly. In some countries, health workers are primarily employed through the government, and wages are set according to pre-determined schedules. Changing these wage schedules can be onerous and require coordination of multiple levels of bureaucracy (Spetz, 2011). Even in the private sector, enactment of wage changes requires organizations to redevelop their budgets, which can allow a shortage to persist while adjustments are made. Such budget changes may be particularly arduous in the face of government budget constraints. Second, the supply of health workers may not easily respond to wage changes. Many health care occupations require months or years of training, creating a delay between when wages rise and when supply can increase (Scheffler *et al.*, 2012). Moreover, training programs may have restricted capacity, due to a lack of financial resources, a shortage of clinical training locations, faculty shortfalls, or other constraints (Spetz, 2012). Any of these circumstances can lead to protracted shortages of health workers.

Shortages have been reported in high-income countries, but tend to be more severe and protracted in middle- and low-income countries (Spetz, 2011). Shortages have been widely reported for physicians, midwives, nurses, psychiatrists, and other mental health workers (OECD, 2013). Shortages can occur even when there is unemployment among the same occupation, due to poor working conditions that reduce workers' interest in employment, bureaucratic problems that slow hiring, and mismatched geographic distributions of jobs and workers (Spetz, 2011). Understanding the factors that influence the supply of health workers and demand for them is necessary to analyze HRH issues and develop policies to ensure adequate HRH for the delivery of health care.

Determinants of the Demand for Human Resources for Health

Need-based demand versus economic demand

Many policy analyses of the health workforce focus on the number of workers "needed." In this context, "need" is usually defined as the number of workers with specific skills to deliver a defined set of health care services to a population (Bruckner *et al.*, 2011; Scheffler *et al.*, 2012; Vujicic, 2014; Scheffler and Fulton, 2014). Determining need is a complex endeavor, and is based as much on demographics and epidemiology as it is on policy priorities. Moreover, while increased health spending is generally associated with better health outcomes, there are diminishing returns at higher spending levels (Anderson and Chalkidou, 2008; Filmer and Pritchett, 1999; Moreno-Serra and Smith, 2011; Nixon and Ulmann, 2006; Savedoff, 2003). The organization of the health care system, the technologies available to support service delivery, and the productivity of workers will shape perceptions of workforce need.

However, an important problem is that need-based demand estimates are separated from information about the budget available to pay for services or the costs of each of the types of health worker that might deliver services. The cost of medical care and the compensation paid to health care providers is ignored in the need-based approach (Scheffler *et al.*, 2008). On a practical basis, a country may not have adequate budgetary resources to hire enough workers to meet perceived needs. Need-based modeling also ignores the importance of wages and other factors in driving the demand for health workers (Scheffler *et al.*, 2012). In the end, the demand for and employment of health care workers is driven more by an economic model than a need-based model.

Figure 6 illustrates the distinction between the economic model and the need-based model. A need-based model might determine the number of nurses is needed to attain the level of health care delivery desired as being the line labeled "Need" and point B. However, the economic model of supply and demand might indicate that the equilibrium employment level of nursing employment is A, with the wage at w*. This equilibrium is notably lower than the need-based goal of B, and thus health system planners might believe there is a shortage. However, to

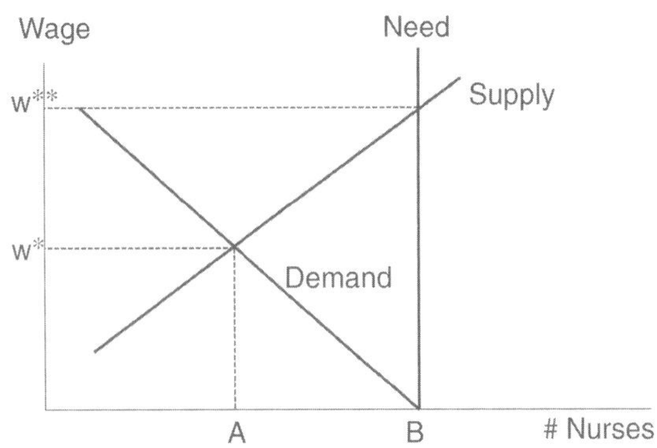

Figure 6. The economic model vs. the needs-based model in health workforce shortages

achieve a supply of B nurses, wages would need to increase to w**, which is well above what the health system can sustain from a demand perspective. This mismatch is a challenge for health system planners.

Assessing the demand for health workers is made more complicated by the potential for providers to induce the demand for their services. A large body of research has found that when the supply of providers is relatively high, there is greater use of health care services beyond what might be "needed" (Delattre and Dormont, 2003; Fuchs, 1978; Gruber and Owings, 1996; Grytten and Sorensen, 2001; Grytten *et al.*, 1995; Sorensen and Grytten, 1999). The underlying theory is that physicians both want to ensure their practice is busy, and they also want to maintain their incomes (De Jaegher and Jegers, 2000). That said, increased health spending is generally associated with improvements in health outcomes, including infant mortality, life expectancy, and disease burden, but there are diminishing benefits as health spending reaches higher levels.

This section reviews the factors that affect the demand for health workers: Population demographics, the burden of disease, income, health insurance, and regulations.

Demand for health care services

The demand for human resources for health is driven primarily by the demand for health care services. Although gains have been made globally in the infrastructure through which health services have been delivered over the past decade, there still are notable gaps in access to services and the continuing need to reduce the burden of communicable diseases such as tuberculosis and HIV/AIDS (Garonna, 2006). Several large countries, including Brazil, China, and the United States, have moved toward providing universal health care insurance and services, and such endeavors will require enhanced investments in HRH (Koon and Mayhew, 2013).

Driving the demand for health care are both short-term and long-term factors. Short-term fluctuations in the need for health services can arise from the emergence of epidemics and natural disasters, which necessitate a concerted rapid response to reduce mortality and morbidity. While contingency plans are important to have in place to address these needs, the long-term demand for health services is associated more closely with durable factors: population demographics and disease burden.

- *Population demographics*

The age distribution of the population plays a central role in driving demand for health services. The health care needs of children are relatively small; investments

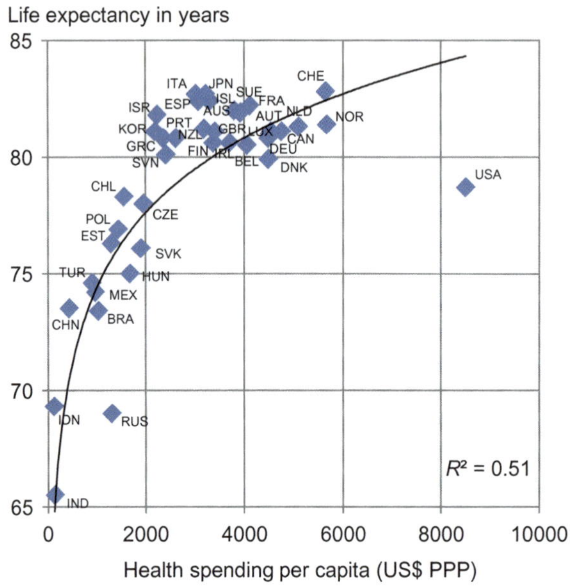

Figure 7. Life expectancy at birth and health spending per capita, 2011
Source: OECD (2013).

in preventive care such as vaccinations can protect their health, and once basic public health investments have been made, severe illnesses are rare among the young. Women of child-bearing age have an increased need for services to ensure that family planning needs are met, and to provide prenatal and birth care (Garonna, 2006). Infant mortality rates have been improving in most countries of the world due to improved basic health care services (OECD, 2013).

These investments in the health of youth have contributed to rising life expectancy. The size of older age groups has risen, and the life expectancy of those who are 65 years old is now another 8.2 years (OECD, 2013). There is a close correlation between life expectancy at birth and health care spending per capita, as seen in Figure 7. This relationship likely works both ways: Greater investment in health care services over the lifespan can increase life expectancy, and those at older ages tend to need more health care services to manage the illnesses and ailments that are correlated with age. Moreover, the growth of the older population is compounded by declining fertility rates worldwide (United Nations, 2013).

Other characteristics of the population also affect the demand for health care services. Gender plays a role because women receive childbirth-related care and they have a life expectancy that is 5.5 years longer than men (OECD, 2013). The education level of the population is also important; greater education levels are associated with better health as well as with longer life expectancy (OECD, 2013).

Disease burden: Communicable and chronic diseases

The disease burden faced by a country is primarily composed of communicable diseases and chronic diseases. The prevalence and severity of these diseases will have a substantial impact on the need for health care services. Conversely, investments in health care can help prevent these diseases and reduce future demand.

Many communicable illnesses such as tuberculosis, malaria, dengue fever, polio, HIV/AIDS, and measles are preventable through public health interventions such as vaccination campaigns, use of mosquito nets, rapid treatment of latent disease (in the case of tuberculosis), and education about the prevention of transmission (in the case of HIV/AIDS). Some such diseases, once contracted, can be challenging to treat. The rising prevalence of medication-resistant tuberculosis strains, e.g., has increased the cost of treating this disease. Coordinated and flexible programs such as the US Global Health Initiative (GHI), have demonstrated the positive impact of targeted efforts, even when there are health workforce shortages. For example, a study of five countries' HIV/AIDS treatment systems found that successful anti-retroviral (ARV) therapy roll-out through the GHI was observed, despite each country having different HRH development and retention problems (Cailhol *et al.*, 2013).

While the burden of communicable disease is dropping and life expectancy is improving, the burden of chronic disease is rising worldwide — primarily among those who live in middle- and high-income countries (OECD, 2013). 7% of people living in OECD member countries had diabetes in 2011, totaling approximately 85 million people; the incidence of diabetes is particularly high among many middle-income countries (Figure 8) (OECD, 2013). At the same time, cardiovascular diseases are the main cause of death among these countries, even though there have been improvements in survival rates after myocardial infarction and stroke (OECD, 2013). These gains, however, have not been uniformly distributed. Within countries, lower-income groups have less access to preventive care and treatment, higher rates of chronic illness, and shorter life expectancies (OECD, 2013). As countries continue to observe a shift in the burden of illness from communicable to chronic diseases, the training requirements of health care personnel also will change (Yamamoto *et al.*, 2012). There also will, for many countries, be competing demands to continue to address the burden of communicable disease among lower-income groups while addressing chronic disease among higher-income groups (Frenk *et al.*, 2010; Arredondo *et al.*, 2005).

The burden of mental illnesses also is substantial, and has not been well-addressed by many countries. Approximately, 10% of the population is estimated to have one or more mental health conditions (OECD, 2013). Access to mental health services is lacking; among OECD countries there were only 15.6

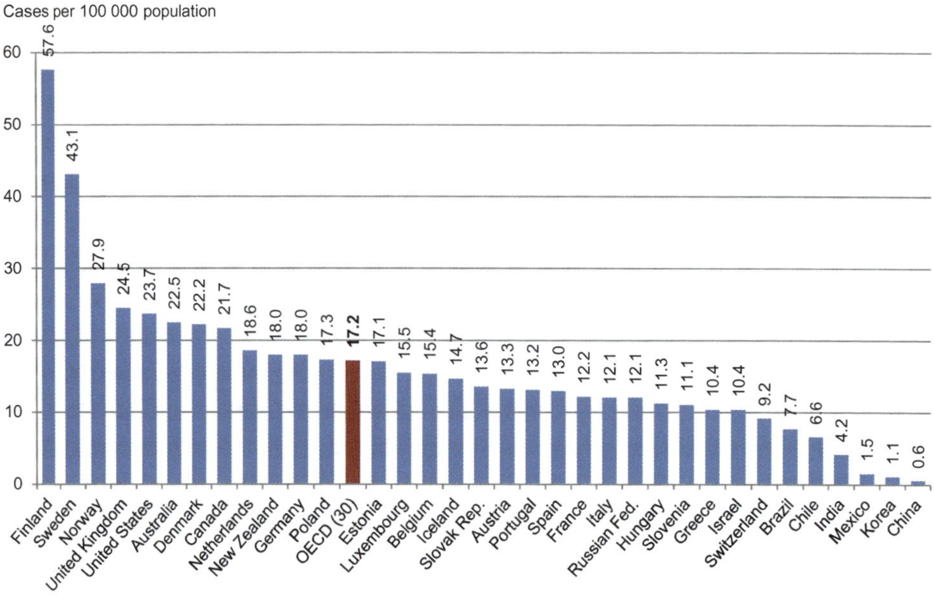

Figure 8. Prevalence estimates of diabetes, adults aged 20–79 years, 2011
Source: OECD (2013).

psychiatrists per 100,000 population in 2011. The highest ratio was in Switzerland, with 45 psychiatrists per 100,000 population, and the lowest was in Mexico, with only 1.2 per 100,000 (OECD, 2013). One need-based analysis determined that there is a shortfall of mental health workers in all low-income countries and 59% of middle-income countries (Bruckner *et al.*, 2011). In general, countries that face a significant disease burden from communicable diseases also tend to have lower mental health system capacities and fewer professionals working in this area (McBain *et al.*, 2012).

- *Income and health insurance*

The relationship between income and the demand for health care services is illustrated by the broad differences in health worker demand across low-, middle-, and high-income countries (Hitiris and Posnett, 1992; Newhouse, 1977). Across middle-income countries, the strongest predictor of variations in health spending is per capita income (Gerdtham *et al.*, 1992a; 1992b). In addition, income is closely connected to the demand for health care *within* countries. Health care is generally thought of as a "normal good," for which demand rises as income rises. Numerous studies have demonstrated that this is true when the income elasticity of health care expenditures is estimated at the population or country level, because income is related to insurance coverage, which fuels investment in new treatments, leading to higher expenditures (Getzen, 2000; Sauerborn *et al.*, 1994; Schwartz *et al.*, 1988). When the elasticity is estimated at the individual level for people that have insurance, then an increase in income does not generate significant additional spending.

The emergence and maturation of health insurance markets also drives demand for health care services. Studies have consistently shown that people with health insurance use more health care services, even after taking into account differences in age, health status, and income (Buchmueller *et al.*, 2005; Cheng and Chiang, 1997; Freeman *et al.*, 2008). Insurance changes the price paid by health care consumers at the time they demand care. Because the price paid at the time of service is lower, demand for services will be higher (Scheffler *et al.*, 2012). The mix of insurance within a country can affect its overall health spending; some research has found that health systems that are more reliant on fee-for-service private reimbursement have greater spending than those with other HRH payment systems such as fixed salaries (Gerdtham *et al.*, 1992a; 1992b). Moreover, the presence and size of user fees for health services can impact demand, with greater effects generally found among lower-income groups (Ching, 1995). These factors will influence the demand for health services, which in turn impacts the need for human resources for health.

Governmental policies

The role of government is to coordinate efforts to address the needs of the population. Identifying health care needs, and developing and implementing plans that address these needs are the reason for governmental policies in human resources for health. Governmental policies in this arena include employment policies and regulatory activities. Some governmental activities are more influential and successful than others.

- *Financing of health employment*

In many countries, the government plays a central role in the financing of human resources for health programs. Government employers can modulate the pay and working conditions of health care jobs to strengthen domestic markets for health care workers and recruit and retain HRH (Mackey and Liang, 2013). However, the governments of resource-poor countries struggle with structural and financial problems that hinder these efforts. The situation in Liberia provides one case study for governmental efforts to rebuild the human resources capacity, where in this case efforts were successful in spite of having low levels of government resources. Although Liberia had endured a 14-year Civil War, the country has enjoyed steady economic growth in the past 25 years. In 2006, the Ministry of Health and Social Welfare (MOHSW) began a concerted effort to increase the size and capacity of its nursing workforce (Varpilah *et al.*, 2011). MOHSW developed the Emergency Human Resources (HR) Plan for 2007–2011 and established a central HR Unit and county-level HR officers. Strategies included increasing and standardizing salaries, mobilizing donor funds to improve management capacity and fund incentive packages in order to retain staff in hard to reach areas, reopening training institutions and providing scholarships to increase the pool of available workers. MOHSW successfully doubled the number of nurses by 2010 (Varpilah *et al.*, 2011).

Governmental efforts are not always successful however. Evidence of corruption and inaction creates challenges for program success in many parts of the world, and this impacts recruitment and retention (Henderson and Tulloch, 2008; Mathauer and Imhoff, 2006; WHO, 2010a). For example, a study of 90 health facilities from the Siraha, Bardiya and Doti districts of Nepal found multiple violations and disregard for policies, and although the decentralization of the health care system has increased ownership at the local level, nepotism and gender and class discrimination remained common problems (Devkota *et al.*, 2013). These factors dampened efforts to recruit and retain health workers.

- *Regulatory policies*

Governments can establish regulations that directly or indirectly affect the demand for human resources for health. Examples include regulations on mandatory retirement policies, employment contracts, and scope of practice regulations (Spetz, 2011).

Mandatory retirement has important impacts on the demand for health workers. The mandated retirement age for public employees in many countries is at age 60 or younger (Dovlo, 2005; Spetz, 2011). Mandatory retirement policies have forced some workers into retirement and led to shortages; e.g., the Fijian government reduced the mandatory retirement age to 55 years in 2009, forcing 110 nurses into retirement. The Fijian Public Service Commission later re-hired some retired nurses in temporary positions at lower pay (Spetz, 2011). In many countries, mandatory retirement from public positions shifts workers from the public to the private sector, as has been documented in Guyana and Russia (Spetz, 2011).

Regulations of the employment contracts with which health workers can be hired can have a large impact on the function of labor markets. An example comes from China, where since 1949 nurse employment and wages were characterized as '*bianzhi*' or "the iron rice bowl," guaranteed by the government. Regulatory and financial reforms began to phase out the '*bianzhi*' nurses and instituted contract-based employment with limited job security and reduced benefits. This change led to an increase in the number of contract-based nurses, along with dissatisfaction among nurses with their remuneration and benefits. Contract-based nurses were more likely than '*bianzhi*' nurses to intend to leave their current positions. Moreover, hospitals with more dissatisfied contract-based nurses were rated lower by patients (Shang *et al.*, 2014).

One of the most important areas of regulation is in the identification of the tasks permitted and prohibited by each type of health worker. These regulations, commonly called "scope of practice" regulations, can limit the roles of health workers, control the shifting of tasks from one cadre of workers to another, and limit options for addressing shortages. Some countries have well-defined roles for each type of health worker. However, in low-income countries that typically have the greatest health care needs and the most severe shortages of workers, the demarcation of the roles of each health care worker group is often less important and less clear. Because African regions have been designated areas of critical shortage by the WHO, with 24% of the global disease burden and 3% of the global health workforce, task shifting has been recommended as a strategy to abate the shortage (WHO, 2008).

Task shifting involves the transferring of control of a set of clinical decisions from one group to another (Ledikwe *et al.*, 2013). Adjustments to the scope of practice of each cadre of worker can increase access to care (Fulton *et al.*, 2011). Clinical officers, medical officers, and nurses with extended training — often characterized as "mid-level providers" — can offer increased access to a full range of services (Fonjungo *et al.*, 2013; Fulton *et al.*, 2011). Deploying and utilizing these workers often requires a change in the regulations regarding scope of practice (Crisp and Chen, 2014).

The delivery of oral health services is one area in which changes in scope of practice and task shifting have been successful in increasing access. Oral health services are insufficient and unevenly distributed in many developing countries, particularly those in Sub-Saharan Africa. Cameroon deployed a mid-level cadre of oral health professionals. Evaluation of this program found that the mid-level providers could safely offer a full scope of dental work, with the exception of treatment for major facial injuries and teaching. This innovation expanded the workforce to add 42 mid-level providers to the supply of four dentists, greatly extending the capacity of the 10 study clinics (Achembong *et al.*, 2012).

As for the case of oral health care services, task shifting is mostly used to target a specific illness or problem, and most evaluations have demonstrated success. A review of studies that tested task-shifting from physicians to nurses targeting HIV in Africa between January 2009 and August 2012 found that nurses' job satisfaction increased with the additional responsibilities, and patient outcomes were comparable (Iwu and Holzemer, 2014). A study in Southern Malawi explored the effectiveness of trained Health Surveillance Assistants (HSA) versus trained volunteer Key Informants in identifying blindness in children. Surprisingly, the volunteer Key Informants were better able to identify blindness in children than HSAs, as HSAs reported not having enough time to make complete assessments (Kalua *et al.*, 2012). Another study showed success using community health workers with on-the-job-training to provide diagnosis and treatment for malaria outside of health care establishments in Senegal (Blanas *et al.*, 2013).

In order for task shifting to be successful, supervision and continuing education are needed. One longitudinal survey in the Bolama Region of Guinea-Bissau explored strategies to address childhood diarrheal disease (Lopes *et al.*, 2014). The Health Region of Bolama initiated a program that used community health workers (CHW) to increase the identification of new cases. Comparisons were made between the cases correctly identified by CHWs when compared to those identified by medical doctors (MDs). Findings suggest that after the training, CHWs significantly improved their ability to diagnose common diarrheal diseases. However, as time elapsed, the concordance between the CHW and the MD practices decreased because the CHWs became less likely to follow treatment algorithms and guidelines (Lopes *et al.*, 2014).

The initial education of health workers needs to be aligned with the tasks they will perform and the health needs of the population. Some countries have found that they could shorten educational programs after a careful analysis of the tasks to be performed by the worker. For example, in Mozambique nurse training was redesigned to speed the graduation rate based on task analysis (Dgedge *et al.*, 2014). The task analysis demonstrated that there was significant task shifting between basic and general nurse cadres, and between maternal and child health nurse cadres, but not much crossover between these groups. Thus, the educational pathways were separated and shortened to 24 months (Dgedge *et al.*, 2014). Some educational reforms have focused on the potential for workers to be trained across multiple professions, potentially with formal cross-accreditation (Saltman *et al.*, 2012). The goal of these approaches is to increase the transferability of human resources to meet emerging needs, by focusing on worker competencies rather than specific professional accreditation. Although these strategies are controversial, they do highlight the importance of all health care workers being prepared to provide patient-centered care, work in interdisciplinary teams, use evidence-based practice protocols, and participate in quality improvement activities (Frenk *et al.*, 2010).

Determinants of the Supply of Human Resources for Health

The supply of human resources for health is determined by the number of people qualified to provide health care services, and their decisions about whether to work and how much to work. Some factors primarily influence the employment decisions of those already qualified to provide health care, such as wages and other compensation, other job attributes, education, age, and family circumstances (Antonazzo *et al.*, 2003; Vujicic, 2014). These factors impact the supply of HRH in the short term. The long-term supply is determined by the factors that affect how many people are qualified to work, such as the extent to which education and training programs are available, migration into and out of the country, and rates of leaving the pool of qualified workers due to disability, burnout and retirement (Antonazzo *et al.*, 2003; Vujicic, 2014).

A simple economic model frames workforce supply in the context of the "stock" of people prepared to work, and the "flow" of people into and out of this stock. Figure 10 depicts this model. On the left side is the flow of people into the health workforce. These people have not yet been prepared to work in health care, and may pursue formal training in health care, training in another field that might be applicable to health care, or no formal training at all. These individuals flow into the stock of the workforce, and the people within this stock make decisions about whether to work in health care, to work in another industry, or to not work at all. If they choose to work, they also decide where to work geographically, whether to work in the public or private sector, and how much to work. The right side of Figure 9 depicts the flow of workers out of the health workforce. People leave the stock of the workforce due to migration, retirement, disability or other reasons.

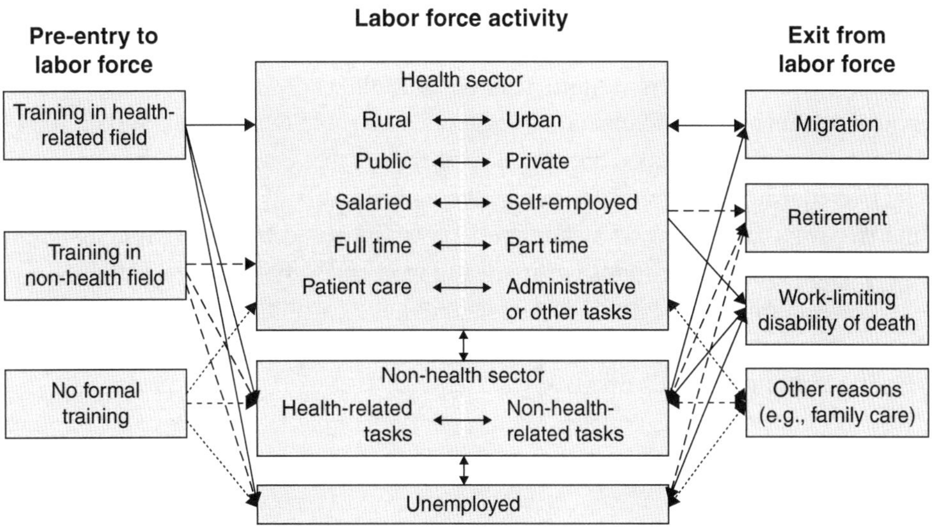

Figure 9. Stocks and flows of health workforce supply

Source: Reproduced, with the permission of the publisher, from Dal Poz *et al.* (2009).

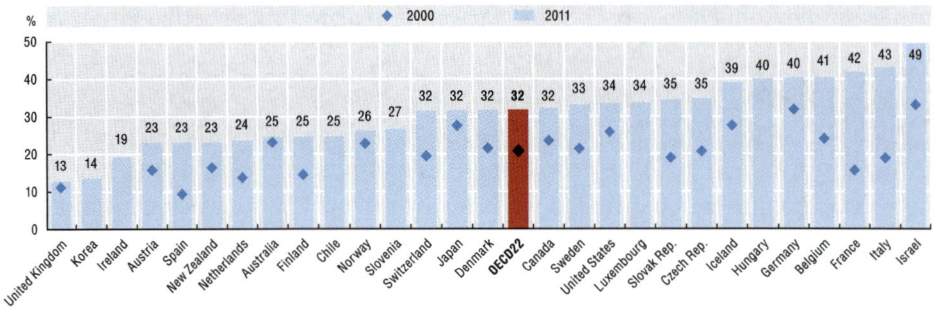

Source: OECD Health Statistics 2013, http://dx.doi.org/10.1787/health-data-en. StatLink http://dx.doi.org/10.1787/888932916838

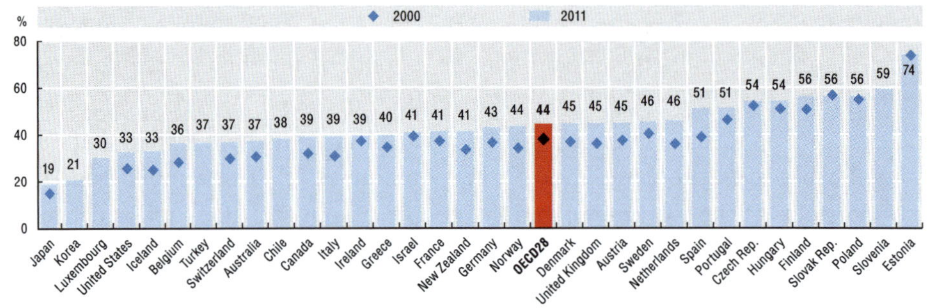

Source: OECD Health Statistics 2013, http://dx.doi.org/10.1787/health-data-en. StatLink http://dx.doi.org/10.1787/888932916857

Figure 10. Age and gender of doctors, 2000 and 2011 (or nearest year)
Source: OECD (2013).

As noted above, there can be an imbalance between supply and demand in a labor market. If demand is lower than supply, wages will be depressed, which may lead to a population of health care workers who do not work in the health industry because other employment is more lucrative or health care employment does not pay enough to compensate for time away from the household (Zurn and Dal Poz, 2004). Policymakers often focus on the supply-side factors that can cause a shortage, such a lack of education programs to train health care workers. It is possible, however, to find that what appears to be a shortage is in truth caused by a lack of demand for workers and/or a lack of funds to hire health workers (Scheffler *et al.*, 2012).

This section delves into three factors that have particular importance in determining the supply of human resources for health: Education and training, demographics, and the rewards of work.

Education and training

Approximately, one million new physicians, nurses and other health professionals are trained world-wide each year, but their distribution and expertise often do not match the diverse needs across the globe. Some countries have no medical schools while others have too many (Frenk *et al*., 2010). Shortages of educational capacity exist most commonly in low-income countries and in rural regions of middle- and high-income countries.

Many countries focus on their education and training infrastructure as a means to address shortages of health care workers (Vujicic and Zurn, 2006). In 2009, the WHO and the President's Emergency Plan for AIDS Relief (PEPFAR) created the *Commission on Education of Health Professionals for the 21st Century* to provide evidence-based guidelines for scaling up education of human resources for health. In 2010, the commission called for an overhaul of global health education, citing a series of social, cultural, structural, organizational, and systems problems (Frenk *et al*., 2010). The commission's recommendations included a set of strategies to engage universities, hospitals, and governmental entities to develop system-wide solutions (WHO, 2011b).

The relevance of future health workers' educational experience is critical. While in school, students must become familiar with the health care problems relevant to their community of interest and become familiar with the equipment used in the clinical settings in which they will work. The mismatch between competencies and expertise acquired in schools and the realities of the work in health care settings has made retention of new graduates extremely difficult (Frenk, 2010; WHO 2011b). The WHO recommends that Ministries of Health and of Education increase collaboration to understand the problems that health workers will most often encounter in the field and develop education that is aligned with population needs (Mullan *et al*., 2011). Guidelines issued by the WHO focus on strengthening relationships between the health care educational system, the health care delivery system, and the public sector to ensure the quantity, quality, and the relevance of health care providers upon completion of educational programs (WHO, 2011b). Some countries have followed these WHO recommendations with notable success. For example, the district government of Bogota, Colombia, initiated a Primary Health Care Strategy to improve health care access in 2004 through expanded HRH capacity, focusing on infant and child health. The program coordinated multiple agencies and educational institutions, and a subsequent evaluation of this coordinated program found that it significantly reduced infant and child mortality in a short period of time (Mosquera *et al*., 2012).

In this context, teaching the most modern, high-technology, approaches to health care may not be a priority. For example, education reform efforts in Rwanda have increased curricula intended to address the country's high rate of childhood mortality and provide care for growing numbers of people with cancer (Binagwaho *et al*., 2013; Shelton and Hodgins, 2014). The European Family Health Nursing Project, which includes representatives from Armenia, Austria, Germany, Italy,

Poland, Portugal, Romania, Slovenia, and Spain, has focused on educating nurses with the core competencies needed to care for these countries' aging populations and rising rates of chronic illness (Martin *et al.*, 2013). In China, many village doctors practice both western and traditional Chinese medicine (Xu *et al.*, 2013).

Some experts have recommended that health education programs focus on specific competencies needed to improve health system performance, rather than strictly following standardized educational programs (Frenk *et al.*, 2010). A review of the quality of health care professional education, including technical and vocational education, determined that having high-quality students from rural and low resource areas, competency-based education, preparation and training of teachers and preceptors, infrastructure and management, and clinical practice sites were the pillars for successful health profession training and education (Johnson *et al.*, 2013).

The selection and recruitment of people who enter health care occupations is important. Many countries have developed cadres of community health workers and clinical officers who originate from the communities in which they work. The intention of this recruitment strategy is to ensure that workers have a deep understanding of local health care issues and can address those issues with a high level of cultural knowledge. For example, Brazil's SUS employs community health workers in every clinic who are residents of the community in which the clinic is located (Buchan *et al.*, 2011). Walter Sisulu University in South Africa has developed programs in which students are recruited from the local community, receive a substantial portion of their training in the community, and then, upon returning to their communities, are evaluated in relation to the health of the community (WHO, 2011b).

Within educational programs, there can be problems associated with poor-quality of teaching and a lack of infrastructure and equipment (Frenk *et al.*, 2010). An evaluation of nursing education in Ghana found that in many programs there are inadequate numbers of faculty and the infrastructure is missing or is insufficient (Bell *et al.*, 2013). In order to expand the supply of laboratory personnel, Ethiopia provided training for new faculty at five universities and purchased supplies and equipment, along with engaging in curricular revisions that included more hands-on practice (Fonjungo *et al.*, 2013). Some countries are leveraging e-learning technologies in order to expand educational capacity, particularly Brazil, India, Egypt, and South Africa (Frehywot *et al.*, 2013).

For some countries, international partnerships have been critical to expanding educational capacity. For example, in order to address a shortage of surgical and perioperative staff in Uganda, several North American and Ugandan institutions created the Global Partners in Anesthesia and Surgery (GPAS) (Lipnick *et al.*, 2013). Between 2007 and 2011, the collaboration doubled the number of people in surgical training and increased the anesthesia staff from 2 to 19 at Mulago Hospital in Kampala (Lipnick *et al.*, 2013). The Rwandan Ministry of Health leveraged funds from the US Emergency Plan for AIDS Relief and the Global Fund to Fight AIDS, Tuberculosis, and Malaria to develop an academic consortium with schools of medicine and nursing in the United States. In three years, the consortium produced 500 physicians, 5,000 nurses, 75 health management graduates, 40 dentists, 20 dental therapists, and 15 dental assistants (Binagwaho *et al.*, 2013).

Demographics and workforce supply

- *Aging*

The age distribution of the population affects not only the demand for health care services, but also the supply of the health care workforce. The health care workforce is aging in parallel with the world's population, raising concerns about the ability of the health care system to replace them as they reach retirement. In 2000, 25% of doctors in the OECD were age 55 or older, and that proportion increased to 30% by 2011 (OECD, 2013) (Figure 11). In Israel, about half of the doctors are over 55 years old (OECD, 2013). The aging of China's population poses a significant challenge for meeting long-term care and health care needs (Glass *et al.*, 2013). Recent analyses from France suggest that nearly 75% of surgeons will retire in the next 15 years (Berger and Mace, 2012; Laskar *et al.*, 2013). According to a survey conducted by the French Society of Thoracic and Cardiovascular Surgery, the expected inflow of practicing surgeons to France is about 18 new residents per year, while the outflow of practicing surgeons is about 17.6 per year between 2013 and 2022 (Laskar *et al.*, 2013), providing little opportunity to meet the needs of a growing population.

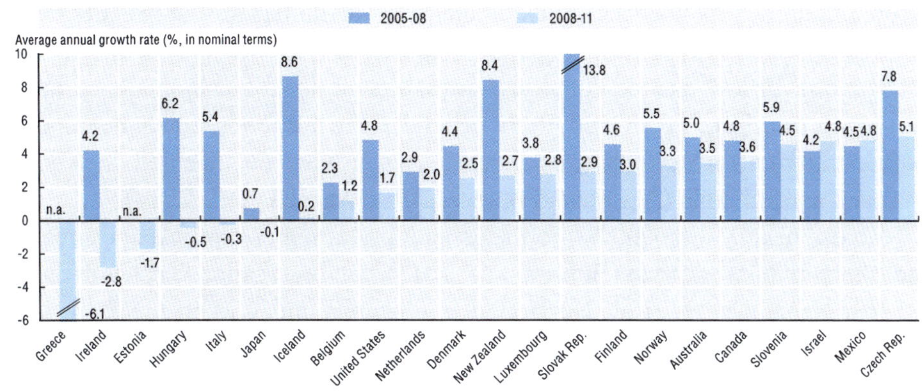

Source: OECD Health Statistics 2013, http://dx.doi.org/10.1787/health-data-en.

StatLink http://dx.doi.org/10.1787/888932917199

Figure 11. Average annual growth of earnings for nurses from 2005 to 2011 (or nearest year)
Source: OECD (2013).

Extending the age of retirement is one strategy some countries are using to maximize the labor force. Recent research from the United States indicates that nurses are working about three years longer on average than they were in 2000, likely due to longer life expectancy and inadequate retirement savings (Auerbach *et al.*, 2014). However, aging health care workers may be affected by age-related sensory and neurocognitive changes, including a decline in processing speed, reduced problem-solving ability and fluid intelligence, impaired hearing and sight, and reduced manual dexterity (Skowronski and Peisah, 2012). A literature review of the effects of shift work on older workers has found that they have shorter and more disturbed daytime sleep between successive night shifts than their younger colleagues (Folkard, 2008). Consequently, these workers are more fatigued and less likely to maintain high levels of performance. Occupational injuries are less frequent in older workers, but when they occur, they are likely to be more serious (Folkard, 2008). Thus, there may be a limit to the extent to which health workers can extend their employment past traditional retirement ages. Moreover, because there are many reasons for retirement, retaining older nurses or delaying their retirement requires a multifactorial approach (Mion *et al.*, 2006).

- *Gender*

There is wide variation in the gender mix of health care workers, both across countries and across occupations. Some professions, such as nursing in most countries and oral dentistry in Brazil, are predominantly comprised of women, while other professions, such as medicine in OECD countries, are primarily filled by men (Abreu *et al.*, 2013). Data on gender have not been consistently collected for health care settings. For this reason, the WHO recommends using census data to analyze the gender distribution in health care occupations. In middle- and high-income countries, women comprise about 75% of human resources for health (all categories combined), although they tend to be concentrated in lower-wage occupations. In low-income countries, women comprise a much smaller proportion of the workforce (WHO, 2009). In general, there are fewer female health care workers in rural areas than urban areas, as has been documented in Kenya, Pakistan, and Ethiopia (Araujo and Maeda, 2013; Wakaba *et al.*, 2014).

Across nearly all countries, job segregation is a major obstacle for equality and safety in the workplace (Bourmpoula, 2012). Job segregation is categorized as either horizontal or vertical. Horizontal job segregation is when there are jobs within the same level of education or status that women are not allowed to pursue. Vertical job segregation, on the other hand, occurs when there is a lack of upward mobility within a career path, such as the problem described as the glass ceiling.

Improvements in the gender distribution of health care occupations are occurring along several fronts. The gender of medicine is shifting with more females becoming doctors. In 2000, 38% of physicians were female in OECD countries; this share rose to 44% in 2011 (Figure 10) (OECD, 2013). In at least nine OECD countries, the proportion of female physicians was higher than 50%; the female share ranges from 19% in Japan to 74% in Estonia (OECD, 2013). Some concern has been expressed that the increase in the share of female physicians only partially increases labor supply, since female physicians tend to work fewer hours than male physicians (Biringer and Carroll, 2012; Delgado *et al.*, 2011; Kletke *et al.*, 1990; Pas *et al.*, 2011; Sarma *et al.*, 2011). Female physicians also are less likely to practice in rural areas, and thus an increase in female physicians could worsen geographic disparities in supply (Wainer *et al.*, 2000).

Women in the health care sector face several disincentives to work. First is that they often are paid less than are men in the same occupations. One study of 10,066 Australian full-time employees within the health sector showed an adjusted wage gap of 16.7% (Vecchio *et al.*, 2013). Significant earnings gaps between genders have been documented for physicians and nurses in numerous countries (Jones and Gates, 2004; Konrad *et al.*, 2012; Lo Sasso *et al.*, 2011; Schumacher, 1997; Seabury *et al.*, 2013; Theurl and Winner, 2011).

The second impediment faced by women in health care occupations is poor access to education. The problem begins with a lack of access to education for girls and women, particularly in developing countries (Ekine *et al.*, 2013; Lutz and KC, 2011; Vishwanath *et al.*, 2011; Sattar, 2012). Challenges in accessing education continue even for those who successfully enter health professions. One study of Chad, Côte d'Ivoire, Jamaica, Mozambique, Sri Lanka, and Zimbabwe found that female nursing and midwifery personnel were significantly less likely than their male counterparts to have received in-service training (Gupta and Alfano, 2011). Some countries have developed training programs specifically targeted to women to address imbalances and increase access to care. In 2004, the government of Ethiopia introduced the Health Extension Program (HEP). This program, intended to expand the delivery of primary care, trained female workers recruited from their villages (Teklehaimanot and Teklehaimanot, 2013). Over 10 years, the program produced over 30,000 Health Extension Workers who are deployed to approximately 15,000 villages and increased health service coverage to 92.1% of the population by 2011 (Teklehaimanot and Teklehaimanot, 2013).

Rewards

The employment decisions of health workers are shaped by the benefits they receive from work, including wages, satisfaction, and personal efficacy, as well as how these benefits compare to those of alternative ways to spend time (Zurn and

Dal Poz, 2004). When employment offers higher compensation and the promise of a high level of satisfaction, workers are more likely to work, and tend to work at a higher intensity.

- *Remuneration*

The remuneration of employees comprises the total compensation, in cash or in kind, paid to employees in return for work performed. Remuneration is the most widely recognized method of incentive to recruit and retain workers (Misfeldt *et al.*, 2014). Remuneration of HRH is often dependent on the economic development of a given country. A study of 194 WHO Member States found remuneration of labor to be the largest expenditure in the health care system, accounting for over 33% of total health expenditures between 2000 and 2010 (Hernandez-Peña *et al.*, 2013). Also between 2000 and 2010, wages increased substantially compared to wages for other worker categories, but they increased less than other health care expenditure categories (Hernández *et al.*, 2009). One study explored the purchasing power variation of Mozambican public sector health workers between 1999 and 2007 (Ferrinho *et al.*, 2012). Results suggest that, on average, purchasing power increased for most health occupations, and the highest percentage increase was observed for the lowest remuneration occupations. These findings contradict a trend seen in middle- and upper-income countries, where health sector pay has deteriorated over the years, with the greatest losses for the poorest workers (Dussault and Buchan, 2014; OECD, 2013).

Among OECD countries, physician remuneration data are segregated by source of income: salary or self-employment and by specialty or general practice (OECD, 2013). There are wide gaps between specialties, with generalists earning less than specialists. For example, in Canada, self-employed specialists earned an average income that was 4.7 times higher than the wages of their salaried counterparts, and three times higher than the wages of self-employed generalists in 2010 (OECD, 2013). A study of 1,982 village doctors in China found that their income was low, and less than half had pensions or expected one (Xu *et al.*, 2013). In most countries, nurse wages are higher than the average wage; however, there is great variation (OECD, 2013). In Luxemburg the average hospital nurse wage was 40% higher than the nationwide average wage, while in Hungary it was 20% lower (OECD, 2013). Prior to the global recession of 2008, a number of countries were concerned with the competitiveness of nurse wages and instituted pay increases (Figure 11). Since the recession, however, several European countries have lowered wages. In Greece, annual salaries for nurses were decreased by 6% between 2009 and 2011 (OECD, 2013).

There is growing interest in using performance-based payment incentives for health care workers. A review of the literature on the effects of these strategies in low- and middle-income countries demonstrated that there is little evidence on the value of this approach to improve productivity or maintain workforce supply (Witter *et al.*, 2013). The review included nine studies from the Philippines, Tanzania, Zambia, Rwanda, Burundi, Democratic Republic of Congo, Vietnam, and China. Interventions varied significantly and results were mixed. The authors noted that the outcomes of performance-based payment depend on the interaction of several variables, including the design of the intervention (e.g., who receives payments, the magnitude of the incentives, the benchmarks upon which payments are based, and how benchmarks are measured), the amount of additional funding offered, other ancillary components such as technical support, and contextual factors, including the organizational context in which the new performance scheme is implemented (Witter *et al.*, 2013).

Non-pecuniary rewards: Working conditions and job status

The non-pecuniary rewards of employment include working conditions and status (social status and preferential treatment) (Hernández *et al.*, 2009). Improvements in these rewards — when well-targeted — can attract new health workers and encourage higher labor supply of the current stock of workers. They also can compensate for lower financial rewards, to some extent. Working conditions include many variables associated with the quality of work life, including access to resources, risk of violence, sanitary conditions, career development opportunities, work–life balance, relationships among employees, and professional autonomy. A meta-analysis that included 13 review articles published between 2000 and 2012 demonstrated that the quality of the working environments had a positive impact on workers' performance, while improvements in workload factors — such as job demand, staffing models, work designs, local practices, employment status, and staff skill mix — were not as effective (Misfeldt *et al.*, 2014).

A large body of research has unveiled dissatisfaction with working conditions among many health workers. For example, a study conducted in Jazan Region of Saudi Arabia assessed the quality of work life among primary health care nurses. Although the research found that the quality of work life had a positive effect on commitment and productivity, there was a great deal of dissatisfaction among respondents with working hours, inability to balance work with family needs, inadequacy of vacation time, poor staffing, management and supervision practices, lack of professional development opportunities, and an inappropriate working environment in terms of the level of security, patient care supplies and equipment, and break-area (Almalki *et al.*, 2012). Another study in India ranked factors that motivate health care workers to remain employed in medical offices in rural areas, finding that job security was the most important factor related to motivation, followed by interesting work, respect, recognition, and wages (Purohit and Bandyopadhyay, 2014). Autonomy of professional labor, defined as control over practice, has been found to be a powerful non-pecuniary incentive for workers (Dingley and Yoder, 2013).

Safety is an important aspect of the work environment, and making the work environment free of violence is a priority to improve recruitment and retention of workers, especially women (Spetz, 2011). Workplace violence, perpetrated by both patients and co-workers, is common in the health care setting in many countries, with nurses often most at risk because of their central role in the delivery of care (Buchan and Calman, 2004). Studies conducted in numerous countries have found high levels of workplace violence and harassment (Hagopian *et al.*, 2009; Henderson and Tulloch, 2008; Kamchuchat *et al.*, 2008; Uzun, 2003a; Uzun, 2003b). A study conducted in Rwanda examined workplace violence in the health sector, and found that over 38% of the health workers interviewed had experienced some form of workplace violence in 1 year, mostly occurring among women (Newman *et al.*, 2011). Negative stereotypes of women; discrimination based on pregnancy, maternity and family responsibilities; and the 'glass ceiling' all affected female health workers' experiences and career paths and contributed to a context of violence (Newman *et al.*, 2011). In addition to these risks, health workers also face health risks associated with infectious disease and have increased risk of quitting due to unsanitary conditions or a lack of adequate protection from life-threatening diseases such as HIV/AIDS (Anderson and Isaacs, 2007; Padarath *et al.*, 2003).

The status of health occupations also is important in determining workforce supply. A study by Ramani *et al.* (2013) explored strategies for retention of health care providers in India where Ayurveda, allopathic medicine and nursing are commonly used by the population. They found that for the allopathic cadre, rural primary care jobs commanded little respect. For individuals working in these settings, greater remuneration and better working conditions are required to offset the low status of the setting. It was proposed that preferential admission to specialist courses in exchange for working at a rural site for a time could be a powerful incentive for this group. The ayurvedic and nursing cadres, on the other hand, considered public sector jobs to have higher status, even in rural areas. For these groups, better salary, working and living conditions could increase recruitment outside the public sector (Ramani *et al.*, 2013).

The Challenge of Health Workforce Geographic Distribution

In nearly every country, there are significant differences in the supply of health workers between urban and rural areas. As seen in Figure 12, about 53% of the world's population lives in urban areas. In contrast, more than three-quarters

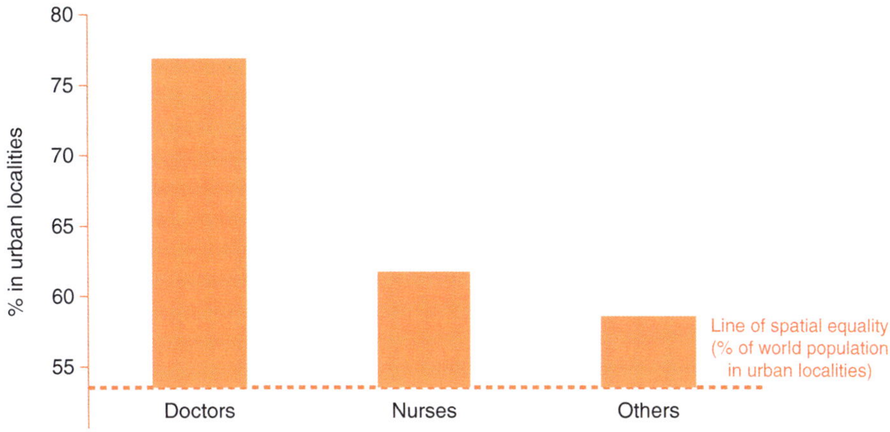

Figure 12. Rural–urban distribution of health providers

Source: Reprinted with permission from World Health Organization. 2006.

of physicians and 60% of nurses live in urban communities (WHO, 2006). The discrepancy between urban and rural supply is particularly notable in Africa. For example, in South Africa 46% of the African population lives in rural areas but only 12% of doctors and 19% of nurses work in those regions (WHO, 2011b).

The uneven geographic distribution of health care workers, both across and within countries, is a primary cause of the lack of health services for many people (WHO, 2011b). Imbalances in the rural and urban supply of workers can be found in low- and middle-income countries (Goss *et al.*, 2014) as well as high income countries (Spetz, 2012). There are also imbalances across countries, which are often associated with the migration of skilled health workers from low-income countries to higher-income countries.

Urban–rural imbalances

Maldistribution of health care workers between rural and urban areas exists in nearly all countries, but this imbalance is acutely felt in the poorer and most isolated regions with the highest disease burden (WHO, 2006; Crettenden *et al.*, 2013). Approximately, 50% of the world's population lives in rural areas, but only 38% of nurses and 25% of physicians serve these areas (WHO, 2006). Rural areas of Africa are particularly undersupplied, where over 40% of the population lives in rural areas but only 12% of doctors and 19% of nurses work in those regions (WHO, 2011b). There are 168 medical schools in Africa but only approximately 10,000 graduates complete the programs each year (an average of

59.5 students per school). Of those who graduate, 22% migrate outside of Africa (WHO, 2011b).

In order to develop strategies to improve the distribution of health workers between urban and rural areas, an understanding of the underlying causes of the imbalance and local workforce needs is required (Ossai *et al.*, 2012). Different demographic and professional groups have different reasons for preferring urban areas; thus, there is consensus that there is not a single solution to imbalances that context is critical, and that interventions must be multifaceted (Araujo and Maeda, 2013). Research on the Indian rural workforce has found that multiple factors lead health workers to remain in rural regions, including geographical and ethnic affinities, rural upbringing, availability of schools, personal values of service, professional interests, co-location with spouses, relations with co-workers, community relationships, and acclimatization with rural life (Sheikh *et al.*, 2012). It is thus not surprising that a study of strategies for the retention of health workers in India found that preferences of employment location were clustered into organizational attributes (salary, infrastructure, career) and contextual attributes (housing, children's development, safety) (Ramani *et al.*, 2013). They found that some worker cadres were more willing to work in rural areas if they received educational incentives, while others were more responsive to salaries, working conditions, and living conditions (Ramani *et al.*, 2013).

Educational interventions to address rural worker shortages typically focus on attracting students to training programs who are likely to want to live in rural areas, and providing significant education and clinical opportunities in rural communities. Some analysts also have recommended curricular changes that include rural health issues (Araujo and Maeda, 2013; Ossai *et al.*, 2012; Rao *et al.*, 2011) and providing continuous professional development for rural health care workers (Keane *et al.*, 2012; Li *et al.*, 2013; Ossai *et al.*, 2012). Research on the nursing workforce has found that pre-selecting students who are more likely to accept positions in rural areas is the most cost-effective intervention, with offering preferential access to workers willing to spend time in rural areas as the next-best option (Lagarde *et al.*, 2012). A cross-sectional study conducted in Ethiopia of 600 medical students confirmed that only 30% of the students would like to practice in rural settings, but those with rural backgrounds were significantly more likely to report interest in rural medical practice (Deressa and Azazh, 2012).

Some regulatory strategies have been used to address rural health worker shortages. Changing the scope of practice of health workers to allow a larger number of workers to provide needed services, and to promote task shifting, can be effective in addressing both general and local shortages (WHO, 2008). Some countries have established policies that require completion of a certain amount of rural service in order to qualify for full licensure as a health worker, while many have developed programs that subsidize education or repay educational loans in return for rural service (Ossai *et al.*, 2012). An analysis of 70 countries with compulsory service requirements identified notable variation in strategies to ensure compliance, including withholding full registration or licensure until rural service is completed, reducing salary if rural practice requirements are not met, and imposing large fines, and there is some evidence that each of these strategies can increase compliance (Frehywot *et al.*, 2010).

A variety of financial incentives, including remuneration, bonuses, and relocation costs, also can effectively support rural recruitment and retention (Ossai *et al.*, 2012). In some countries, such as China, rural health worker incomes are much lower than the incomes of urban workers (Xu *et al.*, 2013); compensation discrepancies have a dampening effect on rural supply. A study of Kenyan nurses determined that nursing students were most motivated to consider rural practice by additional rural allowances and choice in specific rural location (Mullei *et al.*, 2010). However, although wages often are identified as an important factor in rural recruitment and retention, other factors such as job security, work environment, and adequacy of resources often rank higher (Purohit and Bandyopadhyay, 2014). Many studies have demonstrated that financial incentives alone are not enough to motivate health workers to serve in rural areas (Willis-Shattuck *et al.*, 2008).

The professional and personal support available to health workers, which includes living conditions, safe and supportive working environments, appropriate mentoring and supervision, career development programs, creation of a professional network, and public recognition, is important to rural recruitment and retention (Ossai *et al.*, 2012). Recognition is highly influential in health worker motivation, and the availability of adequate resources and appropriate infrastructure can improve morale and retention (Willis-Shattuck *et al.*, 2008). For example, a study of Ghanaian doctors revealed that the workload in rural areas was perceived as greater than in urban locations, and the doctors were also averse to the isolated nature of remote assignments. Doctors were concerned that prolonged rural assignments would lead to career "death" and stressed that mentorship and remote learning centers were needed to support their continuing career development (Snow *et al.*, 2011).

Most rural worker shortfalls have multiple causes, but strategies to remedy them often focus on a single approach. Bundled interventions are more likely to be successful (Dayrit *et al.*, 2010; Lehmann *et al.*, 2008). For example, before 2005 the most common strategy for remedying rural–urban imbalances in India was compulsory rural service bonds and mandatory rural service for admission into post-graduate health education programs. In 2005, a new national strategy was launched that included multiple approaches, including an increase in sanctioned posts for public health facilities, financial incentives, workforce management policies, locality-specific recruitment, and the creation of a new service cadre specifically for public sector employment. The combined strategies effectively increased the number of skilled health workers in rural areas in a short period of time (Sundararaman and Gupta, 2011). There is a need for more knowledge regarding the effectiveness of each strategy that can be used to recruit and retain health workers in rural regions, and new programs should be evaluated rigorously to advance the evidence (Mbemba *et al.*, 2013).

International migration

There is a worldwide migration of health workers from poor to rich countries, which is detrimental to poor countries and benefits both rich countries and the immigrant workers themselves (Aluttis *et al.*, 2014; Buchan *et al.*, 2011). It has been estimated that the migration of workers from resource poor countries to wealthier countries accounts for 40–70% of the health care workforce in the wealthier countries (Mackey and Liang, 2013). An analysis of migration patterns in Southeast Asia identified significant flows of health workers into the comparatively wealthy countries of Singapore and Malaysia, while the Philippines and Indonesia are the main exporters of doctors and nurses in the region (Kanchanachitra *et al.*, 2011). Similarly, research on Nepalese nurses found that most hope to migrate to the United Kingdom, North America, Australia or New Zealand (Adhikari, 2015). A study of Ethiopian medical students found that 53% hoped to migrate to the United States or European countries (Deressa and Azazh, 2012).

The costs of international migration to the sending country include the exacerbation of shortages, the financial loss in the investment in training and education, the financial loss of consumption and tax receipts, decline in morale and commitment among remaining workers, loss of social and human capital, and disruption to health care institutions (Aluttis *et al.*, 2014; Mackey and Liang, 2013; OECD, 2010). There is significant concern about the "brain drain" of low-income countries losing highly-educated, highly-skilled workers through international migration (Mackey and Liang, 2013). The receiving countries benefit from relief of their shortages and tax receipts of foreign workers (Aluttis *et al.*, 2014). Sending countries benefit from the remittances sent by those who migrated, improvements in skills of returnees, and collaborative partnerships between the diaspora and local professionals (Aluttis *et al.*, 2014). Some sending countries, such as the Philippines, have actively promoted the return migration of health professionals. The Philippines Overseas Employment Administration, established in 1995, encourages educated health workers to return with business loans, tax-free shopping for one year, and scholarships (WHO, 2006). Bilateral agreements have been established between some countries to allow students to receive educational and employment experiences abroad for limited amounts of time. This type of agreement, which has been signed between South Africa and the United Kingdom, and between the Philippines and Japan, can provide benefits to both sending and receiving countries (WHO, 2006; Yagi *et al.*, 2014).

A health worker's decision of whether or not to migrate results from forces that push workers to leave their country of origin, and pull workers toward their destinations (Khaliq *et al.*, 2008). Factors that push health workers to consider leaving their country of origin include low pay, political instability, poor working conditions, a lack of opportunity for professional advancement, safety concerns, and low quality of life (Aluttis *et al.*, 2014). Low wages is one of the more important motivators to migrate for health care workers in developing countries, and some countries have implemented wage increases to avert migration. For example, in Ghana it was documented that the number of Ghanaian doctors working abroad declined 10% after 6 years of wage increases (Okeke, 2014). A survey of Ghanaian doctors confirmed that the salary increases reduced migration out of the country. Better career development and postgraduate education opportunities also helped to retain doctors (Lassey *et al.*, 2013; Snow *et al.*, 2011). In addition, difficult working conditions are linked with higher rates of international migration (Buchan and Calman, 2004; Brush and Sochalski, 2007). High unemployment rates for health workers also can drive migration to other countries where there are more jobs available. A study of health worker migration by the WHO found that 27% of respondents reported unemployment as a reason for migration (Munjanja *et al.*, 2005, WHO, 2004); similar findings have been reported in single-country studies (Fang, 2007; Silva and Fernandes, 2008). Strengthening the domestic market for health care workers is critical for retention (Mackey and Liang, 2013). Fair wages and good working conditions that allow workers to function effectively are key efforts necessary to retain workers. However, the governments of resource poor countries struggle with structural and financial problems that hinder these efforts.

Migration decisions are also influenced by factors that pull workers toward other countries. These pull factors are the circumstances migrants will face at their destination, and can include better financial rewards, better facilities and infrastructure, political stability, greater safety, educational opportunities for themselves and their children, professional advancement, and overall quality of life (Aluttis *et al.*, 2014; Khaliq *et al.*, 2008). There are occupational differences in the factors that pull workers to a new country. For example, a study of Portuguese and Spanish physicians and nurses who worked across the border found that Portuguese physicians migrated to Spain for professional development opportunities, higher salaries, and anticipation of better working conditions. However, Spanish nurses were migrating to Portugal simply to have a greater range of employment opportunities (Leone *et al.*, 2013).

- *Global code for recruitment*

The recruitment of human resources for health by rich countries contributes to the shortage of workers in lower- and middle-income countries, and consequently contributes to the bottleneck of health care delivery systems. The 2010 *Global Code of Practice on the International Recruitment of Health Personnel,* signed by all 193 members of the WHO, provides a framework for ethical decision-making regarding international recruitment, and defines practices among sending and receiving countries to decrease the effects of "brain drain" on sending countries (WHO, 2010b). The code supports the rights of individuals to migrate but also proposes agreements between countries to ensure mutual benefit (WHO, 2011a). For example, it suggests that sending countries should be reimbursed for the cost of educating workers and that long-term planning should be considered. Acceptance of the Global Code is voluntary, and the Global Code is not monitored or enforced.

Recent research on the implementation of the WHO Global Code revealed that of 193 countries surveyed, only 56 countries responded to the survey, and 37 of these had taken steps toward implementing the Code. In most countries, the engagement of relevant stakeholders was the first step toward implementation. In 90% of the responding countries, migrant health professionals reportedly enjoy the same legal rights and responsibilities as domestically trained health personnel (Siyam *et al.*, 2013). However, a study of internationally educated nurses employed in the United States found that half had experienced a negative recruitment practice, and that nurses from developing countries were more likely than those from high-income countries to report recruitment practices that violate the Global Code (Pittman *et al.*, 2012).

The Roles of the Public Sector, the Private Sector, and Donor Organizations to Improve Human Resources for Health

In most nations, the development and retention of human resources for health occurs through a blend of public sector programs, private sector actions, and donor organization involvement. The broad role of the public sector is to address the needs of the population, which can be achieved through direct program management or through coordination of private sector and donor activities. The private sector is not beholden to the public in the same way, and therefore tends to focus on specific goals, which often include making a profit. Donor organizations usually approach their work with similar goals as the public sector, but because they are independent, they can autonomously function much like a private organization. Successful human resources for health planning require coordination of the activities of the public sector, private sector, and donor organizations in order to improve health care access, quality, and efficiency.

The WHO has been actively engaged in promoting improved coordination among stakeholders in human resources for health. A key contribution in this area was the publication of *Working Together for Health,* which provided a framework "to get the right workers with the right skills in the right place doing the right thing" (Arredondo *et al.*, 2003). The report acknowledges the impossibility of creating a blueprint for all countries because problems and resources are diverse. Instead, the report offered a context-neutral framework, suggesting the "Working Lifespan" approach. This framework organizes strategies according to the stage of the worker's life they will influence: entry period, workforce period, and exit period. Figure 13 illustrates the framework.

The entry period focuses on preparing sufficient numbers of workers with the skills needed to address health care needs. This includes the building and support of educational institutions, whether public or private, and ensuring that education meets quality standards (Frenk *et al.*, 2010). The licensing and credentialing of health workers, faculty, and schools helps to ensure that standards are achieved.

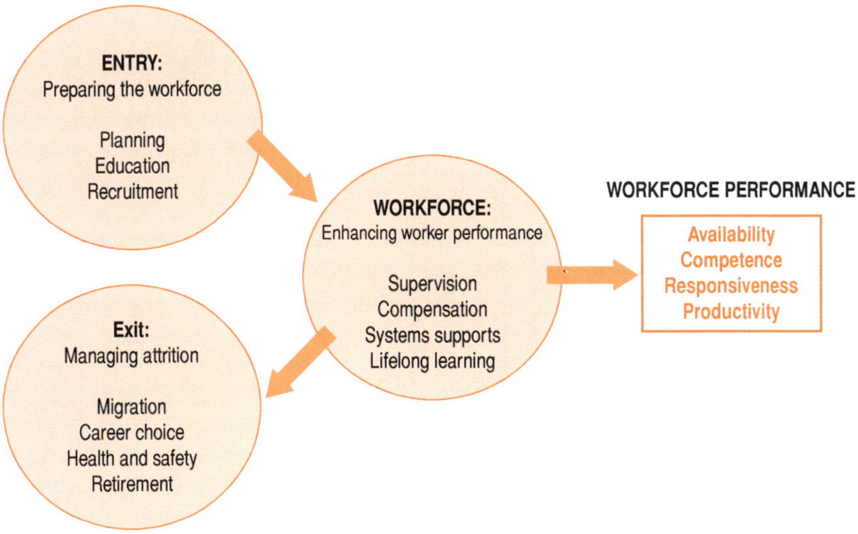

Figure 13. WHO framework for planning for human resources for health

Source: Reprinted with permission from World Health Organization. 2006.

Licensing and credentialing can occur through government agencies or private organizations such as professional boards and societies. The public sector may enact regulations requiring credentialing or accreditation to ensure standards are met. The entry period also includes the recruitment of individuals who are well-suited for health care work to occupations and/or education. Many nations have leveraged both the public and private sectors to implement strategies to improve the entry period. For example, in Brazil, there was a concerted effort to expand access to health care services after a new constitution provided the right to health care. There was a coordinated and sustained effort to scale and skill up the technical workforce, to link curriculum to national health priorities, to provide in-service training, and to encourage teamwork (Buchan *et al.*, 2011). The collaborative education expansions included trade unions, professional organizations, and educational organizations (Buchan *et al.*, 2011). The Ministry of Health provided incentives and guidance to introduce new curriculum that increased not only the number of health workers but also their skills, and provided training in management and multi-professional teamwork. They used "Negotiation Tables" as a vehicle to allow for open and collaborative discussion of labor standards, training needs, and health system needs. Brazil has made substantial progress in increasing access to health workers throughout the country, but still faces challenges with undersupply in some regions of the country.

The workforce period is centered on enhancing the performance of health care workers already employed. This can include establishing policies for health worker staff at public and private health care delivery sites, ensuring that wages are fair and are reliably paid, offering continuing education, and providing resources that the workers need in order to provide care, such as equipment and supplies. These strategies can be developed and implemented by public, private, and donor institutions, and often should be linked to entry-stage initiatives. The Ethiopian Government attempted an innovative approach to revitalization of primary care through a Health Extension Program, in which the government implemented reforms to integrate a new cadre of workers and supply additional resources and infrastructure. Forty new training institutions were established, and the infrastructure of each post was designed to increase access and allow local jurisdictions to maintain their authority over service delivery. There was a simultaneous effort to recruit women from local villages to decrease turnover and address gender inequality (Teklehaimanot and Teklehaimanot, 2013).

The exit period focuses on managing attrition, recognizing that health workers will leave their posts for both planned and unplanned reasons. The efforts needed in this period include managing migration both within regions and internationally, ensuring that career development needs are met to encourage retention, improving health and safety to reduce the impact of infection and violence, supporting workers' family needs, and planning for retirement.

In order to effectively implement national human resources for health plans, countries need to ensure they have good governance practices in place. The WHO recommends that a key role of the public sector is to develop standards of health professional practice and enforce them (WHO, 2006). In addition, good measures of workforce characteristics need to be developed, so that forecasts can be calculated more accurately and the success of programs can be tracked. The WHO encourages countries to collect a minimum dataset and use standardized accounting practices to facilitate the study of human resources for health (WHO, 2006; 2009). At this time, however, many countries do not have such data available, and it is often not standardized or well-documented (Hernández *et al.*, 2009).

There are many examples of successful public–private partnerships to conduct assessment studies for HRH planning. Zambia's National Health Strategic Plan began with an assessment of the concentration of workers across the country and was conducted by the Ministry of Health. Later work leveraged private sector knowledge and data to establish strategies to address attrition and maldistribution of the workforce (Ferrinho *et al.*, 2011). In Kenya, private-sector researchers used national nursing data from the public sector to conduct a geographical analysis of the nursing workforce to establish baseline data on geographic maldistribution and its association with health spending per capita and immunization rates (Wakaba *et al.*, 2014). In some countries, mistrust of the public sector may make it advantageous for HRH planning efforts to be driven by the private sector. For example, a survey of Nepal's governance of human resources for health revealed nepotism and poor compliance with the law, which hindered government-led efforts to improve HRH (Devkota *et al.*, 2013). All nations also should collect evaluative measures, which include data on the availability of health workers, their skills and competencies, and worker productivity. Surveys of health professionals can provide important data, and often are conducted by government entities. The development of human resources for health should be a shared effort of the public and private sectors, and there should also be international cooperation to support cross-country planning (WHO, 2006).

Rapid and uncoordinated changes in the public–private mix of health care systems, however, can be detrimental to health workforce planning and sufficiency. Careful monitoring and planning is needed to avoid disruption of health services. For example, in the late 1990s, Israel began reductions in financing of their highly-regarded health care system, and the private sector grew rapidly. Subsequently, the physician population has grown much more slowly than in the past, and survey data has revealed significant discontent among the physician workforce (Chernichovsky, 2013). China also has experienced notable changes in the public–private mix of the health care system, moving toward greater privatization in 2000 (Tang *et al.*, 2014). After 2000, there was more rapid growth in the health workforce, and a greater share of physicians moved to private hospitals.

Donor organizations can also be an important contributor to the development of HRH policies and the workforce. The WHO, Global Fund, and the GAVI Alliance have funded projects that train health workers and that expand pre-service training capacity by supporting establishment of training facilities, hiring faculty, and support for housing. These organizations also contribute to strengthening governmental HRH policy and planning capacity by providing funding and technical assistance to establish government HRH units, design policies and information management systems, reform health workers' incentive policies, and finance remuneration. These activities provide an opportunity to align and coordinate efforts across agencies and among country-level policymakers, and also provide engaged countries with an international network that emphasizes long-term reforms (Vujicic *et al.*, 2012).

Conclusion

There has been significant progress over recent decades in the development of human resources for health, but there remain severe shortages and substantial maldistribution of health professionals worldwide. Two trends have the potential to exacerbate these problems: Demographic changes and economic development are leading to epidemiologic shifts and a redistribution of the disability burden of diseases. These trends will require health care workers to adapt their skill sets (Crisp and Chen, 2014).

The main demographic change is the aging of the population. Many countries, particularly in East Asia, North America, and Europe, have aging populations and lower birth rates. This trend is causing increases in chronic disease and disability, as well as diseases associated with aging such as cancer. In addition, economic development is driving epidemiologic changes. There is a shift from communicable diseases and nutrition-related illnesses toward non-communicable diseases, including chronic diseases and mental health disorders (Murray *et al.*, 2012).

These aging, epidemiological and disease-burden trends require HRH planners to proactively plan, so the future HRH workforce will meet these demands. Because the health workforce is essential to the provision of health care services, then changes in education, organization, distribution, and remuneration will be needed (Crisp and Chen, 2014; Frenk *et al.*, 2010). Attention must be paid to ongoing problems associated with international migration and urban–rural imbalances. Improvements in data collection, country-level planning, and international coordination will be needed to address local and global health workforce needs and achieve continuing improvement in health status worldwide (Vujicic *et al.*, 2012; WHO, 2006).

References

Abreu MH, Sanglard-Oliveira CA, Jaruche AR, Mambrini JV, Werneck MA, Lucas SD. 2013. A survey of the sociodemographic and educational characteristics of oral health technicians in public primary health care teams in Minas Gerais, Brazil. *Human Resources for Health* 11: 67.

Achembong LN, Ashu AM, Hagopian A, Downer A, Barnhart S. 2012. Cameroon mid-level providers offer a promising public health dentistry model. *Human Resources for Health* 10: 46.

Adhikari R. 2015. Vacant hospitals and under-employed nurses: A qualitative study of the nursing workforce management situation in Nepal. *Health Policy Planning* 30(3): 289–297.

Almalki MJ, Fitzgerald G, Clark M. 2012. Quality of work life among primary health care nurses in the Jazan Region, Saudi Arabia: A cross-sectional study. *Human Resources for Health* 10: 30.

Aluttis C, Bishaw T, Frank MW. 2014. The workforce for health in a globalized context — Global shortages and international migration. *Global Health Action Journal* 7: 23611.

Anand S, Fan VY, Zhang J, Zhang L, Ke Y, Dong, Z, Chen LC. 2008. China's human resources for health: Quantity, quality, and distribution. *Lancet* 372: 1774–1781.

Anderson BA, Isaacs AA. 2007. Simply not there: The impact of international migration of nurses and midwives — Perspectives from Guyana. *Journal of Midwifery and Women's Health* 52: 392–397.

Anderson GF, Chalkidou K. 2008. Spending on medical care: More is better? *Journal of the Medical Association* 299: 2444–2445.

Andre AM, Ciampone MH, Santelle O. 2013. Health care units and human resources management trends. *Rerista de Saúde Públic* 47: 158–163; Discussion 163.

Antonazzo E, Scott A, Skatun D, Elliott RF. 2003. The labour market for nursing: A review of the labour supply literature. *Health Economics* 12: 465–478.

Araujo EC, Maeda A. 2013. How to Recruit and Retain Health Workers in Rural and Remote Areas in Developing Countries. In Lutalo M. (ed.). *Health, Nutrition and Population Discussion Paper.* Washington DC: World Bank.

Arredondo A, Ramos R, Zuniga A. 2003. Economic evaluation of the demand of medical care for mental health in Mexico: Schizophrenia and depression, 1996–2000. *Revista de Investigatión Clinica* 55: 43–50.

Arredondo A, Zuniga A, Parada I. 2005. Health care costs and financial consequences of epidemiological changes in chronic diseases in Latin America: Evidence from Mexico. *Public Health* 119: 711–20.

Auerbach DI, Buerhaus PI, Staiger DO. 2014. Registered nurses are delaying retirement, a shift that has contributed to recent growth in the nurse workforce. *Health Affairs (Millwood)* In press.

Bell SA, Rominski S, Bam V, Donkor E, Lori J. 2013. Analysis of nursing education in Ghana: Priorities for scaling-up the nursing workforce. *Nursing Health Sciences* 15(2): 244–249.

Berger L, Mace JM. 2012. Vascular surgeons in France: An endangered species? *Annals of Vascular Surgery* 26: 1154–1159.

Binagwaho A, Kyamanywa P, Farmer PE, Nuthulaganti T, Umubyeyi B, Nyemazi JP, Mugeni SD, Asiimwe A, Ndagijimana U, Lamphere Mcpherson H, Ngirabega JDE D, Sliney A, Uwayezu A, Rusanganwa V, Wagner CM, NUTT CT, Eldon-Edington M, Cancedda C, Magaziner IC, Goosby E. 2013. The human resources for health program in Rwanda — new partnership. *The New England Journal of Medicine* 369: 2054–2059.

Biringer A, Carroll JC. 2012. What does the feminization of family medicine mean? *CMAJ* 184: 1752.

Blanas DA, Ndiaye Y, Nichols K, Jensen A, Siddiqui A, Hennig N. 2013. Barriers to community case management of malaria in Saraya, Senegal: Training, and supply-chains. *Malaria Journal* 12: 95.

Bourmpoula E. 2012. *Global Employment Trends for Women 2012*. Geneva: International Labour Office.

Bruckner TA, Scheffler RM, Shen G, Yoon J, Chisholm D, Morris J, Fulton BD, Dal Poz, MR, Saxena S. 2011. The mental health workforce gap in low- and middle-income countries: A needs-based approach. *Bulletin of the World Health Organization* 89: 184–94.

Brush BL, Sochalski J. 2007. International Nurse Migration: Lessons from the Philippines. *Policy, Politics, and Nursing Practice* 8: 37–46.

Buchan J, Calman L. 2004. *The global Shortage of Registered Nurses: An Overview of Issues and Actions*. Geneva: International Council of Nurses.

Buchan J, Fronteira I, Dussault G. 2011. Continuity and change in human resources policies for health: Lessons from Brazil. *Human Resources for Health* 9: 17.

Buchmueller TC, Grumbach K, Kronick R, Kahn, JG. 2005. The effect of health insurance on medical care utilization and implications for insurance expansion: A review of the literature. *Medical Care Research and Review* 62: 3–30.

Cailhol J, Craveiro I, Madede T, Makoa E, Mathole T, Parsons AN, Van Leemput L, Biesma R, Brugha R, Chilundo B, Lehmann U, Dussault G, Van Damme W, Sanders D. 2013. Analysis of human resources for health strategies and policies in 5 countries in Sub-Saharan Africa, in response to GFATM and PEPFAR-funded HIV-activities. *Global Health* 9: 52.

Campbell J, Dussault G, Buchan J, Pozo-Martin F, Guerra Arias M, Leone C, Siyam A, Cometto G. 2013. A universal truth: No health without a workforce. *Forum Report, Third Global Forum on Human Resources for Health Recife, Brazil*. Geneva: Global Health Workforce Alliance and World Health Organization.

Chen L, Evans T, Anand S, Boufford JI, Brown H, Chowdhury M, Cueto M, Dare L, Dussault G, Elzinga G, Fee E, Habte D, Hanvoravongchai P, Jacobs M, Kurowski C, Michael S, Pablos-Mendez A, Sewankambo N, Solimano G, Stilwell B, De Waal A, Wibulpolprasert S. 2004. Human resources for health: Overcoming the crisis. *Lancet* 364: 1984–1990.

Cheng SH, Chiang TL. 1997. The effect of universal health insurance on health care utilization in Taiwan. Results from a natural experiment. *Journal of the American Medical Association* 278: 89–93.

Chernichovsky D. 2013. Reforms are needed to increase public funding and curb demand for private care in Israel's health system. *Health Affairs (Millwood)* 32: 724–733.

Ching P. 1995. User fees, demand for children's health care and access across income groups: The Philippine case. *Social Science & Medicine* 41: 37–46.

Crettenden I, Poz MD, Buchan J. 2013. Right time, right place: Improving access to health service through effective retention and distribution of health workers. *Human Resources for Health* 11: 60.

Crisp N, Chen L. 2014. Global supply of health professionals. *The New England Journal of Medicine* 370: 950–957.

Dal Poz MR, Kinfu Y, Dräger S, Kunjumen T. 2007. Counting health workers: Definitions, data, methods and global results. *HRH Discussion Paper Series.* Geneva: World Health Organization.

Dal Poz MR, Neeru G, Estelle Q, Agnes LBS. (eds.). 2009. Handbook on Monitoring and Evaluation of Human Resources for Health with special applications for low- and middle-income countries. Geneva: World Health Organization.

Dayrit MM, Dolea C, Braichet JM. 2010. One piece of the puzzle to solve the human resources for health crisis. *Bulletin of the World Health Organization* 88: 322: A.

Dayrit MM, Dolea C, Dreesch N. 2011. Addressing the Human Resources for Health crisis in countries: How far have we gone? What can we expect to achieve by 2015? *Revista Peruana de Medicina Experimental & Salud Pública* 28: 327–336.

De Jaegher K, Jegers M. 2000. A model of physician behaviour with demand inducement. *Journal of Health Economics* 19: 231–58.

Delattre E, Dormont B. 2003. Fixed fees and physician-induced demand: A panel data study on French physicians. *Health Economics* 12: 741–754.

Delgado A, Saletti-Cuesta L, Lopez-Fernandez LA, De Dios Luna JDE D, Mateo-Rodriguez I. 2011. Gender and the professional career of primary care physicians in Andalusia (Spain). *BMC Health Services Research* 11: 51.

Deressa W, Azazh A. 2012. Attitudes of undergraduate medical students of Addis Ababa University towards medical practice and migration, Ethiopia. *BMC Medical Education* 12: 68.

Devkota B, Ghimire J, Devkota A, Gupta RP, Mahato RK, Thapa N, Shrestha B, Tuladhar P. 2013. Health governance at local level from human resource for health perspectives: The case of Nepal. *Journal of Nepal Health Research Council* 11: 133–137.

Dgedge M, Mendoza A, Necochea E, Bossemeyer D, Rajabo M, Fullerton J. 2014. Assessment of the nursing skill mix in Mozambique using a task analysis methodology. *Human Resources for Health* 12: 5.

Dingley J, Yoder L. 2013. The public health nursing work environment: Review of the research literature. *Journal of Public Health Management and Practice* 19: 308–321.

Dos Reis Moreira, EC, O'Dwyer G. 2013. An analysis of actions to promote health in underprivileged urban areas: A case in Brazil. *BMC Family Practice* 14: 80.

Dovlo D. 2005. Wastage in the health workforce: Some perspectives from African countries. *Human Resources for Health* 3: 6.

Dussault G, Buchan J. 2014. The economic crisis in the EU: Impact on health workforce mobility. In Buchan J, Wismar M, Glinos IA, Bremner J. (eds.). *Health Professional Mobilitly in a Changing Europe.* Copenhagen, Denmark: World Health Organization.

Ekine A, Samati M, Walker J-A. 2013. Improving Learning Opportunities and Outcomes for Girls in Africa. In Ackerman X, Abay NA. (eds.). *2013 Echidna Global Scholars.* Washington DC: Brookings Institution.

Fang ZZ. 2007. Potential of China in global nurse migration. *Health Services Research* 42: 1419–1428.

Ferrinho F, Amaral M, Russo G, Ferrinho P. 2012. Purchasing power of civil servant health workers in Mozambique. *Pan African Medical Journal* 11: 14.

Ferrinho P, Siziya S, Goma F, Dussault G. 2011. The human resource for health situation in Zambia: Deficit and maldistribution. *Humuan Resources for Health* 9: 30.

Filmer D, Pritchett L. 1999. The impact of public spending on health: Does money matter? *Social Science & Medicine* 49: 1309–1323.

Folkard S. 2008. Shift work, safety, and aging. *Chronobiology International* 25: 183–198.

Fonjungo PN, Kebede Y, Arneson W, Tefera D, Yimer K, Kinde S, Alem M, Cheneke W, Mitiku H, Tadesse E, Tsegaye A, Kenyon T. 2013. Preservice laboratory education strengthening enhances sustainable laboratory workforce in Ethiopia. *Human Resources for Health* 11: 56.

Freeman JD, Kadiyala S, Bell JF, Martin DP. 2008. The causal effect of health insurance on utilization and outcomes in adults: A systematic review of US studies. *Medical Care* 46: 1023–1032.

Frehywot S, Mullan F, Payne PW, Ross H. 2010. Compulsory service programmes for recruiting health workers in remote and rural areas: Do they work? *Bulletin of the World Health Organization* 88: 364–370.

Frehywot S, Vovides Y, Talib Z, Mikhail N, Ross H, Wohltjen H, Bedada S, Korhumel K, Koumare AK, Scott J. 2013. E-learning in medical education in resource constrained low- and middle-income countries. *Human Resources Health* 11: 4.

Frenk J, Chen L, Bhutta ZA, Cohen J, Crisp N, Evans T, Fineberg H, Garcia P, Ke Y, Kelley P, Kistnasamy B, Meleis A, Naylor D, Pablos-Mendez A, Reddy S, Scrimshaw S, Sepulveda J, Serwadda D, Zurayk H. 2010. Health professionals for a new century: Transforming education to strengthen health systems in an interdependent world. *The Lancet* 376: 1923–1958.

Fuchs VR. 1978. The supply of surgeons and the demand for operations. *Journal of Human Resources* 13 (Suppl): 35–56.

Fulton BD, Scheffler RM, Sparkes SP, Auh EY, Vujicic M, Soucat A. 2011. Health workforce skill mix and task shifting in low income countries: A review of recent evidence. *Human Resources Health* 9: 1.

Garonna P. 2006. *The Millennium Development Goals: The Way Ahead. A Pan European Perspective.* New York: United Nations.

Gerdtham UG, Sogaard J, Andersson F, Jonsson B. 1992a. An econometric analysis of health care expenditure: A cross-section study of the OECD countries. *Journal of Health Economics* 11: 63–84.

Gerdtham UG, Sogaard J, Jonsson B, Andersson F. 1992b. A pooled cross-section analysis of the health care expenditures of the OECD countries. *Developments in Health Economics and Public Policy* 1: 287–310.

Getzen TE. 2000. Health care is an individual necessity and a national luxury: Applying multilevel decision models to the analysis of health care expenditures. *Journal of Health Economics* 19: 259–270.

Glass AP, Gao Y, Luo J. 2013. China: Facing a long-term care challenge on an unprecedented scale. *Global Public Health* 8: 725–738.

Goss PE, Strasser-Weippl K, Lee-Bychkovsky BL, Fan L, Li J, Chavarri-Guerra Y, Liedke PE, Pramesh CS, Badovinac-Crnjevic T, Sheikine Y, Chen Z, Qiao YL, Shao Z, Wu YL, Fan D, Chow LW, Wang J, Zhang Q, Yu S, Shen G, He J, Purushotham A, Sullivan R, Badwe R, Banavali SD, Nair R, Kumar L, Parikh P, Subramanian S, Chaturvedi P, Iyer S, Shastri SS, Digumarti R, Soto-Perez-De-Celis E, Adilbay D, Semiglazov V, Orlov S, Kaidarova D, Tsimafeyeu I, Tatishchev S, Danishevskiy KD, Hurlbert M, Vail C, St Louis J, Chan A. 2014. Challenges to effective cancer control in China, India, and Russia. *Lancet Oncology* 15: 489–538.

Gruber J, Owings M. 1996. Physician financial incentives and cesarean section delivery. *RAND Journal of Economics* 27: 99–123.

Grytten J, Carlsen F, Sorensen R. 1995. Supplier inducement in a public health care system. *Journal of Health Economics* 14: 207–229.

Grytten J, Sorensen R. 2001. Type of contract and supplier-induced demand for primary physicians in Norway. *Journal of Health Economics* 20: 379–393.

Gupta N, Alfano M. 2011. Access to non-pecuniary benefits: Does gender matter? Evidence from six low- and middle-income countries. *Human Resources for Health* 9: 25.

Hagopian A, Zuyderduin A, Kyobutungi N, Yumkella F. 2009. Job satisfaction and morale in the Ugandan health workforce. *Health Affairs* 28: w863–w875.

Henderson LN, Tulloch J. 2008. Incentives for retaining and motivating health workers in Pacific and Asian countries. *Human Resources for Health* 6: 18.

Hernandez-Peña P, Poullier JP, Van Mosseveld CJM, Van De Maele N, Cherilova V, Indikadahena C, Lie G, Tan-Torresa T, Evans DB. 2013. Health worker remuneration in WHO Member States. *Bulletin of World Health Organization* 92: 808–815.

Hernández P, Torres T, Evans DB. 2009. Measuring Expenditure on the Health Workforce: Concepts, Data Sources and Methods. In Dal Poz MR, GN, Quai E, Soucat ALB. (eds.). *Handbook on Monitoring and Evaluation of Human Resources for Health, with Special Applications for Low- and Middle-Income Countries.* Geneva: World Health Organization.

Hitiris T, Posnett J. 1992. The determinants and effects of health expenditure in developed countries. *Journal of Health Economics* 11: 173–181.

Hoyler M, Finlayson SR, Mcclain CD, Meara JG, Hagander L. 2014. Shortage of doctors, shortage of data: A review of the global surgery, obstetrics, and anesthesia workforce literature. *World Journal of Surgery* 38: 269–280.

Hu Y, Chen J. 2014. How to allocate public health manpower in township health centers in China scientifically and reasonably. *Journal of Biomedical Research* 28: 78–80.

Huang J, Shi L, Chen Y. 2013. Staff retention after the privatization of township–village health centers: A case study from the Haimen City of East China. *BMC Health Services Research* 13: 136.

Iwu EN, Holzemer WL. 2014. Task shifting of HIV management from doctors to nurses in Africa: Clinical outcomes and evidence on nurse self-efficacy and job satisfaction. *AIDS Care* 26: 42–52.

Johnson P, Fogarty L, Fullerton J, Bluestone J, Drake M. 2013. An integrative review and evidence-based conceptual model of the essential components of pre-service education. *Human Resources for Health* 11: 42.

Jones CB, Gates M. 2004. Gender-based wage differentials in a predominantly female profession: Observations from nursing. *Economics of Education Review* 23: 615–631.

Kalua K, Ng'ongola RT, Mbewe F, Gilbert C. 2012. Using primary health care (PHC) workers and key informants for community based detection of blindness in children in Southern Malawi. *Human Resources for Health* 10: 37.

Kamchuchat C, Chongsuvivatwong V, Oncheunjit S, Yip TW, Sangthong R. 2008. Workplace violence directed at nursing staff at a general hospital in Southern Thailand. *Journal of Occupational Health* 50: 201–207.

Kanchanachitra C, Lindelow M, Johnston T, Hanvoravongchai P, Lorenzo FM, Huong NL, Wilopo SA, Dela Rosa JF. 2011. Human resources for health in southeast Asia: Shortages, distributional challenges, and international trade in health services. *Lancet* 377: 769–781.

Kasper J, Bajunirwe F. 2012. Brain drain in Sub-Saharan Africa: Contributing factors, potential remedies and the role of academic medical centres. *Archives of Disease in Childhood* 97: 973–979.

Keane S, Lincoln M, Smith T. 2012. Retention of allied health professionals in rural New South Wales: A thematic analysis of focus group discussions. *BMC Health Services Research* 12: 175.

Khaliq AA, Broyles RW, Mwachofi AK. 2008. Global nurse migration: Its impact on developing countries and prospects for the future. *World Health Population* 10: 55–73.

Kletke PR, Marder WD, Silberger AB. 1990. The growing proportion of female physicians: Implications for US physician supply. *American Journal of Public Health* 80: 300–304.

Konrad AM, Yang Y, Cannings K. 2012. Pay dispersion and earnings for women and men: A study of Swedish doctors. *Gender in Management: An International Journal* 27: 249–270.

Koon AD, Mayhew SH. 2013. Strengthening the health workforce and rolling out universal health coverage: The need for policy analysis. *Global Health Action* 6: 21852.

Lagarde M, Blaauw D, Cairns J. 2012. Cost-effectiveness analysis of human resources policy interventions to address the shortage of nurses in rural South Africa. *Socal Science & Medicine* 75: 801–806.

Laskar M, Spinosi AM, Bendjebla Y, Moreau J, Dahan M. 2013. Are we running out of thoracic or cardiac surgeons? Demography of thoracic and cardiac surgeons in France in 2012. *Interactive Cardiovascular and Thoracic Surgery* 16: 470–474.

Lassey AT, Lassey PD, Boamah M. 2013. Career destinations of University of Ghana Medical School graduates of various year groups. *Ghana Medical Journal* 47: 87–91.

Ledikwe JH, Reason LL, Burnett SM, Busang L, Bodika S, Lebelonyane R, Ludick S, Matshediso E, Mawandia S, Mmelesi M, Sento B, Semo BW. 2013. Establishing a health information workforce: Innovation for low- and middle-income countries. *Human Resources for Health* 11: 35.

Lehmann U, Dieleman M, Martineau T. 2008. Staffing remote rural areas in middle- and low-income countries: A literature review of attraction and retention. *BMC Health Services Research* 8: 19.

Leone C, Conceicao C, Dussault G. 2013. Trends of cross-border mobility of physicians and nurses between Portugal and Spain. *Human Resources for Health* 11: 36.

Li D, Tsui MC, Yuan GZ. 2014. China's new Mental Health Law needs to tackle manpower imbalance of professionals in schizophrenia psychosocial rehabilitation. *The International Journal Social Psychiatry* 60: 410–411.

Li X, Liu J, Huang J, Qian Y, Che L. 2013. An analysis of the current educational status and future training needs of China's rural doctors in 2011. *Journal of Postgraduate Medicine* 89: 202–208.

Lipnick M, Mijumbi C, Dubowitz G, Kaggwa S, Goetz L, Mabweijano J, Jayaraman S, Kwizera A, Tindimwebwa J, Ozgediz D. 2013. Surgery and anesthesia capacity-building in resource-poor settings: Description of an ongoing academic partnership in Uganda. *World Journal of Surgery* 37: 488–497.

Lo Sasso AT, Richards MR, Chou CF, Gerber SE. 2011. The $16,819 pay gap for newly trained physicians: The unexplained trend of men earning more than women. *Health Affairs (Millwood)* 30: 193–201.

Lopes SC, Cabral AJ. De Sousa B. 2014. Community health workers: To train or to restrain? A longitudinal survey to assess the impact of training community health workers in the Bolama Region, Guinea-Bissau. *Human Resources for Health* 12: 8.

Lutz W, KC S. 2011. Global human capital: Integrating education and population. *Science* 333: 587–592.

Mackey TK, Liang BA. 2013. Restructuring brain drain: Strengthening governance and financing for health worker migration. *Global Health Action* 6: 1–7.

Marten R, Mcintyre D, Travassos C, Shishkin S, Longde W, Reddy S, Vega J. 2014. An assessment of progress towards universal health coverage in Brazil, Russia, India, China, and South Africa (BRICS). *The Lancet* 384(9960): 2164–2171.

Martin P, Duffy T, Johnston B, Banks P, Harkess-Murphy E, Martin CR. 2013. Family health nursing: A response to the global health challenges. *Journal of Family Nursing* 19: 99–118.

Mathauer I, Imhoff I. 2006. Health worker motivation in Africa: The role of non-financial incentives and human resource management tools. *Human Resources for Health* 4: 24.

Mbemba G, Gagnon MP, Pare G, Cote J. 2013. Interventions for supporting nurse retention in rural and remote areas: An umbrella review. *Human Resources for Health* 11: 44.

Mcbain R, Salhi C, Morris JE, Salomon JA, Betancourt TS. 2012. Disease burden and mental health system capacity: WHO Atlas study of 117 low- and middle-income countries. *British Journal of Psychiatry* 201: 444–450.

Mion LC, Hazel C, Cap M, Fusilero J, Podmore ML, Szweda C. 2006. Retaining and recruiting mature experienced nurses: A multicomponent organizational strategy. *The Journal of Nursing Administration* 36: 148–154.

Misfeldt R, Linder J, Lait J, Hepp S, Armitage G, Jackson K, Suter E. 2014. Incentives for improving human resource outcomes in health care: Overview of reviews. *Journal of Health Services Research and Policy* 19: 52–61.

Moreno-Serra R, Smith P. 2011. *The Effects of Health Coverage on Population Outcomes: A Country-Level Panel Data Analysis*. London: Business School & Centre for Health Policy, Imperial College London.

Mosquera PA, Hernandez J, Vega R, Martinez J, Labonte R, Sanders D, San Sebastian M. 2012. Primary health care contribution to improve health outcomes in Bogota-Colombia: A longitudinal ecological analysis. *BMC Family Practice* 13: 84.

Mullan F, Frehywot S, Omaswa F, Buch E, Chen C, Greysen SR, Wassermann T, Abubakr DE, Awases M, Boelen C, Diomande MJ, Dovlo D, Ferro J, Haileamlak A, Iputo J, Jacobs M, Koumare AK, Mipando M, Monekosso GL, Olapade-Olaopa EO, Rugarabamu P, Sewankambo NK, Ross H, Ayas H, Chale SB, Cyprien S, Cohen J, Haile-Mariam T, Hamburger E, Jolley L, Kolars JC, Kombe G, Neusy AJ. 2011. Medical schools in Sub-Saharan Africa. *Lancet* 377: 1113–1121.

Mullei K, Mudhune S, Wafula J, Masamo E, English M, Goodman C, Lagarde M, Blaauw D. 2010. Attracting and retaining health workers in rural areas: Investigating nurses' views on rural posts and policy interventions. *BMC Health Services Research* 10 (Suppl)1: S1.

Munjanja OK, Kibuka S, Dovlo D. 2005. *The Nursing Workforce in Sub-Saharan Africa*. Geneva: International Council of Nurses. Available at http://www.icn.ch/images/stories/documents/publications/GNRI/Issue7_SSA.pdf

Murphy JF. 2014. Medical staff retention. *Irish Medical Journal* 107: 4–5.

Murray CJ, Vos T, Lozano R, Naghavi M, Flaxman AD, Michaud C, Ezzati M, Shibuya K, Salomon JA, Abdalla S, Aboyans V, Abraham J, Ackerman I, Aggarwal R, Ahn SY, Ali MK, Alvarado M, Anderson HR, Anderson LM, Andrews KG, Atkinson C, Baddour LM, Bahalim AN, Barker-Collo S, Barrero LH, Bartels DH, Basanez MG, Baxter A, Bell ML, Benjamin EJ, Bennett D, Bernabe E, Bhalla K, Bhandari B, Bikbov B, Bin Abdulhak A, Birbeck G, Black JA, Blencowe H, Blore JD, Blyth F, Bolliger I, Bonaventure A, Boufous S, Bourne R, Boussinesq M, Braithwaite T, Brayne C, Bridgett L, Brooker S, Brooks P, Brugha TS, Bryan-Hancock C, Bucello C, Buchbinder R, Buckle G, Budke CM, Burch M, Burney P, Burstein R, Calabria B, Campbell B, Canter CE, Carabin H, Carapetis J, Carmona L, Cella C, Charlson F, Chen H, Cheng AT, Chou D, Chugh SS, Coffeng LE, Colan SD, Colquhoun S, Colson KE, Condon J, Connor MD, Cooper LT, Corriere M, Cortinovis M, De Vaccaro KC, Couser W, Cowie BC, Criqui MH, Cross M, Dabhadkar KC, Dahiya M, Dahodwala N, Damsere-Derry J, Danaei G, Davis A, De Leo D, Degenhardt L, Dellavalle R, Delossantos A, Denenberg J, Derrett S, Des Jarlais DC, Dharmaratne SD, *et al.* 2012. Disability-adjusted life years (DALYs) for 291 diseases and injuries in 21 regions, 1990–2010: A systematic analysis for the Global Burden of Disease Study 2010. *Lancet* 380: 2197–2223.

Newhouse JP. 1977. Medical-care expenditure: A cross-national survey. *Journal of Human Resources* 12: 115–125.

Newman CJ, De Vries DH, D'arc Kanakuze J, Ngendahimana G. 2011. Workplace violence and gender discrimination in Rwanda's health workforce: Increasing safety and gender equality. *Human Resources for Health* 9: 19.

Nixon J, Ulmann P. 2006. The relationship between health care expenditure and health outcomes. Evidence and caveats for a causal link. *European Journal of Health Economics* 7: 7–18.

OECD. 2010. International migration of health workers. In Organization WH. (ed.). OECD Publishing.

OECD. 2013. Health at a glance 2013: OECD indicators. Available: http://www.oecd.org/els/health-systems/Health-at-a-Glance-2013.pdf

Okeke EN. 2014. Do higher salaries lower physician migration? *Health Policy Plan* 29(5): 603–614.

Ossai EN, Ibiok NC, Chukwuogo O, Umeobieri AK, Aniwada EC, Ugwunna NC. 2012. Rural retention of human resources for health. *Nigerian Journal of Medicine* 21: 138–45.

Padarath A, Chamberlain C, Mccoy D, Ntuli A, Rowson, M, Loewenson R. 2003. Health Personnel in Southern Africa: Confronting maldistribution and brain drain. *EQUINET Discussion Paper Number 3.* Regional Network for Equity in Health in Southern Africa (EQUINET), Health Systems Trust (South Africa) and MEDACT (UK).

Pas B, Peters P, Doorewaard H, Eisinga R, Lagro-Janssen T. 2011. Feminisation of the medical profession: A strategic HRM dilemma? The effects of family-friendly HR practices on female doctors' contracted working hours. *Human Resource Management Journal* 21: 285–302.

Pierantoni CR, Garcia AC. 2011. Human resources for health and decentralization policy in the Brazilian health system. *Human Resources for Health* 9: 12.

Pittman P, Herrera C, Spetz J, Davis CR. 2012. Immigration and contract problems experienced by foreign-educated nurses. *Medical Care Research and Review* 69: 351–365.

Propper C, Venables M. 2013. An assessment of labour's record on health and healthcare. *Oxford Reviews of Economic Policy* 29: 203–226.

Purohit B, Bandyopadhyay T. 2014. Beyond job security and money: Driving factors of motivation for government doctors in India. *Human Resources for Health* 12: 12.

Ramani S, Rao KD, Ryan M, Vujicic M, Berman P. 2013. For more than love or money: Attitudes of student and in-service health workers towards rural service in India. *Human Resources for Health* 11: 58.

Rao M, Rao KD, Kumar AK, Chatterjee M, Sundararaman T. 2011. Human resources for health in India. *Lancet* 377: 587–98.

Saltman DC, Kidd MR, Jackson D, Cleary M. 2012. Transportability of tertiary qualifications and CPD: A continuing challenge for the global health workforce. *BMC Medical Education* 12: 51.

Sarma S, Thind A, Chu MK. 2011. Do new cohorts of family physicians work less compared to their older predecessors? The evidence from Canada. *Social Science & Medicine* 72: 2049–58.

Sattar S. 2012. Opportunities for Men and Women in Emerging Europe and Central Asia. Washington DC: World Bank.

Sauerborn R, Nougtara A, Latimer E. 1994. The elasticity of demand for health care in Burkina Faso: Differences across age and income groups. *Health Policy Plan* 9: 185–192.

Savedoff W. 2003. How Much Should Countries Spend on Health? Geneva: World Health Organization.

Scheffler RM, Bruckner TA, Spetz J. 2012. The labour market for human resources for health in low- and middle-income countries. *Human Resources for Health Observer Issue no. 11*. Available at http://www.who.int/hrh/resources/Observer11_WEB.pdf

Scheffler RM, Fulton BD. 2014. Needs-based estimates for the health workforce. In Soucat A, Scheffler RM, Ghebreyesus TA. (eds.). *The Labor Market for Health Workers in Africa: A New Look at the Crisis.* Washington DC: The World Bank.

Scheffler RM, Liu JX, Kinfu Y, Dal Poz MR. 2008. Forecasting the global shortage of physicians: An economic- and needs-based approach. *Bulletin of the World Health Organization* 86: 516–523B.

Schumacher EJ. 1997. Relative wages and exit behavior among registered nurses. *Journal of Labor Research* 18: 581–592.

Schwartz JB, Akin JS, Popkin BM. 1988. Price and income elasticities of demand for modern health care: The case of infant delivery in the Philippines. *The World Bank Economic Review* 2: 49–76.

Seabury SA, Chandra A, Jena AB. 2013. Trends in the earnings of male and female health care professionals in the United States, 1987 to 2010. *JAMA Internal Medicine* 173: 1748–1750.

Shang J, You L, Ma C, Altares D, Sloane DM, Aiken LH. 2014. Nurse employment contracts in Chinese hospitals: Impact of inequitable benefit structures on nurse and patient satisfaction. *Human Resources for Health* 12: 1.

Sheikh K, Rajkumari B, Jain K, Rao K, Patanwar P, Gupta G, Antony KR, Sundararaman T. 2012. Location and vocation: Why some government doctors stay on in rural Chhattisgarh, India. *International Health* 4: 192–199.

Shelton JD, Hodgins S. 2014. The human resources for health program in Rwanda. *The New England Journal of Medicine* 370: 981.

Silva, Amvad, Fernandes RMP. 2008. *Foreign Nurses in Portugal*. Lisbon, Portugal: Orden dos Enfermeiros.

Siyam A, Zurn P, Ro OC, Gedik G, Ronquillo K, Joan CO C, Vaillancourt-Laflamme C, Dela Rosa J, Perfilieva G, Dal Poz MR. 2013. Monitoring the implementation of the WHO Global Code of Practice on the International Recruitment of Health Personnel. *Bulletin of the World Health Organization* 91: 816–823.

Skowronski GA, Peisah C. 2012. The greying intensivist: Ageing and medical practice — everyone's problem. *The Medical Journal of Australia* 196: 505–507.

Snow RC, Asabir K, Mutumba M, Koomson E, Gyan K, Dzodzomenyo M, Kruk M, Kwansah J. 2011. Key factors leading to reduced recruitment and retention of health professionals in remote areas of Ghana: A qualitative study and proposed policy solutions. *Human Resources for Health* 9: 13.

Sorensen RJ, Grytten J. 1999. Competition and supplier-induced demand in a health care system with fixed fees. *Health Economics* 8: 497–508.

Spetz J. 2011. *Unemployed and Underemployed Nurses Geneva*. Switzerland: International Center for Human Resources in Nursing.

Spetz J. 2012. Health Reform and the Health Care Workforce. *Baker Institute Policy Report*. Houston, TX: James A. Baker III Institute for Public Policy at Rice University.

Sundararaman T, Gupta G. 2011. Indian approaches to retaining skilled health workers in rural areas. *Bulletin of the World Health Organization* 89: 73–77.

Tang C, Zhang Y, Chen L, Lin Y. 2014. The growth of private hospitals and their health workforce in China: A comparison with public hospitals. *Health Policy Plan* 29: 30–41.

Teklehaimanot HD, Teklehaimanot A. 2013. Human resource development for a community-based health extension program: A case study from Ethiopia. *Human Resources for Health* 11: 39.

Theurl E, Winner H. 2011. The male–female gap in physician earnings: Evidence from a public health insurance system. *Health Economics* 20: 1184–1200.

U.S. Bureau of Economic Analysis (BEA). 2011. *Gross Domestic Product (GDP) by Industry Data, Updated December 13: 2011* [Online]. http://www.bea.gov/industry/gdpbyind_data.htm. Available: http://www.bea.gov/industry/gdpbyind_data.htm [Accessed January 7: 2014].

United Nations 2013. World Population Ageing 2013. New York: United Nations.

Uzun O. 2003. Perceptions and experiences of nurses in Turkey about verbal abuse in clinical settings. *Journal of Nursing Scholarship* 35: 81–85.

Varpilah ST, Safer M, Frenkel E, Baba D, Massaquoi M, Barrow G. 2011. Rebuilding human resources for health: A case study from Liberia. *Human Resources for Health* 9: 11.

Vecchio N, Scuffham PA, Hilton MF, Whiteford HA. 2013. Differences in wage rates for males and females in the health sector: A consideration of unpaid overtime to decompose the gender wage gap. *Human Resources for Health* 11: 9.

Vishwanath T, Nguyen N, Do, Q-T, Walker T, Comboni GI, Krishnan N. 2011. Capabilities, opportunities and participation: Gender equality and development in the Middle East and North Africa Region. Washington DC: World Bank.

Vujicic M. 2014. Health Labor Markets in Developing Countries. In Culyer AJ. (ed.). *Encyclopedia of Health Economics, Vol. 1*. San Diego, CA: Elsevier.

Vujicic M, Weber SE, Nikolic IA, Atun R, Kumar R. 2012. An analysis of GAVI, the Global Fund and World Bank support for human resources for health in developing countries. *Health Policy and Planning* 27: 649–657.

Vujicic M, Zurn P. 2006. The dynamics of the health labour market. *International Journal of Health and Planned Management* 21: 101–115.

Wainer J, Carson D, Strasser RP. 2000. Women and rural medical practice. *South African Family Practice* 22: 14–17.

Wakaba M, Mbindyo P, Ochieng J, Kiriinya R, Todd J, Waudo A, Noor A, Rakuom C, Rogers M, English M. 2014. The public sector nursing workforce in Kenya: A county-level analysis. *Human Resources for Health* 12: 6.

Wang Y, Wei S, Li Y, Deng S, Luo Q, Li Y. 2013. Challenges and a response strategy for the development of nursing in China: A descriptive and quantitative analysis. *Journal of Evidence-Based Medicine* 6: 21–33.

WHO. 2006. Working together for health. Geneva: World Health Organization.

WHO. 2008. Task shifting: Rational redistribution of tasks among health workforce teams: Global recommendations and guidelines: World Health Organization.

WHO. 2010a. *Increasing Access to Health Workers in Remote and Rural Areas Through Improved Retention: Global Policy Recommendations.* Geneva, World Health Organization.

WHO. 2010b. WHO Global Code of Practice on the International Recruitment of Health Personnel. Geneva: World Health Organization. Available at http://www.who.int/hrh/migration/code/WHO_global_code_of_practice_EN.pdf.

WHO. 2011a. User's Guide to the WHO Global Code of Practice on the International Recruitment of Health Personnel. Geneva: World Health Organization. Available at http://apps.who.int/iris/bitstream/10665/70525/1/WHO_HSS_HRH_HMR_2010.2_eng.pdf.

WHO. 2011b. Transformative Scale Up of Health Professional Education. Geneva: World Health Organization.

WHO. 2013. *The 2013 update, Global Health Workforce Statistics*. Geneva: World Health Organization.

Willis-Shattuck M, Bidwell P, Thomas S, Wyness L, Blaauw D, Ditlopo P. 2008. Motivation and retention of health workers in developing countries: A systematic review. *BMC Health Services Research* 8: 247.

Witter S, Fretheim A, Kessy FL, Lindahl AK. 2012. Paying for performance to improve the delivery of health interventions in low- and middle-income countries. *Cochrane Database of Systematic Reviews* 15(2): CD007899. Available at http://onlinelibrary.wiley.com/doi/10.1002/14651858.CD007899.pub2/epdf/standard

World Health Organization. Addressing Africa's Health Workforce Crisis: An Avenue for Action. High Level Forum on the Health MDGs, 2004 Abuja. World Health Organization.

World Health Organization. 2014. *Health Workforce* [Online]. Available: http://www.who.int/healthsystems/topics/workforce/en/ [Accessed 30 April 2014].

Xu H, Zhang W, Zhang X, Qu Z, Wang X, Sa Z, Li Y, Zhao S, Qi X, Tian D. 2013. Longitudinal study of rural health workforce in five counties in China: Research design and baseline description. *Human Resources for Health* 11: 17.

Yagi N, Mackey TK, Liang BA, Gerlt L. 2014. Policy review: Japan–Philippines Economic Partnership Agreement (JPEPA) — Analysis of a failed nurse migration policy. *International Journal of Nursing Studies* 51: 243–250.

Yamamoto TS, Sunguya BF, Shiao LW, Amiya RM, Saw YM, Jimba M. 2012. Migration of health workers in the Pacific Islands: A bottleneck to health development. *Asia Pacific Journal of Public Health* 24: 697–709.

Zurn P, Dal Poz MR. 2004. Imbalance in the health workforce. *Human Resources for Health* 2: 13.

Impact and Costs of Pharmaceuticals and Biotechnology

Panos Kanavos
London School of Economics

Prescription pharmaceutical spending accounts for a significant proportion of total health spending, ranging from over a third to just under a sixth in OECD and emerging countries and is the second largest component of health budgets after salaries of health care professionals. Given the peculiarities of pharmaceutical markets (multiple stakeholders, oligopolistic structure, imperfect information and agency) and the multiple — sometimes conflicting — objectives of pharmaceutical policy (macroeconomic efficiency, microeconomic efficiency, quality of care, access, and promotion of industrial policy including R&D investment), governments and health insurers intervene in pharmaceutical markets. Such intervention takes place both on the supply- and demand-side and focuses on a number of key variables, such as the prices of prescription pharmaceuticals, the barriers to entry in individual markets, the behavior of or the choices made by health care professionals (doctors and pharmacists) and the choices patients make. The policy mix in order to satisfy the above policy objectives varies quite dramatically across countries and so does the effectiveness of individual policy measures and the rigor with which they are pursued. This chapter outlines the importance of pharmaceuticals as a health care input, discusses the supply- and demand-side strategies in order to influence prices, volume and expenditure, the various modalities with which they are implemented in different settings, and presents evidence on the impact of such intervention by drawing on the international literature.

Keywords: Pharmaceutical; Regulation; Competition; Innovation; HTA; Access; Efficiency.

Background

Prescription pharmaceuticals are a critical input in health care delivery. Irrespective of the type of health care system financing mechanism in place, the regulation of and intervention in the pharmaceutical market reflects its complex structure, the multiplicity of stakeholders involved, their — often conflicting — interests, the agency behavior and rent-seeking relationships that may develop across the stakeholder community. Additionally, patients today are more informed about their own health and in some cases have been given financial incentives to increase awareness of their pharmaceutical consumption; in a number of settings, patients are also involved in the decision-making process. The media as information providers on health and health care play an increasingly important role in shaping patients' expectations.

Most governments and health insurers face rising pharmaceutical expenditures, often exceeding by far the rate of GDP growth and rising faster that other health care budgets. Additionally, the introduction of an increased number of costly innovative pharmaceutical and biotechnology therapies in recent years offering significant additional clinical benefits in a number of conditions (e.g., immune-oncology) is putting further pressure on budgets and forces governments and health insurers to rethink the policy mix required to maintain an equilibrium between revenue and expenditure.

The role and objectives of governments and insurance funds in regulating markets and deciding on which drugs to cover and how, are complex and diverse. Internationalization and global trends have a growing influence on the provision of pharmaceuticals as well. Facing ever rising health and pharmaceutical care costs, governments and health insurers have a number of objectives, which guide their intervention in pharmaceutical markets: A key objective is macroeconomic efficiency, notably to keep within a global budget and contain its rate of growth. A second objective is technical efficiency by making decisions based on clinical and cost effectiveness principles and obtaining value for money. A third objective is to ensure that prescription pharmaceuticals are both affordable and available and that patient equity is not compromised. Finally, a further objective is quality and appropriateness of care, ensuring that medicines prescribed help achieve the best possible health care outcomes in an equitable manner and improve both the quantity and quality of life for patients, their families and society at large.

The objective of this chapter is 3-fold: first, to discuss the peculiarities of pharmaceutical markets and outline the rationale for intervention by governments and health insurers; second, to analyze approaches used in different settings or by different insurers to manage pharmaceutical spending through supply- and demand-side intervention. And, third, to discuss whether these approaches have had an impact on the pharmaceutical policy objectives outlined above. In meeting these objectives, evidence and examples are used predominantly from OECD countries and where the evidence base allows, from emerging and developing countries.

The chapter is organized as follows: In Section "Pharmaceuticals in the Context of Health Care," we outline the main features of pharmaceutical markets and discuss the rationale for intervention by national governments and/or health insurers. In Section "Intervention in Pharmaceutical Markets," we discuss the supply- and demand-side intervention tools that are available and have been implemented in different settings as well as their different modalities, by drawing on evidence from OECD as well as a number of emerging countries. In Section "Impact of Regulatory Intervention in Pharmaceutical Markets," we discuss the impact these intervention policies have had on key pharmaceutical policy objectives, notably, macroeconomic efficiency, access, microeconomic efficiency improvement and quality of care. Finally, Section "Conclusion" draws the main conclusions.

Pharmaceuticals in the Context of Health Care

In this section, we discuss different aspects of the importance of pharmaceuticals in the context of health care. In particular, we discuss, first, the link between health care and pharmaceutical financing and expenditure by drawing on trends in health and pharmaceutical spending; second, the importance of pharmaceutical R&D and innovation in terms of improving health outcomes; third, market structure of pharmaceutical markets and the type of competition that is likely to emerge; and, fourth, different aspects of regulation, particularly in connection with intellectual property and marketing authorization. We conclude by summarizing some of the peculiarities found in pharmaceutical markets and outline the rationale for intervention by health insurers or governments in different settings.

Health care and pharmaceutical expenditure trends

Both tax and insurance-based (whether public or private) systems face issues of sustainability and an imminent and ever-increasing need to contain growing health care costs, including those associated with pharmaceutical coverage and funding, and to spend scarce resources efficiently. Challenges to sustainability include population ageing, lifestyle choices and their impact (diet, alcohol consumption, exercise), technical innovation, inappropriate variation in clinical practice, resource constraints and increasing public expectations. Both types of systems require procedures for prioritization and efficient use of scarce resources. Despite obvious differences in the organization and delivery of health care, pharmaceutical funding and coverage issues are largely common across developed and emerging countries and, broadly speaking, relate to meeting financial constraints, achieving efficiency in resource allocation and obtaining value for money given the investments made, improving evidence-based policy-making, optimizing (pharmaceutical) regulation, and ensuring that the best possible outcomes are achieved for patients.

Total expenditure on health has risen considerably over the past 20 years across most developed countries, both in absolute terms and as a share of GDP (OECD, 2013), particularly during the 1990s and early 2000s. In many cases, health expenditures are increasing at a faster rate than GDP, and, despite the recent economic downturn, it is likely that this growth will continue due to the ageing population, more expensive technologies and changing expectations for health care services. The relationship between health spending and GDP remains positive. Countries such as Belgium, Austria, the Netherlands, France, Germany, Switzerland, Sweden, the USA, and Canada spend, on average, more on health given their GDP per capita. In contrast, countries such as Luxembourg, Spain, Slovenia, Czech Republic, Hungary, Slovak Republic and Poland spend less on health given their GDP per capita (Figure 1).

In a similar pattern to total health expenditures, total pharmaceutical expenditures have increased in absolute per capita figures and as a proportion of total health expenditure (OECD, 2013). Prescription pharmaceuticals are a significant contributor to total health care spending and can range from less than 10% (e.g., Denmark) to over 30% (Slovakia) (Figure 2). There exists a significant variation in total capita pharmaceutical spending, ranging from as low as \$100 in US PPPs (Egypt) to \$1,000 (USA) (Figure 3). Similar variation exists in total pharmaceutical spending as a percent of GDP, from 0.6% in Algeria to 3.1% of GDP in Greece

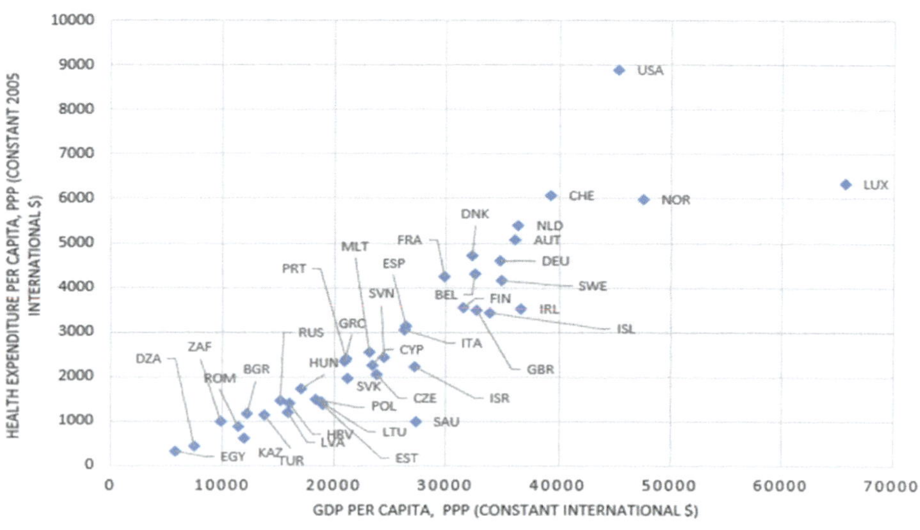

Figure 1. Total health care spending per capita vs. GDP per capita, \$PPP

Source: World Bank Data.

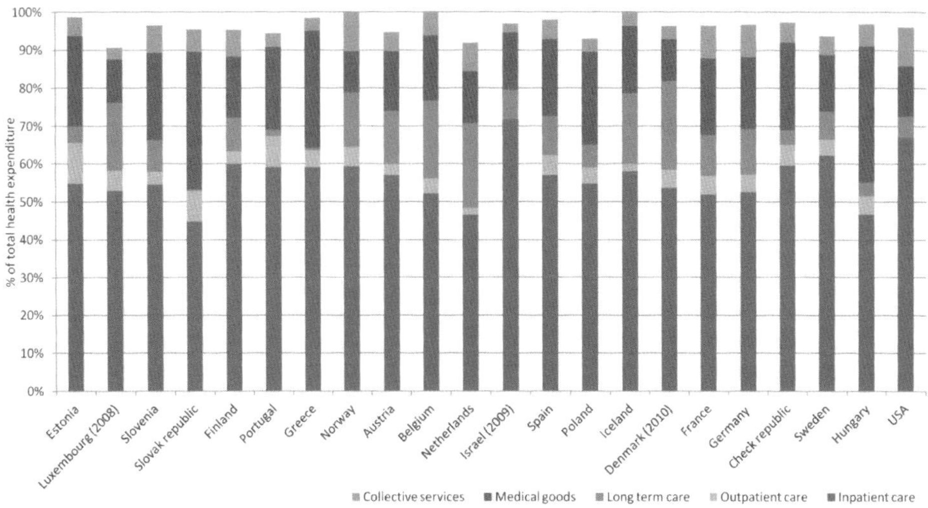

Figure 2. Total health expenditure by function of health care

Source: OECD Health Data: Health expenditure and financing, 2013 and 2014; WHO (2011).

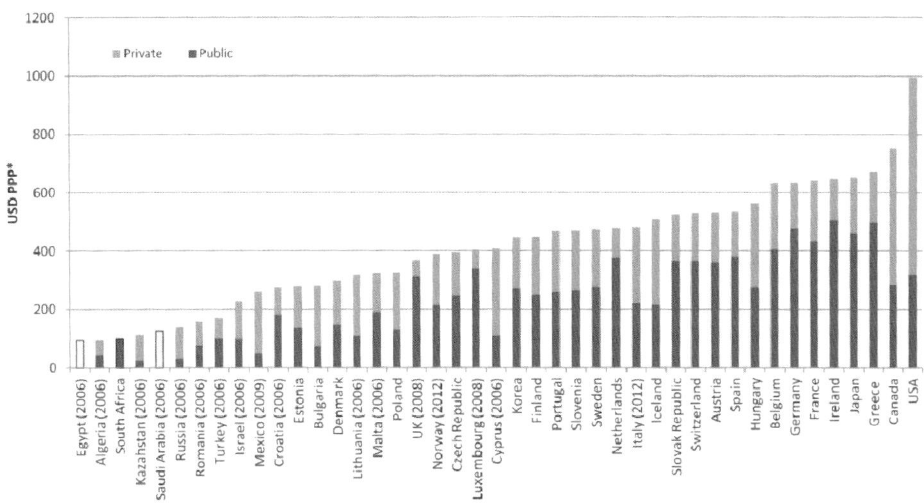

Figure 3. Total pharmaceutical expenditure — per capita (US$ PPP), 2011

Source: 2006 data from WHO World Medicines Situation Report 2011; all others from OECD Health Data 2013 and 2014.

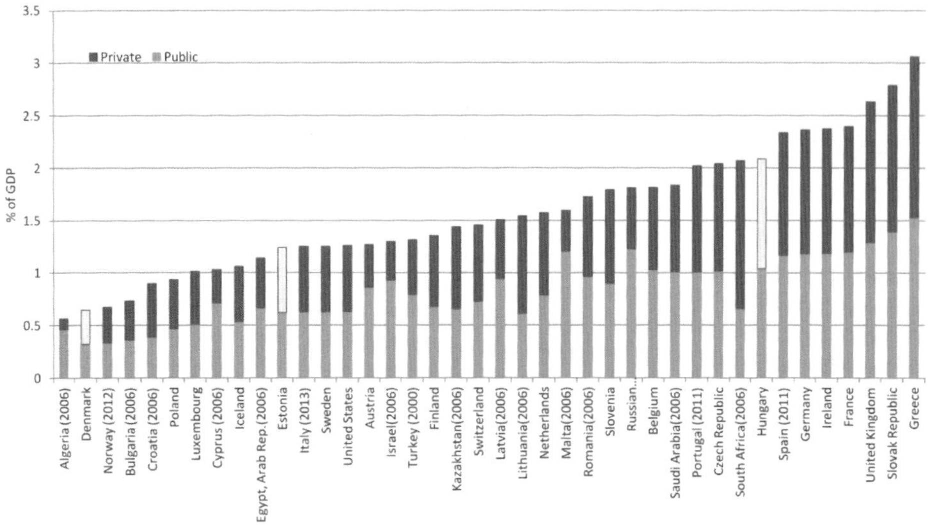

Figure 4. Total pharmaceutical expenditure (Public and Private) — % of GDP

Source: 2006 data from WHO World Medicines Situation Report 2011. All others from OECD Health Data 2013 and 2014.

(Figure 4). There seems to be a similarly positive relationship between pharmaceutical expenditure per capita and GDP per capita (OECD, 2013). Countries like the USA, Canada, Ireland, France, Belgium, Germany, Spain, Austria, and Italy spend proportionally more on pharmaceuticals in per capita terms as share of GDP (i.e., above the regression line), while countries such as Sweden, Finland, Slovenia, Hungary, UK, Czech Republic and Luxembourg spend proportionally less (i.e., below the regression line).

Pharmaceutical expenditures are the third largest component of health expenditures, following hospital and ambulatory care spending (European Commission 2009) and in some cases they are the second largest component of health expenditures. In addition, pharmaceutical expenditures are one of the most identifiable and controllable components of health expenditure. Governments therefore implement a variety of regulatory measures targeting pharmaceutical expenditures for the purpose of controlling overall health care costs.

The importance of pharmaceutical R&D and innovation

The pharmaceutical sector is of great importance for the EU, the USA, and Japan and their manufacturing and knowledge-based economy. In Europe, it directly employs approximately 633,100 people, of which 113,400 work in research and development (R&D). Germany, the UK and France are the largest employers. The United States, by comparison, employ a total of 686,422 directly, with 90,712 people in R&D, including support staff[1], while Japan employs a total of 118,907 people, a figure that has been declining over the past to decades. These figures, however, do not include the thousands of researchers in universities, hospitals and other clinical settings who work closely with the pharmaceutical industry (EFPIA, 2014).

Europe, the United States, and Japan are the world's largest manufacturers and consumers of prescription pharmaceuticals. In Europe, production takes place in several Member States, but the bulk of manufacturing activities is accounted for by only a few (Ireland, UK, France, Germany, Italy, and Spain). Differences can be explained by the size of European countries' domestic markets (Germany, Spain, France, Italy, and UK), but also variable incentive structures to attract manufacturing activities (e.g., low corporate income tax in Ireland).

Pharmaceutical R&D is a critical component of the pharmaceutical sector. Indeed, pharmaceuticals and biotechnology are R&D intensive and indeed the most R&D intensive industry among industrial sectors in terms of the proportion expended on R&D as a percent of net sales (Figure 5).

Aggregate expenditure on pharmaceutical R&D has grown considerably over the past 2 decades. Europe (including Norway and Switzerland) spends slightly

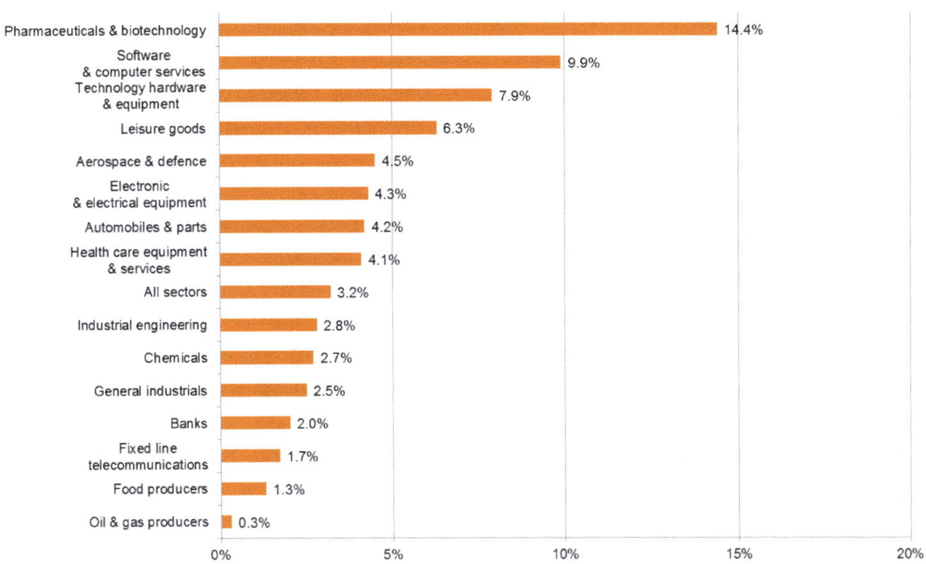

Figure 5. Ranking of industrial sectors by overall sector R&D intensity (R&D as percentage of net sales — 2012)

Source: The 2013 EU Industrial R&D Investment Scoreboard, European Commission, JRC/DG Research and Innovation.

[1]US figures from PhRMA (2010) and there may be slight methodological differences in assessing numbers of those directly and indirectly involved in the industry. European data are from EFPIA (2014).

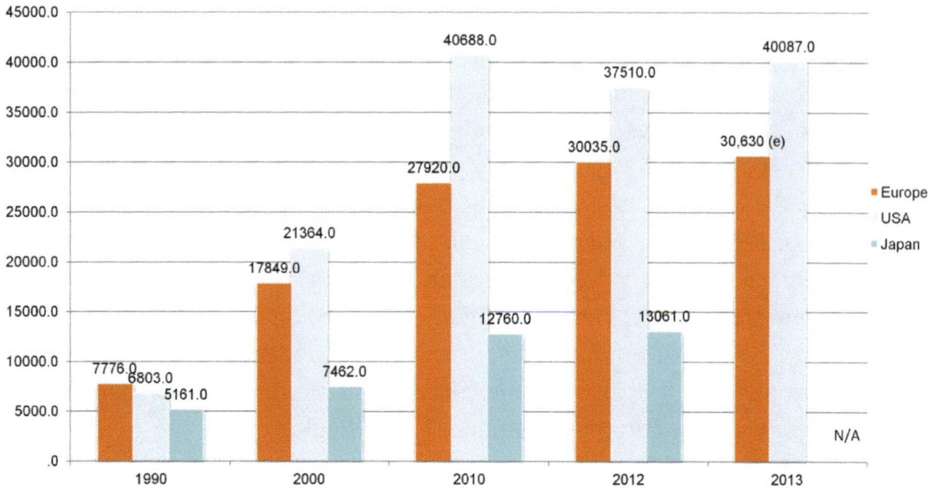

Figure 6. Pharmaceutical R&D expenditure in Europe, USA and Japan (Million of National Currency Units), 1990–2013

Note: e — estimate for 2013.
Source: EFPIA (2014).

less on pharmaceutical R&D (US$30.6 billion in 2013) than the United States (US$40 billion in 2013); both spend significantly more than Japan (US$16,457 million in 2012) (Figure 6). However, in per capita terms, the European figure, which includes Switzerland, is significantly lower than that of the USA or Japan (US$125 in the USA compared with US$145 in Japan and US$63 in Europe). In Europe, R&D activities — particularly basic and discovery research — concentrate in few countries (UK, Germany, France, Italy, Spain, Denmark, Sweden, and Switzerland) that have the infrastructure, scientific critical mass, provide, additional funding mechanisms and a range of direct and indirect financial and non-financial incentives for the location of these activities. Available finance to commercialize intellectual property is also crucial, particularly in the early stages of developmental research. All these factors are necessary requirements to ensure an enabling business environment that stimulates innovation.

There is no apparent direct link between location of R&D activities and prices of pharmaceuticals, perhaps with the exception of the UK, where the local regulatory scheme — the pharmaceutical price regulation scheme (PPRS) — indirectly linking financial incentives for R&D with rate of return on capital employed and, thus, indirectly, with the price of medicines. The rapid growth in the market and research environments in countries such as Brazil and China are contributing to the move of economic and research activities to non-European markets. The geographical balance of the pharmaceutical market — and ultimately the R&D base — is likely to shift gradually towards emerging economies. A key indicator of R&D output is the number of new chemical entities (NCEs) emerging on an annual basis. After a gradual decline during the first decade of the 21st century, the number of NCEs seems to be recovering, with Europe and the USA still being registered as the source of discovery of most NCEs, but in recent years, there have been significant discoveries outside Europe, the USA, and Japan, perhaps pointing to the shifting emphasis in R&D location and the rise of emerging countries as sources of pharmaceutical discovery (Figure 7).

The usefulness of (new) medicines and their value in terms of improved health gain has been studied on numerous occasions at macroeconomic level. Specific classes of drugs have proven to deliver extraordinary value. Evidence on statins, for example, suggests that (a) early initiation of treatment with statins following an acute heart attack reduces the risk of fatal heart disease or a recurrent heart attack by 24%[2]; (b) every dollar spent on statin therapy in heart attack survivors (vs. survivors treated with usual care) has produced health gains valued as high as $9.44; (c) when cholesterol is lowered with statin therapy, the risk of coronary events is reduced by 25% in type 2 diabetes patients[2]; and (d) every additional dollar spent on statin therapy in type 2 diabetics who also suffer from high cholesterol has produced health gains valued at $3. In the case of beta blockers,

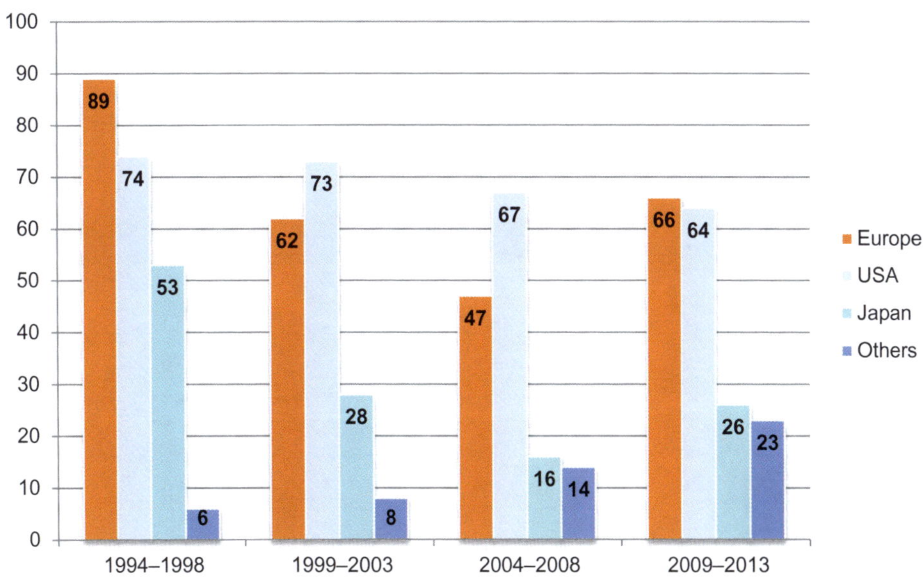

Figure 7. Number of new chemical or biological entities (1994–2013)
Source: EFPIA (2014).

[2]MEDTAP International. 2004. The Value of Investment in Health Care. http://www.medtap.com/Products/HP_FullReport.pdf.

treatment of heart attack patients with beta blockers show a 35:1 return.[2] Additionally, there are even equally impressive examples of ROIs from healthcare innovation: Treatment for heart attacks shows a $7 return on each $1 of investment in new therapies (e.g., thrombolytic drugs, stents, long-term drug therapy) from 1984 to 1998 (Cutler and McClellan, 2001); and improved treatments for low birth-weight infants shows a $6 return for each $1 of incremental investment in new therapies (e.g., special ventilators, artificial surfactants) from 1950 to 1990. Research has also suggested that anti-hypertensive drugs have prevented in excess of 86,000 premature deaths in the US in 2001 among US population aged 40 and older (Cutler *et al.*, 2007).

Pharmaceutical innovation has also transformed the treatment of grievous illnesses, such as cancer, where we have seen significant value delivered at societal and individual patient level. For example, it has been estimated that for the period from 1975 to 2000 cancer drugs have increased the 1-year crude cancer survival rate from 69.4% to 76.1%, the 5-year rate from 45.5% to 51.3%, and the 10-year rate from 34.2% to 38.1% and, in so doing, have increased the life expectancy of the entire US population by 0.4 years. Finally, it has been shown recently that 73% of the 1.74 years increase in life expectancy between 2000 and 2009 was accounted for by innovative medicines (Lichtenberg, 2012) (Figure 8).

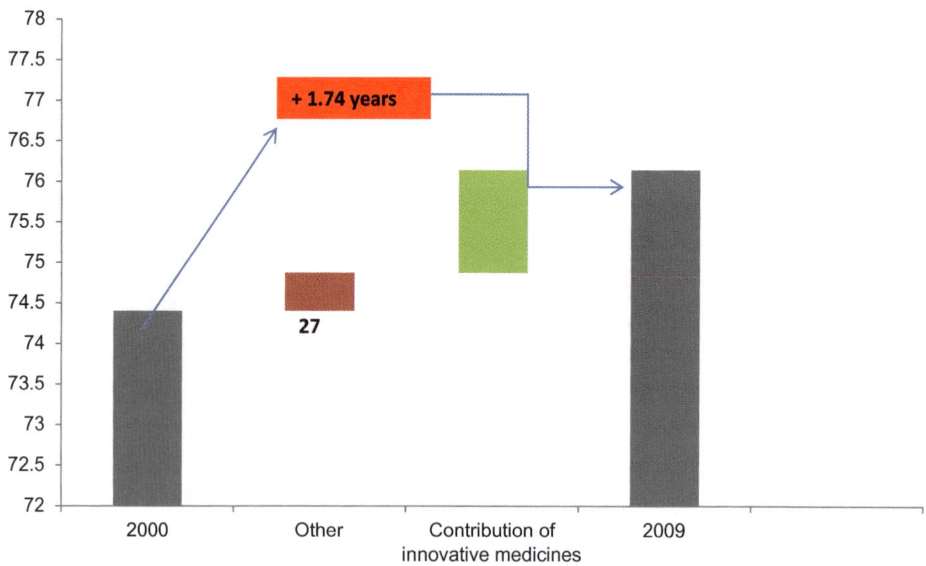

Figure 8. Contribution of innovative medicines to the increase in life expectancy (2000–2009)

Source: Lichtenberg (2012).

Market structure and competition

The structure of pharmaceutical markets is observed to differ depending on the number of firms on the markets, the stage a product is in its lifecycle and whether it is protected by intellectual property, and the ramifications of intellectual property policies. Monopoly, monopolistic competition, oligopoly and (nearly) perfect competition co-exist in different segments of the pharmaceutical market, making it a complex market to analyze from a market structure and competition perspective. Each competition model has consequences in terms of pricing arrangements and social welfare.

The existence of monopoly or monopolistic competition markets can be attributable to intellectual property rights, mainly in the form of patents, data exclusivities and market exclusivity arrangements. Patents reward novel, useful, and non-obvious innovations, and are necessary to promote investment into increasingly expensive drug development. Molecule discoveries are granted a nominal period of market exclusivity for 20 years after filing for a new therapeutic compound in all markets. In some settings, this nominal patent period is further extended by a few years to account for the difference between nominal and effective patent life (OECD, 2013). No other drugs may enter that molecular market for the duration of the patent period. Competitors are still free to develop other compounds for a therapeutic class (e.g., ACE-inhibitors, statins, antacids) under the condition that they do not encroach on the originators patents on the molecule, process, or product. Therefore, it might occur that several differentiated in-patent drugs are available on the market within a therapeutic class, each having market exclusivity at the molecular level due to the monopoly status afforded by patents, but encountering competition from the other monopolists at the therapeutic level. In addition, copyrights are relevant to the issue of monopolistic competition as they can lead to brand awareness and brand loyalty by granting exclusivity to the commercial name of a product (i.e., horizontal differentiation).

Patent protection is tantamount to the award of a monopoly for the period of patent protection. In markets characterized by a single therapeutic alternative, the first entrant in a new therapeutic class has significant first mover advantages in terms of price setting. Follow-on products in the same therapeutic class that are not perfect substitutes but compete on differentiated attributes, are likely to enter

[3] This is the Patent Extension Term in the USA and emerged from the Waxman–Hatch Act of 1984. The same concept is called Supplementary Protection Certificate in the European Union. The difference between nominal and effective patent life arises because of the extensive laboratory and clinical testing required for all molecules in order to arrive at a product that meets certain minimum criteria prior to receiving regulatory approval and becoming commercially available (safety, efficacy and quality).

on price parity with the first in class and compete on market share, unless they can demonstrate superior clinical/therapeutic advantages to the first in class. For first comer therapeutics in a particular therapeutic class, the absence of any direct substitutes enables a firm to underserve a market by engaging in monopoly pricing, by setting marginal revenue equal to marginal cost [MR = MC]. This is observed in in-patent branded drugs and even though other therapeutic alternatives may enter the market offering identical or very similar benefits subject to some differences in quality (e.g., differences in tolerability or side-effect profiles), each patent-protected molecule still maintains unique features because of its therapeutic profile and the brand loyalty associated with it. The only circumstance for direct competition to occur at patent-protected molecule level is through the availability of the same product (and brand) from a parallel channel. This is the case of parallel trade, where distributors, taking advantage of price differences between markets, perform arbitrage and export from low-price markets into high-price markets. In this case, an in-patent originator competes with itself; the distribution channels from factory gate to the retail outlet are slightly different, but the product is always dispensed at the pharmacy. The only reason why a parallel imported medicine can be perceived to be different than the locally-sourced alternative is due to different packaging (Kanavos and Wouters, 2014). The condition allowing parallel trade to take place is exhaustion of intellectual property rights; this can be national, regional or international. Regional exhaustion applies in the case of the European Union in direct compliance with the principle of the free movement of goods.

Monopoly also characterizes markets for orphan indications, where the first product on the market in an approved orphan indication benefits not only from the intellectual property on the molecule, but also on a market exclusivity on the indication which varies between 7 and 10 years depending on the setting. The latter constitutes the only case of institutionalized monopoly in pharmaceutical markets.

Monopolistic competition does not characterize the pharmaceutical market as a whole, but is a form of competition found predominantly at the level of therapeutic class so long as there is notable product differentiation between the different therapeutic options in a given product class. Monopolistic competition is fostered by product differentiation at therapeutic class level and is distinguished by the contrasting organization of the market over time. Non-price related heterogeneity of the products can either be due to *horizontal* product differentiation, where there is some subjective differentiation amongst the products considered by the patients or their agents, such as brand loyalty, or due to *vertical* product differentiation, where an objective optimal mix of characteristics is desired for the drug in question, such as a differentiated side-effect profile which distinguishes it from its competitors, thus creating a natural ordering in the eyes of patients and prescribers. Firms benefiting from product differentiation can be said to have some degree of market power, albeit low, and are thus, strictly speaking, price setters. This indirect privilege accrues mostly to those firms whose products are characterized by vertical product differentiation, although there are settings where horizontal product differentiation attributes provide the basis for differentiation.

In the short run, like monopolistic markets, the firm will independently price a product where marginal revenue equals marginal cost [MR = MC], which is tantamount to the firm's profit maximizing conditions; positive profits will be generated with average revenue being greater than average cost [D = AR > AC]. In the long run, however, entry at the site of positive rents is stimulated, effectively depressing the demand curve (D) to a point of tangency with the long-run average costs (LRAC), and reducing monopoly profits to zero. To assess the degree of market dominance of a firm in a therapeutic class, seller concentration ratios could be employed to present an overall measure of market share, or alternatively, the Herfindahl–Hirschman Index could be constructed using the sum of squared market shares, giving more weight to firms which hold a dominant position in the market. Monopolistic competition can inefficient in two ways: First as P > MC, even in the long run, producing a deadweight loss of producer and consumer surplus, and second from excess capacity, as the output is lesser than that dictated by the lowest point on the LRAC curve.

Perfect competition is seen with more homogeneous products. Product homogeneity is achieved in off-patent markets, where a high number of alternatives, that are bioequivalent to the originator, enter the market. In this context, firms are price takers, no excess monopoly rents are generated, and output approaches the competitive level. In this type of market, patent rights have elapsed and barriers to entry and exit are small. In the case of perfect competition, the firm faces a perfectly elastic demand curve and cannot raise prices at will.

Overall, monopoly and monopolistic competition in the pharmaceutical markets primarily exist in the context of in-patent drugs at the therapeutic class level; in the case of monopolistic competition, product differentiation exists allowing competition to occur with quantities instead of prices. Patents are essential to fostering this type of competition model by providing market exclusivity for a firm to commercially leverage its molecular patents uninterrupted by generics. Firms in these markets are price setters and exercise low degrees of market power, thereby earning monopoly rents in the short run, but, like perfect competition, no economic profits are earned in the long run due to ease of entry form other firms competing at the therapeutic class. Although inefficient, they allow firms to earn returns on their innovations and help ensure funding for investment in future therapies. This discussion does not take into account the existence of intervention — on behalf of insurers — in pharmaceutical markets in order to mitigate the monopoly power of patent protection and market exclusivity. This will be discussed in Section "Intervention in Pharmaceutical Markets" of this chapter.

Regulation in pharmaceutical markets

Regulatory approval (marketing authorization) of new pharmaceutical products is no longer confined to proof of safety, efficacy, and quality only. In recent years, there have been significant developments in the regulatory framework, particularly in the European Union, the USA, Canada, and Australia. Specifically, four developments are worth noting because of their far-reaching implications for the approval of new medicines or the link between the regulatory process and the assessment of value that takes place prior to reaching a decision on coverage. These are, first, the regulatory pathways for orphan designation and the approval of orphan drugs; second, the creation of a pathway for biosimilar products; third, the pathways for accelerated development; and, fourth, the initiation of 'adaptive pathways' in the European context. We examine these and their implications briefly in turn.

- *Orphan drugs*

The Orphan Drug Act (ODA) was passed in the United States in 1983 (ODA, 1983) and was designed to facilitate the development and commercialization of drugs to treat rare diseases, known as orphan drugs. Orphan drug designation does not indicate that the product in question is either safe and effective or legal to manufacture and market in the United States. Instead, the designation means only that the sponsor qualifies for certain benefits from the federal government, such as reduced taxes, enhanced patent protection and marketing rights, including a market exclusivity of 7 year, clinical research subsidies and creating a government-run enterprise to engage in R&D. The EU has enacted similar legislation[4] in which pharmaceuticals developed to treat rare diseases are referred to as "orphan medicinal products". The EU's definition of an orphan condition is broader than that of the USA, in that it also covers some tropical diseases primarily found in developing nations. Orphan drug status granted by the European Commission gives marketing exclusivity in the EU for 10 years after approval. Australia, Japan and, more recently, Canada, have enacted comparable legislation. The overall impact has been positive with several hundred molecules obtaining orphan designation in the above jurisdictions.

[4]Regulation EC/141/2000 of the European Parliament and of the Council on Orphan Medicinal Products. *EC/141/2000* 2000.

• *Biosimilars*

Biosimilars (generic versions of biotechnology products) have been widely and safely used in Europe since 2006. In 2004, the European Commission (EC) passed legislation creating a biosimilars approval pathway. In 2005 and 2006, the European Medicines Agency (EMA) released its first set of biosimilar guidelines, and in 2006, approved its first biosimilar[5,6]. To date, there have been 14 biosimilars authorized, with biosimilar monoclonal antibodies expected soon. The regulatory approval framework for biosimilars requires a rigorous monitoring, tracking, and tracing system, but to date no safety problems with biosimilars have been identified. The EMA requires a stepwise head-to-head comparison between the biosimilar and the reference product to demonstrate similar levels of quality, safety and efficacy. Depending on the similarity of the quality profile, non-clinical and clinical testing may be reduced for biosimilars compared to a new biologic. Any differences in levels of quality between the biosimilar and its reference require the sponsor to satisfactorily explain potential implications of the quality difference on product safety and efficacy. FDA's biosimilar guidance of February 2012 uses a similar approach. The EMA allows biosimilar extrapolation to other indications once the biosimilar has been established as sufficiently comparable to its reference. Extrapolation means inferring conclusions from data using one or more indications to other indications in which there has not been the same analysis. Other aspects of EMA regulation of biosimilars include: Biosimilars shares the same International Nonproprietary Name (INN) as its reference; each biosimilar has a unique brand name or the name of the active substance with the company name; and automatic substitution of brand drug for its Biosimilar is regulated by each member state in the EU. In the USA, The Biologics Price Competition and Innovation Act (BPCIA) of 2009, which was passed as part of the health care reform legislation (Johnson *et al.*, 2011) enacted into law in 2010, authorizes the FDA to establish a long-awaited regulatory pathway for biosimilars. In 2012, the FDA issued draft guidance summarizing the proposed criteria for this pathway.

• *Accelerated development*

In 1992, in response to public concerns that treatments for life-threatening diseases such as HIV/AIDS and many forms of serious cancers were not available soon enough, the FDA enacted programs directed at expediting the development of new medicines through the use of several mechanisms while ensuring requirements for

---

[5] European Parliament and the Council. Directive 2001/83/EC of the European Parliament and of the Council on the community code relating to medicinal products for human use. *2001L0032*2001.

[6] European Parliament and the Council. Directive 2004/27/EC of the European Parliament and of the Council of 31 March 2004 amending Directive 2001/83/EC on the Community code relating to medicinal products for human use. 2004.

demonstrating safety and efficacy were met. These mechanisms include early engagement with the regulator to inform efficient development plans, accelerated review times for marketing applications, and use of flexible trial designs including relying on Phase II trials and surrogate endpoints as evidence to support clinical benefit. Similarly, in 2006, the EMA established the 'conditional marketing authorization' pathway to provide a mechanism for the EMA to authorise medicines based on results from interim clinical evidence only if the treatment is targeted at life-threatening diseases, orphan-designated products, or for use in emergency situations in response to a public health threat.[7] Additionally, an exceptional circumstances program was established by the EMA in 2004 for medicines where it was not possible to collect comprehensive safety or efficacy data because the indications were very rare, and the current clinical understanding was that the collection of evidence was not possible or in conflict with principles of medical ethics.[8] The key features of the approaches around accelerated development by the EMA and the FDA are outlined in Table 1.

A key feature of the pre-approval programs of the FDA and EMA is the use of surrogate endpoints that have a reasonably clear link to clinical benefit. In 2012, the accelerated approval program was amended to allow the FDA to take a broader view on the use of surrogate endpoints; it would allow the use of intermediate clinical endpoints which are endpoints that target an attribute that measures the clinical benefit through other means such as patient-reported outcomes and the evidentiary basis to conclude that the effect is reasonably likely to predict an effect on irreversible morbidity and mortality (FDA, 2013).

While there does not seem to be EMA guidance on the use of surrogate endpoints in the EMA's expedited programs, the EMA has established knowledge sharing partnerships with the FDA since 2003 (Pignatti *et al.*, 2011). For the accelerated approval and conditional marketing authorisation programs, manufacturers are required to complete post-approval confirmatory trials to verify the clinical benefit on a primary or secondary endpoint, ideally in a randomized-controlled setting, or continue to measure the previously studied surrogate or intermediate clinical endpoint for a longer duration (i.e., more mature data set). The initiation of the post approval efficacy studies (PAES) regulation in Europe in late 2014[9]

[7]European Medicines Agency (EMA). Final guidance on conditional marketing authorization (Regulation (EC) No. 726/2004) 2006.

[8]European Commission. Guideline on Procedures for Granting a Marketing Authorization under Exceptional Circumstances pursuant to Regulation No. 726/20042004.

[9]European Commission. Commission Delegated Regulation (EU) No 357/2014 supplementing Directive 2001/83/EC of the European Parliament and of the Council and Regulation (EC) No. 726/2004 of the European Parliament and of the Council as regards situations in which post-authorization efficacy studies may be required. 2014.

Table 1. Expedited programs that influence the evidence generated for medicines that treat serious, life-threatening conditions in Europe and the United States

<table>
<tr><th></th><th>Accelerated approval</th><th>Conditional marketing authorization</th><th>Exceptional circumstances</th></tr>
<tr><td>Agency</td><td>FDA</td><td>EMA</td><td>EMA</td></tr>
<tr><td>Year</td><td>1992, 2012</td><td>2006</td><td>2004</td></tr>
<tr><td>Regulations</td><td>21 CFR, Part 314, Subpart H
21 CFR, Part 314, Subpart E

Section 506 of the FD&C Act, as amended by Section 901 of the FDASIA</td><td>Article 11 of Regulation (EC) No. 507/2006, for products within the scope of Regulation (EC) No. 726/2004</td><td>Article 14(8) of Regulation (EC) No. 726/2004</td></tr>
<tr><td>Purpose</td><td colspan="3">• These programs were developed in response to expectations from patients that promising treatments that target serious, life-threatening or rare conditions where there are no appropriate treatment is currently available are approved prior to a complete marketing application</td></tr>
<tr><td>Eligibility criteria</td><td colspan="3">• Treatment is intended to address a serious condition or life-threatening disease where there are no appropriate treatments
• Reasonable expectation, based on preliminary clinical evidence, that treatment would demonstrate an important improvement over current standard of care (if any)
• Orphan-designated medicines eligible</td></tr>
<tr><td>Additional criteria</td><td>• Justification for choice of surrogate endpoint that can likely predict clinical benefit must be supported by epidemiological, pathophysiological, therapeutic, pharmacologic or biomarkers</td><td>• Can be a medicinal product to be used in emergency situations (i.e., public health threats), as determined by the WHO</td><td>• Current scientific knowledge base and medical ethics would make it unable to collect comprehensive evidence</td></tr>
</table>

(*Continued*)

Table 1. *(Continued)*

	Accelerated approval	Conditional marketing authorization	Exceptional circumstances
Evidence to support approval	• Preliminary clinical evidence will rely on a surrogate endpoint that can likely predict clinical benefit; such as HIV viral load or tumor shrinkage • Evidence can also rely on an intermediate clinical endpoint that is likely to predict clinical benefit and can be measured earlier than irreversible mortality and morbidity; such symptom relief or mobility	• Preliminary clinical evidence demonstrates a positive risk–benefit profile • Treatment fulfills an unmet medical need, i.e., provides an improvement over existing treatments • The benefits to public health of the immediate availability of treatment outweigh risks that additional data is required	• Conditional approval will be granted based on preliminary clinical evidence and if sponsor agrees to specific procedures such as completion of a set of studies to evaluate the safety of the medicine to inform the risk–benefit profile
Obligations under approval	• Conduct ongoing or new post-approval trials to verify clinical benefit that either directly measures the clinical benefit, or measures the surrogate and/or intermediate clinical endpoint for a longer time period (i.e., mature datasets) and can include additional primary and secondary endpoints • Aim is to generate more comprehensive clinical data • Promotional materials used in package leaflets need to be reviewed by the regulatory agency		
Additional obligations	• Submit promotional materials related to product for approval • Approval can be withdrawn if manufacturer disseminates misleading promotional materials	• Specific obligations can include collection of pharmacovigilance data and periodic safety updates • Details on the granting of a conditional approval, details of the proposed studies to be completed and timeframe will be publicly available as part of the EPAR	• Specific procedures relate to the safety of the medicinal product, and to notify the authorities on any incident relating to the use of the product and actions to be taken; this procedures include an EU risk management plan

(Continued)

Table 1. (*Continued*)

	Accelerated approval	**Conditional marketing authorization**	**Exceptional circumstances**
Conditions for withdrawal	• Approval can be withdrawn if post-approval trials are not completed with due diligence or if they fail to confirm clinical benefit		
		• Conditional marketing authorization is valid for 1 year, and can be renewed annually based on the status of specific obligations	• License is valid for 5 years (same as normal approval), and will be renewed depending on the status of the specific procedures

Source: Perampaladas and Kanavos (2015).

outlines the framework and shows the shift from safety-only to safety-and-efficacy studies post approval. The nature, design and parameters of the registration and confirmatory trials receive extensive input from regulators early on in the development cycle to ensure uncertainties around the safety and efficacy of the medicine are addressed.

- *Adaptive pathways*

The concept of adaptive pathways foresees either an initial approval in a well-defined patient subgroup with a high medical need and subsequent widening of the indication to a larger patient population, or an early regulatory approval (e.g., conditional approval) which is prospectively planned, and where uncertainty is reduced through the collection of post-approval data on the medicine's use in patients (EMA, 2015). This approach is particularly relevant for medicines with the potential to treat serious conditions with an unmet medical need, and may reduce the time to a medicine's approval or to its reimbursement for targeted patient groups. It involves balancing the importance of timely patient access with the need for adequate, evolving information on a medicine's benefits and risks. The adaptive pathways approach builds on regulatory processes already in place within the existing European Union legal framework.

Developing the adaptive pathways approach involves early discussion between a wide range of stakeholders to explore ways of optimizing development pathways. These include organizations such as EMA and other medicines regulators, the pharmaceutical industry, health–technology–assessment (HTA) bodies, organizations issuing clinical treatment guidelines, patient and consumer organizations, health care professionals, researchers and academics. In March 2014, the EMA began inviting companies to participate in a pilot project on adaptive pathways, and published a framework to guide discussions on individual pilot studies. The main aim of the pilot is to help develop an understanding of how future adaptive pathways might be designed for different types of products and indications. Companies interested in participating in the pilot are asked to submit ongoing medicine-development program for consideration as prospective pilot cases. These should be experimental medicines in the early stage of clinical development (i.e., prior to the initiation of confirmatory studies). At the time of writing this chapter, it is still unclear as to how adaptive pathways will work in practice as there seems to be some resistance from the side of EU Member States, either in terms of an increased burden of compliance if the scheme is generalized or because some Member States believe that the adaptive pathways process is unnecessary due to alternative strategies that allow for the early introduction of medicines on the market. One such case is the Temporary Authorization for Use

(*Autorisation temporaire d'utilization* — ATU) procedure in France (AFSSAPS, 2001). This procedure is an exceptional measure making available medicinal products that have not yet been granted a Marketing Authorization (MA). The aim of ATUs is to provide early access to new promising treatments where a genuine public health need exists, i.e., in the treatment of patients suffering from serious disease and having reached a situation of therapeutic impasse. This regulatory provision has existed in France since 1994.

Peculiarities of pharmaceutical markets and the rationale for intervention

The pharmaceutical market is a complex market and is characterized by a number of peculiarities. First, patients with the same disease may respond differently to a given treatment. Second, in a normal market, the consumer weighs the costs and benefits and makes an informed decision on the best option. In the pharmaceutical market, patients have insufficient information on their health needs and rely on physicians to make the treatment decision on their behalf. Third, the market can be considered as imperfect and may give rise to moral hazard, considering that in health care systems, a third party payer will cover the cost of prescription medicines wholly or partly. Fourth, pharmaceutical markets are typically characterized by multiple stakeholders, who often have conflicting interests and some of them may display rent-seeking behavior. Fifth, the cost of developing a new product is difficult to assess as it results from years of multidisciplinary research involving multiple projects.

As any market, the pharmaceutical sector is characterized by a *supply-side*, composed of the producers of pharmaceutical products, and a *demand-side*, comprising patients, prescribers (i.e., physicians) and dispensers (i.e., pharmacists) of pharmaceuticals. On the supply-side, patents protect pharmaceutical inventions for a nominal period of 20 years plus a further 5 years maximum a patent extension term, also known as Supplementary Protection Certificate (SPC) in the European context. A period of market exclusivity of up to 11 years — depending on the geography — also applies. During this period, protected inventions benefit from market exclusivity and monopoly or quasi-monopoly power.

On account of the peculiarities in pharmaceutical markets, governments, and health insurers have introduced a number of intervention policies aiming at satisfying a number of policy objectives, notably containing pharmaceutical costs by targeting price, volume, or both, improving efficiency by recommending therapies which provide value for money and ensuring that insured citizens have access to the medicines they need. Action on the supply-side focuses primarily on regulating pharmaceutical prices, both of in-patent and off-patent (generic) products. Specific

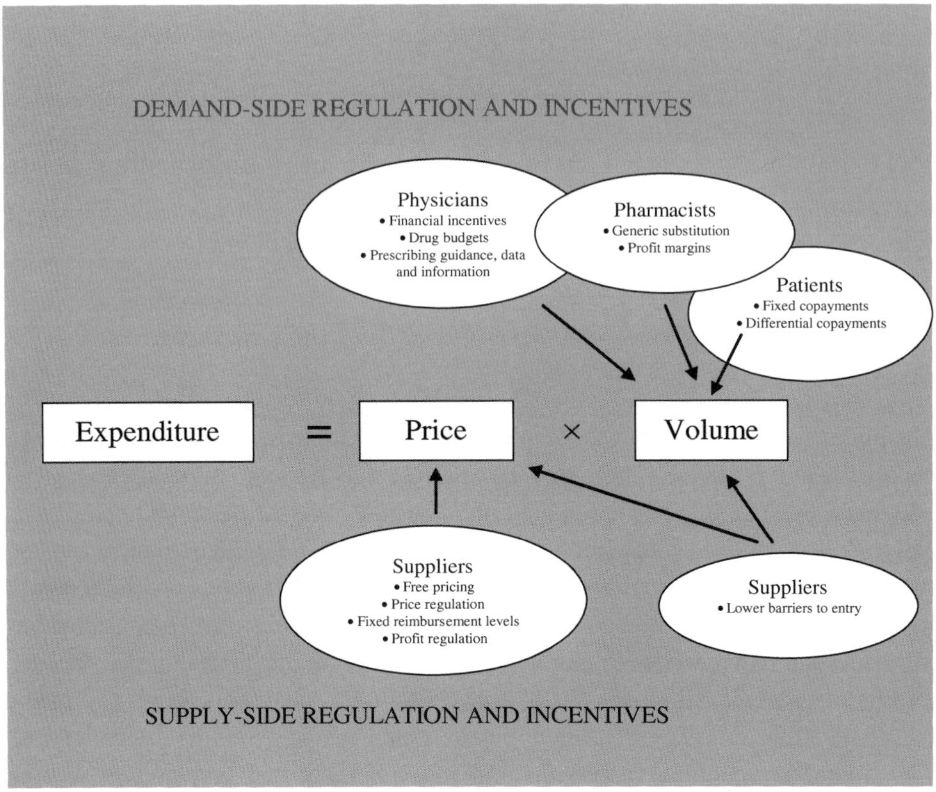

Figure 9. Supply- and demand-side regulatory mechanisms in pharmaceuticals
Source: Mrazek (2001) quoted in Mossialos *et al.* (eds.) (2004).

measures in this context include controls of pharmaceutical prices through different regulatory schemes (i.e., price regulation, fixed reimbursement levels, profit or rate-of-return regulation, among others), and encouragement of price competition by lowering the barriers to entry in pharmaceutical markets. Supply-side action on volume relates to making entry into pharmaceutical markets easier, for instance, by enabling faster entry of generics onto the market place. Action on the demand-side primarily targets volume by implementing policies on physician prescribing (e.g., through financial and non-financial incentives), pharmacy dispensing (e.g., regulation of margins, policies on generic substitution) and patient behavior (e.g., cost-sharing arrangements for different types of medicines) (Figure 9).

Intervention in Pharmaceutical Markets

Intervention in pharmaceutical markets is taking place in order to influence the behavior of key stakeholders. On the supply-side, this includes actions to influence the prices of in-patent and off-patent pharmaceutical products and, in so doing, enable coverage decisions that satisfy key policy objectives for insurers, such as meet a financial target or obtain value for money, whilst at the same time satisfying the interests of patients and manufacturers in terms of access and market entry. In in-patent markets, the rationale is to mitigate the monopoly power of originators; in the latter, the rationale is to ensure that there are gains from patent expiry on the prices of medicines offered by health insurance, or that such gains are maximized. On the demand-side, financial and non-financial incentives are most often in place to ensure that the behavior of prescribers satisfies the objectives of macroeconomic efficiency, cost-effectiveness, quality of care and appropriateness. Key policy measures and strategies on both the supply- and the demand-sides are reviewed and discussed in this section and are summarized in Table 2.

Supply-side intervention: Price determination of in-patent pharmaceuticals

- *Price fixing through external price referencing*

External price referencing (EPR) (also known as international reference pricing) is used extensively in Europe, the Middle East and North Africa, Southeast Asia, and Latin America as a means of list price setting and the price arrived at is usually the maximum price for a pharmaceutical product. Within Europe, 25 of the 28 EU Member States (all except the UK, Germany, and Sweden) use EPR. The fundamental principle behind EPR is that prices in other countries are used to determine the price in a particular market. Usually, a basket of reference countries is used, which differs across countries implementing EPR. Baskets of reference countries can be small (e.g., 3 countries in Slovenia, 4 in the Netherlands or 7 countries in Canada), or large (27 countries in the Czech Republic, 30 in Saudi Arabia, or 36 in Egypt). The average, lowest, or an average of the lowest prices in the basket, is defined as the reference price. EPR is a conceptually simple and relatively effective way in determining maximum originator prices in a particular country. However, it is arbitrary insofar as neither value nor cost are necessarily taken into account. EPR also makes pharmaceutical prices very sensitive to exchange rate fluctuations if prices denominated in different currencies are included in a given basket. This problem arises because of frequent repricing, usually, taking place once or twice annually, in order for a particular country to capitalize on price movements in its basket of reference countries. There appears to be a downward bias on prices due to changes in the exchange rate (Kanavos and Vandoros 2010), which could have adverse effects on investment in innovation. Despite its conceptual simplicity, EPR can be administratively complex. Its complexity is highlighted in Table 3, showing the close interdependencies between European

Table 2. Overview of supply- and demand-side intervention in pharmaceutical markets

Intervention mechanism	Examples of countries employing each mechanism	Key issues
Supply-side: Methods to determine prices of in-patent pharmaceuticals		
Price controls: Administrative or statutory pricing	• All EU Member States except Germany, UK and, to a certain extent, Sweden • Russian Federation, Turkey, South Korea, Brazil, Mexico • Middle East and North African countries	Statutory pricing: Pharmaceutical prices are set on a regulatory basis, chiefly involving external price referencing
External reference pricing	Most EU Member States except UK, Germany, Sweden, Canada, Turkey, Brazil, South Korea, Japan, Egypt, Mexico	Price calculation based on the prices for the same product in other countries ("International Reference Pricing")
Rate of return regulation	UK	Regulates profits of manufacturers on their sales to the NHS or a return on capital employed (ROCE) subject to a threshold and a margin of tolerance thereof
Negotiations and price–volume agreements	France, Italy, Austria, Australia	An agreement between public authorities and manufacturers on price based on a forecast of sales volume
Direct expenditure controls: payback	France, Portugal, Austria	Paybacks relate to industry having to return revenue from excess sales resulting from selling higher quantities than originally agreed with health insurance
Cost-plus pricing	• Still exists in legislation in Spain and Greece, but altogether abandoned • Slovakia • Pakistan, India, Iran, China, Bangladesh	Pricing procedure considers the production cost of a pharmaceutical product as well as other costs such as promotional expenses and a profit margin for fixation of the price (shares are usually expressed as percentage of the cost)

Tendering for off-patent pharmaceuticals in primary care	The Netherlands, Germany, Sweden, Denmark, South Africa	Mechanism whereby a purchaser buys medicines from the pharmaceutical manufacturer that offers the best price. Often, the tender is awarded to a single company with the lowest price, occasionally to two with the two lowest prices. The average duration of a tender cycle is 6–12 months; in Sweden, there is online bidding with prices being updated every 2 weeks
Price capping for generics and linking these to the originator price	Italy, Greece, France	Prices of generics set as a percent of the price of the originator
Supply-side: Reimbursement		
Positive and negative formularies	All countries that have a third-party reimbursement system	Significant variations exist on the size of the positive list/formulary or negative list; in some cases formularies operate at national level, in other cases at regional level or, even, at facility (hospital) level
Internal reference pricing	Germany, the Netherlands, Czech Republic, Italy, Spain, France, Hungary, Austria, South Africa (some insurers), Canada	Price calculation based on the cost of similar treatments for the same indication; it can be at molecular or product category level
Health Technology Assessments (HTA) with emphasis on economic evaluation	UK, Sweden, the Netherlands, Hungary, Poland, Finland, Estonia, Latvia, Lithuania, Canada, Australia, Brazil, Taiwan, South Korea, Mexico, Colombia, Malaysia	Explicit use to inform coverage decisions in many countries, but more generally applied at regional, local or, even, facility level as input to decision-making. In some cases, there is no remit — as yet — for pharmaceuticals, e.g., in Malaysia and Mexico, although this may be changing
HTA with emphasis on clinical benefit assessment	France, Germany	Value assessment is a scientific process, whereby the clinical and safety profile are evaluated against valid comparators; the pricing function becomes a negotiated process between manufacturers and insurers/governments

(*Continued*)

Table 2. *(Continued)*

Intervention mechanism	Examples of countries employing each mechanism	Key issues
Risk-sharing agreements (RSAs)	• Many EU Member States: Belgium, France, Italy, Spain, Sweden, UK, the Netherlands, Poland • South Korea, Malaysia, Brazil (federal and state level), Mexico, Turkey, USA, Canada (provincial level), Australia	RSAs or Managed Entry Agreements (MEAs) can be financial (e.g., Patient Access Schemes [PAS] in the UK), or outcomes-based (e.g., many of the agreements in Italy), or incorporate both financial- and outcomes-related elements (many countries, but mostly in Europe); RSAs are widespread in many OECD countries and are used experimentally or as 'innovations' in Latin America, or East/South-East Asia
Innovative pricing and reimbursement schemes	Italy; Germany, UK, Finland, Australia	— Portfolio deals, whereby manufacturers agree to modulate prices upward in one part of their portfolio, in exchange for reductions in other parts of their portfolio; this should not be confused with bundling, which is discriminatory and, therefore, against competition rules — Disease management
DEMAND-SIDE: Policies towards physicians		
Clinical practice or prescribing guidelines	Most countries that have a third-party payer system in place	Usually stipulating what course of action prescribers should follow and in certain cases, what not to follow. Prescribing guidelines can be effective if linked to e-prescribing tools. They may also be linked to financial incentives/rewards or penalties if physicians are not compliant. Often, there is confusion between prescribing guidance and clinical protocols. The former provide precise guidance to prescribers on what course of action to follow in a particular diagnosis or disease; the latter provide a list of available options in a particular diagnosis or disease.

Mandatory generic prescribing (Prescribing by international non-proprietary name — INN)	UK, Denmark, Estonia	Discrepancy often exists between the scheme being compulsory and its implementation. It is not uncommon for physicians to prescribe by INN, but provide the preferred brand name separately to patients
Financial incentives	Some elements in France, UK	Directly related to salary/reimbursement
Prescription monitoring and audit	Belgium, UK, the Netherlands, France, Denmark, Sweden, Estonia	Random selection of physicians to check prescribing patterns appropriate and inappropriate prescribing
Demand-side: Policies towards pharmacy		
Control of remuneration (e.g., margins, fees)	European countries and Australia; in US and Canada a different model prevails	In some cases part of the remuneration of the distribution chain entails revenue from discounts (e.g., the UK and the Netherlands)
Generic substitution	France, Italy, Spain, Sweden	Extending substitution rights has been a key policy development in many countries over the past decade
Demand-side: Policies towards patients		
User charges	All countries	Different approaches to cost-sharing exist, but their impact on patients is very small with the exception of a few Member States
Encouraging use of Over The Counter (OTC) medicines and "delisting"	UK, Germany, Sweden, the Netherlands, USA, Canada	Definitions of OTC medicines vary across countries, as does the process of delisting from prescription-only status to OTC

Source: The author from the literature.

Table 3. External price referencing in Europe, 2015

		European economic area countries and countries they use as reference																											
		AT	BE	BG	HR	CY	CZ	DK	EE	FI	FR	D	GR	HU	IE	IT	LV	LT	NL	NO	PL	PT	RO	SK	SI	ES	SE	CH	UK
Frequency of use of a particular country as a reference to other countries	AT		✓		✓	✓	✓		✓	✓		✓	✓	✓	✓		✓			✓			✓	✓	✓			✓	
	BE	✓		✓		✓	✓		✓	✓		✓	✓	✓	✓		✓		✓	✓			✓	✓		✓			
	BG						✓		✓				✓				✓						✓	✓					
	CY	✓					✓		✓				✓				✓							✓					
	CZ	✓		✓	✓				✓			✓	✓	✓			✓	✓			✓		✓	✓					
	DK	✓	✓			✓	✓		✓	✓		✓	✓		✓		✓			✓			✓	✓				✓	
	EE	✓		✓			✓						✓				✓	✓			✓			✓					
	FI	✓	✓				✓		✓			✓	✓		✓		✓			✓				✓					
	FR	✓	✓	✓	✓	✓	✓		✓	✓		✓	✓	✓	✓	✓	✓		✓			✓		✓	✓	✓		✓	
	DE	✓	✓			✓	✓		✓	✓	✓		✓	✓	✓	✓	✓		✓	✓			✓	✓	✓	✓		✓	
	GR	✓	✓	✓		✓	✓		✓	✓		✓		✓			✓				✓	✓		✓		✓			
	HU	✓		✓			✓		✓	✓			✓				✓	✓			✓		✓	✓					
	IE	✓	✓				✓		✓	✓		✓	✓	✓			✓			✓				✓		✓			
	IT	✓	✓		✓	✓	✓		✓	✓	✓	✓	✓	✓			✓					✓	✓	✓		✓		✓	
	LV	✓		✓			✓		✓	✓			✓					✓			✓			✓					
	LT	✓		✓			✓		✓	✓			✓				✓				✓		✓	✓					
	LU	✓					✓		✓				✓				✓							✓					
	MT	✓					✓		✓				✓				✓							✓					
	NL	✓	✓				✓		✓	✓		✓	✓		✓		✓			✓				✓		✓		✓	
	NO								✓	✓							✓												
	PL	✓					✓		✓				✓	✓			✓	✓					✓	✓					
	PT	✓		✓		✓	✓		✓	✓		✓	✓	✓			✓							✓		✓			
	RO			✓			✓		✓								✓							✓					
	SK	✓		✓			✓		✓			✓	✓	✓			✓	✓			✓		✓						

Table 3. (*Continued*)

		European economic area countries and countries they use as reference																											
Frequency of use of a particular country as a reference to other countries		**AT**	**BE**	**BG**	**HR**	**CY**	**CZ**	**DK**	**EE**	**FI**	**FR**	**D**	**GR**	**HU**	**IE**	**IT**	**LV**	**LT**	**NL**	**NO**	**PL**	**PT**	**RO**	**SK**	**SI**	**ES**	**SE**	**CH**	**UK**
	SI	✓			✓		✓		✓				✓	✓			✓							✓					
	ES	✓	✓	✓	✓	✓	✓		✓	✓	✓	✓	✓	✓	✓	✓	✓				✓	✓		✓					
	SE	✓	✓			✓	✓		✓	✓		✓	✓				✓			✓				✓					
	CH								✓				✓				✓						✓	✓					
	UK	✓	✓				✓		✓	✓	✓	✓	✓		✓		✓		✓	✓			✓	✓		✓		✓	
	Formula	A	A	L	A	L 4	L^3		L	M	L		A 3+1	L	A	L	L	A –5%	A	L3	L	A	L3	L6	L	L		A	
	Freq(pery)	1*	AL	2	1	0.5	1		1	1	1**		1	AL	AL	AL	1	1	2	1	1	1	—	2	2	1		***	

Source: Kanavos, Nicod, Espin *et al*. (2010).

countries in price-setting through EPR. Such complexity could lead to gaming from the part of manufacturers, for instance in terms of delaying or altogether avoiding launching new products in specific markets, particularly if prices in one market will influence downwards prices in another market or geographical setting. A further issue arising from EPR is that, increasingly, list prices are not reflective of real (transaction) prices between manufacturers and insurers particularly for new and expensive products as the latter are often the subject of negotiation and confidential agreements involving financial- or outcomes-based risk sharing schemes.

- *Price fixing through negotiations, price–volume agreements and paybacks*

Negotiations between manufacturers and public insurers are a common way to set prices of new pharmaceutical products. Negotiations are based on the implicit use of evidence on the therapeutic value of a product and the available funds on behalf of health insurance. Both sides have market power — the manufacturer as a single seller (monopolist) and patent holder and the insurer as single buyer (monopsonist), so prices tend to reflect this balance of power between the two parties. Frequently, prices are fixed based on volume projections (price–volume agreements) and if agreed volumes are exceeded, payback clauses may be in place whereby manufacturers return the excess revenue to health insurers and/or renegotiate prices.

- *Price fixing through cost-plus pricing*

Cost-plus is a pricing method, which helps determine the price of a pharmaceutical product on the basis of its production, administration, distribution and selling costs. Besides the production cost of a pharmaceutical, cost plus takes into account other costs such as promotional expenses and, specifically, a profit margin. Costs of production comprise raw materials, packaging materials and other related costs. In countries such as India, Iran, Slovakia, and China, a markup is added to set ex-factory or retail prices. In Pakistan, the markup is added to the cost of materials and direct labor costs in order to set the retail price. In Bangladesh, the cost of raw materials and packaging materials is multiplied by a factor to calculate retail price. The use of cost-plus pricing as a method of pricing pharmaceuticals has declined over the past few decades partly because it is administratively complex to identify costs for individual pharmaceutical products and partly, because for imported pharmaceuticals, the most important element within a negotiated process between manufacturers and insurers is the product's transfer price. As a result, cost plus pricing is used in a number of developing countries and predominantly to arrive at the prices of locally produced pharmaceuticals.

- *Rate-of-Return Regulation*

Rate-of-return (RoR) regulation is used in the UK to indirectly cap pharmaceutical prices. The PPRS (Pharmaceutical Price Regulation Scheme) is essentially a "profit control" or "rate of return on capital employed" (ROCE) scheme and a voluntary agreement between government and industry, applies to in-patent pharmaceuticals and branded generics and target is manufacturers' profits on sales to the UK National Health Service (NHS) beyond a certain threshold, whilst allowing free pricing and pricing flexibility up to that threshold. The profitability of manufacturers with significant physical capital investment in the UK is determined by ROCE and stands at 21% plus a margin of tolerance. Any excess must be paid back to the UK Department of Health (DH), or prices must be reduced (Department of Health UK, 2013).[10] For manufacturers with insufficient capital base, profitability is gauged through return on sales to the NHS and stands at 6%. Producers can modulate prices based on their portfolio such that any changes are neutral. Within the target ROCE or profit rate, manufacturers have significant freedom in price setting and generous allowances to offset costs against. For example, there are allowances for R&D, promotion and distribution. RoR as applied in the UK is renegotiated every 5 years and is usually associated with a price cut prior to each new agreement coming into force. The most recent PPRS agreement that came into force on 1 January 2014 and is associated with pre-agreed upon increases in pharmaceutical spending (the agreed fixed limit spend will stay flat in 2015 but annual growth will be limited to 1.8% in 2016, with an increase to 1.9% by 2018, which is the final year of the scheme), a clawback for any excess spending and an exemption from growth targets of innovative medicines. The PPRS provides significant financial incentives to manufacturers to invest in R&D.

- *Clinical and cost effectiveness in value assessment*

Economic evaluation is used to determine a pharmaceutical product's cost-effectiveness in relation to a defined set of comparator treatments (pharmaceutical or other). To do so, it encompasses several methods: (1) Cost-effectiveness analysis, (2) cost–benefit analysis, (3) cost–utility analysis, and (4) cost-minimization analysis. The choice of the appropriate method depends on the outcome measures to be evaluated, but generally the use of one method does not necessarily exclude the other. The incremental cost-effectiveness ratio (ICER) then enables to determine whether a drug is cost-effective, as well as its level of therapeutic benefit in relation to its comparator(s). A "cost-effectiveness threshold" or "willingness-to-pay threshold" may be set in this context setting out the upper limit of individual

---

[10] Office of Fair Trading. The pharmaceutical price regulation scheme: An OFT market study. 2007. http://webarchive.nationalarchives.gov.uk/20140402142426/http://www.oft.gov.uk/shared_oft/reports/comp_policy/oft885.pdf.

health care systems' affordability and willingness to pay. Such thresholds determine the maximum additional amount the system is willing to pay for an additional unit of benefit. In Sweden, on the other hand, the willingness-to-pay threshold increases with the severity of the disease.

An alternative method that assesses the value of a new medical technology in terms of its overall therapeutic benefit and safety profile relative to a comparator (best available therapy or standard of care at the time of the comparison) is clinical benefit assessment. In this case, costs are not used to assess the clinical cost effectiveness and the method of clinical benefit assessment provides a ranking of a new technology relative to therapeutic alternatives. Based on this ranking, the value of the new therapy and, ultimately, its price, become the subject of a bilateral negotiation between manufacturers and insurers. France and, to a large extent, Germany pursue a value assessment strategy based on clinical benefit assessment.

- *Value-based pricing*

VBP sets prices based on a value assessment that takes into consideration a wider range of criteria than clinical cost-effectiveness, including the burden and severity of the disease and long-term benefits of the treatment. Notions of "value-based" have developed over the last two decades, and the term is now broadly understood to mean that activities within the health sector should be oriented, organized or funded to maximize health benefits for patients and societies (Paris and Belloni, 2013). VBP in the health sector can be defined as: "The price that ensures that the expected health benefits of a new technology exceed the health predicted to be displaced elsewhere in the National Health Service, due to their additional cost" (Claxton, 2007). This definition implies the use of cost-effectiveness analysis in decision-making. Others have gone further, linking VBP with HTA and suggesting that VBP consists of negotiating prices for new pharmaceuticals based on the value of the drug for the society as assessed through HTA (Husereau and Cameron, 2011). By ensuring access to cost-effective drugs today and incentives for manufacturers to invest in cost-effective products for the future, VBP seeks to provide a sustainable solution to pharmaceutical price regulation. But while it aims to reward innovation, establishing a clear link between the level of innovation and the price is not straightforward.

Although interest in VBP is growing, its practice in European national health authorities is still limited, although one could argue that a wider perspective is taken on value in some health care systems (e.g., Sweden) and attempts have been made to widen the range of criteria used by HTA bodies, for example, through more explicit use of burden of disease or severity and unmet medical need.[11]

[11]Europe WHOW-ROF. Access to new medicines in Europe: Technical review of policy initiatives and opportunities for collaboration and research. 2015. http://apps.who.int/medicinedocs/documents/s21793en/s21793en.pdf.

One proposal for a VBP framework in the context of orphan drugs has been the development of the Transparent Value Framework (TVF), which was developed was developed as part of the Mechanism of Coordinated Access to Orphan Medicinal Products (MoCA-OMP) in the EU Process on Corporate Social Responsibility in the field of pharmaceuticals (Godman *et al.*, 2015). The use of the TVF enables comparison of therapeutic alternatives with similar framework scores to provide future guidance in pricing and reimbursement negotiations; criteria that are considered in this context include the existence of alternatives, the level of unmet medical need, relative effectiveness, the response rate, and the degree of uncertainty. Despite the above, debate is ongoing about the feasibility of implementing the TVF in the decision-making of national reimbursement authorities and further refinement continues.

Supply-side intervention: Price determination of off-patent pharmaceuticals

Branded pharmaceuticals are exposed to competition from generic pharmaceuticals (both branded and unbranded) following patent expiry of the originator brand. Generics are replicas of the original molecule and come to market once intellectual property protection for the original has expired. Generics are sold at a lower price than the originator because generic companies do not incur the associated R&D costs and can enter the market facing a significantly lower entry barrier than the original; specifically, generics need to prove they are bio-equivalent to the original molecule. Although the regulatory requirements governing authorization of generics have been standardized across settings and relate to proof of bio-equivalence, several country-specific policies remain that determine generic drug entry and uptake. The type and scope of generic policies vary considerably across countries, both in terms of pricing and volume. This is translated into significant differences in the share of generic medicines in total pharmaceutical sales in different jurisdictions, as Figure 10 shows from a number of European countries.

Although, strictly speaking, price competition should be expected post-patent expiry as generics enter the market at a discount to the original product, in practice very few countries pursue allow the market to reach an equilibrium based on market forces rather than intervening. Among them are the UK, the USA, Sweden, and Denmark. In the majority of cases, generics are subjected to price interventions by insurers. One of these is price capping and linking generic prices explicitly to the originator product. Another practice is tendering, particularly in outpatient markets, where market size is considerable and the likely impact can be significant. Tendering is pursued by health insurers following the principles reverse auctions and with a view to maximizing the prices offered by all available competitors in a particular molecular market. These two interventionist strategies are discussed in turn.

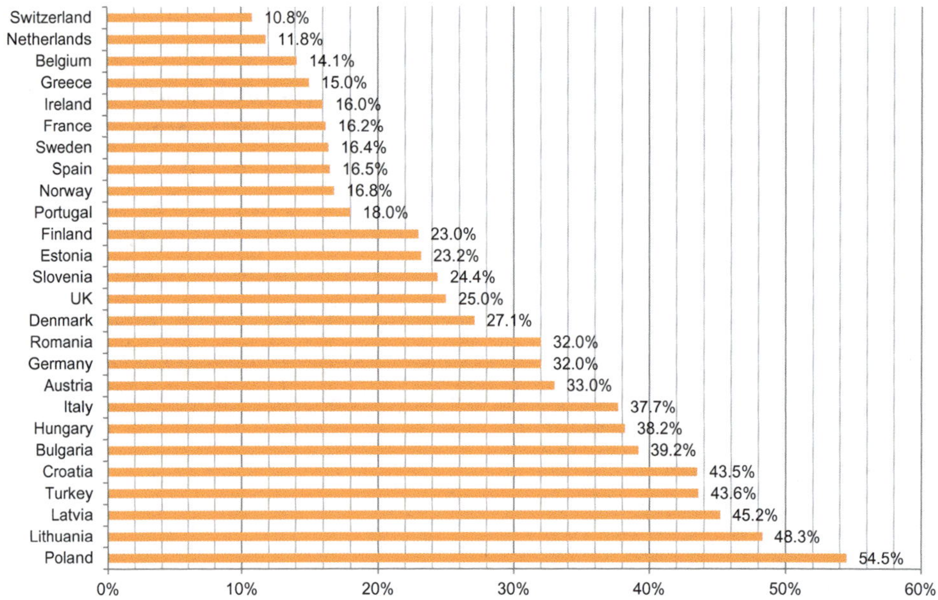

Figure 10. Share (Estimate in %) accounted for by generics in pharmaceutical market sales value (at ex-factory prices) in European countries, 2012

Source: EFPIA (2014).

- *Price caps and price linked to the originator*

Price capping policies in the off-patent pharmaceutical market refer to regulation which sets price ceilings on generic and originator products following originator patent expiry. These policies mirror the situation in the originator market, where maximum prices are established, but also apply in generic markets once the originator product patent has expired. In this case, the regulator is making an assumption about what the price of the generic on the market should be. In principle, price capping aims to contain costs by limiting high drug prices, encourage generic drug use (Brekke *et al.*, 2007) and, because of the capping mechanism, it guarantees a given level of savings to health insurers. Acceptable price levels differ between countries depending on a range of factors including prescribing behavior, utilization trends and budget limits (Mrazek and Mossialos, 2004). Price caps are most often linked to the price of the originator as a maximum allowable percent for the generic. The use of price caps, and prices linked to originators, is not consistent across countries. For example, generic price caps are explicitly linked to originator prices in the UK, Austria, Finland, France, Greece, and Portugal (Carone *et al.*, 2012); In Austria, the price of the first generic must be at least 48% less than price of the originator product on the market, the price of the second generic must be reduced by 15%; and the price of the originator must also decrease by at least 30% within three months of the inclusion of the first generic. In contrast, in Portugal, the price of the first generic competitor must be at least 25% below the price of original product, and the second follower needs to reduce its price by 25% compared to the first follower.[12]

- *Tendering for pharmaceuticals consumed in outpatient care*

Although tendering is a common measure for the procurement of hospital pharmaceuticals, it has not been widely used for out-patient pharmaceuticals (i.e., those consumed in primary care). Recently, tendering has been used for the procurement of out-patient drugs in the Netherlands and Germany (Kanavos *et al.*, 2009). A tender is issued and the lowest price wins the tender and the right to supply the whole market. The terms of the tender and whether a single product can supply the entire market or competitors that can supply at the tender price also have this right are laid out by the body issuing the tender. In the Netherlands, tenders initially (2005) applied to three widely consumed drugs (omeprazole, simvastatin, and pravastatin). In 2008, tenders were expanded to 33 off-patent products. The criterion for defining the winner is the lowest price. As there are different presentations for each product (i.e., strength in mg and number of tablets), tenders apply to the presentation level, therefore, more than one supplier can actually provide the same drug but with different presentations. In Germany, the tendering system is based on rebates, and manufacturers are asked to offer discounts on their initial prices. Tendering is often considered to be a radical measure because in the majority of cases it creates a 'closed formulary' situation where the winner takes the entire market for a pre-specified period of time. If the duration of the period covered by a tender is one year and if competitors do not win a tender in 3 or 4 successive years, they may lose the right to market their product in the country that issues the tender (sunset clause). There are additional issues that tenders raise, for example, what to do with excess stock if a manufacturer loses the tender next time round, or how to deal with stock-outs and delays if manufacturers cannot honour the terms of the tender they have won in a timely fashion. The flipside of course is the competitive prices that are achieved through tenders, as competitors operate in circumstances of asymmetric information.

Supply-side intervention: Tools used to inform coverage decisions

Manufacturers of originator pharmaceuticals retain extensive market power at certain points in time, gained through the patent protection of their products. This allows pharmaceutical companies to make higher profits that cover their R&D

[12] PPRI Network Members (several authors). PPRI/PHIS Pharma Profiles — country specific reports on pharmaceutical systems and policies. Pharmaceutical Pricing and Reimbursement Information (PPRI). 2007–2013. http://whocc.goeg.at/Publications/CountryReports.

costs. However, considering that the regulator cannot fully observe R&D costs (WHO, 2011)[13], it is difficult to assess whether pharmaceutical companies are making excessive profits or not. Moreover, because of the scarcity of resources in healthcare (since healthcare budgets are usually fixed in advance and limited), and of the increasing cost of developing new health care technologies, not all of these drugs can be reimbursed. This has led to the institutionalization of policies to aid coverage decisions, namely which pharmaceuticals to cover, at what price and whether insurees will bear any of the cost on an out-of-pocket basis.

Of the multiplicity of measures regulating reimbursement, four measures are discussed in this section: (1) *Positive/negative formularies*, (2) *internal reference pricing (IRP)*, (3) *health technology assessments (HTA)*, and (4) *performance-based and/or risk-sharing agreements (RSAs)*. These instruments are complementary to the pricing mechanisms discussed earlier, and are designed to influence the sales volume, as well as the prices of the pharmaceuticals that insurers will pay. As a result, therefore, it is not uncommon to expect that there may be a difference between list prices — which are achieved through one or more of the methods outlined in the previous subsections — and reimbursement prices. A positive formulary is a list of all pharmaceuticals that health insurance will reimburse and by how much; IRP sets a maximum reimbursement ceiling among interchangeble products, by promoting cheaper generics; HTA is a method to determine whether a new product has sufficient incremental clinical value or provides value for money in relation to existing comparators and, therefore, can be covered by health insurance; and RSAs attempt to reduce the uncertainty for health insurers, particularly in expensive new products, for instance by only reimbursing manufacturers for all cases where the product proves effective.

- *Positive/negative formulary*

A national formulary contains information on the drugs selected for reimbursement by health insurance. It also includes other related information about the drug, namely the indication or population it is intended for, the different doses and ways of administration, or the circumstances under which the drug is covered or not covered and the relevant co-payments. Formularies can be positive or negative. A positive formulary lists the drugs that are fully or partially covered by the health insurance and is the most common type of formulary used in practice. In contrast, negative formularies list the drugs that are not reimbursed. These can be found in fewer countries (examples are Germany and the UK). The rationale for establishing positive and negative lists is to regulate the utilization of pharmaceuticals, by

[13]R&D costs cannot be fully observed because of (1) the cross-subsidy that exists between successful and unsuccessful products, and (2) uncertainties regarding innovative processes (McGuire *et al.*, 2002).

discouraging physicians from prescribing ineffective drugs, or drugs that are more expensive than other treatment alternatives providing the same level of effect. Strictly speaking, the formulary is a powerful pharmaceutical policy tool. Non-admission to a formulary typically implies that a drug cannot be reimbursed. Formularies can be used to meet drug policy objectives. Occasionally, they are used more aggressively, for example, by selecting one therapeutic option for a given diagnosis, thereby 'closing' the formulary to all other therapeutic options for the same diagnosis and for a given class of products. Prior authorization can also be used, whereby a drug can be prescribed by an authorized physician only if it is authorized by health insurance first.

- *Internal reference pricing*

Internal reference pricing is a commonly employed policy in Europe, Canada, Australia, New Zealand, and as well as in many emerging countries to regulate the level of reimbursement of an off-patent molecule or a therapeutic class. In doing so, health insurance uses generic prices within a product market — usually the lower-priced generics — to set a maximum reimbursement level for a particular product that has generic alternatives. This maximum reimbursement level is the reference price. Products whose price exceeds the reference price are either not reimbursed, or the patient has to pay the difference between the reference price and the actual price of the product out-of-pocket. Usually reference prices are determined at the chemical substance level. This means that the originator and all generics are grouped together. The reference price is usually the lowest or the average of the lowest prices of the group. In some countries (e.g., Germany and the Netherlands), a reference price applies to a therapeutic class, rather than a single molecule. This means that more products are included in the reference group, some of which may be still in-patent. This is used to prevent costs occurring from dispensing so-called "me-too drugs" with very similar therapeutic effects, which are considered to be interchangeable, that are in-patent and are priced much higher than generics of other off-patent molecules of the same therapeutic class.

- *Health Technology Assessment*

Traditionally, reimbursement decisions were based mainly on the drug's efficacy, safety and quality, alongside taking into account other criteria, such as budget impact, severity of illness and, occasionally, industrial policy considerations in a process of negotiation with manufacturers or "behind closed door" discussion. These pharmaceuticals were then included accordingly in the positive or negative formularies. Currently, an increasing number of countries worldwide have introduced HTAs to assess the value of a drug for a specific indication from a medical, economic, and social perspective. HTA agencies can be either regulatory bodies responsible for coverage decisions, or advisory bodies making recommendations on coverage to decision-makers (i.e., Minister of Health).

HTA is increasingly being considered in pricing and reimbursement settings, whereby the costs and benefits of the new drug are weighed against those of an existing therapeutic alternative.[14] Based on the drug's cost-effectiveness (i.e., whether it is more or less cost-effective than its comparator), the price premium over its comparator may be determined and used to set the pharmaceutical's price. In other words, this method enables health systems to determine the value of a drug by assessing its clinical value in relation to costs and against one or more pre-defined comparator drugs. Based on this value assessment, manufacturers are rewarded for the level of innovation they bring to market. These methods are being used explicitly in informing pricing and reimbursement decisions in an increasing number of European countries (e.g., Sweden, Finland, The Netherlands, the UK, Estonia, Latvia, Lithuania, Poland, and Hungary use an assessment of costs and clinical benefits, whereas France uses an assessment of clinical benefit to inform its pricing and reimbursement decisions), North and Latin America (Canada, both at federal and provincial level, Brazil, Colombia, and Mexico) and East and Southeast Asia (South Korea, Japan, Taiwan, Malaysia, among others).

Cost-effectiveness is predominantly not used directly to set prices yet, but it is quite instrumental in determining reimbursement. Importantly, a threshold is used to set the limits of a health system's affordability; for example, the ICER in the UK ranges from £20,000–£30,000 per unit of health gain (as exemplified by the Quality Adjusted Life Year [QALY]), although there are exceptions for instance, the end-of-life criterion, which values life more in the last months of life and, as a result, pushes the ICER upwards. Nevertheless, recent evidence suggests that it could be lower (Claxton *et al.*, 2015).

Other countries use variable or no explicit thresholds, such as Norway and Sweden, where the willingness to pay depends on the severity of the disease area and level of unmet need. Researchers in Sweden estimated the threshold value for a QALY at €45,000 based on individuals' preferences, but for more severe conditions this increased to the region of €100,000.[15] As a result, currently no formal cost-per-QALY threshold appears to exist for new drugs in Sweden. Other

---

[14] A therapeutic alternative is a drug that can be used to treat the same condition. In this case, it is used as the comparator. Different types of comparators exist, such as the current best practice, the cheapest alternative, or the most frequently used.

[15] Europe WHOW-ROf. Access to new medicines in Europe: Technical review of policy initiatives and opportunities for collaboration and research. 2015. http://apps.who.int/medicinedocs/documents/s21793en/s21793en.pdf.

countries have a maximum threshold of up to three times their GDP per capita (e.g., Poland and Colombia, among others).

Without setting explicit thresholds, however, historical data allow for suggestions as to where the line is drawn via a precedent approach, using legal decisions in specific cases to build pressure for moving the threshold up more generally over time. In Belgium, it is thought unlikely that the authorities would reimburse new drugs with an additional cost per QALY of €80,000; an €80,000 per QALY threshold has been reported in the Netherlands, but evidence has shown that for orphan drugs much higher ICERs were accepted (although mainly due to public pressure.[15]

The different way in which HTA is implemented suggests that costs are not always used in assessing the value of a drug. For example in France, value is assessed according to the relative clinical benefit of a drug compared to existing alternatives based on evidence from clinical research. The drug's overall clinical benefit (SMR) is assessed and measured against a series of comparators and this process determines the reimbursability of the new drug. The drug's relative benefit is then ranked on a 5-level scale according to its "level of improvement of the clinical benefit (ASMR)", which is used in the context of pricing decisions. A high score on the relative benefit is likely to allow free pricing subject to the price requested by the manufacturer not being higher than in a basket of four reference countries. Cost effectiveness data may also be requested to support pricing decisions.

- *Risk-sharing agreements*

In many cases, especially for new and expensive medicines, it may be difficult to perform satisfactory HTAs due to the limited amount of available evidence, or that the evidence is subject to significant uncertainty about the health gain the new treatment delivers or its cost effectiveness. In those circumstances, health insurers may decide not to reimburse this drug. However, this is not an ideal solution as it may prevent patients from gaining access to certain promising new therapies. In this context, risk-sharing agreements (RSAs) (also known as performance-based agreements (PBAs) or managed entry agreements (MEAs)) are mechanisms enabling coverage subject to a number of conditions, which may differ depending on the setting, the treatment or the preferences of health insurers. These schemes intend to protect payers, while enabling patients to have access to these innovative medicines under certain circumstances. They can also be used in cases where uncertainties about the appropriate doses or indications exist, or when there is a possibility to offer more enhanced patient access (Espin and Rovira, 2009). Under these circumstances, insurers typically want to minimize their own risks and (a) ensure that the right patients receive the relevant treatment, (b) hedge against

Table 4. Types of risk covered by the different performance-based schemes

	Right patients	Uncertain clinical value	Low cost-effectiveness	Budget overspend
Coverage with evidence development	Yes	Yes	Yes	No
Conditional coverage	Yes	Yes	Yes	Yes
Outcome guarantee	Yes	Yes	Yes	No
Price–volume deal	No	No	No	Yes

Source: P. Kanavos.

uncertain clinical value, (c) address low cost-effectiveness, and (d) ensure a budget cap is observed). Table 4 shows the relationship between risk sharing agreements and the risks involved in each.

A number of currently existing performance-based schemes exist, enabling reimbursement to take place under conditions.

Risk-sharing agreements (RSAs) are the most commonly used. In this case, reimbursement of a new product is determined by one or more options. First, there can be a financial agreement between the insurer and the manufacturer; for example, this could be a price discount, or a price–volume agreement. Second, there can be an outcomes-based agreement, which links reimbursement to the performance of the therapy and whether it delivers the promised benefit; an example of that is an outcome guarantee scheme. And, third, there can be an agreement involving both financial and outcome elements, for example, a discount and an outcome guarantee as well as a budget cap (Ferrario and Kanavos, 2013; 2015). A number of important modalities are outlined below:

- *Coverage with evidence development (CED)*. The product is reimbursed when it is used under controlled circumstances, while developing evidence. For example, the drug can be reimbursed within randomized-controlled trials, or can be recorded in evidence-providing registries. In this case, health insurers are primarily concerned about (a) having insufficient knowledge about who are precisely the right patients for the product, (b) significant uncertainty surrounding the value of the product at the time of reimbursement application and (c) low cost-effectiveness; as a result, the conditions under which it can be reimbursed are very tight and relate to use under controlled circumstances, thus restricting the number of patients benefiting.
- *Conditional coverage (CC)*. Under this scheme, the drug is temporarily covered until it is able to provide evidence on its effectiveness based on a pre-defined set of criteria. If it is unable to achieve the set targets, the manufacturer will

incur price changes or rebates. Similar to the previous case, there are concerns about the overall value of the product and it can be reimbursed only for those who are thought to benefit most; in this case a budget may also be fixed, which if exceeded, the manufacturer is liable for returning the excess.

- *Outcome guarantee (OG)*. When pre-defined outcomes are not realized for individual patients, the manufacturer will bear the full costs or partial costs. In this case, there are concerns about the overall value of the product and it can be reimbursed only for those who respond best to treatment. Contrary to the previous case, budget criteria may not apply.
- *Price and volume (budget) agreements*. If these agreements are not respected, a penalty to the manufacturer will be foreseen. In this case, the primary consideration is to ensure that there is no budget overspend, irrespective of the type of patient benefiting from the product(s) in question.

In addition to RSAs, there are further tools, which help inform reimbursement decisions. Among them are *portfolio deals,* which entail a trade-off between the price or reimbursement price of one product, and the prices of other products in the same company's portfolio. The trade-off can also take the form of discounts on joint volumes. Another tool that has been used in many settings is *disease management* whereby the manufacturer becomes responsible for the management of a disease in certain patients or of a sub-group of the population and guarantees budget savings in return of favorable pricing and coverage. In doing, so the manufacturer cannot discriminate again competitor manufacturers' products.

Demand-side intervention

The pharmaceutical market on the demand-side has certain particularities that need to be addressed. First, patients or consumers do not have the expertise or the knowledge to make choices on the most appropriate treatment, but rely on physicians to make this decision on their behalf ("agency relationship"). Second, since patients usually do not bear the full cost of their treatment, they may tend to acquire a higher amount of more expensive drugs ("moral hazard"). Third, cultural issues in prescribing by physicians and in consumption by patients, can lead to a deterioration of the moral hazard problem: Evidence suggests that over 87% of all patient visits to physicians results in a prescription in Spain, Italy, and France, but this percentage is lower (less than 75%) in the UK, Sweden, and the Netherlands (Kanavos, 2008). Fourth, depending on the type of remuneration pharmacists receive, it may be in their advantage to dispense more expensive drugs even if cheaper alternatives exist. Finally, patients are willing to pay more if they believe that a treatment is better than another. All these peculiarities may result in resources being used inefficiently when purchasing pharmaceuticals, for instance, by prescribing more expensive treatments when cheaper and equally good alternatives exist. In order to avoid this, different regulatory mechanisms targeting patients, physicians, and pharmacists have been introduced. They are discussed in this section.

- *Policies targeting prescribing physicians*

The demand for pharmaceuticals is dictated to a large extent by physician prescribing. Prescribing behavior and decision-making are influenced by several factors including individual characteristics of the physician and patient, industry advertising, and financial and non-financial incentives at work. While studies have found that changing prescribing patterns is difficult and requires a multi-dimensional approach, several policies exist to shape prescribing practices.

A range of policies exist to increase generic market entry and diffusion, including those which encourage or require generic prescribing at the physician level and generic substitution and dispensing at the pharmacist level. The level and scope of generic prescribing policies varies across the EU. For example, while generic prescribing may be mandatory in some Member States, it is simply allowed or encouraged in others. Prescribing procedures also vary in terms of how doctors are allowed to prescribe pharmaceuticals; e.g., whether they are to use the International Non-Proprietary Name (INN), the generic name or only the branded name. Most physicians will prescribe using the brandname unless specifically instructed to use INN, as is the practice in the UK. However, in some Member States, INN prescribing is compulsory in order to minimize the dispensing of branded medicines.

Both financial and non-financial incentives exist to influence prescribing behavior and encourage the prescription of the most cost-effective treatment option. Financial incentives include monetary rewards for achieving prescription targets and remaining within prescription limits. Financial penalties may be enforced for missing targets or exceeding limits. The incentive or penalty structure, as well as the degree of monitoring and the level of enforcement vary between countries that apply these. The German experience is a commonly cited example of the use of pharmaceutical budgets as a method of influencing drug prescription and controlling pharmaceutical costs. In 1993, following negotiations with the German Government, sickness funds and physician associations, it was agreed that if a regional pharmaceutical budget exceeds a maximum expenditure threshold, the physicians would be responsible for the deficit (Ess *et al.*, 2003). While the number of prescriptions initially declined following the implementation of budgetary restrictions, the number began to rise again in 1995. The law was eventually abolished in 2001, following consistent opposition from physicians. In the UK, the fundholding experiment offers interesting insights on the way financial (budgetary) incentives were implemented at the individual general practitioner (GP) level over the 1991–1997 period (Chaix-Couturier *et al.*, 2000; Delnoij and Brenner, 2000); in the UK, the government empowers GPs so that they can make most purchasing decisions directly, by delegating in excess of 75% of the UK NHS budget to them. Other schemes link financial incentives to quality of care improvements, such as the Quality and Outcomes Framework (QOF) in the UK.[16]

Another measure for general cost-containment is the use of prescription monitoring and auditing systems alongside the use of clinical practice guidelines and evidence-based medicine to ensure appropriate prescribing. The goals of monitoring or publishing prescribing behavior include increasing prescribing efficiency, encouraging generic prescribing and, in some cases, verifying adherence to guidelines. Most Member States monitor pharmaceutical prescribing to some extent, but there is variation in the level, frequency and intensity of monitoring. For example, prescription data may be used to compare physician practices and regions within a country, or simply used by individual physicians to monitor their own prescribing habits. In Austria, for example, the most common form of prescribing monitoring is to compare individual prescribing behavior with regional averages (OBIG, 2006). In the UK, prescribing behavior is compared to national and regional levels. Specifically, prescription data on prescription volume and costs for individual GP practices is collated on a national level and statistics are disseminated quarterly to encourage awareness of prescription volume and costs. Individual physicians are notified if they exceed regional averages. Similar systems exist in France, Germany, the Netherlands, Sweden and Italy. Prescription monitoring systems rely on comprehensive electronic medical records, or internet-based databases, such as Denmark's Oridprax, which allow for comparisons at the regional level (OBIG, 2006).

- *Policies aimed at the distribution chain*

Demand-side policies target all stakeholders within the distribution chain, notably manufacturers, wholesalers and retailers. Regulatory interventions include controlling wholesale and retail margins, allowing generic substitution and monitoring price discounts where possible.

Against this background, the structure of the distribution chain (wholesaling and retailing) is characterised by large differences with regards to concentration across countries. Italy has 193 and Spain has 99 wholesalers, while Germany has only 16 and the UK less than 9. However, the top three wholesalers in the UK

[16] Health and Social Care Information Centre (HSCIC). Quality and Outcomes Framework. 2015. http://www.hscic.gov.uk/qof.

control 85% of the market. Finland and Sweden have only two wholesalers each. In a similar vein, the density in retail distribution via pharmacies varies significantly across Member States with some of the Southern Member States (Portugal, Spain, Italy, Greece, and also France) having the highest density of pharmacy networks and some of the northern Member States having among the lowest pharmacy network densities. Horizontal and vertical integration are also regulated in some cases.

Wholesale and retail margins may be progressive, regressive, a fixed percentage of the relevant price or a flat fee. The current practice in the EU nowadays consists of applying either regressive of fixed fee margins. Depending on how they are structured, regressive margins can encourage generic use. Despite recent reductions in distribution margins, the impact of distribution in different Member States can be as high as 50% of a drug's retail price (i.e., the price payable by health insurance). This also depends on whether a drug is an originator brand or a generic and, often, the proportional impact of margins on the retail prices of medicines can be higher for generics than it is for brands.

Generic substitution policies encourage or require that pharmacists dispense the generic version of a medicine when available. Generic substitution varies from mandatory (Sweden) to voluntary (France) to "not allowed" (Austria) (GOEG, 2007–2014; OBIG, 2007). These categories are not static however, as governments alter their policies over time (GOEG, 2007–2014; OBIG, 2007). Generic substitution polices also vary according to the extent to which physicians and patients are allowed to refuse the substitution. In countries such as Sweden the substitution of a generic alternative can be refused by the prescribing physician, but only with medical evidence as justification. Because of the varying degrees of generic prescribing and substitution, there is varied evidence as to the influence of generic substitution on generic utilization. The European Commission (2009) concluded that those Member States that require pharmacists to dispense generic medicines when possible are more likely to have generic entry earlier and achieve higher cost-savings. Moreover, data from Sweden shows that generic substitution has facilitated a drop in market price for generics (approximately 40% since the introduction of substitution in 2002) (GOEG, 2007–2014).

Internal reference pricing systems and generic substitution are methods by which the government encourages the dispensation of generic drugs over more expensive branded medicines. Within the structure of these policies, pharmacists still have considerable market power in the absence of price differences between comparable drugs. Wholesalers or manufacturers, therefore, provide discounts to pharmacies in exchange for dispensing their product, incentivizing the pharmacist to dispense the product with the greatest discount. The difference between the reimbursement price set by the health insurer and the discounted price offered by the wholesaler or manufacturer may be considerable, and the greater the margin between prices, the greater the incentive for pharmacists.

Discounting practices are particularly important in the generic market because the level of discount offered can distinguish one generic from another in a pool of directly comparable, reimbursable drugs. While there are legislated limits on the discounts wholesalers and manufacturers may offer pharmacies, the level and scope of discounts is kept confidential. In a study of the French generic market, for example, it was found that while discounts are related to price, the discounts exchanged are greater than the discount ceilings placed by the government (Kanavos and Taylor, 2007). In a response to discounting practices, and as a method of capitalizing on the cost-saving potential of generic discounts, governments recalculate margins in order to claw back at the pharmacy level discounts.

- *Policies aimed at patients*

Cost-sharing or out-of-pocket (OOP) payments refer to the proportion of health-care and/or pharmaceutical costs borne by the patient. Cost-sharing mechanisms, such as co-insurance[17], fixed fee[18], deductible[19], reference pricing[20], or differential co-pays, have been introduced mainly for two reasons: (a) To ease the public expenditure burden on health, and (b) to address the problem of moral hazard, namely unnecessary or frivolous use. However, the introduction of cost-sharing may generate adverse effects for which appropriate measures need to be implemented. For example, cost-sharing may reduce equity in access if people cannot afford their co-payments. The proportion of OOP as total expenditure on health varies greatly across countries, since different cost-sharing schemes exist in each country but can be significant and in excess of 25% as Figure 11 shows.

---

[17] Patients pay a proportion of the cost of all or most medicines, determined by health insurance. Typically, this is determined by the severity of the illness they treat. For instance, life threatening diseases, such as diabetes, carry a 0% co-insurance.

[18] Patients pay a fixed amount per prescription, irrespective of the cost of medicines they consume. Exemptions typically exist for the chronically ill. A variation of this fixed fee per prescription exists in Germany, where patients pay a fixed fee per pack of medicines.

[19] Under a deductible, patients pay out-of-pocket the entire prescribing costs up to a point in any given year, before their insurance coverage covers anything on top of that beyond that point.

[20] A system, whereby health insurance fixes the maximum reimbursement price, based on a generic medicines (assuming it is available) and if patients desire a higher cost medicine (e.g., the originator) the need to pay the difference out-of-pocket (as is the case in Spain, France, Germany, the Netherlands, Canada, the Czech Republic, among others), or, in some cases, they pay the entire cost out-of-pocket, should they opt for the more expensive option.

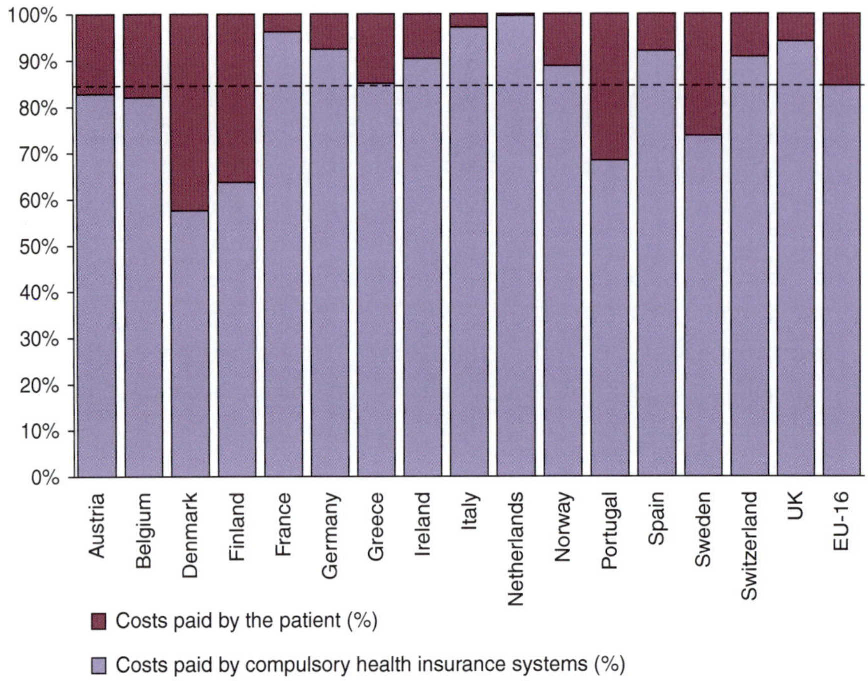

Figure 11. Proportion of pharmaceutical costs paid by health insurance and by the patient in 17 European countries

Source: Kanavos *et al.* (2011) quoted in European Parliament (2011).

Impact of Regulatory Intervention in Pharmaceutical Markets

In this section, we focus on the impact of regulatory intervention on pharmaceutical markets across different settings. In doing so, we examine price differences for prescription pharmaceuticals and their likely causes. We also discuss what the impact is of supply- and demand-side regulation on key pharmaceutical policy objectives, namely cost containment, efficiency and quality of care.

Pharmaceutical price differentials

The issue of price differentials has been discussed extensively in the literature, with different approaches having been used so far (Danzon and Chao, 2000a; 2000b; Danzon and Furukawa, 2008; Kanavos and Vandoros 2011; Kanavos *et al.*, 2013). As different policies apply in in-patent and off-patent markets, price gaps are not the same for these different drug categories. In sum, evidence suggests that significant price differences are observed across countries for in-patent pharmaceuticals. Price variability is also observed in off-patent pharmaceutical markets and seems to be stronger than in in-patent markets. This is a reflection of diametrically opposing approaches to the pricing of generic medicines in different settings.

Whereas some countries fix prices of generics, others have completely deregulated prices. The combination of the two approaches results in price differences, which can be as high as 20:1 in some cases (Kanavos *et al.*, 2011) and if the results of tenders are accounted for, price differences can be even higher. In essence, some countries treat generics as commodities, whereas others treat them as differentiated options to the originator molecule.

With regards to price differences in in-patent originators, Table 5 compares prices of the most selling in-patent originator medicines in a number of key European countries (UK, Germany, France, Switzerland), the USA, Canada, and Australia. Prices are indexed to the US prices (=100) for comparability. For the most selling drugs in these countries over the 2005–2010 period, it shows that there are significant differences between them. The results are confirmed by similar evidence from other settings (Department of Health (UK), 2009).

The factors that account for these differences in the prices of in-patent drugs are several. First, differences may be due to different ways of measurement. As shown on Table 5, the different methods of weighing prices (whether this is

Table 5. Manufacturer and retail price indexes for a sample of originator drugs in 7 countries, 2005, 2007 and 2010

	2005		**2007**		**2010**	
Country	**Country weights**	**US weights**	**Country weights**	**US weights**	**Country weights**	**US weights**
Manufacturer prices						
Australia	86	62	86	53	70	47
Canada	96	62	95	58	81	52
France	77	65	77	55	61	44
Germany	86	105	86	85	74	79
Switzerland	115	109	113	93	85	73
UK	60	46	56	39	46	34
US	100	100	100	100	100	100
Retail prices						
Australia	80	58	86	55	71	49
Canada	92	60	91	56	78	50
France	110	91	105	76	82	61
Germany	99	121	104	103	89	95
Switzerland	139	132	137	112	103	88
UK	81	62	76	53	63	46
US	100	100	100	100	100	100

Source: Kanavos *et al.* (2013).

through weights based on the country of reference [known as Laspeyres index], or the own country weights [known as Paasche index]), result in significant differences between countries. It is important to note that international price comparisons can be significantly affected by the relative level of sales in each country, movement in exchange rates and the proportion (and mix) of pharmaceutical expenditure included in any analysis of international comparisons.

Second, methodological issues around choice of appropriate prices to measure may complicate comparisons even further. Specifically, gaps in price differences are different when considering prices at the ex-factory or retail level. This is because the impact of other stakeholder groups on the formation of retail pharmaceutical prices can be significant. Significant variations exist among countries in the regulation of wholesale and retail margins, although some convergence exists in terms of the type of policy that applies. The differences are attributed to historical patterns in the development of remuneration of the distribution chain, but also to regulating its activities, from opening pharmacies to population criteria in awarding licenses to whether pharmacies or/and wholesalers can integrate horizontally or vertically. In the same context, countries also apply different levels of taxation on prescription pharmaceuticals on the pharmacy price. The difference in prices across countries can be significant simply because of taxation (e.g., VAT) differences: For example, Sweden or the UK apply 0% VAT on prescription pharmaceuticals, whereas Germany applies 19% and Denmark 23%. Figure 12 shows the average price build-up from ex-factory to retail price and the contribution of different stakeholders in this build-up.

A third factor that can explain price differences in in-patent originators across settings is the level of uptake and utilization of new medicines. There appears to

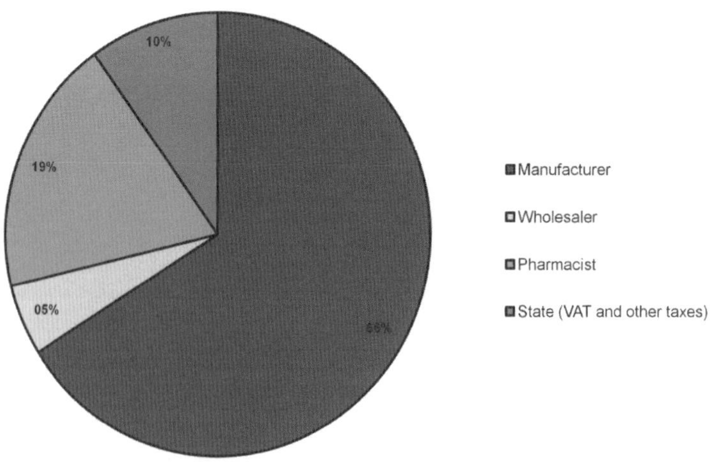

Figure 12. Breakdown of retail price of a medicine, 2012 (%)
Sources: EFPIA (2014).

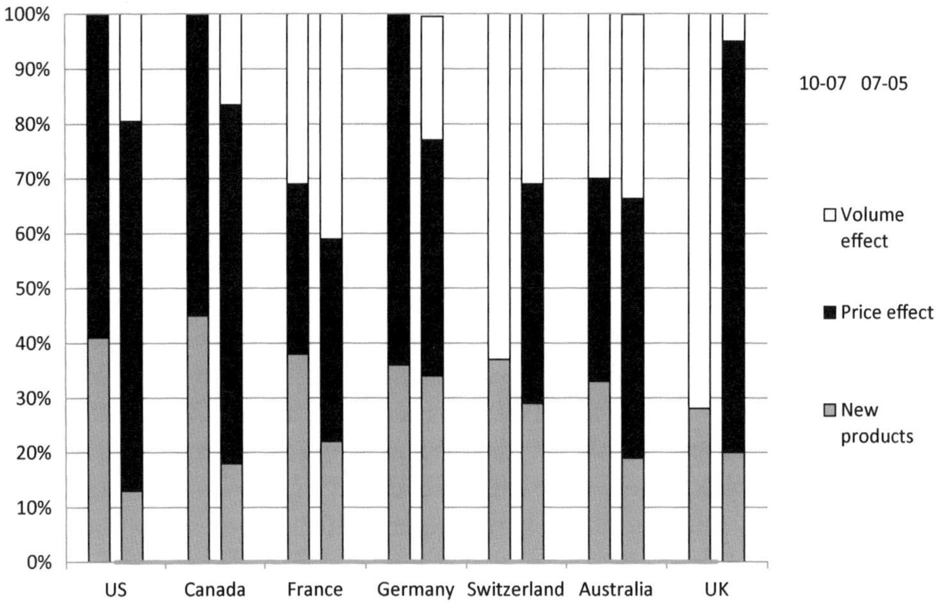

Figure 13. Price, volume and innovation effects on pharmaceutical expenditure between 2007/2010 and 2007/2005

Source: Kanavos *et al.* (2013).

be some correlation between higher prices and the rate of uptake, such that countries with higher levels of uptake and use of new medicines also have higher prices (Figure 13).

Finally, price differences of originators are to a large extent the consequence of different regulatory approaches followed in individual countries. As policies are set individually by each country for all parts of the pharmaceutical supply chain, prices that occur are naturally different, depending on national priorities and approaches to health care, industrial policy and equity considerations. We discuss the different approaches to regulation and their impact in Sections "Meeting pharmaceutical Policy Objectres" and "Access to Medicines at EU Level" for both in-patent and off-patent pharmaceuticals.

Meeting pharmaceutical policy objectives: Cost containment and efficiency

Despite attempts in the literature, it is not possible to attribute price differentials to one single source. It is however likely that the majority of these differences are linked to two factors: differences in economic investment or expenditure on health (associated with GDP); and differences in pricing policy and regulation. The latter are explored in greater detail in this section, as are the implications for cost containment and microeconomic efficiency.

- *Supply-side intervention: Pricing methods for in-patent pharmaceuticals*

Differences in national pricing policies and regulations are partly responsible for observed price differentials in both in- and off-patent markets for several reasons. First, there are fundamental differences between free-pricing and price-controlled systems, which allow different stakeholders, with different interests to control initial price setting. Free-pricing systems, which allow pharmaceuticals to be priced without restriction at launch, may be regulated through other means such as profit control (UK) (Mrazek and Mossialos, 2004), or reimbursement regulation through internal reference pricing and/or use of HTA. Fixed pricing, also referred to as direct price controls, amounts to the setting of fixed maximum prices, which may apply broadly to all medicines whether or not they are reimbursed, or to specific groups of products (for example, reimbursed, inpatient/outpatient, on-patent/off-patent). While the aim is to set prices at a reasonable or affordable level, definitions thereof differ across as well as within countries. They way in which prices are set, i.e., through negotiations (Austria, France, Italy, Portugal, and Spain) or unilaterally by the national authority, affects prices to wholesalers, patients and ultimately to health insurers/governments. Direct price controls may slow price increases or induce lower prices altogether. However, the influence on overall pharmaceutical expenditure may be over-shadowed by increases in expenditures due to volume and the fast uptake of innovative drugs (Mrazek and Mossialos, 2004; Kanavos *et al.*, 2013).

Second, within price-regulated systems, the specific features of individual policies as well as the mix of regulatory measures vary significantly across Member States. Pricing policies and regulatory approaches reflect national priorities in both health and industrial policy, such as containing overall pharmaceutical expenditures or promoting R&D, employment and trade. Third, pricing regulation may be implemented at various stages along the distribution chain, from manufacturer to wholesaler to pharmacist and individual consumer or hospital. Moreover, in several countries, the type and strength of regulation differs between in-patent and off-patent markets. Overall, the main types of pricing methodologies can affect prices of pharmaceuticals differently.

- *External price referencing*

Countries using EPR create a basket including other countries whose prices they wish to use as benchmark. Out of these, they typically select the lowest or the average of the lowest in order to determine the local price. Although EPR can help cost-containment by reducing prices, there are concerns arising from the fact that it is an arbitrary measure targeting prices that ignores other aspects of the market, the particular health priorities in each country and creates uncertainty for the innovative segments of the industry, especially due to the impact of exchange rate fluctuations on reference prices.

EPR can contribute to lower originator drug prices. Price reduction becomes even steeper as most countries adopt the lowest price of all countries in their basket, or the average of the lowest, combined with periodic recalculations, which typically take place annually or, in some cases, more frequently. Additionally, when using EPR, prices are affected by exchange rate fluctuations. Given that the price is that of the lowest or the average of the lowest countries in the basket, exchange rate volatility has been shown to exert downward pressure on prices (Kanavos *et al.*, 2011). Among the unintended consequences of EPR is the reality that manufacturers are likely not to launch a product in a certain country if that country's price influences third countries, or it is likely to be too low and, therefore, encourage parallel exports. Finally, although EPR has been shown to lead to downward price convergence, the evidence that it leads to overall cost containment is scarce.

Overall, EPR can lead to significant uncertainty and cascade effects on prices of prescription medicines, often due to the unintended consequences of factors such as basket design and exchange rate volatility. While pricing is an issue of national competence, countries implementing it may want to consider the wider implications of pricing strategies relying on cross-country comparisons. To that end: (a) The average of all countries in the basket can be used for the determination of the reference price, rather than lowest or average of the lowest; (b) making adjustments for exchange rate fluctuations could help ensure price stability and excluding factors that are exogenous to pharmaceutical price determination; (c) launch delays, due to strategic considerations arising from the knock-on effect of EPR ought to be studied, their extent identified and policies be put in place that discourage such practices, while improving access to medicines.

Rate of return regulation

Rate of return regulation and the way it is currently applied in the UK enables manufacturers to set prices subject to a profit target, which, if exceeded, can trigger price reductions or requirements to return the excess profit to the regulator. The relative price freedom assumed by the scheme could mean that prices are higher than would otherwise be the case, although renegotiations of the scheme are usually associated with price cuts. Assessments of the scheme in the UK based on periodically submitted reports to parliament, suggest that it ensures reasonable prices for the UK National Health Service and a stable and predictable environment for the industry to operate (Department of Health (UK), 2014). UK prices are found to be close to average European prices and often lower. Over the past two years, they have been below that average, due to the depreciation of sterling vis-à-vis the euro. Nevertheless, there is no link between the PPRS and overall cost containment results.

Negotiations

Negotiations have been a common way of setting prices and, by extension, reimbursement levels of new medicines. In this case, payers (health insurance) and manufacturers reach an agreement on the reimbursement price. Although manufacturers are monopolists, monopoly power cannot be exercised to the full because health insurance also has market power, due to its status as a monopsony. Therefore, the price agreed upon is not expected to be unreasonably high or low. Negotiation outcomes are not expected to cause excessive strain on health insurance, or set a price that is extremely low for the manufacturer and discourages future investment in R&D. This way of pricing may implicitly take into account clinical evidence and the therapeutic value of the medicine.

- *Supply-side intervention: Pricing methods for off-patent pharmaceuticals*

Generic price capping

Price caps are set as a method of controlling the prices of both branded and generic pharmaceuticals. In many cases price caps on generics are set according to the price of the originator or branded price. Fixing prices has the potential to provide an alternative to simple cost-based regulation, but is controversial in that the practice of setting fixed prices is subject to bias and may not be completely transparent (Mrazek and Frank, 2004). There remains debate as to whether price caps have successfully facilitated cost-containment as there is mixed evidence on the influence of price fixing on both in-patent and generic drugs (Danzon and Chao, 2000a; Garattini and Tediosi, 2000). For example, a meta-analysis of current literature on the effect of pricing policies found that that generic prices level is higher when price capping regulations are instituted, than without such policies (Puig-Junoy, 2010). Finally, EU-wide study concluded that those countries that do not implement price caps but rely on competitive forces experience faster generic uptake and eventually see generic prices decrease to a greater extent (European Commission, 2009).

Tendering

Tendering, particularly outpatient tendering, is very effective in reducing generic prices in out-patient markets. In the Netherlands, prices decreased as much as 95% following the implementation of tendering (Table 6). This can lead to immediate

Table 6. Impact of tendering on prices of generic products in the Netherlands, 2008–2012

Items	Price				Change in Price		
	May 2008	June 2008	September 2011	February 2012	May–June 2008 (%)	May 2008–Sept 2011 (%)	May 2008–Feb 2012 (%)
Omeprazole tab/cap, 20 mg	€0.36	€0.05	€0.02	€0.02	*–88*	*–94*	*–94*
Alendroninezuur tab, 70 mg	€4.99	€0.36	€0.07	€0.04	*–93*	*–99*	*–99*
Omeprazole tab/cap, 40 mg	€0.65	€0.09	€0.04	€0.03	*–86*	*–94*	*–95*
Paroxetine tab, 20 mg	€0.37	€0.07	€0.03	€0.03	*–82*	*–92*	*–92*
Simvastatin tab, 40 mg	€0.27	€0.04	€0.02	€0.01	*–84*	*–93*	*–96*
Pravastatin tab, 40 mg	€0.54	€0.13	€0.05	€0.03	*–76*	*–91*	*–94*
Simvastatin tab, 20 mg	€0.17	€0.03	€0.01	€0.01	*–85*	*–94*	*–94*
Tamsulosine tab/cap, 0.4 mg	€0.34	€0.07	€0.03	€0.03	*–80*	*–91*	*–91*
Amlodipine tab, 5 mg	€0.19	€0.03	€0.01	€0.01	*–85*	*–95*	*–95*
Citalopram tab, 20 mg	€0.34	€0.04	€0.02	€0.02	*–88*	*–94*	*–94*

Sources: Based on Kanavos *et al*. (2009) and Kanavos *et al*. (2012).

price cuts and savings for health insurance, but, as some evidence from the Dutch setting suggests, these savings must be balanced against losses in the distribution chain, which the Dutch authorities have had to rectify because of the Dutch retail system's reliance on discounts from (generic and other) manufacturers. Tendering does not necessarily pose a threat to innovation, as most substances are already patent expired. However, the sustainability of the generic industry is also important in order to safeguard the future availability of generics. There are concerns that tendering could drive out competition in the long run, especially if it is used for a large variety of products and in many European countries. Some generic producers will not be able to sell their products if they do not win any tenders; exit from the market is then only option. A decrease in the number of generic producers could lead to an increase in generic prices, not necessarily to the level prior to tendering, but part of the price reduction is expected to be offset because of less competition. This could be of some concern to governments, not only from a pricing perspective, but also as part of the EU's industrial strategy and the future of the European generic industry.

Overall Assessment

Overall, both price capping and tendering are considered to be relatively extreme methods of pricing and procurement of generic medicines. While the former helps governments and insurers achieve a saving on their off-patent drug segment, it does not encourage competition and if the cap is set too close to the originator, it does not encourage a shift to generics. Tendering on the other hand can be a harsh measure, although, where it is implemented, the results achieved on prices of generic medicines are truly spectacular. Importantly, decision makers should consider two types of implications: First, the likely competition in subsequent waves of tenders, particularly if many competitors exit the market and the prospect of product shortages; and, second, the implications on other components of the pharmaceutical value chain in case their interests — financial and other — are adversely affected by the conduct of tenders. In this case, corrective measures may need to be implemented, as the case of the Netherlands has suggested.

- *Supply-side intervention: Reimbursement methods*

The advantages and disadvantages of different regulatory reimbursement schemes are discussed hereunder, as well as their impact (direct or indirect) on pricing, cost-containment and innovation. It is important to keep in mind that the principles for an effective reimbursement policy include among others that it: (1) is transparent, (2) allows flexibility to ensure rapid access to new treatments, and (3) is robust in evaluating the drug's clinical benefit and economic impact.

Formularies

Formularies are an effective way to regulate drug utilization and encourage rational use in terms of the choice of the appropriate treatment, dosage, form for a patient, and adequate use. Formularies encourage efficient use of health care resources and may lead to cost savings. For this to take place decision-makers at national, regional or insurance level could consider that clinically and cost-effective treatments remain on formularies, while dis-investment takes place for treatments that are obsolete and less efficacious compared to new ones. Where formularies exist, a more pro-active stance regarding their management could help optimize costs and improve efficiency. Comprehensive guidelines detailing the different scenarios and appropriate treatments to be used (e.g., sub-population, indication, dosage, among others) may increase transparency in processes and thus enable manufacturers to better identify R&D priorities. In turn, this may encourage innovation, increase the number of available drugs and, in fine, foster price competition. Patient and physician input is key for successful formulary design, as it helps minimize discrepancies between recommendations and user behavior. Concerns regarding the lack of flexibility of formularies may be addressed through more frequent reviews. Some countries currently do so on a monthly (Belgium, France) or fortnightly basis (Denmark), to ensure that effective and cost-effective treatment options are available in a timely manner.

Linking product regulation to reimbursement: From efficacy to effectiveness

Reimbursement mechanisms are closely linked to the price of a drug. As a result, it is important to understand the dynamics between pricing and reimbursement regulatory schemes, as well as their impact on the access and affordability of drugs. Occasional delays are observed in achieving reimbursement status. This is often exacerbated by HTAs requiring thorough reviews of the clinical evidence and the associated economic costs of new treatments relative to comparators. There also seems to be discrepancy between the type of evidence requested to manufactures by regulatory authorities on the one hand, and national HTA and/or reimbursement agencies on the other hand. Efforts could be undertaken to mainstream these evidence and information requirements. The recent developments at FDA and EMA level on conditional approval, approval under exceptional circumstances and adaptive licensing (the latter at EMA level), may still have some way to go to become the standard for marketing authorization, but can be tested in practice before becoming generalized. Ultimately, (relative) effectiveness data need to be produced for governments and health insurers to be able to make informed decisions on coverage, as efficacy will no longer suffice.

Internal reference pricing

Internal reference pricing is effective in reducing generic prices in the first instance. However, producers tend to price at or around the reference price, so there is no incentive to deviate from it, unless a different wave of entrants comes to the market offering discounted prices. This relative downward price stickiness has been observed in Germany, France and Italy (Kanavos *et al.*, 2008). Reference pricing may be useful in the short run, after generic entry. However, in order to achieve further price cuts, competition between generics can be more effective. For the latter to take place, there must be enough competitors in the generic market. An alternative would be for competition to be managed, in that health insurance would require an additional discount each time there is new generic entry in a therapeutic market.

Cost-effectiveness pricing, value assessment and multiple criteria to aid decision-making

One of the main issues with cost-effectiveness pricing is the difficulty in assessing the real value of a treatment to patients and to society. This "value" may vary depending on which method was used for its assessment, which costs were included (direct and indirect), and how the benefits were measured. National requirements on the preferred methods used for cost-effectiveness analysis vary across as well as within countries. The conclusion is, therefore, that the value of a drug is subjective, because it depends on many considerations including the method and the perspective (i.e., a payer's or a societal perspective) used for its assessment, as well as the types of costs and benefits considered. As a result, the assessed value may vary accordingly and hence affect pricing and reimbursement decisions. In recent years, there have been attempts to introduce greater transparency in value assessment and a wider range of parameter that capture dimensions of value that traditional cost effectiveness cannot. Techniques such as multiple criteria decision analysis (MCDA) have been suggested as contributing to a more holistic value assessment based on several criteria and by involving a wider range of stakeholders (Marsh *et al.*, 2014; Kanavos and Angelis, 2013). Although prices of new pharmaceuticals are unlikely to decline as a result of using these techniques relative to traditional cost effectiveness, it is likely that decision-makers will seek greater clarify, transparency and comprehensiveness in HTA assessments in the future and this may signal a change in the way value is perceived and assessed.

Coverage recommendations and the use of HTA

Reimbursement decisions determine the level and scope of coverage, including the level of co-payments borne by the patient to gain access to these treatments.

Across countries in the OECD Region, coverage decisions are increasingly based on HTAs. The national formularies then list whether the drug is reimbursed or not. In case where a treatment receives a negative coverage decision, the patient is likely to bear the full cost to gain access to this treatment, thus limiting the affordability and access to this treatment. In theory, HTAs should be more or less homogeneous at least within the same region. In reality, however, substantial variations in recommendations have been identified across countries, even in circumstances where policy objectives are similar. This is impacting on the affordability and access to these treatments for those with negative or delayed coverage decisions, as well as on price levels depending on whether HTAs are used directly or indirectly as a price setting or reimbursement scheme.

HTA recommendations compiled over several years from six different agencies illustrate these differences, with a special focus on central nervous system (CNS) drugs, cancer drugs, and orphan drugs. In the case of CNS treatments for example, only 24% received consistent recommendations from all six agencies, while the remaining 76% got a mix of positive and negative recommendations.[21] The number of drugs and the indications appraised also varied across countries (Figure 14). The same trend was identified in cancer treatments as well as in orphan drugs.

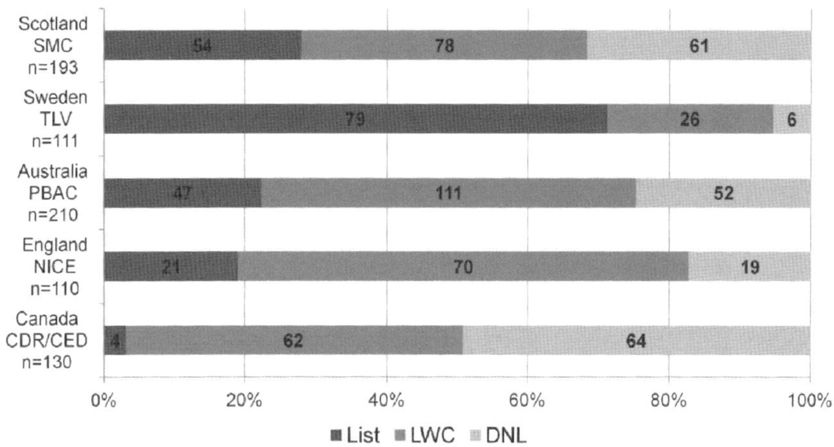

Figure 14. HTA similarities and differences in recommendations in 5 countries, 2010

Source: Kanavos *et al*. (2010). EuroObserver, December.

[21]HTA recommendations per drug and per indication are divided into three levels: (1) Positive recommendation, where the treatment is reimbursed as applied for, (2) positive recommendation with criteria, where the treatment is reimbursed with restrictions (i.e., to a subgroup of the population, or when prescribed by a specialist), (3) negative recommendation, when the treatment is rejected for reimbursement.

Several reasons exist for these variations. First, the selection criteria of the drugs for which an HTA is conducted differ across agencies. In the UK, for example, all drugs are potentially reimbursable once they receive a market authorization; of the drugs that are approved each year, only a fraction are appraised by NICE, its HTA body, based on a series of selection criteria, including need and likely high impact on NHS resources. In contrast, all drugs are appraised in France and Australia, and all newly licensed drugs and new indications are appraised in Scotland. In countries where not all drugs are appraised periodically, a risk exists that some of the drugs reimbursed that haven't been appraised are not cost-effective.

Second, the duration of HTA processes may delay access to certain treatments, especially in countries where these processes are longer (i.e., 32 to 56 weeks in the England vs. 17 to 18 weeks in Sweden). Negative recommendations may cause additional delays, since most often the manufacturer will appeal against the decision and/or resubmit its application. When price negotiations are included in the HTA process, additional delays may also be incurred. However, the timeliness of HTAs may on one hand give patients faster access to promising technologies, but on the other may be based on earlier evidence that may induce uncertainties in the appraisals. It is important that balance is maintained in this regard.

Third, there is limited amount of evidence available, and, in particular, a lack of long-term data resulting in uncertainties and gaps in the evidence. In the case of cancer drugs, HTA agencies may respond in a number of ways when faced with these uncertainties, all of which can vary across countries: (1) By focusing on a sub-group population or a narrowed-down indication for which the evidence is more certain, (2) by including indirect comparisons or expert opinions to supplement the evidence, (3) by deferring the decisions until further evidence is available, (4) by rejecting the application, (5) by pressuring the manufacturer to decrease its prices, or (6) by implementing RSAs (Pomedli, 2010; Kanavos *et al.*, 2010).

In other cases, as seen mostly in cancer and orphan drugs, positive recommendations (including positive with criteria) were granted in particular cases, although there was a high level of uncertainty in the evidence. This was often seen in cases where few or no other alternative treatments exist, when patient need is high and the severity of the disease is significant (Pomedli, 2010; Van den Aardweg, 2010).

Diverging interpretation of the same evidence has also shown to cause differences in HTA outcomes. For example, when assessing the efficacy of a treatment against schizophrenia, different weights and permutations of the type of evidence considered were identified. Some agencies considered mainly the primary clinical endpoint, whereas others chose the primary and secondary endpoints, the latter including a measure for quality of life. Moreover, different economic models and comparators were used for a same drug and same indication. As a result, considering all the above in addition to the uncertainties emerging from cost-effectiveness pricing discussed earlier, many reasons for diverging interpretations of the same evidence may exist resulting in possible differing HTA outcomes (Nicod and Kanavos, 2012).

Fourth, the lack of transparency in the processes may also impair manufacturers in their applications, for whom the submission requirements may not be clear, resulting in possible negative appraisals. Moreover, the level of stakeholder involvement has also shown to be limited, with potentially negative impacts on HTA decisions or recommendations (Drummond *et al.*, 2008).

Finally, the effective implementation of HTA recommendations has also shown to be variable depending on the advisory or regulatory role of the HTA agency. In the case of Sweden, where the national HTA agency is a regulatory body whose decisions are to be adopted by the county councils, not all county councils are able to afford all reimbursement decisions, thus resulting in national differences as far as reimbursed treatments are concerned.

Overall, HTAs are complex processes with many stages and involving many stakeholders. One should keep in mind that at each stage different factors may influence HTAs outcomes, thus affecting the affordability and accessibility of these treatments. Different initiatives have been implemented at international and EU level to work on improving HTAs. In Europe, for example, the EUnetHTA collaboration is an initiative launched in 2008 aiming to develop an effective and sustainable HTA collaboration in Europe, through: (1) Reducing duplications of efforts and improve the efficiency in the use of resources; (2) increasing the impact of HTA in EU Member States; (3) strengthening the link between HTA and health care policymaking; and (4) supporting countries with little experience in HTAs.[22] These initiatives intend to harmonize or standardize the HTA processes so to improve their level of transparency, quality and comprehensiveness, and facilitate the extraction of relevant information that can then be transferred cross-border.

The impact of RSAs

The number of RSAs has proliferated in recent years, particularly in Europe, North America and Australia, and they are increasingly implemented in emerging countries (Figure 15). For example, there are already cases of RSAs in Turkey, South Korea and Brazil, whereas the countries such as Malaysia, Mexico and Colombia, among others, are examining their introduction. A recent study suggests that the most common RSAs among European countries are price–volume agreements (PVAs), accounting for 39% of total RSAs (used extensively in Italy,

[22] European Network for Health Technology Assessments. Overview of results. 2009.

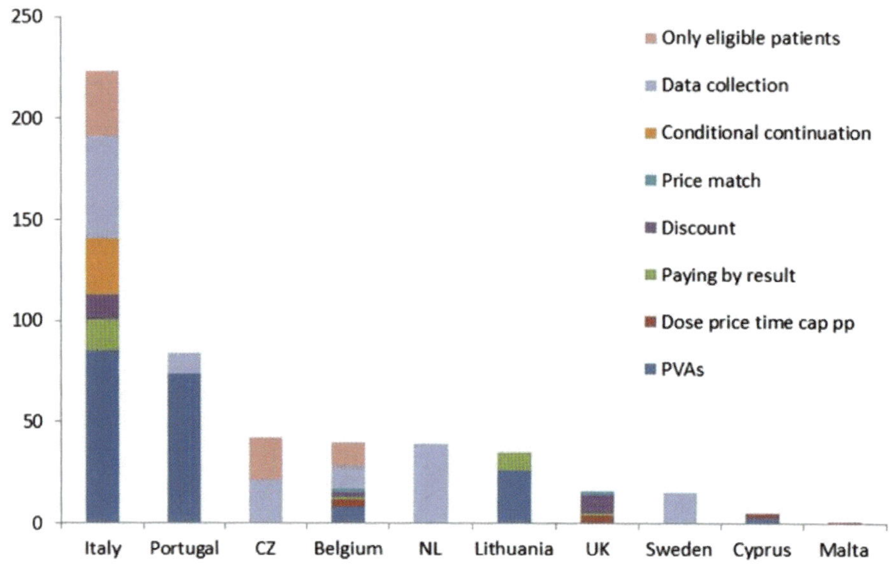

Figure 15. Types of MEAs in European countries, 2013
Source: Ferrario and Kanavos (2013).

France and Portugal, among others), followed by requirements for data collection (29%), particularly in Italy, the Czech Republic, the Netherlands and Sweden and limiting access to eligible patients only (13%) (Ferrario and Kanavos, 2013). Furthermore, conditional continuation (6%) is frequently used in Italy; discounts (5%) are prevalent in Italy and England; and payment-by-results arrangements (5%) are used in Italy and Lithuania. Evidence shows that RSAs are increasingly used in reimbursement decisions for orphan drugs (Morel *et al.*, 2013).

RSAs are often used for high-cost patented drugs, for which there is limited evidence of effectiveness in a non-controlled environment and of their long-term effects. A significant proportion of RSAs (37%) surround antineoplastic and immune-modulating agents (Morel *et al.*, 2013). An evaluation of all 42 patient access schemes (the designation used for RSAs in the United Kingdom) that the Scottish Medicines Consortium (SMC) had engaged up to April 2012 confirmed that most of the schemes focused on antineoplastic products, followed by medicines for musculoskeletal diseases, infectious diseases, eye diseases and diseases of the central nervous system. While drawing on incentives from both financial and health outcome-based RSAs, most of these patient access schemes were simple financial-based schemes involving discounts or rebates as opposed to more complex financial schemes involving, for instance, price capping or performance/outcome-based schemes (Wladysiuk *et al.*, 2013).

RSAs offer the possibility of negotiating a more favorable price for a treatment characterized by significant uncertainty and, thereby, enable access to patients, subject to confidentiality of some of the arrangements. However, the burden of managing RSAs relies on the complexity of an agreement; notoriously, payment for performance and coverage with evidence development schemes have been among the most burdensome to implement. Early research findings in 2009 showed that 73% of United Kingdom hospitals did not have the capacity to manage current schemes (Williamson, 2010). The administrative burden, lack of communication and concerns with passing on savings were highlighted as key issues with some of the schemes for cancer drugs in the United Kingdom. Meanwhile, some of these agreements have been changed to simple discount schemes, and all new agreements the department of health has engaged since 2011 are either simple discounts or free stock agreements. In this context, greater flexibility around the time limits for processing claims was deemed crucial and good communication between key stakeholders important (Adamski *et al.*, 2010; Williamson, 2010).

An analysis of strengths, weaknesses, opportunities and threats highlighted that among RSAs' strengths is their ability to help address post-licensing uncertainty and to enable access to innovative treatments in a context of uncertainty (Ferrario and Kanavos, 2013; 2015). In general, RSAs offer more flexibility than other pricing methods, and combine both financial and nonfinancial elements to address different issues. Further, RSAs can help increase the evidence base of the therapy in question by agreements such as coverage with evidence development. Pure financial agreements such as price/dose capping and price match help improve the cost-effectiveness of a new intervention. This enables health care payers to control the impact on budgets better, improve use and increase access to medicines. Similarly, RSAs enable manufacturers to obtain reimbursement for drugs that otherwise would be rejected.

Despite these strengths, several weaknesses remain: First, there is little evidence to support the claimed benefits of RSAs in practice and the extent to which some of the challenges involved in RSAs affect the financial outcome. Second, lack of transparency in the agreements implemented, their objectives and evaluation of their impact prevents cross-country learning and limits patients' ability to engage in RSA processes. The opportunities for RSAs are many. Many countries collect useful data but few leverage this opportunity, and continuity in collecting the data is often lacking. Countries could benefit from increasing efforts to re-evaluate the effectiveness of the drugs, streamline post-marketing studies with data collection requirements as part of RSAs and adaptive licensing, increase transparency in agreements and create formal channels for involvement of patient representatives.

Finally, countries must be cautious not to adopt RSAs as quick fixes or *ad hoc* solutions that are not integrated into a comprehensive process for introducing new medicines, but should ensure that MEAs are used with long-term perspectives in mind. Health authorities must be careful not to allow for "playing the system".

- *The effectiveness of generic policies*

The significant increase in pharmaceutical expenditure over the past 20 years, both in absolute terms and as a percent of total health spending has forced governments and health insurers to look for options to curb the rate of growth of pharmaceutical spending. Generic medicines can play an important role in curbing rising pharmaceutical costs and their cost-saving potential is significant as they provide both a lower-priced option for prescribers and patients and a tool to drive-down prices of originator drugs. Evidence suggests that across OECD countries over 65% of the pharmaceutical market comprises off-patent medicines (Kanavos, 2008) and this share is likely to be higher in emerging and developing countries. Consequently, a robust generic policy should be impactful in terms of both macro- and micro-economic efficiency. Governments and health insurers implement combinations of supply-, proxy demand- and demand-side policies aiming to increase the diffusion and use of generics as well as maximize their price effect. Through competition after loss of exclusivity of the originator (patent expiry, expiry of data exclusivity period), generic drug entry and diffusion are expected to influence both the price and volume share of branded products (Garattini and Tediosi, 2000; Danzon and Furukawa, 2003).

There are two important considerations, however, with regards to the implementation of a robust generics policy. The first is that such a policy comprises a set of measures and metrics spanning the entire spectrum of pharmaceutical policy, from elements of intellectual property rights protection all the way to direct or indirect incentives for patients on drug selection. The second is that the structures must be in place for governments or health insurers to link the different components in an integrated, yet coherent, policy framework. Table 7 outlines the range of policies followed by seven key OECD countries and shows the significant range between supply-side and demand-side measures. Whereas the range of options on both the supply- and the demand-side is significant, the emphasis is often on the supply-side. Yet, if generic policies are to be successful, it is crucial that the demand-side operates in a way that is acceptable to key stakeholders. For example, if there is little information to patients about generics, it is unlikely that they will consider it to be a viable treatment option, despite what health care professionals may tell them. Additionally, incentive structures do need to be aligned. For example, progressive markups of paying pharmacies would never encourage generic substitution. The issue of quality is absolutely critical in this context. If patients and/or health care professionals perceive generics to be of inferior quality that the originators, they will never be prescribed or used. It is, therefore, crucial that regulatory standards

Table 7. Generic pharmaceutical policies in 7 OECD countries, 2015

Policy measure	**UK**	**Germany**	**France**	**Italy**	**Spain**	**USA**	**Canada**
Supply-side policies							
Bolar-type regulation	✓	✓	✓	✓	✓	✓	✓
Robust regulation for the proof of bioequivalence, biosimilarity and GMP standards enforcement	✓	✓	✓	✓	✓	✓	✓
Market exclusivity of first generic						✓	
Price cap linked to originator prices[1]	✓		✓	✓	✓		
Free pricing for (most) generics	✓	✓				✓	✓
Internal reference pricing (molecular)[2]		✓	✓	✓	✓		✓
Internal reference pricing (therapeutic)[2]		✓					
Tendering in outpatient markets		✓					
Managed competition[3]							
Proxy demand-side policies							
Promoting Generic prescibing[4]	✓	✓	✓		✓	✓	✓
Compulsory generic prescibing[5]	✓						
Explicit prescribing guidance (can be linked to incentives or targets)	✓		✓			✓	
Prescribing monitoring and audit[6]	✓	✓	✓	✓	✓	✓	✓
Generic substitution at pharmacy[7]		✓	✓	✓	✓	✓	✓
Flat fee combined with regressive margin for pharmacies		✓	✓	✓	✓		
Flat fee per prescription at pharmacy level	✓					✓	✓
Discounting allowed at pharmacy level[8]	✓		✓			✓	✓
Clawback in operation[9]	✓						
Demand-side policies							
Differential co-payments[10]						✓	
Co-insurance[11] or flat fee[12]	✓	✓	✓	✓	✓		✓

Notes: [1] Refers to the Maximum Price Scheme (MPS) in the UK, which applies to a limited number of generic medicines, as per the regulation of 1999. In the other countries where it applies, generics are subject to an official maximum (list) price, which cannot be exceed a certain proportion of the branded price. It is a command-and-control measure designed to guarantee savings by switching to a generic product.

(Continued)

Table 7. (*Continued*)

[2]The Reference Price is the maximum amount that health insurance will pay for a particular product. The dates of introduction differ considerably by country, as does the definition of what reference pricing clusters encompass and the extent to which such clusters can include in-patent products (molecules). Molecular reference pricing refers to all available options for a given molecule and constitutes a narrow definition of reference pricing, whereas therapeutic reference pricing refers to the clustering of molecules within a therapeutic class (e.g., statins) and reimbursing a generic from the available options. Therapeutic reference pricing may include options (molecules), which are still covered by a patent.
[3]Refers to the stepwise reduction of the maximum price, (e.g., 5% or 10%) if additional generic entry occurs.
[4]Generic prescribing is not compulsory, but is in some way promoted by health insurance. This is usually combined with reference pricing and the latter implies that patients will need to be informed about cheaper as well as more costly choices.
[5]Generic prescribing is compulsory as a policy, unless there are no generic alternatives available, or unless the physician believes the originator drug should be dispensed; the policy usually also applies to in-patent products, where physicians are required to prescribe by international non-proprietary name (INN).
[6]Although all countries report prescribing monitoring and audit, there is significant variability in how that takes place in each country. In the majority of cases, prescribing audit concerns only prescribing outliers; occasionally, it may lead to sanctions to those found to consistently over-prescribe relative to their peers.
[7]This refers to the extent to which pharmacists are allowed to substitute for a cheaper product (generic) if the physician has prescribed by brandname. Substitution rights have been extended since the mid- to late-1990s in many OECD countries and apply more extensively as opposed to "emergencies only," or "subject to physician approval", although some physician autonomy still exists if the "dispense as written" box on the prescription exists and has been ticked.
[8]Reflects the extent to which discounts are officially allowed and practiced, in addition to officially set margins.
[9]Refers to health insurance retrieving part of the discount given from manufacturers or wholesalers to pharmacies.
[10]Co-payments may vary according to the type of drug being dispensed. For example, generics usually attract a lower co-payment compared with the branded version of the same medicine. This type of cost-sharing has been in operation for a long time in the USA and was implemented in Germany in 2007, as a means of encouraging generic use.
[11]As they apply, with exceptions for certain categories of insurees, in France and Spain.
[12]This is a flat fee per prescription (for instance, as it applies in the UK or some regions in Italy), or a flat fee per pack (for instance, as it applies in Germany).

Source: P. Kanavos.

around proof of bioequivalence or proof of biosimilarity or good manufacturing practice (GMP) are robust and are enforced. One typical problem that many developing and several middle income countries face is that their regulatory agencies are weak and/or do not have the resources to enforce what is already in legislation.

Despite the above range of policies outlined, the performance of individual health systems on the range of generic policies applied is inconclusive. The literature on the influence of generic competition on originator brand name prices and market share is somewhat divided. While some studies (Caves *et al.*, 1997; Wiggins and Maness, 2004), have found that the price response to generic entry is as expected, in that originator prices decline following generic entry, others have found that prices of originator brands may rise upon generic entry (Frank and Salkever 1997; Regan, 2008; Vandoros and Kanavos, 2013). In addition, while increased competition between generic producers has been found to decrease prices of generic drugs, the price of branded drugs is not necessarily reduced by increased generic competition (Dalen *et al.*, 2006). It has also been shown that originator brand manufacturers do not respond to generic market entry by decreasing prices, but rather generic entry may correspond to a decrease in the speed of originator price increase (Grabowski and Vernon, 1992; Rizzo, 1999). Evidence also suggests that manufacturers will often not compete on price once generic competitors enter the market (Frank and Salkever, 1997; Cook *et al.*, 1998). Similar concerns exist about the price levels achieved and the rate of price decline following generic entry. The literature points to significant price declines after generic entry (Grabowski and Vernon, 1992; Rizzo, 1999; Cook *et al.*, 1998); yet it has been argued that different forms of regulation may have an effect on the amplitude of such a price decline and the generic market share (Danzon and Chao, 2000b; Grabowski and Vernon, 1992; Glowicka *et al.*, 2009). The interface between competition and regulation seems to lead to different pricing outcomes across countries; for example, whereas price variation for originator brands in ambulatory markets was found to be 2- to 3-fold between highest- and lowest-priced country, price variation for generics was found to be 5- to 20-fold between highest- and lowest-priced country (Kanavos *et al.*, 2011).

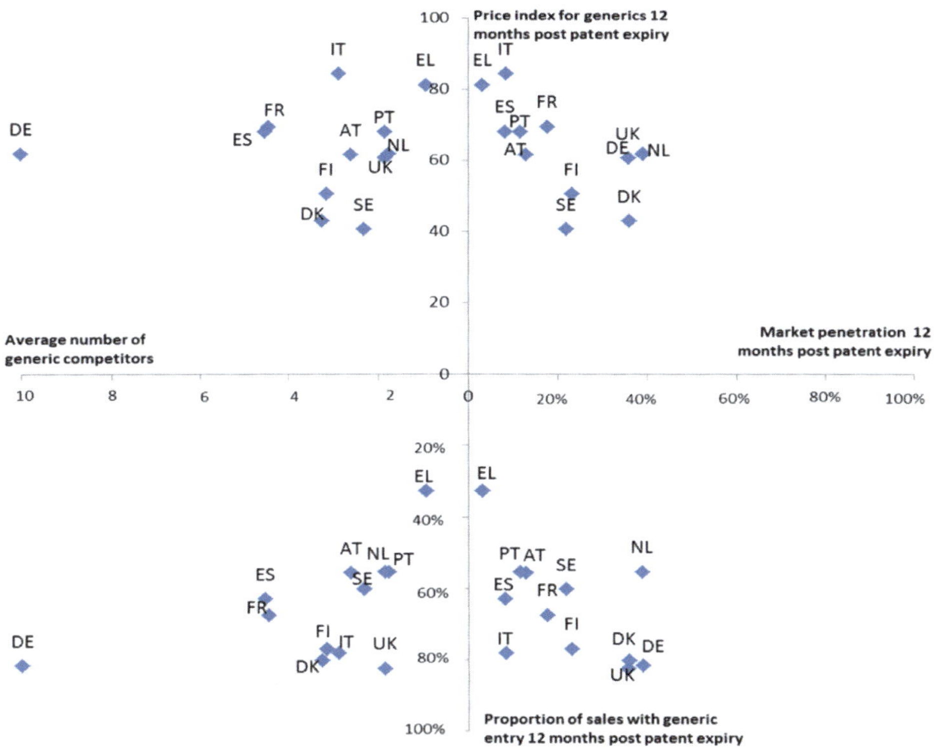

Figure 16. Summary of generic policy performance indicators across 12 EU Member States
Source: Kanavos (2014). *Health Policy.*

In a recent study, an attempt was made to summarize a set of performance indicators that would be meaningful and would capture the performance of generic policies in a number of European settings (Kanavos, 2014). The indicators comprise of: (a) the availability of generics post-patent expiry, which is linked to the time delay to generic entry, (b) the number of generic competitors at different points post-patent expiry, (c) the price developments for originators and generics post-patent expiry, and (d) the amplitude of generic penetration at different points post-patent expiry. Optimal performance would suggest that price declines should be really steep and fastest, while generic penetration should be fast and capture a significant share of the product market. This framework was subsequently tested across 12 EU countries and Figure 16 shows how each country fared with regards to these indicators. It appears that very few perform well across the range of indicators proposed and that those who perform best also have in place a coherent set of policy measures to capture the potential of generics. A further finding is that there are still savings to be had even in those circumstances where decision makers believe that these are maximized. Overall, generic penetration is greater in countries with free pricing systems, yet countries could benefit from employing both demand- and supply-side policies to reduce generic prices and decrease the time to generic entry. Relaxing supply-side regulation on generic medicines, particularly in large markets, may also contribute to price reduction.

Other measures for inclusion of new medicines into reimbursement

Increasingly, governments and health insurers are resorting to additional measures in order, on the one hand, to address high and increasing costs, while on the other to offer the opportunity of access to new compounds that address (significant) unmet medical need, but whose clinical and/or cost-effectiveness evidence is debatable. In this context, there have been initiatives, such as the special fund for orphan drugs in Scotland (to enable access to high-cost orphan medicines), the cancer drugs fund in England (which includes cancer medicines that have been cost-ineffective by NICE, but are available on a patient-by-patient basis) and similar approaches in Belgium. In a similar fashion, countries such as France and Germany consider the benefit of a new orphan medicine as "given", if the fiscal impact of each orphan does not exceed €30 million and €50 million, respectively. If it does, then a complete assessment will need to take place. These approaches highlight the need by governments and health insurers to have a sense of predictability in pharmaceutical expenditure.

At the same time, some countries have formalised procedures allowing access to novel therapies very early on and, in some cases, before marketing authorization is granted. One such regulatory provision is the temporary authorization for USA (ATU) in France, which has existed since 1994. ATUs have made it possible to treat tens of thousands of patients per year, several months before MA. The diseases most frequently concerned are cancers, infectious diseases such as AIDS, and neurological diseases. For example, all the new antiretroviral drugs have been available in France by ATU an average of 12 months before the MA decision, for around 6000 patients per medicinal product. Since 1994, more than 400 medicinal products have been the subject of applications for an ATU and a benefit/risk ratio assessment. These may concern medicinal products already authorized abroad or drugs that are still under development (AFSSAPS, 2001).

Access to medicines at EU level

Access to medicines is determined by two factors, first, the affordability of medicines, which is the extent to which health insurance covers the (pharmaceutical) needs of patients in an adequate manner and at affordable cost; and, second, the availability of prescribed medicines (or the medicines of choice) at appropriate outlets. The implications of these two dimensions and their relevance to prices are discussed below.

- *Affordability*

Co-payments

The affordability of pharmaceuticals varies across countries as a result of the variance in national GDP, GDP per capita and available health budgets. The affordability of a drug at the patient level is dependent on the extent to which a drug is covered by the health insurer, combined with the cost-sharing burden placed on the patient. Patient co-payments for pharmaceuticals are a form of direct cost-sharing meant to mediate demand and/or generate revenue for the health system.

The introduction of co-payments may reduce demand for health services, while pharmaceutical co-payments may reduce the demand for essential drugs, and even more so for discretionary or symptomatic drugs (Rubin and Mendelson, 1995; Brook *et al.*, 2006). The same studies found, however, that cost-sharing systems reduce the demand disproportionately amongst the poor. As a response, there are exemptions for various groups including children, the elderly and those with low-income. Moreover, because the burden of co-payments will be most disenfranchising for those with lower levels of health, there are further exemptions for certain types of pharmaceuticals. For example, many countries provide drugs treating chronic and fatal diseases free of charge.

Evidence on the likely impact of co-payments on affordability in developed countries is scarce, but there are indications that such an impact exists. A recent WHO study suggests that high co-payments are restricting drug affordability and availability. Specifically, at 43% effective prescription-only medicines (POM) co-payments in Estonia seem to be higher than in most other EU countries and are posing an affordability barrier; the majority of medicines dispensed are subject to some form of co-insurance and about 50% of all prescriptions dispensed are subject to a 50% co-insurance. Treatments for a number of chronic diseases are subject to a 25% co-insurance (75% coverage), whereas differential co-payments also exist depending on the provider visited (whether the patient visits a GP or a specialist) (Kanavos *et al.*, 2009). Interviews with stakeholders suggest that high prices of (new) medicines pose a significant affordability problem to health insurance systems in several EU Member States and can also expose patients to high and unaffordable co-payments.

Overall, the use of co-payments as a cost-containment method remains an issue of debate considering its potential influence on affordability and thus access to pharmaceuticals, especially for vulnerable populations. Co-payments must be set at a level that does not restrict access but which promotes rational drug use. It is suggested that a reduction in the level of co-payments could be achieved by promoting rational drug use, cost-effective prescribing and patient awareness of cheaper therapeutic options at the pharmacy.

Coverage decisions by HTA bodies

The impact of a negative HTA recommendation is substantial in terms of pricing, R&D incentives and access to a given treatment. Substantial differences in terms of coverage recommendations and decisions from HTAs have been reported. Minimizing such differences in recommendations requires significant effort and may have significant implications for access.

Not all HTA agencies assess all the drugs reimbursed. Since their role is to identify ineffective and cost-ineffective treatments as well, it is important to understand how many of these "cost-ineffective" treatments are still being reimbursed and to what extent the amount spent on these treatments is used inefficiently. It could hence be useful to assess all drugs that are reimbursed, either periodically or each time a new treatment in the same therapeutic class comes onto the market (although the latter option would be somewhat costly).

HTAs are most often based on the treatment's clinical-cost-effectiveness. Measurement of costs and effects determines the HTA outcome. Efforts could be made to understand costs from both a health service and a societal perspective, by taking into account the direct and indirect costs from the treatment. When measuring effects, aspects such as effect on the quality of life of the patient or the severity of the disease could be considered in addition to efficiency.

Early communication and collaboration between HTA agencies and manufacturers may help to improve the reimbursement application and result in possible better HTA outcomes. In a similar direction, monitoring potential launches of new medicines (Horizon Scanning) could be of value to all governments as well as institutions by providing knowledge and understanding of the types of treatments that are likely to emerge in the mid- to long-term.

Gauging the long-term clinical impact of new treatments is most important for European society and, probably an issue of supra-national competence. Whereas the evidence on which marketing authorization and coverage are decided rests on efficacy, it is important to understand how treatments work in the community (i.e., effectiveness). In a number of priority areas, where additional evidence may be required, nation-wide registries could be fostered to help inform the process of decision-making. For this to take place, initiatives would be beneficial regarding methodologies and priority areas.

The implementation and impact of HTA depends greatly on whether the HTA agency is a regulatory or advisory body. In the latter case, it is essential that the recommendations are communicated in a clear, simple and transparent way, to enable well-informed decision-making. In addition, clear guidelines on HTA procedures and requirements may improve the quality of the clinical and economic evidence as well as manufacturer compliance, thus reducing information costs. Further, transparency in the appraisals is likely to encourage stakeholder compliance with associated recommendations.

- *Availability*

The availability of medicines is dictated by supply- and demand-side factors, such as levels of drug use, overall expenditure on medicines, drug prices, as well as more wide-ranging factors including market structure, regulatory policies, and cultural practices. As a result of variation in these factors, drug availability varies between countries. In this context, it is important to distinguish between the number of authorized pharmaceuticals and the number of authorized pharmaceuticals actually available on the market. In many countries, notably Portugal, Greece and Austria, the number of available pharmaceuticals is smaller than the number of authorized pharmaceuticals (GOEG, 2007–2014). Research has also revealed this is the case in many countries in Eastern Europe, where new products are not being launched by manufacturers. Such differences between authorized and available pharmaceuticals may be the result of three issues: First, drug companies apply for drug authorization but do no not market the drug in each country, fearing that price regulation by means of EPR will jeopardize their pricing strategies elsewhere and, in the European context, this could also lead to parallel trade; second, for generic products, several applications for the same product are often submitted by business consultancies, in order to be sold to generic companies once authorisation is received; and third, not all forms and pack sizes of pharmaceuticals products will be marketed in each country. While data availability issues complicate direct comparisons, it has been found that the number of medicines available varies across the EU, with the greatest number available in Germany and the UK, with the least available in the Scandinavian countries (Folino-Gallo *et al.*, 2001). Three main concerns for drug availability, relate to the availability of drugs in small markets, the potential for parallel trade, the delay in concluding reimbursement negotiations and the lack of availability of generic alternatives.

Access to pharmaceuticals in small markets

Despite the growth in pharmaceutical consumption over the past 20 years, overall access to pharmaceuticals is significantly lower in smaller markets. Such limited access is a result of several factors influenced by historical context, national budgets, and reimbursement policies on the supply-side, as well as local market size, and national language on the demand-side. For example, the additional costs of translation of information and labelling of medicinal products, may not in the long-term, appear profitable enough for pharmaceutical companies to apply for, or renew, their market authorization. Regulatory bodies are not necessarily in a position to force manufacturers to market any medicinal products, nor are there legal instruments allowing them to handle and solve such situations. Issues of pharmaceutical availability due to expired market authorization can be overcome by policies which allow physicians or professional bodies to request and procure drugs from other countries for individual patients. While this is a likely solution there are two significant barriers: First, application processes can be cumbersome and time consuming and, second, the affordability of the drug may be compromised as unauthorized drugs may not be considered for reimbursement and patients will have to pay out-of-pocket.

Differential pricing and parallel trade

Pharmaceutical price regulation has led to significant price differences. In circumstances where arbitrage is allowed — due to exhaustion of IP rights, whether this is national, regional or global — parallel trade takes place. In the European Union, where regional exhaustion of rights exists, parallel trade has also perceived as a cost-containment mechanism by policymakers in some countries, and this practice has in some cases been encouraged (West and Mahon, 2003; Kanavos and Costa-Font, 2005). For example, in the Netherlands, health insurance would share any price difference between locally sourced and parallel traded products with pharmacists; in Germany quotas were used to force pharmacists to sell parallel-traded drugs, although this is no longer the case.

Evidence suggests that parallel trade does not lead to significant savings for health insurance, as parallel traded products are usually priced at the same level or very close to the corresponding locally sourced ones (Kanavos, 2008; Kanavos and Costa-Font, 2005).

In practice, profits accrue to the supply chain, and little or no savings accrue to health insurance (Kanavos, 2008). It has also been shown that parallel trade does not necessarily trigger price competition that would lead to a sustainable price reduction and equilibrium; therefore, locally sourced products are not priced at lower levels as a result of parallel trade (Kanavos and Vandoros, 2010).

One of the unintended consequences of parallel trade is that it can lead to shortages in exporting countries, due to medicines being exported to countries where prices are higher. This has had an impact on availability and access in exporting countries and there have been cases (e.g., in Greece) of temporary export bans in order for the market to stabilize. Further, it has been suggested that parallel trade can be a threat to innovation and lead to significant welfare losses (Danzon, 1998; Bordoy and Jelovac, 2003; Rey, 2003; Ganslandt and Maskus, 2004; Szymanski and Valletti, 2005), as it reduces the expected profits from an innovative product. A further issue arising from parallel trade is the likelihood of counterfeiting. Parallel traders often repackage medicines in order to help sell them in the destination countries. However, this increases the threat of counterfeiting. Repackaging can give the opportunity to criminals to disguise counterfeit medicines (Davies, 2009).

Delays in pricing and reimbursement negotiations

Delays in pricing and reimbursement negotiations can act both as a disincentive for innovation and as a barrier to access by leading to differential availability between countries. For example, within the EU, the time elapsing between market authorisation by the European Medicines Agency (EMA) and accessibility (date of completion of pricing/reimbursement) ranges from 101 to 403 days (Ashworth *et al.*, 2002; Bloor and Freemantle, 1996)[23] and can have an impact on access and availability in many Member States. HTAs are often carrying a significant part of the burden in this context, particularly those processes that are 'consultative' in nature, as they can delay considerably access to new products.

Generic drug availability

Overall access to and affordability of pharmaceutical treatments is influenced by the availability of cheap generic alternatives to expensive branded drugs. Generic

[23] Excludes Germany and the UK.

availability can be examined by the level of generic competition, the time delay to generic entry and demand for generics as dictated by physicians and pharmacies. Very frequently, the cheapest alternative is not available at the pharmacy; under these circumstances, a more expensive medicine will be dispensed, at a higher cost to the patient and, possibly, health insurance. Evidence suggests that the optimal window of opportunity to capitalize on generic availability is the period 1–3 years after patent expiry, beyond which alternative therapeutic options may attract the interest of practicing physicians.

In addition to the proportion of molecules and sales facing generic competition, another component of the generic market that influences availability is the time delay to market entry; that is the time elapsed between originator patent expiry and patient access to a generic alternative. In Europe, the European Commission's Inquiry into the Pharmaceutical Sector (European Commission, 2009) concluded that it takes on average seven months for generic medicines to become available, which, if reduced could result in an additional 20% savings on pharmaceutical expenditure. While time delays are influenced by several factors, the role of pharmaceutical companies and some of the strategies they employ may inhibit early entry and delay generic penetration. These strategies include the creation of "patent clusters" (strategic patenting), prolonging patent litigation and lodging complaints to national authorities claiming patent right violations (European Commission, 2009).

- *Concluding remark on access*

Access to new medicines is often hindered or delayed by HTA processes, which is also impacting the price of these medicines. Faster access to promising treatments is enabled with rapid completion of HTAs and speedy implementation of the recommendations. This can also result in potentially large savings, by a faster and more efficient allocation of resources. In reality, processes in some agencies are longer (i.e., 32–56 weeks in the UK) than in others (17–18 weeks in Sweden). When price negotiations are included in the HTA processes, this may create further delays. Conversely, HTA recommendations that are issued earlier rely on a less evidence. Striking the right balance involves enabling fast access to treatments as well as the production of sufficient evidence for reliable HTA.

Both availability and affordability are influenced by explicit decisions to fund (or not) a particular medicine based on the medicine's cost and willingness-to-pay by competent health authorities in a particular health system. Several countries examining precisely the same clinical and economic evidence may come up with opposite funding/reimbursement decisions. Varying eligibility criteria also seem to be creating a differential rationing situation, which impacts patient access on affordability grounds.

Availability and affordability may also depend on decisions made at regional level, following initial guidance or recommendation to fund a particular treatment at national level. Based on this, it is possible for certain regions in one Member State to adopt a new treatment that has received a positive HTA recommendation, while others reject it, thus creating an uneven playing field within a Member State. Differential outcomes of this type may need to be carefully examined.

Incentives and physician performance

The influence of demand-side policies on physician performance in many EU Member States is limited and complicated by several factors including: (1) Generic prescribing and financial and non-financial incentives are relatively new in many Member States, or have undergone significant changes since their initial implementation, (2) prescribing policies vary significantly across Member States, (3) such policies are often implemented simultaneously with other organizational restructuring or supply-side policies, and (4) the evaluation is constrained by a lack of comprehensive information systems tracking prescriptions.

The evidence available from the UK, Germany and France, provides a basis for some broad conclusions and further research in the area. In the UK, studies have found that while the introduction of fundholding and financial incentives led to containment in the overall prescribing costs, it was not accompanied by similar improvements in the quality of prescribing. Conversely, financial incentives could be directly linked to increased quality and appropriateness of prescribing. The size of financial incentives is not correlated with the magnitude of change or improvement in costs or quality of prescribing. Therefore, further research is needed to clarify the relationship between the size, and character of incentives, which are required to effectively alter prescribing behavior (Ashworth *et al.*, 2002). In Germany, budgetary restrictions implemented in 1993 initially caused a substantial decline in the number of prescriptions. Prescription levels quickly returned to their previous levels, following sluggish policy implementation and enforcement, although it is suggested that they led to a 10% savings on the drug budget (though this cannot be attributed to demand-side policies alone, especially considering studies suggesting that physicians may have shifted costs by referring more patients to hospitals (Bloor and Freemantle, 1996). In France, surveys suggest that the system of guidelines attached to small financial incentives or penalties has reduced prescribing of certain drugs, even though more rigorous analysis is still required.

The evidence, albeit limited, indicates that incentives can work, but that several components require further scrutiny. It is, therefore, suggested that the following areas be investigated further: First, the aims and targets of each demand-side policies and the desired impact on performance must clarified; second, more comprehensive follow-up systems must be implemented to accurately record change in prescribing costs and behavior; and third, transparent measurement tools must be developed to assess physician performance. This research is necessary to identify both the intended and unintended impact of demand-side policies on physician behavior.

Conclusion

This chapter has demonstrated that there are many different approaches to regulating pharmaceuticals in different settings that affect public policy objectives to control costs while also aiming to improve efficiency, quality of care, access and equity.

Governments and health insurers are faced with rising pharmaceutical expenditures but have taken widely divergent approaches to addressing these. Some policies aimed at enhancing quality of care, efficiency or access may decrease the ability to contain the rate of growth of expenditures. Rising expenditures in themselves may not be a problem if they are accompanied by economic growth, health gain and/or by a similar rise in revenues to governments or health insurers. In practice, the added health gain for added expenditure is often unclear and liable to subjective interpretation. The discussion in this chapter has highlighted that no single policy approach acts without a trade-off on the impact along the key policy objectives (macroeconomic efficiency, technical efficiency, quality and equity in access), in addition to competing trade-offs between the objectives of the policies themselves.

Many of the measures presented and discussed in the preceding sections were found to have some impact on costs and cost containment. However, the extent of any cost savings or their sustainability over the longer term is variable — this is the case, for example, of external price referencing or of HTAs and their application in different settings. In other cases, the cost-saving potential of interventions is questionable; this was the case, for example in cost effectiveness pricing and risk sharing agreements. In the majority of cases the cost savings generated by any one policy are either limited or short-term. The most effective approaches work best when combined with other policy measures. For instance, price fixing alone has a limited effect, but it is more successful when policies are applied to the volume side of the expenditure equation as well.

As health systems have become increasingly risk-averse and increasingly demand certainty about the effectiveness of resources allocated to specific uses, risk-sharing and other certainty-enhancing mechanisms can offer insights into government/insurer and supplier behavior, while enabling (selective) access to costly treatments. It is more likely than not that the quality of the evidence required in the future in order to make an informed decision about coverage will increase significantly. This is also predicted by changes in regulatory approvals and the conduct of some of the pivotal clinical trials in real life settings in the near future.

At the same time, it appears that health systems have not exhausted opportunities to generate savings on existing budgets. This can be achieved either through action on the supply-side, for example, by exerting pressure on prices of generics, or/and by promoting further demand-side policies that result in greater generic penetration. The latter can be achieved by refining the incentive structures of health care professionals and patients, as well as having the appropriate monitoring and enforcement mechanisms in place.

Importantly, it appears that health systems will need to make important resource allocation decisions in the near future. If health gains from new and novel treatments increase substantially, it will become necessary to dis-invest faster in other components of the health care system. Typically, health care budgets, whether in pharmaceutical, ambulatory or in-patient care, are characterized by both inertia and silo effects. The recent improvements in pharmaceutical care delivery and the expected improvements in health care outcomes may imply that inertias and silo budgeting may need to be done away with.

Acknowledgments

In writing this chapter, I have benefited from conversations, inputs and comments from many colleagues and am grateful for their feedback and support: Aris Angelis, Alessandra Ferrario, Hanne Bak-Pedersen, Elena Nicod, Julien Gagnon, Kumar Perampaladas, Olivier Wouters, and Sotiris Vandoros. I am grateful to Erica Visintin for excellent research assistance. All outstanding errors are my own.

References

Adamski J, Godman B, Ofierska-Sujkowska G, *et al.* 2010. Risk sharing arrangements for pharmaceuticals: potential considerations and recommendations for European payers. *BMC Health Service Research* 10: 153.

Agence Francaise de Securite Sanitaire des Produits de Sante (AFSSAPS). 2001. Temporary Authorisations for Use (ATUs). http://agence-tst.ansm.sante.fr/html/pdf/5/atu_eng.pdf.

Ashworth M, Golding S, Shephard L, Majeed A. 2002. Prescribing incentive schemes in two NHS regions: Cross sectional survey. *British Medical Journal* 324(7347): 1187–1188.

Bloor K, Freemantle N. 1996. Lessons from international experience in controlling pharmaceutical expenditure. 2. Influencing doctors. *British Medical Journal* 312(7045): 1525–1527.

Bordoy C, Jelovac I. 2003. Pricing and welfare of parallel imports in the pharmaceutical industry. *MERIT.* Vol Research Memoranda 004. Maastricht: Maastricht Economic Research Institute on Innovation and Technology.

Brekke KR, Konigbauer I, Straume OR. 2007. Reference pricing of pharmaceuticals. *Journal of Health Economics* 26(3): 613–642.

Brook R, Keeler E, Lohr K, Newhouse J. 2006. The Rand Health Insurance Experiment. *Research Brief.* http://www.rand.org/pubs/research_briefs/RB9174.html.

Carone G, Schierz C, Cost XA. 2012. Cost containment policies in public pharmaceutical spending in the European Union. *Economic Papers* http://ec.europa.eu/economy_finance/publications/economic_paper/2012/pdf/ecp_461_en.pdf.

Caves RE, Whinston MD, Hurwitz MA. 1991. Patent Expiration, Entry, and Competition in the United-States Pharmaceutical–Industry. *Brookings Papers on Economic Activity* 1–66.

Chaix-Couturier C, Durand-Zaleski I, Jolly D, Durieux P. 2000. Effects of financial incentives on medical practice: Results from a systematic review of the literature and methodological issues. *International Journal for Quality in Health Care* 12(2): 133–142.

Claxton K. 2007. Oft, Vbp: Qed? *Health Economics* 16(6): 545–558.

Claxton, K, Martin, S, Soares, M, *et al.* 2015. Methods for the estimation of the National Institute for Health and Care Excellence Cost-effectiveness threshold. *Health Technology Assessment* 19(14): 1–503, v–vi.

Cook A, Acton JP, Schwartz E. 1998. How increased competition from generic drugs has affected prices and returns in the pharmaceutical industry. *Washington, DC: Congressional Budget Office.*

Cutler DM, Long G, Berndt ER, *et al.* 2007. The value of antihypertensive drugs: A perspective on medical innovation. *Health Affairs (Millwood)* 26(1): 97–110.

Cutler DM, McClellan M. 2001. Is technological change in medicine worth it? *Health Affairs (Millwood)* 20(5): 11–29.

Dalen DM, Strom S, Haabeth T. 2006. Price regulation and generic competition in the pharmaceutical market. *European Journal of Health Economics* 7(3): 208–214.

Danzon PM, Chao LW. 2000a. Cross-national price differences for pharmaceuticals: How large, and why? *Journal of Health Economics* 19(2): 159–195.

Danzon PM, Chao LW. 2000b. Does regulation drive out competition in pharmaceutical markets? *Journal of Law & Economics* 43(2): 311–357.

Danzon PM, Furukawa MF. 2008. International prices and availability of pharmaceuticals in 2005. *Health Affairs (Millwood)* 27(1): 221–233.

Danzon PM, Furukawa MF. 2003. Prices and availability of pharmaceuticals: Evidence from nine countries. *Health Affairs (Millwood)* Suppl Web Exclusives: W3–521–536.

Danzon PM. 1998. The economics of parallel trade. *Pharmaeconomics* 13(3): 293–304.

Davies J, Taylor D. 2009. Reducing the threat of medicines counterfeiting in the EU. *School of Pharmacy, University of London, London.*

Delnoij D, Brenner G. 2000. Importing budget systems from other countries: What can we learn from the German drug budget and the British GP fundholding? *Health Policy* 52(3): 157–169.

Department of Health (UK). 2013. The Pharmaceutical Price Regulation Scheme. https://www.gov.uk/government/uploads/system/uploads/attachment_data/file/282523/Pharmaceutical_Price_Regulation.pdf.

Department of Health (UK). 2009. The Pharmaceutical Price Regulation Scheme: Tenth Report to Parliament. https://www.gov.uk/government/uploads/system/uploads/attachment_data/file/300301/PPRS_Twelfth_Report_to_Parliament_-Final.pdf.

Department of Health (UK). 2014. The Pharmaceutical Price Regulation Scheme: Twelfth report to Parliament. https://www.gov.uk/government/uploads/system/uploads/attachment_data/file/300301/PPRS_Twelfth_Report_to_Parliament_-Final.pdf.

Drummond MF, Schwartz JS, Jonsson B, *et al.* 2008. Key principles for the improved conduct of health technology assessments for resource allocation decisions. *International Journal of Technology Assessment Health Care* 24(3): 244–258; Discussion 248–362.

Espin J, Rovira, J. 2009. *Risk Sharing for Pharmaceuticals: Terminology, Classification and Experiences*. EMINet Report, European Commission, Brussels.

Ess SM, Schneeweiss S, Szucs TD. 2003. European healthcare policies for controlling drug expenditure. *Pharmacoeconomics* 21(2): 89–103.

European Parliament and the Council. 2000. Regulation EC/141/2000 of the European Parliament and the Council on Orphan Medicinal Products. EC/141/2000.

European Parliament and the Council. 2001. Directive 2001/83/EC of the European Parliament and of the Council on the community code relating to medicinal products for human use. *2001L0032001*.

European Parliament and the Council. 2004. Directive 2004/27/EC of the European Parliament and of the Council of 31 March 2004 amending Directive 2001/83/EC on the Community code relating to medicinal products for human use.

European Commission. 2006. Guideline on Procedures for Granting a Marketing Authorization under Exceptional Circumstances pursuant to Regulation No. 726/20042004.

European Medicines Agency (EMA). 2006. Final guidance on conditional marketing authorization (Regulation (EC) No. 726/2004).

European Commission. 2009. Pharmaceutical Sector Inquiry. http://ec.europa.eu/ Accessed 28 October 2010.

European Commission. 2013. *The 2013 EU Industrial R&D Investment Scoreboard*: European Commission, JRC/DG Research & Innovation.

European Federation of Pharmaceutical Industries and Associations (EFPIA). 2014. The Pharmaceutical Industry in Figures — Key Data 2014. Brussels. Available from: www.efpia.eu/uploads/Modules/Mediaroom/figures-2014-final.pdf.

European Medicines Agency (EMA). 2015. Adaptive Pathways. http://www.ema.europa.eu/ema/index.jsp?curl=pages/regulation/general/general_content_000601.jsp.

Ferrario A, Kanavos P. 2015. Dealing with uncertainty and high prices of new medicines: A comparative analysis of the use of managed entry agreements in Belgium, England, the Netherlands and Sweden. *Social Science & Medicine* 124: 39–47.

Ferrario A, Kanavos P. 2013. Managed Entry Agreements for Pharmaceuticals: The European Experience. http://eprints.lse.ac.uk/50513/. Accessed 19 November 2014.

Folino-Gallo P, Walley T, Frolich JC, Carvajal A, Edwards IR. 2001. Availability of medicines in the European Union: Results from the EURO-Medicines project. *European Journal of Clinical Pharmacology* 57(6–7): 441–446.

Food and Drug Administration (FDA). 2013. Accelerated Approval Programme. http://www.fda.gov/Drugs/ResourcesForYou/HealthProfessionals/ucm313768.htm.

Frank RG, Salkever DS. 1997. Generic entry and the pricing of pharmaceuticals. *Journal of Economics & Management Strategy* 6(1): 75–90.

Ganslandt M, Maskus KE. 2004. Parallel imports and the pricing of pharmaceutical products: Evidence from the European Union. *Journal of Health Economics* 23(5): 1035–1057.

Garattini L, Tediosi F. 2000. A comparative analysis of generics markets in five European countries. *Health Policy* 51(3): 149–162.

Glowicka E, Lorincz S, Pesaresi E, Romero LS, Verouden V. 2009. Generic Entry in Prescription Medicines in the EU: Main Characteristics, Determinants and Effects. Brussels: European Commission. Pharmaceutical Sector Inquiry. http://ec.europa.eu/competition/sectors/pharmaceuticals/inquiry/staff_working_paper_part1.pdf. Accessed 18 July 2014.

Godman B, Malmstrom RE, Diogene E, *et al*. 2015. Are new models needed to optimize the utilization of new medicines to sustain healthcare systems? *Expert Review of Clinical Pharmacology* 8(1): 77–94.

GOEG. 2007–2014. Pharmaceutical Pricing and Reimbursement Information (PPRI) — Country Reports. Vienna, Austria. Accessible from: http://whocc.goeg.at/Publications/CountryReports.

Grabowski HG, Vernon JM. 1992. Brand loyalty, entry, and price-competition in pharmaceuticals after the 1984 drug Act. *Journal of Law & Economics* 35(2): 331–350.

Health and Social Care Information Centre (HSCIC). 2015. Quality and Outcomes Framework. http://www.hscic.gov.uk/qof.

Husereau D, Cameron C. 2011. Value-based pricing of pharmaceuticals in Canada: Opportunities to Expand the role of health technology assessment? http://www.cfhi-fcass.ca/SearchResultsNews/11–12–16/8eeaf655-b2b6–4c39-a909–6854acfea850.aspx. Accessed 26 November 2014.

Johnson JR, Ning YM, Farrell A, Justice R, Keegan P, Pazdur R. 2011. Accelerated approval of oncology products: The food and drug administration experience. *Journal of the National Cancer Institute* 20 103(8): 636–644.

Kanavos P, Angelis A. 2013. Multiple criteria decision analysis for value based assessment of new medical technologies: A conceptual framework. *LSE Health Working Papers* 33.

Kanavos P, Costa-Font J, Seeley E, Zweimuller J. 2008. Competition in off-patent drug markets: Issues, regulation and evidence. *Economic Policy* (55): 500–544.

Kanavos P, Costa-Font J. 2005. Pharmaceutical parallel trade in Europe: Stakeholder and competition effects. *Economic Policy* (44): 751–798.

Kanavos P, Ferrario A, Nicod E. 2012. Tender systems for outpatient pharmaceuticals in the European Union: Evidence from the Netherlands and Germany. http://progenerika.de/wp-content/uploads/2013/02/Anlage-2_Tendering-Report-EMINET-13OCT2012-FINAL.pdf.

Kanavos P, Ferrario A, Vandoros S, Anderson G. 2013. Higher US branded drug prices and spending compared to other countries may stem partly from quick uptake of new drugs. *Health Affairs (Millwood)* 32(4): 753–761. doi: 10.1377/hlthaff.2012.0920.

Kanavos P, Nicod E, Espin J, van den Aardweg S. 2010. *Short- and Long-term Effects of Value-Based Pricing vs. External Price Referencing*. http://ec.europa.eu/enterprise/sectors/healthcare/files/docs/valuebased_pharmapricing_012010_en.pdf.

Kanavos P, Nicod E, van den Aardweg S, Pomedli S. 2010. Special Issue on Health Technology Assessment.

Kanavos P, Nicod E, van den Aardweg S, Pomedli S. 2010. The impact of health technology assessments: An international comparison. *Euro Observer* 12(4):1–7. http://www.euro.who.int/_data/assets/pdf_file/0007/127798/EuroObserver_Vol12_No4_Winter_2010.pdf.

Kanavos P, Schurer W, Vogler, S. 2011. *EMINet Report on the Pharmaceutical Distribution Chain*. Brussels: DG Enterprise.

Kanavos P, Seeley E, Vandoros S. 2009. Tender systems for outpatient pharmaceuticals in the European Union: Evidence from the Netherlands, Germany and Belgium. EMINet Report, European Commission, Brussels.

Kanavos P, Taylor D. 2007. Pharmacy discounts on generic medicines in France: Is there room for further efficiency savings? *Current Medical Research and Opinion* 23(10): 2467–2476.

Kanavos P, Vandoros S, Irwin R, Nicod E, Casson M. 2011. Differences in costs of and access to pharmaceutical products in the EU.

Kanavos P, Vandoros S. 2010. Competition in prescription drug markets: Is parallel trade the answer? *Managerial and Decision Economics* 31(5): 3265–3338.

Kanavos P, Vandoros S. 2011. Determinants of branded prescription medicine prices in OECD countries. *Health Economics Policy Law* 6(3): 337–367.

Kanavos P, Wouters OJ. 2014. Pharmaceutical parallel trade: Legal, policy, and economic issues. In: Culyer AJ (ed.). *Encyclopedia of Health Economics*. San Diego, USA: Elsevier; pp. 20–28.

Kanavos P. 2014. Measuring performance in off-patent drug markets: A methodological framework and empirical evidence from twelve EU Member States. *Health Policy* 118(2): 229–241.

Kanavos P. 2008. Does pharmaceutical parallel trade serve the objectives of cost control? *Eurohealth* 14(8): 22–26.

Kanavos, P, Vandoros S, Habicht J, De Joncheere K. *Review of the Estonian Pharmaceutical sector: Towards the Development of a National Medicines Policy: Final Report*. Copenhagen: WHO Regional Office for Europe; 2009. https://extranet.who.int/iris/restricted/handle/10665/107271.

Lichtenberg FG. 2012. Pharmaceutical innovation and longevity growth in 30 developing OECD and high-income countries, 2000–2009. *NBER Working Paper No. 18552.*

Marsh K, Lanitis T, Neasham D, Orfanos P, Caro J. 2014. Assessing the value of healthcare interventions using multi-criteria decision analysis: A review of the literature. *Pharmacoeconomics* 32(4): 345–365.

MEDTAP International. 2004. The Value of Investment in Health Care. http://www.medtap.com/ Products/HP_FullReport.pdf.

Morel T, Arickx F, Befrits G, *et al.* 2013. Reconciling uncertainty of costs and outcomes with the need for access to orphan medicinal products: A comparative study of managed entry agreements across seven European countries. *Orphanet Journal of Rare Diseases* 8: 198.

Mossialos E, Mrazek M, Walley T. 2004. *Regulating Pharmaceuticals in Europe: Striving for Efficiency, Equity and Quality.* Open University Press.

Mrazek M, Frank R. 2004. The off-patent pharmaceutical market. In Mossialos EMM, Walley T. (eds). *Regulating Pharmaceuticals in Europe: Striving for Efficiency, Equity and Quality.* Open University Press.

Mrazek M, Mossialos E. 2004. Regulating pharmaceutical prices in the European Union. In Mossialos E, Mrazek M, Walley T (eds.). *Regulating Pharmaceuticals in Europe: Striving for Efficiency, Equity and Quality.* Geneva: World Health Organization.

Nicod E, Kanavos P. 2012. Commonalities and differences in HTA outcomes: A comparative analysis of five countries and implications for coverage decisions. *Health Policy* 108(2–3): 167–177.

Office of Fair Trading. 2007. The pharmaceutical price regulation scheme: An OFT market study. http://webarchive.nationalarchives.gov.uk/20140402142426/http://www.oft.gov.uk/shared_oft/reports/comp_policy/oft885.pdf.

Organisation for Economic Co-operation and Development (OECD). Health Data 2013.

Osterreichisches Bundesistitut fur Gesundheitswesen (OBIG). 2007. Pharmaceutical Pricing and Reimbursement Information (PPRI). October 2010.

Osterreichisches Bundesistitut fur Gesundheitswesen (OBIG). Surveying, Assessing and Analysing the Pharmaceutical Sector in the 25 EU Member States. 2006. http://ec.europa.eu/competition/mergers/studies_reports/oebig.pdf. Accessed 29 October 2010.

Paris V, Belloni A. 2013. Value in pharmaceutical pricing. *OECD Health Working Paper.* 63. http://dx.doi.org/10.1787/5k43jc9v6knx-en. Accessed 24 November 2014.

Perampaladas K, Kanavos P. Comparing FDA and EMA approaches to accelerated development: Implications for access and assessment in Europe. *MIMEO* 2015.

Pharmaceutical Research and Manufacturers of America (PhRMA). 2010. Pharmaceutical industry profile: 2010. Washington, DC: PhRMA.

Pignatti F, Gravanis I, Herold R, Vamvakas S, Jonsson B, Marty M. 2011. The European Medicines Agency: An overview of its mission, responsibilities, and recent initiatives in cancer drug regulation. *Clinical Cancer Research* 17(16): 5220–5225.

Pomedli S. 2010. HTA and access to cancer medicines. *Euro Observer,* 12(4): 1–71. http://www.euro.who.int/_data/assets/pdf_file/0007/127798/EuroObserver_Vol12_No4_Winter_2010.pdf.

Puig-Junoy J. 2010. Impact of European pharmaceutical price regulation on generic price competition: A review. *Pharmacoeconomics* 28(8): 649–663.

Regan TL. 2008. Generic entry, price competition, and market segmentation in the prescription drug market. *International Journal of Industrial Organization* 26(4): 930–948.

Rey P. 2003. The Impact of Parallel Imports on Prescription Medicines. *MIMEO.*

Rizzo JA. 1999. Advertising and competition in the ethical pharmaceutical industry: The case of antihypertensive drugs. *Journal of Law & Economics* 42(1): 89–116.

Rubin RJ, Mendelson DN. 1995. Cost sharing in health insurance. *New England Journal of Medicine* 333(11): 733–734.

Szymanski S, Valletti T. 2005. Parallel trade, price discrimination, investment and price caps. *Economic Policy* (44): 705–749.

US Congress. 1983. Orphan Drug (ODA), Public Law. No. 97-414, § 527(a), 96 Stat. 2049.

Van den Aardweg S. 2010. HTA of orphan drugs across six countries: Fair, flawed or failing? *Euro Observer* 12(4): 1–7. http://www.euro.who.int/_data/assets/pdf_file/0007/127798/EuroObserver_Vol12_No4_Winter_-2010.pdf.

Vandoros S, Kanavos P. 2013. The generics paradox revisited: Empirical evidence from regulated markets. *Applied Economics* 45(22): 3230–3239.

West P, Mahon J. 2003. Benefits to Patients and Payers from Parallel Trade. http://archives.who.int/prioritymeds/report/append/8210ParallelTradeReport.pdf.

Wiggins SN, Maness R. 2004. Price competition in pharmaceuticals: The case of anti-infectives. *Economic Inquiry* 42(2): 247–263.

Williamson S. 2010. Patient access schemes for high-cost cancer medicines. *Lancet Oncology* 11(2): 111–112.

Wladysiuk M, Tabor A, Godman B. 2013. 'HTA for Crisis': Sharing experiences during the 7th EBHC Symposium. *Expert Review Pharmacoeconomics & Outcomes Research* 13(1): 47–49.

World Bank.2012. World Development Indicators. Health expenditure per capita, PPP (constant at 2011 international $). Available at http://data.worldbank.org/indicator/SH.XPD.PCAP.PP.KD.

World Health Organization. 2011. *World Medicines Situation Report 2011.* Geneva: WHO.

Technological Innovation in Health Care: A Global Perspective*

Sheila Smith

Centers for Medicare & Medicaid Services

This chapter describes the relationship between health policy, medical innovation, and health care spending from a global perspective. The results of estimation of the relationship between international variation in health systems characteristics and growth in spending attributable to medical innovation (using a residual-based method) suggest that variation in health systems characteristics play a relatively minor role in explaining variation in the contribution of medical technology to spending growth across countries and time — although this result is notably clouded by measurement issues. However, the analysis presented in this chapter does find strong support for a decline in the common contribution of medical technology to growth in health spending across a broad range of countries and time periods. Estimation based on a 14-country sample implies that the declining contribution of medical technology generates a reduction in the trend rate of growth in constant dollar per capita health spending of 1.1 percentage points (relative to an average growth rate of 3.2%) between 1970 and 2012. A causal link between the deceleration in spending on medical technology and changing health systems characteristics cannot be explicitly demonstrated, but is consistent with theoretical expectations of the effects of broad changes in methods of coverage and payment for new technologies over this period. The chapter concludes with policy considerations regarding the potential implications of slower growth in health care spending on new technology from a social welfare perspective.

Keywords: Medical Technology; Innovation; Diffusion; Health Care Policy; Medical R&D; Health Care Spending Growth.

*The views and conclusions expressed here are those of the author and do not necessarily represent the views of the Centers for Medicare & Medicaid Services or the US Government.

Introduction

The focus of this chapter is on the relationship between health policy, medical innovation, and health care spending at a global level. Medical innovation expands the menu of treatment options available to improve health outcomes and potentially improves the efficiency and effectiveness of existing forms of medical care. New, more effective, treatment options for medical care are undisputedly a good thing in and of themselves. The rapid increase in the capabilities of medicine has spurred a consistent increase in the share of resources that societies are willing to allocate to the purchase of medical care, as compared to alternative areas of consumption.

Research broadly confirms that this rapid expansion in health care spending has been "worth it" overall (Cutler and McClellan, 2001). To paraphrase William Nordhaus, if given the choice between increases in non-health consumption since 1960 versus the advances in medical capabilities since this time, most would find this a difficult choice (Nordhaus, 2002). To provide a rough sense of scale, it is estimated that medical advances between 1960 and 2012 generated incremental value of about $17,000 per person (constant 2012 dollars), well in excess of the increase in health care spending over this period in the United States (close to $8,000 per person).[1] While great uncertainty is associated with any such estimate, a consensus exists that the value derived from medical innovation is a substantial net positive over the costs.

However, it is also widely acknowledged that these benefits of medical advances occur in the context of health systems that are characterized by a great deal of inefficiency. Indeed, if new medical technologies are systematically introduced at a rate greater than can be justified by their relative costs and benefits, then this implies that inefficiency can grow over time. Near universal insurance coverage in advanced economies means that patients pay for only a small fraction of the costs of their own care at the point of purchase, which creates incentives for overconsumption, both for existing forms of medical care and for new technologies at the margin (moral hazard). The complexity of medical care and uncertainties about its benefits in terms of improved health means that patients usually do not understand the nature of the care they receive or how it

---

[1]Nordhaus concluded the value of the implied increase in health status for the United States between 1900 and 1995 was approximately equal to the value of the increase in total non-health consumption over this period. Applying this assumption to updated data, the increase in real per capita non-health consumption between 1960 and 2013 was $16,998 (2012 dollars) based on data for personal consumption expenditures and consumer price deflator from the Bureau of Economic Analysis (US Department of Commerce), while the increase in health care spending per capita over this period was $8,041 (US Department of Health and Human Services).

benefits them. Physicians and other medical providers make choices on behalf of patients, but incentives inherent in methods of payment may distort these decisions. Thus, there is only a weak link between the actual care provided, and that which a given patient would choose if given complete knowledge of benefits and full responsibility for costs.

The design of payment methods for providers attempts to strike a difficult balance between incentives that encourage use and are relatively insensitive to costs, and those which discourage overuse and risk withholding beneficial care. The high degree of uncertainty surrounding the value of health outcomes associated with medical treatments makes the choice of cost-effective treatment options difficult, even aside from questions of payment incentives. Health care markets function poorly in allocating medical care in a way that aligns benefits with costs in most cases. These weaknesses are accentuated in the case of new medical procedures (and to a somewhat lesser extent) for new drugs and medical devices, as clinical evidence of health benefits will be more limited. Permissive policies for coverage and access minimize the chance that beneficial care will be withheld, and encourage research toward the development of new technology — at the cost of higher health care spending. Restrictive policies accept a higher threshold for access to new technologies, and potentially discourage medical innovation — as a tradeoff for lower health care spending.

Given the dominance of the public sector in financing medical care, particularly in advanced economies, these issues necessarily fall within the scope of health policy. Where markets function poorly in producing outcomes that are in line with consumer preferences, public- and private-sector institutions effectively act as agents and intermediaries, both on behalf of patients, and for the entire pool of people who collectively contribute to fund the provision of medical care. Health policy choices gradually shape the structure of health systems and can be expected to influence the way new technologies are introduced to the system and the rate at which they diffuse.

Health policy has numerous objectives. These include issues of equity and access to care as well as concerns about access to new technologies, all of which must necessarily be balanced within a limited pool of resources. The availability of new technology has long been acknowledged to be a double-edged sword — while the capabilities of medicine continue to expand, technology also acts as a key driver of health care spending growth. As such, technological change exacerbates budgetary strains in both the public and private sector. The need for cost-containment becomes increasingly compelling in light of recent slow economic growth, and motivates the heightened focus on introducing new technologies in a way that is cost effective. The impact of the 2008 financial crisis and the extended period of slow economic growth that has followed have imposed tight constraints on overall government budgets for a broad range of countries. The Euro-Area debt crisis has compounded these issues for the affected countries.

Given the increasingly large magnitude of health care spending within government budgets, growth in health spending crowds out other priorities for public spending in an increasingly visible way. High levels of government debt have limited the ability to fund spending through deficits, while the dynamic implications of a rising tax burden for economic growth crimp the ability to increase the size of government budgets relative to the economy as a whole. For the period 2000–2011, the share of total government expenditures allocated to health care increased by 1.2 percentage points (out of a total of 35.6% of government spending accounted for by health care) based on a broad sample of 29 OECD countries (OECD, 2013). The increased share going to fund health care was offset by decreases in all other areas except social protection (which includes pensions). Areas accounting for a reduced share of public spending included defense (–0.4 percentage points), housing and community amenities (both –0.5 percentage points), education (–0.3 percentage points), and public order and safety and environmental protection (both –0.1 percentage points).

One outcome of the increasing pressure on public budgets for health care has been an increasing effort to introduce new technology in a cost-effective way. A broad range of countries have expanded and formalized the role of health technology assessment (HTA) in determining which new technologies will be covered, in determining pricing, and in evaluating the treatment of new technologies within the diagnosis-related group (DRG) based systems that determine payment in most countries.

In evaluating the relationship between technological change in medicine and health policy, it is clear that feedback effects occur in both directions. Health policy has responded to the availability of new technology by attempting to build institutional capabilities that filter the introduction of medical innovation in a way that is cost effective — balancing benefits against costs. We can also reasonably expect to see the effect of this growing emphasis on cost-effectiveness exerting an increasing influence on the direction of medical research, and ultimately on the characteristics of technologies that are developed. In sum, the flow of medical technology is determined endogenously as a function of the characteristics of health systems, which are shaped by health policy initiatives (Weisbrod, 1991; Weisbrod and LaMay, 1999).

In its most fundamental sense, medical technology is knowledge, and knowledge is global in nature. Medical research and development is highly concentrated in a handful of advanced economies, but the direction of this research can be expected to respond to demand for health care in markets throughout the world.

This is most clearly the case for pharmaceuticals, which are primarily developed and marketed by private firms that are global in scale and for-profit in nature. The increasing use of HTA and price negotiation in important markets for drugs shapes the research agenda for these firms. The direction of innovation for medical and surgical procedures has a much larger public-sector and academic role, which can be expected to dampen its responsiveness to market incentives. Yet even here, increasingly selective coverage decisions, and the way that procedural innovations are treated within DRG-based systems can be expected to influence the potential for diffusion, and will thus be a factor in determining research priorities.

The primary focus of this chapter is the empirical estimation of how variation in health policy across a range of countries has influenced health care spending growth attributable to medical innovation and technology. This question is relevant to the effects of the evolution of health policy over time, and the effects of variation in health systems across countries for relative rates of adoption and diffusion of medical technologies. This focus is an admittedly one-sided perspective on the relationship between health policy and medical technology; it concentrates solely on the costs of technology, while ignoring the value of the improved capability of medicine for health outcomes which is the motivating force for the adoption of technology. However, the context that this perspective provides should fill a useful gap in the existing literature, which has tended to focus on the effects of health policy on the adoption and diffusion of individual technologies for the treatment of narrow diagnoses at a micro-level. For example, the diffusion of medical technology in the treatment of heart attacks in inpatient settings has been fairly exhaustively studied (Bech *et al.*, 2008; Cutler *et al.*, 1998; Moise, 2003). This approach has produced a rich and detailed picture of variation in the adoption and diffusion of a handful of important diagnoses and technologies. However, it is also a partial and piecemeal picture with a selective focus that has been heavily influenced by data availability. The conclusions of this research cannot easily be generalized. The objective of the approach presented here is to provide context at the macro-level that should be relevant to the assessment of whether health policy initiatives directed toward medical innovation have been successful from the limited perspective of cost-containment.

We define *medical technology* as the scientific, technological, and clinical state of knowledge of medical products, processes, and procedures that defines the potential set of treatment options for medical care (Rettig, 1994). The *effects* of medical technology on the composition of medical care are distinct from this state of knowledge. The effect of medical technology will be a function of a number of different factors that determine the willingness and ability to pay for these forms of treatment; these factors include the effects of health policy. The contribution of medical technology to health spending growth will be determined by the rate of uptake and diffusion of new options for medical treatment, combined with their relative price in comparison with existing forms of care. The uptake and diffusion of medical technologies is a function of their characteristics, and of the preferences of consumers within the constraints imposed within the health systems that guide the availability of these options.

The work presented in this chapter is largely empirical. The analysis has two key objectives. The first of these is to estimate the trend in the contribution of medical technology to growth over time for a broad cross-section of countries. The question addressed is whether the contribution of medical technology to growth in health spending has tended to slow over time in response to a broad tendency towards the adoption of health policy that generally exhibits increasing restrictiveness in the coverage of new medical technologies. The approach used is rooted in methods of national growth accounting and is similar to the approach used previously to estimate a range for the contribution of medical technology to growth for the United States (Newhouse, 1992; Smith *et al.*, 2009). The second objective is to estimate the relationship between the resulting estimates of the contribution of technological change to growth to variation in health systems characteristics, both over time, and across countries.

The conclusions of this analysis point strongly to a change in the contribution of technology to growth in health spending over time. The effect of technological change on health spending growth appears to decline gradually over time, and the magnitude of this decline is larger than would be predicted on the basis of global investment in R&D. These results hint at a shift towards the development of more cost-effective technologies, consistent with incentives implied by a growing emphasis on cost effectiveness in the expanded application of HTA and trends in payment incentives away from fee-based systems.

Conclusions on the relationship between variation in growth in health care spending across countries, and broad health systems characteristics (that reflect the cumulative effects of health policy decisions) are weaker and more ambiguous. Broadly, two types of systems show a marginally significant tendency toward a reduced contribution of medical technology to growth. One such type of health system is characterized by a combination of integrated delivery of health care with binding budget constraints, while the second involves a greater reliance on consumer cost-sharing at the point of purchase. This suggests that there may be more than one effective alternative for slowing the impact of medical technology on health care spending.

Medical Technology and the Demand for Health Care: An Endogenous System

Medical innovation produces new medical procedures and products through the process of research and development. This expansion in the capabilities of medicine influences demand for health care — and therefore also effects expectations of future growth in health care spending. Expectations for the risk of incurring health care costs drives demand for health insurance coverage, including influencing preferences on the nature and generosity of coverage. The conditions and payment methods associated with health insurance coverage feedback as a determinant of demand for health care, including any restrictions on coverage or incentives for the purchase of medical technology. Completing this endogenous feedback loop, the current and expected willingness to pay for medical technologies determines the incentives to invest in R&D that leads to the development of new technology. This system defines the health care "quadrilemma" defined by Burton Weisbrod more than 20 years ago (Weisbrod, 1991). Figure 1 illustrates the dynamics of this model.

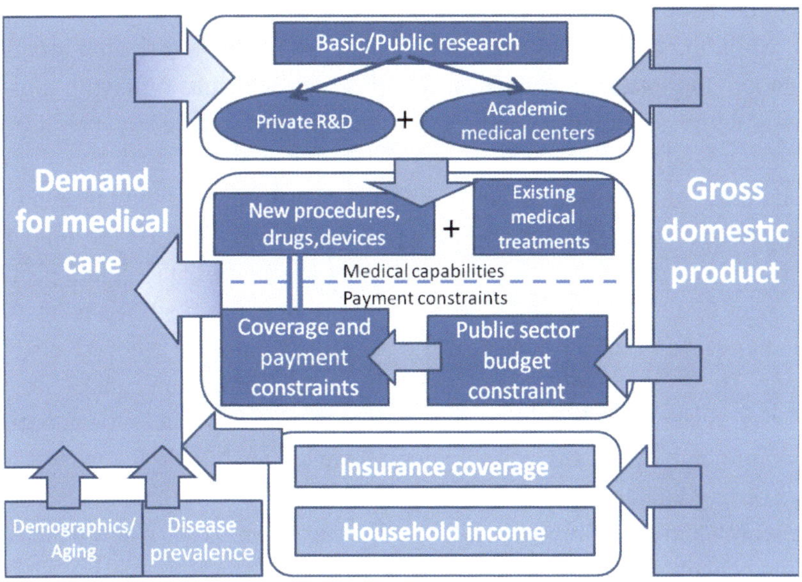

Figure 1. The health care quadrilemma

Source: Based on Weisbrod (1991).

The dynamics of this model of the role of technology in the health system play out differently depending on the nature of the health system in question. In countries with integrated health systems, where government manages both overall financing of care and its delivery, there tends to be little or no choice on the terms of the conditions of insurance coverage that determine access to technology. Thus, the interaction between demand for medical technology and the nature of insurance coverage occurs at a highly aggregate level, and in a public context. Within a system such as the National Health Service (NHS) in Britain, change in coverage of technology must occur through public pressure on the government authorities that establish the ground rules for coverage, or through a change in the control of government in response to election results (promising to expand access and increase spending or vice versa).

Within a system that is characterized by a choice of private insurance, such as the United States, some of this effect of demand for coverage of medical technology can occur through a shift in demand between health plans that offer more or less generous coverage. However, even in the United States, which is known for the unusually large role played by private insurers, a substantial part of the constraints on access to technology are channeled through the public sector. The coverage decisions of Medicare strongly influence the course chosen by private payers, while the design and pricing decisions of Medicare are also broadly followed by private insurers. Thus, even in this case, decisions on health policy that nominally address public spending generate spillover effects for private payers, thus packing a larger punch than might initially be evident.

Regardless of the level at which the feedback between individuals and insurers occurs, public demand for access to medical technology will be the fundamental underlying determinant of the constraints that are placed on spending on these technologies by public or private payers. Ultimately, insurers — at any level — are intermediaries who act on behalf of the pool of consumers who are covered by insurance. The role of health policy in coverage determinations, placement within DRG-based systems, and pricing for new technologies influences the adoption and diffusion of newly launched technologies. However, in shaping the market for currently diffusing technology, health policy also establishes the incentives that determine research and development priorities. The current market for new technologies, including constraints on access and pricing decisions, can be expected to influence the future direction of medical innovation. Whether the effect of policy that imposes constraints on the diffusion of technology is a net positive or negative for social welfare will depend on the specifics of constraints that are established.

Two stages of health policy impacts on medical technology:

(1) *Current effects*: How does health policy influence the use and pricing of new technologies that are currently available and in the process of diffusion?

(2) *Dynamic effects*: How have the effects of health policy on use and pricing of technologies influenced the pace and direction of medical research?

What determines the pace of medical innovation and its direction? There are three basic institutional sources for medical research and development (R&D): Public research organizations, academic medical centers, and private industry (pharmaceuticals, medical devices, and biotechnology). The divisions among these organizations have been muddied to some extent by the growth in collaborative research projects that extend across these boundaries, reflecting both the increasingly interdependent nature of procedural, pharmaceutical and device innovation. However, medical research can still be broadly delineated based on the type of innovation: Surgical and medical procedures are developed by medical researchers and clinicians in non-profit or public institutions on what remains a lightly-regulated, somewhat *ad hoc* basis. The diffusion of procedure tends to rely on the availability of specialized medical skills to perform the procedure and (in some cases) ability to make capital investments in equipment and facilities. Procedural innovations are generally not patentable, so there is no residual claimant who benefits from their expanded use.

Efforts to constrain the adoption and diffusion of medical technology attempt to discriminate on the basis of comparative effectiveness, and to an increasing extent, cost-effectiveness. The presence of substantial inefficiency inherent in the current delivery of medical care suggest at least the potential for slowing health spending growth while continuing to benefit from a substantial part of what innovation has to offer for medical care. However, this endeavor is not without risks. Medical innovation is a complex and intertwined process. Innovations that initially appear unpromising in the early stages may experience a later breakthrough that will alter their dynamics Gelijns and Rosenberg (1994). A number of currently successful drugs were resurrected from earlier failed candidates (Chambers *et al.*, 2015). Research into rare diseases often leads to a more nuanced understanding of the body's processes that translate into progress in other areas (Chambers *et al.*, 2015). It is when a technology is at the early stage of diffusion that health policy has the most control over its prospective use in practice. However, this is also a point at which uncertainty about potential benefits and side effects is the greatest and where the nature of the technology itself may still be evolving. Also relevant to the impact of health policy, but more difficult to address, is the issue of heterogeneity in patient populations. A blanket decision on coverage and pricing based on an evaluation of an average for costs and benefits associated with a given technology will ignore the natural variation in the response of individual patients to different therapies (Basu *et al.*, 2011).

The empirical estimation of the impact of health policy on the contribution of medical technology to health spending growth presented in this chapter will attempt to evaluate both the current period impact of policy (based on variation across countries), and also the dynamic effects of policy on the effects of health technology (based on variation over time) in terms of the implications for health care spending growth at the national and international level. It is worth reiterating that conclusions for health care spending are looking at one outcome of a complex system, and that this perspective does not address the benefits of access to new technologies in decreased mortality and improved quality of life. An answer to the question of whether policy has tended to slow growth in spending on new medical technology does not answer the question of whether this effect is a net positive for social welfare.

Effects of Health Policy on Technology

Health policy can be defined as a menu of tools used by central and regional governments that set the ground rules for health care markets. The characteristics of the health system are shaped by past policy choices. Presumably, the broad intent of health policy is to maintain consistency with the underlying preferences of citizens for health care *a priori* — i.e., the choices that consumers would make given the knowledge of the full costs and benefits of treatment. Indeed, the utility-based analysis that is relied upon for much of HTA explicitly intends to maximize social welfare.

Policy actions influence the uptake and diffusion of new medical technologies through five main channels: (1) coverage determinations, (2) capital investment, (3) payment methods (e.g., bundled vs. fee-based), (4) pricing, and (5) public budgets.

These channels for policy are not separate in their effects; decisions on coverage and payment methods are often accompanied by determinations of pricing. Countries that establish binding aggregate budget constraints will also make decisions on coverage, payment methods, and pricing associated with individual technologies. The scope of medical care influenced through these channels is also very different. Coverage determinations primarily impact only a relatively small number of technologies, with most of the attention devoted to drugs and medical devices (although the scope of this process has tended to expand over time). Capital investment is a necessary precondition for many medical interventions; the decision to invest in facilities thus opens the door to a stream of future expenditures. Payment incentives and pricing are broad in the scope of their application and tend to have interdependent effects.

The process of coverage determination is most straightforward for newly launched pharmaceuticals and medical devices. Regulatory approval requires a substantial body of clinical evidence, which can then be applied to further assess the potential costs and benefits for coverage and pricing determination. In many countries, this process not only involves the evaluation of clinical evidence to determine whether the new product offers a significant improvement over existing standards of care, but also rest on questions of cost-effectiveness. In a number of countries, the determination is also based on the question of cost-effectiveness as a joint function of the relative price and the incremental improvement to health status implied by the evidence. Increasingly, institutions conducting coverage determinations on behalf of public payers are asking for evidence that demonstrates clinical effectiveness relative to existing therapies (rather than merely relative to a placebo) as a condition of coverage.

Cost-effectiveness is currently not explicitly a factor in Medicare coverage decisions within the United States. However, recent research concludes that even in the case of Medicare, coverage decisions have become far more restrictive over the past 20 years despite the absence of an explicit acknowledgement of cost effectiveness as a factor in the process (Chambers *et al.*, 2015).

Gradations of coverage approval may include restrictions on indications to selected patient populations or temporary coverage of the technology for the purpose of compiling additional evidence. A second important issue often involves the placement of the new technology within the context of existing DRG-based systems. The diffusion of the technology may be encouraged through add-on payments secured as a condition of its application, or (less aggressively) through increased payments for the entire DRG category where the use of the technology is indicated.

Research suggests that pressures on coverage and pricing are significantly reducing the rate of return on investment in R&D for pharmaceuticals, for drugs that have been brought to market in recent years (Berndt *et al.*, 2015). Indeed, for drugs introduced between 2005 and 2009, researchers found that the pharmaceutical industry experienced a slightly net negative economic rate of return (insufficient to fully cover the costs of capital). Given a lengthy period required to complete R&D and clinical testing, and to receive regulatory approval, these recent new drugs are the result of research decisions initiated 10 to 15 years earlier. The constraints on coverage inherent in current policy will influence the rate and flow for drugs brought to market a decade or more from now.

The objectives inherent in current methods of coverage and pricing determination are (1) significant advances in clinical outcomes relative to current treatment protocols and (2) an effective price on this improvement in health status that falls within an acceptable range. In broad terms, these goals seem far from objectionable. However, the difficulties are not so much in the concept as in the implementation. The quality of the data upon which coverage decisions are made varies. This is most clearly the case in contrasting pharmaceuticals (and medical devices) with medical and surgical procedures. Conditions of regulatory approval ensure that new pharmaceuticals undergo clinical trials which imply a substantial body of evidence to evaluate their effectiveness. Evidence on new procedures is far more limited and ambiguous. New procedures are not patented, they tend to evolve significantly as they go through stages of experimentation, and the outcomes achieved are likely to be conditional on the skill of the practitioner. These limitations reflect the more informal gestation of these technologies and mean that it is far more difficult to make an informed decision until these technologies have to some extent already diffused. Yet these interventions tend to be costly. Research on heart attacks show that most of the increase in spending growth for this diagnosis reflects the increased use of surgical interventions as opposed to medical management (Cutler *et al.*, 1998).

Decisions on coverage should be made in a way that is consistent with underlying consumer preferences. Yet, there is no such thing as an average willingness to pay — preferences among consumers for which technologies should be approved and what price should be paid will necessarily differ. Some set of decisions must be made at the aggregate level, and a substantial fraction of those covered will disagree. Given a new and effective treatment for an existing disease or condition, public pressure will push toward its availability. We see this effect, for example, in the difficulties that Britain's National Health Service has encountered with new cancer drugs that exceed current thresholds for approval. In coverage determinations, Britain's National Institute for Health and Care Excellence (NICE) applies an approximate threshold for cost effectiveness in terms of incremental cost per quality-adjusted-life-year (QALY) that excludes coverage for a number of new cancer drugs.[2] In response to public outcry generated in sympathy to cancer sufferers who could not obtain access to the new therapies, a new Cancer Drugs Fund was introduced that applied laxer standards for cost-effectiveness relative to those applied to other new drugs considered for coverage (Cook, 2014). Of course, one might say that the real question is not how much a drug costs per QALY, but rather how much the people who fund the insurance pool (in this case British taxpayers) are willing to pay for it. The real task for the public and private organizations that make these determinations is to discern this willingness to pay.

Recent growth in global pharmaceutical R&D has been roughly flat (average annual growth of 1.8%), following a period of rapid growth from 2000 to 2009 (average annual growth of 11.9%). This suggests that pharmaceutical companies have been responding to lower rates of return by reducing their investment in R&D. The incentives inherent in tighter coverage and payment policies might also be expected to encourage a shift in the nature of innovation toward fewer

[2] A QALY is a standard measure used to integrate the health benefits due to longer life and improved quality of life in a single indicator.

incremental, "me-too" drugs that offer little additional benefits over existing therapies, and more new drugs that offer more substantial benefits relative to available alternatives (and are therefore widely approved for coverage).

Ironically, one such product is Sofusbuvir (Sovaldi), a Hepatitus C drug that is reportedly a true medical breakthrough in the treatment of the disease, with substantially higher cure rates and fewer side effects. Sovaldi has gained fame largely due to the high price of a course of treatment (combined with a large population of candidates for treatment) despite the fact that the estimated cost per QALY for the therapy ($26,000) is within the range usually considered acceptable (Liu *et al.*, 2014). The ongoing public debate in the wake of the Sovaldi phenomena can be expected to influence health policy, which may ultimately factor into decisions on future R&D spending.

An additional powerful channel for influencing the adoption and diffusion of new technology is through capital investment decisions. Some of the most expensive medical innovations are dependent upon investment in capital equipment within hospital facilities. For example, the current standard of care for a heart attack patient entering an emergency room involves the provision of angioplasty within 90 minutes of arrival at the hospital. However, the provision of this procedure requires the availability of a cardiac catheterization laboratory. Effectively, the determination to invest in widespread availability of this capability is the necessary condition for the diffusion of this technology. The HealthBasket research project examined standards of treatment for common conditions including heart attack across a range of countries within the European Union. They found that variation in the provision of PTCA to heart attack patients was standard in Germany, France, and Italy, spottily available in the UK, and virtually unavailable to any patients in relatively lower income European countries such as Greece and Spain (Bech *et al.*, 2008).

The effects of policy on new medical procedures will be felt through the use of global budgets or supply-side constraints on capital investment. The international expansion of Diagnosis Based Groups (DRGs) for inpatient payment, while seemingly targeted to reduce incentives for intensive forms of treatment for low-value cases, is less likely to influence the volume of major procedures, since they are often the basis for DRGs. However, the determination of pricing for the DRGs that incorporate new medical technologies will also be an important issue for diffusion. Sufficiently generous pricing may allow for diffusion to occur even in the absence of add-on payments (Shih and Berliner, 2008).

Methodology

The empirical analysis presented in this chapter applies at a national level, across countries and across time. As mentioned, the basic objective of this analysis is to determine the effects of technological change in medicine in a way that is applicable at the national and international level. This objective is partly a reaction to a perceived gap in the existing literature that addresses cross-national variation in medical technology and health systems.

Both medical technology and health policy are difficult to define and measure in a way that allows for generalized comparisons over time. It is possible to identify differences in the use of technology at a highly specific level (e.g., what is the standard treatment protocol for a specific medical condition in different countries?). It is possible to identify differences in health systems at a fairly broad level (e.g., integrated national health system versus mixed public payment/private insurance) or a very specific level (e.g., is there a technology add-on payment for the provision of drug-eluting stents in the provision of angioplasty).

As mentioned, the result is that the empirical literature that addresses the impact of variation in health policy on the adoption and diffusion of medical technology at an extremely specific level. The scope of analysis is effectively dictated by the limitations of the data. In particular, these studies are limited to a consideration of (1) high-volume conditions with a clear diagnosis, treated largely in inpatient settings where data on treatment patterns is more easily available, and (2) brief periods of time. The most thoroughly studied diagnosis/setting by far is the treatment of heart attacks in inpatient settings. Two important examples of such research are the studies based on the TECH project and the Euro-Area HealthBasket project (Moise, 2003; Busse *et al.*, 2008). These were two data-intensive projects that worked through identifying set of common diagnoses and compiling extensive records on the treatment provided in acute care settings. The results of these studies are both fascinating and useful. However, by the fragmentary nature of the view that this produces of the health system, and particularly because this analysis is limited to effectively a point-in-time perspective, this literature has a limited amount to say about the development and diffusion of medical technology within health systems over time, and across countries over time.

The approach that is applied in this study has, perhaps, the opposite character; it is estimated at the most aggregate level. The methodology used has a long history with roots in national growth accounting. Effectively, the contribution of medical technology is estimated by controlling for other factors contributing to growth. The residual growth is attributed to technology. This method has been applied previously to estimate the contribution of medical technology to growth for individual countries based on time-series data (Newhouse,1992; Smith *et al.*, 2009; Australian Productivity Commission, 2005).

This is a difficult task at the national level, because it is hard to ensure that the analysis has effectively identified and accounted for all factors that contribute to growth. The challenge is far harder when working with cross-country time-series data, because comparable cross-country data is limited. Simply put, it is *not* possible to control for the factors that contribute to variation in health care spending to a degree that would allow us to compare the contribution of changing medical technology to *levels* of health spending for individual countries (e.g., France vs. Australia). However, it is arguably possible to calculate a residual for *growth* in health care spending over time in a way that allows conclusions to be drawn on the changing contribution of medical technology, and to evaluate whether this trend in growth bears a relationship to health system characteristics.

There are two key reasons to develop an approximate set of estimates of the contribution of medical technology to health care spending growth across countries. First, key health systems characteristics vary at a national level. Regulatory approval, and usually major coverage determinations as well, are made at the national level. The definition of the categories that form the basis for payment within DRG-based systems is also determined at a national level. The breadth and pricing for DRG categories increasingly influences the diffusion of technologies in an inpatient context. If the objective is to evaluate the link between health systems and the role of medical technology, then an estimate of the contribution of medical technology at the national level is necessary.

Second, a critical issue for policymakers concerns public-sector budgeting, which rests on an understanding of the factors that drive health care spending. This perspective also benefits from a macro-level, time-series perspective. Granted, the objective of health policy with regards to technology is not to slow its adoption, but to guide decisions on adoption and provide appropriate incentives for diffusion so that limited resources can be deployed more efficiently. However, from a budgetary perspective, it is useful to know whether evidence suggests that health policy efforts have reduced the growth in spending on medical technology, even in the absence of answers on the broader questions of social welfare.

The empirical analysis presented has two parts:

(1) Estimate the contribution of changing medical technology to growth in health spending across a broad cross-section of countries over time.
(2) Evaluate the relationship between variation in the contribution of medical technology to health spending growth and health systems characteristics.

Using a broad cross-section of countries over a time period extending over decades has an additional advantage for our objective; medical knowledge is global in nature. If the tendency for health care spending to grow faster than the economy as a whole is in fact due to the expanding capabilities of medicine, then this should produce a trend that will be shared across all of the countries in our pooled cross-sectional time-series dataset. The broader the country sample, and the longer the time dimension, the more likely that the many country specific and temporary effects that we cannot fully control for will be uncorrelated, thus allowing the identification of the common trend.

The approximate contribution of technology to health spending growth is estimated based on panel data for two sets of countries:

(1) World Health Organization (WHO): 162 countries, 1995–2011.
(2) Organisation for Economic Cooperation and Development (OECD):
    (a) 29 countries, 1995–2011.
    (b) 14 countries, 1970–2011.

A model is estimated with health care spending growth as the dependent variable across a sample of countries and over time. The objective is to explain variation in health care spending growth as a function of factors that are major drivers of health care spending. The residual (unexplained) variation in growth is attributed to the role of changing medical technology. In terms of estimation methods, this approach is similar to the large body of literature that addresses international variations in health care spending based on pooled panel data (Gerdtham and Jonsson, 2000). However, the focus of most of this literature is on international variation in *levels* of health spending. Here, a similar approach is applied to variation in *growth rates*. As discussed below, the estimation of the model in terms of growth rates is critical for the validity of this approach as applied to the role of technological change.

In terms of methodology, this approach is most comparable to a study of international variations in health care spending by Barros (1998). The Barros study is not generally referenced as a source on the relationship between health systems characteristics and medical technology, because the author does not describe it as such. However, the approach is highly applicable to this question. Indeed, Barros suggests a tentative conclusion on the contribution of technology as a side-note to the study's general discussion of estimation results, stating that "it is worth noting that the unexplained residual amounts to roughly 30% of growth in health care spending."

The Barros estimate of 30% is below Newhouse's estimate that technology residual accounts for "at least half" of growth in real per capita health care spending rising costs in the US, and at the low end of the range (27–48%) found in the later re-estimation of the technology residual in Smith *et al.* (2009). The difference in the conclusions reflects both the subject data and the methodology. Newhouse (1992) and Smith *et al.* (2009) conclusions were based on a set of parameter estimates used to characterize the sensitivity of health spending to a range of factors. These parameter estimates were based on separate empirical findings from the health economics literature based on differing data and methodology (for example, price and insurance elasticities were based on the conclusions of the Rand Health Insurance Experiment). In contrast, Barros' conclusion was based on an econometric estimate — his residual was the common time trend across all of the countries pooled in his sample. The same will be true of the results of the analysis presented below.

A second issue for the attribution of the residual concerns the likelihood of an interaction effect between aggregate national income and the introduction and diffusion of medical technologies. Analysis of data on international variation in treatment patterns compiled for the TECH Research Network found a systematic tendency for technologies to be introduced earlier and to expand more rapidly in countries with a relatively higher level of GDP per capita[3] (Jonsson and Eckerlund, 2003). Based on the assumptions in the Newhouse (1992) methodology, such an income–technology interaction effect would be incorporated entirely within the residual — which was intended to establish an upper bound on the contribution of medical technology to growth. However, within the methodology applied here the effect would be effectively divided between the two factors: Partially attributed to income, partially to technology. This would cause the residual estimated based on the current methodology to be lower than the Newhouse (1992) estimate.

As mentioned, the model is estimated based on two different datasets, with different countries included in the samples. Each of these datasets has advantages and disadvantages. First, we use time-series cross-sectional data compiled by the World Health Organization (WHO), which maintains a system of National Health Accounts (NHA) that document health spending by source of financing based on a broad range of country-specific secondary sources (Poullier *et al.*, 2002). The data cover both an extended period of time (1995–2012), as well as a very broad cross-section of countries. This database includes health spending per capita, gross national income (GNI), the out-of-pocket (OOP) share of health spending, public share of health spending, as well as demographic data on the composition of populations by age.[4]

The 17 year sample from 1995 to 2012 is a shorter time period than might be optimal if we want to dampen the effect of economic cycles and one-time events on trend. However, this disadvantage is offset by the breadth and heterogeneity of the country sample, which (excluding countries with substantial gaps in the time series) covers 162 countries. The sample includes a substantial number of

[3]The TECH Research Network was an international collaborative effort to compile comparable micro-level data on the composition of treatment at a detailed level for a range of common diagnoses across a broad range of countries.

[4]Documentation for the database notes the use of imputation to fill in missing values for some years and concepts where there are gaps in source data, however, the data does not include imputation flags, so the extent of this practice is unclear.

countries from every continent in the world, and includes a broad cross-section of low- and middle-income countries.

In contrast, the OECD database is fairly homogeneous — covering only countries in the top tier of the income distribution used by the WHO for classification. However, the OECD data offers a major advantage for the objective of evaluating the relationship between the role of medical technology and the health systems' characteristics. Independent research efforts have produced a broad set of proxies that classify health systems within many of the OECD countries according to their characteristics. These measures can be used to test whether there is any relationship between the estimated contribution of medical technology to growth, and the cross-country variation in health systems that result from differing paths on health policy.

In addition to the ability to classify health systems' characteristics in a way that can be incorporated econometrically, the OECD database has the advantage of a substantially longer time-series history for a range of countries, allowing us to look at the composition of growth in health care spending over a period from 1970–2012. The process that leads from research and development to initial introduction of new technologies, to (in some cases) investment in the necessary expertise and facilities and equipment required to support the new technologies, to the diffusion of the technology through the patient population that may benefit from it occurs over a number of years. A longer period of time will also help to ensure enough variation to screen out short-term country-specific effects and therefore better identify the common trend attributable to the role of technological change. Lastly, the ability to estimate the contribution of technology over such an extended period will allow us to more effectively test whether this contribution has changed over time.

Identifying drivers of health care spending growth

Only a few factors that contribute to levels of health spending change persistently over time — thus influencing health care spending growth in a systematic way. Key factors that contribute to growth in health spending on a continual basis over time include:

- Aggregate income growth.
- Demographic shifts in the age–gender composition of the population.
- Changes in insurance coverage.
- Growth in relative medical prices.
- Medical innovation.

The dependent variable in the model is constant dollar growth in health care spending per capita. Ideally, the model should include variables for each of the major factors that drive growth in health care spending. Any factors that cannot be defined as variables in the model will by definition be included in the residual unexplained variation in growth. The critical question for the application of this approach here is whether it is possible to control adequately for the effects of factors other than medical innovation that can be expected to influence health spending growth, so that the effects of medical technology will be the dominant influence captured within the residual over time.

As mentioned, many factors that influence health spending do not exert an effect in a continuous, persistent way over time. Rather, the impact is likely to be specific to each individual country and nonrecurring or episodic in nature. Examples might include epidemics, weather conditions, and shortages of certain types of health professionals, or cultural or economic factors that are idiosyncratic to individual countries. The effects of such factors should appear primarily in variations specific to those countries. Such effects are unlikely to be correlated across countries or time for such a broad sample as that being used for this estimation. If we can assume that the factors that we cannot explicitly control for are distributed largely independently across countries, this should allow us to estimate the relative importance of the handful of factors that do systematically influence health care spending growth over time for all countries.

Consistent international panel data for health spending per capita, aggregate income (proxied by gross domestic product, or GDP), and the age composition of the population are available across a broad range of countries. The role of insurance is usually represented by a proxy defined by OOP share of health spending, a concept for which data are also available for a broad range of countries.

Relative medical price inflation

There is no available source for internationally comparable data on relative medical prices. A series of health care purchasing power parity (PPP) indexes is compiled by the OECD, however, these indexes are widely considered to be inconsistent and very incomplete in their coverage. The key issue is that many public health systems do not rely on market prices. Thus, part of the reason for the lack of data is that health systems with public-sector delivery of medical care simply do not have market-determined prices outside of those paid for drugs and devices purchased from private firms. Second, the measurement of medical prices is a uniquely difficult issue, even when the issue is confined to the construction of a time-series within a single country. Attempts to develop price measures that are applicable across countries continue to find a degree of variation that seems implausible. Prices necessarily reflect the allocation of high fixed costs across patients, and methods for performing this allocation are not consistent. Where available, price measures also often reflect some degree of implicit cross-subsidization, and may not capture the actual transaction prices in light of variable discounting from reported prices.

Much of the variation in health expenditures that is attributable to relative medical prices is cross-sectional in nature. Variation in the relative use of health expenditures in comparison with the inputs used to produce medical care (physician visits, nurses, hospital bed-days, prescriptions) support this conclusion (Anderson *et al.*, 2003). Variation in capital intensity, in intensity per bed-day, the mix of services provided, and in relative productivity precludes the use of these measures as a reliable proxy for relative price on a cross-sectional basis. However, we are primarily looking at cross-country variation in growth rates rather than levels, and for this purpose, measures of price are far less important.

From the perspective of relative growth, there are two factors that mitigate the lack of medical price data. Relative medical prices are determined by relative input prices and relative productivity growth. We are attempting to control for factors other than technological change that influence health care spending. This means that we are interested in a measure of price growth that reflects productivity growth from the perspective of production efficiency for existing forms of medical care. This contrasts with research that addresses price measurement based on the increased valuation placed on the improvement in health outcomes associated with new technology (Cutler *et al.*, 1998).

William Baumol's model of unbalanced growth implies that relative medical price inflation will be a function of economy-wide productivity growth (Baumol, 1967; 1993). If so, this suggests that a substantial part of the variation in relative medical prices may actually be captured by variation in real per capita GDP. Real per capita GDP is a measure of output. However, at the aggregate level, the growth in income to factors of production must equal the growth in output. This allows us to use real per capita GDP as a proxy for income. However, if labor force participation is roughly constant over the long run, growth in real per capita GDP will also be an approximate measure of growth in labor productivity. Growth in economy-wide wages can be expected to track average growth in labor productivity over the long-run. Labor market competition should ensure that the wage rates in industries with relatively lower productivity growth must keep pace with areas where productivity growth is faster.

The implication is that relative growth in health sector wages should be correlated with real per capita GDP. Data on relative compensation for health care providers drawn from the OECD Health Database can be used to test this hypothesis. We use average wage rates for registered nurses (RNs). The sample of countries (26 countries) where this data is available is by far the largest and probably the most internationally comparable from a skill-mix perspective. We estimate a pooled regression of real wage growth for RNs as a function of a constant, and current and lagged growth in real per capita GDP (all variables in log differences) using generalized least squares (GLS). This covers the period from 1994–2011, but is unbalanced, with a total of 202 observations. We find that growth in real per capita GDP is a strongly significant predictor of international variation in relative wage growth for RNs for our sample of 26 countries, with an estimated elasticity of 1.3. This suggests that relative wages for health providers are a function of economy-wide labor productivity growth, but tend to grow at a systematically faster pace. This potentially reflects the fact that the health care workforce is relatively highly skilled in comparison with the economy as a whole, and is also growing more rapidly, potentially bidding up wages for a limited pool of skilled personnel. In sum, growth in real wages are correlated with real per capita GDP, which can be expected to capture some part of their contribution to growth in health care spending in our estimation of the effect of technology.

In addition to growth in relative input prices, a second factor that contributes to relative growth in relative medical prices is relative productivity growth. Baumol's model suggests that the unavoidably labor-intensive, customized nature of medical services is likely to make it more difficult to achieve gains in the efficient production of health care, similar to sectors such as education. This suggests that improvements in productive efficiency (for example) for a diagnostic consultation with a general practitioner will be hard to achieve. If productivity growth in the production of medical services is consistently low, then relative productivity growth — which drives relative medical price inflation — should be a function of economy-wide productivity. There is a small empirical literature that addresses this hypothesis, which provides empirical support for the relationship implied by the Baumol model in the case of the health care sector (Hartwig, 2008).

In sum, our assumption in estimating a bound for the contribution of technology to growth is that cross-sectional time-series variation in real per capita GDP growth will not only capture income effects, but will also likely act as a proxy to capture some part of the variation in growth that is attributable to relative medical price inflation as well. Certainly, there will be variation in relative medical price inflation across countries that will not be captured by this method. This variation will be included in the residual growth used to estimate an upper bound for the contribution of medical technology to growth. If the relative productivity-driven effects hypothesized by Baumol are captured by the inclusion of real per capita GDP, then medical technology should be the critical remaining driver of growth for the long-term trend in growth embodied within the regression residual.

Dynamic issues in the link between medical technology and GDP: Accounting for lags

The rate at which new technologies are adopted and diffuse into medical practice across countries has been shown to be a function of income levels. We can expect this causal link to appear with a substantial lag. Practical access to many innovations requires investment in specialized equipment and facilities, and/or access to specialists with scarce expertise. This linkage is widely acknowledged in the health policy literature, and has been the subject of analysis at the micro level as well. (Anderson and Slade, 1999; Lambooij *et al.*, 2010). Investment in specialized health facilities and equipment requires planning and budgetary allocation, whether it occurs in the public or private sector. Such investment tends to begin in major population centers and spread over a period of years. There are also substantial lags in the diffusion of new technologies that stem from informational costs. Medical practice patterns are characterized by a great deal of inertia. Part of this reflects simply the time costs of learning about new treatment options. Part of it reflects the fact that procedural innovations often require expertise that cannot easily be transferred without personal instruction.

In particular, the sensitivity of uptake to the characteristics of the specific technology is that there is an interaction effect between technological change and national income levels. In a broad sense, the adoption of a technology will occur only when aggregate income levels have passed a certain threshold. The corollary to this interaction effect is that, for the high-cost capital and skill-intensive the process of the diffusion of technologies will be extended over long periods of time, as lower income countries will not invest in these expensive technologies when there are many more urgent medical needs that remain to be addressed within a limited budget.

This dynamic in clearly seen in the case of coronary artery bypass grafts (CABGs), a technology that has been used in practice since the late 1960s that has fully diffused in higher income countries, however, for middle- and lower-income countries it is still in the process of diffusion (OECD, 2014). This effect can also be seen in international variations in percutaneous transluminal coronary angioplasty (PTCA). PTCA has been shown to greatly improve survival from AMI (heart attack) if provided within a narrow 90 minute window following the onset (Keeley *et al.*, 2003). However, the treatment requires the immediate availability of a cardiac catheterization laboratory and a surgical team to perform the procedure. This is therefore a very costly treatment option. The result can be seen in patterns of international diffusion: In several high income countries, including the US, France, and Switzerland, the capability for PTCA has now fully diffused from a technical perspective, there is little additional benefit from further expansion

— in fact use of the procedure has flattened or declined. However, in low to middle-income countries, this technology is accessible in only a few urban centers. The fact that uptake and diffusion are a function of income has stretched out the process of diffusion over decades.

Model Specification

The dependent variable in the model is real per capita health expenditures (h_t), and the independent variables are real per capita GDP (y_t) and OOP share of health spending (i_t). The effects of population aging are estimated based on over the share of the population that is over 65 years of age.[5] Thus, the adjustment for demographic effects is incorporated in the dependent variable of the model based on an index (d_t) rather than econometrically estimated. All variables are expressed in log differences (growth rates); ε_t is the usual error term.

All variables are defined as log differences (growth rates) in the specification that we use for estimation.[6]

$$\Delta \ln h_t - \Delta \ln d_t = \beta_0 + \sum_{n=0}^{T} \beta_{t+n} \Delta(\ln y_{t-n}) + \gamma \ln i_t + \varepsilon_t . \tag{1}$$

The constant term in Eq. (1) provides a measure of an upper bound for the exogenous contribution of medical innovation to growth in health spending. This should give us a measure of the relative importance of medical innovation for growth in health spending over time and across countries. However, as mentioned above, in addition to this exogenous component of the contribution there is likely to be a substantial contribution for the uptake and diffusion of medical technology that is a function of aggregate income. Since we have no instrument for the contribution of medical technology that allows us to estimate this interaction effect, we can only say that this interaction effect will be included in the contribution to growth from aggregate income.

---

[5] An index for the impact of shifts across demographic age-groups on growth in real per capita health care spending was calculated for all countries and time periods. This index relies on the assumption of a constant base-year distribution of health care spending per capita across four broad age cohorts (0 to 15 years, 16 to 64 years, 65 to 79 years, and 80 years and older). The base-year distribution is drawn from research by Hagist and Kotlikoff (2005), who compile data from national sources for 10 countries for the years 2000–2001. Growth in the share of spending for each age cohort is multiplied by the base-year distribution for relative per capita spending for that cohort, and aggregated across all age cohorts to produce the index of the effects of demographic shifts on health care spending.

[6] We tested the variables h_t and y_t for stationarity based on the Im–Pesaran–Shin Test for unit roots in panel data. We find that both series are non-stationary in log-levels, but are stationary in first differences (I(1)). However, this issue is moot, since conceptually, our interest is in variation in growth rates in any case.

The residual that is used to define the contribution of technology separately is estimated based on three datasets. The first of these is a sample of 162 countries that with a comprehensive global scope compiled by the World Health Organization (WHO) and Global Health Observatory (GHO) (WHO and GHO, 2014). The second dataset is a sample of 29 countries drawn from the OECD Health Data (OECD, 2014). The third dataset is also drawn from the OECD health database, but is selected with the intention of estimating the model based on a long time-series of balanced panel data. We estimate the same model specification based on each of these datasets.

The objective in estimating the model based on the WHO dataset rests on the extremely broad and heterogeneous set of countries in the sample. The variability in the characteristics of the health systems in this large and broad dataset should allow us to test the validity of the proposed methodology for estimating the contribution of medical technology to health care spending growth. As discussed above, our ability to control for the impact of non-technology factors is sharply limited by the availability of data. Yet the variables that we do have are arguably the ones that are most vital for the purpose, allowing us to estimate the effects of aggregate income, insurance coverage, and demographics on growth. With the exception of relative medical price, these are the key variables that we expect to drive growth in health spending on a consistent basis over time, because they are the only factors that change continuously across all countries over time. While innumerable factors will influence health spending levels, if these effects are not correlated they will not influence coefficient estimates, although any net effect on growth over the entire time period will be captured in the residual. Within this highly heterogeneous sample, a common trend will be more clearly attributable to the changing state of medical knowledge, since this is the one factor that is clearly global in nature.

All variables are extracted from the WHO Global Health Observatory website, with the exception of the population over the age 65, which was pulled from data compiled by the World Bank. Excluding countries where the available time-series was short, our panel consists of data for 162 countries, most of which have near complete data for the period from 1995–2012. The dependent variable $\Delta \ln h_t$ is the log difference of real per capita health care expenditure growth, converted to US dollar terms using PPPs, and deflated to constant 2005 US dollar terms. As a measure of aggregate income (y_t) Gross National Income (GNI) is used. GNI is equal to the sum of a nation's gross domestic product (GDP) plus net income from outside of the country.[7] The proxy for insurance coverage (i_t) is the out-of-pocket share of health spending.

[7] For most nations the difference between GDP and GNI is not large. Income flowing into the country tends to be roughly balanced by payments flowing out of the country. But in selected countries GNI

Results of Estimation

1. Results of estimation based on WHO dataset

Estimation of residual growth based on countries in the WHO dataset produces results for the sensitivity of health care spending to variations in income and insurance coverage that are highly consistent with past empirical literature. The estimated elasticity with respect to income is 0.9, and the estimated lag structure associated with this effect is long, extending over a period of 8 years. This elasticity estimate is at the low end of estimates based on national-level data, which range from about 0.9 to 1.6. This reflects the effect of the much broader and more heterogeneous country sample, and the fact that this specification is estimated based on growth rates (rather than in levels, as is the case with most similar specifications) (Gerdtham and Jonsson, 2000).[8]

The elasticity of health care spending with respect to insurance coverage (average OOP share of spending) is –0.2, comparable to estimates generated by the Rand Health Insurance Experiment based on very different methodology and data (Manning *et al.*, 1987). The estimated contribution of medical technology to growth in health care spending that is implied by the residual is 19% of the total growth. This is below the low end of the estimated range found by Smith *et al.* (2009). However, this difference reflects the fact that the Smith *et al.* study estimates incorporates an estimate for a positive interaction effect between income growth and technological change. Excluding the effects of this interaction effect, the residual estimated here falls within a comparable range. This estimate is also lower than the estimated 30% share of health spending growth attributed to medical technology by Barros (1998) — a result that likely reflects both the difference in sample, and the inclusion in this model of the effects of OOP share of spending (which accounts for an estimated 6% of growth) and an differing representation of demographic change. After accounting for these differences, the parameters and implied composition of the factors contributing to growth are reasonably in line with past estimates.

---

can be quite different from GDP. For example, Ireland is a popular location for foreign companies, who tend to repatriate profits to an extent that more than offsets income flows from overseas. Thus GDP overstates income for Ireland. However, for many low-income countries benefit from a net flow of income from their nationals who are employed in other countries; thus GDP understates aggregate income. The latter case is relevant for a number of countries in the WHO sample.

[8] An additional relevant difference in the specification is the exclusion of fixed effects specific to country and time period (2-way fixed effects). Since these fixed effects tend to be positively correlated with variations in the income variable, their inclusion tends to reduce the coefficient on the income variable.

Table 1. Decomposition of real per capita health spending growth for WHO sample[a]
(US dollars, converted from national currency units based on PPPs: World Health Organization (WHO) 162-country sample, 1995–2012)

	Contribution to growth (percentage points, annual growth)	Share of growth (%)
Aggregate income growth (Including income–technology interaction effect)	2.2	62.8
Insurance coverage (OOP share of spending)	0.2	5.8
Demographic shifts	0.4	12.4
Residual (Medical technology + other factors)	0.7	19.0
Real per capita health spending (mean growth rate)	3.5	100.0

Notes: [a]Share of growth attributed to each factor is the unweighted mean contribution to growth across all countries in the sample. The share of growth for each country is based on parameters generated by the estimation of Eq. (1), using a log-based decomposition of growth over the entire sample period.
Source: Author's calculations.

The WHO database is global in scope, and includes countries that are extremely heterogeneous in the characteristics of their health systems, as well as in the economic, demographic and social context. A common residual trend in health spending growth across such a broad sample must reflect a common factor that provides a plausible explanation that can apply globally, independent of system characteristics. From a theoretical standpoint, medical innovation is the only plausible candidate for this role.

The estimated contribution to growth of medical technology based on the residual also tends to decline over time (a time trend added to the regression specification is negative and significant). This declining trend is consistent with what we would expect to see if the effects of health policy have tended to either slow the rate at which new technologies are introduced and at which they diffuse. However, we cannot explicitly show any causal link between trends in health policy and this declining residual, so this result is only suggestive.

2. Results of estimation based on OECD dataset

OECD 29-country sample, 1995–2012

Results of estimation for the OECD 29-country sample over 1995–2012 show an income elasticity of 1.2 and an OOP price elasticity of –0.1. The effect on spending growth due to the share of population over age 65 years is controlled for within

Table 2. Decomposition of real per capita health spending growth for OECD sample[a] (US dollars, converted from national currency units based on PPPs: Organisation for Economic Cooperation and Development (OECD), 29-country sample, 1995–2012)

	Contribution to growth (percentage points, annual growth)	Share of growth (%)
Aggregate income growth (Including income–technology interaction effect)	2.5	65.7
Insurance coverage (OOP share of spending)	< 0.1	0.5
Demographic shifts	0.4	10.6
Residual (Medical technology + other factors)	0.9	23.2
Real per capita health spending (mean growth rate)	3.8	100.0

Notes: [a]Share of growth attributed to each factor is the unweighted mean contribution to growth across all countries in the sample. The share of growth for each country is based on parameters generated by the estimation of Eq. (1), using a log-based decomposition of growth over the entire sample period.
Source: Author's calculations.

the dependent variable, which is real per capita health care spending adjusted for the estimated effect of variation in the demographic (age and gender) composition of the population. Compared with a mean growth rate of 3.8% for the OECD sample of 29 countries, this implies a contribution of medical technology to growth of 23%.

In comparison with the WHO sample, we note three key differences. The income elasticity is higher (1.2 vs. 0.9), but both estimates fall within a range that is consistent with past research. The elasticity with respect to OOP price is smaller in magnitude than for the WHO sample (–0.08 vs. –0.16). This is not surprising given that cost-sharing in this sample is much lower on average and less variable across countries. The mean rate of growth in the OOP share for this country sample is also very small, with the result that the estimated contribution of changing insurance coverage — at least over this time period — is negligible. In addition, cost-sharing in the OECD countries tends to be in the form of small, relatively minor payments that are waived for patients at low income levels and are accompanied by annual caps on OOP responsibility, whereas in the many low and middle-income countries that are included in the WHO sample, cost-sharing may mean that the patient is responsible for the entire cost of treatment. Thus, it is reasonable to expect to see a relatively smaller impact of cost-sharing at the margin for the relative higher-income countries in the OECD sample. The estimated share of growth attributed to medical technology here is 23%, somewhat higher than the 19% estimated for the WHO data sample. For this sample as well, we continue to find a statistically significant negative trend in the estimated contribution of medical technology to growth.

OECD 14-country sample, 1970–2012

The same model was estimated over a longer time-series for a cross-section of 14 countries where we have data for the period 1970–2012. Time-series for OOP spending are not available over this period, so this variable is not included in the model. The results of estimation showed a larger income elasticity (1.4) than in the shorter and more recent OECD sample (1.2), a significantly greater weight on longer lags on income growth, and a lower contribution to growth attributed to medical technology (18% of growth in real per capita spending). This lower contribution is largely a function of the higher income elasticity, which probably reflects a correspondingly larger positive interaction effect between income growth and technology uptake and diffusion.

For the model estimated over this sample as well, a time trend is negative and highly significant, implying that the contribution of medical technology declined by 1.1 percentage points between 1970 and 2012. Relative to the mean rate of growth in real per capita health spending of 3.2% over this period, this is a substantial reduction in trend. Note, however, that this estimated time trend is much shallower than the trend estimated based on either the WHO sample or the OECD sample for 1995–2012.

Chart 1 shows a comparison of the residual contribution to growth based on the three different samples, including the trend effect, based on (1) the WHO database for 170 countries, 1995–2012, (2) the OECD database for 29 countries, 1995–2012, and (3) the OECD database for 14 countries from 1970–2012 (excluding OOP spending growth).

Evaluating the decline in the estimated contribution of medical technology to growth

Based on a comparison of the rate of decline across results of estimation for the three alternative samples, the trend for the 1970–2012 sample appears more plausible from the perspective of a long-term decomposition of growth in real per capita health spending.[9] The substantially longer sample period (42 years vs. 17 years) arguably provides a much more defensible basis for the estimation of a

[9]While we omitted the OOP share from this regression for lack of a longer time-series, we would expect that variable to have a net positive effect on growth over time, since insurance coverage tended to expand over this period. Thus our residual is biased against finding a negative trend in residual

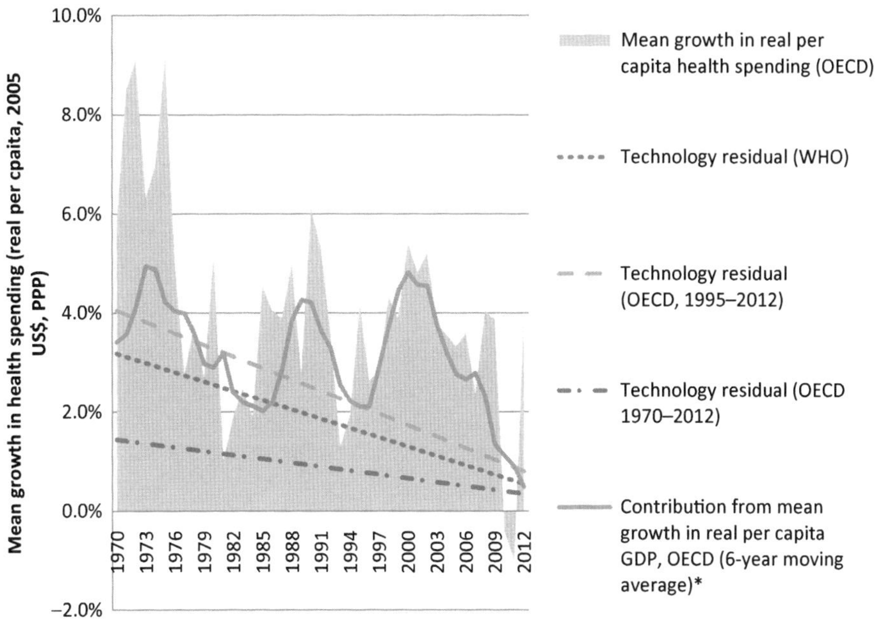

Chart 1. Estimated contribution to growth in health spending from income and medical technology

Notes: * The coefficient of 1.4 used to represent the estimated contribution of aggregate income growth to spending is based on the estimation for the OECD sample for 1970–2012. The growth rate in real per capita health spending shown is the cross-sectional mean for this sample (unweighted).
Source: Author's calculations.

trend in the contribution of medical technology over time. The longer history is less likely to be subject to shared shocks that may influence all countries in the sample. Notably, the effects of the 2008 financial crisis were global in scope and may potentially have influenced health spending across a cross-section of countries.

We can also see that growth in real per capita health spending exhibits long cycles of approximately 10–20 years from trough to trough. This implies that (1) trends in health spending growth cannot be defensibly evaluated based on periods of less than about 20 years as such periods capture only a part of a full cycle, and (2) an assessment of factors that change slowly, such as health care institutions really requires more than a single cycle. For example, the most recent ten years of data from 2002 to 2012 extend from a cyclical peak to just past a cyclical trough. A valid evaluation of long-term trend must take this cycle into account. A relationship estimated from 1995–2012 encompasses roughly one full

growth. However, the longer time-frame probably also plays a role in explaining the slower trend estimated based on this longer time span.

growth cycle. Regressions estimated from 1970–2012 include three such cycles, thus providing a much stronger basis for capturing a full picture of the role of factors such as technological change that exert an influence across these cycles. The presence of a significant trend in the broad and heterogeneous country samples for the WHO and OECD data for 1995–2012 validates the attribution of the shared trend to the role of changing medical technology. However, the rate of change in the contribution of technology to long-term growth in health spending is probably better captured based on the smaller OECD country sample for 1970–2012.

As mentioned in the introduction to this chapter, the *effects* of medical technology on health care utilization and spending are distinct from advances in the state of knowledge that defines technological change in medicine. The effects of medical technology on health care spending will be a function of a number of different factors that determine the willingness and ability to pay for these forms of treatment. One possible explanation for the declining contribution of medical technology to growth in health spending is that this deceleration does not reflect a slowdown in the rate of innovation — the actual generation of new treatment options — but rather a declining rate of uptake and diffusion of innovations. One possible way to distinguish between these two explanations is to evaluate the rate of change in medical technology (as state of knowledge) explicitly based on R&D expenditures, as a proxy for the innovation that is generated by R&D. If the productivity of R&D expenditures remains constant over time, then this variable should be an effective proxy for the state of medical knowledge.[10] If we continue to see a decline in the residual used to estimate the impact of medical technology on health spending growth after controlling for growth in R&D expenditures over time, this would suggest that we are actually seeing a decline in the rate at which new treatment option are introduced and diffuse, rather than a slowdown in the rate of innovation itself.

Data are available from the OECD on total R&D spending for most OECD countries and some non-OECD countries, covering the period from 1981–2013 — although with some gaps in the data. The vast majority of medical research is

[10]There are three major issues with using R&D expenditures as a proxy for technological change. First, we must assume that the productivity of R&D expenditures in generating medical advances is constant both across countries and over time. Second, we expect the impact of R&D to occur with long and variable lags. Medical and surgical procedures, which are lightly regulated, may begin to diffuse into practice soon after their initial development — although limited by determinations of insurance coverage. Pharmaceutical R&D, however, generates new products only with very long lags, spanning 10 or more years (Berndt *et al.*, 2015). Third, it is likely that R&D expenditures will be an endogenous function of real GDP at the country level. However, while the effects of R&D may have a more immediate and stronger effect in the country where research is performed, medical innovation should be global in nature, independent of the original source of medical advances in the long-term.

conducted in the developed countries that dominate our OECD sample, although a rising share is performed in Asia.

The inclusion of growth in R&D expenditures to the basic model specification control is an attempt to explicitly control for the effect of advances in medical technology. The specification with this added variable was estimated based on the OECD sample of 14 countries where we have complete data for health spending and GDP for the period from 1970–2012. The source for R&D expenditures is the OECD Health Database (OECD, 2014). Medical knowledge is global in nature, defining the set of options for medical treatment that is independent of geographic location. Thus, the effects of medical innovation in any country in our sample should presumably reflect progress in medical knowledge and the development of new methods of treatment based on R&D across all countries. In short, we want an R&D spending concept that approximates a global aggregate. We approximate a global aggregate based on the 40 countries covered by the OECD data for R&D expenditures.[11]

The basic model for the 14-country OECD sample was estimated including the global R&D variable. We find that the coefficient on this broader R&D spending variable is positive as expected, statistically significant, and of a substantial magnitude. However, the negative time trend in the estimated contribution of medical technology to health care spending remains, and the magnitude of the decline is approximately equivalent to the deceleration that is seen in the model without the R&D variable.[12] Adding the global R&D expenditures variable to the WHO panel regression produces broadly similar results; the variable is positive and significant, however, the trend towards deceleration in the residual remains significant. This result suggests that slower growth in health care spending attributed to medical technology may more likely reflect the adoption and diffusion of

[11] A number of these countries have a limited historical time series. We winnow the country sample to 22 countries that cover most of this period. For countries such as Australia and Switzerland, where data are available periodically, rather than for every year in the sample, we interpolate linearly between sample years. This 22-country sample accounts for close to 90% of R&D spending within the 40-country sample, however, this declines to 70% by 2012, reflecting rapid growth in countries that have not historically been strong in medical research (particularly China). As mentioned, the role of countries not included in our 22-country aggregate grows rapidly over the period from 1992–2012. If global R&D is in fact an important determinant for growth in health spending, then the exclusion of these countries will distort the estimated relationship for the later part of our estimation period. To correct for this, a new series was constructed based on the assumption that the share of R&D spending for these 18 countries remains constant at 11% of the total over the period 1981–1992. This allows us to extrapolate the 40-country aggregate backwards by splicing the growth for the 22-country aggregate.

[12] The explanatory power of the R&D comes partially from a lower average for the residual attributed to the effects of medical technology over the entire period from 1970–2012, and partially from a lower-income coefficient.

new treatment options, rather than an actual slowdown in the rate of medical innovation in the sense of an expanding menu of options for treatment.

3. Estimation of relationship between health policy variables and contribution of medical technology to health care spending growth

The next stage is to estimate the relationship between the contribution of medical technology and health systems characteristics. The measures of the variation in health systems characteristics used for this purpose are drawn from a typology developed by Joumard *et al.* at the OECD. This typology was based on the results of the recent OECD Survey of Health Systems Characteristics conducted in 2008–2009 (Joumard *et al.*, 2010). This source has the advantage of a recent, detailed dataset that classifies a broad range of national health systems.

From the perspective of evaluating different approaches to managing the adoption and diffusion of technologies, the Joumard typology is also appealing in its choice of a defining dimension for categorizing gradations of variation systems' characteristics. Health systems are defined along a spectrum defined by a health system's relative reliance on market-based methods vs. regulatory-based (command and control) methods. Market reliance is determined based on the presence and extent of a role for private insurers (either in basic or supplementary coverage), the role of competition (e.g., user choice of insurers and/or medical providers), the use of provider incentives to influence the volume and quality of care provided (e.g., DRG-based systems), and the use of patient cost-sharing. At the other end of the spectrum, the main alternative to a market-reliant system is a system that is dominated by public payment and delivery of services, where the levers for cost control rely on a combination of regulation and a central or regional budgeting process. The clusters defined along this spectrum are shown in Figure 2.

For the purpose of our analysis of panel data, we aggregate these country clusters to produce four categories, rather than six, in light of the relatively small number of cross-country observations available to help estimate the relationships between health care spending growth and health systems characteristics.

These four categories are:

1. Basic health insurance coverage through private insurers: (1) from Figure 2.
2. Basic insurance coverage provided through the public sector, but a substantial role for supplementary private coverage: (2) and (3) from Figure 2.

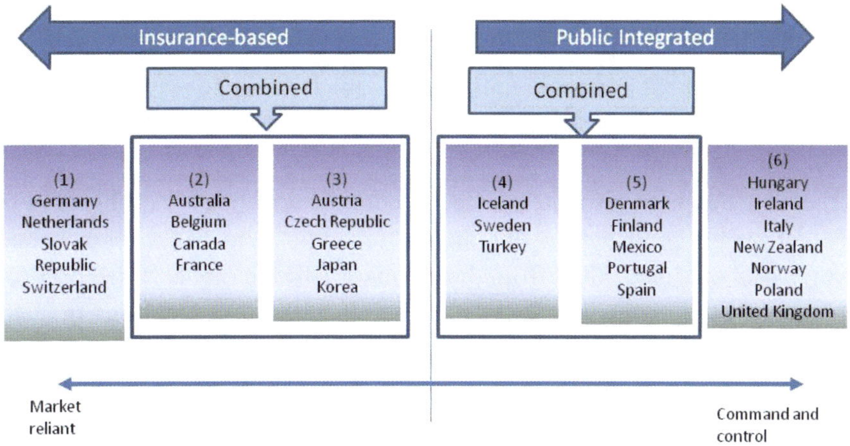

Figure 2. Country clusters of health systems with similar characteristics
Source: Joumard *et al.* (2010).

3. Public sector integrated system with some reliance on market mechanisms and soft budget constraints: (4) and (5) from Figure 2.
4. Public sector integrated health systems with little or no reliance on market mechanisms and strict budget constraints: (6) from Figure 2.

Estimation of the health care spending model incorporating these additional variables for the characteristics of the health systems shows that they are associated with substantial effects on health care spending growth. These effects are in a consistent direction and relative magnitude across the spectrum from the market-based side of the spectrum to the command and control end. After controlling for the effects of aggregate income and OOP share of spending, the estimated incremental impact of health system characteristics on health spending levels is shown below:

1. Private insurance for basic coverage (+15.5%).
2. Supplementary private insurance, in addition to public basic coverage (+0, reference category).
3. Public integrated system, with some reliance on market-mechanisms and relative soft budget constraints (−1.8%).
4. Public integrated system, little or no cost-sharing, strict budget constraints (−8.5%).

The clear message of this estimation is that systems on the market-based end of the Joumard spectrum exhibit relative faster growth in health spending than would be predicted based on income levels and cost-sharing, while those on the command and control end of the spectrum exhibit slower than anticipated growth in health spending. This does not address the relationship between medical technology and health system characteristics, but it does give us a baseline to look at as a comparison point.

The next step is to estimate a model where the dependent variable is defined as the estimated contribution of medical technology to health care spending growth, based on the residual from the estimation of the model based on Eq. (1). The results of the estimation show that the clusters of national health systems based on the Joumard *et al.* spectrum are not significantly related to cross-country variation in health spending growth attributable to medical innovation at standard levels of statistical significance. However, there is one suggestive result; the countries identified as integrated public health systems with strictly binding budget constraints show slower growth in the contribution of technology to health spending growth with a level of confidence of 75%. This result suggests that countries in this category take up new technology more slowly, reducing growth in real per capita health care spending by about a tenth of a percentage point annually.

On the whole, however, the results of estimating these two models with the Joumard *et al.* health system variables implies that variation in health care spending growth (1) is systematically related to health system type, but (2) is not systematically related to the effects of changing medical technology based on our estimates.

In addition to testing the explanatory power of the country clusters defined along the Joumard *et al.* spectrum, we separately estimated the effects of each individual health system characteristic that was compiled in the OECD Health System Survey. The original data on which these measures are based is largely binary (i.e., yes or no answers to survey questions) (Paris *et al.*, 2010). This detailed data is used by Joumard *et al.* to construct a series of variables for health system characteristics that reflect the strength of the perceived effect on a scale ranging from 1 to 6 (Joumard *et al.*, 2010). Results for each of the health systems variables are shown in Table 3.

The health systems variables that are statistically significant (or close to significant) are:

(1) The reliance on general practitioners (GPs) as gatekeepers (-).
(2) Global budget constraints (-).
(3) Decentralized (regional) control of health systems (-).
(4) Breadth of basic insurance coverage (-).
(5) Depth of basic insurance coverage (-).

Table 3. Estimates of the contributions of health system characteristics to health care spending growth

Dependent variables: Country-specific estimates of the contribution of medical technology to growth in real per capita health spending based on residuals from pooled regression (as shown in Table 1).

Variables	Coefficient	Standard error	*t*-statistic
Private provision	0.00094	0.00127	0.74
Volume incentives	0.00032	0.00148	0.22
Regulation of provider prices	0.00065	0.00178	0.37
User information	0.00152	0.00143	1.07
Supply constraints: workforce and equipment	−0.00038	0.00130	−0.29
Choice among providers	0.00053	0.00086	0.61
Gate-keeping	−0.00109	0.00075	−1.46
Price signals on users	0.00433	0.00327	1.33
Choice of insurer	−0.00018	0.00096	−0.19
Insurer levers	0.00031	0.00116	0.27
Over-the-basic coverage	−0.00136	0.00105	−1.29
Priority setting	−0.00006	0.00161	−0.03
Budget constraint	−0.00158	0.00085	−1.85
Regulation of prices paid by third-party payers	0.00063	0.00231	0.27
Decentralization	−0.00153	0.00101	−1.52
Delegation	0.00339	0.00183	1.85
Consistency	0.00058	0.00115	0.51
Breadth	−0.01132	0.00416	−2.72
Scope of coverage	0.00426	0.00561	0.76
Depth of coverage	−0.01103	0.00461	−2.39

Source: Author's calculations from OECD 29-country dataset.

We estimate a combined regression including all of these variables. In this estimation, gatekeepers, decentralization of the health system, and depth of coverage become more clearly insignificant. We are left with two variables; the use of global budget constraints and the breadth of coverage (results not shown). The explanatory power of the use of global budgets for health care spending is significant at the 10% level. This is consistent with our results based on regression for countries using the Joumard *et al.* spectrum.[13]

[13]The significant negative coefficient on breadth of coverage is unexpected. Breadth of coverage measures the fraction of the population that has basic insurance coverage. The implication of the

Conclusion

The empirical analysis in this chapter has addressed the relationship between growth in health care spending attributable to medical innovation (on the one hand), and health systems characteristics intended to control health care spending while maintaining quality of care (on the other hand). This analysis has proceeded in two stages: (1) estimate the contribution of medical technology to growth in real per capita health spending based on the attribution of an econometrically-estimated residual, and (2) estimate the relationship of growth in this technology-residual to cross-country variation in health systems characteristics.

The estimation of the technology residual based on pooled cross-country panel data for growth in real per capita health spending produced estimates of the contribution of medical innovation to growth that are plausible in their magnitude on average, and in their path over time. Coefficients that capture the contribution of aggregate income and insurance coverage to growth are reasonably consistent across the WHO dataset and the smaller OECD dataset.

Where conclusions differed between the two datasets (slightly higher income elasticity, lower elasticity for OOP share, smaller residual), these conclusions seem highly consistent with what we know of the shared characteristics of the countries in the OECD relative to the countries in the WHO sample. Estimates of the share of growth in real per capita health spending that is explained by the residual were 18% (OECD 14-country sample, 1970–2012), 23% (OECD 29-country sample, 1995–2012) and 19% (WHO 162-country sample, 1995–2012). These estimates appear somewhat low in comparison with previous estimates that concluded that the contribution of changing medical technology fell within a range of 27–48% (Smith *et al.*, 2009). However, this difference reflects interaction effects between income growth and technological change; part of the contribution of technological change is explained by income growth (richer countries tend to introduce new technologies at an earlier stage and to place fewer constraints on their diffusion). This technology-related effect is thus captured within the contribution attributed to income growth.

The significance of a global aggregate for R&D spending as an explanatory variable for health spending growth — and its role in explaining part of the

estimated negative coefficient is that universal coverage slows growth in real health care spending per capita, and more specifically, for the rate of uptake and diffusion of new medical technology. This seems implausible. A closer look at the data shows that virtually all of the countries in this sample have near-universal basic insurance coverage; the only exceptions are Mexico and Turkey. These two countries are very different in multiple characteristics from the rest of the sample. A reasonable interpretation is that the significant negative coefficient on this variable reflects an omitted variable that is relevant to growth for these two outliers over the sample period.

residual contribution, provides additional supports for the interpretation of the growth residual as a measure of the contribution of medical innovation to growth. The continued presence of a declining trend in the estimated contribution of medical technology to growth in health care spending suggests that this trend may reflect slower uptake and diffusion of new technologies, rather than a slower pace of medical innovation.

The second stage of empirical estimation evaluated the link between the estimated contribution of medical technology to growth and health systems' characteristics. Findings showed no significant relationship, indicating that growth attributable to changing medical technology is not sensitive to cross-national variation in health systems based on the four broad types defined here.

Estimation of the relationship of the contribution of medical technology to health policy variables at a more detailed level did produce some significant conclusions, including a negative relationship with the share of general practitioners as a share of the physician workforce, and with the requirement that general practitioners act as "gatekeepers." Those two results combined point to the importance of the role of physician specialists in the uptake and diffusion of new technologies — a plausible result. A second significant result was the slower growth attributable to medical technology in systems characterized by global budget constraints; again, this is a result that seems in line with expectations.

The strongest and most consistent result based on this approach was the implied slowdown in the contribution of medical technology to growth over time. This slowdown was significant in all of the country samples and time periods considered. Particularly in the case of the extremely broad and heterogeneous WHO country sample, this is a very strong result. Such a trend in growth for a single country, or even for a set of relatively homogeneous countries that dominate the OECD sample, could reasonably be attributed to some shared omitted variable that influenced health spending growth over the 1995–2012 period. There are few factors that could possibly explain a trend in growth that is shared across all of the 162 countries in the WHO sample over an extended period.

Based on the OECD 14-country sample for 1970–2012, the decline in the contribution of medical technology reduced growth in health care spending growth in 2012 by 1.1 percentage points as compared to 1970, and by 0.5 percentage points as compared to 1995. The cumulative implications of this deceleration for the health care share of government budgets are substantial. Cross-sectional analysis suggests that tight control of budgets for health spending at a central level, combined with restrictions on access to specialist physicians plays some role in explaining variation in this contribution across countries at a point in time. However, the magnitude of the effects accounted for by these factors is relatively small in comparison with the deceleration in the contribution of medical technology to health care spending over time. While this may partially reflect the difficulty in measuring institutional and organizational change, it also suggests that the more important factors explaining the slowdown over time are likely to be factors that (1) are shared across all countries in the sample, and (2) fall outside of the set of systemic characteristics that we have been able to evaluate explicitly. One explanation consistent with the pattern of results that we see in the data is the potential for a dynamic effect of cost-containment on the *focus* of medical research. Medication innovation must pass through an increasingly restrictive gauntlet in the form of coverage determinations and restrictions across a broad range of countries that (1) account for a disproportionate share of research, and (2) account for a disproportionate share of the market for medical innovations.

Within the model framework proposed by Weisbrod, we could expect the types of medical technology that are developed to reflect an assessment of the size and profitability of the potential market for innovations (Weisbrod, 1991). Thus, we would expect to see a shift in the targets of medical research to encourage a greater emphasis on the cost-efficiency of innovations that are under development. If the broad range of cost containment policies that are implemented at the national level are indeed influencing spending growth through an impact on the nature of medical technology, then we would not expect to see this effect in cross-country variation — because it would apply to all the countries in our sample. Where we would expect to see such an effect is in a deceleration in the contribution of medical technology to growth in health spending over time. This prediction is consistent with the results of our estimates, which show just such a decline.

This deceleration in the contribution of technology to growth in health care spending is persistent and long-term in nature. In other words, these results imply that we have already seen some "bending of the curve" for health spending from a global perspective. Logic suggests that this deceleration reflects a combination of supply-side and demand-side factors. On the demand-side, we see a broad-based change in the way that these technologies are introduced and diffused through patient populations across multiple countries in the sample. On the supply-side, we can expect a greater priority placed on the objective of cost effectiveness in selecting targets for research and development — that ultimately influences the types of medical technology that are being launched.

The net effects of slower growth in health care spending on new technology from a social welfare perspective depend on how these effects have been achieved. Given the known inefficiencies in the provision of health care, we can hope that some of the slower growth in spending on technology reflects expanding new treatment options in a way that is well targeted, to encourage provision to patients where evidence suggests benefits are likely to be relatively high. However, widely used policy tools — including limitations on access from coverage determinations based on HTA, incentive effects associated with DRG systems, and limitations on access to specialists — remain blunt in their application, directed as they usually must be too large and heterogeneous patient populations. Policy tools that rely on an assessment of average costs and benefits have a difficult time in dealing with treatments that offer substantial health benefits to a minority of patients, with the potential for broader diffusion to patients whose benefits are small. From a dynamic perspective, there are will also be costs in terms of advances in medical knowledge foregone, of medical technologies not pursued due to the perception that a sufficient market does not exist for these treatment options. Given the reality of limited resources this is inevitable — all paths cannot be pursued. However, these tradeoffs do argue for policy options that maintain some flexibility in determining access to new technologies, as opposed to a more rigid top–down approach.

References

Anderson G, Reinhardt U, Hussey P, Petrosyan V. 2003. It's the prices, stupid: Why the United States is so different from other countries. *Health Affairs* 22: 89–105.

Australian Productivity Commission. 2005. *Impact of Advances in Medical Technology in Australia, Research Report.* Melbourne Productivity Commission.

Barros PP. 1999. The black box of health care expenditure determinants. *Health Economics* 7(6): 533–544.

Basu A, Jena A, Philipson T. 2011. The impact of comparative effectiveness research on health and health care spending. *Journal of Health Economics* 30(4): 695–706.

Baumol W. 1967. Macroeconomics of unbalanced growth: The anatomy of urban crisis. *American Economic Review* 57(3): 415–26.

Baumol W. 1993. Health care, education and the cost disease: A looming crisis for public choice. *Public Choice* 77(1): 17–28.

Bech M, Christiansen T, Dunham K, Lauridsen J, Lyttkens C, McGuire A, and the TECH Investigators. 2008. The influence of economic incentives and regulatory factors on the adoption of treatment technologies. *Health Economics* 17: 1114–1132.

Berndt E, Nass D, Kleinrock, M, Aitken M, 2015. Decline in economic returns from new drugs raises questions about sustaining innovations. *Health Affairs* 34: 245–252.

Busse R, Schreyogg J, Smith PC. 2008. Variability in healthcare treatment costs amongst nine EU countries — Results from the HealthBasket Project. *Health Economics* 17: S1–S8.

Chambers J, Chenoweth M, Cangelosi M, Pyo J, Cohen J, Neumann P. 2015. Medicare is scrutinizing evidence more tightly for national coverage determinations. *Health Affairs* 34: 253–26.

Cook, C. 2014. How much is a year of life worth? *BBC Newsnight* August 29.

Cutler D, McClellan M. 2001. Is technological change in medicine worth it? *Health Affairs* 5: 11–29.

Cutler D, McClellan M, Newhouse JP, Remler D. 1998. Are medical prices declining? Evidence from heart attack treatments. *Quarterly Journal of Economics* 113(4): 991–1024.

Enthoven A. 1980. *Consumer Choice Health Plan: The Only Practical Solution to the Soaring Cost of Medical Care*. Reading, PA: Addison-Wesley.

Finkelstein A. 2007. The aggregate effects of health insurance: Evidence from the introduction of medicare. *Quarterly Journal of Economics* 122(1): 1–37.

Gelijns A, Rosenberg N. 1994. The dynamics of technological change in medicine. *Health Affairs* 13(3): 29–45.

Gerdtham U, Jonnson B, 2000. International Comparisons of Health Expenditure. In Anthony Culyer, Joseph Newhouse (eds.). *Handbook of Health Economics: Volume 1A*, Elsevier.

Hagist C, Kotlikoff LJ. 2005. Who's going broke? Comparing Growth in Public Healthcare Expenditure in Ten OECD Countries, National Bureau of Economic Research, *Working Paper No*. 11833: 29.

Hartwig J. 2008. Has health capital formation cured 'Baumol's Disease'? — Panel Granger Causality Evidence for OECD Countries, *KOF Working Papers* No. 08–206.

Jonsson B, Eckerlund I. 2003. Why Do Different Countries Spend Different Amounts on Health Care? In Stephane Jacobzone (ed.). *A Disease-Based Comparison of Health Systems: What is Best and at what Cost?* OECD.

Joumard I, Hoeller P, Andre C, Nicq C. 2010. *Health Care Systems: Efficiency and Policy Settings*. OECD.

Keeley EC, Boura JA, Grines CL. 2003. Primary angioplasty versus intravenous thrombolytic therapy for acute myocardial infarction: A quantitative review of 23 randomised trials. *Lancet* 361(9351): 13–20.

Liu S, Watcha D, Holodniy M, Goldhaber-Fiebert JD. 2014. Sofosbuvir-based treatment regimens for chronic, genotype 1 hepatitis C virus infection in U.S. incarcerated populations: A cost-effectiveness analysis. *Annals of Internal Medicine* 161(8): 546–553.

Manning W, Newhouse J, Duan N, Keeler E, Leibowitz A, Marquis S. 1987. Health insurance and the demand for medical care: Evidence from a randomized experiment. *American Economic Review* 77(3): 251–277.

Moise P. 2003. The Technology–Health Expenditure Link. In Stephane Jacobzone (ed.). *A Disease-Based Comparison of Health Systems: What is Best and at what Cost?* OECD.

Newhouse JP. 1992. Medical care costs: How much welfare loss? *Journal of Economic Perspectives* 6(3): 3–21.

Nordhaus WD. 2002. *The Health of Nations: The Contribution of Improved Health to Living Standards*. *NBER Working Paper* 8818.

OECD. *Health Statistics 2014*. http://www.oecd.org/health/healthdata. [14 June 2014].

OECD 2013. Structure of general government expenditures, in *Government at a Glance*, OECD.

Papanicolas I, Smith PC. 2013. International Comparisons of Health Systems. In *Health Systems Performance Comparison*, European Health Observatory, pp. 75–112.
Paris V, DeVaux M, Wei L. 2010. *Health Systems Institutional Characteristics: A Survey of 29 OECD Countries*, OECD Health Working Papers 50.
Poullier JP, Hernandez P, Kawabata K. 2002. *National Health Accounts: Concepts, Data Sources, and Methodology*. World Health Organization.
Rettig RA. 1994. Medical innovation duels cost containment. *Health Affairs* 13(3): 7–27.
Shih C, Berliner E. 2008. Diffusion of new technology and payment policies: Coronary stents. *Health Affairs* 27: 1566–1576.
Smith S, Newhouse J, Freeland M. 2009. Income, insurance, and technology: Why does health spending outpace economic growth. *Health Affairs* 28(5): 1276–1284.
Weisbrod, B. 1991. The health care quadrilemma: An essay on technological change, insurance, quality of care, and cost containment. *Journal of Economic Literature* 29(3): 523–552.
Weisbrod BA, LaMay CL. 1999. Mixed signals: Public policy and the future of health care R&D. *Health Affairs* 18(2): 112–125.
World Health Organization (WHO), Global Health Observatory (GHO). http://www.who.int/gho/en [18 June 2014].

Primary Care: Effectiveness and Costs

Tor Iversen
University of Oslo

This chapter reviews the payment and organization of primary care, with an emphasis on primary care providers (PCPs). We draw a distinction between two frameworks. The first framework, related to a low density of PCPs in the community, assumes that a PCP considers not only the patient in front of him, but also the entire community of patients. Here we find that capitation, fee-for-service (FFS) and combinations of the two all encourage the delivery of a small number of services to each patient. A policy implication appears to be that in a society with a low density of physicians, general health insurance, and physicians who consider the community of patients, the payment system does not greatly influence the volume of health services provided to each patient. The other framework assumes that the PCP, if he is part of a rich society with a high density of PCPs and general health insurance, only considers the health of the individual patient. Under this situation, FFS is predicted to encourage a more service-intensive practice style and capitation a less service-intensive practice style. Our theory predictions are broadly supported by empirical studies.

Keywords: Primary Care Physicians; Payment Schemes; Effectiveness; Costs.

Introduction

Primary health care aims to be the population's first encounter with the health system. However, what precisely constitutes primary health care is not so clear. The Institute of Medicine defines primary care as "the provision of integrated, accessible health-care services by clinicians who are accountable for addressing a large majority of personal health-care needs, developing a sustained partnership with patients, and practicing in the context of family and community" (IOM, 1994,

p. 15). The World Health Organization (2008) further develops this definition and considers reforms in the direction of primary care to involve:

- The predominant type of first-contact provider should be shifted from specialists and hospitals to generalist primary care teams in close proximity to where a person lives.
- Primary care providers (PCPs) should be made responsible for the health of all the members of a well-identified population.
- Through stronger administrative authority and purchasing power, PCPs should be empowered to coordinate the various inputs of specialized, hospital and social services.
- PCPs should be person-centered.
- Primary care should be comprehensive and reach the full essential benefits package, from promotion through to palliation, for all age groups.
- Primary care should provide continuity. This means that information for individuals should be recorded over the life-course, and transferred between levels of care in cases of referral and to a primary-care unit elsewhere when people relocate.
- PCPs should be a regular entry point. This means that measures should be taken to ensure that providers know their clients and vice versa.

Starfield (1998) sums this up by defining the "four pillars" of primary care as: (1) First contact with the health-care system; (2) continuity of care over time; (3) concern for the whole patient rather than a disease or part of the patient; and (4) coordination of care.

The role primary health care plays varies between systems. Macinko *et al.* (2003) score the OECD countries according to indicators that reflect the "four pillars" of primary care during the period 1975–1995. They find considerable, yet quite stable variation over time. They also find that the total score on the primary care indicators is negatively associated with overall mortality and several kinds of cause-specific mortality when they control for other macro-level variables that are likely to have an impact on mortality. The study does not claim that primary care is the cause of reduced mortality.

An important and much discussed issue is whether or not primary care is a substitute for specialized care and hence, whether it has the potential of being overall cost saving. In this review, we comment on both the outcome issue and the cost-saving issue.

The main topic of our review is about payment systems for PCPs and what characteristics existing payment systems seem to have with regard to achieving specific efficiency targets within primary care. The appropriate payment system is an important policy question in the discussion about primary care reforms in many countries. Hopefully, this review of theoretical and empirical studies will contribute to the debate on the characteristics of different payment types. We also comment upon the connection between primary care and specialist care in terms of referrals and possible cost-shifting.

Handbooks that have investigated physician behavior and published reviews of PCPs have inspired this review. Central references are McGuire (2000), Scott (2000), Léger (2008), McGuire (2011), Rice (2012), Chandra *et al.* (2012), and Iversen and Lurås (2012).

The structure of this chapter is as follows. Section "Characteristics of Regulation and Types of Payment for PCPs" describes types of primary care regulation including common payment types for PCPs. Section "An Economic Approach to Effectiveness in Primary Care" presents an economic approach to efficiency in primary care. Section "An Illustration of the Predicted Effect of FFS and Capitation on the Volume of PCP Services" presents a theory framework from which we derive the characteristics of the payment types. Section "The Empirical Research Literature on Characteristics and Effects of Payment Systems in Primary Care" reviews empirical literature of the characteristics of the payment types. Section "Implications for Health Policy" draws policy implications.

Characteristics of Regulation and Types of Payment for PCPs

A classification of primary care systems consists of several dimensions:

- Regulation of entry, practice location, and mode of provision.
- Regulation of provided quality.
- Regulation of revenue/payment scheme for PCPs.
- Regulation of PCPs' role in patients' access to primary care and specialized health care; in particular, whether or not PCPs act as gatekeepers to specialized care.

We use the information from Paris *et al.* (2010), who present the Organisation for Economic Cooperation and Development (OECD)'s survey among member countries in 2010 to describe the countries' relative standings on the dimensions described above. With regard to regulation of practice location and mode of provision, we see from Table 1 that there is considerable variation among the countries. About 70% of the countries do not have practice-location regulations. Without regulation of practice location, a PCP is free to set up his practice anywhere he wants. The dominant mode of provision varies between public centers and private solo practice or group practice. From Table 1, we see no clear relationship between regulation of practice location and dominant type of practice.

A revenue/payment scheme relates both to who is paying the provider and to the service components that are paid for. A PCP can be paid both by the patient

Table 1. Predominant modes for the provision of primary care services and payment for primary care physicians

Country	Regulation of where to locate a practice	Predominant mode of provision for primary care services	Primary care physicians payment	Bonus for PCP	If so, targets related to
Australia	No	Private group practices	FFS	Yes	Preventive care, Chronic disease
Austria	Yes	Private solo practices	FFS/Cap	No	
Belgium	No	Private solo practices	FFS	Yes	Chronic disease
Canada	No	Private group practices	FFS	No	
Czech Republic	No	Private solo practices	FFS/Cap	Yes	Preventive care
Denmark	Yes	Private group practices	FFS/Cap	No	
Finland	No	Public centers	Salary/Cap/FFS	No	
France	No	Private solo practices	FFS	No	
Germany	Yes	Private solo practices	FFS	No	
Greece	No	Private solo practices	Salary	No	
Hungary	Yes	Private solo practices	Cap	Yes	
Iceland	No	Public centers	Salary	No	
Ireland	No	Private solo practices	FFS	No	
Italy	Yes	Public centers	Cap	Yes	Preventive care, Chronic disease
Japan	No	Private clinics	FFS	Yes	Preventive care, Chronic disease
Korea	No	Private solo practices	FFS	No	
Luxembourg	No	Private solo practices	FFS	No	
Mexico	Yes	Public centers	Salary	No	
Netherlands	No	Private group practices	FFS/Cap	No	
New Zealand	No	Private group practices	FFS/Salary	Yes	Preventive care, Chronic disease
Norway	Yes	Private solo practices	FFS/Cap	No	
Poland	No	Private clinics	Cap	Yes	Preventive care, Chronic disease
Portugal	No	Public centers	Salary	Yes	Preventive care, Chronic disease
Slovak Republic	No	Private group practices	Cap	No	

(*Continued*)

Table 1. (*Continued*)

Country	Regulation of where to locate a practice	Predominant mode of provision for primary care services	Primary care physicians payment	Bonus for PCP	If so, targets related to
Spain	No	Public centers	Salary/Cap	Yes	Preventive care, chronic disease
Sweden	No	Public centers	Salary	n.a.	
Switzerland	Yes	Private solo practices	FFS	No	
Turkey	Yes	Public centers	FFS/Salary	Yes	Preventive care
United Kingdom	No	Private group practices	Salary/Cap/FFS	Yes	Preventive care, chronic disease, patient satisfaction

Source: Paris *et al.* (2010).

directly and by a private or public payer that operates on behalf of the patient. In many countries, a PCP is paid by a mix of private or public payer contributions and patient co-payment, often with an annual cap on patient co-payments. Countries vary with regard to the kind of primary care for which patients are expected to make OOP payments. Some countries require a co-payment on physician visits, other countries require a co-payment on medicines, and some require a mix of small co-payments on many items.

A revenue/payment system for PCPs can involve several components:

(A) *Input-based components*: Payment is related to the cost of the factors of production. In these systems, the payer reimburses the cost of inputs including physicians' and other personnel's time in addition to purchased inputs in the production, such as laboratory fixed and disposable equipment and cost of facilities. An extreme version, that is very rare nowadays, would be that the PCP writes an invoice where he lists the costs of all resources involved in an encounter.

(B) *Fee-for-service (FFS) components*: Payment is based on the number and type of services provided. Paid services under this system are often consultations (may vary based on the length and type of consultation), diagnostic examinations including laboratory tests, and other procedures. Minor surgery may, for instance, sometimes be done in a primary care setting. Unlike under type (A), a PCP who, for some reason is slow in performing a diagnostic test, would not be reimbursed for the extra time under FFS.

(C) *Episode-based components*: Payment is based on the number of treatment episodes. A treatment episode may consist of many encounters between a PCP and a patient, or it may consist of few. Variation in treatment practices may involve variation in the number of consultations during a treatment episode among PCPs. Under (C), the number and composition of services during a treatment episode are not compensated individually. There is a fixed sum per episode of illness or treatment, for instance, for a flu episode. The payment is the same irrespective of whether the physician visits the patient at home or sees the patient in the physician's office.

(D) *Capitation-based components*: Payment is based on the group of people a PCP takes responsibility for. In many systems, the population has the opportunity to have a designated PCP. The PCP then has an obligation to provide care for his assigned patients, and a patient often has an economic incentive to visit his PCP as opposed to others. For instance, there may be an additional copayment if the patient visits another PCP (except for getting a second opinion). Under this system, PCPs often receive a monthly fixed amount (capitation fee) per patient on their list, irrespective of whether a patient requires services during the period. The capitation fee may be equal for each patient or it may be adjusted for a patient's health state and expected demand for services (risk-adjusted capitation fee).

(E) *Fixed payments per period*: Payment is a fixed practice allowance to cover a portion of the estimated cost of running a practice or a fixed salary that a PCP receives as part of an employment contract.

(F) *Extended practice budgets*: The PCP pays part of the cost of specialized care for his patients. A PCP is generally a patient's gate to specialized health care. By requiring the PCP to pay some portion of patients' cost in specialized health care, the PCP has an incentive to take not only his own costs into account, but also the costs that are generated in other sectors of health care over which the PCP has some influence by way of referral. Variants of extended-practice budgets have been introduced in several countries — for instance, in England through so-called fundholding practices.

(G) *Pay-for-performance*: Payment depends on the achievement of performance-targets. Pay-for-performance (P4P) schemes, introduced around 2000, aim to reward improvements on measurable quality indicators that a PCP is able to influence. This may include processes that are supposed to influence patient health positively, such as regular check-ups for patients with chronic diseases and regular measurement of blood pressure for patients with hypertension. It may also include results in terms of the health improvements that the PCP is supposed to be able to influence, for instance blood pressure levels for patients with hypertension.

In practice, payment systems are often a mix of several of the components explained above. Table 1 shows a snapshot of payment systems for PCPs in OECD countries around 2010. From Table 1, we see that countries with predominantly public primary care systems mainly rely on salary as the payment method. However, some of these countries have a mix of salary with FFS and capitation. Italy, meanwhile, relies on capitation only. In countries with private solo or group practice, there is a mix of capitation and FFS. Table 1 also contains information about whether there are bonus payments available for achieving targets related to quality of care. At the time of the survey, we see that just under half of OECD countries had such pay-for-performance payment schemes in place. Quality targets typically relate to preventive care, chronic disease management and patient satisfaction.

The last dimension in the classification of primary care systems relates to the regulation of patients' access to health care. We also include the opportunity to choose a PCP under this heading, as having the opportunity to choose makes it possible to access particular PCPs. In the second column of Table 2, we see that, in most countries, patients have free choice of PCP. In the third column of Table 2, we see that countries vary with regard to the requirement of having a regular PCP. In some countries it is compulsory and in other countries it is financially encouraged (for instance by means of reduced copayments), while in about half of countries it is neither compulsory nor financially encouraged.

Table 2 also shows regulation of access to specialized care. This type of regulation aims to have an appropriate division of tasks between primary care and specialized care. In about half of the countries, a referral from a PCP is compulsory in order to access specialized care. On the other end of the spectrum, in about one fourth of the countries included in Table 2, there is neither gatekeeping in terms of direct regulation nor financial incentives in place to guide specialized care decisions.

An important weakness of Paris *et al.* (2010) is that the US did not respond. A reason might be that provision of primary health care in the US is too heterogeneous to fit into the table columns. Rice *et al.* (2013) recently did a review of the US health system. They draw on challenges in primary care, as summarized by Bodenheimer and Pham (2010). Rice *et al.* (2013) report several venues for the delivery of primary care. A major one is a physician's private clinic. Another primary care venue is the public or non-profit community health center, which provides access to primary care for low-income, uninsured, and minority populations. There are also government-sponsored clinics for the military, prison, migrant and homeless populations. Urban public and teaching hospitals may also have outpatient clinics for primary care services. A small number of integrated care systems, such as Kaiser Permanente, provide primary care as part of their integrated

Table 2. Regulation of primary care services

Country	Choice Of PCP	Registration with a primary care physician	Referral to access secondary care	May prices differ across providers?
Australia	Free	No obligation and no incentive	Financially encouraged	Prices may differ
Austria	Incentives	No obligation and no incentive	No obligation and no incentive	No price or unique price
Belgium	Incentives	Financially encouraged	Financially encouraged	Prices may differ
Canada	Free	No obligation and no incentive	Compulsory	No price or unique price
Czech Republic	Free	No obligation and no incentive	No obligation and no incentive	No price or unique price
Denmark	Limited	Compulsory	Compulsory	No price or unique price
Finland	Limited	No obligation and no incentive	Compulsory	No price or unique price
France	Free	Financially encouraged	Financially encouraged	Prices may differ
Germany	Free	Financially encouraged	Financially encouraged	No price or unique price
Greece	Incentives	No obligation and no incentive	No obligation and no incentive	Prices may differ
Hungary	Free	Financially encouraged	Compulsory	n.a.
Iceland	Free	No obligation and no incentive	No obligation and no incentive	No price or unique price
Ireland	Free	No obligation and no incentive	Financially encouraged	Prices may differ
Italy	Free	Compulsory	Compulsory	No price or unique price
Japan	Free	No obligation and no incentive	No obligation and no incentive	No price or unique price
Korea	Free	No obligation and no incentive	No obligation and no incentive	No price or unique price
Luxembourg	Free	No obligation and no incentive	No obligation and no incentive	No price or unique price
Mexico	Limited	No obligation and no incentive	Compulsory	No price or unique price
Netherlands	Free	Compulsory	Compulsory	Prices may differ

(*Continued*)

Table 2. (*Continued*)

Country	Choice Of PCP	Registration with a primary care physician	Referral to access secondary care	May prices differ across providers?
New Zealand	Free	Financially encouraged	Compulsory	Prices may differ
Norway	Free	Compulsory	Compulsory	No price or unique price
Poland	Free	No obligation and no incentive	Compulsory	No price or unique price
Portugal	Limited	Compulsory	Compulsory	No price or unique price
Slovak Republic	Free	Compulsory	Compulsory	Prices may differ
Spain	Limited	Compulsory	Compulsory	No price or unique price
Sweden	Free	No obligation and no incentive	No obligation and no incentive	No price or unique price
Switzerland	Free	Financially encouraged	Financially encouraged	No price or unique price
Turkey	Free	No obligation and no incentive	No obligation and no incentive	Prices may differ
United Kingdom	Limited	Financially encouraged	Compulsory	No price or unique price

Source: OECD (2010).

systems. Most primary care physician private practices are physician-run and/or owned. Rice *et al.* (2013) report that most are small: 32% of primary care physicians are in solo practice and 46% are in practices with two to five physicians. The majority is paid fee-for-service (FFS) with capitation payment surviving only in few states, such as California (Bodenheimer and Pham, 2010). During the mid-1990s, health maintenance organizations (HMOs) often based their care structure on the PCPs as gatekeepers and an increase in the supply of PCPs was reported. From the late 1990s, HMOs and the primary care gatekeeper model were in decline.

According to Bodenheimer and Pham (2010) the wide and growing income gap between PCPs and specialists, coupled with the challenging work life of primary care physicians, has led to problems with recruiting US medical graduates into primary care careers, resulting in problems with access to primary care. There are several policy initiatives to increase the supply of PCPs. Some of them are related to the Affordable Care Act (ACA) — the health care reform law enacted in

2010. Also, new types of organizations may favor primary care (Bodenheimer and Pham, 2010). For instance, the Patient Centered Medical Home (PCMH) is an initiative to reduce the fragmentation of primary care. Characteristics, among others, are that each patient has an ongoing relationship with a PCP who directs the medical team and coordinates a patient's various medical needs. Also, Accountable Care Organizations (ACOs) are a method of care coordination initiated by the ACA in 2010. ACOs are groups of providers in an area including primary and specialty care physicians, hospitals and others, who coordinate their care for Medicare patients.

An Economic Approach to Effectiveness in Primary Care

We present the following with regard to an interpretation of effectiveness and cost in primary care from an economic perspective.

At the individual level, the uncertainty regarding future health states is one basic characteristic of health. Severe illness may require a substantial cost in order to regain a previous health state. Risk-averse individuals would like to insure against the financial consequences of future health care costs. Health care insurance means that an uncertain future expense is exchanged with smaller regular expenses corresponding to the insurance premium. Hence, the purpose of insurance is to make possible a substantial reduction in patient co-payment at the point of use.

The welfare gain of financial protection comes at a cost of potential inefficiency at the point of health care consumption (Léger, 2008). Because health care insurance implies a patient copayment smaller than the marginal cost of providing a service (limited demand-side cost sharing), patients have an incentive to demand more care than the socially optimal level of care (*ex-post* moral hazard). An important purpose of the payment system for primary care physicians is to help achieve the optimal level of care for patients by means of supply-side cost sharing. Supply-side cost sharing (Ellis and McGuire, 1993) means that PCPs are not fully paid for the marginal cost of providing services. Hence, they have an incentive to take marginal costs into account when they decide the volume and composition of services to provide to their patients.

Suppose that a patient's health is a function of disease severity (θ) and the number received of an unspecified health service (q):

$$h(\theta, q)$$

$h(\theta, q)$ is assumed to be concave in q.

Social efficiency requires that the marginal health benefit of a service $h_q(\theta, q)$ equals the marginal cost, c, of providing the service. To obtain the optimal number of services is defined as the first efficiency concern. We denote the socially optimal number of services by q^*. If patient payment corresponds to the marginal cost of providing the service (no insurance), patients are expected to demand services to the point where the marginal health benefit equals the marginal cost for the patient, which now equals the marginal cost to society. Hence, considered from the *ex-post* position (after the occurrence of illness), the quantity of the health service corresponds to social efficiency. However, since the patient carries the financial risk, there is a welfare loss for risk-averse individuals, and full patient payment at the point of use is not socially optimal from the *ex-ante* (before the occurrence of illness) position. The socially optimal co-payment from the *ex-ante* position should then balance the optimal level of service provision *ex post* against the degree of financial protection that insurance should provide.

So far, we have implicitly assumed that patients decide the quantity of health services similar to the quantity of other goods and services they demand. However, several studies show that patients primarily initiate their contact with the health system during an episode of illness. Having contacted a physician office or a hospital, their further choices depend on the advice the physician provides. A crucial question is then whether the physician payment system may play some role in moving the quantity of service from the patient's optimal volume q^{**} (corresponding to $h_q(\theta, q) = 0$ with full insurance) when there is no co-payment towards q^* (corresponding to $h_q(\theta, q) = c$) that correspond to the socially efficient volume of care.

A second component of social efficiency in primary care relates to the incentives for physicians to reduce costs. Above, we reasoned as if marginal cost is a constant. A more reasonable assumption is that the provider is able to influence the marginal cost by exerting cost-reducing effort. Examples of cost-reducing effort are investment in electronic systems for scheduling of appointments and setting up electronic communication between the PCP and patients for the handling of minor issues. Effort implies a cost, so the provider would rather not exert the effort if it does not pay off in terms of a greater revenue or patient benefit. The socially optimal level of cost-reducing effort is derived from the condition that the marginal cost-reduction should equal the marginal cost of exerting cost-reducing efforts.

Providing optimal quality of care is a third concern of social efficiency. Quality is costly in the sense that the provider's time and effort are required. Socially optimal quality is characterized by the condition that marginal cost of providing quality should equal the willingness to pay for the health that the marginal quality provides.

A fourth efficiency concern relates to the division of tasks between PCPs and specialists. For some tasks, it is clear that specialized health care is needed because PCPs cannot contribute the necessary specialized competencies and equipment. Most surgeries and cancer treatments are examples. But within many areas, there are grey zones — tasks that could be performed at either level of care. Often, cost would be lower in a primary care setting due to lower cost of personnel and equipment. On the other hand, diagnostic accuracy and treatment results might be better in specialized health care simply because of the expertise in a particular field. Hence, for the socially optimal division of tasks between the two levels, health improvements of transferring tasks to specialized care must be balanced against the additional cost of transferring a patient from primary care to specialized care.

A fifth concern relates to selection of patients. Primary care typically caters to individuals who have a variety of health conditions. Some individuals are more costly to care for than others. A patient with a chronic disease such as, for instance, chronic obstructive pulmonary disease (COPD) or Type II diabetes would require more time and attention from a PCP than a healthy 30-year-old male who hardly ever visits a physician's office. An important concern then, is that the organization and revenue system(s) of primary care should be set up to prevent patient selection of any kind; i.e., to avoid that a PCP prefers to cater to the healthy and avoid the unhealthy or the other way around.

An Illustration of the Predicted Effect of FFS and Capitation on the Volume of PCP Services

Different payment schemes may have different levels of properties in helping to achieve the five social targets outlined in Section "An Economic Approach to Effectiveness in Primary Care". Here, we elaborate on this issue by using the economic approach to study the different properties of FFS and capitation in achieving the optimal volume of care.[1]

Assume a physician objective function V:

$$V = \delta[A + (R + Fq)n - c(nq)] + (1 - \delta)nh(\theta, q)$$
$$c'(nq) > 0, \quad c''(nq) > 0, \tag{1}$$

where n is the number of patients the PCP takes responsibility for, and q is the number of services (only one type of service in this simplified example). We assume no patient co-payment, so all income to the physician comes from the insurance institution. We allow the payment system to be a mix of many components. A is a fixed practice allowance (fixed revenue to cover some of the fixed costs of running a practice), R is a flat capitation payment (a fixed annual payment for each regular patient) and F is FFS. The cost function is $c(\ )$ and is assumed to be convex. The physician's opportunity cost of time is included in the cost

[1] A somewhat more detailed elaboration of the model is found in the Appendix.

function. The PCP is a partial altruist in the sense that he both cares for the profit with weight δ and for the total health benefits of his patients (weight $1-\delta$). The formulation of the patient health term implies that the PCP not only has concern for the health of the individual patient but for the entire group of patients for whom he has responsibility. Later, we shall see that the distinction between assuming responsibility for an individual patient or for the entire group of patients has important policy implications. The physician's decision variables are the preferred number of regular patients and the number of services provided to each patient (all patients are assumed to have equal characteristics).

We can now distinguish between four payment systems which have the components from Section "Characteristics of Regulation and Types of Payment for PCPs" and occur in the real world:

A: Pure FFS ($F > 0, A = 0, R = 0$).

B: Pure capitation ($F = 0, A = 0, R > 0$).

C: Combination of practice allowance and FFS ($F > 0, A > 0, R = 0$).

D: Combination of capitation fee and FFS ($F > 0, A = 0, R > 0$).

The optimal number of patients and services from the physician's perspective is found by maximizing Eq. (1) with respect to n and q. The following is an explanation of the main results. We refer readers interested in technical details to the Appendix.

These are the results according to payment system:

A. The optimal number of services from the physician's perspective under FFS is smaller than the optimal number of services from the individual patient's perspective and equal to the minimum number that is considered to be acceptable by the profession. The reason for this somewhat unusual result under FFS stems from the combination of concern for the entire population of patients and the concavity of the health function. Concavity implies that the marginal health benefit of services is declining and less than the average benefit. Again, this means that it is more rewarding in terms of the total health benefit to provide services to an additional patient compared to providing more services to already serviced patients. From a health policy interpretation, this means that social responsibility (obligation to take the entire community into account) encourages the PCP to provide (few) services to many patients.
B. Under capitation, it is always more profitable to provide few services to many patients than to provide many services to few patients. Hence, in this case, the physician's profit interest also pulls in the direction of few services. The

optimal number of services from the physician's perspective is similar to what it is under FFS, and equal to the minimum number that is considered to be acceptable by the profession.

C. Because both FFS and capitation imply a minimum number of services, combinations of the two components (system D) and combination of FFS and practice allowance (system C) imply the same minimum number of services as the pure systems.

We arrive at the conclusion that when physicians care for the total health of the population, their optimal service intensity to the individual patient is independent of the payment system they are offered, and at a minimum level. The reason for this somewhat unusual conclusion is that physicians are assumed to care for the entire population of patients (see again Eq. (1)) and not only the patient in from of him. That physicians care for the total health of the population is perhaps typical for societies with a low density of physicians. The opportunity cost of providing many services to one particular patient is then visible in terms of the suffering of other patients who do not obtain access to physician services.

In societies with higher physician density, every individual is covered and the physician may then perhaps shift attention to the individual patient in front of him. The revised objective function is then:

$$V = \delta[A + (R + Fq)n - c(nq)] + (1 - \delta)h(\theta, q)$$
$$c'(nq) > 0, \quad c''(nq) > 0. \tag{2}$$

Again, we find the first-order condition for an interior solution by maximizing V with respect to n and q. We can distinguish between the effects of the different payment systems on the volume of service provision:

A. Under FFS, the physician's income is independent of whether many services are provided to few patients or few services are provided to many patients. He would then provide the number of services that maximize a patient's health, i.e., the number of services that implies that the marginal benefit of health services is equal to zero ($h_q'(\theta, q) = 0$). The number of services is then greater than the optimal number from the social perspective, as the marginal cost of health services is not balanced against the marginal health effect.

B. Under capitation, the physician's profit motive pulls in the direction of a minimum number of services. This concern is balanced against the concern for the patient, and an interior solution implies a number of services greater than the minimum and smaller than the optimum from the patient's perspective.

Table 3. Predicted number of services under alternative payment systems varies with physician objectives and environments ($\underline{q}$ is minimum number of services)

	$0 < \delta < 1$		
	Without n in utility function		**With n in utility function**
	Sufficient patients	**Shortage of patients**	
A. FFS	$q = q^{**}$	$q > q^{**}$	$q = \underline{q}$
B. Capitation	$\underline{q} \leq q < q^{**}$		$q = \underline{q}$
C. FFS/Practice allowance	$q = q^{**}$	$q > q^{**}$	$q = \underline{q}$
D. FFS/Capitation	$\underline{q} \leq q < q^{**}$	Greater than with no shortage	$q = \underline{q}$

C. Under the combination of practice allowance and FFS, the number of services is similar to the number under pure FFS, as the practice allowance (a fixed sum irrespective of the service provision) does not impact on the balance between profit and patient health.
D. Under the combination of FFS and capitation, the FFS component makes it more profitable to provide services than under pure capitation, but still, it is most profitable to provide the minimum number to many patients. However, because the physician also takes account of patient health, the optimal number of services from the physician perspective is greater than under pure capitation.

Table 3 sums up the optimal number of services from the physician perspective under alternative payment schemes.

In Table 3, the column "shortage of patients" needs some explanation. Remember that under FFS, the physician would provide to a patient the number of services that maximizes the patient's health benefit (q^{**}). The optimal number of patients from the physician perspective is then determined such that the marginal income of a patient equals the marginal cost of providing services to that patient. With a shortage of patients, the number of patients who would like to receive care from the PCP is smaller than the physician's optimal number. In order to increase the income, patients are provided with an additional number of services beyond q^{**}. That would not have happened if the physician could have his optimal number of patients, because he could then provide each patient with the number of services that maximizes health without losing income. Under pure capitation, a shortage of patients has no consequences for service provision because the physician cannot increase his income by providing more services.

The first efficiency concern in Section "An Economic Approach to Effectiveness in Primary Care" is to obtain the optimal number of services. The second efficiency concern defined in Section "An Economic Approach to Effectiveness in Primary Care" is the provision of cost-reducing effort by the PCP. In the model, this aspect was ignored because cost was assumed to depend only on the total number of services provided by the PCP. In general, the provider has an incentive to provide optimal cost-reducing effort as long as the increased profit that results from cost-reducing effort accrues to the PCP.[2] This result is further elaborated on in Zweifel *et al.* (2009, Chapter 10).

A third efficiency concern mentioned in Section "An Economic Approach to Effectiveness in Primary Care" is related to quality of care. Whether or not FFS and capitation encourage high quality care depends on how volume of care is related to health benefit. In the model set out in Eqs. (1) and (2), there is a functional form between services and health benefit that implies a certain number of services that maximizes patient health. In the formulation of Eq. (2), inferior quality is predicted under capitation because of too few services because the PCP is not paid for providing services. With FFS, patients are predicted to receive the number of services that maximize their health. If the PCP experiences a shortage of patients, he has an economic incentive to produce inferior quality because of too many services. Several authors (Newhouse, 1996) have therefore suggested that a mix of capitation and FFS is appropriate for providing optimal quality.

Capitation may have quality-enhancing properties if PCPs compete for patients and patients are informed about quality. Patients would then switch PCP if the present PCP provides poor quality. Gravelle (1999) and Gravelle and Masiero (2000) study theoretically the properties of capitation contracts in providing high-quality health care. In Gravelle (1999), profit-maximizing PCPs compete for patients who are informed of a PCP's level of quality. An increase in the capitation fee makes the marginal patient more valuable to PCPs and encourages them to increase quality in their competition for patients.

That patients have a correct perception of health care quality is a dubious assumption to make, and is modified in a two-period theory model by Gravelle and Masiero (2000). Patients already listed with a PCP have experience with that PCP and are assumed to have perfect knowledge of that particular PCP and imperfect information about the others. Again, an increase in the capitation fee is shown

[2]In a multi-period context, it might be more complicated because cost reductions today may result in fee reduction in the future.

to increase the equilibrium quality as it becomes more valuable for the PCP to provide high quality care to prevent patients from switching.

In his review of physician agency, McGuire (2000) assumes that quality is non-contractible in the sense that it cannot be used as a basis for payment. Pay-for-performance (P4P), however, makes some elements of quality contractible. Some authors, inspired by Holmstrom and Milgrom (1991), argue that P4P influences the allocation of resources in favor of contractible quality measures (for instance, regular check-ups for patients with chronic diseases) at the expense of non-contractible quality measures (for instance, showing empathy during the consultation). Kaarbøe and Siciliani (2010) find that reliance on P4P is socially optimal when there are complementarities between the contractible and the non-contractible types of quality. For instance, investment in information technology may reduce the physician's cost of providing both the contractible and the non-contractible types of quality. When the two dimensions are substitutes, for instance because they compete for the physician's time, less P4P is generally recommended, although there are some exceptions.

A fourth efficiency concern is related to the division of tasks between primary care and specialist care. In the literature, it seems a general conclusion that capitation encourages a high referral rate and FFS encourages a smaller referral rate. Barros and Martinez-Giralt (2003) study theoretically the effect of the payment system on referrals from PCPs. Even if treatment costs are partially compensated, the effort to reduce referrals to hospitals is at the minimum value under capitation because of an externality resulting from the referral decision. If primary care and specialist care are integrated under a joint-management and capitation payment, the number of referrals is expected to decline because the referral decision is now internalized. In Iversen and Lurås (2000), a PCP both chooses his preferred number of patients and the referral rate. Capitation encourages a higher referral rate to specialist services and more regular patients on their rosters for primary care services than under the FFS scheme, because a higher income then can be obtained for the same effort. Hence, because of the referral externality, the PCP shifts costs to the specialist sector and the results are similar to what Barros and Martinez-Giralt (2003) find from their model.

Several authors have recently been interested in gatekeeping and to what extent payment systems can encourage efficient gatekeeping. Allard *et al.* (2011) distinguish between PCPs according to their degree of altruism and ability. They show theoretically that under capitation, PCPs have an incentive to refer often, irrespective of degree of altruism and ability. Under FFS, less altruistic, yet able, PCPs have an incentive to treat patients on their own, while more altruistic, and also less able, PCPs are expected to refer all patients. The remaining PCPs, i.e., those with a high diagnostic ability and a moderate sense of altruism, have an incentive to base their decision (either treat or refer the patient) on the outcome of their presumably accurate diagnosis. Jelovac (2014) sums up these results and relates them to other studies.

Iversen and Ma (2011) and Godager *et al.* (2015) study the effect of an increase in the number of gatekeeping PCPs on the referral rate under a mixed FFS and capitation system. Based on their model, they find that increased competition among gatekeeper PCPs has two effects that pull in opposite directions. On the one hand, increased competition reduces the marginal value of leisure, encouraging PCPs to reduce referrals and do more diagnostics and treatment on their own. On the other hand, increased competition for patients strengthens the patients' bargaining power, making it easier for patients to initiate a referral.

The last concern mentioned in Section "An Economic Approach to Effectiveness in Primary Care" is about selection of patients and potentially inferior access for patients with poor health and need for many services. Capitation payments may imply incentives for selection behavior, i.e., for PCPs to increase capitation income by selectively trying to attract healthy people with few health care needs to their lists. With imperfect risk adjustment of capitation payment, FFS may be required to prevent PCPs from cream-skimming (selecting the healthiest patients). Newhouse (1996; 2002) suggests a mixed (blended) reimbursement scheme involving both FFS and capitation, which can be seen in many countries (for instance in the UK, the Netherlands, Denmark, and Norway).

The Empirical Research Literature on Characteristics and Effects of Payment Systems in Primary Care

Effects on quantity of health services

Scott (2000) sums up the empirical literature on the effects of organization and payment systems in primary care. He takes a broad perspective and reviews studies of patient choice of physician, referral behavior, quantity and quality of services provided. He finds mixed results from the reviewed studies, although FFS often resulted in a greater number of services compared with capitation and salary. The same applies to Rice (2012) who reviews studies that were published after Scott did his review. Rice (2012) also finds several studies that fail to find that FFS results in an expanded number of services compared with other payment types.

Gosden *et al.* (2000) present a systematic review of studies of FFS, capitation and mixed systems. Due to strict selection criteria, only four studies, involving a total of 640 PCPs and 6,400 patients are considered. The authors find that FFS resulted in more primary care visits/contacts, visits to specialists and diagnostic and curative services, but fewer hospital referrals and repeat prescriptions compared with capitation. Compliance with the number of visits recommended by clinical guidelines was higher under FFS compared with capitation payment.

van Dijk *et al.* (2013) evaluate the change in the remuneration system for General Practitioners (GPs) in the Netherlands in 2006. The change involved going from separate remuneration systems for socially insured consumers (capitation) and privately insured consumers (FFS) to a combined system of capitation and FFS for both groups. The authors predicted that introduction of FFS for socially insured consumers should result in an increase in physician-initiated contact rates for this group. The empirical study finds a higher increase in physician-initiated utilization for the socially insured consumers compared with privately insured consumers. This was most apparent in persons aged 25–54.

Devlin and Sarma (2008) use the 2004 Canadian National Physician Survey and analyze the number of patient visits per week provided by family physicians in alternative forms of remuneration schemes. They find that FFS physicians conduct more patient visits relative to physicians under the other types of remuneration schemes that were examined. They also find that family physicians self-select into different remuneration regimes based on their personal preferences and unobserved characteristics.

In Norway, PCPs are paid by a mix of capitation and FFS. There has been some debate about whether PCPs who experience a smaller number of patients than their preferred number, i.e., they experience a shortage of patients, are likely to provide a greater number of services compared with PCPs with their preferred number of patients. Iversen and Lurås (2000) and Iversen (2004) study the quantity of services that GPs provide in a mixed-capitation and FFS payment system. Physicians who experience a shortage of patients are predicted to increase the number of services they provide to each patient in order to increase their income. The empirical analyses show that GPs who experience a shortage of patients have higher incomes per listed person than GPs with the preferred number of patients. Grytten and Sørensen (2008) argue that GPs with a deficit of registered patients on their lists treat more patients who are not registered (external patients) than GPs with a surplus of registered patients. They do not find that a shortage of patients is associated with a greater number of services to registered-list patients.

It is methodologically difficult to identify the causal effects of payment components based on observational studies. To analyze the influence of FFS and capitation, Hennig-Schmidt *et al.* (2011) perform a controlled laboratory experiment where medical students were asked to decide on the quantity of medical services. They find that patients are overserved under FFS and underserved in capitation. The authors conclude that patients who need few medical services are better off under capitation, whereas patients with a high need for medical services benefit more from physicians paid by FFS.

Physicians are likely to vary in their degree of altruism. Godager and Wiesen (2013) employ data from the Hennig-Schmidt *et al.* (2011) experiment to estimate physician altruism, i.e., the weight that physicians attach to patients' health benefits. They find substantial variation in the degree of physician altruism.

Effects on the quality of health services

Sorbero *et al.* (2003) find that patients with chronic conditions and capitated primary care physicians are 36% more likely to switch physicians than similar patients with physicians paid on an FFS basis. The study points to the possibility that quality may be compromised under capitation.

To estimate the effect of capitation on time spent with patients, Melichar (2009) makes use of an empirical model that accounts for the selection of physicians into different financial arrangements. Fixed effects regression results reveal that physicians spend less time with their capitated patients than with their non-capitated patients. The author concludes that he cannot rule out the possibility that capitated patients may receive lower quality of care in outpatient settings than do non-capitated patients, but another possibility is that capitation may also lead doctors to eliminate unnecessary services from their routine without affecting health outcomes.

An important question is whether P4P has contributed to better quality care. In short, the US studies find some positive effects, although not overwhelming in magnitude. Damberg *et al.* (2009) do a survey-based study of the results of the largest P4P programs and find that, although physician organizations have increased their investments in quality-improving technologies after the introduction of P4P, breakthrough quality improvements are not reported. Mullen *et al.* (2010) study the effect of P4P on physician medical groups that contract with a large network HMO. By means of difference-in-differences models, they compare the performance of medical groups under P4P with the performance of medical groups not using P4P. They find some positive effects on rewarded quality measures, in particular on some screening procedures, and no spill-over effects on non-rewarded quality dimensions. The authors conclude that they find neither evidence of major improvement in quality nor notable disruption in care resulting from P4P.

Other authors find more positive results for P4P. In the UK, a P4P scheme called the Quality and Outcomes Framework (QOF) was introduced in 2004/2005. Under the QOF, practices are awarded 'points' for delivering services that are based on best available evidence of effectiveness. There are four domains: clinical, organizational, patient experience and additional services where the clinical domain accounts for 65% of the maximum available points. Sutton *et al.* (2010) study the effect of QOF on general practices in Scotland. Patients are split into two groups — one group having a chronic disease that is targeted by QOF and the other group having a chronic disease that is not targeted. Furthermore, a distinction is made between quality indicators that are covered under QOF and quality indicators that are not. The authors are, in particular, interested in studying spill-over effects to quality indicators that are not under QOF (unincentivized indicators). They find both positive effects on incentivized indicators for the target groups and positive spill-over effects on the similar indicators for the non-targeted group. There are also spill-over effects from the incentivized indicators to the unincentivized indicators for the targeted group. The effects seem to increase with greater rewards.

Scott *et al.* (2009) study the effects of a P4P program on quality of care in diabetes management in Australia, and they find that the program has the effect of increasing quality of care measured by the indicator Haemoglobin testing (HbA1c). Bruni *et al.* (2009) and Iezzi *et al.* (2014) study the effect of a similar program for general practices in Italy, and report that the program significantly reduces the probability of hyperglycaemic emergencies for patients included in the program.

Scott *et al.* (2011) summarize, by means of a systematic review, the studies of effect of financial incentives on the quality of health care provided by PCPs. Seven studies are included in the review. Six of the seven studies show positive, but modest, effects on quality of care for some primary outcome measures, but not all. One study found no effect on quality of care. The authors find that poor design led to substantial risk of bias in most studies. None of the studies addressed issues of selection bias as a result of the ability of primary care physicians to select into or out of the incentive scheme or health plan.

Similar to unadjusted capitation, P4P entails an incentive to select healthy patients. First, if practices in deprived areas spend excessive effort to reach quality targets because of patient characteristics, deprived areas may experience more problems in attracting physicians because it is more costly for PCPs to attain the targets there. However, Doran *et al.* (2008) find that under QOF, the gap between the achievement of quality targets in the least deprived and the most deprived areas has declined since the introduction of QOF. Second, there may be incentives to falsify reports and select certain patients for reporting. PCPs are allowed to exclude a maximum proportion of their patients (exception reporting) from quality reporting. Here, results of studies from the UK seem to vary somewhat. While Doran *et al.* (2008) find that rates of exception reporting have generally been low, with little evidence of widespread gaming, Gravelle *et al.* (2010) find results that show gaming both with regard to reporting disease prevalence and exceptions.

Effects on referrals and utilization of specialized health services

For many years, the organization and financing of primary care in the UK has contained an element of global capitation. During the first initiative, the fundholding system, the Health Authority delegated an annual budget to larger general practices (fundholders) and made them responsible for purchasing elective procedures at hospitals for their listed patients. Gravelle *et al.* (2002) and Dusheiko *et al.* (2006) study the effect of the UK fundholding scheme on hospital elective-admission rates. They predict that the abolition of the fundholding system promotes the number of admissions among the previous fundholders to increase because of the decline in the marginal cost of an admission. Dusheiko *et al.* (2006) show that the abolition of fundholding increased the ex-fundholders' admission rates for the elective admissions they previously paid for, between 3.5% and 5.1%, and conclude that gatekeeping practices will reduce their elective admissions by a modest, but not negligible, amount when confronted with a budget and explicit prices. Croxson *et al.* (2001) find similar results with data from the introduction of the fundholding system.

Propper *et al.* (2002) study the effect of fundholding on hospital waiting times in the UK. The results indicate that when fundholding PCPs paid for their patients' care, they were able to secure a reduction in waiting times of about 8% for their patients relative to all other patients. Dusheiko *et al.* (2004) use the opportunity offered by the abolition of the voluntary fundholding regime, and they find a significant non-trivial negative effect on waiting times for chargeable elective treatments and also for some treatments that were non-chargeable during the fundholding regime. Hence, some spill-over effects from chargeable to non-chargeable treatment were found. Starting in April 1999, the fundholding system was replaced by Primary Care Groups that were later transformed into Primary Care Trusts (PCT) that all practices in a particular area must join. The White Paper published by the UK government in July 2010 sets out the opportunities for consortia of GP practices to take on the power and responsibility to commission the great majority of NHS services for their patients (Clinical Commissioning Groups).

Iezzi *et al.* (2014) investigate the impact of implementing diabetes management programs with financial incentives in the Italian Region Emilia-Romagna in 2003–2005. They focus on avoidable hospitalizations for diabetic patients for whom PCPs receive additional payments that exceed capitation. Their findings indicate that, at sample averages, an increase of €100 of the financial incentives paid per GP is expected to reduce the number of diabetic Ambulatory Care Sensitive Conditions (ACSCs) by 1%, or about 100 cases when projected on the entire region.

The health economics literature on the possible impact of primary care capacity on secondary health services is small but growing. Using US data, Baicker and Chandra (2004), and Chernew *et al.* (2009) find that the percentage of primary care physicians in a market is negatively associated with Medicare's reimbursement per beneficiary. The reason may be less use of expensive specialist health care with a higher proportion of PCPs. Chernew *et al.* (2009), however, find no correlation between the percentage of primary care physicians and the growth in Medicare spending.

Bradley Wright and Ricketts III (2010) use area-level data to show that within a location, a higher density of primary care physicians is associated with less inpatient admission and emergency room visits. Fortney *et al.* (2005) present results from a natural experiment at the US Department for Veterans Affairs, in which the number of primary care facilities was increased in some districts but not in others. Using a difference-in-differences analysis of longitudinal data and instrumental variables to correct for potential endogeneity problems, they find that an increase in primary care encounters is associated with a decrease in specialty medical encounters. Fortney *et al.* conclude that primary care is a substitute for specialist health care. With survey data at the individual-patient level, Atella and Deb (2008) study whether primary care physicians and secondary specialists are substitutes or complements. They estimate a structural simultaneous equation model where visits to different types of physicians are endogenous. When unobserved heterogeneity is appropriately accounted for, they find that PCPs and specialists are substitutes. If primary care services are less expensive than specialist health care, an expansion of the number of PCPs would then have a potential in reducing total health care costs.

In a mixed capitation and FFS system, Iversen and Ma (2011) study PCP referrals to radiology services. In their model, the PCPs are partially altruistic, and compete for patients. The results show that even if the PCP does not directly benefit from referring a patient to radiology services, a PCP operating in a competitive market refers more. This happens because the PCP may provide more treatments to a patient after the radiology referral, but also because a referral may increase patient satisfaction which may help the PCP to retain patients and also to attract new patients to the list. Empirical analyses support this theoretical result. Godager *et al.* (2014) take these results further by analyzing a mix of survey data and register data at the individual level of patients and PCPs. The empirical results suggest that competition has negligible or small positive effects on referrals overall. Hence, these results do not support the policy claim that increasing the number of PCPs reduces secondary care.

Beales and Smith (2012) examine the published evidence on the role of primary health care in controlling the cost of specialized health care. They emphasize the three fundamental functions of primary care that may contribute to this objective: Reducing or delaying the onset of disease; reducing the use of specialist care once a clinical condition has been identified; and reducing the intensity of use of specialist care once a need for such care has arisen. The authors conclude that there is little persuasive evidence on the macro benefits of primary care spending, and — with a few exceptions — the micro evidence is small scale and inconclusive, although there are indications of promising policy options for future experimentation. They find that whatever the intervention under scrutiny, there are some further policy-design issues that must be satisfied if the initiative is to stand any chance of success.

Implications for Health Policy

The previous sections have elaborated on payment and organization of primary care with emphasis on PCPs. Section "Characteristics of Regulation and Types of Payment for PCPs" briefly described regulation and payment schemes for PCPs in the OECD countries. Section "An Economic Approach to Effectiveness in Primary Care" presented our understanding of an economic approach to effectiveness and cost in primary care. Section "An Illustration of the Predicted Effect of FFS and Capitation on the Volume of PCP Services" outlined theory-based predictions of the properties of main payment schemes, and Section "The Empirical Research Literature on Characteristics and Effects of Payment Systems in Primary Care" described results of empirical studies of the effects of payment schemes. We now discuss possible implications for health policy that might be drawn from the previous sections.

The theory section draws a distinction between two frameworks. Within the first framework, we assume that the PCP considers not only the patient in front of him, but the entire community of patients. This framework is related to a low density of PCPs in the community. In order to serve most of the patients, the number of services to each patient has to be strictly rationed. Within this framework, we find that capitation, FFS and combinations of the two encourage a small number of services to each patient. A policy implication seems to be that in a society with a low density of physicians, general health insurance and physicians who consider the entire community of patients, the payment system does not greatly matter for the volume of health services provided to each patient.

Within the other framework, we assumed that the PCP only considered the health of the individual patient. An interpretation of this framework is a rich society with high density of PCPs and general health insurance. All patients are then covered by a PCP, and there is no particular motivation to reach out to everyone. Within this framework, theory predicts a difference between payment systems with regard to the volume of health services provided. In particular, we predict that FFS will encourage a more service-intensive practice style, and we predict that capitation will encourage a less service-intensive practice style. While we expect that FFS will provide more than the optimal number of health services from a social efficiency point of view, we expect that capitation will provide fewer services than optimal from a social efficiency point of view. These hypotheses are broadly supported by the results from the empirical studies described in Section "The Empirical Research Literature on Characteristics and Effects of Payment Systems in Primary Care". As referred to in Section "An Illustration of the Predicted Effect of FFS and Capitation on the Volume of PCP Services", influential authors have suggested that a mix of FFS and capitation perhaps encourages the approximate optimal number of services from the society's perspective. However, not much is known about the optimal composition of FFS and capitation in a mixed system. Here, the other efficiency concerns defined in Section "An Economic Approach to Effectiveness in Primary Care" would also be involved.

A mix of capitation and FFS may also have some favorable properties with regard to the fifth efficiency concern mentioned in Section "An Economic Approach to Effectiveness in Primary Care". Because risk adjusted capitation is unlikely to be perfect, there may be an economic incentive for the PCP to choose the healthy rather than the unhealthy individuals. FFS compensates for (some of) the additional costs attached to unhealthy individuals and hence, dampens the incentive to favorable risk selection by the PCP.

There are diverging conclusions from the research literature about whether capitation or FFS is preferable for the quality of services provided. Again, some authors have suggested a mix of capitation and FFS to balance the dangers of underprovision or overprovision. Also, pay-for-performance may have an important role as a component of a payment system for PCPs. Although the results from empirical studies presented in Section "The Empirical Research Literature on Characteristics and Effects of Payment Systems in Primary Care" are somewhat mixed, the potential of the method is likely to be better understood as more health systems start to experiment and evaluate the effects of pay-for-performance on health policy goals.

In the previous section, we addressed the socially optimal division of tasks between primary health care and specialist health care. The issue is also high on the political agenda in most countries. There is no strong empirical evidence that systems with PCPs as gatekeepers to specialized health care are associated with smaller overall health care cost than systems without PCPs as gatekeepers. More empirical studies are needed. Results from both theoretical and empirical studies suggest that capitation at the level of PCP encourages a high referral rate to specialist health care. Fundholding (extended capitation that also includes the cost of some specialist care) as practiced in the UK, seems to have potential to restrict the number of patients referred from the PCP to specialist care. A PCP practice will then also carry the financial risk attached to the number and types of referral. For small practices this risk may be considerable and has to be compensated in order to attract physicians to primary care. Extended capitation gives an incentive for PCPs to merge and create larger practices to better handle financial risk. There may also be an incentive for vertical integration to ensure an optimal allocation, from a system perspective, that both include primary care and secondary care. These aspects seem to be important for the integrated care approaches of both the PCMH and ACOs, as described in Section "Characteristics of Regulation and Types of Payment for PCPs." With more integrated care, primary health care will perhaps be a less distinct entity compared with what we observe in many countries today. An increasing share of the population with chronic diseases that require coordinated effort from both primary care and specialized care pulls in the same direction. An important challenge for governments is to initiate experiments and controlled trials that make it possible to transmit knowledge across countries about which innovations seem to be working and which innovations do not.

References

Allard M, Jelovac I, Léger PT. 2011. Treatment and referral decisions under different physician payment mechanisms. *Journal of Health Economics* 30: 880–893.

Atella V, Deb P. 2008. Are primary care physicians, public and private sector specialists substitutes or complements? Evidence from a simultaneous equations model for count data. *Journal of Health Economics* 27: 770–785.

Baicker K, Chandra A. 2004. The productivity of physician specialization: Evidence from the Medicare program. *American Economic Review* 94: 357–361.

Barros PP, Martinez-Giralt X. 2003. Preventive health care and payment systems. *Topics in Economic Analysis & Policy* 3(1): 1–21.

Beales S, Smith PC. 2012. The role of primary health care in controlling the cost of specialist health care. In Iversen T, Kittelsen S (eds.). Challenges in health care financing and provision. *Nordic Economic Policy Review* 2(2): 153–186.

Bodenheimer T, Pham HH. 2010. Primary care: Current problems and proposed solutions. *Health Affairs* 29: 799–805.

Bradley Wright T, Ricketts III C. 2010. The road to efficiency? Re-examining the impact of the primary care physician workforce on health care utilization rates. *Social Science & Medicine* 70: 2006–2010.

Bruni ML, Nobilio L, Ugolini C. 2009. Economic incentives in general practice: The impact of pay-for-participation and pay-for-compliance programs on diabetes care. *Health Policy* 90: 140–148.

Chandra A, Cutler D, Song Z. 2012. Who ordered that? The economics of treatment choices in medical care. In Pauly MV, McGuire TG, Barros PP (eds.). *Handbook of Health Economics*, Volume 2. Elsevier Science: Amsterdam, 397–432.

Chernew ME, Sabik L, Chandra A, Newhouse JP. 2009. Would having more primary care doctors cut health spending growth? *Health Affairs* 28: 1327–1335.

Croxson B, Propper C, Perkins A. 2001. Do doctors respond to financial incentives? UK family doctors and the GP fundholder scheme. *Journal of Public Economics* 79: 375–398.

Damberg CL, Raube K, Teleki SS, de la Cruz E. 2009. Taking stock of pay-for-performance: Candid assessment from the front lines. *Health Affairs* 28: 517–525.

Devlin RA, Sarma S. 2008. Do physician remuneration schemes matter? The case of Canadian family physicians. *Journal of Health Economics* 27: 1168–1181.

Doran T, Fullwood C, Kontopantelis E, Reeves D. 2008. Effect of financial incentives on inequalities in the delivery of primary clinical care in England: Analysis of clinical activity indicators for the quality and outcomes framework. *Lancet* 372: 728–736.

Dusheiko M, Gravelle H, Jacobs R. 2004. The effect of practice budgets on patient waiting times: Allowing for selection bias. *Health Economics* 13: 941–958.

Dusheiko M, Gravelle H, Jacobs R, Smith PC. 2006. The effect of budgets on doctor behaviour: Evidence from a natural experiment. *Journal of Health Economics* 25: 449–478.

Ellis RP, McGuire TG. 1993. Supply-side and demand-side cost sharing in health care. *Journal of Economic Perspectives* 7: 135–151.

Fortney JC, Steffick DE, Burgess Jr JF, Maciejewski ML, Petersen LA. 2005. Are primary care services a substitute or complement for specialty and inpatient services? *Health Services Research* 40: 1422–1442.

Godager G, Iversen T, Ma Ch-T A. 2015. Competition, gatekeeping, and health care access. *Journal of Health Economics* 39: 159–170.

Godager G, Wiesen D. 2013. Profit or patients' health benefit? Exploring the heterogeneity in physician altruism. *Journal of Health Economics* 32: 1105–1116.

Gosden T, Forland F, Kristiansen I, Sutton M, Leese B, Giuffrida A, Sergison M, Pedersen L. 2000. Capitation, salary, fee-for-service and mixed systems of payment: Effects on the behaviour of primary care physicians. *Cochrane Database of Systematic Reviews 2000*, Issue 3. Art. No.: CD002215. DOI: 10.1002/14651858.CD002215.

Gravelle H. 1999. Capitation contracts: Access and quality. *Journal of Health Economics* 18: 315–340.

Gravelle H, Masiero G. 2000. Quality incentives in a regulated market with imperfect information and switching costs: Capitation in general practice. *Journal of Health Economics* 19: 1067–1088.

Gravelle H, Dusheiko M, Sutton M. 2002. The demand for elective surgery in a public system: Time and money prices in the UK National Health Service. *Journal of Health Economics* 21: 423–449.

Gravelle H, Sutton M, Ma Ch-T A. 2010. Doctor behaviour under a pay for performance contract: Treating, cheating and case finding. *Economic Journal* 120: F129–F56.

Grytten J, Sørensen R. 2008. Busy physicians. *Journal of Health Economics* 27: 510–518.

Hennig-Schmidt H, Selten R, Wiesen D. 2011. How payment systems affect physicians' provision behavior — An experimental investigation. *Journal of Health Economics* 30: 637–646.

Holmstrom B, Milgrom P. 1991. Multitask principal–agent analyses: Incentive contracts, asset ownership, and job design. *Journal of Law, Economics and Organization* 7 (special issue): 24–52.

Iezzi E, Bruni ML, Ugolini C. 2014. The role of GP's compensation schemes in diabetes care: Evidence from panel data. *Journal of Health Economics* 34: 104–120.

Institute of Medicine. 1994. Defining Primary Care: An Interim Report. Committee on the Future of Primary Care. Washington, DC, National Academies Press.

Iversen T. 2004. The effects of a patient shortage on general practitioners' future income and list of patients. *Journal of Health Economics* 23: 673–694.

Iversen T, Lurås H. 2000. The effect of capitation on GPs' referral decisions. *Health Economics* 9: 199–210.

Iversen T, Lurås H. 2012. Capitation and incentives in primary care. In Jones A (eds.). *The Elgar Companion to Health Economics*, Second Edition. E. Elgar Publishing, Cheltenham, pp. 280–288.

Iversen T, Ma Ch-t A. 2011. Market conditions and general practitioners' referrals. *International Journal of Health Care Finance and Economics* 11: 245–265.

Jelovac I. 2014. Primary Care, gatekeeping and incentives. In Culyer AJ. (ed.): *Encyclopedia of Health Economics*, Volume 3. Elsevier Science: Amsterdam, pp. 142–145.

Kaarbøe O, Siciliani L. 2010. Multi-tasking, quality and pay for performance. *Health Economics* 10: 225–238.

Léger PT. 2008. Physician payment mechanisms. In Lu M, Johnsson E (eds.). *Financing Health Care. New Ideas for a Changing Society*. Wiley-VCH Verlag: Weinheim, pp. 149–176.

Macinko J, Starfield B, Shi L. 2003. The contribution of primary care systems to health outcomes within Organisation for Economic Cooperation and Development (OECD) countries, 1970–1998. *Health Services Research* 38: 831–865.

McGuire TG. 2000. Physician agency. In Culyer AJ, Newhouse JP (eds.). *Handbook of Health Economics*, Volume 1. Elsevier Science, Amsterdam, pp. 461–536.

McGuire TG. 2011. Physician agency and payment for primary medical care. In Glied S, Smith PC (eds.). *The Oxford Handbook of Health Economics*. Oxford: Oxford University Press, pp. 602–625.

Melichar L. 2009. The Effect of reimbursement on medical decision making: Do physicians alter treatment in response to a managed care incentive? *Journal of Health Economics* 28: 902–907.

Mullen KJ, Frank RG, Rosenthal MB. 2010. Can you get what you pay for? Pay-for-performance and the quality of healthcare providers. *RAND Journal of Economics* 41: 64–91.

Newhouse JP. 1996. Reimbursing health plans and health providers: Efficiency in production versus selection. *Journal of Economic Literature* 34: 1236–1263.

Newhouse JP. 2002. Pricing the Priceless. A Health Care Conundrum, Cambridge MA: The MIT Press.

Paris P, Devaux M, Wei L. 2010. Health systems institutional characteristics: A survey of 29 OECD countries. *OECD Health Working Papers No*. 50. OECD, Paris.

Propper C, Croxson B, Shearer A. 2002. Waiting for hospital admissions: The impact of fundholding. *Journal of Health Economics* 21: 227–252.

Rice T. 2012. The Physician as the Patient's Agent. In Jones A (ed.). *The Elgar Companion to Health Economics*, Second Edition. E. Elgar Publishing: Cheltenham, pp. 271–279.

Rice T, Rosenau P, Unruh LY, Barnes AJ, Saltman RB, van Ginneken E. 2013. United States of America: Health system review. *Health Systems in Transition* 15: 1–431.
Scott A. 2000. Economics of general practice. In Culyer AJ, Newhouse JP (eds.). *Handbook of Health Economics*, Volume 1. Amsterdam: Elsevier Science, pp. 1175–1200.
Scott A, Schurer S, Jensen PH, Sivey P. 2009. The effects of an incentive program on quality of care in diabetes management. *Health Economics* 18: 1091–1108.
Scott A, Sivey P, Ait Ouakrim D, Willenberg L, Naccarella L, Furler J, Young D. 2011. The effect of financial incentives on the quality of health care provided by primary care physicians. *Cochrane Database of Systematic Reviews 2011*, Issue 9. Art. No.: CD008451. DOI: 10.1002/14651858.CD008451.pub2.
Sorbero MES, Zwanziger DAW, Muhamel JD, Weyl N. 2003. The effect of capitation on switching primary care physicians. *Health Services Research* 38: 191–209.
Starfield B. 1998. Primary Care: Balancing Health Needs, Services, and Technology. New York: Oxford University Press.
Sutton M, Elder R, Guthrie B, Watt G. 2010. Record rewards: The effects of targeted quality incentives on the recording of risk factors by primary care providers. *Health Economics* 19: 1–13.
van Dijk CE, van den Berg B, Verheij RA, Spreeuwenberg P, Groenewegen PP, de Bakker DH. 2013. Moral hazard and supplier-induced demand: Empirical evidence in general practice. *Health Economics* 22: 340–352.
WHO (2008). The World Health Report 2008 — Primary Health Care (Now More Than Ever).
Zweifel P, Breyer F, Kifmann M. 2009. Health Economics. Heidelberg London New York: Springer Dordrecht.

Appendix

Socially efficient volume of services[3]

The consumer's utility function is

$$U(H, X),$$

where

H is health state

X is consumption

and $\dfrac{\partial U}{\partial H} > 0,\ \dfrac{\partial^2 U}{\partial H^2} < 0,\ \dfrac{\partial U}{\partial X} > 0,\ \dfrac{\partial^2 U}{\partial X^2} < 0$ and $\dfrac{\partial^2 U}{\partial H \partial X} > 0,$

[3]This set-up is inspired by Léger (2008).

Consumer's health is assumed to be a declining function of disease severity θ and an increasing and concave function of the amount of medical treatment, q. θ has a known distribution function, $\Gamma(\theta)$.

$$H = h(\theta, q)$$

$$\frac{\partial h}{\partial \theta} < 0 \; \frac{\partial h}{\partial q} > 0 \; \frac{\partial^2 h}{\partial q^2} < 0.$$

The health technology is assumed to be known to the consumer.

$(1-d)$ is the probability of disease

A patient's expected utility:

$$EU = dU(H^0, \mathrm{I}) + (1-d)\int_\theta U(h(\theta, q), X) d\Gamma(\theta),$$

$$X = I - pq,$$

H^0 is health in the healthy state.

I is state independent income.

p is co-payment by the patient.

q is quantity of health services.

X is consumption of an aggregate of other goods.

Price of X equals one.

A consumer, who is ill with severity θ, chooses q by maximizing:

$$U(h(\theta, q), I - pq).$$

The first-order condition for an interior solution gives:

$$\frac{U'_h h'_q}{U_X} = p, \tag{A.1}$$

that tells us that the marginal rate of substitution between health services and consumption should equal relative cost.

Equation (1) defines demand for medical care as a function of disease severity and cost:

$$q = q(\underset{+}{\theta}, \underset{-}{p})$$

Paying the full price of medical care at the point of use implies a considerable financial risk for the consumer. Risk-averse consumers certainly prefer insurance offered at an actuarially fair premium.

Actuarially fair insurance is:

$$\alpha = (1-d)\int_{\theta} p^{*} q(\theta, p) d\Gamma(\theta),$$

where p^* is the market price of medical care under perfect competition.

Patient budget constraint with insurance:

$$I = X + \alpha.$$

If illness severity was verifiable and contractible, we have:

$$\alpha = (1-d)\int_{\theta} p^{*} q(\theta, p^{*}) d\Gamma(\theta).$$

But with full insurance and illness severity non contractible, we have:

$$\frac{U'_h h'_q}{U_X} = 0,$$

That is health care is demanded until marginal health benefit is zero.

Actuarially fair insurance has to reflect this over-consumption:

$$\alpha^{**} = (1-d)\int_{\theta} p\theta^{*} q(\theta, p^{*}) d\Gamma(\theta).$$

Ex-post moral hazard may result in some individuals choosing to be uninsured and carrying the risk themselves.

The inefficiency arises because it is not possible, or at least very expensive, to make an insurance contract with reimbursement that depends on illness severity.

Hence, patient co-payment has to be maintained to move towards optimal consumption of health care

$$\frac{U'_h h'_q}{U_X} = \gamma p.$$

Hence, there is a trade-off between excessive consumption of medical care and the patient's financial risk.

We can illustrate the demanded number of services with constant cost per service equal to c.

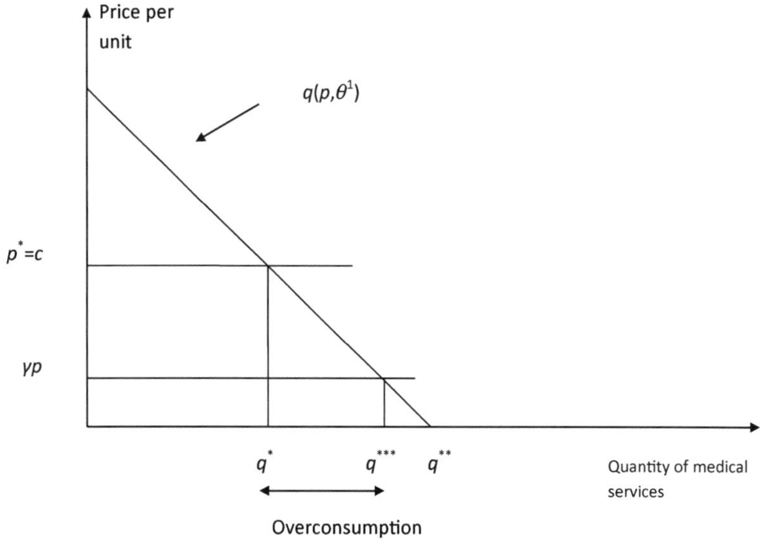

Supply-Side Rationing by Means of the Physician Payment System

We now examine whether the physician payment scheme can move the number of provided services in the direction of the social optimum quantity q^*. If so, supply-side rationing can relieve the patient from the financial risk that co-payments imply.

Assume a physician objective function:

$$V = \delta[A + (R + Fq)n - c(nq)] + (1 - \delta)nh(\theta, q)$$
$$c'(nq) > 0, \; c''(nq) > 0.$$

n is no. regular patients. We assume $n > 1$.

q is number of services.

There is no patient co-payment.

δ is profit weight in the utility function.

The physician cares for patient health (weight $1-\delta$) — i.e., partial altruism or professionalism is assumed.

A is fixed practice allowance.

R is capitation payment; i.e., fixed annual payment for each regular patient.

F is fee for service (FFS).

A is a practice allowance; i.e., fixed revenue to cover (some of the) fixed costs of running the practice.

θ is disease severity.

We assume increasing marginal cost of providing care. The physician's time cost is included in the cost function.

Decision variables are n and q.

Four types of systems:

A: Pure FFS ($F > 0, A = 0, R = 0$).

B: Pure capitation ($F = 0, A = 0, R > 0$).

C: Combination of practice allowance and FFS ($F > 0, A > 0, R = 0$).

D: Combination of capitation fee and FFS ($F > 0, A = 0, R > 0$).

Let us first explore the effects of the payment components when $\delta = 1$ — no concern for patient health:

$$V = A + (R + Fq)n - c(nq).$$

With pure FFS it is only the total number of services provided, nq, that counts and the first-order condition (FOC) requires that F equals marginal cost of providing services.

Under capitation there is no incentive to provide services and the minimum quantity, $\underline{q}$, will be provided.

Assume now that physicians have preferences for total health gain patients may have. Then:

$$V = \delta[A + (R + Fq)n - c(nq)] + (1 - \delta)nh(\theta, q).$$

A: Pure FFS ($F > 0, A = 0, R = 0$)

$$\frac{\partial V}{\partial n} = \delta q[F - c'(nq)] + (1-\delta)h(\theta,q) = 0$$

$$\frac{\partial V}{\partial q} = \delta\,[F - c'(nq)] + (1-\delta\,)h'_q(\theta,q) \le 0.$$

Divide through by q:

$$\frac{\partial V}{\partial n}\bigg/ q = \delta[F - c'(nq)] + \frac{(1-\delta)h(\theta,q)}{q} = 0$$

Then:

$$\frac{\partial V}{\partial q} = \delta[F - c'(nq)] + (1-\delta)h'_q < 0$$

as

$$\frac{h(\theta,q)}{q} > h'_q(\theta,q) \text{ as h() is concave,}$$

this implies $h'_q(\theta, q) > 0$ and $q = q < q^*$ where q is the minimum quantity compatible with the professional standard.

The concern for the total number of patients makes it more rewarding to provide few services to many patients than to provide many services to a small number of patients.

B: Pure capitation ($F = 0, A = 0, R > 0$)

$$V = \delta\,[Rn - c(nq)] + (1 - \delta)nh(\theta, q)$$

$$\frac{\partial V}{\partial n} = \delta\,\left[R - c'(nq)q\right] + (1-\delta\,)h(\theta\,, q) = 0.$$

Divide through by q and rearrange:

$$-\delta\,c'(nq) + (1-\delta\,)\frac{h(\theta\,, q)}{q} = -\delta\,\frac{R}{q} < 0$$

$$\frac{\partial V}{\partial q} = -\delta\,c'(nq) + (1-\delta\,)h'_q(\theta\,, q) \le 0$$

Then:

$$\frac{\partial V}{\partial q} = -\delta c'(nq) + (1-\delta)h'_q(\theta,q) < 0.$$

As

$$\frac{h(\theta,q)}{q} > h'_q(\theta,q) \text{ as h() is concave,}$$

this implies

$$h'_q(\theta, q) > 0 \text{ and } q = \underline{q} < \underline{q}^*.$$

C: Combination of practice allowance and FFS ($F > 0, A > 0, R = 0$)

$$\frac{\partial V}{\partial n} = \delta q[F - c'(nq)] + (1-\delta)h(\theta,q) = 0.$$

Divide through by q:

$$\frac{\partial V}{\partial n}\bigg/ q = \delta[F - c'(nq)] + \frac{(1-\delta)h(\theta,q)}{q} = 0$$

$$\frac{\partial V}{\partial \underline{q}} = \delta\,[F - c'(nq)] + (1-\delta\,)h'_q(\theta\,,q) \le 0.$$

Then:

$$\frac{\partial V}{\partial q} = \delta[F - c'(nq)] + (1-\delta)h'_q(\theta,q) < 0$$

since

$$\frac{h(\theta,q)}{q} > h'_q(\theta,q) \text{ as } h() \text{ is concave,}$$

this implies

$$h'_q(\theta, q) > 0 \text{ and } q = \underline{q} < q^*.$$

D: Combination of capitation fee and FFS ($F > 0, A = 0, R > 0$)

$$\frac{\partial V}{\partial n} = \delta\big[(R + Fq) - c'(nq)q\big] + (1-\delta)h(\theta,q) = 0.$$

Divide through by q and rearrange:

$$\delta\left[F - c'(nq)\right] + (1-\delta)\frac{h(\theta,q)}{q} = -\frac{\delta R}{q} < 0$$

$$\frac{\partial V}{\partial q} = \delta\left[F - c'(nq)\right] + (1-\delta)h'_q(\theta,q) \leq 0.$$

Then:

$$\frac{\partial V}{\partial q} = \delta\left[F - c'(nq)\right] + (1-\delta)h'_q(\theta,q) < 0$$

since

$$\frac{h(\theta,q)}{q} > h'_q(\theta,q) \text{ as } h() \text{ is concave.}$$

This implies

$$h'_q(\theta,q) > 0 \text{ and } q = \underline{q} < q^*.$$

So in the case when a physician has a preference for the total health benefit generated, even pure FFS systems will generate a low level of services.

Assume now that there is some concern for the individual patient's health:

$$V = \delta[A + (R + Fq)n - c(nq)] + (1 - \delta)h(\theta,q).$$

A: Pure FFS ($F > 0, A = 0, R = 0$)

$$V = \delta[Fqn - c(nq)] + (1 - \delta)h(\theta,q)$$

$$\frac{\partial V}{\partial n} = \delta q\left[F - c'(nq)\right] = 0$$

$$\frac{\partial V}{\partial q} = \delta n\left[F - c'(nq)\right] + (1-\delta)h'_q(\theta,q) = 0$$

implies

$$h'_q(\theta, q) = 0$$

$$q = q^{**} > q^*.$$

Incentive to provide more than the socially optimal number of services, q^*.

B: Pure capitation ($F = 0, A = 0, R > 0$)

$$V = \delta[Rn - c(nq)] + (1 - \delta)h(\theta,q)$$

$$\frac{\partial V}{\partial q} = -\delta\, nc'(nq) + (1-\delta)h'_q(\theta,q) \leq 0$$

implies $h'_q(\theta, q) > 0$ and $\underline{q} \leq q < q^{**}$.

The concern for the patient could make number of services greater than the minimum amount, although the minimum amount maximizes income.

C: Combination of practice allowance and FFS ($F > 0, A > 0, R = 0$)

Implies $h'_q(\theta, q) = 0$ and $q = q^{**} > q^*$.

D: Combination of capitation fee and FFS ($F > 0, A = 0, R > 0$)

$$V = \delta[(R + Fq)n - c(nq)] + (1 - \delta)h(\theta,q)$$

$$\frac{\partial V}{\partial n} = \delta\left[(R + Fq) - c'(nq)q\right] = 0.$$

Divide through by q:

$$\delta\left[F - c'(nq)\right] = -\frac{\delta R}{q} < 0$$

$$\frac{\partial V}{\partial q} = \delta n\left[F - c'(nq)\right] + (1-\delta)h'_q(\theta,q) \leq 0$$

implies $h'_q(\theta, q) > 0$ and $\underline{q} \leq q < q^{**}$, but greater than under pure capitation.

Summing up:

Provided number of services under alternative payment systems varies with physician objectives and environments.

	$\delta = 1$		$0 < \delta < 1$		
				No *n* in utility function	
	Sufficient patients	**Shortage of patients**	***n* in utility function**	**Sufficient patients**	**Shortage of patients**
A. FFS	only total *qn* determined	$q > q^{**}$	$q = \underline{q}$	$q = q^{**}$	$q > q^{**}$
B. Capitation	$q = \underline{q}$	$q = \underline{q}$	$q = \underline{q}$	$\underline{q} \leq q < q^{**}$	
C. FFS/Practice allowance	only total *qn* determined	$q > q^{**}$	$q = \underline{q}$	$q = q^{**}$	$q > q^{**}$
D. FFS/Capitation	$q = \underline{q}$	$q > \underline{q}$	$q = \underline{q}$	$\underline{q} \leq q < q^{**}$	Greater than with no shortage

Health Systems Performance

Peter Berman

Harvard School of Public Health
Boston, USA

Health systems account for more than 10% of the global economy. Citizens and policymakers ask, "what are we getting for this large expenditure?" Answers to this question require defining, measuring, and comparing health system performance. This chapter reviews recent conceptual and empirical developments that attempt to address this demand. Defining health system performance requires thinking about what we want and expect from a health system, and valuing these outcomes. Health system performance encompasses of several different types of outcomes. Simple, single-dimensional measures performance fail to represent multiple outcomes well. This introduces complexity into the definition and measurement of health system performance. Elements of this complexity are summarized in this chapter, along with the efforts of analysts in different countries and globally to develop approaches that capture complexity but are also tractable for analyzing health system performance. A key question for policymakers is, what determines performance and differences in performance between countries and within countries? Politics suffuses efforts to define performance problems and set directions to remedy them. The functioning elements of health systems are explored, including their financing and payment, regulation, and delivery mechanisms, as well as citizen and provider behavior. These elements determine the results. They make up much of the content of health system reforms, whose ultimate objective is to improve performance. As health needs and health system capabilities evolve, so too will our notions of performance. This is a rich area for current and future research and action, to which health economics has and will make important contributions.

Keywords: Health Systems; Health and Development; Health Policy; Health System Strengthening and Reform; Health System Performance.

What is Health Systems Performance and Why Do We Care?

All human societies value health. All devote, often considerable, resources to the attainment and maintenance of health. In 2012, worldwide, health accounted for 10.1% of total global economic activity (WHO, 2014).

These resources devoted to health and the ways in which they are organized and function, within some definitional parameters, can be considered to be the health system. The World Health Organization (WHO) defines the health system as "all the organizations, institutions and resources that are devoted to producing health actions," which are "all activities whose primary purpose is to promote, restore, or maintain health" (WHO, 2000). While one can quibble about the precise boundaries of such systems and how to delineate their components and processes, the existence and social importance of health systems is hard to dispute.

Nation–states are the dominant mode globally of organizing societies and are usually clearly and distinctly defined. This leads to consideration of national health systems as a unit of analysis. Of course, there are often potentially interesting and substantive variations within nations as well as linkages across nations. The term "health systems" is used with many different meanings. For example, a local organization, which runs multiple ambulatory care clinics, can be called a health system. A firm, which integrates hospitals and primary care providers, can be called an "integrated health system" (Shortell and McCurdy, 2009). Much has also been written about "district health systems." This chapter will focus on national health systems, with occasional digressions of interest.

The *Oxford Dictionaries* define performance as "An action, task, or operation, seen in terms of how successfully it was performed" (*Oxford Dictionaries*, 2015). Health systems are a social means to achieve desired ends, the foremost of which is health. An important advance in our thinking about health systems has been the recognition that their purpose is not simply one of attaining and maintaining health. Health systems achieve other desirable social outcomes. These include protection against the uncertain future burden of potentially high-cost medical needs due to ill health (often summarized with the notion of "financial risk protection") and providing people some degree of security, caring, and respect for their persons (often summarized as "citizen satisfaction" or "responsiveness"). Health systems can also be a means to correct inequalities or disparities in society, which necessitates that some attention be devoted to questions of distribution and fairness or equity.

It is because health systems are means to achieve ends, because these ends are highly valued, and because health systems are costly whereas social resources are limited, that concerns about health system performance — how successfully health systems achieve their goals — arise. Citizens and governments ask these fundamental questions concerning health system performance: How is our health system doing in producing the desired results? How well is it doing in relation to the resources being used? How well is it doing in comparison to other health systems? What could be done so that it performs better?

These questions have both evaluative and managerial elements — citizens and their institutions seek to assess the health system as well as to improve it. These questions and their answers are also profoundly political, an aspect discussed further in the following paragraphs.

These are difficult questions and it is important to say at the outset that there are no universally accepted answers to how to measure health system performance, how to explain it, or how to improve it. There are, however, useful and to some extent generalizable insights that have arisen from efforts to answer these questions. The questions are vital, and the efforts being made to address them are current and relevant.

This chapter discusses some key elements and recent results of efforts to assess and improve health system performance. It begins with a careful discussion of defining health system performance and the questions of ethics or values that underpin such definitions. The section on "Health Systems Performance Goals" investigates problems that arise in measuring the components of health system performance. The section on "Measuring Health System Performance" examines comparative health systems performance measurement across countries and over time. Some aspects of the politics of health system performance measurement are then discussed. Recent innovations in measurement and analysis are reviewed. The chapter concludes with observations on the work that has been done on health systems performance to date and ideas for the future.

Health Systems Performance Goals: Conceptual and Ethical Considerations

With health systems as the means to achieve some set of desirable social ends, inquiry about performance means inquiry about how successful systems are in achieving those ends. Then, what are those ends? Or, to elaborate the question further: What outcomes should be included in a useful definition of those ends? What are some examples of health system outcomes that have been proposed as elements of performance, and what can be learned from different ways in which these outcomes have been defined?

Goals of health systems

The 2000 World Health Report (WHO, 2000); Roberts *et al.* (2008) Getting Health Reform Right: A Guide to Improving Performance and Equity, developed with the World Bank (Roberts *et al.*, 2008); and the 2002 OECD Report on "Measuring

Up: Improving Health System Performance in OECD Countries" are three relatively recent international and influential efforts propose to a widely acceptable set of health systems goals or outcomes for countries. Other similar examples include Smith (2002) and Wait (2004). Their conclusions and the frameworks they proposed were broadly similar, but with some interesting differences that highlight useful distinctions.

All three asserted that health system goals should represent outcomes that are valued for their own sake (intrinsically-valued), and not primarily as means to achieve other goals (instrumentally-valued), although that does not preclude health system outcomes from contributing to other consequences that are not of primary relevance to health systems.

For example, much effort may be devoted to improve the likelihood that clinical services will achieve the health improvement outcomes they are technically able to achieve when performed correctly. Such improvements in "technical quality" or "clinical efficacy" are beneficial and desirable, but they are not desired intrinsically or as ends in themselves. Rather, they are desired as instruments to improve people's health, or health outcomes. Better quality of health care is not an ultimate goal or outcome of the health system, but rather an intermediate one that contributes to an ultimate or final goal, health.

Figure 1 places the frameworks put forward by WHO, Roberts *et al.*, and the OECD side-by-side. Let us compare their commonalities and differences.

All three frameworks include multiple categories along both the vertical and horizontal axes of these tables shown in Figure 1. Framing health systems goals in this way, especially by WHO, was profoundly consequential. For, while it would seem non-controversial that a goal of health systems is to improve health (the first horizontal dimension), the notion that there are health system goals other than improving health that merit equal acknowledgement had not been so clearly and officially stated by the world's recognized arbiter of norms and standards for health.

Health system goals in relation to components for assessment			**OECD proposed health system performance framework**			**Ultimate outcomes: Health system performance**		
	Average level	Distribution		Average level	Distribution		Average level	Distribution
Health improvement	✓	✓	Health improvement/ outcomes (+)	✓	✓	Health status	✓	✓
Fairness in financial contribution	✓	✓	Financial contribution/ health expenditure (-)	✓	✓	Financial risk-protection	✓	✓
Responsiveness to expectations	-	✓	Responsiveness and access (+)	✓	✓	Satisfaction	✓	✓
				Efficiency	Equity			
Source: Adapted from Murray & Frank (2000)			*Source*: Adapted from *Measuring Up: Improving Health System Performance in OECD Countries* (2002)			*Source*: Adapted from Roberts *et al.* (2008)		

Figure 1. A Comparison of international health system performance frameworks.

And what are the other goals? The second horizontal dimension recognizes that health systems play a key role in determining the economic situations of people and households experiencing ill health. Reducing the financial risk to people in their pursuit of health represents another intrinsic goal of health systems, separable from the goal of improving their health.

The third horizontal dimension captures aspects of the human experience of ill health and interactions with the health system. Its presence indicates the view that people value for its own sake a positive experiential outcome, apart from whether it improves health or protects against financial risk.

The three frameworks also differ in their characterization of these dimensions. For the first dimension related to health, WHO uses the term "health improvement," Roberts *et al.* use "health status," and the OECD seems to include both as "health improvement/outcomes." There is a distinction between "improvement" and "status" as goals, with the former implying a change from a previous condition and the latter implying a state of being. Such differences may be important in assessing performance, for example when level of health and change in health would represent different degree of success.

For the second dimension, the terms are also different. "Fairness in financing" embodies an ethical judgment which may allow for differences in view; whereas "financial risk protection" and "financial contribution/expenditure" are more neutral concepts which may allow more objective measurement.

For the third dimension, WHO describes it as "responsiveness of the health system to people's legitimate expectations." whereas Roberts *et al.* (2008) uses the term "citizen satisfaction." This is an important difference that represents two somewhat distinct value positions that will be highlighted further below. "Legitimate expectations" implies a normative, externally determined standard of how health systems should affect people. For example, who determines what are legitimate, in contrast to illegitimate, expectations? "Citizen satisfaction" implies no such standard, but rather leaves it up to the users of the health system to assess the degree to which they find their interaction with the system satisfactory. The OECD framework combines the dimensions of "responsiveness" and "access."

Returning to Figure 1, the vertical axis also contains two dimensions. The first of these is the average level of attainment — for the purposes of this discussion that means, for example, the national average level of the health, fairness or risk protection in financing, and responsiveness or satisfaction dimensions as proposed in each framework. The second dimension is labeled "equity" by OECD and "distribution" by WHO and Roberts *et al.* (2008). Both terms refer to differences in the allocation of the desired outcome within the nation's population. Here again, a seemingly small but telling distinction. "Equity" implies fairness and a value judgment that must be made about what are more or less acceptable differences.

"Distribution" leaves that judgment undefined and explicitly allows measures of performance to differ according to what dimensions of distribution may be important, such as income, gender, age, and geography to give a few examples.

These examples highlight an important fundamental issue in determining health system goals. Is there, and should there be, a universal norm of goals that all health systems should seek to achieve? Or should it be largely left to nations to determine their goals and thereby their own definitions of health system performance? A common set of goals is clearly useful. It is a necessary basis to be able to make consistent comparisons of countries' overall health systems performance, although comparisons across single common dimensions would still be possible. It makes deeper analysis of the determinants of that performance more widely applicable. WHO's World Health Report 2000, which ranked all countries in terms of a composite index of health systems performance, is a well-known example of this approach, which involved complex measurement and a weighting of 5 dimensions shown in Figure 1.

However, a universal framework also has some disadvantages. It may exclude goals that are of importance to some countries and include goals not of importance to all countries. It also risks imposing values on national assessments through measurement or weighting that may not be acceptable or appropriate in a particular country.

The widespread adoption of versions of the frameworks above, as well as recent adoption of global resolutions in favor of universal health coverage (UHC), would support the conclusion that there is some potential for universal frameworks for health system performance goals with some flexibility for national interpretation.

Ethical underpinnings of goals and goals determination

Since health systems goals reflect the ends that societies desire health systems to achieve, any determination about what those ends are necessarily implies value judgments about which outcomes are important to society and which are not. And since it is now recognized that multiple goals may be needed, any exercise of assessing performance entailing multiple dimensions implies that there will need to be other value judgments in determining the relative importance of different goals. There are two issues then to consider: How countries might differ in terms of their values (and the consequences of these differences in goal-setting), and how countries can (or should) recognize these values and reflect them in national goals for health systems.

In proposing a national process for planning health system reform, Roberts *et al.* (2008) advocate that planners should begin with an understanding of the desired performance outcomes for a national health system. They provide a useful taxonomy of ethical concepts that help form the basis of different views on health systems goals.

To summarize this taxonomy (readers are encouraged to refer to Roberts *et al.* (2008) Chapter 3 for further details), there are three foundational ethical perspectives that are common reference points for health system goals. It is important to note that a particular goal may be supported by more than one of these perspectives — that is, the individuals' values may draw on more than one of these perspectives simultaneously.

> *Liberalism*: *"The critical concept for liberals is rights — claims that all individuals can make on each other by virtue of their humanity. Liberalism, focuses on rights and opportunities, on where people start, not on where they end up .... The frequent claim that citizens have rights to health care — or even health itself — reflects liberal concerns." (Roberts et al., 2008)*

> *Utilitarianism: "Utilitarianism, says that we should judge a policy by its consequences ... . This approach generally assumes that 'the end justifies the means.' It says we should judge a policy by asking how it affects the individuals in a society and pick the option that most improves the sum total of their well-being." (Roberts et al., 2008)*

> *Communitarianism: "Communitarianism, states that what matters is the kind of society that public policy helps create and the kind of individuals who live in it ... This theory argues that the character of a community depends on the character of the individuals who compose it. The state, therefore, should ensure that individuals develop good character and help produce a good society." (Roberts et al., 2008)*

And how do (or should) such perspectives and the goals they engender be expressed in the formation of national goals for health system performance? Here again surfaces a rich debate with strong ethical dimensions. Broadly, one can distinguish two streams of thinking.

The first stream focuses on reference to recognized universal norms. Take, for example, the United Nations International Covenant on Economic, Social, and Cultural Rights, which states that all people have a right to the highest attainable standard of health. This covenant has been signed by 162 nations globally, has been interpreted by some as entailing a legal obligation on countries to assure universal coverage of health care.

A second stream focuses more on the process of expressing national values and then determining goals as a consequence of this expression. One view of this is that it takes place through democratic participation in a representative electoral process — that is, elected officials represent the values of the citizens who elect them and can be turned out of office if they fail to express these values. Of course, fair electoral processes are not universal and may malfunction. And what of the values of those who lose elections and the people who voted for them?

Domains of health system performance			
United Kingdom	Canada	Australia	USA (Institute of Medicine)
• Health improvement • Fair access • Effective delivery of appropriate health care • Efficiency • Patient/carer experience • Health outcomes of NHS care	• Acceptability • Accessibility • Appropriateness • Competence • Continuity • Effectiveness • Efficiency • Safety	• Effectiveness • Appropriateness • Efficiency • Responsiveness • Accessibility • Safety • Continuity • Capability • Sustainability	• Safety • Effectiveness • Patient-centeredness • Timeliness • Efficiency • Equity

Source: Table created based on Arah *et al.* (2003) review and analysis of national framework documents from each country.

Figure 2. Country-specific health systems performance frameworks.

Daniels and Sabin (2002) have written extensively concerning conditions of processes to increase fairness in social decisions about priorities and allocations. He notes that there is "no consensus on principled solutions to a family of morally controversial rationing problems" and that, drawing on the earlier work of John Rawls, "in the absence of such a consensus, we should rely on a fair process for arriving at solutions ... and for establishing the legitimacy of such decisions." He proposes several conditions that could be followed by societies to assure an "accountability for reasonableness" in resolving value-based problems in setting priorities for health and health care.

One can see in these discussions the tension between supporting a universal and common set of goals and supporting a more flexible, locally-driven process of goal setting. Indeed, following the publication of WHO's 2000 Report, the Organisation for Economic Cooperation and Development (OECD) commissioned papers and a conference on "Improving Health System Performance in OECD Countries" (OECD, 2002). The report of that meeting highlights that countries may come up with their own outcomes frameworks for health systems performance. An analysis by Arah *et al.* (2003) summarizes some of the different criterias and terminologies employed in different countries, as shown in Figure 2. The paper also provides examples of the wide range of performance indicators used in different countries to monitor these criteria.

Measuring Health System Performance

Having discussed the question of what health systems performance means, the next challenge is how to represent or measure the state of performance.

Since it is widely agreed that performance assessment needs to reflect multiple dimensions, analysts have to address the question of whether to develop a single composite index of performance or to present individual measures of the components of performance. Even familiar single measures — such as life expectancy at birth, a widely used measure of health — often actually represent more complex combinations of cause-specific outcomes as well as different causal mechanisms that have been summarized into a single indicator. This is even more true for more complex health attainment indicators, such as disability-adjusted life expectancy (DALE) or disability-adjusted life years (DALY) lost (Anand and Hanson, 1997; McKee, 2001).

The considerations relevant to the choice of whether to use single index measures or multiple index measures are well developed in the literature on multiple attribute analysis (Keeney and Raiffa, 1993; Yoon and Hwang, 1995). They won't be further examined in detail here. Complex composite indicators are difficult for laypersons to understand and may embed specific ethical viewpoints in a "black box" of aggregated measures. This may make fully informed and transparent social choice more difficult to achieve.

Figure 3 presents two examples of recent health systems performance analyses using a single performance index figure (WHO, 2000) and multiple indicator comparisons (Davis, 2007; Davis *et al.*, 2007; Davis *et al.*, 2014; and The Commonwealth Fund Commission on a High Performance Health System, 2006).

In the first example, WHO analysts developed measures of 5 components of their health systems performance framework from Figure 1. They gave weights to these individual measures, modified them to incorporate estimated effects of large differences across countries' levels of income and education, and produced a composite overall performance index used to rank all countries normalized from 0 to 1.

Overall health system performance in members states, WHO indexes, estimates for 1997

Rank	Member State	Index
1	France	0.994
2	Italy	0.991
3	San Marino	0.988
4	Andora	0.982
5	Malta	0.978
6	Singapore	0.973
7	Spain	0.972
8	Oman	0.961
9	Austria	0.959
10	Japan	0.957

Source: *The World Health Report* (2000)

Health Care System Overall Country Ranking, 2013

	AUS	CAN	FRA	GER	NETH	NZ	NOR	SWE	SWIZ	UK	US
Overall Ranking	4	10*	9	5	5	7	7	3	2*	1*	11*
Quality Care	2*	9	8	7	5	4	11*	10*	3	1*	5
Effective Care	4	7	9	6	5	2*	11*	10*	8	1*	3
Safe Care	3	10*	2*	6	7	9	11*	5	4	1*	7
Coordinated Care	4	8	9	10*	5	2*	7	11*	3	1*	6
Patient-Centered Care	5	8	10*	7	3	6	11*	9	2*	1*	9
Access	8	9	11*	2*	4	7	6	4	2*	1*	9
Cost-Related Problems	9	5	10*	4	8	6	3	1*	7	1*	11*
Timeliness of Care	6	11*	10*	4	2*	7	8	9	1*	3	5
Efficiency	4	10*	8	9	7	3	4	2*	6	1*	11*
Equity	5	9	7	4	8	10*	6	1*	2*	2*	11*
Healthy Lives	4	8	1*	7	5	9	6	2*	3	10*	11*
Health Expenditures ($)/ Capita, 2011**	3800	4522	4118	4495	5099	3182	5669	3925	5643	3405	8508

Notes: *Includes ties. ** Expenditures shown in US$ PPP (purchasing power parity); Australian $ data are from 2010.
Source: Calculated by The Commonwealth Fund based on 2011 International Health Policy of Sicker Adults; 2012 International Health Policy Survey of Primary Care Physicians; 2013 International Health Policy Survey; Commonwealth Fund *National Scorecard 2011*; World Health Organization for Economic Cooperation and Development, *OECD Health Data, 2013* (Paris OECD, Nov 2013); adapted from *Davis et al.*, 2014.

Figure 3. Recent applications of health systems performance analysis, single performance index versus multiple indicators comparison.

Figure 3 shows the top ten countries ranked in this way. This approach has the advantage of producing a clear ranking or "league table" of countries' performance, based on the analysts' decisions about measurement and weighting. However, it also disguises a lot of contributing information about within-country and between-country differences across the contributing indicators.

In the second example, analysts at the Commonwealth Fund collected a set of widely used performance measures for a number of high-income countries and displayed them as a multiple-attribute scorecard. This approach draws attention to differences between measures and presents a more nuanced picture — a specific country may do better on some measures than on others. It also emphasizes that, in comparing countries, there may be different patterns of health system performance attainment, with some countries doing better on some dimensions and some countries doing better on others.

In such multiple-attribute comparisons, it may be difficult to say whether one country's health system performance is better than another's. This can only be done by applying weights to the different measures and creating a single index, bringing us back to the problems of what are the weights and who decides. This may be avoided when one country's attributes are "dominant" over other countries — that is, it performs better on all the measures. This is rarely the case and made less likely by more complex sets of measures. The ambiguity inherent in this type of presentation can be enlightening, but it often doesn't answer the simple question of whether one country's health system is performing "better" than another's. This is a question that citizens and politicians often pose, even if scholars and analysts feel it may be too simple.

As the Commonwealth Fund example shows, looking into the multiple components involved in overall health system performance can quickly lead one to investigate measures of narrower domains of performance than just looking at the whole health system using broad definitions of ultimate outcomes. Most of the chapters in the OECD Report "Measuring Up" (OECD, 2002) are devoted to examining measurements and comparisons of elements of broader performance domains such as consumer perceptions of quality, differences in health outcomes for different diseases, and technical quality of care in hospitals and long-term care facilities. The United States Agency for International Development (USAID) has also produced a "Health Systems Assessment Approach: A How-To Manual" (Islam, 2007), which is a rich compendium of possible variables describing the different components of a health system, but which would be hard to associate with outcomes in any systematic way. This may help guide analysts to specific sources of data, but provides little guidance on overall performance assessment.

Two useful insights on measurement can be drawn from these resources and numerous other experiences evident in the literature on this topic. First, there is clearly a difference between measuring performance in some holistic sense and measuring indicators of performance or things that contribute to performance. The latter is certainly much more tractable. But a great deal of care should be taken in generalizing about overall health system performance based on a set of specific indicators that measure a health system's various parts. Specific initiatives can improve performance in one area of health system functioning while they may worsen performance in another, for example, when they draw scarce resources to one disease or treatment while reducing resources for another, affecting overall health outcomes and country health systems (see for example, debates in World Health Organization Maximizing Positive Synergies Collaborative Group, 2009; Shiffman, 2007; Biesma *et al.*, 2009). Or, improvements in meeting the needs of some citizens may lead to relative neglect of the needs of others, affecting distribution of benefits (see for example, Arnst, 2007). Both examples could result in divergence between specific examples of within-system performance improvement and overall systems performance improvement.

Second, measures of overall performance outcomes like health status, financial protection, and citizen satisfaction can be difficult to make or obtain. They may also be insensitive to short-run changes. As a result, there has been greater attention to what Roberts *et al.* (2008) refer to as "intermediate outcomes" — measures of access, quality and production efficiency. These factors are more easily measurable and responsive to intervention. They clearly contribute to the intrinsic goals of health systems, but they are not themselves equivalent to those goals.

Another area of concern in measurement is the influence of non-health system factors in producing the outcomes identified as performance goals, and the ability of performance frameworks to capture these factors. Failing to consider the non-health system causal determinants of outcomes can lead to incorrect attribution of performance attainment, either positive or negative, to the health system. Some examples of these determinants include a country's income level; its geographic location (e.g., more or less exposure to certain environmental causes of ill health such as vector-borne diseases); cultural characteristics affecting, for instance, patterns of collective action and responsibility and health-related behaviors; and effort on social determinants of health that improve health outcomes independent of the effect of health care services (Bradley and Taylor, 2013).

To correctly attribute health outcomes and other performance outcomes to health systems requires some effort to capture the effects of these confounding factors. There is also a related counterfactual question, which is what the country outcomes would be in the absence of a health system. These questions will be discussed in the section on "Comparing Performance Across Countries and Across Time".

Comparing Performance Across Countries and Across Time

One of the main uses of national health system performance measurement is to enable comparisons between countries or comparisons of the same country at different points in time, in order to assess national progress. Comparisons offer the promise of answers to questions that are often on the minds of health policymakers, such as why their country isn't doing as well as another; what performance they should expect in their country if they are able to make progress; whether their efforts to improve performance have yielded the desired results; and whether the pace of their progress is sufficient given others' experience.

In many countries, there is also a rich agenda focused on improving performance for different parts of the national health system, for example, for regions, services addressing different population groups, or diseases. Many of the same approaches apply for such "within country" performance analyses, although definitions of objectives, measures, and change instruments may be more granular and are not the focus of this chapter.

As discussed in the previous section, a key consideration is determining which type of measures should be used to make such comparisons. In addition to the problems discussed above, complex composite measures of health system performance can introduce unobserved sources of variability in measures that may make them less reliable as metrics of comparison or change. A familiar example of this is an indicator such as average life expectancy. Two countries with similar life expectancies can differ substantially in cause-specific mortality or distribution of life expectancy across different groups. Simpler measures, in the form of indicators of specific elements of performance, can be attractive as an alternative. But simpler measures introduce other problems. For example, within a single country, performance is typically good on some measures and less good on others. How can one combine this variation in performance into an overall composite measure? This problem becomes even more difficult when comparing across countries where there will be different mixes of performance measurement across countries in addition to that within countries. There are no universally-accepted solutions to these problems. The second-best solution is transparency regarding measures being used and honest debates about the trade-offs represented by the variations in performance.

Figure 4 presents one example from the OECD's recent Report "Health Care Systems: Efficiency and Policy Settings" (OECD, 2010). This figure groups countries according to a set of common institutional health system characteristics (discussed further in the next page). For the displayed set of performance indicators, there is large variability both between and within groups.

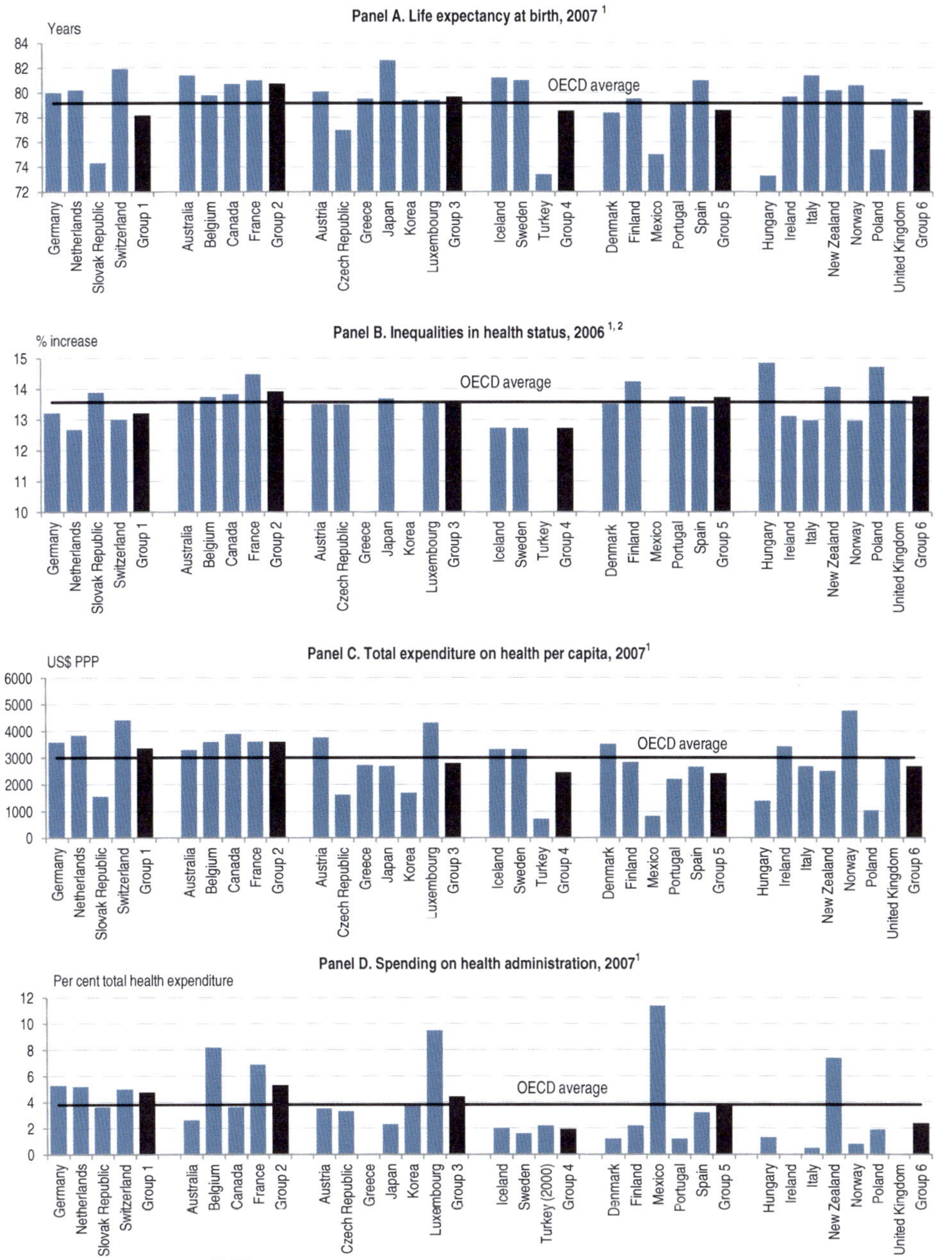

1. Or latest year available.
2. Measured by the standard deviation in mortality ages for population older than 10.

Figure 4. Variability in health system performance indicators, OECD countries, 2007.

Source: OECD (2010), p. 141.

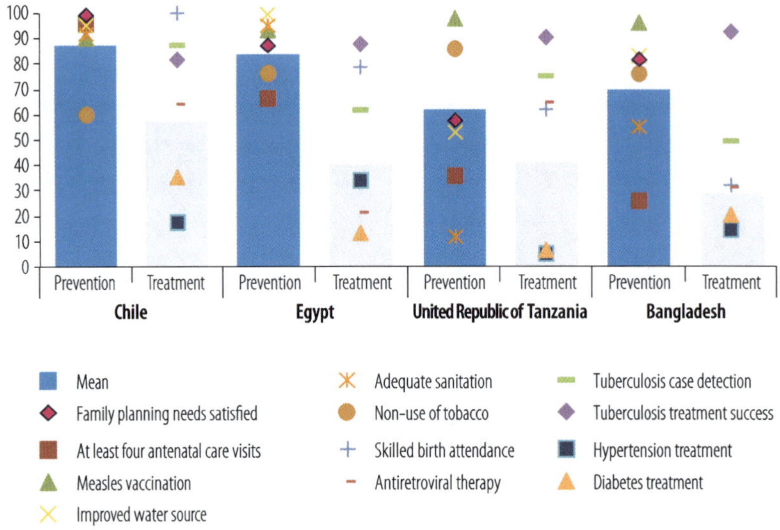

Figure 5. Service coverage rates for six illustrative prevention interventions and six illustrative treatment interventions for four countries.

Source: "Monitoring Progress Towards Universal Health Coverage [UHC] at Country and Global Levels" (WHO and WB, 2014).

Figure 5 presents another example from the proposed WHO–World Bank measures for "Monitoring Progress Towards Universal Health Coverage [UHC] at Country and Global Levels" (WHO and WB, 2014).

In this example, a WHO and World Bank working group has proposed a set of service coverage indicators to represent country attainment in that dimension of UHC (a proxy for health status outcomes) and another set of indicators in the same publication is presented for out-of-pocket health payments to represent attainment in financial protection.

This figure compares 4 lower- and middle-income countries (Chile, Egypt, United Republic of Tanzania, and Bangladesh) in terms of coverage levels for 6 preventive and 6 treatment interventions that are proposed as global methods for monitoring progress in achieving UHC. For each country, high levels of coverage are achieved for some services and lower levels of coverage for others. Any statement about overall coverage achievement can only be made if these individual indicators are aggregated — requiring (again) a weighting of some kind. Otherwise, one cannot make any definitive statement about one country performing better than another — for example, the simple question of which country is doing better in achieving UHC at a particular point in time — unless there is clear dominance which, interestingly in this example, is not the case for either prevention or treatment interventions separately or combined.

A further challenge is likely to occur when these indicators are monitored over time. One should expect that they will not all improve at the same rate and that improvement rates will vary across indicators and countries — some performance outcomes may even get worse. It will be difficult to make straightforward statements about each country's progress toward UHC from an indicator-based framework.

Another dilemma is the risk that when international organizations monitor selected simple indicators of performance it can distort national priorities. Policymakers and system managers may focus their efforts on improving the few indicators that are being measured, perhaps to the detriment of other important elements of performance. This issue has been raised repeatedly in relation to the Millenium Development Goals (MDGs) for both external and domestic health financing. For example, the concept of "neglected tropical diseases" has highlighted relative underfinancing for some health outcomes not explicitly cited in the MDGs (Smith and Taylor, 2013). Concerns about "displacement" have been raised, for example, whether the scale-up in funding for HIV/AIDS has reduced attention by external funders to other important health problems (Lordan *et al.*, 2011) or whether the scale-up in external health aid for lower income countries may have displaced domestic financing which would be addressed to other priorities not emphasized in the global aid agenda (Lu *et al.*, 2010). It is important, however, to note that the accusation of "distortion" implies that policymakers may be induced to do things which do not accord with their own independent priorities, a proposition which is difficult to prove. All measures of performance embody some set of preferences for some outcomes relative to others.

The Politics of Health System Performance

While a great deal has been written about the technical aspects of health system goal-setting, indicator definition, and measurement, Roberts *et al.* (2008) remind us that "decision-makers confront ethical and political issues throughout the reform cycle," which they suggest begins with defining ultimate and intermediate outcomes and their relative importance in overall performance goals. Berman and Bitran (2011) also highlight the critical role of clear definition of desired outcomes in developing an analysis of health system performance. Many debates about how well a health system is performing or the performance differences between health systems are actually not "technical," but rather, debates about politics and values.

Smith *et al.*, note in their concluding chapter (Smith *et al.*, 2009, Chapter 6.1) "the immensely political nature of any attempt to measure performance" given "its power to challenge vested interests within the health system" (p. 698). They list among the relevant interest groups taxpayers, voters, patient groups, clinical professionals, insurers and other purchaser organizations, provider organizations, pharmaceutical companies, governments, geographical interests, age groups, and social groups (based on, for example, income or ethnicity). In short, all citizens have an interest in setting goals and allocating resources for health, and there are many vehicles for expressing these interests. Analysts enamored of technical or quantified measures promote the social value of "rational" decision-making, transparency, and accountability for improving health system performance. But the interests of powerful groups in society fundamentally mediate these concepts. Such groups seek to assure their gains and minimize their losses from such analyses and their policy consequences.

The contrast between proposals from international sources, like the WHO, for setting health system performance goals (Figure 1) and those that emerge from national deliberation processes (Figure 2) is one illustration of how local politics trumps more generalizable technical analysis in this field. Analysts' frameworks are useful inputs to national discussions, but the results in terms of how goals are actually defined, which goals are included for national assessment of health system performance, how they are measured, and what weights are given to different elements are all intensely driven by local politics, interests and values. One recent example of this is the conflict in the United States about whether states should accept federal subsidies to expand enrollment in health insurance for the poor through the Medicaid Program. Federal subsidies for expanding Medicaid enrollments under the U.S. "Affordable Care Act" have been rejected by 22 out of 50 states as of February 2015 (http://obamacarefacts.com/obamacares-medicaid-expansion/) with a number of state governments expressing concerns about the future fiscal burden on state budgets of Medicaid expansion should federal subsidies be removed in the future (http://www.usnews.com/debate-club/is-medicaid-expansion-good-for-the-states).

While these observations are often repeated, less is said in the literature about what can be done to influence these processes. Roberts *et al.* (2008) emphasize in Chapter 4 the need for political skill among health system reformers to influence the political processes affecting problem definition rather than simply awaiting the outcome and note that analysts framing problems primarily in technocratic terms are often poorly equipped or reluctant to engage in such political processes. Indeed, they argue that successful reforms to improve health system performance often build on years of skillful political and policy shaping. They advocate a systematic process of applied political analysis to understanding the positions and interests of different stakeholders and to influence them. Leatherman (OECD, 2002) provides a detailed description of some key stakeholder groups, links them to specific issues within health system performance measurements, and suggests some approaches for how stakeholder groups might be influenced. Gonzalez-Rossetti and Bossert (2000) uses 3 case studies in Chile, Colombia and Mexico to describe how the political economy context, policy process, and policymakers' political strategies, specifically the use of "change teams," enabled health policy reform. Fox and Reich (2013) provide an overview of how the political economy shaped the development of national health insurance schemes using both successful and unsuccessful examples of health financing reform.

Challenges and Innovations in Measurement and Comparison

As the preceding sections have shown, there have been a variety of approaches taken to address the challenges of defining goals, creating different measures of performance, and developing comparisons and benchmarks that can be used by policymakers and analysts. This section will explore three important problems that arise in analyzing health system performance and some recent efforts to address them. The three problems are:

- How to address the counterfactual question of what health outcomes (or other performance indicators) would be in the absence of the health system. (In the sense that the difference between no health system and the current situation could be used as a measure of the health system's contribution to performance outcomes.)
- Whether and how to compare performance in countries that differ greatly in terms of health systems environments — for example, different national income and education levels.
- How to explain differences in health system performance and how to do so in ways that would be useful to health policymakers.

Thinking about a "baseline" for health systems performance

If one estimates measures of health system performance at any particular point in time, the results reflect not only the contributions of the health system at that time or recent period, but also the accumulated contributions from the past. Clearly, the "baseline" against which to measure these contributions is not zero — all citizens would not cease to live in the absence of the health system. This problem, then, is how to capture that baseline so that measures of health system performance can reflect only the actual contribution of the health system to outcomes. The baseline will differ in countries with very different external environments (see the next section for further discussion on that).

This problem was raised in the WHO volume of technical papers, which followed the World Health Report 2000. Tandon *et al.* (2003) noted that to define health system efficiency, "... adjustment is made for the fact that output would not be zero in the absence of a modern health system." As shown in Figure 1, the WHO composite health system performance index has 5 elements, which are weighted in the overall index to a normalized value of 100. To take account of this adjustment to represent the counterfactual case, Tandon *et al.* (2003) report that 2 of the 5 components, fairness in financial contribution and responsiveness distribution are given "full scores," that is, treated as if there is full equality, since "a non-existent system treats everyone totally equally." Conversely, two other components, health inequalities and responsiveness level, are given "zero" scores, "since a non-existent health system would clearly be completely unresponsive and although health inequalities would exist in the absence of a health system with respect to the health system's goal of reducing inequalities, zero progress can be claimed."

In short, Tandon *et al.* (2003) focused on estimating a baseline level of health attainment as the main source of variability in a no-health-system case. This was done for a baseline period around 1900, with an equation that estimated "a minimum-frontier production function" for health-adjusted life expectancy (HALE) simply as a function of literacy across countries at that baseline period.

Comparisons involving very heterogeneous countries

It may be interesting to compare both absolute and relative health system performance between countries. For absolute comparisons, it would make sense to control for very large contextual or environmental differences between countries by comparing rather similar countries. One could, for example, compare countries such as Germany and the United Kingdom in terms of a set of agreed upon outcome measures, combined in a weighted composite index, and concludes that one performed better than the other. The difference in their scores could be interpreted as a measurement of the differences in their performance. Because Germany and the United Kingdom are not, apparently, very dissimilar countries, this type of comparison would have a certain degree of face validity.

But what if one was comparing Germany and Bangladesh? Because of the large differences between these two countries in determinants of health system performance measures, such as income and education, this absolute comparison seems inappropriate. Of course, health system performance will differ between these two countries. Rather, it may be more interesting to ask how well does these countries do relatively, given their very different conditions and constraints. Tandon *et al.* (2003) also explored this question. Adjustments for such differences were included in the scores and rankings reported in the World Health Report 2000.

Measuring and comparing the absolute health attainment of countries may be interesting. But it is also useful to consider how well countries do relative to their

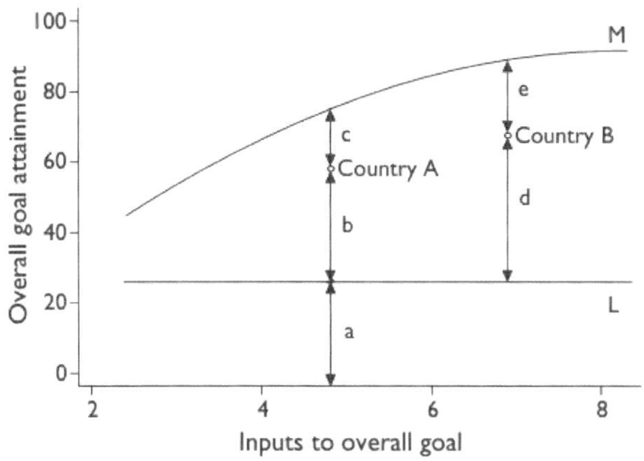

Figure 6. Defining health system efficiency

Source: Evans *et al.* (2003).

baselines, that is, their capacities and constraints. This introduces the notion of health system efficiency. This was represented by Evans *et al.* (2003) in Figure 6. The two countries shown, A and B, have very different levels of capacity, reflected in different quantities of inputs on the horizontal axis. They achieve different levels of goal attainment, shown on the vertical axis. The curve M represents the overall relationship across all countries between inputs and outputs — for example, health expenditure per capita as a simple index of inputs. Country B's overall performance is clearly better in absolute terms than Country A. But which country's health system is more efficient in translating inputs into outputs? In this figure, both countries are shown to be equally efficient in goal attainment relative to the resources they are using.

Policymakers are often interested in the question of how their country is doing relative to other similar countries — for example, in terms of income, education, social and environmental conditions — but may find comparisons of absolute performance between very dissimilar countries of little interest. However, they are interested in their relative performance to dissimilar countries if one can control for the differences in their conditions.

Tandon *et al.* (2003) pose the question of how one can estimate something like the M curve in Figure 6 as optimal performance at different levels of inputs. They explore this using health expenditure per capita as an index of inputs. If such measurement is possible, one may then be able to interpret the distance between a country's actual performance and their "best possible" performance (represented in this case as the link between outcomes and a simple measure of resources used, but more complex formulations are possible) as a measure of relative performance, and what could possibly be attained given their country constraints and conditions.

Morena-Serra and Smith (2012) explore this type of analysis using data envelopment analysis (DEA), a quantitative technique widely used to estimate efficiency in production. They use several measures of performance as outcomes, such as immunization coverage attained and levels of out-of-pocket expenditures. These include both health care coverage and financial protection measures. But they do not create a single weighted composite index. They also use multiple measures of inputs. They conclude that the analysis they did with DEA may be most useful as an "exploratory tool" which can help identify countries in different relative positions. This can then be used to explore in more detail the specific conditions of those countries. They find a wide range of efficiency ratings across countries that is difficult to interpret due to significant data problems as well as limited theoretical guidance on what the relationships between inputs and outputs should be.

What explains differences in health systems performance?

Comparisons are useful to highlight differences, yet these differences give rise to the question of why they exist. If one knows what the health system factors are that cause differences in performance, the next question would be about what actions could be taken to influence these factors and result in better performance.

Much of the analysis of the determinants of health system performance has been at the level of highly aggregate variables. The distinction between health-system specific factors that determine performance outcomes and factors not specific to health systems is a useful one. In terms of health-system specific factors, perhaps the most widely cited is spending on health. Generally, the focus tends to be on financial and physical inputs to health systems, such as funds, human resources, and pharmaceuticals and supplies (Islam, 2007). For country-level factors not specific to health systems, analysis has tended to focus on aggregate variables reflective of general conditions in the national environment such as income, education, geographic conditions, and governance.

These types of analyses often produce similar results. They may find significant relationships between inputs and outcomes across countries with very different levels of the causal variables of interest, but when comparing countries with similar levels of these variables, there is often a wide dispersion, suggesting that some of the most commonly considered inputs — for example, health expenditures per capita or human resource availability — have limited predictive value to explain levels of outcomes within groups of similar countries. The chart in Figure 7 is an example of this — initially developed in the *World Development Report of 1993* (World Bank, 1993) and re-estimated here by Berman and Bitran (2011).

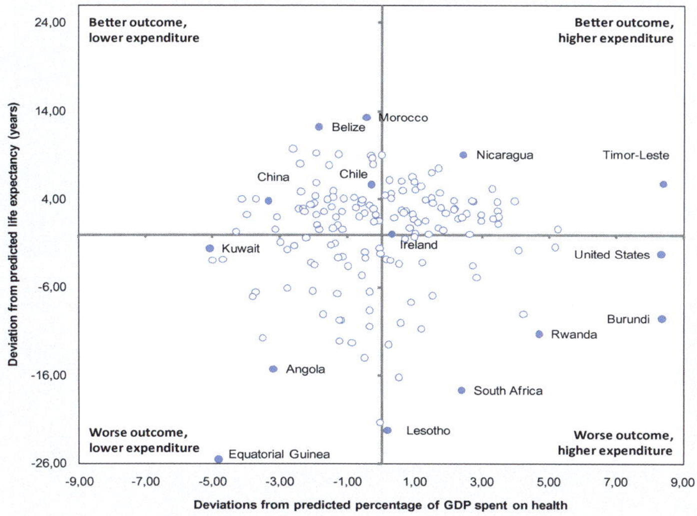

Figure 7. Relationship between health expenditure and life expectancy

Source: Berman and Bitran (2011).

The figure shows the relationship between health expenditure and life expectancy across a large number of countries, controlling for national income and education levels. If health spending strongly explained life expectancy, most countries would be in the lower left or upper right quadrant of the chart. Instead, they are dispersed throughout. An analysis of performance changes in countries over time finds similar dispersion. There is definitely a strong trend of improving health over time with growth in income and education, but countries with similar starting points may diverge substantially from this overall trend. This suggests that factors other than inputs and environment are important for outcomes. What those factors are and how they operate to improve health systems performance are key questions inspiring the emerging field of health systems analysis.

Results like this suggest that explanations of health system performance attainment are still at a rudimentary stage. Roberts *et al.* (2008) propose a framework of 5 health system "control knobs" defined as domains of health system policies, which, if modified, may produce changes in performance. These five "control knobs" are financing, payment, organization, regulation and persuasion. However, they are cautious in concluding that solutions that work in one country can simply be adopted in another — providing, rather, "conditional guidance" and the counsel to adapt, not adopt.

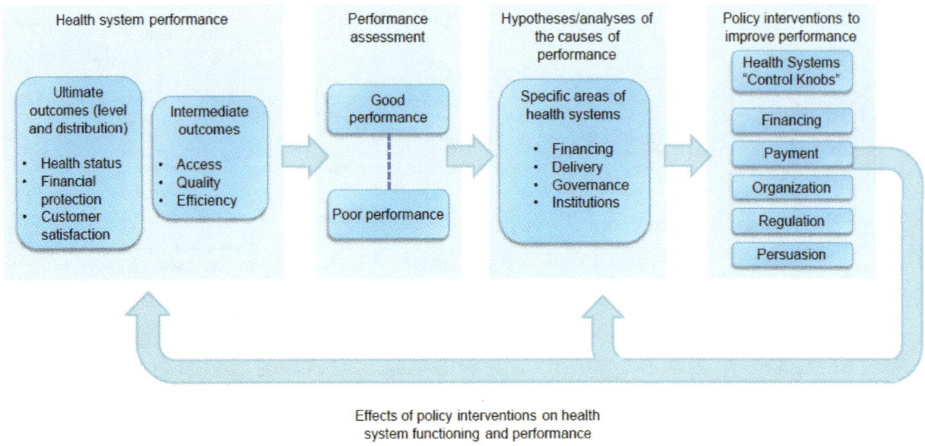

Figure 8. Logic framework for health system analysis
Source: Berman and Bitran (2011).

To better address this question of what explains differences in performance and what countries can do to improve performance, better measures of the processes that translate health system inputs into outcomes are needed. Berman and Bitran (2011) proposed a framework (Figure 8) which embeds analysis of the causes of performance problems as a step linking outcomes (health system performance) with potential strategies or interventions to improve performance (control knobs).

Recent work by the OECD (OECD, 2008; Joumard *et al.*, 2010; Paris *et al.*, 2010) provides some promising movement in this direction. OECD analysts have begun defining "institutional characteristics" of health systems, systematic descriptors of coverage, financing, and delivery arrangements that logically lie between inputs and outcomes. Applying these definitions enables a richer development of typologies of health system arrangements that can be associated with performance and perhaps ultimately better understanding of cause–effect relationships.

Conclusion

Citizens, politicians, policymakers, and other stakeholders often ask "how good is the health system in my country?" This simple question provides the foundation for much more extensive inquiry and for demands for change and action.

This chapter frames the question as one about health system performance. It unpacks the question and argues that it is hardly simple. Much has been written to provide answers. Embedded in these answers, and in the evidence and argumentation that underpins them, are challenging issues of social values and preferences, political power and influence, and complex research and analytical results. Mostly, these complexities lie below the surface of public and academic discussion. But they profoundly influence those discussions. Conscientious observers and participants in health system reform debates should understand these complexities and refer back to them regularly for clearer thinking. Some key areas of focus which emerge from this review are:

Ground analysis of health system performance in honest thinking about health system goals, including questions of distribution. There is no perfect method for capturing citizens' preferences for the different outcomes resulting from health system performance. No health system succeeds in doing everything that everyone wants to be done, so trade-offs and hard choices are inevitable. Clear understanding of the implications of such choices is important for making better choices.

Measure extensively around intermediate outcomes related to access, quality, and efficiency, including their distribution. Measurement around high-level health systems goals is important. But it may not be very sensitive to short-term improvements in health system performance and is often not practical to measure for more specific components of health systems. Intermediate outcomes like access, quality, and efficiency and their distribution can be linked analytically to higher-level goals, but it should be the main focus of measurement for performance improvement efforts.

Health systems can be improved by improving their parts, but the parts do not automatically equal the whole, so be aware of (and prepared for) possible unintended consequences from partial strategies. As health systems become more developed, much analysis of performance focuses on specific diseases and interventions (e.g., diabetes or chemotherapy for cancer) or specific sub-groups in populations (e.g., women of a certain minority group or teenagers). Such analysis leads to specific initiatives to improve outcomes for these "parts" of the health system. Improving the parts can improve the whole and can have positive spillover effects on other parts, but it can also have negative unintended consequences on other parts. Keep the whole in view when working on the parts.

Link strategies to improve health system performance to the intermediate outcomes and goals they will affect in a logic- and evidence-based causal analysis. Considering the "why" of health system performance levels and differences is an essential step for proposing the "how" of performance improvement. Techniques of diagnostic inquiry and root cause analysis, with constant critical inquiry, are essential for sound policy and strategy.

Question evidence. Learn and adapt from the experience of others. National and sub-national contexts are varied, and that variation matters for improving performance. However, all lessons do not have to be learned anew. When adopting evidence and intervention strategies from others, be prepared to adapt to national and local conditions.

Design is important, but don't forget implementation. A common response to analysis of health system performance is the proposal of reforms to improve it. Reform development often overemphasizes the technical design and underemphasizes the constraints and demands of effective implementation. Critical assessment of health system capacities is a key step, which, if neglected, can set back efforts at improving system performance.

References

Anand S, Hanson K. 1997. Disability-adjusted life years: A critical review. *Journal of Health Economics* 16(6): 685–702.

Arah OA, Klazinga NS, Delnoij DMJ, Ten Asbroek AHA, Custers T. 2003. Conceptual Frameworks for health systems performance: A quest for effectiveness, quality, and improvement. *International Journal for Quality in Health Care* 15(5): 377–398.

Arnst, K. 2007. "A Gender Gap in Cancer" *Bloomberg Business Week*, 13 June 2007. http://www.businessweek.com/stories/2007-06-13/a-gender-gap-in-cancerbusinessweek-business-news-stock-market-and-financial-advice.

Berman P, Bitran R. 2011. Health Systems Analysis for Better Health Systems Strengthening. HNP Discussion Paper, The World Bank, Washington, DC.

Biesma RG, Brugha R, Harmer A, Walsh A, Spicer N, Walt G. 2009. The effects of global health initiatives on country health systems: A review of the evidence from HIV/AIDS control. *Health Policy and Planning* 24(4): 239–252.

Bradley EH, Taylor LA. 2013. *The American Health Care Paradox: Why Spending More is Getting Us Less*. Public Affairs: New York.

Daniels N, Sabin J. 2002. *Setting Limits Fairly: Can We Learn to Share Scarce Resources*. Oxford University Press: Oxford.

Davis K. 2007. *Learning from High Performance Health Systems around the Globe*. The Commonwealth Fund: New York.

Davis K, Schoen C, Schoenbaum SC, Doty MM, Holmgren AL, Shea K, Nicholson JL. 2007. *Mirror, Mirror on the Wall: An International Update on the Comparative Performance of American Health Care*. The Commonwealth Fund: New York.

Davis K, Stremikis K, Squires D, Schoen C. 2014. *Mirror, Mirror on the Wall: How the Performance of the U.S. Health Care System Compares International*. The Commonwealth Fund: New York.

Evans DB, Murray CJL, Tandon A. 2003. Health System Efficiency: Time, Attribution, and Multiple Indicators. In Murray C, Evans D. (eds.). *Health Systems Performance Assessment*. World Health Organization: Geneva, pp. 699–703.

Fox AM, Reich MR. 2013. Political Economy of Reform. In: Preker AS *et al.* (eds.). *Scaling Up Affordable Health Insurance*. World Bank: Washington, DC.

Gonzalez-Rossetti A, Bossert TJ. 2000. *Enhancing the Political Feasibility of Health Reform: A Comparative Analysis of Chile, Columbia, and Mexico*. LAC Health Sector Reform Initiative.

Islam M. (Ed.) 2007. *Health Systems Assessment Approach: A How-To Manual*. Submitted to the U.S. Agency for International Development in collaboration with Health Systems 20/20, Partners for Health Reformplus, Quality Assurance Project, and Rational Pharmaceutical Management Plus. Arlington, VA: Management Sciences for Health.

Joumard I, André C, Nicq C. 2010. *Health Care Systems: Efficiency and Institutions*. Organisation for Economic Cooperation and Development: Paris.

Keeney RL, Raiffa H. 1993. *Decisions with Multiple Objectives: Preferences and Value Trade-Offs*. Cambridge University Press.

Lordan G, Tang KK, Carmignani F. 2011. Has HIV/AIDS displaced other health funding priorities? Evidence from a new dataset of development aid for health. *Social Science and Medicine* 73(3): 351–355.

Lu C, Schneider MT, Gubbins P, Leach-Kemon K, Jamison D, *et al.* 2010. Public financing of health in developing countries: A cross national systematic analysis. *Lancet* 375: 1375–1387.

McKee M. 2001. *The World Health Report 2000: Advancing the Debate*. European Regional Consultation on Health Systems Performance Assessment. Copenhagen: WHO Regional Office for Europe, pp. 3–4.

Morena-Serra R, Smith PC. 2012. *An Exploratory Application of Data Envelopment Analysis to Health Services Coverage and Access*. Results for Development Institute: Washington, DC.

Murray, CJL, Frenk J. 2000. A framework for assessing the performance of health systems. *Bulletin of the World Health Organization* 78(6): 717–731.

Organisation for Economic Co-Operation, and Development. 2002. *Measuring up: Improving Health System Performance in OECD Countries*. OECD Publishing.

Organisation for Economic Co-Operation, and Development. 2008. *Institutional Indicators for the Analysis of Health-System Performance: Conceptual Framework*. OECD Publishing.

Organisation for Economic Co-Operation, and Development. 2010. *Health Care Systems: Efficiency and Policy Settings*. OECD Publishing.

Oxford Dictionaries 2015. (http://www.oxforddictionaries.com/us/definition/american_english/performance).

Paris V, Devaux M, Wei L. 2010. Health Systems Institutional Characteristics: A Survey of 29 OECD Countries. *OECD Working Papers* 50. OECD Publishing.

Roberts MJ, Hsiao W, Berman P, Reich MR. 2008. *Getting Health Reform Right: A Guide to Improving Performance and Equity*. Oxford University Press: New York.

Shiffman J. 2007. Has donor prioritization of HIV/AIDS displaced aid for other health issues? *Health Policy and Planning* 23(2): 95–100.

Shortell SM, McCurdy RK. 2009. Integrated health systems. *Information, Knowledge, Systems Management* 8(1): 369–82.

Smith PC. 2002. Measuring health system performance. *The European Journal of Health Economics* 3(3): 145–48.

Smith PC, Mossialos E, Papanicolas I, Leatherman S (eds.). 2009. *Performance Measurement for Health System Improvement: Experiences, Challenges, and Prospects*. Cambridge University Press.

Smith J, Taylor EM. 2013. MDGs and NTDs: Reshaping the global health agenda. *Plos Neglected Tropical Diseases.* DOI: 10.1371/journal.pntd.0002529.

Tandon A, Lauer JL, Evans DB, Murray CJL. 2003. Health System Efficiency: Concepts. In Murray C, Evans D. (eds.). *Health Systems Performance Assessment*. World Health Organization: Geneva, pp. 683–692.

The Commonwealth Fund Commission on a High Performance Health System. 2006. *Why Not the Best?: Results from a National Scorecard on US Health System Performance*. The Commonwealth Fund: New York.

Wait, S. 2004. *Benchmarking: A Policy Analysis*. Nuffield Trust.

World Bank. 1993. *World Development Report 1993: Investing in Health*. World Bank: Washington, DC.

World Health Organization. 2000. The World Health Report. *Health Systems: Improving Performance.* World Health Organization: Geneva.

World Health Organization. 2014. *Global Health Observatory* [online]. Available: http://www.who.int/gho/health_financing/total_expenditure/en/ [Accessed Nov 19 2014]

World Health Organization Maximizing Positive Synergies Collaborative Group. 2009. An assessment of interactions between global health initiatives and country health systems. *Lancet* 373: 2137–2169.

World Health Organization, World Bank Group. 2014. *Monitoring Progress Towards Universal Health Coverage at Country and Global Levels.* WHO Press.

Yoon PK, Hwang CL. 1995. *Multiple Attribute Decision Making: An Introduction*. Sage Publications.

Pay for Performance in Health Systems: Theory, Evidence and Case Studies

Jed Friedman
The World Bank

Richard M Scheffler
University of California, Berkeley

Pay-for-performance (P4P) is an emerging payment mechanism that, unlike previous mechanisms, remunerates health providers based on performance in order to increase efficiencies in health systems. P4P designs vary by healthcare settings, health measures, the form of reward, and the basis for reward. Countries around the globe are developing P4P designs specific to the needs of their citizens, leading to numerous forms of P4P programs with diverse measures and disparate outcomes. Despite P4P program prevalence, P4P has been yet to be comprehensively evaluated, making it difficult to assess overall P4P effectiveness. Results from OECD countries show that P4P programs have galvanized payers and providers to better measure health care quantity and quality. Select low-income countries have implemented P4P at a national level, strengthening health system capacity through collection and analysis of population health data. Early research at all country income levels reveals that there is promise to improve healthcare efficiencies through P4P, but more research must be conducted in order to know the optimum payment incentive and channel for payment distribution, as well as the most effective means to change provider behavior.

Keywords: Pay-for-Performance; P4P; Health Results Based Financing.

Introduction and Motivation

Dominant modes to finance health care include input-based contracts, fee-for-service, and capitation-based payments. Whatever the chosen mode of financing, the health financier ultimately cares about producing the best health possible conditional on the resources available and so the efficiency of health spending is a key concern.

It is with this focus that various health systems have begun in recent years to experiment with payment mechanisms intended to improve efficiency in the health system by conditioning a proportion of total payment on the achievement of pre-specified measures directly relevant for the creation and maintenance of a healthy population. At times this payment is conditioned on health outcomes themselves. The explicit link of health payments to health achievements is commonly termed pay-for-performance (P4P). This chapter reviews recent developments in P4P, the forms that P4P take around the world, and the emergent evidence on their relative effectiveness (or ineffectiveness). This chapter also discusses the reasons and conditions when a P4P mechanism may be preferred to other forms of financing, as well as the challenges to consider when designing and implementing such a system.

P4P through the lens of economic theory

Why might a health financier choose P4P as one form of payment? A standard economic framework that often motivates the P4P approach is entitled the "principal–agent" model, where a principal (in this case the purchaser of health services) delegates, perhaps through a formal contract, to an agent (in this case the provider of health services). While a seemingly straightforward contractual arrangement, complications in this relationship arise if the objectives of the principal and agent differ or if the available information to the agent is different from that of the principal. In principal–agent theory, both the degree of differential information between principal and agent and the ability of the principal to monitor the output and effort of the agent determines the most effective type of contract. In situations when it is difficult to fully monitor the effort of the agent but not the outputs of that effort, and when the agent may have private information on the local health production process that the principal doesn't have, it can be optimal to reward the agent on the basis of performance and the achievement of pre-specified outputs (see Savedoff and Partner (2010) for a general discussion of this framework).

Another relevant feature of the principal–agent contract is the fiduciary risk imposed on the agent by the principals. If too small a proportion of total compensation is made available to the agent through a performance contract it may not be sufficient to encourage the effort required to meet the targets. On the other hand, if too large a proportion of total compensation is made contingent on performance this may introduce too much risk for the agent and lead to demotivation, high stress, and possibly lower performance and higher staff turnover. Hence a key determinant for a P4P program is the optimal proportion of total payment channeled through the P4P mechanism. While this optimal proportion is context specific, little theoretical or empirical work to date has been able to inform the process, and programs often determine this proportion on an *ad-hoc* basis.

One key area of health delivery with which there has been much recent application of P4P approaches, especially in OECD countries, concerns the quality of care. The following section "Major Health Care Payment and Incentive Schemes" discusses these theoretical issues in further detail from the framework of a P4P scheme for health care quality.

Major health care payment and incentive schemes

Today, most health care providers are not rewarded for improving quality. The traditional methods for paying physicians, such as salary, fee-for-service or capitation, pay for the quantity of care and not quality. For example, a fee schedule common to many insurance systems only pays for the unit of service, not the quality of said service or whether it improves intermediate health outcomes. Capitation payments (paying per person enrolled in practice) leave quality assessment up to patients, assuming that they can change practice if quality is inadequate. In hospitals, even new payment methods like diagnostic-related groups (DRGs), which pay a fixed amount per patient based on diagnosis (to adjust for case mix), do not formally measure quality of care.

Some believe that competition between providers will drive up quality by allowing patient choice, but competition alone does not solve the perennial problem of information asymmetry between physicians and patients, and also between physicians and payers. Assessing quality requires information (such as hospitalization rates, nosocomial infection rates, and overall effectiveness of treatments) that is beyond what patients can know at reasonable cost. In the production of quality care, provider effort is surely an important input, however effort cannot be directly observed by the payer although in principal a P4P mechanism can focus on the observable quality measures directly related to provider effort. In fact, determining what constitutes quality and devising appropriate measurements is a prerequisite for designing effective P4P schemes.

Financial incentives and risk shifting

Figure 1 presents a progression of shared risk between providers and payers for healthcare costs. A fee-for-service scheme reimburses providers as often as they provide services, which subjects the payers to a greater financial risk of paying often and more for services, with little financial risk for providers. Per diem pays a provider a set amount per patient for each day the patient is in the providers care.

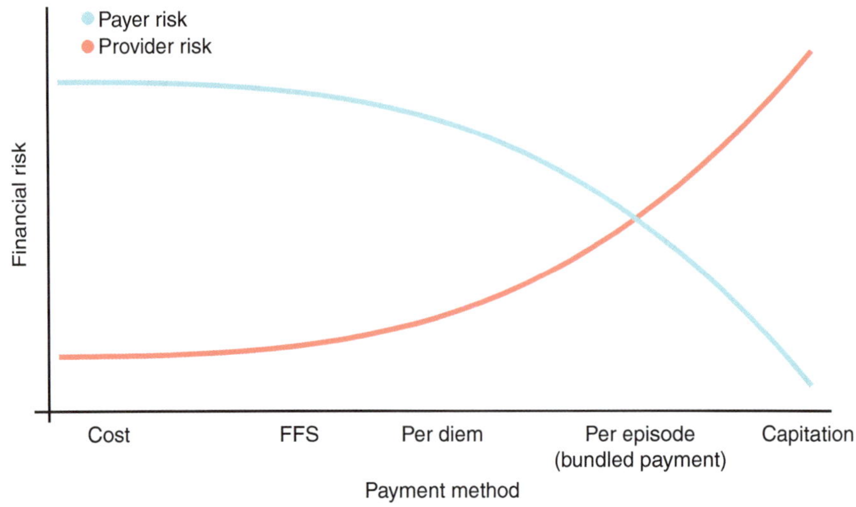

Figure 1. Financial risk of care for provider and payer, by payment method
Source: Frakt and Mayes (2012).

The risk still remains mostly on the payer, as the shared cost through co-payments from the patient will cover the difference of the per diem and the actual cost. With bundled payment, providers face the risk of delivering care to patients within the episode. However, if the providers administer care at a lower rate, they share the surplus. In the same manner, providers who receive payment through capitation also keep the surplus, as the provider is given a fixed payment per member per month. However, the provider faces risk of financial losses if the patient mix is predominantly sick and the cost of providing their care is higher than the capitated payment.

Pay for performance gives providers more financial incentives without necessarily adding risk, as long as the incentivized health achievements are under the control of the provider. The only risk falls on those providers who perform poorly, which could lead to improved quality if the desire to avoid risk induces providers to improve quality or to exit the market. Pay for performance can be combined with any payment system and attempts to redistribute risk within a given payment system with the aim to improve the efficiency and quality of care.

Emergence of P4P

Various P4P schemes formally measure quality of care and pay for it. There are now many new examples in OECD countries and beyond that are attempting to explore a new frontier in payment systems that incorporate quality. Though the evidence is still insufficient to draw definitive conclusions, results from P4P schemes suggest what common sense would tell you: That quality of care increases when you pay for it. Paying for preventive and public health services appears to be particularly effective and can increase coverage of cancer screening, vaccination rates, etc. (Cashin *et al.*, 2014). Often, primary care physicians neglect preventive services such as screening for cancer, measuring blood pressure and treating it, counselling patients to stop smoking or to improve their diet. The most successful P4P programs pay additionally for providing these services or reaching some target. These programs generally show significant increases in the use of these important public health interventions that are likely to maximize health gain.

P4P is also useful in offering incentives for the prevention and care co-ordination of chronic diseases like diabetes. It can ensure that diabetics undertake important preventive tests and also help encourage co-ordination between diabetes specialists, often based in hospitals, and primary care providers.

One of the critical issue that has bedeviled P4P programs is monitoring the quality indicators. In many instances, information on quality is not routinely collected. Therefore, part of the P4P program is to collect information, requiring potentially costly up-front investment in computers, training, and software. In addition, there is generally no culture for physician practices to report clinical indicators and they need to be cajoled into providing the information. Many programs pay physicians incentives for providing the information, including funding to computerize their record keeping. These up-front costs are often larger than the savings generated in the short run (Cashin *et al.*, 2014).

P4P systems typically cost more in the first couple of years, but may return this investment over time as the system works and people become healthier. Furthermore, cost savings may occur in other parts of the system. For example, better preventive care in primary care leads to decreases in hospitalizations. In unitary systems like the UK National Health Service (NHS), the single purchaser, in this case the Department of Health, internalizes this type of cross savings. In multipayer systems, however, assessing the savings is more difficult, since the payer may not realize the benefits. Whether P4P actually saves money will partly depend on whether the long-term cost savings can be internalized by the body that introduced the P4P scheme. But the more important question is not if it saves money, but whether it improves quality commensurate to its costs, in other words, whether or not it achieves value for money.

Another complication with the introduction of P4P is that it can be hard to know for sure whether quality of care has improved, or whether the system is merely adjusting to reporting on quality; P4P systems often require new collection of quality data that did not exist before, but it may be that physicians were providing high quality care, but not reporting on it. It is also difficult to know if P4P schemes improve efficiency because this assessment requires the long-term collection of costs across the health system.

Most of the P4P schemes also suffer from limited evaluation, particularly in the use of control groups, making it difficult to draw conclusions. However, the experience of P4P schemes in a number of countries is that they do appear to increase the quality of care. The experience of California primary care P4Ps suggests that it can be used to incentivize important public health interventions like screening for cancer, immunization, smoking cessation, etc., that are highly cost effective and some of the best buys in health care (Robinson *et al.*, 2009; Yegian and Yanagihara, 2013). This model was replicated in Brazil and a similar model was used in Rwanda (Borem *et al.*, 2010) that also demonstrated increased use of preventive and public health services. This last example of Rwanda also indicates, particularly for low- and middle-income country (LMIC) health systems, that P4P can also be applied to the quantity of health care (in terms of number of services delivered) as well as the quality of care.

All told, the relative effectiveness of a P4P scheme will depend on numerous factors related to the information differential between the payer and provider, the additional financial risk (if any) introduced by the scheme, and the cost or ability of the payer to accurately monitor the incentivized health measures. A recent Cochrane review of the effectiveness of various P4P programs in LMICs found results to vary but also highlighted several other factors that affect P4P performance, including the specific intervention design, funding, and other ancillary variables such as organizational culture, technical support availability and country-specific health context (Witter *et al.*, 2012).

P4P Program Design Framework

To show how P4P programs are typically designed and implemented, a general P4P program framework is presented in Figure 2. The framework includes measures, the basis for the reward, and the reward. Quality and efficiency are the two major categories of measures. These are also known as supply-side P4P measures, because they are provider-based measures related to health care delivery (Scheffler, 2008; Scheffler, 2010a, b).

The first component of a P4P scheme is the measurement of quality — the first box in Figure 2. The quality measures follow a well-known paradigm of structure, process, and outcomes (Donabedian, 2005). Structure refers to the health care setting, including the facility, equipment, supplies, pharmaceuticals, information technology, and human resources. When P4P programs reward structure, it is often for investments in information technology. Process, broadly defined, are the procedures used to provide health care services, including practice guidelines,

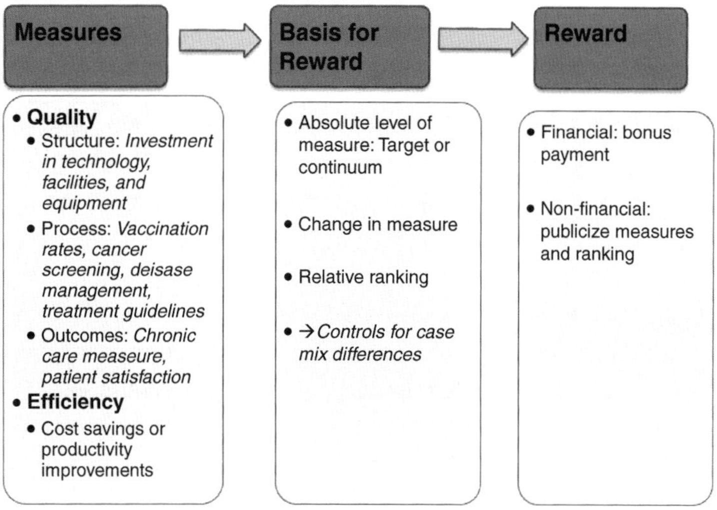

Figure 2. General framework for P4P programs
Source: Authors of this Chapter.

disease management protocols, and vaccination and screening rates. P4P programs often use process measures like whether a child was fully vaccinated or a woman screened for breast and cervical cancer as quality measures.

Outcome measures are the most difficult to include in a P4P design and rarely include mortality or morbidity, in part because these outcomes are not fully under the control of the health provider. For example, survival for breast cancer that has not spread beyond the breast is now commonly assessed over more than 10 years and it is difficult to reward providers for outcomes that take place so far in the future. As a result, measuring quality depends more on intermediate outcomes such as blood pressure, blood sugar, and cholesterol levels.

Efficiency measures focus on costs. For example, a physician's performance may be measured by the number of inpatient days per 1,000 enrollees or the ratio of outpatient procedures occurring at a hospital versus a lower-cost health care facility. These measures ideally should be adjusted for case mix, since the severity of patients' illnesses is one of the main determinants of cost. Often, age and sex are used for case-mix adjustment, but these can be insufficient, and more complex case adjustment classification systems are needed to adjust for differences in patient severity. For example, if one practice had all healthy young people and the other had old diabetics, it would not be surprising that the first practice would have better efficiency-related outcomes than the other (See also Volume 1, Chapter 6 of this Handbook, *Global Risk-Adjusted Payment Models*).

P4P schemes differ between high- and low-income countries. In high-income countries, particularly those that use fee-for-service health care payments, the problem is constraining the ever-increasing demand for health services when those greater number of services are not strongly related to ultimate health outcomes. However, in many low-income countries with longstanding NHSs (often referred to as the Public-Integrated Model), where health personnel are civil servants, there is often underutilization and lack of coverage of key public health interventions like immunization and antenatal care. Here, the goal is to increase utilization, particularly for high-priority services as well as to increase quality. The classic example for low- and middle-income countries (LMICs) is the Rwanda P4P, where the scheme paid for a list of priority services (see Basinga *et al.*, 2011). Other example measures include rewarding physicians to work in the public sector instead of the private sector (e.g., Turkey) or to diagnose patients with tuberculosis (China).

In fact, any measure can be selected for use in a P4P program, from narrow vertical disease program goals, like increasing vaccination, to broader goals like improving primary care. In P4P programs like the Quality Outcome Framework (QOF) in the United Kingdom, many different disease-specific goals are combined into a single composite measure (Dixon *et al.*, 2011).

Rewarding providers

The second box within Figure 2 is the basis for reward. The primary categories used to base the reward include the absolute level of the measure, a change in the level, or the relative ranking. First, the absolute level reward could be based on achieving a target, such as achieving an 80% vaccination rate, or based on a continuum (e.g., as done in QOF, once the minimum threshold is reached). A target rate may not be optimal from the programmatic perspective, because those who start near or are already above the target will receive a reward with little to no improvement. And those who begin far below the target will likely need a large incentive to exert effort to reach the target. Alternatively, the reward may be based on a change in the measure over time, such as how a provider's breast cancer screening rate has changed from a pre-determined baseline. In a case like this, the magnitude of improvement is rewarded. Finally, rewards can be based purely on relative performance or rankings — i.e., a practice is given a reward for being in the top 10% ranking. This payment basis has some appeal since the random variation in incentivized outcomes for all providers can be controlled for if the random variation affects all providers in an equal manner. For any of the reward bases, it is important to control for case mix differences in order to reduce provider's incentive to avoid high-need patients and to better control for outcomes outside of the provider's control, thus reducing the required risk premium.

The third box within Figure 2 is the reward, which may be financial, non-financial, or a combination of both. Rewards are often a bonus or lump sum payment or they can be a proportional increase in the rate of payment or reimbursement. A non-financial reward can entail publicized provider rankings based on different measures. Although public rankings are not directly financial, they can become financial if patients or insurers use the rankings to determine which provider to visit or contract with.

Under either model, a direct reward to individual health care workers is harder to structure due to potential case mix differences, higher monitoring costs, and lower reliability when a particular individual treats a small number of patients for a given measure. For example, particular individual providers may see an above-average share of patients with complex conditions or patients that require intensive treatment. Adjustments are often difficult to make because of the lack of data and the cost to collect the data. When the effort of each worker cannot be monitored or measured individually, a worker might tend to reduce his effort, because his reward is mostly based on the efforts of the other workers — the shirking problem. This will be particularly true when the reward is equally distributed among workers.

Another concern about P4P schemes is equity. Often, the best practices with the best physicians are located in wealthier areas serving wealthier and more educated populations. These are the types of people who immunize their children, do not smoke, are not overweight, and follow medical advice. In poor areas, patients are less educated and often do not come to the doctor's office and yet have greater health needs. One of the concerns about paying for performance is that it could reward the practices that are already doing well and increase inequities in the health system. It is important to monitor any P4P scheme for equity and to pay attention in the design to avert unintended consequences for equity while promoting efficiency (See also Volume 1, Chapter 11 of this Handbook, *Inequalities and Inequities in Health and Health Care*).

Payment models

Figure 3 shows the two primary payment models used to distribute payments. The first type involves the payer paying the medical group or institution (e.g., hospital or primary care clinic) directly, and these entities then decide how to distribute the payment to individual health care workers. The second type involves paying the individual workers directly. Most P4P programs pay rewards to the medical group or institution, because they are better able to determine how to best distribute the payment among health care workers, as they have more information than the payer. Other challenges with individual-based payments are mentioned in the previous section. In some cases, when a medical group or institution is paid by multiple payers, such as a public payer, private insurer, and individual patients, the incentives may not align because rewards are based on different measures.

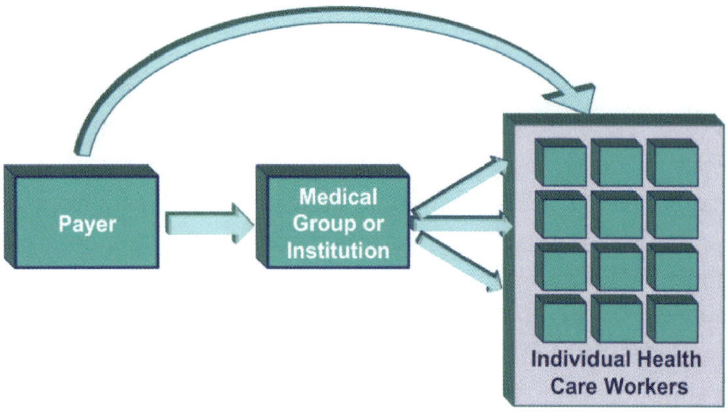

Figure 3. P4P reward payment models

Source: Authors of this Chapter.

P4P Experience and Design Features Around the World

P4P programs in OECD countries

A recent OECD survey has found P4P programs to be common within and across many OECD countries. The information on provider P4P programs in OECD countries is based on the OECD Survey on Health System Characteristics 2008–2009 (hereafter "OECD Survey") and the authors' research for the United States (Borowitz *et al.*, 2010; Paris *et al.*, 2010). The OECD Survey was sent to the 30 member countries in October 2008; Chile was excluded because it became an OECD member after this date. All countries, except Sweden and United States, responded by February 2009. The survey included 81 questions designed to collect qualitative information on health care coverage and provision as well as resource allocation and governance. The survey questions on provider P4P programs asked whether programs existed in primary care, specialty care, and hospitals, as well as which measures were used in each area. Another set of survey questions asked about the modes of payment to primary care physicians, specialists, and hospitals.

Figure 4 summarizes the OECD Survey results on provider P4P programs and the predominant mode of payment to primary care physicians, specialists, and hospitals, while Figure 5 reports these results on a country-by-country basis. P4P programs were reported to exist in 19 of 30 OECD countries, including incentive schemes at the following levels of care: primary care physicians (14), specialists (10), and hospitals (7). For primary care physicians and specialists, most bonuses were for quality of care targets such as preventive care and management of chronic diseases. For hospitals, most bonuses were for processes, but some were also for outcomes and patient satisfaction.

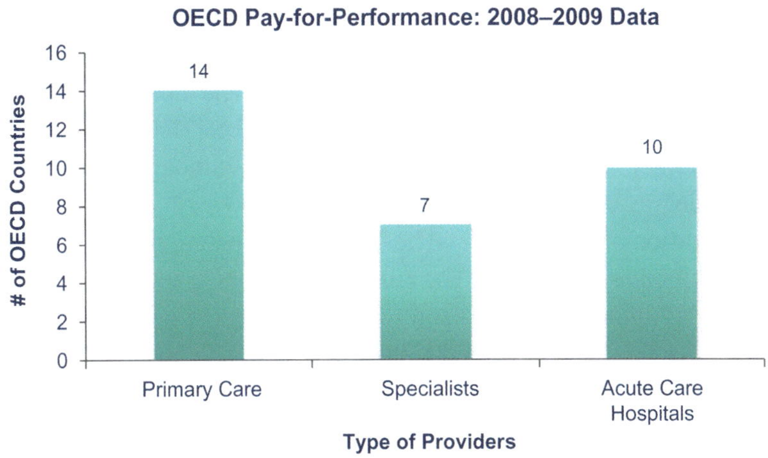

Figure 4. OECD survey results

Source: Authors of this Chapter.

Countries	Primary Care	Specialists	Acute Care Hospitals
France	Yes	Yes	Yes
Korea	Yes	Yes	Yes
Netherlands	Yes	Yes	Yes
Spain	Yes	Yes	Yes
United Kingdom	Yes	Yes	Yes
United States	Yes	Yes	Yes
Australia	Yes	No	Yes
Chile	Yes	Yes	No
Portugal	Yes	No	Yes
Sweden	Yes	No	Yes
Czech Republic	Yes	No	No
Hungary	Yes	No	No
Luxembourg	No	No	Yes
Mexico	Yes	No	No
New Zealand	Yes	No	No
Count	14	7	10

Figure 5. OECD countries with P4P

Source: Authors of this Chapter.

As might be expected, there is significant variation among countries. Countries such as Belgium, Japan, Turkey, the United Kingdom, and United States report P4P in all three sectors (primary care, specialists, and hospitals). In contrast, Austria, Denmark, Finland, France, Germany, Greece, Iceland, Norway, and Switzerland do not report having any P4P programs, although this absence may reflect some degree of underreporting.

The proportion of physicians and hospitals participating in P4P programs was only reported for a few countries. The proportions for each sector were as follows: Primary care: Belgium (90%), Poland (80%), and United Kingdom (99%); specialty care: Poland (5%) and United Kingdom (68%); and hospitals: Luxembourg (9%). The share of the physician and hospital earnings represented by the bonus payment was only reported for a few countries, and they were generally 5% or less, except for the United Kingdom. The bonus shares for each sector were as follows: Primary care: Belgium (2%), Poland (5%), and United Kingdom (15%); specialty care: Poland (5%); and hospitals: Belgium (0.5%) and Luxembourg (1.4%). These data are a beginning, and clearly further data is needed in order to understand the attributes of these P4P programs.

Primary care targets

There are 14 countries from the OECD survey with primary care P4P. As shown in Figure 6, the majority of the countries use primary care targets that relate to

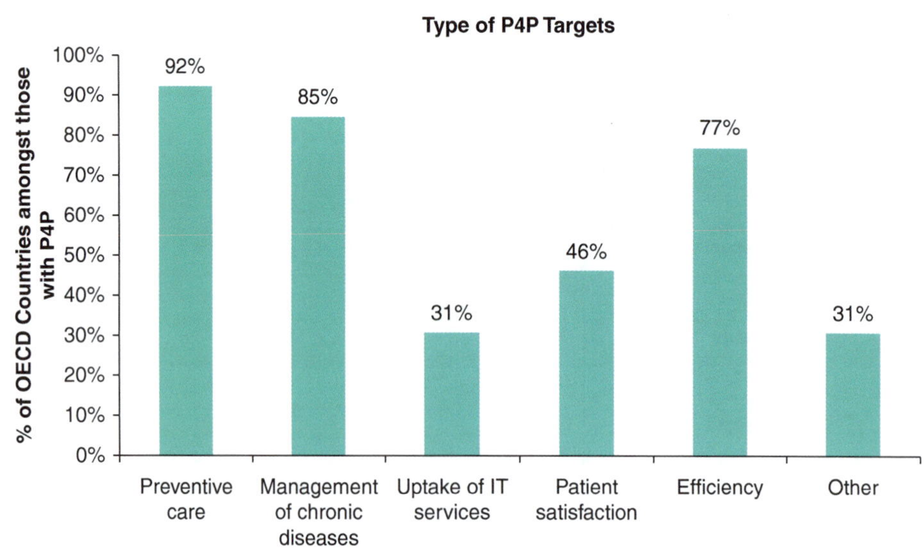

Figure 6. OECD primary care types of performance targets

Source: Authors of this Chapter.

preventive care, management of chronic disease, and efficiency. All of the countries, except Korea and Czech Republic, use more than one of these types of targets. For primary care physicians, the predominant payment mode and number of countries by mode were as follows: fee-for-service (11), capitation (4), salary (4), and a mixture (10). For specialists in outpatient settings, the results were as follows: fee-for-service (11), salary (9), and a mixture (9). For specialists in inpatient settings (not shown), the predominant mode was salary. For hospitals, the results were as follows: payment per case/diagnosis-related group (7), prospective global or line item budget (5), and a mixture (17), which mostly included a mix of payment per case/diagnosis-related group and prospective global budget. No clear patterns emerge between the existence of provider P4P programs and a country's predominant payment mode.

Measures to evaluate performance

As reported in Figure 7, the majority of OECD countries with P4P programs are using preventive care, management of chronic diseases, and efficiency measures. The majority of countries are also using three or more measures to evaluate

Countries	Preventive care	Management of chronic diseases	Uptake of IT services	Patient satisfaction	Efficiency	Other
Sweden	1	1	1	1	1	0
United States	1	1	1	1	1	0
Chile	1	1	0	1	1	1
France	1	1	1	0	1	0
Mexico	1	1	0	1	1	1
Portugal	1	1	0	1	1	0
United Kingdom	1	1	0	1	1	0
Australia	1	1	1	0	0	1
Hungary	1	1	0	0	1	0
Spain	1	1	0	0	1	0
New Zealand	1	1	0	0	0	0
Czech Republic	1	0	0	0	0	1
Korea	0	0	0	0	1	0
Count	**12**	**11**	**4**	**6**	**10**	**4**

Figure 7. OECD primary care types of performance targets by country

Source: Authors

Countries	Absolute measure	Change over time	Relative ranking
Sweden	1	1	1
United States	1	1	1
Korea	0	1	1
New Zealand	1	1	0
Spain	1	1	0
Australia	1	0	0
Chile	1	0	0
Czech Republic	0	0	1
France	0	1	0
Hungary	1	0	0
Mexico	0	0	1
Portugal	1	0	0
United Kingdom	1	0	0
Count	9	6	5

Figure 8. OECD primary care measurements of targets
Source: Authors of this Chapter.

performance. In terms of performance metric, Figure 8 makes clear that absolute metrics are the most common (with 9 of 14 countries adopting absolute metrics for at least some performance payments) while change over time and relative ranking metrics also appear in six and five countries, respectively.

Primary care payment flow

Figure 9 summarizes the primary care payment flow in OECD countries. The payment flows of the bonuses differ by country and can go directly to the individual physicians or to the organization (e.g., physician group) and are adopted at almost equal rates. Nine countries pay individual physicians directly, and seven countries pay an organization (e.g., a physician group). Australia, Portugal and the US use both mechanisms.

P4P programs in LMICs

Parallel to the growth in P4P programs in OECD countries, LMICs have also witnessed a rapid increase in experience with P4P. Rwanda was one of the first

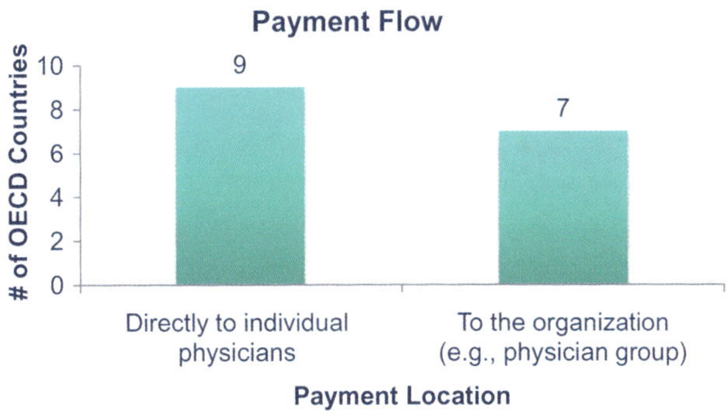

Figure 9. OECD Primary care payment flow

Source: Authors of this Chapter.

LMICs to adopt P4P, with a national pilot that began in 2008. Designed to confront the typical health system challenges faced in the LMIC setting, the Rwanda program focused on incentivizing health providers at the primary and secondary levels to increase the quantity of services provided to the population (Sekabaraga *et al.*, 2011). This took the form of an introduced fee-for-service schedule focused on prioritized health services, mostly related to maternal and child health. After initially promising results from the evaluation of the pilot, the P4P was scaled up to the national level and similar models were adopted in several other LMICs on a pilot basis. Figure 10 relays the spread of pilot P4P programs that were either implemented or planned for implementation by the end of 2014.

While every national pilot contains unique features, many have followed the same basic structure of the initial Rwanda P4P design. Distinctive features include:

- A fee-for-service schedule with a focus on a fixed, tractable number of maternal and child health services. (Figure 11 lists the services and fee schedules as adopted by the Zambian P4P pilot implemented from 2011–2014.) The motivating goal behind this design feature is to incentivize the quantity of service in order to increase access and utilization.
- While the fee schedule largely focuses on the quantity of services, quality of health care is directly addressed through a summary measure of assessed quality of care, with assessments typically conducted by provider-peers or higher-level supervisors in the health system. The most common means to assess quality is through a balanced scorecard approach that attempts to assess care across multiple dimensions — both structural and process — in a comprehensive fashion. The balanced scorecard generates a summary score

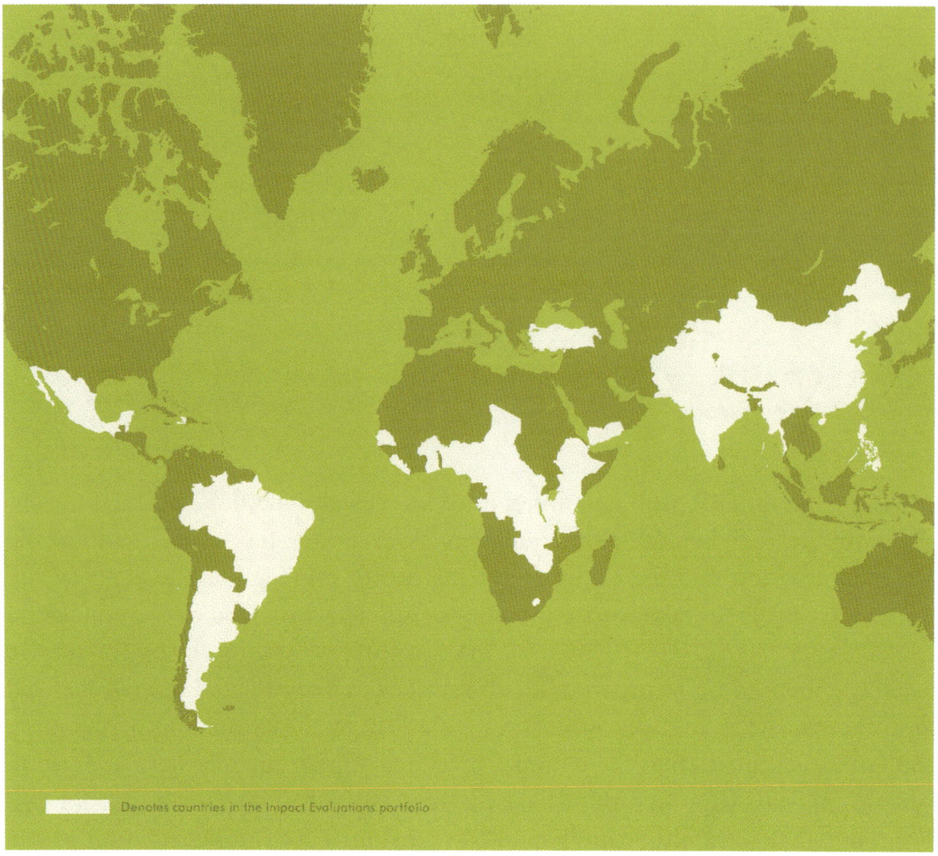

Figure 10. LMICs with known pilot P4P programs, planned or implemented by 2014
Sources: Information from the 2014 Report, Health Results Innovation Trust Fund, http://www.hritfreport.org/.

that is then used to scale the P4P payments earned under the fee schedule. Higher summary quality scores will result in significantly higher payments. One key goal of the quality assessment, besides increasing provider attention to quality issues, is to galvanize health facilities to apply the P4P earnings towards quality-enhancing investments that in turn should yield even higher returns in the following round of quality assessment. Figure 12 presents the example of the Balanced Scorecard instrument as used in Rwanda, the dimensions of quality assessed, the relative weights given to each dimension, and the means of assessment.

- For the above iterative mechanism to result in higher quality, the incentivized clinic or hospital should have the autonomy to allocate retained earnings toward investments that are particularly effective given their local context and specific health situation. For this reason, P4P programs in LMICs also typically

Nos.	Indicators	Fee (ZMW)
1	Curative Consultation	1.00
2	Institutional Deliveries by Skilled Birth Attendant	32.00
3	ANC prenatal and follow up visits	8.00
4	Postnatal visit	16.50
5	Full immunization of children under 1	11.50
6	Pregnant women receiving 3 doses of malaria IPT	8.00
7	FP users of modern methods at the end of the month	3.00
8	Pregnant women counselled and tested for HIV	9.00
9	No. of HIV pregnant women given NVP/AZT	10.00

Figure 11. Fee-for-service schedule from the Zambian P4P pilot program, 2011–2014

Sources: Chansa *et al.* (2015).

	Services	Weight	Share of weight allocated to structural components	Share of weight allocated to process components	Means of assessment
1	General administration	0.052	1.00	0.00	Direct observation
2	Cleanliness	0.028	1.00	0.00	Direct observation
3	Curative care	0.170	0.23	0.77	Medical record review
4	Delivery	0.130	0.40	0.60	Medical record review
5	Prenatal care	0.126	0.12	0.88	Direct observation
6	Family planning	0.114	0.22	0.78	Medical record review
7	Immunization	0.070	0.40	0.60	Direct observation
8	Growth monitoring	0.052	0.15	0.85	Direct observation
9	HIV services	0.090	1.00	0.00	Direct observation
10	Tuberculosis service	0.028	0.28	0.72	Direct observation
11	Laboratory	0.030	1.00	0.00	Direct observation
12	Pharmacy management	0.060	1.00	0.00	Direct observation
13	Financial management	0.050	1.00	0.00	Direct observation
	Total	1.000			

Figure 12. Balanced Scorecard Dimensions and relative weights given to select quality dimensions, Rwanda, 2008–2010

Source: Basinga *et al.* (2011).

increase the degree of autonomy in financial and hiring decisions granted to participating facilities.

- Finally, with the focus on informational flows of services provided, assessed quality scores, and payments, P4P programs place increased emphasis on a health system's reporting system which often result in investments in the comprehensiveness and accuracy of the Health Management Information System (HMIS) and other monitoring systems. These investments may result in widespread benefits to all actors in the health system through an increase in the availability and quality of data.

P4P Country Case Studies

This section presents select case studies of P4P programs in more detail.

United Kingdom: Quality and outcomes framework

The Quality and Outcomes Framework (QOF) is the largest P4P scheme in the world. It began in 2004 and is a voluntary incentive pay program for general practitioners with almost universal participation, with 99.8% of patients registered in England enrolled in participating GP practices. The objective of the QOF is to reward GP practices for how well they care for patients, not just how many patients they have on their list.

The QOF contains four main areas, known as domains: Clinical, organizational, patient experience and additional services. Each domain contains indicators that define the specific process or outcome that practices participating in the QOF are asked to achieve for their patients. For example, one of the clinical indicators for coronary heart disease (CHD) is the percentage of patients with CHD who are currently treated with a beta blocker (unless a contraindication or side effects are recorded). Clinical indicators are based on the best available evidence of the effectiveness of interventions in primary care.

The points are converted into monetary incentives by a conversion factor. In 2004, there was a maximum total of 1,050 points, and each was worth GBP76 (US$133). Currently, 146 indicators are used to determine 1,000 points covering clinical quality, organizational quality, and patient experience. Each point is worth GBP126.77. To illustrate how the QOF works, consider the example of the quality indicator for asthma, which is based on the percentage of patients with asthma who have had an asthma review in the previous 15 months. No points are awarded until the review rate reaches 25%, and the maximum number of points, 20, is awarded once the review rate reaches 70%. For review rates between 25% and 70%, the number of points earned linearly increases as the review rate increases.

In 2004–2005, the median general practitioner earned 1,003 points of the 1,050 points available, or 95.5%, which was much higher than expected. When QOF was negotiated, it was presumed that the average would be approximately 75% but it ended up at over 90%. QOF increased the gross average income of general practitioners by GBP23,000 (US$40,200); before QOF, general practitioners typically earned GBP70,000–GBP75,000 (US$122,000–US$131,000) (Doran *et al.*, 2006). Because of the large payout, the 2006/2007 minimum thresholds were all increased, and some of the maximum thresholds were increased as well.

It is difficult to determine whether health care quality improved as a result of the QOF, because there were no clear counterfactual groups — almost everyone participated. However, Campbell *et al.* (2009) analyzed data before and after the QOF was initiated and found the rate of improvement in the quality of care initially increased for asthma and diabetes, but not for heart disease, and by 2007, the rate of improvement had slowed for each condition. There is also some evidence that the program has improved equity of outcomes. However, importantly, they also found that quality of those aspects of care that were not linked to an incentive had declined for asthma or heart disease.

One of the criticisms of the QOF was the process for determining which diseases and interventions would be included in the QOF. It was felt that this should not be political, but a technical exercise, and responsibility was shifted to the National Institute for Health and Clinical Excellence (NICE), which began overseeing a new independent and transparent process for developing and reviewing QOF health and clinical improvement indicators beginning 1 April 2009. The relative priority of these topics for inclusion in QOF would then be considered by an independent advisory committee, formally known as the Primary Care Quality and Outcomes Framework Indicator Advisory Committee. Each recommended indicator will be accompanied by a suite of supporting information — for example, on when new and renewed indicators should be reviewed and on the cost-effectiveness evidence to inform their financial value.

New Zealand: Performance-based management

New Zealand started its Performance-based management (PBM) program in 2006 within its Primary Health Organizations (PHOs), which are non-profit organizations that provide primary health care services (Buetow, 2008). By January 2007, 81 PHOs, which represented over 98% of New Zealanders, enrolled in the PBM program. The PBM setup payment was NZD 20,000 per PHO plus 60c per enrolled member. There was a guaranteed minimum payment of NZD 1.00–1.50 per enrollee for PHOs entering the PBM program before December 2007. A maximum payment of NZD 6 per enrollee could be obtained if all targets were achieved, which include clinical indicators (60%), process indicators (10%), and financial indicators (30%). The clinical indicators include, for example, vaccinations for children and elderly, cervical smears, and breast cancer screening. The process indicators include, for example, ensuring access for those with high needs. Last, the financial indicators include, for example, pharmaceutical and laboratory expenditures. The payments are made to the PHO, who then decide how to distribute funds to individual health care workers. Based on a survey of 29 PHOs, they reported better clinical care co-ordination and data management as a result of PBM.

Argentina: Plan Nacer

Plan Nacer, the Argentinian P4P program for its national health system, conditions health financing from the central government to provinces on the basis of: (a) enrollment of uninsured populations into the program and (b) select population health indicators. The uninsured population in Argentina is substantial and the responsibility for coverage of this population rests with the provincial health systems. Plan Nacer was designed to provide coverage for 14% of the uninsured, based on age and pregnancy status. The program covers uninsured pregnant women during pregnancy and up to 45 days after birth, as well as uninsured children up to six years of age.

The program was first launched in 2004 in the nine provinces of northern Argentina that were most affected by Argentina's 2001 economic crisis, then expanded to the rest of the country in 2007. Enrollment grew rapidly, with 82% of the eligible population in the Northern provinces participating in the program just four years after its start.

Plan Nacer gives additional health financing beyond standard administrative budgets in the form of an $8 payment per enrollee per month. Of this amount, up to $3 is reserved conditional on the achievement of specified maternal and child health targets — there are 10 indicators in all including the early detection of pregnancy (defined as the first prenatal visit before the 20th week of pregnancy), and infant birth weight over 2500 grams.

In turn, the provinces receive these resources and then pay affiliated clinics for a listed 80 prioritized maternal and child health services on a fee-for-service basis. The services were selected as those particularly effective for improving maternal and child health outcomes, and the facility payments are permitted to be used at the discretion of the participating clinics to improve the quality of services. Permitted expenditures include infrastructure and equipment investments as well as staff recruitment and staff incentives.

Using administrative data and a difference-in-difference analytic framework, Gertler and Giovagnoli (2014) find that Plan Nacer improved the quantity of services, as exhibited by a greater number of total prenatal visits, the quality of services, as measured by higher likelihood of pregnant women receiving tetanus toxoid vaccines and lower likelihood of cesarean sections, and improved birth outcomes, specifically a 19% reduction if the probability of low birth weight and a 74% reduction in neonatal mortality.

Gertler and Giovagnoli (2014) also find some evidence of a low-level crowding out of service availability for non-beneficiaries — which is a possibility with the overall increase in service utilization given the fixed number of facilities — but not to a sufficient degree to affect health outcomes.

Zimbabwe: Health results based financing project

The P4P program in Zimbabwe, known as the Zimbabwe Health Results Based Financing (ZHRBF) Project, was piloted in two rural districts in 2011 and then expanded to 16 other districts — roughly one-third of the country — in 2012. The program was introduced to all primary health clinics and hospitals in the participating districts with a fee schedule for 16 services at the primary clinic level and six at the hospital level. All incentivized indicators were already routinely collected through the Zimbabwe HMIS. Quarterly facility payments were scaled according to an aggregate quality score as measured through a balanced scorecard.

The ZHRBF was implemented against a background of rapid gains in service coverage and improving health outcomes as the country recovered from its 2008–2009 crisis. Nevertheless, as summarized in Friedman *et al.* (Forthcoming), the rate of increase in targeted health indicators in the P4P districts was faster, and this differential in improvement represents the causal effect of the ZHRBF following the evaluation design planned before the implementation period.

Impact estimates include a 13 percentage point increase in the in-facility delivery rate for pregnant women, a 12 percentage point increase in post-natal coverage, and significant improvements in the quality of select services, in particular the quality of antenatal care (ANC). However not all service coverage saw increases, especially services that already had high coverage at baseline, such as overall ANC coverage.

United States: Multiple examples of P4P

In the United States, P4P programs are pervasive and include a wide variety of payers, such as private insurers, large employers, Medicare, and Medicaid. The programs have generally had a low impact, because the bonus has been a low percentage of provider revenues. For example, the California Pay for Performance Program is perhaps the largest P4P program in the United States in terms of bonuses paid. As of 2009, it included eight commercial HMO health plans, covering 11.5 million enrollees, and approximately 230 physician groups with 35,000 physicians. Between 2003 and 2007, the plans paid US$264 million in bonuses, which represented only 2% of the physician groups' revenues. The goal was for the payment levels to be 10%; however, plans have been reluctant to increase the percentage until there is stronger evidence on improved quality. The program started with 13 measures in three domains, and has expanded to 68 measures in five domains, including the following with their associated weights: clinical quality (40%), patient experience (20%), IT-enabled systems (20%), coordinated diabetes care (20%) and resource use and efficiency (with a separate incentive pool).

Clinical performance improved an average of 3 percentage points per year, with groups who had the lowest baseline improving the most, particularly for HbA1c screening for diabetics — a good measure of diabetic control (Robinson *et al.*, 2009). The largest change was groups adopting specific IT activities, which increased an average of 7 percentage points per year. The non-financial incentives included publicizing the rankings, for example, for the top 20% and the most improved. These amount to indirect financial incentives, because public recognition has been used by physician groups in their advertising and marketing materials. In summary, provider groups are still motivated to participate in this P4P scheme, but health plans are less motivated because quality improvements are not large, which is likely due in part because of the low P4P payments which are only 2% of total income, which may not be sufficient to motivate providers.

- *Medicare has many small-scale P4P demonstration programs in place*

The Centers for Medicare & Medicaid Services (CMS) is involved in many P4P demonstration projects. However, as compared to its approximate US$420 billion budget in FY2009 for Medicare, the P4P program payments of approximately US$40 million are very small (Tanenbaum, 2009). Two of these programs are addressed here.

In order to increase the collection and reporting of quality measures, Medicare's Physicians Quality Reporting Initiative began in 2007 and pays physicians an additional 2% of their allowed charges for reporting quality measures to CMS (James, 2012). In 2007, the physician participation rate was 16% (Porter, 2008).

The Physician Group Practice (PGP) Demonstration began in 2005 and included ten PGPs as well as control groups (Trisolini *et al.*, 2008). The demonstration included both quality and efficiency measures. The 32 quality measures were drawn from CMS's Doctor's Office Quality (DOQ) project, focusing on measures from five health condition modules: coronary artery disease, diabetes, heart failure, hypertension, and preventive care. One of the diabetes measures, for example, is the percentage of diabetics who received an HbA1c (blood sugar) test at least once per year.

For each quality measure, PGPs must satisfy at least one of three targets: (1) The higher of either 75% compliance or, where comparable data are available, the mean value of the measure from the Medicare Health Plan Employer Data and Information Set (HEDIS); (2) the 70th percentile Medicare HEDIS level (again, where comparable data are available); or (3) a 10% or greater reduction in the gap between the level achieved by the PGP in the demonstration's base year and 100% compliance in Year 1. The first two targets are threshold targets, while the third is an improvement-over-time target. The initial results show some promise. All groups achieved target performance levels on at least seven of 10 diabetes quality measures.

The PGP can also receive a payment based on efficiency or cost savings. For each PGP, Medicare savings from the Demonstration are calculated by comparing actual spending to a target: the PGP's own base year per capita expenditures trended forward by the comparison group's expenditure growth rate. The PGP and comparison groups' case mixes are adjusted to account for differences in the type of patients treated. The PGP is eligible to receive 80% of the savings that are above a 2% savings threshold. Two out of ten physician groups had at least 2% lower Medicare spending growth rates as compared to control groups.

- *US Physicians support P4P, with certain conditions*

73% of US physicians support financial incentives for quality, if the measures are accurate (Casalino *et al.*, 2007). However, a vast majority (70%) do not think measures of quality are accurate. Only 32% of US physicians support public reporting of individual physician's performance. Over 80% are concerned that measuring performance will cause physicians to avoid high-risk patients.

Issues and Challenges with P4P Design and Implementation

One key design challenge, especially in OECD countries, has to do with setting an adequate incentive level. P4P recipients need to receive a large enough incentive percentage to change behavior resulting in higher quality of health care provided. If incentives are too low, health providers may not respond to the program at all. Typically, 5% of total income is not enough to change behavior (as indicated in some OECD case studies); rather, incentive percentages of 15 to 20% are needed. On the other hand, the incentive level can also be set too high if the desired behavior change can also be achieved at a lower level. In this case, the P4P program can be more cost effective at lower incentive levels.

Some key implementation issues with pay for performance that arise in many contexts include: shirking, case mix, and multiple payers. Shirking arises when people rely on the good work and high performance of others, while working minimally themselves. Pay for performance also requires an adequate mix of patients. The case mix is necessary to ensure one provider does not have sicker or tougher patients than others; risk adjusting the patient populations is important. Hence, there is a need for an up-to-date, high-powered risk adjustment model to appropriately compare doctors to one another and health entities to similar health entities. Additionally, medical groups and institutions often have multiple payers, especially in the US Different payers could have different pay for performance systems, which could make it difficult for medical groups to meet all performance goals and thus makes P4P planning and implementation challenging.

The quality of implementation is also critical to the success of a P4P program, especially when the P4P scheme is new and not yet familiar to participating health professionals. Huillery and Seban (2014) review a pilot P4P program in the Democratic Republic of Congo (DRC) that failed to achieve any measurable gains in service utilization or quality. A key factor in the inability of this program to spur gains in targeted outcomes appears to be various implementation failures, most notably interruptions in the regular payment schedule and an overall decrease in funding to participating facilities. Clearly, for a P4P program to have a chance at success, participating institutions and health personnel must expect that realized achievements would actually result in receipt of the incentives earned.

The findings from the DRC also indicate another potential concern with P4P programs, albeit one not yet supported by a preponderance of empirical evidence, and that is that the introduction of explicit financial rewards for health activities may place undue emphasis on the "extrinsic motivation" of health workers to perform, perhaps to the detriment of a worker's "intrinsic motivation" and long-term sustainability of health system performance. These concerns are often cited as a possible negative effect of P4P but, to date, rigorous field-based evidence on this issue is sparse. Box 1 discusses the issue in more detail and reviews the available evidence.

Another potential issue with P4P is the "crowding-out" of effort away from non-incentivized indicators, which will occur if total effort is already close to a maximum level and the shift of greater attention to prioritized activities results in a de-emphasis on other health functions. This possibility is discussed further in the next section.

Finally, since remuneration under P4P can be based on self-reported information — as is often the case in LMIC settings — a P4P program must consider the possibility of health providers inflating service counts or related "gaming" behavior in order to maximize compensation (Ireland *et al.*, 2011). To dissuade such behavior, P4P programs often develop robust systems of data verification, including the use of third party independent audit. Box 2 reviews this evidence on the ability of data verification schemes to reduce the likelihood of "gaming." While at least somewhat effective in reducing the tendency to deliberately misreport, data verification schemes are not inexpensive and often constitute an important subcomponent of the overall cost of the program.

Box 1. Health worker intrinsic motivation and P4P

Economists have long noted that price mechanisms can be effective at modifying human behavior. Psychologists classify this aspect of behavior motivation as extrinsic motivation, meaning that the behavior is induced by external pressure. In contrast to extrinsic motivation, psychologists posit intrinsic motivation as arising from within the individual. These long-standing concepts are often attached to discussions of public sector pay reform and, more recently, P4P. A common concern voiced in discussions of P4P is that incentivizing the provision of care at the provider level will result in less care or lower-quality care as the extrinsic motivation from the incentives "crowds out" the intrinsic motivation to do good or be respected by peers. To the extent that intrinsic and extrinsic motivations co-exist and respond to changes in the regulatory environment such as varying incentive levels, this is largely an empirical question.

Findings from psychology and the relatively new field of behavioral economics possibly suggest that performance bonuses backfire, particularly for cognitively challenging tasks. This evidence includes:

- About 56 college undergraduates who were given puzzles to solve were less successful when offered monetary reward than when given verbal reinforcement or no reward at all (Deci, 1971).
- Paying for blood donations actually reduced the quantity of blood donated (Uptom, 1973).
- Swiss volunteers reduced the time spent in volunteer activities once they were offered payment for the same activities (Frey and Goette, 1999).
- Parents in Israel were more likely to pick their children up late from school once fines were imposed (as opposed to social disapproval) for late-pick-ups (Gneezy and Rustichini, 2000)
- Both MIT students and villagers in India solved fewer complex puzzles when offered large incentives than when offered either small incentives or no incentives (Ariely *et al.*, 2009).
- A meta-analysis of 128 studies concludes that incentives reduce intrinsic motivation especially when incentives are task-contingent and tangible (i.e., non-verbal) (Deci *et al.*, 1999).

Note that virtually all of this evidence consists of contrasting a non-incentivized control group with (some form of) incentivized treatment group. Indeed, the Deci *et al.* meta-review mentioned in the last bullet point above

(*Continued*)

Box 1. (*Continued*)

is explicitly restricted to studies that involve an experimental group compared to a no-reward control group. While there is surely much to learn, in general, from research that experimentally introduces incentives into a previously non incentivized environment, the implications for P4P are not particularly clear.

Note that health workers are *already* in an environment where incentives are used to induce behavior. P4P reform is only a change in the *form* of incentive. To be more precise, P4P reform is a movement along the contingency axis of incentive type. In developing countries, P4P typically involves a switch from what is termed engagement- to completion-contingency incentives (i.e., a change from incentivizing the beginning versus the completion of a task), while in OECD health systems the switch is more typically from completion- to performance contingency (i.e., a change from completing a task to doing it well).

Why is this distinction important? The *Deci et al.* meta-analysis finds *no difference* in the negative effect of incentives on intrinsic motivation whether they take the form of engagement- or completion- or performance-contingency. Given this summary of the literature, it is not clear *a priori* how P4P may affect intrinsic motivation.

It is certainly possible that P4P reform may reduce the intrinsic motivation of health workers, at least in some contexts. But there is little current evidence that directly speaks to this issue — another recent meta-review that looks at P4P in the public sector reviews 46 relevant studies but none of these studies directly investigates public sector P4P because "experimental studies are less numerous in the public sector" (Weibel *et al.*, 2010). The future direction of research in this area is clear, but there is little evidence till date.

Box 2. Verifying the performance in P4P: Deterrence of "gaming" and current knowledge gaps in effective practice

P4P reward indicators are often self-reported. There is a clear challenge to linking rewards to a self-reported indicator: the temptation for incentivized health providers to inflate gains and misreport. P4P schemes often need a verification mechanism to deter such behavior known, as "gaming."

Gaming is a real concern, at least in certain contexts, for P4P. Take, as an example, the reporting of British doctors under the comprehensive P4P of the QOF in the UK (Gravelle *et al.*, 2010). To calculate the payment tied to a

(*Continued*)

Box 2. (*Continued*)

particular indicator, the QOF scales the ratio according to indicator-specific threshold triggers. One such indicator is the ratio of heart disease patients whose blood pressure has recently been measured at less than 150/90, in relation to all heart disease patients registered with the practice. As the clinical quality indicators are ratios, the QOF P4P aims to nudge practitioners to increase the numerator. However, the QOF also gives some leeway to how doctors report the denominator since they can declare certain patients to be ineligible and except them from the calculation. Ineligibility is largely a doctor's judgment call based on various grounds such as the patient having refused treatment or failed to attend scheduled appointments. This incentive form creates a nonlinear function of compensation that practitioners can in principle learn to navigate. For example if, in the first year of the QOF, a clinic does not reach the desired threshold then in future years it may be tempted to except more patients from the denominator. Clinics that have already reached the upper threshold and believe they can stay there have less incentive to game in subsequent years.

There is indeed some evidence of differential reporting behavior in the QOF by the initial level of quality. Gravelle *et al.* (2010) estimate the 2005 exception rate for clinics who in 2004 exceeded the upper threshold at 7.2%. In contrast, the 2005 exception rate for clinics who were under the threshold in 2004 is 8.6%. This increase is certainly slight, but also precisely estimated. Taken together, it appears that UK doctors did deliberately misapply the exception criteria, although the magnitude of such gaming is small in this instance.

The risk of third-party audit is the most common approach to dissuade gaming and induce veracity in self-reporting. Two fairly recent studies highlight the effectiveness of the audit approach. The announcement of intensified audits for hospitals in Buenos Aires led to a 15% reduction in input prices paid by hospitals when the risk of audit was at the highest point (Di Tella and Schargrodsky, 2003). When audit risk receded to an intermediate level, procurement prices rose a bit but were still 10% lower than the pre-crackdown prices. A recent multi-year audit experiment conducted with Danish taxpayers found that the income subject to third-party reporting — the vast majority of income in Denmark — is reported extremely accurately by tax payers. However self-reported income (from all sources) was under-reported by an average of 37% (Kleven *et al.*, 2011). The experience of an audit has a strong positive impact on self-reported income the following year.

The risk of audit can dissuade gaming behavior, but the Danish tax study also points to the importance of third-party reporting of health indicators to

(*Continued*)

Box 2. (*Continued*)

deter gaming. For P4P, third-party reporting may be feasible in select settings through mechanisms such as an independent population survey, although the cost-effectiveness of this approach is likely to be limited. Innovative institutional arrangements, such as the joint liability of independent reporting units, may also be able to approximate third party reporting in settings where independent survey is not unfeasible.

In other settings, there may be no cost-effective alternative to verification through audit. However, if using an audit approach, there are numerous operationally relevant questions in a P4P context that need to be resolved, including: What is the most effective form of audit, what is the most effective frequency of audit, and how severe should sanctions be for deliberate misreporting? Currently, while theory provides some guide, there is little empirical evidence and only a few recent studies that address these questions. One possibility to investigate is whether unpredictable audit likelihood or fuzzy audit trigger thresholds are more effective than standard auditing approaches (Bevan and Hood, 2006).

P4P Mechanisms Create Behavioral Change Through Six Factors

Previous sections have reviewed various designs of P4P programs around the world and presented emergent evidence on their relative effectiveness. This section turns to a comprehensive framework to summarize the channels through which P4P schemes result in behavioral change on the part of providers.

To begin, note that payers do not have complete information when setting the incentives of P4P programs. Furthermore, because P4P programs incur monitoring and risk premium costs, the new mix of services produced under P4P may result in either a higher or lower level of health. The new health level depends on six key factors: Health-increasing substitution, health-decreasing substitution, provider surplus extraction, net externalities, monitoring costs, and risk premium costs.

Figure 13 plots these six factors in a stylized manner to show their potential impact on health as a function of the share of a provider's revenue that is based on P4P (or, alternatively, the share of a worker's wage based on P4P). Health could be based on various measures, such as clinical indicators, patient self-reported health, or quality-adjusted life years. The health measure could be based on an average patient or on disadvantaged patients (e.g., health of 10th percentile or average health of a sub-group of patients, based on race, ethnicity, or geographical location).

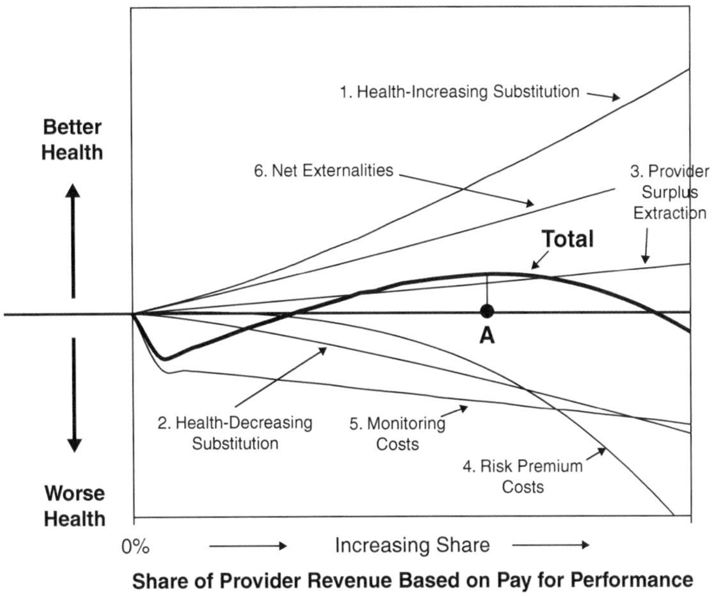

Figure 13. Key factors of P4P that influence health: An illustration

Source: Authors of this Chapter.

The net effect of the six factors is summed in the curve labeled "Total," and is from the payer's perspective, with point A marking the P4P incentive level expected to maximize health. The figure shows that as the share of provider's revenue that is based on P4P increases, health increases up to a point, and then begins to decrease as the risk premium cost begins to dominate. Next, we discuss the primary purpose of the figure, define the counterfactual condition that a P4P program is being compared to within the figure, and explain why the horizontal axis is the share of provider's revenue that is based on P4P.

The primary purpose of the figure is to decompose P4P's impact on health into the key channels through which it acts. This allows researchers to better understand the causal factors behind observed health changes under P4P. The relative contribution and shape of each line are based on theoretical and empirical studies and will vary between settings and contexts; more work is clearly needed to fully understand these relationships.

Most P4P programs use new funds to pay for bonuses, risk premium costs, and monitoring costs. Those funds could have been spent in other ways. For example, the funds could have been used to increase the payment rates under the existing payment model, hire additional staff, purchase equipment, or build a facility. In order to isolate the impact of the incentives from the funding increase, the health impact on Figure 13's vertical axis is in reference to an unobserved counterfactual condition, that is, if those new funds were being used to increase payment rates under the existing payment model. For empirical studies, the counterfactual condition can be proxied by randomizing which providers receive the new funding and incentives versus only the new funding (e.g., see Basinga *et al.*, 2011 for Rwanda).

In Figure 13, the horizontal axis is the share of provider's revenue that is based on P4P, because the size of the incentive is a key P4P design issue. The share that will maximize health depends on health system characteristics, such as the payment model, administrative controls, and the potential to increase efficiency, as well as other features of the contract, such as monitoring level, decision-making authority, job design, and asset ownership. To date, P4P programs' bonus payments have almost always been less than 10–15% of a payee's revenue, and often less than 5% (Rosenthal and Dudley 2007; Paris *et al.*, 2010).

Factor 1: Health-increasing substitution

Health-increasing substitution occurs when more efficient services and inputs (including enhanced effort) are substituted for less efficient ones. For example, as more rewarded flu vaccinations are provided, fewer curative flu services are needed. The health care services provided, in conjunction with other inputs (e.g., patient behaviors, patient genetics, and the environment), produce health. In Figure 13, health-increasing substitution is assumed to start with a gradual slope, because the incentive must be larger than the marginal cost to act on the incentive. For example, surveys of physician groups in California report that the incentive must be at least 5% of total compensation to motivate significant change (Rebhun and Williams, 2009). Once those fixed costs are absorbed, the slope of the line increases. We assume a linear slope, but it may increase at a different rate, depending on the provider's cost of effort to provide different services.

Factor 2: Health-decreasing substitution

Health-decreasing substitution, a form of "crowding-out," occurs when less efficient services and inputs are substituted for more efficient ones. This can occur when an agent performs multiple tasks encompassing multiple sub-tasks (Holmstrom and Milgrom, 1991). It is impractical to include P4P incentives for each sub-task, and some sub-tasks are either unobserved or difficult to measure. Therefore, the agent may substitute effort from unobserved and unmeasurable non-rewarded sub-tasks (e.g., counseling), which may be relatively more efficient for health production, toward the rewarded sub-tasks (e.g., record keeping). For example, in the United Kingdom's QOF, some providers report recording specific clinical activities rewarded under the P4P program has reduced the time available to listen to patients' concerns (Maisey *et al.*, 2008). A payer's knowledge of the health production function is assumed to be less than a provider's knowledge, increasing the potential that incentives lead to health-decreasing substitution. In Figure 13, health-decreasing substitution is assumed to mirror health-increasing substitution, because it has similar properties. If the P4P measures are well designed, then the magnitude of health-decreasing substitution will be less than the magnitude of health-increasing substitution, and there will be a net positive impact on health related to substitution.

Factor 3: Provider surplus extraction

Provider surplus extraction is the difference between the provider's profit (or health worker's utility, including time not devoted to work) under the counterfactual condition versus the profit (or utility) under P4P. If given a choice, an average provider, with respect to efficiency, will prefer not participating in a P4P program if it will receive the mean P4P payment (i.e., the counterfactual condition), even when its level of effort is low. The surplus that the payer extracts from the provider can be used to purchase additional health care services. The surplus extraction will vary across providers. For example, surplus extraction will be greater from an inefficient provider, because the P4P bonus payment will likely be low. This may cause these providers to exit the market, resulting in P4P having a sorting function (Lazear, 2000). On the other hand, surplus extraction will be less from an efficient provider, because the P4P bonus payment will likely be high. Worker surpluses are significant in low-income countries, where absenteeism and dual-practice are common (Chaudhury *et al.*, 2006). From society's perspective, provider surplus extraction is a distributional issue, not an efficiency issue. However, from the payer's perspective, the extracted provider surplus can be used to improve health through increased provider effort. In Figure 13, provider surplus extraction is assumed to be linearly related to a provider's share of revenue based on P4P. The magnitude of this slope will be context specific and depend on the amount of existing provider surplus.

Factor 4: Net externalities

A P4P program is designed to change the mix of services and inputs used, based on providing incentives for specific indicators. In addition, a P4P program may change the mix of services and inputs, because the P4P program modifies organizational norms and decision-making processes. The changes in the mix of services and inputs from these modifications are defined as externalities, because the mix changes are the result of influences beyond the specific indicators. For example, a positive externality may be generated, because P4P implementation may modify the governance of the organization and educate providers on the latest clinical practice guidelines. The program may improve decision-making, through the analysis of the data generated by the P4P program, which may have a positive effect on other services that are not tied to incentives. Negative externalities are also possible. For example, a P4P program may cause workers to become less team-oriented, if the P4P is designed so that they compete with each other for bonuses. In Figure 13, net externalities are assumed to be positive and to be related to investments in monitoring, because increased investment in monitoring systems is likely to yield these externalities. The shape of the externality curve is an empirical question that will be context specific. In both the UK and New Zealand, for example, improved data systems are considered to have wider beneficial effects on overall quality of care (Galvin, 2006; Martin, Jenkins and Associates Limited, 2008).

Factor 5: Monitoring costs

A P4P program will incur set-up and ongoing monitoring costs because it is dependent on data-driven payments. These costs will be in addition to the monitoring costs of the existing payment model. These costs reduce the budget available to purchase health care services, resulting in lower health. In Figure 13, monitoring costs include a fixed part when P4P is introduced. As more revenue is subject to P4P, more monitoring will likely be required to prevent cheating and improve the measurement accuracy, which reduces unnecessary financial risks to the provider.

Factor 6: Risk premium costs

A risk-averse provider (as most providers are assumed to be) will require a risk premium to participate in the program if the P4P payment is subject to factors beyond the provider's control. And for a given measure and degree of provider's control over that measure, the risk premium will need to increase as the share of compensation subject to P4P increases. The risk premium cost reduces the budget available to purchase health care services, resulting in lower health. A provider's risk can vary substantially, from relatively low risk for clinical quality process measures to higher risk for clinical outcome measures. In Figure 13, the risk premium is assumed to increase at an increasing rate as the share of a provider's revenue based on P4P increases. This shape is based on providers (or workers) being almost risk neutral when the stakes are small and who become more risk averse when a larger proportion of income is at stake (Arrow, 1971; Rabin, 2000).

Factor summation

Two of the aforementioned factors positively affect health: Health-increasing substitution of health care services and inputs as well as provider surplus extraction. Three factors negatively affect health: Decreasing substitution of health care services and inputs, monitoring costs, and risk premium costs. The final factor, net externalities, includes impacts beyond the specific P4P indicators, such as data systems and governance, which could positively or negatively affect health, depending on their benefits and costs. When a health policy maker considers the design of a P4P program, how all six of these factors will respond to the program in the specific health setting need be considered in order to fully understand the potential impact of the program. It is hoped that future research on P4P programs will be able to directly assess the influence of these separate factors on provider behavior in order to develop more optimal P4P program designs suited to the specific context in which it will operate.

Summary of P4P Evidence

There have been various systematic reviews of P4P program effects, and Eijkenaar *et al.* (2013) synthesize the findings from 22 systematic reviews. In OECD countries, there are mixed results of the success of pay for performance programs. Many programs often lack a research design to identify P4P effectiveness, particularly in the long run. Some evidence suggests that incentives were often not strong enough — one US study found that an increase in payments triggered the desired behavioral response while the initial lower payment level did not (Mullen *et al.*, 2010). As the prevalence of P4P programs continues to increase, for both private and public health providers, the emergent evidence base should be far more comprehensive in the future. In LMIC countries, recent years has seen rapid growth in national level P4P programs. The preliminary evidence from a handful of rigorous studies is largely positive but not universally so.

More research is needed to understand how P4P performs in diverse settings and at various levels of the health system. Some tentative conclusions from the Eijkenaar *et al.* (2013) review of systematic reviews concludes that P4P appears to be more effective when incentivized measures have relative room for improvement and are easy to track; when incentives are directed at individual health providers or small groups; when rewards are based on providers absolute performance; and when the program is designed collaboratively with providers.

Little attention till date has been given to possible adverse outcomes such as gaming or reduced intrinsic motivation of health workers. Furthermore there is relatively little research on the cost-effectiveness of P4P programs when compared with alternative uses of the health funds — one recent analysis argues that QOF payments are potentially cost-effective for most of the nine evaluated measures yet the substantial resources embodied in administration costs were not included in this analysis (Walker *et al.*, 2010). Future research will hopefully be able to identify not only the net impact of P4P on health, but also its cost effectiveness and the precise behavioral channels through which P4P is most effective.

P4P Policy Issues and Main Conclusions

P4P programs have been widely introduced across OECD countries, yet the research designs to evaluate them are often inadequate to provide a definitive answer about the effect of P4P programs on quality and costs (Rosenthal *et al.*, 2006).

There are only a handful of examples of rigorously evaluated P4P programs, and one of the first examples comes from a surprising source: The Rwandan P4P Program. The lesson from the Rwanda P4P is not the type of incentives used, but rather the proper approach to evaluation, which allows the isolation of the effect of P4P from other reforms. Indeed, as the Rwandan experience is replicated in other countries, it is likely that soon there will be much better evidence on "what works" for P4P in LMICs than in OECD countries. This evidence will include not only assessments of effectiveness but also cost-effectiveness.

However, even with limited evaluation in OECD countries, the initial results of P4P programs can be promising and have galvanized payers and providers to better measure health care quantity and quality (Rebhun and Williams, 2009). There appears to be growing evidence that incentivizing priority public health interventions like cancer-screening works, and P4P also works in getting physicians to follow evidence-based guidelines for chronic conditions such as diabetes and cardiovascular disease. But there are still challenging measurement and design issues.

Measures of quality of care will improve. Yet this will continue to be a difficult area since quality is multidimensional, includes clinical effectiveness but also patient experience, and outcomes are difficult to measure, particularly for individuals. Basing P4P on ultimate health outcomes presents the additional challenge that they do not appear in the population for a long time. Given these constraints, paying for quality will continue to require better methods of measuring quality of care. Furthermore, the impact of P4P schemes has often been limited because, aside from a few notable exceptions such as the UK QOF, the size of the incentives has been small.

In the LMIC setting, P4P mechanisms can be seen as a form of strategic purchasing by linking payments to defined services or targets. Thus, it has the potential to strengthen national capacity through the collection and analysis of information designed for the purpose of improving population health. However, additional challenges arise in these settings, as many P4P pilots are financed with donor support, and the financial sustainability of these programs are an open question even if they do prove to be an effective tool for health financing. Front line health clinics can grow to depend on P4P as a major source of revenue, especially in countries where P4P is used to formally replace patient user fees. Therefore, financial sustainability remains a key challenge for many P4P programs.

While P4P is intended to deliver improvements in technical and allocative efficiency in the health sector, P4P schemes are not the only means to achieve this. In some areas, an alternative to supply-side incentives is to affect the demand for services. Patient incentive programs are becoming more prevalent, growing out of conditional cash transfer programs developed for education programs, such as those used to encourage school attendance (Fiszbein *et al.*, 2009). The possible gains from combining P4P with demand-side initiatives need to be explored, as well as to what degree these two approaches are substitutable if the health payer is concerned with increasing service quantity (See also Volume 1, Chapter 9 of this Handbook, *Incentivizing Health Care Utilization and Health Outcomes*).

There is still a lot to learn about how and when P4P programs work. What is the ideal level of payment incentive to change provider behavior? Through which causal channels does P4P operate most effectively? How should payments be distributed? If OECD countries currently implementing P4P schemes can organize proper evaluations, then other high-income countries can learn what works, and all countries can benefit from real improvements in health care quality and efficiency in the future.

References

Ariely D, Gneezy U, Loewenstein G, Mazar N. 2009. Large stakes and big mistakes. *The Review of Economic Studies* 76(2): 451–469.

Arrow KJ. 1971. The theory of risk aversion. In *Essays in the Theory of Risk-Bearing*, North-Holland, Amsterdam, pp. 90–120.

Basinga P, Gertler PJ, Binagwaho A, Soucat AL, Sturdy J, Vermeersch CM. 2011. Effect on maternal and child health services in Rwanda of payment to primary health-care providers for performance: An impact evaluation. *The Lancet* 377(9775): 1421–1428.

Bevan G, Hood C. 2006. What's measured is what matters: Targets and gaming in the English public health care system. *Public Administration* 84(3): 517–538.

Borem PE, Alves Valle M, Silva Montiero De Castro R, Kenzou Fujii A, Lioza de Oliviera Farias F, Liete Gastal C, Connor. 2010. *Project Brazilian Pay-for-Performance Case Study.* UNIMED-Belo Horizonte Physician Cooperative. Bethesda, MD: Health System 20/20 Project, Abt Associates.

Borowitz M, Scheffler RM, Fulton B. 2010. Improving value for money in health by paying for performance. *Organisation for Economic Co-Operation and Development. Value for Money in Health Spending*.

Buetow S. 2008. Pay-for-performance in New Zealand primary health care. *Journal of Health Organization and Management* 22(1): 36–47.

Campbell SM, Reeves D, Kontopantelis E, Sibbald B, Roland M. 2009. Effects of pay for performance on the quality of primary care in England. *New England Journal of Medicine* 361(4): 368–378.

Casalino L, Elster A, Eisenberg A, Lewis E, Montgomery J, Ramos D. 2007. Will pay-for-performance and quality reporting affect health care disparities? *Health Affairs* 26(3): 405–414.

Cashin C, Chi Y, Smith P, Borowitz M, Thomson S. 2014. Paying for performance in health care. Implications for health system performance and accountability. Open University Press, European Observatory on Health Systems and Policies Series. [Online] Available: Http://www.euro.who.int/en/about-us/partners/observatory/publications/studies/paying-for-performance-in-health-care.-implications-for-health-system-performance-and-accountability.

Chansa C, Das A, Qamruddin J, Friedman J, Mkandawire A, Vledder M. 2015. Linking results to performance: Evidence from a results based financing pre-pilot project in Katete District, Zambia. *Discussion Paper No*. 98265, The World Bank.

Chaudhury N, Hammer J, Kremer M, Muralidharan K, Rogers FH. 2006. Missing in action: Teacher and health worker absence in developing countries. *The Journal of Economic Perspectives* 20(1): 91–116.

Deci EL. 1971. Effects of externally mediated rewards on intrinsic motivation. *Journal of Personality and Social Psychology* 18(1): 105.

Deci EL, Koestner R, Ryan RM. 1999. A meta-analytic review of experiments examining the effects of extrinsic rewards on intrinsic motivation. *Psychological Bulletin* 125(6): 627.

Di Tella R, Schargrodsky E. 2003. The role of wages and auditing during a crackdown on corruption in the city of Buenos Aires. *Journal of Law and Economics* 46(1): 269–292.

Dixon A, Khachatryan A, Walace A, Peckham S, Boyce T, Gillam S. 2011. The Quality and Outcomes Framework (QOF): Does it reduce health inequalities? *Final Report*. NIHR Service Delivery and Organisation Programme.

Donabedian A. 2005. Evaluating the quality of medical care. *Milbank Quarterly* 83(4): 691–729.

Doran T, Fullwood C, Gravelle H, Reeves D, Kontopantelis E, Hiroeh U, Roland M. 2006. Pay-for-performance programs in family practices in the United Kingdom. *New England Journal of Medicine* 355(4): 375–384.

Eijkenaar F, Emmert M, Scheppach M, Schöffski O. 2013. Effects of pay for performance in health care: A systematic review of systematic reviews. *Health Policy* 110(2): 115–130.

Fiszbein A, Schady NR, Ferreira FH. 2009. *Conditional Cash Transfers: Reducing Present and Future Poverty*. World Bank Publications.

Frakt AB, Mayes R. 2012. Beyond capitation: How new payment experiments seek to find the 'sweet spot' in amount of risk providers and payers bear. *Health Affairs* 31(9): 1951–1958.

Frey BS, Goette L. 1999. *Does Pay Motivate Volunteers?* University of Zurich, Institute for Empirical Research in Economics.

Friedman J, Mutasa R, Mafaune P, Nyameru R, Das A. Forthcoming. The Impact of Zimbabwe's Health Results Based Financing National Pilot on Utilization and Quality of Care. *World Bank Policy Research Working Paper.*

Galvin R. 2006. Pay-for-performance: Too much of a good thing? A conversation with Martin Roland. *Health Affairs* 25(5): W412–W419.

Gertler PJ, Giovagnoli PI. 2014. Rewarding provider performance to enable a healthy start to life: Evidence from Argentina's Plan Nacer. *World Bank Policy Research Working Paper*, (6884).

Gneezy U, Rustichini A. 2000. Fine is a price. *Journal of Legal Studies*, *29*, 1.

Gravelle H, Sutton M, Ma A. 2010. Doctor Behaviour under a pay for performance contract: Treating, cheating and case finding? *The Economic Journal* 120(542): F129–F156.

Holmstrom B, Milgrom P. 1991. Multitask principal–agent analyses: Incentive contracts, asset ownership, and job design. *Journal of Law, Economics, & Organization* 7: 24–52.

Huillery E, Seban J. 2014. *Performance-Based Financing, Motivation and Final Output in the Health Sector: Experimental Evidence from the Democratic Republic of Congo* (No. 2014–12). SciencesPo Department of Economics.

Ireland M, Paul E, Dujardin B. 2011. Can performance-based financing be used to reform health systems in developing countries? *Bulletin of the World Health Organization* 89(9): 695–698.

James J. 2012. Health policy brief: Pay-for-performance, *Health Affairs.* [Online] Available: Http://www.healthaffairs.org/healthpolicybriefs/brief.php?brief_id=78.

Kleven HJ, Knudsen MB, Kreiner CT, Pedersen S, Saez E. 2011. Unwilling or unable to cheat? Evidence from a tax audit experiment in Denmark. *Econometrica* 79(3): 651–692.

Lazear EP. 2000. Performance pay and productivity. *The American Economic Review* 90(5): 1346–1361.

Maisey S, Steel N, Marsh R, Gillam S, Fleetcroft R, Howe A. 2008. Effects of payment for performance in primary care: Qualitative interview study. *Journal of Health Services Research & Policy* 13(3): 133–139.

Martin, Jenkins and Associates Limited 2008. *Evaluation of the PHO Performance Programme: Final Report.* Martin, Jenkins and Associates Limited: Auckland.

Mullen KJ, Frank RG, Rosenthal MB. 2010. Can you get what you pay for? Pay-for-performance and the quality of healthcare providers. *RAND Journal of Economics* 41(1): 64–91.

Paris V, Devaux M, Wei L. 2010. *Health Systems Institutional Characteristics: A Survey of 29 OECD Countries*, *OECD Health Working Papers*, No. 50, OECD Publishing.

Porter S. 2008. Preliminary Report Offers First Glimpse of Quality Reporting Progress, AAFP. Available at: www.aafp.org/online/en/home/publications/news/news-now/practice-management/20080305pqrireport.html.

Rabin M. 2000. Risk aversion and expected-utility theory: A calibration theorem. *Econometrica* 68(5): 1281–1292.

Rebhun D, Williams T. 2009. The California pay for performance programme: The second chapter measurement years 2006–2009. *California: Integrated Healthcare Association.*

Robinson J, Williams T, Yanagihara D. 2009. Measurement of and reward for efficiency in California's pay-for-performance program. *Health Affairs* 28(5): 1438–1447.

Rosenthal MB, Landon B, Normand ST, Frank R, Epstein A. 2006. Pay for performance in commercial HMOs. *The New England Journal of Medicine* 355: 1895–1902.

Rosenthal MB, Dudley RA. 2007. Pay-for-performance: Will the latest payment trend improve care? *Journal of the American Medical Association* 297(7): 740–744.

Savedoff WD, Partner S. 2010. Basic economics of results-based financing in heath. *Results-Based Financing for Health.* Washington, DC: World Bank. http://www.rbfhealth. org/ rbfhealth/system/files/RBF% 20Economics.pdf.

Scheffler RM. 2008. *Is there a Doctor in the House?: Market Signals and Tomorrow's Supply of Doctors.* Stanford University Press.

Scheffler R. 2010a. Pay for Performance (P4P) Programs in Health Services: What is the Evidence? *World Health Report (2010) Background Paper*, 31.

Scheffler R. 2010b. Improving Value for Money in Health by Paying for Performance. In *OECD Health Policy Studies Value for Money in Health Spending* (pp. 105–122). OECD Publishing.

Sekabaraga C, Diop F, Soucat A. 2011. Can innovative health financing policies increase access to MDG-related services? Evidence from Rwanda. *Health Policy and Planning* 26(Suppl. 2): ii52–ii62.

Tanenbaum SJ. 2009. Pay for performance in Medicare: Evidentiary irony and the politics of value. *Journal of Health Politics, Policy and Law* 34(5): 717–746.

Trisolini M, Aggarwal J, Leung M, Pope G, Kautter J. 2008. The Medicare Physician Group Practice Demonstration: Lessons learned on improving quality and efficiency in health care. *The Commonwealth Fund.*

Uptom WE. 1973. *Altruism, Attribution, and Intrinsic Motivation in the Recruitment of Blood Donors* (Doctoral dissertation, Cornell University, August).

Walker S, Mason AR, Claxton K, Cookson R, Fenwick E, Fleetcroft R, Sculpher M. 2010. Value for money and the quality and outcomes framework in primary care in the UK NHS. *British Journal of General Practice* 60(574): e213–e220.

Weibel A, Rost K, Osterloh M. 2010. Pay for performance in the public sector — Benefits and (hidden) costs. *Journal of Public Administration Research and Theory* 20(2): 387–412.

Witter S, Fretheim A, Kessy FL, Lindahl AK. 2012. Paying for performance to improve the delivery of health interventions in low- and middle-income countries. *Cochrane Database of System Reviews* 2(2): CD007899.

Yegian J, Yanagihara D. 2013. Value based pay for performance in California. *Integrated Healthcare Association*, Issue No. 8, pp. 1–5.

Medical Tourism

Johanna Hanefeld and Richard Smith
London School of Hygiene and Tropical Medicine
Thinakorn Noree
International Health Policy Program, Ministry of Public Health, Nonthaburi

The past 10 to 15 years has seen a substantial rise in the number (or at least the perception) of patients traveling for medical treatment, often to exotic or long-haul destinations; it is this latter element that has lent popular press especially to use the somewhat pejorative term *medical tourism.* A rapid increase in research focused on the issue over the past five years suggest a more complex and nuanced medical tourism market, including specific regional patterns and a rise in South-to-South medical tourism, than previously assumed. Despite the rise in medical tourism and concomitant interest in the issue, there are no formal mechanism for monitoring the volume and flows of medical tourists. At the same time, no international regulation or standards exist safeguarding patients who travel. As a result, data on economic and health systems impact has been limited to date. Equally, understanding of industry structure, patient motivation and experiences is partial. This chapter explores the available empirical evidence on medical tourism, depicts its rise and considers data from recent research by the authors, on Thailand and on the United Kingdom, to investigate the shape and impact of medical tourism today.

Keywords: Medical Tourism; Trade in Health Services; Health Systems; Thailand; UK.

Introduction

Patients traveling for medical treatment is not a new phenomenon. During the 18th and 19th centuries, wealthy Europeans would travel to 'take the waters' in spa towns in Hungary, the Crimea region and other places. Looking back even further, even in antiquity people would travel to consult healers or spiritual leaders in search of health and cure (Smith and Puczko, 2009). Thus, the fundamental principle of people traveling to access treatment is not new (Connell, 2008).

Yet, the past 10 to 15 years has seen a substantial rise in the number (or at least the perception) of patients traveling for medical treatment, often to exotic or long-haul destinations; it is this latter element that has lent popular press especially to use the somewhat pejorative term *medical tourism,* which we define here as patients traveling abroad with the explicit intention of seeking medical treatment and with the intention to pay for it. Several countries, including Thailand, Singapore and India have positioned themselves as providers of health care to incoming patients (Noree *et al.*, 2014; Chanda, 2011). Trade in health services, including medical tourism (termed the consumption of medical services abroad) is covered by the World Trade Organizations' (WTO) General Agreement on Trade in Services (GATS), which also covers telemedicine, foreign direct investment in health and the movement of health workers (Smith *et al.*, 2009). GATS provide a formal framework under which health services can be traded. Countries which sign up to GATS agree to open their health sector to trade under conditions set out by the WTO, which include general non-discrimination rules for foreign investors and overall provide the reassurance of an international regulatory framework of the WTO. Simply put, GATS is intended to regulate and simplify trade in health services, including medical tourism, by providing overall guidance for trade. However, it is important to note that GATS is very general and does not focus specifically on health trade, thus it does not extend to any specific regulation of the content of services traded, for example quality of health services provided, or patient safety.

Although there is a perception of a vast increase in patients traveling to obtain health care, reliable estimates of the numbers of patients traveling are scarce, as patients often travel outside the public sector and organize their own travel. However, case-study data certainly point to an increase in medical tourism over the past decade, even if it is not to the magnitude that some (often industry-sponsored) reports suggest (Hanefeld *et al.*, 2013a; Lunt *et al.*, 2014). The availability of cheaper air travel allowing patients to travel with relative ease and at low cost, paired with greater communication through the internet which allows providers from one country to directly market themselves to patients in another have been cited as reasons for this observed increase (Lunt *et al.*, 2010). Other key features associated with medical tourism have been the concurrent rise and growth of mass consumerism, a greater emphasis on patient choice, and increasing financial constraints on public health systems. As a result of these characteristics, medical tourism has been portrayed very much as a 'sun, sand and surgery' phenomenon where empowered consumers from high-income countries travel to access cheaper health services in low and middle income countries (Lunt *et al.*, 2013; Mazzaschi, 2011; Imison and Schweinsberg, 2013). Wealthy patients from the Gulf States — Bahrain, Kuwait, Oman, Qatar, Saudi Arabia, and United Arab

Emirates — have also represented a visible section of the medical tourism market, with patients either traveling to access treatment farther afield for higher quality (Lunt and Mannion, 2014), or within the region to access treatment not available within their own countries (Siddiqi *et al.*, 2010).

Yet, despite these perceptions of medical tourism, there is increasing evidence of a more complex and nuanced medical tourism market (Connell, 2013). Several scholars have highlighted the issues of patient mobility within the European Union (EU) (Legido-Quigley *et al.*, 2012; Glinos *et al.*, 2012), where legal challenges relating to patients' travel between different national health systems have led to an EU Directive on patient mobility (Legido-Quigley *et al.*, 2011). The Directive regulates medical travel between Member States and it stipulates that EU citizens have the right to seek treatment in an EU Member State other than the country where they are ordinarily resident. However, the Directive also provides several important caveats. These include that treatment must be shown to be unavailable within a reasonable timeframe at home and receiving treatment in another Member State has to be agreed in on in advance by the patients' resident health system. The Directive has come into force in late 2013, and given the different conditions for patients seeking treatment, the extent to which it will lead to an increase in patients traveling is yet unclear. It is worthy to note that the Directive does not deal with emergency care i.e., when an EU citizen accidentally falls sick while in another EU Member State, this is provided for separately.

Other research has highlighted the regional nature of medical tourism (Osterle *et al.*, 2009). For example, US citizens may be more likely to travel to Costa Rica for cosmetic surgery, while UK patients may seek similar procedures in Poland or other European countries, Austrian patients seek dental care in Hungary, while Chinese travel for plastic surgery to South Korea. This is clearly not the only determinant of medical travel as patients do travel long distances as well in search for treatment. However, these regional patterns suggest geographic proximity can be a factor in decision to travel for treatment (Hanefeld *et al.,* 2015). Research also suggests an increase in South-to-South medical tourism which has been largely ignored or underreported to date (Crush and Chikanda, 2015; Crush, 2012; Ormond, 2013). These findings highlight that in addition to the more commonly perceived consumers traveling in search for better or more affordable treatment from high to middle and low-income countries, there is equally an increased movement of people from low-income and middle-income countries in search of treatment unavailable to them in their country. In sum, medical tourism refers to a wide spectrum of patients traveling in search for treatment.

This chapter will explore the current period of medical tourism, setting out its shape, size and specific characteristics. Initially drawing on current literature to identify a clear definition of medical tourism vis-a-vis other forms of patient mobility, the chapter then outlines the role of marketing and communication in medical travel, patient experiences, including risks and types of procedures for which patients travel, and patient motivation and health system effects.

Definitions

As evident from the background, mobility relating to treatment may in some cases be distinct from the phenomenon of medical tourism. Different scholars have offered a variety of definitions relating to the travel of patients or treatment of patients who are not normally resident in the country where they are treated, and these are often fluid. Medical tourism excludes several categories of people receiving treatment abroad, including expatriates (people temporarily resident in another countries where they may require and receive medical care), and tourists visiting a holiday destination who fall ill and as a result require medical treatment (usually by accident and/or emergency).

The term cross-border medical care often refers more narrowly to patients traveling across borders within a single geographic region, which may be governed by a formal agreement for reciprocal care. For example, within the European Union pilot initiatives have explored how tertiary facilities could provide care regionally, even where this may cross a national boundary (Wismar *et al.*, 2011). Equally, cross-border care is a term often used when referring to the clinics along the Mexican–United States border, which serve Mexican migrants to the US who return to Mexico to access medical care (Horton and Cole, 2011). While definitions of cross-border care overlap with those of medical tourism — for example, Wismar *et al.* offer a definition for cross-border care identical to medical tourism — where people speak of cross-border medical care, this often refers to care within a region that encompasses more than one country and medical tourism to patients moving across regions, although there is clearly overlap between the two terms.

Moreover, most medical tourism research distinguishes between medical tourism and health and wellness tourism — commonly seen as excluding actual medical treatment and relating more to spa treatments. Over the past year, health tourism has in some instances been used to refer to patients traveling with the intention of obtaining treatment they may not be entitled to for free in an illicit manner (Arie, 2013). This kind of perceived 'welfare scrounging' has formed part of public policy debates within the EU with the term *health tourists* being used to differentiate those wishing to obtain services illicitly for free from *medical tourists* who are seeking services with the intention to pay (Hanefeld *et al.*, 2013b).

Others have emphasized the intent of travel for treatment as important in definitions of medical tourism (Thompson, 2011). Researchers in particular from the fields of anthropology and sociology have referred to *medical migrants* where patients travel in search of treatments not available to them in their country of origin. This lack of availability may relate to high regulation of the treatment or lack of expertise in their home country. Common examples are where patients travel for experimental treatments such as stem cell therapy, or treatments associated with gender reassignment (Thompson, 2008). *Medical migrants* or *medical migration* are terms used to accentuate a lack of choice by some patients who travel in search of treatment. Academic literature has highlighted these as distinct to the consumerist element that is captured in many definitions of *medical tourism*.

In sum, there is a relatively common definitional use of the term medical tourism which refers to patients traveling abroad with the explicit intention of seeking medical treatment and with the intention to pay for it.

Marketing and Communication

Medical tourism, to a large extent, takes place where individuals choose to travel to purchase services from a private provider (Hanefeld *et al.*, 2014). As a result, communication and marketing, specifically through the internet, has played a central role in the development of the medical tourism industry, including by enabling private providers to market themselves to patients in other countries (Lunt *et al.*, 2010).

Communication and marketing in medical tourism serves several functions. Many patients — including potential medical tourists — go online to seek either diagnosis, information or a second opinion while also considering going abroad (Lunt and Carrera, 2011). Given this function, the lines between advice, information and marketing are often blurred. A key role here is that of web-based support forums, where future and past patients come together to discuss benefits of treatment. In many cases, patients also discuss and recommend physicians and clinics. This informal feedback, an electronic 'word of mouth' function, is critical to medical tourism as there is no clear system of accreditation, quality control or referral. As a result, providers seek to market themselves online to patient and support groups.

In addition to information and web-based forums is providers' direct marketing to patients, with many clinics and hospitals having a website or online presence directly aimed at attracting patients from abroad. Reviews of websites marketing medical tourism have been conducted by several researchers (Nassab *et al.*, 2010; Lunt and Carrera, 2011; Horsfall *et al.*, 2013). Common findings from across these studies include the limited attention the websites give to follow-up care (as low as 4%) and risks associated with procedures (Mason and

Wright, 2011). Moreover, websites aimed at attracting patients from abroad often provide information on logistics such as accommodation and transport. Findings also highlight that accreditation or qualifications of clinicians, while listed in some cases, take less prominence than the testimonies of past patients.

Personal recommendations are a key feature of the medical tourism industry in the absence of clear global regulation or quality indicators, and these inform the industry's structure. A specific, common component of this is the medical tourism facilitator (Snyder *et al.*, 2011). These are brokers situated in the patients' country of origin, who organize logistics, liaise with patients and facilitate their treatment. In very many cases these are themselves former patients (Lunt *et al.*, 2013; Holliday *et al.*, 2013) who then begin working for a clinic to help identify further patients. The role of these brokers or facilitators ranges from organizing the travel and treatment to taking on roles closer to friends or treatment buddies, who in some cases can act as an important cultural bridge for the patients when abroad.

Linkages between clinicians in both origin and destination countries are an additional bridge between potential patients and providers. For example, clinics and providers abroad may offer an initial consultation or follow-up through a clinician in the country where patients' originate. In several cases, providers of medical tourism based abroad also recruit through their networks, often gained where they may have trained or have worked for a period. For example, where a doctor from India may have practiced or worked in the United Kingdom (UK) in the past, this often provides a link to a UK clinic which then refers private patients to him or her (Lunt *et al.*, 2013). While this is not practice within the public sector, such as the UK NHS, it is more common where patients seek private care in their home country.

Patient Experiences, Histories, Risks and Disease

Recent research findings have highlighted that industry structure and specificity also exist, depending on the types of treatment for which patients travel (Hanefeld *et al.*, 2015). While many countries have sought to attract medical tourists for high-end procedures, including heart and orthopedic surgery (Leng, 2010; Pachanee and Wibulpolprasert, 2006), actual evidence of patient data of medical tourists who have traveled remains limited, albeit some new data from Thailand is now forthcoming (see discussion later in the chapter). Where evidence is available, it suggests that common treatment types for which patients travel include cosmetic and bariatric surgery, fertility treatment and dentistry, as well as more high-end, specialist procedures. Closer examination of tourists traveling by treatment type reveals distinct industry characteristics and differing motivations for patients in their decisions to travel for treatment.

For example, recent research on patients traveling for dental treatment from the UK, highlighted that this appeared to have been primarily motivated by the cheaper cost of treatment abroad, greater perceived availability of treatment in other countries as well as perceived greater expertise by dentists abroad (Hanefeld *et al.*, 2015). This confirms the earlier research on dental tourists in Europe, which identified Hungary as a destination seen to combine quality and availability of dentists at low cost (Osterle *et al.*, 2009).

This contrasts with patients who travel for fertility treatment. Published literature highlights fertility tourism as an area for which people travel and which has attracted attention by scholars exploring different aspects of medical tourism, including patient motivation (Hanefeld *et al.*, 2014; Inhorn, 2011; Whittaker and Speier, 2010; Culley *et al.*, 2011). There seem to be several 'regional' markets for fertility tourism, with patients in the EU traveling to Spain or Eastern Europe and others, including patients from North America, traveling to India for surrogacy (Whittaker and Speier, 2010). Despite geographic differences, fertility tourists commonly travel: to access gametes (donor sperm or oocytes) which may not be available in their country of residence or to circumvent regulations that may limit or prohibit treatments they are able to receive under law. For example, in France same-sex couples are legally prohibited to have fertility treatment, leading to many female same-sex couples to travel to neighboring Belgium to access donor sperm (Van Hoof *et al.*, 2015). This includes patients seeking to avoid age or medical restrictions on fertility treatment, or patients seeking certain treatments that are not available to specific sections of the population based on religious or societal grounds (Culley *et al.*, 2011; Inhorn, 2011). It extends to patients seeking gamete donations from individuals from shared ethnic or religious backgrounds. For example, patients from the Middle East may travel for anonymity, but also specifically seek Middle Eastern donors (Inhorn, 2011). In some cases, research also highlighted the search for anonymity as one of the factors motivating fertility tourists' travel. In addition to availability, regulation and the search for anonymity, cost also was highlighted as a key factor in determining the final destination of fertility tourists (Culley *et al.*, 2011).

Medical tourism is often associated or portrayed in popular media in relation to cosmetic procedures, specifically exploring aspects of consumer culture and tourism (Holliday *et al.*, 2013; Lunt *et al.*, 2010). This is likely to be because the majority of cosmetic surgery procedures are elective, and therefore most readily fit into the image of medical tourism as a commercial phenomenon. Where empirical research has been conducted, this does suggest that cosmetic patients travel for treatment and that the cost of treatment plays an important role in motivating people to travel abroad (Smith *et al.*, 2012; Nassab *et al.*, 2010; Noree *et al.*, 2014). Recent research focused on outbound UK medical tourists highlighted that, in many cases, cosmetic tourism represented the first journey abroad for patients (Holliday *et al.*, 2015).

Bariatric surgery is a further procedure where evidence suggests patients travel abroad to access treatment (Hanefeld *et al.*, 2015; Snyder and Crooks, 2010). Motivation here, similar to the cosmetic tourists, does relate to cost, as bariatric surgery is still often considered an elective procedure (NCEPOD, 2012; Birch *et al.*, 2010). In addition, as bariatric surgery is a comparatively new field of practice in many countries, research identified expertise of the surgeon in particular as a motivating factor for why patients travel for bariatric surgery (Hanefeld *et al.*, 2015).

While treatment-specific motivation emerges from the medical travel literature, other factors, such as proximity and trust, also appear important. These factors are in particular evident in explaining why people from minority groups or migrants may travel to return to their country of origin to access treatment and care (Lee *et al.*, 2010; Laugesen and Vargas-Bustamante, 2010). These 'diaspora patients' may be motivated by lower cost, but many cases may choose to travel at personal expense to access treatment available to them for free in their country of origin.

So, while there are clear differences in motivation of patients to travel, mainly related to the type of treatment sought by patients, factors such as cost, availability and expertise are common across conditions, even where these are weighed differently. Glinos *et al.* summarized these motivations into a framework explaining patient movement based on availability, affordability, familiarity and perceived quality of health care services (Glinos *et al.*, 2010).

Beyond providing an explanation for patient travel, understanding their motivation has been critical to understanding the structure of the medical tourism industry (Hanefeld *et al.*, 2015). Given the unregulated and informal nature of the industry, personal networks have emerged in several studies recently published as essential to understanding why patients chose a particular provider and why certain providers work in specific medical tourism destinations (Lunt *et al.*, 2014; Holliday *et al.*, 2015; Hanefeld *et al.*, 2015). These different studies highlighted how networks of former and prospective patients are critical to patients traveling, for example, for cosmetic and bariatric surgery. They not only provide the opportunity for exchange of practical information, such as recommendations of a specific provider (Hanefeld *et al.*, 2015), but also act as a source of information, by sharing their lived experience of treatment abroad, for patients considering treatment (Holliday *et al.*, 2015). Social media and the ongoing support provided by current and former patients appear particularly important in fertility treatments and cosmetic and bariatric surgery. For these treatments and procedures, the information function fulfilled by these personal, often online networks is particularly important as patients may not have been in prior contact with physicians in their country of origin but rather decide on a course of treatment at least in part as a result of the information they received online. Clinics and providers seeking to attract tourists from abroad have tapped into this by recruiting or collaborating with former patients to become facilitators.

Countries such as Thailand and Malaysia that seek to promote themselves as medical tourism destinations may also have formal facilitators in key source countries, who arrange the logistics of treatment and travel for patients (Snyder *et al.*, 2011). However, the role of the patient facilitator is a distinct feature of the industry, even though the role may vary by type of treatment.

Lunt and colleagues identified three types of medical tourism market structure: (a) consumer-driven, where an individual patient decides on a selected provider based on information, for example, through the internet, and arranges travel and treatment by themselves; (b) facilitator-enabled, where a facilitator or broker manages the details of treatment and travel; and (c) networked provision, which is the more integrated type of medical tourism where former patients or facilitators have a role linking support to the provision of treatment, i.e., providing a blurring between patient and provider and adding the social relation as a key element (Lunt *et al.*, 2013).

Risks and Regulation

Risk of complication is inherent in all medical treatment and care. However, there are specific risks associated with patients travelling to access services in another country. These risks are particularly important to consider when examining the economic impact of medical tourism and patient welfare. Risks include malpractice and medical complications, which often emerge after a patient has returned to their country of origin. There are reports of complications from cosmetic surgery experienced by patients who traveled abroad for treatment, who then needed follow-up treatment after they returned home to address those complications (Miyagi *et al.*, 2012). This issue came into focus in Europe at the end of 2011, when a French company had to recall faulty breast implants that were found to have an unusually high rupture rate, resulting in a high number of patients resident in countries other than France affected by the recall. In the UK alone, it was estimated that around 42,000 women required removal of faulty implants, paid for by the public health system. This scandal highlighted the risks involved, the costs that can arise for the public health system from patients traveling abroad to access treatment privately, and it gave an indication of the scale of the issue (Smith *et al.*, 2012).

In addition, risks may be confounded by language barriers, as patients may have a more limited understanding of the information they are being presented when they speak a different language than the provider (and, similarly, providers may have more difficulty understanding the patient). This can also extend to patient records, which may be incomplete or in a different language, making it harder for clinicians treating returning medical tourists to adequately address complications (Crooks *et al.*, 2010). When complications require further treatment, it is also likely to incur additional costs, and here further challenges arise. In the absence of clear regulation or reciprocal agreement, redress through legal systems is a challenge and in many cases not a realistic avenue for patients to seek compensation for the costs of medical complications (Vick, 2012). Additional risks are posed where patients who travel act as vectors of disease. Several cases of disease outbreaks have been documented related to a returning medical tourism patient, including an outbreak of NDM1 bacteria in the UK and a separate unrelated outbreak due to a medical tourist in Singapore (Kumarasamy *et al.*, 2010; Rogers *et al.*, 2011). While these are isolated cases of reported problems, and it is not clear whether medical tourists have a higher risk than average travelers, of contracting and then spreading an infection, they demonstrate broader risks to public health that can result from medical tourism.

What these risks, as well as the experiences of patients who have traveled, underline is the absence of clear international regulation and guidance governing medical tourism or associated industries. There are some international bodies, foremost the Joint Commission International (JCI), that offer accreditation for facilities providing services for patients from other countries. However, these are not governmental or intergovernmental bodies, but commercial ventures that offer accreditation at a comparatively high cost, which makes it an unfeasible standard for smaller providers, such as individual clinics, seeking to attract medical tourists. A review of provider websites offering medical tourism services highlighted that the vast majority of these providers were not accredited to an international standard (Horsfall *et al.*, 2013). In addition to a lack of regulation of actual facilities, there is currently no restriction on advertisements by providers or on the information they must provide, for example, in relation to the risks or aftercare that must be provided. This is a clear gap in regulation given the inherent information asymmetry between doctors and patients (Lunt *et al.*, 2013).

Health System Effect

Overall, data on actual system level effects of medical tourism on systems, such as income, health workers, and patients is not available or collected in a systematic way. However, there are a small number of case studies which have explored this, focused on the economic and equity effects of medical tourism for destination countries (Lautier, 2008; NaRanong and NaRanong, 2011; Siddiqi *et al.*, 2010). There are several ways in which medical tourism impacts the health systems of originating and destination countries. Where data exist, these suggest a small positive effect of medical tourism on GDP growth and suggest a negative effect in terms of equity of recipient country health systems as health workers move from public sector provision to serve incoming patients in the private sector at higher wages. Medical tourism has also been seen to raise the cost of treatment where out-of-pocket payments exist, as medical tourists have the ability to pay higher fees. This has shown to increase fees for service overall (NaRanong and NaRanong, 2011). These issues have come into focus particularly where the flow of medical tourism has been from comparatively rich countries in the North to poorer countries in the South, which may be facing pre-existing health system challenges, such as health worker shortages. Such potentially negative effects of course have to be balanced against the overall economic benefits from medical tourists' health and tourism expenditures.

On the other hand, medical tourism may help use excess capacity within health systems or help improve learning curves and specialization in countries with smaller populations. Additionally, medical tourism has been seen by recipient country governments as a way of raising foreign currency reserves, such as in the case of Thailand (Pachanee and Wibulpolprasert, 2006). However, no data exist on whether governments which aimed to raise foreign exchange through medical tourism have reinvested such capital into their health systems.

Attention and research on the health system effects of medical tourism on origin countries (where patients come *from*) has primarily concentrated on the risks related to infection and complications, as indicated above. A series of papers published in medical journals has reported outcomes from patients who have traveled for treatment. These included the rate of complications and the costs that arose from medical emergencies that had to be addressed by the public health systems in the patients' countries of origin (Miyagi *et al.*, 2012; McKelvey *et al.*, 2009; Melendez and Alizadeh, 2011; Hanefeld *et al.*, 2013a). However, little consideration has been given to the cost savings arising from patients traveling abroad, including savings on future health care expenditure.

The potential for medical tourism to have both negative and positive impacts on health systems highlights the importance of considering and actively planning for medical tourism rather than leaving it to unmanaged organic growth. This raises questions of governance, including whether, for example, specific and regulated bilateral trade may be a way to harness such positive potential while controlling for the potential risks (Martinez Alvarez *et al.*, 2011). Governance and the management of medical tourism with a view to maximizing positive health system impacts has thus far only been researched to a limited extent and remains underexplored.

Case Study: UK Medical Tourists

The UK, like many publicly-funded universal health care systems has, over the past decade, experienced a series of contractions in its funding base, resulting in increased rationing of services that are available for free to its citizens through its National Health Service (NHS) (Pollock *et al.*, 2012). The UK, as a center of clinical excellence with a long-standing history of private medicine in places such as Harley Street, has historically also been a destination for patients seeking medical care. This has included wealthy patients from the Middle East and Gulf States visiting the UK for treatment (Lunt *et al.*, 2014). The squeeze in public finance has meant that, since the 1990s, government policy has progressively focused on the expansion and potential for income from marketing the NHS globally, including famous specialized hospitals such as Great Ormond Street Hospital for Sick Children or Moorfields Eye Hospital. This has generated initiatives such as the global arm of the NHS — *NHS Global-*, partnering with hospitals in the Middle East to attract patients and generate funding (Lunt *et al.*, 2014). Recent changes in UK legislation that support these efforts include lifting a previously imposed cap on private patient numbers, making it possible for hospitals to increasingly attract medical tourists as private patients paying for private services received within the NHS (Hanefeld *et al.*, 2013a).

At the same time, increasing waiting times and increasing mobility may be a contributing factor to the trend of UK patients traveling abroad to access treatment. Analysis of the International Passenger Survey, a survey conducted with a random sample of passengers entering and exiting the UK, revealed that over the past decade, a growing number of patients have traveled to access treatment abroad, with an estimated 63,000 patients leaving the UK for treatment in 2010, up from a suggested less than 10,000 a decade earlier (Hanefeld *et al.*, 2013a). The increasing number of patients traveling abroad from the UK appears corroborated by reports and case studies by UK physicians reporting treatment of complications in returning medical tourists in recent years (McKelvey *et al.*, 2009; Miyagi *et al.*, 2012). Authors analyzed available data to estimate the costs and savings the UK NHS has realized due to medical tourism, focusing on key areas for which UK patients are seeking treatment abroad, such as cosmetic, bariatric and fertility treatment. The analysis was informed by qualitative interviews with 77 UK patients who had traveled abroad for treatment. Authors calculated the NHS costs incurred from treating complications that arose from services that UK residents received through medical tourism. It included the savings from patients who traveled for treatment which they would have ordinarily been entitled to in the UK, and savings from likely future health and social care expenditures where data were available. The results highlighted a net cost resulting from UK fertility tourists who traveled abroad for treatment (Hanefeld *et al.*, 2013a), due in large part to clinical data from the UK showing an increase in multiple births among patients returning from treatment abroad when compared to the UK (McKelvey *et al.*, 2009). These, in turn, are associated with higher rates of complications during pregnancy and an increased need for medical care during pregnancy. Equally, cosmetic tourism, which in the UK is mostly not funded through the public health system, resulted in a costs, as patients return with complications such as infections (Miyagi *et al.*, 2012). On the other hand, research revealed that bariatric patients frequently traveled for surgery, which likely resulted in net savings both in terms of health expenditure and in terms of future costs averted (Hanefeld *et al.*, 2013a).

The assessment of economic impact of outbound medical tourism on the NHS is based on case study evidence and restricted to one health system. Yet, it highlights the potential for medical tourism to have both positive and negative health system impacts. These findings suggest that medical tourism should be one option considered by health system planners and decision-makers when thinking about financing and efficient use of capacity. Rather than focusing solely on potential negative effects, these findings suggest possible positive consequences as well.

Case study: Thailand

Thailand has marketed itself as a medical tourism center since 2003 and is considered one of the world's foremost destinations for medical tourism. The reason for this heavy promotion of foreign patients is that they are a significant source of foreign earnings. For instance, NaRanong *et al.* estimated that revenues from medical tourists would be the equivalent of 0.4% of Thailand's gross domestic product. However, there is considerable concern expressed within the health community about such expansions of services for foreign patients, both within Thailand and amongst the global health community more generally. Concerns have focused on the equity impact of medical tourism in destination countries, where health systems may be weak and limited resources are diverted toward care for lucrative patients from abroad. Past research from Thailand has revealed a negative impact on equity through health workers moving into the private sector and an increase in fee-for-service as public sector prices follow increased fees in the private sector.

Estimates by the Thai government, which have been widely reported, have suggested that more than 1 million international patients visit Thailand per year.

To better understand and further assess this issue, the authors undertook a cross-sectional survey of all medical tourists in five private Thai hospitals, comprising 911,913 electronic patient records. Hospitals were purposively selected, and account for 63% of international patients visiting Thailand. This is the first ever and largest study globally assessing medical tourism based on actual patient data (Noree *et al.*, forthcoming 2016).

Results of the research indicate that only 167,000 medical tourists visited Thailand in 2010. Also contrary to popular opinion, only 30% of medical tourists were from high-income countries in North America and Europe (most were from the Middle East and South East Asia), and most patients traveled for small procedures rather than major and expensive surgery. Medical tourists were also shown to be particularly profitable, spending significantly more on tourism activities than regular tourists. No negative consequences for the health system were identified.

The results of this recent work are in some ways surprising: there were fewer tourists, fewer tourists from high-income countries commonly assumed to be source countries, and no large-scale negative effects on the health system. It also underlines the nuance emerging from the research. A greater number of patients are traveling from middle- and low-income countries, regional trends are present in the medical tourism market, and current data limitations have limited our understanding of the impact of medical tourism on health systems.

Conclusion

Having examined the different facets of medical tourism, it is evident that data limitations — mainly due to a lack of regulation and the fact that medical tourism primarily takes place in the private sector — pose limits to the ability to quantify the volume and direction of medical tourism. This restricts a full assessment of the economic contribution of medical tourism to destination countries' economies and of its health system impacts. It also limits the extent to which policymakers can plan to minimize negative effects and maximize positive effects of patients traveling for treatment.

Yet, a rapidly growing body of scholarship highlights several clear trends, directions for further research and — most importantly — areas for policy action. Where data exist, it points to clear growth in the number of patients traveling for treatment. Even if closer examination of available sources seems to indicate that some estimates cited within the literature provide an inflated picture, medical tourism looks set to grow. In addition, the empirical evidence suggests that South-to-South medical tourism is a far more common phenomenon than previously assumed. Moreover, there seem to be a number of specific markets, such as within regions or focused on for example cosmetic procedures, rather than one large and uniform phenomenon of medical tourism. This deserves greater attention: It highlights that the impact of medical tourism is likely to be context specific, and suggests that policies aimed at regulating and addressing challenges arising from medical tourism, or indeed fostering this type of exchange, will need to address these specificities, making it even more important for different regional patterns to be better understood.

Where case studies exist, they highlight the potential for costs and benefits arising from medical tourism for both destination and for originating health systems, underlining need to consider these in a more nuanced way than have been to date.

Evidence, including from a case study of UK outbound medical tourism, confirms the risks associated with medical tourism, including especially risks of medical complications once a patient returns to their country of origin following treatment. These findings provide a clear imperative for international action to regulate medical travel, starting with clear information for patients. Given the global nature of this phenomenon — even where there are regional characteristics — regulation by a body such as the World Health Organization is needed. Indeed, the creation of a new regulatory authority at global level may be warranted to deal with trade in health services, as is stronger regulation and oversight at the national level within individual countries. This should include guidelines on information that must be provided to patients, minimum standards, and guidance for policymakers on how to integrate medical tourism considerations into health systems planning. Finally, the globalization of health care suggests the space for an international body representing patients to ensure that their interests are protected in light of the largely unstructured but growing medical tourism market.

References

Arie S. 2013. Are migrant patients really a drain on European health systems? *British Medical Journal* 347: f6444.

Birch DW, Vu L, Karmali S, Stoklossa CJ, Sharma AM. 2010. Medical tourism in bariatric surgery. *The American Journal of Surgery* 199: 604–608.

Chanda R. 2011. India–EU relations in health services: prospects and challenges. *Global Health* 7: 1.

Connell J. 2008. Tummy tucks and the Taj Mahal? Medical tourism and the globalisation of health care. In Woodside A, Martin D, (eds.). *Tourism Management: Analysis, Behaviour and Strategy,* CABI, Wallingford, UK, pp. 232–244.

Connell J. 2013. Contemporary medical tourism: Conceptualisation, culture and commodification. *Tourism Management* 34: 1–13.

Crooks VA, Kingsbury P, Snyder J, Johnston R. 2010. What is known about the patient's experience of medical tourism? A scoping review. *BMC Health Services Research* 10: 266.

Crush J. 2012. Patients Without Borders: Medical Tourism and Medical Migration in Southern Africa. *Southern African Migration Programme.* Johannesburg.

Crush J, Chikanda A. 2015. South–South medical tourism and the quest for health in Southern Africa. *Social Science & Medicine* 124: 313–320.

Culley L, Hudson N, Rapport F, Blyth E, Norton W, Pacey AA. 2011. Crossing borders for fertility treatment: motivations, destinations and outcomes of UK fertility travellers. *Human Reproduction* 26: 2373–2381.

Glinos IA, Baeten R, Helble M, Maarse H. 2010. A typology of cross-border patient mobility. *Health & Place* 16: 1145–1155.

Glinos IA, Doering N, Maarse H. 2012. Travelling home for treatment and EU patients' rights to care abroad: Results of a survey among German students at Maastricht University. *Health Policy* 105: 38–45.

Hanefeld J, Horsfall D, Lunt N, Smith R. 2013a. Medical Tourism: A Cost or Benefit to the NHS? *PLoS ONE* 8: e70406.

Hanefeld J, Lunt N, Smith R. 2013b. Paying for migrant healthcare. *British Medical Journal* 347: f6514.

Hanefeld J, Lunt N, Smith R, Horsfall D. 2015. Why do medical tourists travel to where they do? The role of networks in determining medical travel. *Social Science & Medicine* 124: 356–363. Doi:10.1016/j.socscimed.2014.05.016.

Hanefeld J, Smith DR, Lunt N, Horsfall D. 2014. What do we know about medical tourism — a review of the literature with discussion of its implications for the UK NHS as an example of a public health care system. *Journal of Medical Travel* 21(6): 410–417.

Holliday R, Bell D, Cheung O, Jones M, Probyn E. 2015. Brief encounters: Assembling cosmetic surgery tourism. *Social Science & Medicine* 124: 298–304.

Holliday R, Bell D, Jones M, Hardy K, Hunter E, Probyn E, Taylor JS. 2013. Beautiful face, beautiful place: relational geographies and gender in cosmetic surgery tourism websites. *Gender, Place & Culture* 1–17.

Horsfall DG, Lunt N, King H, Hanefeld J, Smith RD. 2013. The impact of the internet on medical tourism. *In*: Botterill, D, Pennings, G. (eds.). *Medical Tourism and Transnational Health Care.* London: Palgrave Macmillan.

Horton S, Cole S. 2011. Medical returns: Seeking health care in Mexico. *Social Science and Medicine,* 72 (11): 1846–1852.

Imison M, Schweinsberg S. 2013. Australian news media framing of medical tourism in low- and middle-income countries: a content review. *BMC Public Health* 13: 109.

Inhorn MC. 2011. Globalization and gametes: Reproductive 'tourism,' Islamic bioethics, and Middle Eastern modernity. *Anthropology and Medicine* 18(1): 87–103.

Kumarasamy KK, Toleman MA, Walsh TR, Bagaria J, Butt F, Balakrishnan R, Chaudhary U, Doumith M, Giske CG, Irfan S, Krishnan P, Kumar AV, Maharjan S, Mushtaq S, Noorie T, Paterson DL, Pearson A, Perry C, Pike R, Rao B, Ray U, Sarma JB, Sharma M, Sheridan E, Thirunarayan MA, Turton J, Upadhyay S, Warner M, Welfare W, Livermore DM, Woodford N. 2010. Emergence of a new antibiotic resistance mechanism in India, Pakistan, and the UK: A molecular, biological, and epidemiological study. *The Lancet Infectious Diseases* 10: 597–602.

Laugesen MJ, Vargas-Bustamante A. 2010. A patient mobility framework that travels: European and United States–Mexican comparisons. *Health Policy* 97: 225–231.

Lautier M. 2008. Export of health services from developing countries: The case of Tunisia. *Social Science & Medicine* 67: 101–110.

Lee JY, Kearns RA, Friesen W. 2010. Seeking affective health care: Korean immigrants' use of homeland medical services. *Health & Place* 16: 108–115.

Legido-Quigley H, Glinos IA, Baeten R, Mckee M, Busse R. 2012. Analysing arrangements for cross-border mobility of patients in the European Union: a proposal for a framework. *Health Policy* 108: 27–36.

Legido-Quigley H, Passarani I, Knai C, Busse R, Palm W, Wismar M, Mckee M. 2011. Cross-border healthcare in the European Union: clarifying patients' rights. *British Medical Journal* 342.

Leng CH. 2010. Medical Tourism and the State in Malaysia and Singapore. *Global Social Policy* 10: 336–357.

Lunt N, Carrera P. 2011. Systematic review of web sites for prospective medical tourists. (Special Issue: Health and medical tourism.). *Tourism Review* 66: 57–67.

Lunt N, Hardey M, Mannion R. 2010. Nip, tuck and click: Medical tourism and the emergence of web-based health information. *Open Med Inform J* 4: 1–11.

Lunt N, Horsfall D, Exworthy M, Smith R, Hanefeld J. 2013. Market size, market share and market strategy: Three myths of medical tourism. *Policy and Politics* 42(4): 597–614.

Lunt N, Jin K, Horsfall D, Hanefeld J. 2014. Insights on medical tourism: markets as networks and the role of strong ties. *Korean Social Science Journal* 1–19.

Lunt N, Mannion R. 2014. Patient Mobility in the Global Marketplace: A Multidisciplinary Perspective. *International Journal of Health Policy and Management* 2: 155–157.

Martinez Alvarez M, Chanda R, Smith RD. 2011. The potential for bi-lateral agreements in medical tourism: A qualitative study of stakeholder perspectives from the UK and India. *Globalization and Health* 7.

Mason A, Wright KB. 2011. Framing Medical Tourism: An Examination of Appeal, Risk, Convalescence, Accreditation, and Interactivity in Medical Tourism Web Sites. *Journal of Health Communication* 16: 163–177.

Mazzaschi A. 2011. Surgeon and Safari: Producing valuable bodies in Johannesburg. *Signs* 36(2): 303–312.

Mckelvey A, David AL, Shenfield F, Jauniaux ER. 2009. The impact of cross-border reproductive care or 'fertility tourism' on NHS maternity services. *BJOG: An International Journal of Obstetrics and Gynaecology* 116: 1520–1523.

Melendez MM, Alizadeh K. 2011. Complications from international surgery tourism. *Aesthetic Surgery Journal,* 31(6): 694–697.

Miyagi K, Auberson D, Patel AJ, Malata CM. 2012. The unwritten price of cosmetic tourism: An observational study and cost analysis. *J Plast Reconstr Aesthet Surg* 65: 22–28.

Naranong A, Naranong V. 2011. The effects of medical tourism: Thailand's experience. *Bulletin of the World Health Organization* 89: 336–344.

Nassab R, Hamnett N, Nelson K, Kaur S, Greensill B, Dhital S, Juma A. 2010. Cosmetic tourism: public opinion and analysis of information and content available on the Internet. *Aesthetic Surgery Journal* 30: 465–469.

NCEPOD. 2012. Bariatric Surgery: Too Lean a Service? UK.

Noree T, Hanefeld J, Smith R. forthcoming 2016. Medical tourism in Thailand — facts not fiction. *Bulletin of the World Health Organization.*

Noree T, Smith R, Hanefeld J. 2014. UK medical tourists in Thailand — they are not who you think they are. *Globalisation and Health*.

Ormond M. 2013. *Neoliberal Governance and International Medical Travel in Malaysia,* London, Routledge.

Osterle A, Balazs P, Delgado J. 2009. Travelling for teeth: characteristics and perspectives of dental care tourism in Hungary. *British Dental Journal* 206: 425–428.

Pachanee C-A, Wibulpolprasert S. 2006. Incoherent policies on universal coverage of health insurance and promotion of international trade in health services in Thailand. *Health Policy and Planning* 21: 310–318.

Pollock AM, Price D, Roderick P, Treuherz T, Mccoy D, Mckee M, Reynolds L. 2012. How the Health and Social Care Bill 2011 would end entitlement to comprehensive health care in England. *Lancet* 379: 387–389.

Rogers BA, Aminzadeh Z, Hayashi Y, Paterson, DL. 2011. Country-to-country transfer of patients and the risk of multi-resistant bacterial infection. *Clinical Infectious Diseases* 53: 49–56.

Siddiqi S, Shennawy A, Mirza Z, Drager N, Sabri B. 2010. Assessing trade in health services in countries of the Eastern Mediterranean from a public health perspective. *International Journal of Health Planning & Management* 25: 231–250.

Smith M, Puczko L. 2009. *Health and Wellness Tourism,* Oxford, Elsevier.

Smith R, Lunt N, Hanefeld J. 2012. The implications of PIP are more than just cosmetic. *The Lancet* 379: 1180–1181.

Smith RD, Chanda R, Tangcharoensathien V. 2009. Trade in health-related services. *Lancet* 373: 593–601.

Snyder J, Crooks VA. 2010. Medical Tourism and Bariatric Surgery: More Moral Challenges. *The American Journal of Bioethics* 10: 28–30.

Snyder J, Crooks VA, Adams K, Kingsbury P, Johnston R. 2011. The 'patient's physician one-step removed': the evolving roles of medical tourism facilitators. *Journal of Medical Ethics* 37: 530–534.

Thompson C. 2008. Medical Tourism, Stem Cells, Genomics: EASTS, Transnational STS, and the Contemporary Life Sciences. *East Asian Science, Technology and Society: an International Journal* 2: 433–438.

Thompson C. 2011. Medical migrations afterword: Science as a vacation? *Body and Society* 17: 205–213.

Van Hoof W, Pennings G, De Sutter P. 2015. Cross-border reproductive care for law evasion: A qualitative study into the experiences and moral perspectives of French women who go to Belgium for treatment with donor sperm. *Social Science & Medicine* 124: 391–397.

Vick L. 2012. The perils of cosmetic surgery/medical tourism. *Clinical Risk* 18: 106–109.

Whittaker A, Speier A. 2010. "Cycling overseas": care, commodification, and stratification in cross-border reproductive travel. *Medical Anthropology* 29: 363–383.

Wismar M, Palm W, Figueras J, Ernst K, Ginneken Van E. 2011. *Cross-border Health Care in the European Union,* Copenhagen, WHO.

Public–Private Partnerships

Pedro Pita Barros* and Rui Sousa Monteiro†
**Nova School of Business and Economics, Universidade Nova de Lisboa, Campus de Campolide, 1099-032 Lisboa, Portugal*
ppbarros@novasbe.pt
†Senior Public–Private Partnerships Specialist, World Bank, 1818 H Street NW, Washington, DC 20433, USA

Public–Private Partnerships (PPPs) are long-run contracts between a public entity and a private partner for delivery of a good (infrastructure) and/or service otherwise carried out under traditional public sector rules and procedures.

PPPs involve project selection, tendering procedures to select the private partner, and contract execution. Each phase has risks and challenges.

The value of the PPP lies in the ability of the private partner to deliver outcomes. The private partner needs to face the right incentives, determined by transfers of risk. The incentives need to ensure a whole-life costing view.

Selection of good projects is essential. A bad project will not be made good because it is a PPP. Political biases toward too many projects are to be recognized.

The tendering should select the best private partner to obtain value-for-money (VfM) and set monitoring and (eventual) renegotiation conditions.

The contract will likely have renegotiations, as knowledge and technology evolve; will have to deal with monitoring of outcomes; will face public scrutiny of government payments and control of quality in the service.

Selecting, organizing and executing a PPP contract is more demanding to the public sector, as an organization, than is usually expected. A PPP's success requires clear rules, transparency in all phases and a high degree of professionalism by public sector officials.

Keywords: Public–Private Partnerships; Economic Incentives; Political Governance.

What are Public–Private Partnerships?

Definition

Public–Private Partnership is a term that covers different meanings. We will focus here on an economics-driven definition: A public–private partnership (PPP) is a long-term contract between a public entity and a private partner, initiated by the public sector, to provide a service that would be otherwise directly provided by the public sector. This definition builds on the ones proposed by the European Commission and the World Bank.

The two main features, from an economic perspective, of a PPP contract are its long-term nature (often 20, 30 years or more) and a level of risk transfer to the private partner higher than under traditional public procurement. There are several other definitions of a PPP, including the ones from the European Commission:

> Private Public Partnership "refers to forms of cooperation between public authorities and the world of business which aim to ensure the funding, construction, renovation, management or maintenance of an infrastructure or the provision of a service." (European Commission, 2004, p. 3)

and from the World Bank:

> "A long-term contract between a private party and a government agency, for providing a public asset or service, in which the private party bears significant risk and management responsibility." (World Bank, 2012, p. 11)

PPP contracts are long-term, incomplete (in a precise sense defined below), and complex. Their long-term nature implies they are subject to technological, demographic, commercial and political change over the course of the contract. These two aspects of the long-term contract, incompleteness and complexity, will be discussed at length as they are associated with several problems that have been found in PPPs in health care.

Another idea that will be thoroughly discussed is that PPP contracts are tools, and their efficiency and adequacy are subject to conditions to work. In particular, the role of risk transfer will be addressed.

PPPs in health care usually involve people from many different professions, to whom a major barrier is the use of the same term to mean very different things. Harding details the definition of health care PPP used by three different professional "tribes" (Harding, 2012). For the tribe of economists and financial analysts, PPPs are an instrument to "mobilize private actors to invest capital in delivery of health services and products." The focus is on the ability to raise private funding for public sector projects. The "health services tribe" sees PPPs as a "long-term contract for services (may include use of public assets)," the delivery of health care is at the core. Finally, for the "global health tribe," a PPP is an "on-going relationship to work together on health sector issues of common interest" to private entities and the government. Each group focuses on a different angle of the same instrument. Noting these several interpretations, we want to emphasize the issues associated with the creation and management of a long-run contract.

The long-term nature of the PPP contract is directly connected to its object — the useful life of physical assets to be built under the contract, either with or without direct operation of the assets that provide services.

Bundling and private finance

The long-term contract of PPP is set for the design, construction, finance, maintenance and (in some variants) operation of a public asset. A first issue is the extent of participation of the private partner. Bundling these activities is at the core of the contractual scheme.

The goal is forcing a commitment, by the private partner, on the performance of the asset during the life of the contract, inducing a **whole-life approach** to the project, and so optimizing both capital investment and maintenance plans.

When the PPP includes operation of clinical activities, the expectation is that private management is able to deliver the service more efficiently, a claim still to be subject to empirical testing.

The credibility of that commitment is established by **private finance** — allocating to the private partner the responsibility for financing the project. Private capital (own capital, or debt) should be high enough for acting as "hostage capital," and so the funding of the project (through user-fees, government payments, or a mix of them) should be spread over the life of the contract, always keeping some private capital at risk, and so a strong incentive for high performance of the asset. In the health care sector, PPPs tend to be paid by transfers from the public partner and not using fees by users on the service provided (patients in the case of health care) (EPOS — Health Management, Health and Economics, 2013).

The assumption is that the PPP operator, having private capital at stake, will prepare the design of the infrastructure and the maintenance plans in a way that will minimize the cost of reaching the prescribed levels of service provision and performance.

The resulting efficiency savings should be able to more than compensate for the added cost of capital. Private capital is subject to corporate and/or project risk, higher than the cost of public debt. This is a central aspect, often misunderstood, in PPPs. The transfer of risk from the public to the private partner has an extra cost relative to public debt financing that can only be compensated by savings introduced by the private partner. For this to occur, the private partner needs to face the adequate incentives, which requires bearing risk (more on this in the following sections). A typical example is the private partner to bear the construction cost risk of new facilities. By paying a fixed price for the availability of infrastructure, the risk associated to higher or lower costs, and controlled to a large extent by the private partner, is transferred from the public sector to the private sector — but the performance risk is also transferred to the private partner, meaning that the option of reducing costs by "cutting corners" will not be available, but only the option of managing and controlling the cost of a high performing infrastructure. Note that the interest is not in the risk transfer *per se* but in the incentive it induces for efficiency of the private partner.

The long-term perspective

Traditional public procurement can be done in a variety of ways: hospital design and construction may be procured together (*design–build* contracts) or separately; public agencies may even design the hospital in-house; maintenance may be provided in-house or procured periodically. PPP procurement bundles all these activities, implying not only signing a **long-term contract**, but also preparing a **long-term business plan** based on which the public authority will decide on the contractual model and on detailed contractual provisions.

By locking the private partner into a long-term contract, the public partner is also locking itself into that relationship. Dissolving the partnership is always a possibility, but it will have a significant cost — that high cost, accepted by the public authority, signals its commitment to the partnership and reduces incentives for opportunistic behavior.

Being long-term, PPP contracts are incomplete because there is uncertainty regarding the future states of the world. Not all contingencies can be predicted. Thus, by necessity PPP contracts will be incomplete. In addition, gains will result from innovations the private partner can bring (an issue we will take up later) — this means allowing flexibility in the contract and avoid it to be over-prescriptive. Thus, by design, the contract will be incomplete in some parts (which is reflected in clauses that mention, typically, a variant of "managing according to the best practices and the National Health Services rules"). Any hospital business plan will be influenced by **technological and demographic change**, and also by health policy. Future health policies are likely to change current characteristics of every health system, such as the configuration of the health system; the range of hospital service lines to be supplied; referral rules between the hospital and other hospitals, primary care centers, and long-term units; user-fees and any other fees; and even the way production is measured, and performance is defined. It is virtually impossible that the initial business plan is executed exactly as planned, as uncertain events unfold.

While in several other areas PPPs have been proven effective (and possibly even efficient) ways for delivering infrastructure and services, **PPPs for hospitals and health care** are still in an experimental phase, with several models being implemented and tested. Different incentives schemes are used in the PPP-hospitals currently in operation.

How long should a contract be in order to balance the need for whole-life costing and the perceived hardships linked to contractual commitment, is still an issue. And the inclusion of clinical services is being tested, as it significantly changes the nature of the contract — different performance indicators, different reward schemes, different step-in rights allocated to financing parties, possibly dual terms for infrastructure and services, etc., but it also reduces the opportunities for conflict (and potential fiscal cost) coming from the interface between public and private management, and enlarges the scope for gains to both parties.

Hospital PPPs must be compared not only to the alternative procurement modes for public hospitals but also to alternative modes for service provision. These include buying from the market, or using competitive schemes for managing service provision (delegating responsibility for hospital infrastructure to service deliverers, or not).

PPPs in health care started in the early-1990s in the UK, at the time called Private Finance Initiative (PFI). Since then PPPs have spread to other countries, both developed and emerging economies. The existence of 30-year and longer-term contracts means that only in a decade from now a full assessment of completed cycles of PPP contracts can be done. Meanwhile partial evaluations were performed in several countries. Of course, failure early on implies a negative overall assessment, while full success can only be determined at the end of the contract (even if mid-way reviews are positive).

The hospital-PPP models currently in place cannot be fully assessed, in terms of efficiency or sustainability — being long-term, none of them lived a complete cycle. There are some partial assessments, focusing on the initial years. The inner structure of those models needs to be understood, and some of their characteristics and properties should be identified, in order to improve contract design, contract management, and health-policy design and implementation.

The rest of this chapter will cover these issues.

Types of PPP in Health Care

Health care has a specificity that impacts the way PPPs are defined. Health care delivery is a service subject to considerable uncertainty regarding future technology, and interruption of service is generally a major concern for the public partner.

Health care service delivery covers different types of activities, with broad categories traditionally being primary care, specialized and acute hospital care, and long-term care. Specific services within each of these broad types of care can be contracted in a PPP regime. Most existing PPPs in health care are associated with hospitals.

PPPs in health care are currently present in many countries. A good source on PPPs in the health care sector is DLA Piper (2009), where a systematic review of PPPs in Europe is carried out. Some countries' PPPs include the construction and management of clinical activities (for example, Portugal), others are essentially infrastructure-only PPPs (for example, UK, France, Germany), and some have both types (Spain and Italy). The international experience shows that countries with a national health service funded through general taxation use PPPs more intensively, as they substitute for immediate public investment. From DLA Piper, we see that the UK, Italy, Spain, and Portugal rank high in intensity of PPPs and all of these countries have a national health service. In the developing world, we also find increasing interest in the use of PPPs, with projects being launched in all continents in countries such as Brazil, India, Nigeria, Peru, South Africa, and Turkey, among others. For developing countries, PPPs are often seen as a quick way to build health care infrastructure under tight Government funding.

The basic model

The basic model for hospital PPPs deals mainly with infrastructure, and includes no clinical services. These contracts are design-build-finance-maintain (DBFM) contracts, with some also including certain equipment (typically imaging or non-medical equipment) and the provision of several non-clinical services (cleaning, catering, security, laundry, utilities management).

The United Kingdom, Italy, and France have a large number of operational PPP hospitals under these schemes. The largest program for PPP hospitals is the British Private Finance Initiative (PFI), using a model where the public sector procures the building and operation of infrastructure by a private partner that brings investment against a stream of future rental payments. The PFI model changed over time but maintained some basic characteristics, such as the absence of clinical services in the range of services to be provided by the private partner. The 121 British health care PFI projects signed from 1992 until the end of 2013 (including more than 70 hospitals over the two decades, almost all currently in operation) present (HM Treasury, United Kingdom, 2014) a capital value of £11.8 billion. Italy has more than 50 PPP hospitals, with a capital value close to €4 billion, almost all of them already operational. France implemented more than 50 of these PPP schemes, also almost all operational.

This model — we may call it "**accommodation**", "**basic**", or "**infrastructural model**" interchangeably — has also been adopted in other countries in Europe and elsewhere, such as Canada, Germany, Mexico, and Spain. Peru, South Africa, and Turkey are also preparing large infrastructural PPP programs for hospitals.

The perceived lack of value-for-money in including non-clinical services in this type of contract (National Audit Office, United Kingdom, 2010) led gradually to a larger focus on infrastructure, with the last contracts signed in the United Kingdom streamlined to the DBFM core, with no services included other than maintenance of the infrastructure.

The private partner is usually rewarded through a periodic government payment — a unitary payment for design, construction and maintenance, adjusted to the actual performance — plus the payment of (non-maintenance) services effectively provided. Adjustment to performance means that contracts specify bonus and penalties according to targets for indicators of performance — most commonly penalties linked to underperformance.

In the infrastructural model, each hospital has a non-PPP management structure in charge of the provision of clinical services (usually public managers, but sometimes a non-governmental organization), and a PPP management structure for the activities included in the contract. As many activities (for instance, cleaning, catering, security) are outsourced to specialized providers, several activities will have three monitoring entities — the service provider who is managing provision, the private infrastructure operator who is monitoring the outsourced activities and will pay PPP penalties in case of underperformance, and the public hospital managers who are monitoring the contract and managing health care provision. Clinical workers may, or may not, have the status of public employees, according to the particular contract set. For new facilities, PPP contracts can more easily implement private sector contracting rules. When the PPP is for renewal or substitution of existing public sector capacity, clinical workers transferred from old to new facilities most often keep public employees' status.

The full-service model

Another PPP model for hospitals integrates all hospital services in a PPP contract — we term it the "**full-service model**". The first experiments were done in Australia (Latrobe hospital, in the State of Victoria) and Spain (Alzira hospital, in the Region of Valencia) and, for different reasons, failed in their initial design. The Latrobe hospital reverted to public management. The Alzira hospital was renegotiated and is now operating under private management, but with payments from the public to the private partner significantly higher than initially contracted. The renegotiation actually implied a termination of the first contract by the public partner and a new procedure won by the initial private partner (more on the Alzira experience below; see also (EPOS — Health Management, Health and Economics, 2013); (EXPH (EXpert Panel on effective ways of investing in Health), 2014)).

Despite these initial setbacks, several full-service PPP hospitals are currently operational in Spain and Portugal, plus a few scattered outside of Europe (for instance, one in Lesotho, another in Brazil).

There are three different subtypes of full-service PPP contracts: One based on the **payment of availability and services**, another based on a **lump-sum payment** for a certain range of services, and still another based on **per capita payments**, based on the population of a pre-defined catchment area.

PPPs can also include the provision of primary care facilities and the operation of primary care clinical activities — a primary care center, a set of primary care centers, or even a set of satellite primary care centers. Alzira and the other PPP hospitals in Valencia manage the primary care centers in their vicinity (Marín-Ferrer and Rosa-Torner, 2007); the Queen Mamohato Lesotho contract includes three gatekeeping centers, called "filter clinics" (Boston University, 2013), acting as gatekeepers to the hospital, treating the less severe cases; and the Government of Bahia is considering adding a primary care facility to the Subúrbio contract.

PPPs in the full-service model may involve one or two special purpose vehicles, or SPVs. In the latter case, the infrastructure provider SPV will receive a separate payment from the public partner, protecting its debt from clinical risk, and allowing different time horizons for the infrastructure component (longer period) and for clinical services management (shorter time span). The two SPVs will be separate legal entities, although closely connected. Most participants in one of these legal entities will also have a participation in the other. Some specialized private partners may participate only in one. For example, building companies will be an important partner for the infrastructure SPV and may decide to be out of the clinical activities SPV. The two SPVs may have different time horizons, for example 30 years for infrastructure and 10 years for clinical activities. Under a single SPV, the longer period of infrastructure prevails over clinical activities operations, and risks related to infrastructure and to operation of clinical activities are shared, by definition.

The partial model

Sometimes the PPP encompasses only part of the infrastructure, within a more general facility — e.g., a radiotherapy unit, or an imaging unit, or a hospital sterilization unit, or a building for accommodating inpatients.

This model is widely used in developing countries for solving widespread needs on radiotherapy or hemodialysis, both inside and outside the framework of the hospital system — Pakistan procured independent dialysis facilities, Bahia (Brazil) is procured a network of hospital imaging/diagnosis centers.

It is also used in high-income countries. France used the partial PPP model for a wide range of hospital needs: a sterilization unit in the university-hospital of Amiens, a certified High Environmental Quality building at the Pitié-Salpêtrière hospital in Paris, a long-term inpatient care center at Arras, and a building for children and maternal care at the university-hospital of Caen.

Non-PPP variants

Contracting with the private sector can also be done with different modes that do not constitute a Public–Private Partnership in the sense defined above. South Africa implemented "co-location" hospitals, which are private hospitals that provide several services as "public hospital", with different pricing and quality than the remaining services provided as a private hospital. The co-location approach reduces the investment costs of the private side, and increases supply of services while retaining both public and private hospitals as separate entities.

India signed "land for beds" contracts, under which the government would provide land (a scarce good in India) in major cities for private entities to build private hospitals where a specific number of beds would be reserved for free treatment of poor people (typically BPL people, "below the poverty line" people, or lower-caste people). There is evidence that those free-service provisions are not being implemented, due to poor contract specification (for instance, not specifying that medicines and consumables are to be provided free originates charges that effectively repel poor patients) and insufficient monitoring by public authorities (Raman and La Forgia, 2013).

Economic Rationale for PPP

The choice of a PPP should be based on a sound economic motivation. A main concept in the justification for a PPP is **value for money** (Burger and Hawkesworth, 2011). The central notion in economics is opportunity cost, which demands identification of alternative courses of action. In the case of a PPP project, there are two important decision involving explicitly the notion of opportunity cost: The selection of the project (should it be done, or not — (Organisation for Economic Co-operation and Development (OECD), 2013) calls this "absolute value-for-money assessment") and comparing the use of a PPP against an alternative way of carrying out the project (for example, traditional public sector procurement — OECD calls this "relative value-for-money assessment").

The building blocks for the economic rationale of PPPs

Value for money. The term *value-for-money* (VfM) has acquired a precise meaning in the PPP context. It means the difference between the net present value of doing the project under the PPP contract and going it under traditional public procurement. Assuming that benefits are the same over the life cycle of the project whatever model is selected, the actual comparison is between the net present value of costs under the PPP and under traditional public procurement. The assumption simplifies the process, as benefits do not need to be defined in a precise way and computed. The assumption is supported in the view that rules of access under the public system of health care facilities and treatment provided are set irrespective of the nature of the specific provider delivering these services. The cost of doing the project with a traditional public procurement procedure is known as the "Public Sector Comparator" in the PPP-related literature.

The underlying assumption is obviously simpler to maintain in the accommodation PPP than in the full-service PPP, as in the latter different management of clinical activities may have a direct impact in benefits to the patients. The relevant economic notion of costs includes more than just production costs. It includes transaction costs and externalities produced. Computation of *value-for-money* has therefore several methodological challenges in producing estimates that approximate the economic costs.

Performance. Critical to the success of a PPP project is the ability to define volumes of service and performance levels in a way that is simultaneously politically acceptable and contractible (i.e., measurable up to a degree of certainty that can be presented to a court, if needed).

When that ability exists, and when expectations regarding the future service needs (after considering probable and possible impacts from technological, demographic, commercial, and political change) can be reasonably established, PPPs can be considered as a potentially effective and efficient procurement mode, aligning the private profit motivation with the public interest. The ability to measure performance is another central element of a successful PPP project. Performance is defined in terms of quantitative indicators of treatment provided as well as quality indicators of care and of process of delivery.

Service provision. The whole-life costing approach implies the internalization of future maintenance (and refurbishment/renewal) costs, designing investment and maintenance plans in an optimal way. This internalization, if extended to operational activities, leads to higher potential efficiency savings — the range of operational activities that can be included in a PPP contract is related to the various sources of change affecting the project over the long-run, reducing the ability of the private partner to commit on providing certain services, and the ability of the public partner to commit on demanding services. Services subject to more uncertain variation in the future are less likely to be considered in a PPP.

Guaranteed maintenance. Because PPPs imply transferring the responsibility for maintenance to the private partner, they are a convenient way for guaranteeing future maintenance. Current Government budgeting processes do not allow for the (credible) long-term allocation of public funds for asset maintenance, leading to fluctuations on maintenance levels and a suboptimal maintenance trajectory in non-PPP projects, with inherent higher costs and lower performance.

At the end of the contract, physical assets of a PPP are transferred to the public sector. This creates an end-of-period moral hazard effect in terms of private partner keeping investment up to maintain quality of assets until the end of the active life of the PPP project. As the contract approaches the end and facilities have to be returned by the private partner to the public sector, the incentive to save on maintenance costs mounts. It needs to be counteracted with an appropriate set of contractual incentives — a common one is an easier early termination during the final years, with lower break-up costs for government.

Bundling and whole-life costing

A core efficiency driver in a PPP mechanism is bundling design, construction, and maintenance (or even operation) of an infrastructure (e.g., a hospital) under a single contract.

First, by transferring to a single private consortium the responsibility for these activities under a fixed price, the PPP contract creates a very strong incentive for designing and building the infrastructure in such a way that minimizes the cost of obeying a contractually agreed set of quality and performance requirements — the private partner is supposed to do a whole-life costing of the project, over the term of contract, balancing the marginal impact of initial investment vs. ulterior investments and maintenance/operational costs. Setting a fixed price in the PPP contract to pay for delivery of services results from a deliberate choice to provide efficiency incentives (see below the discussion on the payment system).

As we will discuss later, the relevance of this whole-life costing depends on the range of activities that will be managed (and paid for) by the private partner over the term of the contract. Monitoring of the contract by the public party is required to ensure that cost savings are not obtained through lower performance or lower quality of care provided.

Second, this whole-life costing exercise, done under competitive pressure, during the procurement process, creates the conditions for government (or the public-sector procuring agency) to pay the efficiency price for the contract (and so for the range of services included).

Third, the contractual allocation of responsibilities allows for the private partner to react to the environment, and to the results of its own actions, in a way that, in each moment, minimizes the whole-life cost of the project conditional on past actions (namely sunk costs on infrastructure and equipment). Therefore, economic efficiency is supposed to arise from the contractual responsibility the private partner assumes regarding paying for any extra costs needed for delivering the contracted quality and performance, as well as from its right to benefit from any realized savings.

Whole-life costing implies optimizing the trade-off between capital expenditure and the cost of future maintenance over the life of the project, in order to obtain a certain level of performance with minimum cost.

Whole-life costing and infrastructure operation. Infrastructure is critical because of its typical large size, implying large sunk costs — that is the reason for PPPs to include at least infrastructure maintenance as private-sector responsibility (and so a reason for PPP contracts to be long-term contracts).

PPPs should be compared to design-build contracts — short-term contracts through which a private consortium is hired to design and build an infrastructure according to contractually specified quality standards.

Design-build contracts are much simpler contracts where the contractor does not have a long-term performance commitment. They may be the most efficient solution when it is quite easy to contractually define quality standards. But when those standards are hard to define, or difficult to monitor, submitting private bidders to a competitive selection process implies an implicit invitation for corner-cutting solutions to be adopted, and so are a recipe for low performance, for higher operational costs, and for cost overruns.

One of the reasons for the adoptions of a PPP program for hospitals in Portugal was the experience with design-build in the 1980s (e.g., Hospital de Leiria, Hospital Amadora-Sintra), leading to poor quality of adopted solutions (e.g., low-quality non-clinical equipment, very small waiting room in the pediatric emergency ward) and to consequent cost overruns associated with the additional work and cost needed to adjust infrastructure to the level of demand.

In order to induce the private partner to use economic rationality in designing and building infrastructure (and selecting equipment), but without cutting corners, PPPs allocate to that partner the long-term responsibility for the performance of that infrastructure — and so at least the responsibility for maintenance is included in the contract.

Of course, increasing the range of responsibilities allocated to the private partner changes the incentives and consequently the expected efficiency of the adopted solutions. Basically, the PPP contract, through definition of quality indicators and how they will be measured and evaluated, internalizes an externality related to the quality of infrastructure (including design and architecture) and its impact in future maintenance and operations.

Full transfer of responsibilities for the operation of the infrastructure maximizes the expected efficiency of whole-life costing — at least in a stable environment, with no major change to the contractual quality and performance requirements.

This is a typical solution for roads, a highway concession for instance, also adopted for hospitals. For a hospital it means a concession for designing, building, and operating a public hospital according to the National Health Service rules. But in the case of hospitals, two major characteristics are visibly different from the road case. While in the case of a road there is a legitimate expectation that cars will still use rubber tires (or wheel surfaces made from similar materials) for a very long period, in the case of an acute hospital there is an expectation of significant technological evolution, both in medical equipment and in the way patients are operated and treated. More, the exact features of this technological evolution cannot be predicted accurately. Medical knowledge and technological possibilities evolve often in unpredictable directions.

Also, a road concession can be managed as a stand-alone project, while the hospital needs to be managed in the context of the health system, with a set of referral links (with primary care centers, lower- and higher-complexity hospitals, specialized treatment centers, long-term care units, and so on), and possibly under a managed-demand system that may reallocate excess demand from one unit to another.

Allocation of all operational responsibilities to a private partner (as experienced in several PPP solutions in Spain, Portugal, Brazil, and Lesotho) maximizes the internalization of the impacts of investment and design decisions (at the inception and during the life of the contract). But, in the case of hospitals, the main drawbacks are the difficulty the private sector faces in forecasting hospital technology and management, and the difficulty the public sector faces in committing to a set of performance requirements in a context where the needs of the health system will change significantly over time. So full-service PPPs for hospitals require complex incentive mechanisms — and the country examples that currently exist include different models with widely different incentive mechanisms.

Role of risk allocation

The public sector can, in general, borrow more cheaply than the private sector. This raises the immediate question why PPP have economic rationale.

The key insight is that risk transfer happens to introduce incentives for efficiency to the private party. Efficiency gains from the private side means savings in costs large enough to pay for the additional cost of funding and, at the same time, to have a lower payment by the public sector relative to what would be the direct construction (and eventually operation) of the infrastructure by the public sector.

Thus, risk allocation is an instrument and not an objective of the PPP from an economic perspective. This means that a PPP should not be assessed by how much risk it transfers between public and private sectors but what is the incentive effect of each risk transfer and what impact does it produce.

Numerous risks have been identified with PPP projects. Project risks have here the meaning of uncertain aspects that may materialize in a different way than expected in the baseline scenario used to set the PPP contract. Common risks (or uncertainties) identified in most PPPs include demand uncertainty (volume of demand may vary with changes in demographic and health trends in the population), construction cost uncertainty (positive or negative shocks in costs), operating risks (management inefficiencies, human resources issues, etc.), and financial risks (interest rate changes, funding unavailability).

The contract has to set the way these risks are allocated. The payment rule adopted needs to be consistent with assignment of risks. These risks vary from setting to setting, and risk allocation and payment rules will be different from contract to contract. It is usual for contracts to report, explicitly or implicitly, the risk sharing matrix. Risk allocation should be done taking into consideration the ability of each side to bear the risk (and the cost of it) and the incentive properties of risk allocation.

The transfer of risk in the PPP contract influences its cost to the public sector. By reducing the risk to the private partner, the contract may allow the private partner to find loans at better rates. Since revenues to the private partner are secured by contract with a public partner, creditors may see them as a safe stream of revenues and thus provide better interest rate on loans. The uncertainty does not disappear completely, at least on contractual grounds, as the Government (the public partner) may not bail out the private partner in case of severe financial problems. The absence of bail out does not mean necessarily interruption of service, as contracts usually allow, under certain extreme conditions, the public partner to take back the facility.

In practice, taking back a PPP project has seldom been done, and if done by decision of the public partner, it may result in compensatory payment to the private partner. Often, difficulties with PPPs in terms of financial results end in formal, or informal, contract renegotiations. An example of taking back a PPP was the decision about the Centre Hospitalier Sud-Francilien (CHSF) at Corbeil-Essonnes (France). In 2014, the French Government decided to take back the concession after a period of permanent conflict between the management of the hospital and the construction company Eiffage (putting an end to a PPP that started in 2011 and should last until

2041). The decision was based on the perception of lower cost of construction and maintenance under public management than under a PPP, with support from a report of the French Court of Auditors. In addition, the political debate was going against the PPP on ideological grounds. Whether, or not, they are right about the lower maintenance costs under public management only time will tell.

Similarly, the Chilean Government decision, in 2014, to stop the PPP hospital program (canceling the awards in progress and all projects being launched for tender) is not clearly based on economic facts. It is being perceived as influenced by ideological bias and by unions' pressure. The Chilean Government refrained from taking back the hospital concessions already being implemented due to high financial costs involved.

The balance of risk allocation within a PPP can be influenced by the stakeholders and their interests. In countries where financial entities play a strong role in the economy and economic decision-making, stakeholder influence will be more present. Strong financial entities (mostly, banks) that provide the funds for the PPP pressure for a less extensive risk transfer to the private partner as a way to reduce the cost of loans given and to provide more certainty to creditors. However, this reduces the incentives for efficiency in the PPP, decreasing the interest in the project. Thus, more influential creditors as stakeholders may lead to a risk allocation that keeps more risk in the public sector, at the cost of less powered incentives for efficiency by the private partner, which was (or should be) the driving force for gains associated with the PPP versus the traditional public procurement alternative.

This effect is consistent with options taken in some PPPs (e.g., in Portugal) but there is not a systematic review of the role of financial institutions as stakeholders in determining risk allocation and the success of the PPP.

The interest rate differential between public and private borrowing may not be large because governments are the main payers of PPP services in the health sector. Moreover, failing PPP projects are often "nationalized" by Governments — that is, Governments end up assuming the management of facilities and its costs to avoid interruption of the service to the population. Since the transfer of risk to the private party of a PPP increases its costs of funding, the gains from the PPP must originate from some other source than pure risk bearing and the motivation for the risk transfer must lie in other motives than risk bearing. As Governments have a lower cost of funding than private entities, and risk-transfers to the private partner of the PPP do not decrease its cost of funds, the gains from a PPP cannot result from the different risk bearing costs of the two parties. The rationale is that risk transfer to the private partner creates incentives for higher efficiency in construction and maintenance (and operation of clinical activities, if included in the PPP contract). This higher efficiency creates savings that allow to pay higher funding costs, pay management services by the private partner and still have a lower payment by the public sector than doing the project directly, as described in the following section.

The incentive role of risk transfer

The PPP contract provides a different set of incentives for efficiency when compared with traditional public procurement. These different incentives are often expected to result in shorter times to build the infrastructure and in lower operational costs, either of maintenance or of operation of clinical activities (whether included or not in the PPP). The decisions regarding the infrastructure design may affect costs of clinical activities. And different incentives for public or private management of clinical activities may be put in place. Moreover, a private operator for clinical management activities may have more freedom in human resources policies and procurement rules than a public entity. Also, it may introduce organizational innovations that provide better care at lower cost. Finally, the private party is less prone to cost overruns than the public sector due to more credible monitoring and control of works.

To highlight the role of risk transfer as an incentive mechanism, take the thought experiment of doing a PPP without any risk transfer from the public to the private sector. In this case, the public sector will pay to the private side whatever cost is invoiced, which has then a clear incentive to build costs to get a higher payment. The risk transfer, by paying a fixed, pre-determined, amount for the project provides an incentive to the private party to have low cost, as any dollar saved is a dollar earned. Indexation of the payment value to inflation does not change the incentive properties of the contract and it is a common adjustment. Of course, lump-sum payment introduces an incentive to cut too much on costs if the contract does not provide an adequate specification of the project that can be *ex-post* verified. There is no systematic account of which PPP contracts resulted in losses or in profits to the private partner. Information from different countries and PPP suggests a mixed situation. Some PPPs have resulted in handsome payments to private partners. Other PPPs involved losses, and handing over the PPP to the Government was avoided in several cases by renegotiation of the PPP.

The contractual payment system, from the public to the private partner, adopted in the PPP will influence its performance. This is particularly true for PPPs including clinical activities, as the diversity of payment mechanisms may lead to very different results. Take the demand addressed to a health care facility under a PPP contract. When patients have to pay some user charge or copayment, the demand will be different, and so will the revenues received by the private contractor.

Under full insurance provided to the population and payment according to the number of episodes or people treated, the PPP operator will want to serve as many patients as possible as often as possible. However, if a capitation payment is set, with a yearly amount paid for population in a designated catchment area, the incentive is to keep people away eventually lead them to other health care providers, meaning that penalties for mobility of patients looking for treatment elsewhere need to be introduced. Low quality of care concerns can also arise, and need to be addressed with auditing and monitoring.

Thus, the same PPP contract may yield different outcomes, both in financial terms and in quality of care terms, depending on the payment model designed for clinical activities.

The basic model has less variety of payment mechanisms, as the main objective is to repay the initial investment.

The role of incentives is performed by the payment rule, and a fixed payment rule provides a stronger incentive for cost reduction while at the same time imposing more uncertainty to the provider of the project. Cost reimbursement does remove the uncertainty to the private party contracted to execute the project (or at least removes the possibility of negative outcomes). Thus, providing incentives for an efficient operation implies shifting risk to the provider. This is the case not because of risk sharing between the parties but to induce different decisions by the private party.

Governments are better bearers of risk than individual companies. In terms of raising funds to pay for the project, such difference translates into interest rates in public debt being smaller than interest rates on private funding. Thus, for the same efficiency level in carrying out the project, the public entity faces lower costs than a private firm, just due to funding costs.

The gain from using the PPP depends on the ability of the private sector to be more efficient, not just because there is a risk transfer. Also, the procedure to set the payment should seek to ensure that it is as low as possible, from the perspective of the public sector. Reducing the risk to the private party, which can be done by introducing some cost reimbursement component, reduces the incentives to efficiency effort. This, in turn, means lower gain from using a PPP model.

A simple illustration of how payment mechanism rules define both risk allocation and incentives comes from the choice between payment by capitation and payment by episode of treatment for a hospital PPP. Both types of payment rule are prospective payment and provide incentives for cost operation efficiency. Payment by capitation allocates the risk of demand volume to the private partner operating the PPP while payment by episode of treatment allocates that same risk to the public payer. Whenever volume of demand is independent of actions of any of the two parties, the decision is to be taken on the basis of ability to bear risk. However, if actions by one of the sides can influence the volume of demand then the incentives created need to be factored-in. Suppose that prevention actions by the PPP operator can reduce significantly the number of episodes of treatment. Under a capitation payment, the PPP operator has a strong incentive to perform prevention activities. It will save costs of treatment without hurting the revenues of the PPP. On the other hand, under a payment by episode of treatment, there is no incentive for prevention activities, as success will mean a lower level of revenues. Thus, the allocation of demand volume risk has a central role in defining the incentive for prevention activities by the PPP operator.

Risk allocation and payment rules are closely related, and they are defined based on risk-bearing costs and incentives created. It also forces a clear definition of the objectives to be achieved by the PPP so that "instruments" like risk allocation can be established in the best way to achieve these objectives. It is worth repeating once more that risk allocation is not an objective of the PPP contract, it is an instrument of the parties and it is an instrument defined by the contractual rules agreed by the parties.

Choosing a model

The choice of one of the two main PPP models, basic or full-service, is not an obvious one. There is no clear-cut rule to say that a certain PPP/service should be provided under one or another model. There are, nonetheless, some guiding principles.

Recalling that, at heart, a PPP gain comes from better control and management by the private side facing the appropriate incentives (usually set by the transfer of risk), the advantage of a basic or a full-service model can be cast in terms of their contribution to the potential gains of the PPP.

While savings in the building and maintenance result mainly from design and architecture, savings in clinical activities management result from better managed services, with a focus on human resources management. For clinical activities management, the critical asset for success is the medical staff.

Some governments have adopted PPP contracts where the private partner is responsible for the design, construction, and maintenance of a hospital, and also for the provision of a set of equipment and services: for instance, imaging and diagnostic equipment, radiotherapy equipment, and dialysis equipment; the provision of electricity, gas, heating, water, medical gases, and medical vacuum; and the provision of security, cleansing, laundry, and catering services — so-called soft services. This may also include the provision of information systems and information and communication services in general.

Many PPP hospitals followed this infrastructure plus non-clinical services modality, but the largest PPP programs have gradually moved from more inclusive models to plainer models and have converged towards a bare design-build-maintain model (as a reaction to the growing incidence of the interface issues described in the next few paragraphs). A large spectrum of possibilities has been covered by the existing diversity in PPP contracts.

The rationale for adding some soft services to the accommodation PPPs relies on both the internalization of design impacts (for instance, having the private partner responsible for cleaning will induce it to design hospitals that are easier to clean) and the reduction of interface risks (for instance, avoiding conflicts between the cleaning manager, claiming poor design, and the maintenance manager, claiming sub-standard cleaning). However, adding soft services to the PPP contract presented in most cases a requirement for a periodic scheme for reviewing the cost of those services or supplies, within a long-term contract where the cost of the core design–build–maintain activities would be paid for according to a pre-determined annual rate (fixed, or automatically adjusted according to an agreed index, e.g., the consumer price index, or the health care component of it).

Adding services would expectedly add to the internalization of impacts. Still, it would not fully align the private sector with (clinical) hospital management needs and goals. Why should the private partner make early replacements of equipment rapidly turning obsolete, if it would not benefit from the resulting operational savings, or from resulting health improvements? Why should the private partner continuously adjust its service provisions to the changing needs of the clinical operator, if it would not benefit from it, but simply incur in change costs?

For the non-full-service PPP models, interface risks are expected to arise, with variable intensity and impact — small or large differences, between private and public partners, in the appraisal of contractual performance, or on the need for action. Whenever two control and command structures coexist within the same physical space and address complementary activities, such differences are expected to happen and need to be managed. They may happen, for instance, in the perceptions of the need for preventive or corrective maintenance, in the coordination of clinical activities with cleaning or catering activities, or in the actions needed for preventing contamination.

Under the full-service model, the gains from the PPP include the ones resulting from better management of clinical activities. Thus, the scope for gains from the PPP seems to be larger under the full-service model.

The scope for gains is also influenced by the PPP design. Suppose that the public sector provides a very detailed project for the infrastructure component, leaving little room for own decisions by the private side. Then the gains from the PPP will be relatively small and even perhaps uninteresting to the private side. The full-service model, by adding the gains from better management of clinical activities, may elicit more interest from the private sector. Another crucial aspect is the ability to write a contract with fewer open issues. The type of service to be delivered may be standardized, in which case the future much more predictable and amenable to inclusion in the contract. A more incomplete contract (in the economic sense of the term) makes it more likely that future, costly renegotiations will take place.

Adding clinical activities to the infrastructure PPP introduces more uncertainty in the contract. For example, the uncertainty about future technology and future health care needs introduce more incompleteness in the PPP contract when clinical activities are included. It also means that a long-term PPP contract is more attractive in terms of contractual completeness when it includes only standard procedures, not frontier procedures or research and teaching activities.

There are forces for and against the full-service PPP model (versus the basic model). The inclusion, or not, of clinical activities in the PPP will depend on the strength of each advantage and disadvantage and on the weight attached to them. It comes as no surprise that different countries have opted for different models, although to the best of our knowledge, there is no systematic review of the option selected against the elements described above.

An important aspect in the discussion of the full-service compared to the basic model is the relative size of each component of the contract. It is often the case that a single year of costs in clinical activities can be similar to, if not larger than, the cost of construction. This makes the clinical activities management a more important cost, over the project life cycle, than the construction cost.

Clinical activities are also far less predictable in the medium- and long-term than infrastructure costs. Thus, both quantitatively (level of costs) and qualitatively (uncertainty about future costs), the clinical-activities component of a health care provider embody a higher risk than construction and maintenance. On the other hand, the scope for savings to be gained due to higher efficiency is larger when clinical activities are included in the PPP contract, making it more attractive.

A different issue to address is the question of how to set contracts within the second type of design (Barros and Martinez-Giralt, 2009), with both construction and management of clinical activities included in the PPP. A PPP of this type usually involves two contracts, or two Special Purpose Vehicles: A contract with the institution in charge of the construction and maintenance of the hospital; and a contract with the entity in charge of clinical activities. One of private parties will be responsible for the subcontracting of the soft facilities, thus yielding two variations of the contracting set-up, according to which contract includes the latter. That is, soft facilities can be included either in the construction and maintenance contract or in the contract for management of clinical activities. The term 'soft facilities' describes the infrastructural support services, such as laundry, catering, cleaning, security, parking, and waste management.

In the absence of cost externalities from design and construction to the management of clinical activities, a PPP arrangement where soft facilities are subcontracted by the private party taking the contract for clinical services management is best. When the externality arising from the investment in infrastructure affects only the level of quality of the "soft facilities", and not the cost of providing clinical services, then the contract for infrastructure construction and maintenance should include these "soft facilities" within its scope.

On the one hand, clinical managers are probably in a better position to monitor the quality of soft facilities provision; on the other hand, we should not disregard the need for functional integration between soft and hard facilities and heavy equipment that may allow for less costly operation and better coordination.

Since typically soft facilities activities (such as laundry, food catering, cleaning, security, and waste disposal) are contracted out, the question of which contract they should be allocated to can be seen as which party (clinical activities management or hard facilities management) entails smaller distortions in subcontracting such soft facilities provision.

The basic trade-off is between a better monitoring role performed by clinical activities management over the quality of soft facilities provision and the internalization of infrastructure investments impact on the costs of providing clinical services and on costs of providing quality in soft facilities output (Barros and Martinez-Giralt, 2009). This latter aspect reflects the belief that a well-thought-out hospital design facilitates clinical activities and lowers the cost of providing quality in non-medical services (the so called soft-facilities).

Additional incentive schemes

By definition, private partners will be highly focused on obtaining profits — the PPP engine is precisely aligning their profit motivation with the public interest (through the contract provisions and effective contract management). Selecting an able and efficient private operator is critical for having a partner that **can** obtain profit without needing to resort to rent-seeking activities (such as unnecessary renegotiation of contract terms, attempts to lower quality of service under the contract terms, and efforts to increase revenue by doing more health care of low benefit to patients). But even an able and efficient private operator will not refrain from obtaining extra profits by exploring its strong points and the weak points of the public partner.

Diverting costs to other health care providers, or having those costs paid by the public partner as extra work, is an issue contracts and contract managers must face. Increasing service provision — translating extra-efficiency in higher volume, not lower cost — is another relevant issue.

Avoiding cream skimming. PPP contracts are output-based — but payment mechanisms, if they are to be manageable, cannot avoid some simplifications. Those simplifications will imply that the revenue–cost differential, for each output, will be different, creating an incentive for the private provider to select the more profitable patients. In every PPP contract, some activities will not be considered in the agreed package — and in full-service PPPs some patients are expected to be transferred to or from other health care facilities.

Full-service PPPs may pay for a certain volume of clinical services, or pay for services actually delivered according to a DRG-weighted formula. Fixed-volume contracts create an incentive for serving lower-cost patients. DRG-weighted formulas, if not updated regularly, may create significant variation in the revenue/cost ratio for different items. Even if regularly updated, and reflecting efficiency prices for each item, the cost structure of the incumbent private provider will always create some bias in favor of some patients, and against others.

Capitation-based full-service PPPs (such as the so-called "Alzira model" in use in Spain), serving a well-defined geographical area, require a particular incentive scheme that guarantees they preferentially serve the local population, while being able to serve non-local population if they do it efficiently. We should note that, although the "Alzira model" is used by health systems where the freedom to choose the health care provider is institutionalized, the contracts establish the private provider as a local 'preferred provider,' a quasi-monopolist, and so a compensatory incentive scheme is needed. A common scheme is requiring the private provider to pay (using National Health Service rates) for treatment the local population receives in other hospitals (creating incentive for the private operator to provide service, and to provide it with high-enough quality for the local population to use local services instead of non-local); and to allow them to serve non-local population (being paid a percentage of the National Health Service rates).

A clear definition of the range of clinical services that the private provider should offer is critical for the success of a full-service PPP. Also critical is a full set of protocols for accepting patients and for the transfer of patients to and from other health care providers (i.e., other hospitals, specialized facilities, primary care facilities, long-term care facilities, and ambulatory care), as well as proper screening of emergency ward patients (using the Manchester color protocol to screen patients at the point of entry, for instance, and defining clearly how the patients classified in the green and blue colors in this protocol are to be treated).

Containing demand fostering. Due to working in a different (less bureaucratically constrained) management framework, and to the profit-motivated economic rationality that is expected to guide its activity, PPP hospitals are expected to be more efficient. That efficiency may be translated into lower cost of service provision, or into higher volume of service provided. Government contracting authorities typically guarantee payment for a certain hospital capacity (usually measured in terms of beds, surgical theaters, and equipment, not in terms of output-delivery capacity), so the added private-sector efficiency creates overcapacity and a pressure towards adding volume, not lowering global cost.

If not dealt with appropriately in the contract (and through careful contract management), this pressure may jeopardize the success of the project, if not the fiscal sustainability of the PPP program. Per-capita contracts are supposed to be more resilient to this kind of pressure. The Portuguese model uses a managed-offer scheme, with yearly negotiated expected volumes of production, and the private-partner ability to unilaterally establish those volumes of production within a pre-defined range based on past production — and that scheme was resilient enough to survive the 2008–2014 fiscal crisis in Portugal.

Other contracts (e.g., Subúrbio in Bahia (Brazil), and Queen Mamohato hospital in Lesotho) prescribe a lump-sum payment for a certain volume of production — but the private-sector drive to deliver higher volumes of production, in a context of high non-served demand, has created successful pressure for increases in actual production, implying a growing fiscal effort to pay for those contracts.

Avoiding public-policy traps. Containing unpredicted profit-seeking moves by private providers, and so containing the cost of a PPP project, is important. But sometimes it is helpful to realize that some incentives can be mitigated but not fully contained — and rigid containment rules may have unintended consequences. The case of emergency services is a relevant one: While the contract may establish (negotiated or unilaterally declared by the public authority) upper limits on the volume of inpatient or outpatient services to be provided in each period, and correspondent penalties for non-compliance, the same should not be done regarding emergency services, where such limits would not be credible — no government would afford to face news saying that a public hospital has stopped attending emergency cases. Inpatient and outpatient care other than emergency care do not face this public pressure as patients are diverted to other facilities or forced to wait longer. For that case, screening rules (admission protocols) may mitigate the issue.

A Political Economy View of PPP

Previously, we discussed the economic reasons to have a PPP. Other motivations may be present. A common motivation pointed out as present is the PPP benefit of deferred budgetary impact for the government. This claim is starting point of this section.

Political motives

The creation of the PPP can have at its roots political motives by the public decision makers. The most obvious political motive that can be identified is the ability of a PPP to defer to the future the costs of current investment. The same, of course, is also done by issuing debt to finance public investment. The major difference, from a political point of view, is that carrying the investment by the Government will be reflected in the current budget deficit, a variable usually under close scrutiny by economic agents. Moreover, several countries have adopted, in the last couple of decades, budget rules committing to controlled budget deficits, imposing a cost for politicians of breaking it or even making the public investment unfeasible. A PPP provides a way to defer the current investment cost into the future, without being reflected in current budget deficits.

This political motive for a PPP as a way to spread investment costs to the future without showing it in current budget deficits is mainly associated with the investment cost, as paying for operation can be present if the new PPP substitutes for existing health care delivery. Whenever the PPP makes a new range of services available, or extends the volume of services, provided, then some future impact on budget spending will occur although not necessarily different from doing the project as public investment.

A second political motive linked to the Government budget impact for the use of a PPP is the value that may be attached to the certainty of health spending. By shifting (and paying) risk to the private partner, the political agent can have more certainty about public spending. This risk allocation does not reflect necessarily optimal risk sharing between public and private agents.

A third political motive is driven by political ideology favoring private management over public management, regardless of whether this is based on evidence.

One should expect efficiency to be part of the rationale for political decision-makers to propose PPPs. Unfortunately that seldom occurs, due to political myopia, with the main rationale for PPPs being effectiveness and "the creation of fiscal space," a misconception, as only efficient PPPs create fiscal space. The non-efficiency rationales deal with effectiveness (making the service available) and fiscal limbos.

On the first, effectiveness, the PPP incentive mechanisms are very powerful in terms of credible commitment for fast delivery of PPP projects (fast, if the PPP preparation and procurement processes do not create too much delay). The efficiency mechanism implicit in PPPs calls for delayed payment of infrastructure, in order to keep private money at stake (as discussed earlier).

Take now the issue of fiscal limbos. Because the current fiscal and financial reporting practices allow for government commitments regarding payments not to be recognized in government books, although they are also not recognized in private sector books, PPPs can currently be relegated to an accounting limbo, therefore allowing for a fiscal black hole for PPPs. We should note that recent public sector accounting standards (e.g., IPSAS-32) call for PPPs to be reported in public accounts — but only Germany and perhaps a few other countries have implemented them. Thus, recent trends in accounting standards for the public sector may mitigate this limbo effect in the future.

PPP as a commitment device

The PPP project can work as a commitment device for bureaucrats to ensure future budget streams for maintenance of infrastructure. Under traditional procurement to build the project, the department or entity running the new infrastructure will have to ask every year funds from the Government budget to pay for maintenance and operation of the infrastructure. The PPP project transforms the yearly budget negotiation into a contract that secures such funds in the future to pay to the private partner.

The PPP contract works as a credible commitment to implement a project. PPPs can also be a way for private partners to "capture" governments or to ensure future risk-free profits. By Government capture we mean the inability of Governments to politically recognize failure of a PPP, opting for renegotiation of conditions to avoid taking over the project from the private partner. This capture will often result in economic rents, that is, profits that are above the level required to the keep the private partner in the PPP project. From the private partner perspective, conditional on the actual risk allocation resulting from the project, the PPP may guarantee a steady and safe flow of revenues. The legal enforcement of a PPP contract makes it a credible commitment device.

Governance of PPP

A PPP is government initiated. The government, meaning the public sector, needs to be equipped to deal with the three main steps associated with a PPP: Assessing the opportunity for a PPP (which requires looking at costs and benefits), selecting the private partner (which includes ensuring an adequate tendering process) and managing the contract during its life-time (monitoring and enforcing the contract and managing changes).

The public sector also has other players that interact with the PPP, to a larger or smaller extent, according to each country's institutional framework. Other typical public sector stakeholders are Courts of Auditors and Parliaments.

For example, the Parliament plays a large role in PPP oversight and decision-making in the UK. But also public health care providers under traditional public-sector management may look closely at PPPs, both to learn and to compare performance.

Relevant stakeholders can also be found in citizens, academia, private partners that were not selected, media, etc.

Bringing a PPP from idea to life involves a series of steps — each of them helps to shape the PPP and its success. First, identifying, assessing, and selecting projects; then structuring and procuring them; later, for a long period, managing the contract, fiscal liabilities, change and renegotiation; and finally managing contract termination.

In summary, a PPP involves different phases: (1) Start of the process, involving project selection (project identification, cost–benefit analysis, prioritization, and sustainability checking) and the decision (and justification) on doing a PPP; (2) detailed definition of objectives and scope of the PPP by the public side, resulting in a detailed specification of the project, where detailed means that enough information is supplied to potential interested private parties; (3) pre-qualification and attracting interest of private entities; (4) tendering procedure; (5) final negotiation (if predicted in the rules of the tendering procedure); (6) contract close and financial close; (7) construction of the infrastructure; (8) operation and maintenance; (9) end of contract and transfer of facilities back to the public sector; and (10) *ex-post* evaluation of the project. During the term of a PPP contract there may occur some renegotiation, driven by exogenous changes in public policy, need for additional services, need for clarifying or correcting the contractual arrangement (e.g., redefining performance indicators), or by mere private partner's opportunism when economically stressed.

The success of the PPP in each phase conditions its success in subsequent phases. A badly designed tendering procedure may not attract the best candidates, the ones able to deliver higher savings, and a higher cost to the public sector of doing the project will result. And, if the project requirements are not clearly presented, and so cost expectations are not sound enough, a very strong bidding stage can also result in a higher likelihood of financial trouble for the private partner as it may have committed to a very low price to do the project.

Assessing and selecting PPP projects

The start of a PPP requires, from the public partner, detailed work in **project identification**, a **cost–benefit analysis** on the merits of the project and an assessment of its **sustainability** in terms of public finance. Good project selection is crucial. A project with a low social value will not be made good just because it is done under a PPP. Thus, health care authorities need to ensure (a) that the project has positive net social value, (b) that it is a priority project, and (c) that it is fiscally sustainable. Selecting high-social-value projects is not enough — governments need to prioritize projects and check their fiscal sustainability, considering potential costs, benefits and risks.

The PPP is just one of the instruments that can be used to carry out a valuable project — the selection of a project should consider the alternatives to carry it out. We could say that projects should be first assessed and approved (based on their own merits in terms of serving the needs of the populations), and then the procuring authority should decide on the implementation mode, comparing the several possible traditional modes and the several possible PPP modes. But in practice health care authorities need to be aware that those different modes present different costs, benefits and risks, and so the selection of projects and the decision on implementation mode will be intertwined.

Procuring the contract

Once a project has strong backing in terms of the social value that it will generate, the next steps are detailing the PPP scheme and preparing the **draft contract**, and then selecting the private partner.

The health care authority needs to define the objectives and scope of the PPP, resulting in a detailed specification of the project, where detailed means that enough information needs to be supplied to potential interested private entities. By enough information we mean information that allows private entities to build their business cases and assess how much savings they can achieve if they are selected to do the project.

A competitive selection process is often seen as the best way to select the private partner at the lowest cost to the public partner — lowest cost for the quality intended by the procuring authority. For a competitive selection process to produce good results it needs to attract several candidates interested to become partners — this requires transparent and well-crafted rules for decision in the tendering procedure.

The tendering procedure usually takes the format of an auction, with different options being available. Sometimes, a two-stage procedure is used, in which a first phase defines a smaller set of candidates (say, two final candidates) and then a second phase allows the selected candidates to make a best-and-final-offer, with a possible closing negotiation phase of the exact contractual clauses of the PPP.

At this point, the stage of selection of the private partner ends and the execution of the PPP contract begins. After the contract signature, the next step is the construction of the infrastructure — then follows the period of maintenance and operation of the facility, also called the active-life period.

Managing the contract

The contracts governing Public–Private Partnerships are complex and detailed contracts, requiring both day-to-day oversight and a strategic approach whenever contract renegotiations are requested (by either side).

A crucial element in a PPP is the technical ability of the Government (or the relevant public sector entity) to manage the contract.

Specific knowledge is involved, in particular when clinical activities are included in the PPP. Auditing and monitoring reports are necessary and relevant but do not substitute for a close, permanent, oversight (which is often set and regulated by the contract).

Building expertise in the technical staff of the public sector and being able to retain it under aggressive hiring by the private sector is a key challenge in the governance model of a PPP. An overall social-value assessment of doing a PPP contract must weigh in the additional costs of building and maintaining the technical expertise by public sector staff.

Research and reports on the performance of PPPs put a strong emphasis on the monitoring requirements of contract management, the most visible component of contract management, and the one most closely linked to contractual provisions. But, for public authorities, contract management presents three main components: monitoring the services and implementing the contract, partnering with the private operator, and managing change and public-sector risks.

Monitoring and enforcing standards of performance (including quality) requires contract management capabilities by the public sector. When a system of payments and penalties according to contractual indicators is in place, enforcing it may face difficulties to the public contractor.

The output of the contract involves, in health care, aspects that are difficult to control. Defining performance in terms of health improvement to the population is arguably quite difficult to do in an objective and verifiable way. Still, performance has to be monitored, and contracts should define penalties to be applied to poor performance. The idea is not to reduce the costs to the public sector by application of penalties but to ensure adequate performance for the payment set under the contract. Powerful aids in this monitoring are the existence of audits and the disclosure to the public of project performance.

The need for a close relationship between the public and the private partners of a PPP has led to the creation of the position of "contract manager" to actively act on behalf of the public partner in several projects. The contract manager needs to oversee day-to-day aspects of the contract implementation but it also needs to have a strategic view of the partnership over the long run.

Renegotiation

Long-term contracts subject to uncertainty and contract incompleteness are prone to renegotiation. Renegotiation may alter considerably the value of the contract for either partner. Renegotiation procedures need to be included in a PPP contract in a clear way, as it will determine future bargaining power of the parties. It is important to define who can initiate a renegotiation and how a renegotiation is organized.

Renegotiation may occur for several reasons. The more frequent ones are: (1) demand of service beyond those planned in the contract under fixed payment, which increases costs but does not change revenues to the private partner, and (2) a desired change in service conditions by the public partner, namely introduction of new technologies or treatments.

The first renegotiation motive, demand for services above those planned under fixed payment, means that financial balance of the private partner is at risk for reasons beyond its control. Consequently, a renegotiation of the contract should reinstate "fair" conditions of operation to the private partner. Of course, it is open for discussion which elements are influenced by whom. To illustrate two extreme situations, consider in turn the case where demand for a health care facility is determined by its quality relative to other public sector alternatives. A private partner by investing in quality may trigger an increase in demand for its services above planned and use it to ask for extra payment through a renegotiation procedure. In this example, the renegotiation is driven by the actions of the private partner.

Suppose now that under the same circumstances, it is the public partner that lowers the quality of alternatives, driving demand to the PPP facility. Not allowing a renegotiation in this situation opens a way for the public partner to "expropriate" gains from the private partner by diverting demand. In this latter case, it is the public partner actions that trigger the renegotiation process.

A few months after the start of its operation, the Subúrbio Hospital in Bahia (Brazil), faced an unexpected change: The local municipality, perceiving the high quality of service provided by the state hospital, closed down its two neighboring primary care facilities, inducing a sudden increase in hospital demand, simultaneous with a decrease in the case-mix. This created additional demand to the PPP hospital, triggered by decisions of the health authority and being exogenous to the private partner in the PPP.

The importance of renegotiation in the outcome of the PPP is especially true for the introduction of new technologies. The contract may define the default position of each partner regarding new technology. It is different whether the default is mandatory introduction of the innovation in a PPP activity, with a pre-defined price (for example, the same price or cost of the public hospitals with that technology) or the public partner has to convince the private partner with a newly negotiated price, as the private partner has the right to refuse the new technology.

Renegotiation is not always formal. Sometimes it takes the form of a complete re-tendering of the project (in the case of "La Ribera" in Spain, the new 'tender' had a single bidder due to the way it was conceived, see EXPH (2014)), but in many cases it is mainly an agreement on the interpretation of the contract, the way it measures production, or the way performance indicators are quantified.

Fiscal management

Beyond the direct effect of approving a PPP project individually, there is a "portfolio effect" resulting from accumulation of public sector payment commitments, a form of public debt. Moreover, it decreases Government's spending flexibility. It forces business cycles fluctuations to be accommodated in public finances by the other public spending. The future implications of this Government budget inflexibility seem to be usually ignored when deciding each PPP *per se*, as only the accumulation of PPPs will cause the issue to arise. OECD, in its *Principles for Public Governance of Public–Private Partnerships* (OECD, 2012), states that "in line with the government's fiscal policy, the Central Budget Authority should ensure that the project is affordable and the overall investment envelope is sustainable," suggesting that the investment expenditure budget should be based on medium and long term fiscal projections and regularly updated.

Besides payment commitments, PPPs bring also fiscal risks for government, through explicit or implicit contingent liabilities. Unilateral changes by the public authorities, force majeure, or private operator bankruptcy, are examples of events that may impact the fiscal position of government. That is why OECD recommends (OECD, 2013) that PPPs should be included and explained in the budget reports, even where they do not directly affect the public finances.

Terminating the contract

The end of the contract typically involves the transfer of facilities to the public sector or to a new private operator competitively selected, and an *ex-post* evaluation of the project, including identification of lessons and recommendations.

When the contract is approaching its term, close monitoring is required — growing incentives for the private partner to cut investment and deplete the assets will need to be counteracted. Thus, for the public partner, the involvement has a different nature at the start, at the execution, and at the end of the PPP project.

The role of private stakeholders

The diversity and complexity of tasks involved in PPPs imply that the private partner is typically a consortium of private firms with different primary activities — usually one or more health care companies, and one or more construction or engineering companies.

The definition of the PPP type also determines the crucial private stakeholders. Under an infrastructure-only PPP, the contribution of the private partner lies in the ability to design, build and operate the infrastructure efficiently. The key resources the public sector looks for in the private partner are the knowledge to build the facility in time and under budgeted cost and being able to perform maintenance of the infrastructure efficiently. Construction companies are the main candidates to fulfill these requirements adequately.

On the other hand, under a full-service PPP, management of clinical activities becomes the crucial aspect. The private partner needs to have a good record and experience in the management of clinical activities as the savings obtained in this activity will be the main source of gains to the PPP — the cost of design, construction, and equipment is typically less than the cost of service delivery for a single year.

The ability of the private partner to build within the deadline and without cost overruns the health facility is of course important but it is no longer the main issue. Thus, the private partner will most likely come from organizations with expertise in health care management and delivery. These will be different partners from the building and construction companies that are interested in the infrastructure-only PPPs.

In full-service PPPs, shareholding power is in the hands of health care firms: health care groups control all Portuguese PPP hospitals (UTAP, 2014), Promédica Patrimonial controls Prodal Saúde that runs Subúrbio Hospital (Bahia, Brazil) (Carrera, 2012), Tsepong (Pty) Ltd. controls Queen Mamohato Hospital (Lesotho) (PwC — PriceWaterhouse Coopers, 2013), while construction companies typically put up the remaining capital. In Subúrbio Hospital — a PPP created after the main building had already been built — the secondary partner is an engineering company, relevant for maintenance and operation.

But in accommodation PPPs, shareholding power is in the hands of construction companies (e.g., Eiffage in the Centre hospitalier sud-francilien, France), with health care companies as minority shareholders or simply absent. The first assessment of those contracts (MNAIH — Mission Nationale d'Appui à l'Investissement Hospitalier, 2007) notes that the bidding consortia were typically the major construction companies associated with their own specialized maintenance and engineering companies.

This influence of health care companies in full-service PPPs, and of construction companies in accommodation PPPs is highly relevant for understanding the kind of issues and conflicts that arise during the operation of PPP hospitals. That influence is also felt during the procurement process, where bidding consortia mimic the legal entity that they are expected to create if awarded the contract. And, of course, having health care companies, or construction companies, leading the complex process of presenting a proposal for a PPP-hospital (including a concept for the hospital and a draft technical project) will lead to different results.

The PPP project has several stakeholders involved: The Government, or a public agency, as public partner; the private partner that will carry out the project, which will be different for each type of PPP; the funding creditors, mainly banks; the health professionals; taxpayers; and, patients. The relative importance and role of each of them will vary with the specific details of the PPP.

In the discussion of PPPs, an often-ignored stakeholder is the institution involved in funding the PPP. Most of the attention is on the contract, but who is involved in the financing process is also of interest as it may influence the resulting contract. In large economies, with a well-developed banking system, private banks are usually behind the financial arrangement to fund the PPP.

In most developing countries, the financing side often involves development banks or public banks. Building up the financial component of funding the PPP will face tension with the incentive role of risk transfer. Transferring more risk to the private partner tends to raise the cost of funding and the institutions providing the funds may demand less risk transfer to keep the cost of funds low. But doing so also decreases the efficiency incentives provided by the transfer of risk and less gains from the PPP will be generated and distributed. Whenever the funding bodies have influence over the PPP design, it is more likely to see less risk transfer.

An example of this is the participation of regional savings banks in the "Alzira" PPP (Valência, Spain), which in practice internalized in the public sector the risks that are usually transferred from the public payer to the private partner. The regional savings banks are controlled by the regional Government, who will provide help in case of need. The Regional Government that acts as public partner is simultaneously managing the regional savings banks that fund private investors.

PPP within the Health System

Health system design and PPPs

The existence of a PPP has more implications to the health system than mere ownership of hospital facilities and management, especially in the context of public health systems. The existence of PPPs requires first of all, as mentioned before, the ability of the public sector to adequately manage the long-term contract involved. But it also demands clarification on how the health care unit under the PPP contract interacts with other providers in the health system.

A PPP in health care is usually integrated into a health system. The design of the health system as a whole influences the gains and opportunities associated with the PPP. The demand for services provided by the PPP is influenced, if not determined, by the health system design. This is naturally more important in the full-service PPP, as clinical services management may directly impact the demand for that facility's services. For infrastructure-only PPPs, coordination within the health system is largely done by the public partner managing the facility.

Take as a prime example the case of a full-service PPP for provision of hospital care. The demand of services directed to the hospital will include referrals from other health care units in the system, either primary care units or other hospitals. It may also be the case that the PPP hospital sends back patients to primary care after treatment or even takes decisions to induce self-selection of cases (more complicated, and, costly cases) into other hospitals (for example, building a reputation of not treating certain costly cases).

Some of these relationships can be addressed controlled by carefully crafted and monitored contract rules, by adequate payment systems and careful monitoring of performance indicators included in the contract. Referrals from the PPP hospital to other hospitals in the public network will likely obey rules and penalties for undue referrals that are in included in the contract. The possibility of inducement of self-selection of patients into other areas requires that care given to patients supposed to be treated in the PPP hospital is traced in the health system. An adequate relationship with primary care is also facilitated by a carefully designed payment system to primary care and the PPP hospital.

The PPP hospital may also have an incentive to divert demand from other health care units if the payment system rewards positively more activity.

Thus, the PPP cannot be seen and assessed in isolation from the remaining elements of the health system. In some models, the externality effects between primary care activities and hospital activities are internalized by including primary care services under the full-service PPP.

For example, a PPP hospital with a fixed yearly payment based on capitation will have an incentive to develop mechanisms and relationships that treat people at primary care when it is feasible to do so, avoiding the hospital cost, while a primary care service paid by a global budget (fixed wage for health professionals) have an incentive to refer more patients to the hospital. But a fee-for-service payment in primary care would align the interests of both the hospital and primary care services in treating more patients in primary care, though not necessarily by keeping the population healthier through primary prevention activities.

A different incentive is created if the PPP hospital receives extra payment for additional activity. The capacity defined in the PPP design will also matter when the PPP is inserted into the health system. Whenever slack capacity exists in the PPP health care provider, it will attempt to serve more demand (especially in a full-service PPP).

PPPs may have an impact on a country's health system through the inputs market, in particular the health care labor market. A PPP project managed by a private entity may offer opportunities to scarce skilled health professionals, especially in the case of full-service PPP. The impact upon the health system and in particular, upon the public provision of health care that may exist in the country, will ultimately depend on the rules applied to dual practice in the country. When working in a PPP (private sector position) and having another job in the public health care system is not incompatible, the PPP may enlarge the potential remuneration of health professionals and help retain health professionals in the public system. On the other hand, if dual practice is not allowed, the PPP may deplete the public health care system of these professionals and create staffing problems to (other) public providers of health care. As in other types of effect, the impact of a PPP will be conditional on its size and on the particular rules of the health system.

Integrating PPPs in the management of the health system

Contract managers establish the link between private operators and public authorities. But sound management of a PPP program implies some changes in the management of a national health system — in fact, those changes are perhaps critical for the success of a PPP program.

Health care PPPs present an opportunity (and an invitation) for improving the strategic management of national health systems. Countries adopting PPP procurement are typically countries with some kind of national health system, where government assumes a coordinating role and somehow influences directly health services supply, and indirectly its demand (through referrals and price-setting).

Signing a PPP contract, *per se*, improves the volume and quality of **available information**, as the private operator must provide volume and performance data, and those data (and the information system that provides data) must be audited.

Some PPP contracts are based on **benchmarking** mechanisms, forcing public authorities to improve the collection of data from other nodes of the health care system.

PPP hospitals, having long-term contracts with some kind of target capacity, must have a set of protocols for **patient referrals**, inducing the need for a proper management of those referrals, expectedly according to capacity and relative cost of the system nodes.

Above all, the use of private providers creates a long-term constraint on public policy (the financial commitment to pay for infrastructure availability and for a set of services), requiring an effort to extract benefits out of that long-term relationship. That implies some type of **strategic management** of the health system, in order to "adjust" health care supply and health care demand according to the relative cost of service provision and according to the priorities on health care policy.

More often than not, public sector health care providers would benefit, for their own efficiency of operation, from being subject to the same rules regarding information, benchmarking mechanisms, patient-referral protocols and strategic management as applied to PPP health care units. The presence of PPPs did not generally create movements to make public sector providers subject to those same rules. Some influence can be detected in particular countries. In Portugal, the clinical management PPPs of Hospital Amadora-Sintra in the late 1990s created a discussion that led to the pilot experiment in pure public sector hospitals of a management model with more procurement and human resources management freedom, later on (in 2003) expanded to roughly half of the public hospitals and nowadays to almost all of them.

Results, Opportunities, and Challenges

Success and failure. It is still soon to present a verdict on PPPs for health care — or on the main contractual models used for the implementation of those PPPs. Most general statements on PPP success or failure lack sufficient economic or clinical evidence, instead being driven by preconceptions, ideology, or group interests.

Success and failure may also coexist, depending on how success and failure are defined in light of the different components of the 'public interest.' For instance, a project may deliver the expected services at efficiency costs and with adequate quality, but negatively affecting the public purse through strong service volume growth — in an extreme case challenging fiscal sustainability. Or, a project may deliver efficiently, but its procurement may have biased project structuring in some way.

So, even with full disclosure of evidence on health care PPPs, the weights allocated to the different appraisal components that lie within the realm of 'public interest' will allow for a reasonably broad range of final assessments. So, more important than the final verdict will be the assessment of several different facets of PPPs.

Most published evidence relates to the **effectiveness** of PPPs — their ability to deliver proper infrastructure and equipment, their ability to deliver good-quality clinical services. But, more relevant than effectiveness, should be the **efficiency** of PPPs. Efficiency, here, should not be simply the short-term efficiency in the use of public resources (i.e., Do PPPs provide the lowest cost for government to provide a certain volume of service at a certain level of quality?, or Do PPPs provide the best service delivery for a certain cost?), but mainly the long-term efficiency in the provision health care as appraised by society (i.e., looking at the cost of service provision, not simply the cost to government). For a PPP model to be sustainable, we need efficiency in the use of public resources **plus** private-sector profitability. This implies that the cost of providing health care services through PPPs be lower than the costs of alternative delivery modes, for a certain quality standard. Quality standards based on measurable indicators can be part of contract norms, triggering penalties if not met.

But efficiency is not enough if health care authorities are not able to **manage** the PPP contracts and the effects of change upon them — endogenous change (such as pressure for opportunistic renegotiation, or pressure for policy changes that may impact PPP efficiency) and exogenous change (such as demographic or technological change).

We are also concerned with the ability of government to **fund** projects' costs in the short and long term. Even if each project is well designed, well implemented and well managed, the PPP framework may create incentives for too many projects to be approved, challenging fiscal sustainability.

Comparing PPPs to what? Infrastructure has a poor track record in terms of implementation delays and cost overruns — Flyvbjerg presents motives that could explain that, namely the misrepresentation of projects' costs and benefits, in order for each project promoter to increase its chances of seeing it approved (Flyvbjerg, 2007). PPPs, because of their whole-life-costing approach, and because of the due-diligence process required by private financing, typically present reduced (or no) construction delays and reduced (or no) cost overruns — but that happens after a lengthier procurement process and a more careful cost-assessment process, incorporating the expected costs of design and construction 'surprises.' So, reduced construction delays do not mean faster implementation of the project, and absence of cost overruns does not imply that the project is cheaper. Of course, the added certainty on cost and on commissioning dates does present value to the budgetary process and to health care system management, but a full cost-benefit analysis should be applied.

Many reports (for instance, the Boston University 2013 report on Lesotho Hospital (Boston University, 2013)) describe extensively the health gains obtained with the PPP. Comparing new hospitals with old hospitals is fine, but not the point here — we are concerned with comparing the PPP management of those projects with the alternative management by public entities under separate contracts or in-house delivery to achieve the same goals.

In what relates to infrastructure and equipment, comparing new to old is not relevant — what is relevant is comparing what the PPP is bringing, and at what cost, to what could be achieved with alternative procurement modes.

Disclosing the evidence. PPPs bring to public procurement a healthy focus on outputs and results: the availability of facilities and equipment, and the provision and cost of health care services (not what was spent on doctors and other health care professionals, or what was spent on construction or acquisitions). When government is paying for specific services (e.g., cleaning, catering, laundry, security), the focus is on performance and cost of those services.

That output focus presents an opportunity for authorities to use PPPs as benchmarks for health care delivery — and in several cases, PPP contracts use incentive mechanisms where each project is compared to a reference set of comparable public hospitals.

This focus on performance is somehow correlated to some institutional reforms, for instance the creation in 2009 of ANAP (*Agence Nationale d'Appui à la Performance des établissements de santé et médico-sociaux*) in France, merging several entities including the former health care PPP Unit — among many other activities with hospitals and regional health authorities, ANAP hosts an Observatory of Hospital Construction Costs and is currently researching on life-cycle optimization of maintenance and periodic renewals of hospitals.

However, actual reporting on performance and cost is scarce — most health care authorities do not publish data on performance, and data on costs are usually aggregated. In its 2010 report on PFI-hospital performance (National Audit Office, United Kingdom, 2010), the British Audit Office notes, after presenting the evidence on cleaning and catering, that it could do that analysis for 2008–2009 or 2009–2010 because "the NHS stopped collecting the data" — and it notes that it had no data for the other services.

Poor disclosure may simply reflect poor performance management. The British Audit Office reports that only 28% of the regional health authorities reported having management systems satisfying the six criteria defined by the Office for a good performance management system (reports problems, identifies performance, identifies deductions, identifies actions to improve performance, ensures problems are dealt with, provides timely reports) (National Audit Office, United Kingdom, 2010).

Identifying lessons from experience. Learning from past experiences, and from experiences abroad, does happen in some countries, but typically evaluation of PPP experiences is surrounded by a veil of secrecy. What is published is usually focused on the effectiveness of the project or program — not on its efficiency — and does not encompass all the costs of the project.

In the United Kingdom, according to its government (HM Treasury, 2012), the Public Finance Initiative program "has become tarnished by its waste, inflexibility and lack of transparency". In France, the Court of Audits recent report on PPP hospitals (Cour des Comptes, France, 2007) concludes that they were procured in a rushed way, the potential advantages attributed to PPPs were poorly explored, and financial issues were not sufficiently taken into account. Being the two largest hospital PPP programs in the world, these announcements, combined with a plethora of anecdotes, are creating a bad reputation for hospital-PPPs. But the vast majority of those PPP contracts are still in place, with the hospitals fully operational, and many of them performing similar or better than other public hospitals. (National Audit Office, United Kingdom, 2010) In many cases, the waste is already incurred, as a sunk cost, when the contract was signed, as decisions about (over) capacity, for example, are already taken.

There are other countries that engaged in hospital PPP procurement that have not had the same negative results — for instance, the Canadian provinces report the absence of the major problems affecting European projects.

Full-service PPPs seem to be more resilient than infrastructure-only PPPs. In Brazil, Lesotho, Spain, Portugal, health care authorities praise performance in those hospitals — they face a few challenges, but the public perception is widely different, and hospital-PPP reputation is not tarnished.

Around the world, many countries are currently procuring or preparing hospital PPP projects, so it is highly relevant to identify lessons from the experience, to identify results from the different models, and to determine if and how they can be improved.

Most of these perceived results of the PPP experience in hospitals are not published, resulting from direct contacts with PPP practitioners (e.g., procurement managers and experts, hospital managers, contract managers, auditors).

One advantage attributed to PPP projects is the ability to deliver quickly the infrastructure and associated health care services. Some estimates point to a cost benefit analysis of PPP of circa 30%, on the one hand, and roughly in-time completion of projects (on average 3.4% ahead of time), which compares with 23.5% delayed projects under traditional public procurement, on the other hand (Raisbeck *et al.*, 2010).

There is, however, no evidence from other countries that systematically corroborates these results. This is particularly true when assessing realized costs of PPP contracts in several countries. Often opacity of accounting procedures and lack of proper measurement preclude a rigorous assessment of realized costs. This opacity in itself is an indication that expected costs savings associated with the PPP project did not materialize in line with predictions.

Besides costs of the project and speed of completion, other dimensions of impact from PPPs have been identified.

Rigidity is a complaint commonly related to accommodation PPPs (but not to full PPPs) — it is usually presented in the context of managerial change, sometimes in the context of technological change. The new PPP policy (HM Treasury, 2012) of the British government refers to PFI's "inflexibility," noting that "PFI contracts have been insufficiently flexible during the operational period, so making alterations to reflect the public sector's service requirements has been difficult" and adding that PFI had been used "in sectors and projects where there was insufficient long term certainty on the future requirements of services; or where fast-paced technological changes made it difficult to establish requirements for the long term".

In France, ANAP's 2013 Report presents, as the first condition for opting for the PPP procurement mode, "perfectly stable" capacity needs defined for many years, noting that program changes during the design and construction phases are a major source of disruptions potentiating cost overruns for the public partner (ANAP, 2013).

Lack of VfM is now recognized in the British case, in what relates to soft services attached to accommodation PPPs.

Typically full-service PPPs do not suffer from those same challenges: the private partner is operating the hospital itself and so commercial and technological changes are endogenous issues, to be decided according to economic rationality; and soft services are also managed under the same rationality. Of course, innovations that present dubious health effects, or that are too costly, will tend not to be adopted by the private operator.

Demand pull is to be expected in contracts where the private partner faces demand risk. Up to a certain level of demand, this serves the public interest — but above that level, budgetary and public health issues are raised. Pulling too much demand to a PPP hospital may divert patients from other public units — and create a fiscal challenge when the public purse is paying services to thc private operators and paying public operators for idle capacity. Or it could simply increase service provision up to a point of fiscal unsustainability. But demand pulling may also create health concerns whenever users are being offered "excessive" care, for instance offered imaging services that create welfare-reducing scare over non-threatening potential diseases — the Health System should also manage those cases.

Value for money and the public sector comparator. The use of VfM comparisons (or computation of the public sector comparator) is not widespread. Within a set of European countries using PPPs in the health sector, only a minority of countries (3 out of 9)[1] do report their computation of VfM using the public sector comparator. (On the role of VfM, see Boardman *et al.* (2010) and the references therein.)

While Portugal uses the public sector comparator as a reference level for checking the budgetary framework requirement that only allows for the use of

[1]Portugal, United Kingdom and the Czech Republic vs. Spain, Germany, Romania, Italy, France and Finland.

private finance when the PPP project is cheaper than the non-PPP solutions, many other countries follow the British VfM methodology and use it for deciding between the PPP and non-PPP options. Recently, in the sequence of an Audit Office report on VfM (National Audit Office, United Kingdom, 2013), the United Kingdom recognized that "the quantitative assessment tool has encouraged procuring authorities to compare a PFI solution against a conventionally funded — and in some cases undeliverable — alternative, rather than consider alternative contracting approaches", and consequently withdrew the VfM methodology (HM Treasury, United Kingdom, 2012) in 2012, introducing a "qualitative VfM" (World Bank, 2013) — in parallel, the project assessment methodology now requires a broader assessment of possible alternatives, namely:

> "At the outset, during strategic outline stage of project development, a long list of options should be generated and considered at a high level and a short list selected for more detailed analysis. The maintenance and smarter use of existing assets should be considered as a "de minimis" option. Where this is insufficient, options should be considered for targeted action to tackle network stress points or develop networks on a small scale. Where appropriate, large-scale transformational projects that are part of a clear long-term strategy can also be considered. Demand management can apply to any of these options and should be considered." (HM Treasury, United Kingdom, 2011)

The main criticism regarding the now-abandoned VfM methodology was its mechanical approach to assessment, using the 'right' assumptions for obtaining the desired result, and taking it as a black box instead of using it to understand costs, benefits, and risk. It was not uncommon to have the model run repeatedly, changing the assumptions until the desired result was obtained — sometimes the PPP option was adopted because the quantitative model presented a tiny advantage in favor of the PPP option, without pondering this quantitative advantage with the governance issues related to a long-term contractual commitment. Following this methodology, many countries did implement their own quantitative assessment, in many cases so sophisticated that no one really understood it, reinforcing its use as a black box.

A report recently published by the Treasury Committee of the British Parliament added evidence on this, reaffirming that the quantitative VfM "had features which served to advantage PFI in the comparison with conventional procurement" and noting that:

> "Key assumptions in the model were not supported by empirical evidence. [...] Despite Treasury guidance that the model should not be a 'pass-or-fail' test, many project teams did not provide sufficient explanation of the underlying rationale for their choice of contracting approach. [...] While the model compared PFI to

'conventional procurement,' it did not enable the comparison of other contracting approaches with PFI. For the six projects we looked at it was not always clear what was meant by conventional procurement. In two of those cases 'conventional procurement' was not considered by the project team to be the next best alternative, so in those cases the model could not indicate whether or not PFI was the cheapest approach available. The Treasury recognizes that in some instances where the model was used, the conventional option to which PFI was compared was in fact undeliverable. [...] Project teams' ability to gain additional benefit from using the model was hindered by the lack of visibility of the model's workings. Many of the assumptions were hard-wired into the model and most of the workings were hidden. While this made it easier for those reviewing the use of the model, it also meant project teams were less able to explore the way their assumptions and estimates interacted and affected the project. [...] We would like to see modelling used more intelligently. This requires models to be designed in such a way that they aid a project team's understanding of their project and allow the team to explore the relationships between the project's various elements. [...] We would like to see project teams treat models as just one element, set alongside other factors, which informs their judgment about which contracting approach offers best value for money." (Treasury Committee, House of Commons, United Kingdom, 2014)

The current debate on quantitative VfM (and the need for developing qualitative approaches) in the context of "comparative VfM", should not divert us from the critical need for a sound "absolute VfM" (cost–benefit analysis) or from the need for some kind of qualitative exercise in that context.

On the role of the public sector comparator in the VfM quest, Gouveia and Raposo compute, for two Portuguese PPP hospitals, the expected cost of infrastructure construction and the cost of operation of clinical activities (**Unsupported source type (Misc) for source Gou12.**). While in one case, the value used for the public sector comparator is in line with expected cost (*Hospital de Cascais*), in the other case the public sector comparator shows a considerable upward bias (almost double the cost of clinical activities). Competition in the bidding stage for selection of the private partner brought the value closer to the predicted cost.

Public sector comparator

		Lower	**Mean**	**Upper**	**PSC**	**Bid**
H. Cascais	Infrastructure	66	69	73	80.7	359
	Clin. activities	324	345	367	328.05	
H. Braga	Infrastructure	121.77	146.14	184.32	200.00	794
	Clin. activities	361.91	418.25	483.51	986.00	

Notes: Braga is a teaching hospital. Bid = winning bid in tendering procedure. Unit = million €.
Source: (**Unsupported source type (Misc) for source Gou12.**).

Thus, competition in the tendering phase may help achieve VfM, making the ability to attract competitors to the tendering stage a feature for a successful PPP.

Competition does not depend only on the number of competitors — in Portugal, three main health care groups fighting for contracts that could bring them a reputation in the market, induced much higher competition than the three major public-works firms that in France were bidding for health care projects (MNAIH — Mission Nationale d'Appui à l'Investissement Hospitalier, 2007).

Project effectiveness

Effectiveness means the ability of project to deliver the service specified in the contract. Evidence on effectiveness comes mainly from official reports. According to the British supreme auditors (National Audit Office, United Kingdom, 2010), "most [hospital] contracts are performing satisfactorily or better and meeting the expectations of Trusts [the health authorities]" and "there is strong enough evidence to say that most contracts are delivering the value for money expected of them." Looking at the details in that report, one can see that only 67% of the trusts (i.e., two-thirds) report satisfaction with their contracts — and only 11% rated all their services as better than 'satisfactory.' Regarding maintenance, 14% of the trusts rated performance as "less than satisfactory." The only services for which performance was assessed were cleaning and catering — and for them there is no significant difference between PFI and non-PFI hospitals.

In Portugal, with respect to effectiveness, the four PPP hospitals are delivering their services as any other public hospital. An early PPP contract, the Amadora-Sintra hospital, was also considered to be delivering services according to the contract. The Amadora-Sintra hospital was a particular PPP as the construction was done by the public sector and only at a later stage the management of clinical activities (and responsibility for the building, equipment, and their maintenance) was set as a public–private partnership. The contract was signed in late 1995 and the private management started operating by the end of the first quarter 1996. A first evaluation was done just after two years and half, concluding with an assessment of a better performance by the PPP than the one of a comparable hospital in the Lisbon region.

Later on, in 2001, a second evaluation was performed by the Lisbon regional health administration, which points to an advantage for the public hospital (non-PPP). This view on the relative effectiveness of the PPP was challenged by the Minister of Health, although the supporting documentation was never published. Existing information points to a biased comparison as for the public hospitals analysis was based on official budget and not actual expenditures (which have been regularly well above the official budget) (Barros and Gomes, 2002). Another evaluation was made by (Simões, 2004), concluding in favor of more effective results from public management with more entrepreneurial-like rules over the PPP model, which was nonetheless better than traditional public management. In 2008, the Government took the decision to end the PPP by political motives (public hospitals should have public management), effective from start of 2009. An interesting fact is the recent decision to re-tender the PPP contract for the Physical Rehabilitation Center in Algarve, that had reached its term — that decision was based on the quality and volume of service provided, as well as its efficiency (savings with that contract were estimated at 10% of the cost for the National Health Service — see UTAP's report (section 2.4) (UTAP — Unidade Técnica de Acompanhamento de Projetos, 2014).

Innovation in management

An important aspect of the PPP is how it manages and promotes innovation, either technological or in health care delivery organization. There are two moments in which this issue appears. One is, of course, at the design of the infrastructure. The architecture of the health care facility may reflect innovative ways of organizing health care and define different pathways for patients. The second moment is during operation of the PPP. Naturally, this second aspect is attributable to the PPP only under the full-service PPP. A nuance on the first moment of managing innovation is the approach of "procurement for innovation" adopted by the Karolinska Institute (Sweden) in the PPP contract for its new hospital. In this case, the PPP contract is set to satisfy a future need of the contracting agent, a need that cannot be completely specified at the start. The private partner and the contracting entity need to collaborate to develop the innovations required to satisfy the health care needs. The focus is therefore on the probability of finding the intended innovation. The contract is about satisfying a health care need, and the way to do it is unspecified in the contract as the objective is to find an innovation to do it (EXPH (EXpert Panel on effective ways of investing in Health), 2014). Partnership, therefore, goes well beyond financial flows and monitoring of *ex-ante* specified performance criteria.

Compared to full-service PPPs, accommodation PPPs present a reduced scope for innovation — still, designing the contract on the basis of outputs is supposed to create enough scope for innovation. The evidence, however, points toward a reduced innovation rate in accommodation PPPs. The analysis of the first ten hospital PPPs in France finds, for all of them, poor innovation characteristics — both in terms of architectural and functional innovation — presenting as a main cause the highly prescriptive nature of the contractual requirements (instead of purely functional programs) and risk-avoidance by private operators (all of them public-works firms, not health care providers) (MNAIH — Mission Nationale d'Appui à l'Investissement Hospitalier, 2007).

Reacting to the issues with the first set of accommodation PPP hospitals procured by the federal government of Mexico, the State of Mexico decided to be more prescriptive in the procurement of its own accommodation PPP hospitals, notwithstanding the recognition that this would reduce the scope for innovation.

By comparison, full-service PPPs tend to be less prescriptive — Portugal underwent significant effort to purge overly prescriptive requirements from its Requests for Tender, allowing bidders to develop their own functional programs based on the procurement agency minimal requirements, basically the capacity to serve the needs of a certain population (historically documented for several years).

From the point of view of the public agent, another relevant issue is how the innovation achieved within the PPP can be made to spillover positively to other health care units of the health system. Managing innovation, within the context of a PPP, occurs at multiple stages: In the design and architecture definition of the PPP, in the operational phase (in the full-service PPP), and in the lessons learned and spillover effects from innovations eventually produced by the PPP.

Efficiency in resource allocation

While supposedly subject to an *ex-ante* evaluation of expected efficiency (in many cases biased, as referred to above), that efficiency is seldom assessed after procurement — as the British Audit Office (National Audit Office, United Kingdom, 2011) noted, "although most PFI projects are delivering the services expected, we have previously highlighted the lack of systematic ongoing value for money evaluation by departments of operational PFI projects"; worse, the same report notes that procuring authorities fail to specify the essential cost and operational data needed for that evaluation, and concludes that "there is no clear data to conclude whether the use of PFI has led to demonstrably better or worse value for money than other forms of procurement." Based on that report, the Public Accounts Committee of the Commons concluded that

> "There is no clear evidence to conclude whether PFI has been demonstrably better or worse value for money for housing and hospitals than other procurement options. In many cases local authorities and Trusts chose the PFI route because the Departments offered no realistic funding alternative." (Committee of Public Accounts, 2011)

The real assessment of PPP efficiency should come from the comparison of PPP provision costs (for the private operator) with alternative provision modes.

Using government costs — i.e., what government is paying for the services — is misleading: what we need to compare is the net value for society, not simply for government. A government may temporary save some money, or obtain higher quality, using a contract that, *ex-post*, is not profitable for the private operator — but if most private operators are experiencing losses, then (a) the society may be experiencing losses and should discontinue the PPP model, and (b) the model will not be replicable in the future for lack of private-sector profitability. Efficiency may take several dimensions and be assessed according to several metrics. The main efficiency effects are as follows.

Defining costs and cost overruns. The definition of "cost overrun" is more difficult than it may seem. For instance, National Audit Office (U.K.) reports need to be duly interpreted. When it says, for instance, that there are "no significant cost overruns for the range of activities included in the contract," it could mean that all significant additional costs are related to activities not included in the contract — excessive costs for small changes, very large costs for large changes. Sometimes what is not said becomes as important as what is actually stated.

Evaluating efficiency: infrastructure quality. Typically both infrastructural and full-PPP contracts deliver good-quality infrastructure, if not high-quality infrastructure. Those are the conclusions of the British NAO and the French ANAP.

However, several complaints regarding infrastructural PPPs suggest that corner-cutting behavior that affects design-build contracts can also affect PPP contracts, implying that the PPP-developed hospital infrastructure may not be a complete fit for its intended purpose. Examples include the first PFI hospitals in the UK and in Mexico, which had long patient walking paths inside the building and other issues, or the largest PPP hospital in Italy, in Mestre, with air-conditioning failures resulting from the "natural ventilation" proposed by the private partner. In Mexico, the result of this lack of fitness-for-purpose was a higher degree of public-sector control over the hospital design, leading to a potential loss of whole-life-costing efficiency.

Evaluating efficiency: infrastructure costs. We know that, 'for the set of activities included in the contract,' British PFI hospitals do not present significant cost overruns — but lower cost overruns do not mean low cost. Evidence points towards higher infrastructure costs due to the higher assumption of risk by the private operators, but more efficient decisions by the private partner should bring costs down, leaving ambiguity to whether, or not, final infrastructure costs are higher.

In many cases, PPPs come with an upgrade in the quality of hospital infrastructure (and service), so it is difficult to establish relevant comparators.

There is evidence that change orders in infrastructural contracts (where the public sector authority or a third party is providing clinical services) have led to significant over-costs: Changing some large imaging equipment could cost millions in adapting the building, a simple additional electrical socket in the wall could cost 700 pounds (most of it as compensation for the additional cost of cleaning and maintaining the wall during the term of the contract). In some cases, British authorities were procuring changes (e.g., refurbishing a surgical theater) with other contractors, outside the scope of the PFI contract, in order to avoid the huge cost of having it done by the PPP operator. Change orders in France created significant cost overruns and notorious conflict situations.

In full-PPP contracts, the interface between PPP operator and contractors is a private business, not affecting public-sector costs.

Evaluating efficiency: Non-clinical services. The British experience demonstrated no advantage in the inclusion of non-clinical services in accommodation PPP contracts (National Audit Office, United Kingdom, 2010). Accordingly, over time we can observe a gradual reduction in the services included in successive PPP contracts signed in the United Kingdom, up to a point where no service (besides infrastructure maintenance) was included in the most recent contracts. The current British PPP policy prescribes that no services should be included in PF2 contracts: "services, such as cleaning and catering, will be excluded from the contract and provided separately through shorter term contracts in order to provide the public sector with the flexibility to alter service specifications over time" (HM Treasury, United Kingdom, 2012).

British PFI contracts included non-clinical services for the full term of the contract, providing for a review of those services every few years, either through benchmarking or through market consultation. The British Audit Office confirmed that "cleaning, laundry and portering costs are about the same whether delivered through PFI or not" (National Audit Office, 2010).

Evaluating efficiency: Clinical services quality. The Portuguese PPP hospitals present a perceived good quality, as do the Spanish ones. The first PPP hospital of Bahia, Brazil (Subúrbio Hospital) is perceived as having a quality much higher than the other public hospitals, and even higher than most private hospitals in the state. Lesotho's Queen Mamohato Hospital also presents a quality much higher than the previous hospital (PwC, 2013). Thus, PPP hospitals that include clinical services seem to deliver higher quality than comparable public sector hospitals. The question that remains to be answered is what is the value and cost of such quality increases. Quality measures range from patient satisfaction surveys to indicators detailed in contracts, with reference to process quality.

Evaluating efficiency: Clinical services cost. Portugal's PPP hospitals were procured for a cost below the public sector comparator (in one case significantly below, although that may be due to definition of an overly high value for the public sector comparator in the first place) and are experiencing no cost overruns.

In the case of Lesotho, Queen Mamohato Hospital (its central hospital) is currently costing government twice the cost of the former central hospital (now decommissioned). That fact creates fiscal sustainability issues but it does not imply inefficiency, as the current volume of service is larger and the quality higher. Bahia's Subúrbio hospital (Brazil) is presented by the state government as being an efficient one, from the viewpoint of the public sector — but the private operator is facing losses that may imply renegotiation or failure.

Flexibility in the long run

Being long-term contracts, PPPs need to provide enough flexibility for accommodating both external environment and policy changes. Contract models may preclude such flexibility — but poor contract management, or a disconnection between public policy and the reality of business ventures, may also create rigidities that prevent the alignment of private interest and public policy.

Non-clinical service issues. The UK stopped its PFI program several years ago, after procuring a large number of PPP hospitals. Recently the British Treasury had strong words for the PFI program — the PF2 policy document refers to the "waste" and "rigidity" of PFI (HM Treasury, United Kingdom, 2012); the National Audit Office (NAO) criticized too large a transfer of resources to the private sector (internal rates of return in the range between 50 and 70% per year for the first few projects), and recently concluded there was no VfM in the service components of PFI contracts. In practice, the UK had already moved towards keeping those non-clinical services out of PFI contracts. France, prior to stopping its PPP hospital program, had also decided to reduce the range of non-clinical components.

The state government of Mexico (to distinguish from the government of Mexico) has recently contracted PPP hospitals with non-clinical services included, under a risky scheme where imaging equipment is included, as well as provisions for its replacement during the life of the contract, 25 years, by new equipment with the same characteristics. The government is insisting that it will force doctors and managers to keep the same equipment for the life of the contract, but no health professional believes that those contracts will not be renegotiated in order to upgrade equipment.

Including non-clinical services in an infrastructural PPP creates interface risks — all the potential for conflict associated with rent-seeking coming out of having two (or more) management structures inside the same building. First, all risks affecting current activities will create opportunities for one of the parties to gain something at the expense of the other — for example, the contamination of a surgical theater may result from clinical negligence or from poor maintenance. Second, any new clinical needs may have an impact on the need for non-clinical services, inducing rent-seeking behavior in a PPP operator not subject to competitive pressure.

Clinical service issues. The main potential issue, when addressing clinical services, is the compatibility of a long-term contract with the need for flexibility in public policy. The Portuguese PPP hospital contracts have a ten-year term for the clinical component, but Spanish contracts have a much longer term. A shorter term for clinical services allows potential substitution for another provider to keep pressure for efficiency of current private partner. At the same time, it does create an incentive to take decisions that "lock-in" the current partner (for example, by investing in a particular organizational culture that increases the costs of other management teams of taking over operations in the future).

Efficiency in procurement

It is useful to consider a broad separation between the tendering phase and the contractual phase of the partnership. Assessments of a PPP success in each phase have different criteria, and what happens in the tendering phase will condition what can be expected in the second phase (contract operation).

On the tendering phase, the success of the PPP is assessed according to two main dimensions: speed of the selection process, from having the decision to launch a PPP up to contract signature; and the price of the PPP, which is dependent on how many private entities the tendering procedure was able to attract and how eager they were to compete for the contract. A fast procedure with a low cost (price to be paid by the public party) is considered, usually, to be a good outcome.

The outcome in the first phase will then condition the second phase, after contract signature. A low price set in the tendering phase will make the private party more sensitive, in the contractual phase, to negative shocks in its profitability. A low initial price may trigger more easily renegotiations of contract due to financial vulnerability of the private party.

Under the full-service model, which includes both infrastructure and clinical activities, the Portuguese PPP have less impressive financial than clinical results. This was a direct consequence from the competitive tendering procedure, as aggressive bidding took place, bringing the final price well below the public sector comparator. A lower price to be paid by the public entity is better for the public budget but carries a higher risk of losses to the private partner.

Affordability

The UK is now realizing that they did procure too many hospitals, and possibly too large — several PPP hospitals were inaugurated with a few floors closed ("mothballed") for lack of need for them. The largest PFI hospital, and one of the largest British hospitals, the St. Barts in London, has one floor mothballed, its associated Heart Hospital has two floors mothballed (Building.co.uk, 2010). Many UK health trusts are facing financial difficulties, with some of them claiming that they are cutting service provision in order to be able to serve the financial commitments regarding PPPs — meaning that services are being cut in order to pay for hospital space and equipment that is idle. Some people even say that optimal public policy would advise closing down one or two of the recent PFI hospitals — but that this move is not done simply for its political implications.

In France, PPP hospitals created several high-visibility issues, due to conflict between hospital management and private partners over the quality of construction and the quality of services provided, leading even to hospital directors quitting, and to the early termination of a major contract in 2014. Due to the perceived "rigidity" of contracts, the government decided a few years ago to stop the PPP program. But currently there is evidence that the government procured PPP hospitals that were too large — government officials say that because they were PPPs (i.e., projects to pay later, not with current budgetary resources), doctors and managers asked for much more space and equipment than needed, actually much more than what will be needed in the future.

The budgetary rigidity imposed by PPP contracts will take its toll in future public sector accounts, as the PPP contracts accumulate, particularly in the lower phases of the business cycle when governments may receive lower revenues.

Another challenge to affordability comes from private-sector efficiency itself — in full-service hospital PPPs the efficiency of service provision tends to be translated into continuous growth of health care offer, allowing starved demand to be served, and so continually increasing the total cost of service delivery in those hospitals. This is a process going on in the Lesotho and Subúrbio hospitals, with no mechanisms for credibly containing this effect — but not in the Portuguese hospitals, where a managed supply mechanism is embedded in the contracts, allowing for an annual negotiation of maximum supply of health care, and for unilateral determination of it by the public partner within a certain interval contractually prescribed.

When the fiscal challenge comes from exuberant efficiency, an opportunity is created for health care reform: Instead of containing the production in the PPP units, the solution may be reducing production in less efficient hospitals (or even closing them), increasing the overall efficiency of the health care system.

Lesotho's case raises an interesting question: Can PPPs be used as a tool for enlarging the Health budget, by creating an upward pressure that the Ministry of Finance cannot resist?

By creating effective delivery of health care services, users will provide support; by demonstrating efficiency, private operators will gain bargaining power upon the Ministry of Finance — then the private operator may press for increases in service provision, solving public needs but creating fiscal stress. Regardless of whether PPP payments are included in the budget of the Ministry of Health or outside it, this pressure may force an increase in the Health care budget, or induce diversion of financial resources from other health expenditure, or even lead to the collapse on the contractual relationship — analysts may emphasize the 'correction' to the Health care budget brought by the PPP, or for budgetary diversion, or its potential for jeopardizing fiscal sustainability. The actual health care and fiscal impact will depend on the size of the initial under-funding of health care, and on government capacity for managing fiscal commitments and health care policy.

Project selection

Affordability issues are closely linked to project selection — including the number, size and location of projects. As Hellowell notes in his statement to the Commons' Treasury Committee (see its report on PF2 (HM Treasury, United Kingdom, 2014; Committee of Public Accounts, 2011), PPP project selection (in the UK) was significantly biased by the "PFI Credits" that created an advantage for PPP projects, exacerbating the budgetary incentive to pursue private finance. The "PFI Credits" regime was removed by the British Treasury — but, as Hellowell notes, health care authorities still have a strong incentive to pursue PPPs (even when non efficient) due to constraints on departmental capital budgets and the current reporting framework: the new public sector accounting standards (IPSAS-32) eliminated the off-balance status of most PPPs, but public debt in Europe is reported according to statistical rules, the Eurostat rules, and those rules follow a different criterion, more permissive regarding classifying PPP as "private assets."

Project selection may also be affected by something common in other types of PPPs: Decision makers proposing as PPPs some low-social-value projects but with high political visibility, the ones they know that will not be approved during the budgeting process when compared with alternative uses of public resources. Projects procured under conventional modes need to compete for limited budget resources, while PPP projects will be paid out of future budgets not yet at stake. Political and budget myopia in the selection of PPPs is a serious risk.

A third reason for biasing project selection is the mere reflection of risk-avoidance by public managers: selecting projects and designing them in such a way that risks are shifted to the private partner, regardless of its efficiency, as a way for avoiding managing the risks that should be kept in public hands.

These two last factors biasing project selection are fostered by frameworks where PPPs do not follow the usual public investment management process, having instead a separate assessment channel (as happened in the United Kingdom until recently, and as happens in most countries), and where relative value-for-money (comparing the PPP option with other procurement options) is more relevant than absolute VfM (cost–benefit analysis).

Final Remarks

The existing data related to performance of PPPs compared with 'conventional public procurement' is insufficient, allowing no conclusions regarding dominance of one approach over the other.

PPPs have been used for accelerating the construction of health care facilities, and expanding services. This advantage seems to have been realized. But private parties' investment has to be paid, at a higher cost than public funding (due to the risk premium associated with private funds).

There is no single answer to the question of whether PPPs are beneficial, or not. The success of a PPP in delivering the desired service in terms of time, quality and cost depends on the conditions of each country, in particular of the quality of the public sector in project selection and monitoring, as well as the design of the particular PPP.

To increase the odds of a successful PPP, the contract needs to avoid over specification by the public partner, as the private partner needs to find more efficient ways to achieve the desired goals. Only through a more efficient operation can the private partner provide simultaneously lower disbursement by the public partner, higher financial costs and its own profit.

Currently there are many experiments on PPP contracts for hospitals, in several countries, using a few different contractual models — they are experiments because their ultimate success can only be established after their normal termination, many years into the future. For now, we can say that a few of them failed and the vast majority demonstrated effectiveness in infrastructure and service delivery — but their efficiency is not proven, and that efficiency will depend critically on the quality of contract management and on the environment (particularly the technological, demographic and political environment).

Existing health care PPP contracts span different countries in several continents, different legal systems (e.g., common law and civil law systems), different procurement regimes, and different contractual models. These contracts deserve adequate research, in order to appraise them according to the fitness of private partners, the fitness of the contractual model, and the fitness of the contract management and health system management by public authorities.

References

ANAP. 2013. *Les partenariats public–privé des établissements de santé et médico-sociaux: Conditions techniques de recours aux PPP*. [Online] Available at: http://goo.gl/iVsBI8 [Accessed 8 November 2014]. Agence Nationale d'Appui a la Performance des etablissements de santé et medico-sociaux, France.

ANAP. n.d. *Agence Nationale d'Appui a la Performance des établissements de santé et médico-sociaux, France*. [Online] Available at: http://goo.gl/1wmZZO [Accessed 8 November 2014].

Barros PP, Gomes JP. 2002. *Os Sistemas Nacionais de Saúde da União Europeia, Principais Modelos de Gestão Hospitalar e Eficiência no Sistema Hospitalar Português*. http://goo.gl/QqsczX.

Barros PP, Martinez-Giralt X. 2009. Contractual design and PPPs for hospitals: Lessons for the Portuguese model. *European Journal of Health Economics* 10(4): pp. 437–453.

Boardman A, Greenberg D, Vining A, Weimer D. 2010. *Cost Benefit Analysis: Concepts and Practice*. (4th Ed).

Boston University. 2013. *Endline Study for Queen Mamohato Hospital PPP: Final Report*. [Online] url: http://goo.gl/ePfBhG Available at: http://goo.gl/zaIN8T [Accessed 08 November 2014].

Building.co.uk, 2010. *Floor at UK's most expensive PFI hospital remains empty*. [Online] Available at: http://goo.gl/mtpfTx [Accessed 8 November 2014].

Burger P, Hawkesworth I. 2011. *How to attain Value for Money: Comparing PPP and traditional infrastructure public procurement*. url: http://goo.gl/IQ3zv0.

Carrera M. 2012. *Parceria Público–privada na saúde no Brasil: Estudo de caso do Hospital do Subúrbio de Salvador — Bahia*. Fundação Getúlio Vargas, Escola de Administração de Empresas de São Paulo.

Committee of Public Accounts. 2011. *PFI in Housing and Hospitals: Fourteenth Report of Session 2010–11*. [Online] Available at: http://goo.gl/nyaaLS [Accessed 8 November 2014].

Cour des Comptes, France. 2007. *France, Les partenariats public–privé du plan Hôpital 2007: Une procédure mal maîtrisée*. [Online] Available at: http://goo.gl/oVLTJW [Accessed 8 November 2014].

EPOS — Health Management, Health and Economics. 2013. *Analysis for an evaluation of the Public–Private Partnerships in health care delivery across EU*. report EAHC/2011/Health/20. http://goo.gl/vx3f3n.

European Commission. 2004. *Green Paper on Public–Private Partnerships and Community Law on Public Contracts and Concessions*. Brussels. url: http://goo.gl/MAqnxb.

EXPH (EXpert Panel on effective ways of investing in Health). 2014. *Health and Economic Analysis for an Evaluation of the Public–Private Partnerships in Health Care Delivery across Europe*. [Online] Available at: http://goo.gl/Trui2H [Accessed 8 November 2014].

Flyvbjerg B. 2007. Policy and planning for large infrastructure projects: Problems, causes, and cures. *Environment and Planning B: Planning and Design* 34: 578–597.

Harding A. 2012. *The many definitions of public-private partnership in the health sector*. [Online] Available at: http://goo.gl/L7Mblr [Accessed 08 November 2014].

HM Treasury, United Kingdom. 2011. *Valuing infrastructure spend: Supplementary guidance to the Green Book*. [Online] Available at: http://goo.gl/u4stxg [Accessed 8 November 2014].

HM Treasury, United Kingdom. 2012. *A new approach to public private partnerships*. [Online] Available at: http://goo.gl/29geI2 [Accessed 8 November 2014].

HM Treasury, United Kingdom. 2014. *Private Finance Initiative Projects*. [Online] Available at: http://goo.gl/dE8Y6G [Accessed 8 November 2014].

International Federation of Accountants, 2011. *International Public Sector Accounting Standard 32 — Service Concession Agreements: Grantor (IPSAS)*. [Online] Available at: http://goo.gl/5Fbj4M [Accessed 8 November 2014].

Marín-Ferrer M, Rosa-Torner A. 2007. *Las nuevas formas de gestion sanitaria: Modelo Alzira*. http://goo.gl/76ReI8. (in Spanish).

MNAIH — Mission Nationale d'Appui à l'Investissement Hospitalier. 2007. *Le Partenariat public–privé Hospitalier: Une première évaluation*. http://goo.gl/vKaIjs.

National Audit Office, United Kingdom. 2010. *The performance and management of hospital PFI contracts*. [Online] Available at: http://goo.gl/5Mliab [Accessed 08 November 2014].

National Audit Office, United Kingdom. 2011. *Lessons from PFI and other projects*. [Online] Available at: http://goo.gl/O1ZFLs [Accessed 8 November 2014].

National Audit Office, United Kingdom. 2013. *Review of the VFM assessment process for PFI: Briefing for the House of Commons Treasury Select Committee*. http://goo.gl/I4w0Dm.

Organisation for Economic Co-operation and Development, OECD. 2012. *Principles for Public Governance of Public–Private Partnerships*. http://goo.gl/lLX6K7.

Organisation for Economic Co-operation and Development, OECD. 2013. *Draft Principles of Budgetary Governance: First orientations for a set of core standards and principles*. http://goo.gl/ApFx5h.

PwC — PriceWaterhouseCoopers. 2013. *Health System Innovation in Lesotho — Design and early operations of the Maseru public–private integrated partnership*. Healthcare public–private partnerships series, No. 1 Executive Summary. http://goo.gl/iKacdk.

Raisbeck P, Duffield C, Xu M. 2010. Comparative Performance of PPPs and traditional procurement in Australia. *Construction, Management and Economics* 28(4): pp. 345–359.

Raman V, La Forgia J. 2013. *PPP hospitals in India: A comparative analysis of purchasing arrangements and performance*. Washington DC: World Bank.

Simões J. 2004. A avaliação do desempenho de hospitais. *Revista Portuguesa de Saúde Pública* 4: 91–120.

Treasury Committee, House of Commons, United Kingdom. 2014. *Private Finance 2: Tenth Report of Session 2013–14, Vols. I e II*. [Online] Available at: http://goo.gl/2IktN6; http://goo.gl/KbWW2H [Accessed 8 November 2014].

UTAP — Unidade Técnica de Acompanhamento de Projetos, 2014. *Boletim Trimestral PPP — 4° Trimestre de 2013*. [Online] Available at: http://goo.gl/tcXQVM [Accessed 8 November 2014].

UTAP. 2014. *Unidade Técnica de Acompanhamento de Projetos*. [Online] Available at: http://www.utap.pt [Accessed 07 November 2014].

World Bank. 2012. *Public–Private Partnerships Reference Guide*. [Online] Available at: http://goo.gl/NQRz2Z.

World Bank. 2013. *Value-for-Money Analysis — Practices and Challenges: How governments choose when to use PPP to deliver public infrastructure and services*. [Online] Available at: http://goo.gl/9rYUpc.

Translational Health Economics

Wolf Rogowski and Jürgen John
Helmholtz Zentrum München,
German Research Center for Environmental Health, Germany

Maarten IJzerman
University of Twente, Netherlands

Translational health economics (THE) can be defined as the use of theoretical concepts and empirical methods in health economics to bridge the gap between the decision to fund and use a new health technology in clinical practice (the backend of translational medicine) and the decision to invest into its development (the front end of translational medicine). This chapter provides an overview of this emerging area of research and discusses limitations and research needs.

Theoretical concepts and empirical methods for three aspects of THE are presented: First, to analyze "value" for a potential health technology and to apply or to further develop methods for scrutinizing value propositions related to the decision to initiate a translation process; second, to analyze "uncertainty" and to apply or to further develop methods for generating evidence about a health technology's value early on; and third, to analyze barriers of information and motivation in the cooperative process of translation as well as institutions to overcome these. Rather than the traditional concept where health economic evaluations inform health care decision makers about established technologies with established evidence, THE seeks to integrate the development of innovations, and to provide links to health care business perspectives and decisions.

Keywords: Translational Health Economics; Translational Medicine; Early Evaluation; Innovation; Cost-effectiveness.

Background

Innovations in health care have contributed to increased life expectancy and quality of life in recent decades (Cutler and McClellan, 2001; Lichtenberg, 2005; Lichtenberg, 2012; Philipson *et al.*, 2012). Now that the "lower-hanging fruits" of medical discoveries, i.e., those that were relatively easier to find and develop like antibiotics, have been successfully translated into clinical care and saved millions of lives, biomedical research and development (R&D) is becoming increasingly challenging. International collaboration of highly specialized researchers is necessary to take today's complex technologies, such as new applications of personalized medicine (Rogowski *et al.*, 2009b), into practice. However, doing so involves large expenditures, which could be invested elsewhere. In 2012, worldwide biomedical R&D spending amounted to US$268.4 billion (Chakma *et al.*, 2014).

Challenges of translational medicine

Unfortunately, despite huge investments, only a few of the promising biomedical research findings have indeed been further developed and used in health care practice (Contopoulos-Ioannidis *et al.*, 2003). R&D is a risky undertaking, and a large number of technologies that are fully developed do not succeed in health care markets (Markiewicz *et al.*, 2014). The combination of high costs for R&D and high numbers of development failures leads to a situation where the societal costs per newly developed medical technology are substantial. For new pharmaceuticals, the costs associated with R&D have been assessed by a number of empirical studies, with estimates ranging from US$92 million cash (US$161 million capitalized) to US$883.6 million cash (US$1.8 billion capitalized) per successfully developed drug (Morgan *et al.*, 2011).

Therefore, companies investing in biomedical R&D increasingly scrutinize their portfolios to justify the profitability of their development projects to their shareholders. If the expected benefits of translating their R&D into clinical practice cannot easily be turned into expected company profits, the question about public funding of R&D arises. Nearly 40% of biomedical R&D spending is funded from public sources (Chakma *et al.*, 2014) and the multitude of national programs, such as the National Institutes of Health in the US as well as multi-national programs such as the European Union's Horizon 2020 Program[1], are examples of public policy initiatives to take up this challenge of research funding. However, as with current debates about health care expenditure in general, there is an increased understanding that public funds for research are also limited and research investments should lead to health improvements in a cost-effective manner.

The awareness of the need to improve the flow of knowledge from research settings to clinical practice (from "bench to bedside") has been introduced under the term "translational medicine" (TM). TM has become an omnipresent term in the medical literature — publications related to this subject matter have risen from around 0 in the 1990s to over 100 per year in the following decade (Keramaris *et al.*, 2008). Besides being a relevant topic for medical research, it is increasingly recognized that other disciplines may contribute. For example, extensive reviews

[1] See: http://ec.europa.eu/programmes/horizon2020/ (accessed 18 January, 2014).

in epidemiology (Khoury *et al.*, 2010) and public health (Ogilvie *et al.*, 2009) have addressed how the lenses of research methods developed by these disciplines can be used to clear up and expand the hazy road of new discoveries as they move from bench to bedside.

Contributions not only from epidemiology and public health, but also from economics are increasingly considered. From an economic perspective, TM can be seen as a process characterized by sequential, interactive decisions about whether or not an investment in translation should be initiated and/or continued (Rogowski *et al.*, 2008; Ijzerman and Steuten, 2011).

At the beginning of a translation process, typically, there is an idea, based on a scientific result or a technical achievement. As a first task of successful translation, public and private funders of R&D need to understand whether and where further developing and implementing this idea could provide value in health care. This requires determining how the value of innovation can be defined — a mutually acceptable understanding for all involved stakeholders (research funders, industry, health care payers, patients, and citizens or the insured) about what the ultimate aims of R&D are, and how the costs associated with research can be related to that value. Also, it requires understanding how this value can be quantified in monetary terms so that it can be compared with the costs associated with further developing and delivering this value to patients.

Second, once a translation process has been initiated, those who are in charge of developing and providing the technology (e.g., the R&D project and market access managers) as well as those in charge of funding it (e.g., public payers and agencies for health technology assessment) need to address the inevitable uncertainty about whether the technology's costs and effects in health care practice do indeed match the hypothesized value proposition. This requires a shared understanding of uncertainty as well as empirical methods to decrease decision uncertainty as early as possible during the translation process. Having this in place at an early stage can help avoid unnecessary efforts of further developing technologies that are not considered worthwhile. When the development phase is finished and the product is entering clinical practice, methods of evidence generation can overcome evidence barriers to market access.

Third, besides the new health technology itself, the translation process within which it is selected and further developed is of interest, particularly for those who make decisions about research and innovation policy. Successful selection, development and provision of new technologies that will be considered valuable requires societal cooperation: Successful interaction between a large number of highly specialized players from different disciplines (e.g., biology, medicine, economics, law) and settings (e.g., private companies, research institutions, government agencies). However, the different stakeholders involved are likely to have diverging interests about how to allocate the large amounts of research and health care funding. Additionally, there may be not only high objective uncertainty about a new technology's performance, but also private information which may create subjective uncertainty and be used by single players to promote their interests. Therefore, societal collaboration in TM can fail very easily. Improving the process of TM thus also requires a theoretical understanding of such problems and uncertainties surrounding information and motivation of individual stakeholders, as well as empirical evidence about the relevant characteristics of existing TM processes and their impact on selection, development and implementation of medical innovations.

Definitions

Supporting the process of decision-making in translational medicine, translational health economics is an emerging field of research which addresses three complementary fields from a health economics perspective. Translational health economics (THE) can be defined as the use of theoretical concepts and empirical methods in health economics to bridge the gap between the decision to fund and use a new health technology in clinical practice (the back end of translational medicine) and the decision to invest into its development (the front end of translational medicine). This includes (1) analyzing "value" for a potential health technology and applying or further developing methods to scrutinize value propositions related to the decision to initiate a translation process; (2) analyzing "uncertainty" and applying or further developing methods for generating evidence about a health technology's value early on, to accelerate project abort or market access; and (3) analyzing barriers of information and motivation in the cooperative process of translation as well as institutions to overcome these to facilitate successful selection, development and implementation of health technologies that are valuable to health care systems and patients. THE thus supports forward translation (from R&D project to health technology) through backward translation (health technology decision criteria to R&D project selection).

The tangible end product of successful translation is a health technology available in practice — which can be defined as the "drugs, devices, and medical and surgical procedures used in health care, and the organizational and supportive systems within which such care is provided" (Assessment, 1978; Banta, 2003). More generally, technology can be defined as a combination of aims (problems) and means (solutions) (Hauschildt, 2004, p. 5). Even if "health technology" is frequently associated with complex therapeutics, such as drugs with long and expensive R&D processes, THE is, like TM, neither restricted to a single clinical area nor to a specific type of product or process it generates. It can relate to very different solutions to existing problems in medical service provision, including "low-tech" approaches to improve patient health, such as a new weight loss program for diabetics, as well as organizational innovations such as reimbursement by diagnosis-related group, risk adjustment schemes, or performance-related pay arrangements.

The term "translational" involves a notion of novelty that is distinct from "normal" health technology assessment. Generally, different definitions can be used to determine novelty, e.g., the degree of novelty (disruptive vs. incremental innovation) or the fact that it is the first use (by anyone in the world, by a country, or by a single institution) (Hauschildt, 2004, p. 5). In a narrow view of "early evaluation" following the definition of the International Network of Agencies for Health Technology Assessment, this could be understood as an evaluation of technologies at development stages starting from initial idea generation up to Stage I of clinical trials (Markiewicz *et al.*, 2014). In a broad view, also the diffusion of medical technology and public health impact could be included like in frameworks where potential individual health benefit is seen as the last step of translation (Drolet and Lorenzi, 2011). Here, novelty is understood as "novel for the health care provider" and a technology which is standard in academic centers may still be novel for a practicing physician in the countryside. In the following, as an attribute of a health technology, "translational" is understood to imply significant novelty however defined, but focusing on development stages prior to a situation where the preconditions for well-informed national coverage decisions are met (particularly sufficient evidence as to whether or not the technology fulfills a health care payer's coverage criteria).

A more specific characteristic of THE than the technology development stage is that it takes a process view, analyzing the value chain in which the novel technology is developed and assessing the associated barriers and information necessary for progression. It includes all steps that must be taken, from idea and hypothesis of potential health benefit to market access and care delivery.

Outline of this chapter

The following sections provide an overview of how health economic concepts and methods can be used to build a bridge between the benefit obtained from funding a translated idea (a health technology) back to the initial decision to invest in its translation. The chapter is structured according to the three areas of investigation mentioned above, without claiming that these provide a conclusive overview of the field:

1) How can the value of a potential new medical technology be established to inform the initiation of a translation process?
2) How can evidence of an emerging health technology's value be established as early as possible during the translation process?

3) How can the translational value chain be optimized, given its highly cooperative nature and the multiple barriers of information and motivation which need to be overcome?

For each of these questions, an overview of theoretical considerations is presented, followed by an overview of empirical applications. The discussion section addresses strengths and limitations of the presented answers to the questions above and outlines areas in need of further research.

1. Establishing the value of a potential technology prior to translation

The first question of a translation process is whether the initial investment in research should be made at all. In order to compare the costs to be invested in research with the potential benefit, the technical idea or biological achievement which serves as starting point needs to be transferred into a value proposition. Most likely, everyone will consent to the statement that an intervention which gives sight to the blind or the ability to walk and dance to the paralyzed would be valuable. However, for many other aspects, disagreement is likely to prevail — for example, how much statutory health insurance funds should pay for such an intervention; or, how to value only small improvements in sight and mobility. This is further complicated by the fact that the technology' potential attributes of value are still subject to modification during the development process so that value needs to be established for hypothetical health technologies.

Theoretical considerations about the value of medical innovation

"Value" is a term which relates to different concepts in moral philosophy, and can even be used in a broad sense to encompass moral philosophy in general (Schroeder, 2012). Economic theories of value develop a theoretical basis for ranking different policy choices. For choices of health technologies, they allow estimating the willingness to pay for a health technology (i.e., the cost at which funding a technology is ranked equally to not funding it).

There are two major theories of value in health economics, welfarism and extra-welfarism (Brouwer *et al.*, 2008). Welfarism is the most developed theory of value in economics and the default understanding of value that economists typically learn during their education. Extra-welfarism, on the other hand, emanates from more recent attempts to formalize concepts of value found in the practice of health policy decision-making. It is thus less theoretically elaborated but more relevant for reimbursement decision-making.

Neoclassical welfarism

Neoclassical welfarism assumes that "value" only can be determined in terms of individual preference rankings. Typically, it is additionally assumed that an individual's preference rankings satisfy the axioms of rationality, such as completeness and transitivity; only the affected individual is relevant for valuing utility; and utility information is not comparable across individuals. Individuals choose to acquire their preferred bundle of goods at the market, and the amount an individual is willing to pay for a good represents its value in terms of other goods the individual is willing to give up instead (Boadway and Bruce, 1984, p. 2; Sen, 1979; Brouwer *et al.*, 2008). In this view, only the Pareto criterion can be used to rank policy choices: A situation is preferred if at least one person is better off and no-one is made worse off after the choice. The Pareto criterion is frequently extended by compensation criteria, the best known but theoretically problematic one is that a social state is preferred also if, at least, the winners could hypothetically compensate the losers and then everyone would be better off (Kaldor, 1939; Hicks, 1939; Blackorby and Donaldson, 1990).

The welfarist view is tightly connected to welfare economic theorems about the functioning of markets: If perfect markets prevail, profit-maximizing activities of individual market participants are assumed to be guided by input and output prices, which ultimately depend on the consumers' willingness to pay (WTP) to produce a Pareto-optimal combination of goods and services oriented at consumer preferences (Boadway and Bruce, 1984, p. 3). In the absence of perfect markets, market decisions can be simulated by means of cost-benefit analysis, where individuals are asked for their WTP in hypothetical choices. Introducing a new technology can then be said to be desirable if WTP exceeds its costs. Both in market choices and in cost-benefit analysis, WTP is a measure for evaluating health technologies, which is well-founded in welfarist economic theory (MacIntosh, 2010, p. 11 ff.).

Generally, the welfarist theory of value can also be applied to the acquisition of health care services and health insurance (Grossman, 1972; Zweifel *et al.*, 2009). However, in the practice of health economic evaluation conducted by public health care payers, the customers' (patients' or insurers') WTP plays only a minor role in the measurement and valuation of benefits. Few coverage decision makers who specify preferred outcomes in their guidelines for health economic evaluation allow WTP and typically, WTP is not the preferred outcome measure.[2]

Extra-welfarism

This is likely to be the case because the neoclassical welfarist evaluation framework for evaluating medical technology involves principles which are at odds with

[2]See: http://www.ispor.org/peguidelines/index.asp, accessed on 28 December 2013.

frequently held intuitions about the fair allocation of health care resources. In particular, individual WTP is not generally considered an acceptable criterion for allocating health care resources because it depends on ability to pay. Instead, it can be claimed that health care should be allocated independent of individual wealth, on the basis of criteria such as medical need (Brouwer *et al.*, 2008).

Responding to this criticism of welfarism, extra-welfarism extends the evaluative space beyond individual utility. One concept of particular relevance is that the aim of health care is to improve health in an objectively measurable manner (for example, in quality-adjusted life years, QALYs) rather than to maximize the individuals' subjective utility derived from health care (Culyer and Newhouse, 2000; Brouwer *et al.*, 2008). Even if QALYs can also be applied to a welfarist foundation (Weinstein and Manning, 1997), in their most explicit use by the English National Institute of Health and Care Excellence (NICE), they are seen as a preference-based measure for the extra-welfarist aim of meeting health care needs or improving health (National Institute for Health and Clinical Excellence, 2008).

An important motivation for the development of an extra-welfarist approach is to include explicit considerations about allocative efficiency in cases where the Pareto principle alone appears to be an insufficient basis for policy choices (Sen, 1999). One possible view, which has frequently been taken in extra-welfarism, is that the more medical need that can be ameliorated with a given bundle of resources, the better, regardless of individual WTP and regardless of whom the health gains accrue to. An efficient allocation is therefore one which maximizes the overall QALYs gained from constrained health care resources (Culyer *et al.*, 2007). Also other attributes ethically relevant attributes can be included into the concept of social value such as concerns for severity or equity, even if there are still a number of methodological challenges which remain to be resolved (Wailoo *et al.*, 2009).

It should be noted that, while the term "extra"-welfarism has been based on the assertion that it incorporates measures which extend beyond utility alone, it has also been criticized for being too narrow in scope compared with traditional welfarism (Birch and Donaldson, 2003). This is because it focuses on selected, ethically justified attributes which can be determined in some interpersonally comparable manner, such as gains in quality-adjusted life expectancy with pre-specified dimensions for measuring quality of life — which necessarily omits other aspects that may be relevant for some individuals in their preference orderings.

Corresponding with extra-welfarist considerations of medical need and health benefit, objective scientific evidence that a medical intervention is effective at improving health outcomes is a key criterion of health care coverage decisions worldwide (Rogowski *et al.*, 2008). The extent to which coverage decision-makers specify how additional health benefits and additional costs of a health care technology are balanced so that an explicit willingness to pay threshold λ can be determined differs between jurisdictions. For example, the English and Welsh NICE quite explicitly specifies a λ of £20.000–£30.000 per QALY based on considerations of opportunity costs (McCabe *et al.*, 2008). The value of a new medical intervention can then be quantified as net (monetary) benefit (NB), depending on incremental health effects (ΔE), incremental costs (ΔC), and the threshold value λ (Briggs *et al.*, 2006, p. 128 ff.):

$$NB = \Delta E \cdot \lambda - \Delta C. \quad (1)$$

This value of the new technology needs to be appraised alongside other social value judgments such as to avoid unfair discrimination which are to be considered deliberatively in decision making (National Institute for Health and Clinical Excellence, 2008)

As the other extreme, health care coverage decision-makers like the Federal Joint Committee in Germany or Medicare in the US refrain from making any statement on WTP but officially advance the view that all technologies which are proven as effective and regarded as necessary will be funded (Rogowski *et al.*, 2008). This reluctance to explicitly address willingness to pay may reflect politicians' reluctance to withhold health care based on the argument that it is too expensive; it is politically more acceptable to argue that care for which effectiveness has not been established and thus is unnecessary is rejected (Garber, 2004). Ethically, the use of cost-effectiveness thresholds has been criticized on the grounds that the idea that health care should maximize any consequence like health gains, conflicts with the non-consequentialist ethical view that fair resource allocation involves respecting the dignity of the patients equitably (Klonschinski, 2014). The work on extra-welfarist theories of value in health care is still ongoing, and these issues remain to be resolved.

Theories of value and the evaluation of a novel health technology

Assessing the potential value of a new health technology requires an understanding of the different concepts of value. To determine whether a new health technology provides additional value from the perspective of public health care payers, it is not sufficient to investigate whether patients have preferences for an intervention — even if this is a necessary condition of market success because a treatment cannot be applied if it is rejected by patients. It needs to be demonstrated that it improves health in terms of patient-relevant endpoints, compared with existing care (e.g., reduced pain or decreased mortality, rather than only evidence of benefit in terms of immediate endpoints such as a change in some laboratory parameter).

If the payer explicitly specifies WTP like in the case of NICE, this can be used to value the health gains. In the absence of explicit WTP estimates, the lower bound of the value of the new technology is given by $-\Delta C$ (i.e., the solution of Eq. (1) for $\lambda = 0$), which corresponds with a price markup at which the technology would still be cost neutral because it leads to cost savings elsewhere in the health care system (e.g., due to reduced adverse events). However, it has to be noted that such price markups that result in cost neutrality may not exist, and the technology would have to be priced negatively to be cost-saving across the health care system. This could be the case, as a hypothetical example, in the case of technologies that lead to substantial gains in life expectancy for those with a costly chronic disease. A payer's WTP may depend upon many determinants in addition to cost-effectiveness (such as valuations of the extent of patient benefit, treatment alternatives, guideline recommendations, number of patients and budget impact, but even political visibility of the patient group). Therefore, innovators must rely on crystal ball prognoses — for example, based on prices currently paid for similar health technologies in the same clinical area.

Cost savings that arise from using the new technology can serve as an indicator of value when the ultimate customer of a health technology is a health care provider like a hospital rather than the patient or the health care system — e.g., in the case of an innovation which increases the efficiency of surgical procedures. Also, if a technology is marketed directly to a single sickness fund which may primarily be interested in reducing costs rather than expanding services, cost savings may be the most important evidence source of value. The value proposition of an innovation would then include an understanding of the costs associated with a care pathway from the perspective of the tentative contract partner, and the impact the innovation is likely to have on these costs.

In the health care markets of many wealthier countries, the largest part of health care expenditure is funded by national health care systems, statutory sickness funds or other health insurance. It can be argued that in social security systems and welfare states, the value of health care derives from the basic goals of responsible payer institutions, such as providing equitable and efficient health care (Brouwer *et al.*, 2008). Therefore, the concept of value oriented at individual market acquisitions may be of less relevance here. However, value as considered in neoclassical welfare economics is of increasing relevance for services offered in the intermediate area between publicly funded health services and services traditionally offered on free markets. Interventions that increase the comfort of care or improve patients' general wellness and satisfaction are examples of services that are likely to be valuable to patients, even without tangible health benefits. Here, individual WTP may be the most relevant measure of value in the business case of a new medical technology.

Value for money from the perspective of the health care payer[3] (which includes the patient in case of out-of-pocket co-funding) may be seen as a necessary condition for a health technology to be used in clinical practice. The business cases in terms of cost savings for health care providers or, potentially, single sickness funds illustrate that this also needs to translate to value for money of single stakeholders in terms of adequate reimbursement so that the service can be offered in a financially sustainable manner. However, as a sufficient condition for the technology to be used, it also needs to meet the preferences of the different stakeholders involved in service provision. For example, a new surgical procedure may need to be easy to use for the surgeon, or a new cancer drug may need to be easy to administer for the oncologist. Besides determining value for money, preference elicitation methods also can play a role in assessing whether this sufficient condition is met.

Empirical approaches

For the decision to invest into the translation of a medical idea into a health care technology, it is important not only to know whether the technology would be valuable from a health care system perspective and fit with the preferences of those who would be in charge of implementing it; it is also relevant to know whether developing and offering the technology would be profitable from a business perspective. To complement traditional instruments such as business planning and investment analysis, decisions to invest in health care markets may benefit from additional tools such as early modeling. Furthermore, quantitative methods to analyze preferences and usability as well as qualitative deliberation may be needed to complement model-based analyses by aspects that cannot easily be incorporated into a value function for the health care system.

Using Early Models to Link Value from the Health System to the Business Perspective

Even if there is no evidence of effects and costs of the new intervention as it is still in the idea stage, health economic modeling can provide relevant information for this task. In a simple form, early modeling involves the development of a basic, deterministic decision-analytic model in which the hypothetical new intervention is added to the existing comparators as an additional scenario. This allows exploring room for improvement stemming from the new intervention and its

[3] That is, that a technology is associated with positive net benefit. See Formula (1).

potential impact on costs and effects of care, and provides substantial information needed for assessing attractiveness from a company perspective (Koerber *et al.*, 2013).

Typically, the company perspective on an innovation is evaluated within a business plan. Key elements of a business plan include: A specification of the product or service and how it generates value; a market analysis, where the market size is estimated and the most attractive segments identified; a competitor analysis which assesses existing solutions to the problem being offered by other companies, and how the new product or service is different or better; and a marketing strategy of how the product or service is priced and how it will be delivered to its user (Butler, 2014; Valentin, 2015).

Information about the potential value of a new technology can be derived from an early modeling process that predicts health-related quality of life within the health states that are modified, and the costs associated with them. The market analysis can be informed by data on baseline epidemiology in existing models; information about competitors and their performance can be found in the comparators included in these models. Pricing benchmarks can be derived from reimbursement rates of the existing care in the target area (Koerber *et al.*, 2013). In a context of value-based pricing (Gregson *et al.*, 2005; Sussex *et al.*, 2013), these pricing benchmarks can be further refined once a model has been established. For example, the model can be used to establish minimum performance thresholds of how effective a technology must be in terms of health outcomes so that the investor's price target is met or, given the current estimate of benefit, what a value-based price would be. Also, the model allows an analysis of where in the care process the new technology is likely to provide the most valuable contribution, by analyzing different application scenarios. If a novel treatment mechanism (for example, by a drug) has several different applications (for example, that it could be applied to different diseases), early modeling may also be used to inform manufacturers about the best possible sequence of market access of these different applications (Hartz and John, 2008; Koerber *et al.*, 2013). From an investment perspective, translating the idea into a health care technology is profitable if the discounted expected stream of revenues less variable costs exceeds the expected costs of investing in the translation. Value-based prices from early models can provide an important input to calculations of the investment's net present value for different uptake scenarios.

The analysis of profitability from a business perspective can also be suitable to determine when public funding may be needed to realize a translational project that is likely to be valuable from a societal perspective but not profitable from a business one. This can be the case, for example, if a new technology like a new biomarker could provide substantial health benefit but, due to early publication and thus limited patentability, as well as low prices for diagnostics, the value-based price necessary to amortize the investment cannot be obtained. In such a situation, no manufacturer — or others working in applied research — would have the incentive to further develop the technology without public support.

Empirical Methods to Assess Multi-dimensional Value

Using early models on the basis of formalized objective functions implies that these capture the aspects of value that are most relevant for the coverage decisions. However, there may be situations where standard measures of value in health care, such as health-related quality of life measured by questionnaires like the EuroQol[4] and valued by national tariffs, are not sufficient to achieve a new technology's use in clinical practice. Instead, besides the aspects formally relevant for health care coverage, additional attributes of technologies may be important to meet stakeholder preferences or achieve usability, for example, the process within which an intervention is applied to the patient, or the ease of use of a new surgical tool.

Generally, a number of empirical methods can be used to assess these aspects. First, standard empirical methods used in the social sciences (such as questionnaires, focus groups, ethnography or context-related qualitative surveys) can be applied to elicit views of users and patients. Furthermore, structured frameworks (such as usability tests, the think-aloud method, heuristic evaluation or cognitive walkthrough) have been developed to assess the usability of new technologies. Additionally, methods to incorporate user preferences into technology design have been developed (these include the lead user method or participatory design). In the context of developing health technologies, early dialogue with public payers is also a relevant approach (Bartelmes *et al.*, 2009; Hartz and John, 2008).

These methods can be combined using systematic methods of multi-criteria decision analysis (MCDA). MCDA encompasses a broad range of techniques to assist decision-making involving multiple criteria, by identifying the criteria, weighing and prioritizing the criteria, and finally providing a framework to summarize the information about the different possible decision options (Devlin and Sussex, 2011; Ishizaka and Nemery, 2013; Belton and Stewart, 2003).

---

[4]EuroQol is one example of a generic instrument for measuring health-related quality of life. It uses the five dimensions of problems with mobility, self-care, usual activities, pain/discomfort, and anxiety/depression (see www.euroqol.org).

MCDA originates from operations research and decision sciences, but has been introduced into the field of health technology assessment to guide benefit–risk assessments and decisions on reimbursement. MCDA criteria weights can be obtained through different formats, for example within a group decision-making process where a consensus among all participants is sought about how important the single attributes should be in the decision whether or not to fund a health technology (Hummel *et al.*, 2014). Given that these methods can be used to support the dialogue between technology developers and tentative users or decision-makers, and given that not only the criteria and weights but also complementary considerations can be shared, these methods are particularly suited for early assessment of value, and a number of examples of this have been reported in the literature (Hilgerink *et al.*, 2011; Ijzerman and Steuten, 2011).

An alternative group of approaches to elicit preferences that has received much attention in recent health economics literature is conjoint analysis, in particular discrete-choice analysis (DCE). Conjoint analysis is a statistical method which allows estimating the relative weight certain attributes carry in choices about alternatives with two or more attributes. In conjoint analyses, a product such as a health technology is disaggregated into different attributes which are assumed to be of key importance for its evaluation (for example, its health effects, its costs, and the severity of the condition it addresses). Survey respondents are asked to choose from hypothetical products which are characterized by different levels for these attributes (for example, comparing one technology that provides a health gain of one month at a cost of €1,000 to a patient with highly severe disease with another technology that provides a health gain of 6 months at a cost of €500 to a patient with a mild disease). By regression analysis, the relative weight of each attribute level for the overall choice is estimated. Conjoint analysis can be used to estimate WTP for different tentative product designs, assuming that hypothetical market choices are the most valid basis for value judgments about new health technologies (de Bekker-Grob *et al.*, 2012; Bridges *et al.*, 2011; Reed Johnson *et al.*, 2013). Alternatively, it can also be used to elicit value judgments about the weight of decision criteria, based on extra-welfarist considerations (Severin *et al.*, 2013). Examples of using conjoint analysis for the early evaluation of medical technologies have been reported in the literature (Sanders *et al.*, 2011; Ijzerman and Steuten, 2011). For an overview, please refer to de Bekker-Grob (2012) and Weernink *et al.* (2014). Even if a number of empirical methods exist for estimating value functions, it is likely that a need for complementary, qualitative considerations will always remain.

Furthermore, for the entity that invests in the development and translation of a novel technology, aspects other than the private profitability of the investment project or the cost-effectiveness from a societal perspective may be relevant. For strategic private investors, additionally relevant issues may be, for example, whether the development of the technology is of importance for other projects or whether it allows them to enter a certain medical market. From the perspective of public research funders, additional aspects of value may need to be considered, such as establishing or re-activating new companies, effects on employment, or international recognition. This is because, apart from health policy, they also have industry or other social policy objectives on their minds (Salter and Martin, 2001; Yazdizadeh *et al.*, 2010).

Health care decision-makers often represent institutional rather than individual perspectives. To establish a novel technology in an environment where the notion of value is different among multiple stakeholders, modeling and predicting value can hardly be done using current utility theory. A suitable theoretical framework is yet missing, and the search for methods beyond standard economics may prove to be helpful.

2. Establishing evidence of value during the translation process

The previous section illustrated how economic models and scenario analysis can be used to determine a new technology's potential value without evidence about the technology *per se*. However, at early stages of development, a new technology's effectiveness and costs are highly uncertain. Once the decision to develop a product or service has been made, product managers as well as those acquiring the product require more information about the true effectiveness and costs associated with the product's use in clinical practice. The concept of gates between development stages has been proposed as a way to conceptualize the process of development, where at different development stages, evidence about the technology's effectiveness and costs relative to the initial value hypothesis must be provided to initiate the next development step (Cosh *et al.*, 2007; Ijzerman and Steuten, 2011).

In such a process, early modeling to develop a value proposition can be seen as only the first step to value-based translation. Additionally, rather than only manipulating few parameters in scenario analyses of more simple early models, it may be desirable to have an understanding of the uncertainty of all parameters simultaneously. This brings us to the second challenge in THE and the second step in value-based translation: Establishing evidence of the emerging technology's value as early as possible in the translation process (Sculpher *et al.*, 1997).

Theoretical considerations about the value of further evidence

There are different theoretical frameworks to address the problem of decision uncertainty and the generation of evidence, frequentism and Bayesianism, which we will discuss in the following sections.

Frequentist and Bayesian considerations about the generation of evidence

The most widely shared methodological paradigm for generating evidence in health care is frequentism. Frequentism is tightly connected to a school of thought in the philosophy of science called "critical rationalism," which is deeply influenced by the work of Sir Karl Raimund Popper. It holds that knowledge cannot validly be generated through induction from observed "facts," because all observation involves potentially erroneous beliefs and subjective perceptions. Instead, evidence generation involves conjecture and refutation: Science proceeds by generating hypotheses and by trying to falsify them. Frequentist hypothesis testing provides a well-developed and widely used approach to apply this philosophical position in statistical practice (Allmark, 2004).

Frequentist methods regard values of interest such as the incremental effect of a new technology as a fixed (but unknown) quantity. Statistical inference assesses whether the value observed in empirical data is likely to evolve from the play of chance only (the null hypothesis), or whether this null hypothesis can be refuted because the probability of obtaining a result at least as extreme as the observed one is below a pre-determined level of significance (Bland and Altman, 1998). Hypothesis testing is tightly linked to the challenge faced by health care payers: They have to distinguish between medical interventions which meet the payer's criteria for coverage (or the legally required criteria for coverage) and those that do not, so that patients covered under the scheme have a claim to the appropriate interventions. Given this link and the widespread acceptance of frequentist statistical methods, coverage decisions are frequently based on results of statistical significance testing, in particular, regarding the criterion of medical effectiveness (Rogowski *et al.*, 2008; Rogowski, 2010).

Bayesian methods are based on a different perception of unknown quantities, such as the incremental effects and costs of an emerging technology: These quantities are assumed to have probability distributions that express our prior knowledge or beliefs about them. Evidence generation can add additional knowledge to generate posterior distributions (Bland and Altman, 1998).

In the area of pharmaceuticals, where the costs of translation processes have been studied most extensively, clinical trials contribute more than half of the total costs of developing new technologies in recent studies (Morgan *et al.*, 2011; Paul *et al.*, 2010). Therefore, the question arises of how much and which kind of evidence collection during the process of TM is worth the expenses for applied research.

Bayesian value of information analysis

Assuming that value from a health care system perspective can be formalized in terms of an objective function, Bayesian value of information (VOI) analysis provides concepts which can be applied to derive answers to the question of what evidence is worth the cost. VOI is based on a conceptual framework that distinguishes between two distinct decisions in a health technology assessment process: Whether to adopt or reimburse a technology, and whether to invest scarce resources into an improvement of the evidence base for that technology (Claxton, 1999). VOI analyses estimate the value of additional evidence collection in terms of the projected costs of a wrong decision being made based on existing evidence of effectiveness and cost-effectiveness and the probability that collecting further evidence will alter decisions. The expected value of perfect information (EVPI) represents the expected cost of uncertainty related to a decision problem, i.e., as the opportunity cost of a potential error. It can be interpreted as the value of additional information which would eliminate all uncertainty on the model parameters (Claxton *et al.*, 2002; Griffin *et al.*, 2007).

Formally, the EVPI is measured in terms of net benefit (NB, as defined in Eq. (1) is $\Delta E \cdot \lambda - \Delta C$). The EVPI for an individual patient equals the difference between the expected value under certainty about the model parameters θ and the expected value of the decision based on the current evidence:

$$\text{EVPI} = \text{E}_\theta \max_j \text{NB}(j, \theta) - \max_j \text{E}_\theta \text{NB}(j, \theta). \quad (2)$$

Under full information, the net benefit $\text{NB}(j, \theta)$ is maximized over the alternative strategies j for each realization of the model parameters, and the expected value is taken over the distribution of θ [$\text{E}_\theta \max_j \text{NB}(j, \theta)$]. In contrast, under uncertainty, the decision-maker chooses a strategy to maximize the expected net benefit over the parameter distribution [$\max_j \text{E}_\theta \text{NB}(j, \theta)$] (Rogowski *et al.*, 2009a).

The EVPI presents the upper bound of potential value of further research. To determine the cost-effectiveness of a specific design for collecting further evidence, expected value of sample information (EVSI) needs to be calculated. Both EVPI and EVSI can be calculated for the decision as a whole and for single (subsets of) parameters (Briggs *et al.*, 2006, p. 201 ff.). The VOI needs to be multiplied by the total number of patients affected by the decision — the number of patients per year multiplied by the number of years the information generated remains useful (discounted). Different time horizons can be applied which range from a short term of a few years up to an infinite time horizon (Philips *et al.*, 2008).

Decision-analytic considerations can inform not only the question of whether or not a value proposition is sufficiently strong to justify the initiation of a translation process, but also the question of how much evidence should be collected to confirm this value proposition. For example, from a VOI perspective, investments into further research are more likely to be worthwhile if a larger group of patients is affected, if uncertainty is higher, if the expected cost-effectiveness is close to the threshold value, and if the costs of research are lower (Rogowski *et al.*, 2012).

However, it would be a misunderstanding of the potential of VOI analysis to assume that any investment into further evidence generation where the expected VOI exceeds the expected costs of evidence generation would always increase the chances to make a correct decision on the technology under development. The particular study might well increase the decision uncertainty, as the reduction in parameter uncertainty could be associated with a more precisely estimated distribution of NB, but simultaneously with a shift of that distribution. This could be the case if the new study reveals that the cost-effectiveness of the technology is closer to the cost-effectiveness threshold than previously expected; despite a more precise estimate, the probability of making a wrong decision may then be higher.

Further Considerations

In addition to VOI considerations, from a decision analytic perspective, the net benefit (NB) forgone if a cost-effective technology is not applied is relevant, as well as the costs of reversing the decision if a technology is introduced that is not cost-effective in practice (Griffin *et al.*, 2007). Besides these technology characteristics, the characteristics of the payer are also relevant, in particular the payer's authority to initiate research, to withdraw a technology and to influence its price and thus its cost-effectiveness (Walker *et al.*, 2012).

Based on characteristics of both the technology itself and the payer, recommendations about an optimal decision on a medical innovation can be derived: to reject or grant coverage (and potentially revise the decision later), to cover the technology only within research settings or if complemented by research (to inform the decision to adopt or reject), and/or to influence the price of the technology at the time of the first coverage decision or later (in particular, to ensure that its price can be reduced if the technology turns out not to be cost-effective from the payer perspective) (Walker *et al.*, 2012).

If no probabilistic model is available for applying VOI methods, deterministic sensitivity analysis can provide some guidance for planning and designing clinical trials. For example, they can help identify key areas of uncertainty for which further evidence is required and shed light on relevant comparators. Sensitivity analyses can also provide information about which study parameters are of particular importance for establishing cost-effectiveness (Hartz and John, 2008).

As in decisions about the technology's net benefit, further considerations may need to be included in the decision to generate additional evidence about a new health technology's value. These include, for example, controversial nature of proposed technology; disease burden, variation in rates of use; the relevance of the disease or target condition to current regional or national health policies and/or priorities; and other ethical, legal, and psychosocial implications associated with the new technology (Noorani *et al.*, 2007; Pluddemann *et al.*, 2010). Public funders may consider further issues in their prioritization of scarce resources within life sciences research budgets, such as the opportunity to develop tools and instruments that can also be used for other scientific purposes, training doctoral students or researchers regarding topics of future relevance; or they may consider equity issues that may give special priority to interventions for patients with orphan diseases (Banzi *et al.*, 2011; Salter and Martin, 2001; Mindell *et al.*, 2008).

Empirical approaches

The standard approach to decrease uncertainty about new health technologies from the viewpoint of clinical epidemiology is to conduct clinical studies. In the case of relative effectiveness, randomized controlled trials (RCTs) are the gold standard of evidence collection. As illustrated above, VOI methods can be used to inform the design of clinical trials (Claxton *et al.*, 2004; Claxton and Sculpher, 2006). Recent reviews of VOI studies indicate a number of applications already, but also point out that usefulness for decision-makers needs to be improved (Tuffaha *et al.*, 2014, Steuten *et al.*, 2013). Evidence from clinical studies is also an important input to health economic analysis and good decision-analytic modeling practice requires incorporating the best available evidence (Philips *et al.*, 2006). However, decisions to continue translation or to use the technology may have to be made in the absence of adequate information from clinical studies about all relevant parameters. Additionally, assessing value for money involves including evidence about resource consumption associated with the technology's use in practice. Given that the focus of THE is on early generation of evidence beyond standard methods (e.g., standard clinical trials used for drug market approval and economic evaluations used for final coverage decisions), complementary fields of research that address questions of early evaluation are of particular relevance in THE.

Generally, a number of methods for early technology assessment are available to update the initial estimate of value (Banta and Vondeling, 1994; Bartelmes *et al.*, 2009). Approaches of particular relevance are described in the following sections: First, the elicitation of expert beliefs to generate first evidence of relative effectiveness and the update of such priors on the basis of early clinical trials; second, the generation of evidence within managed-entry agreements — contracts between manufacturers or providers and health care payers about the conditional coverage of new health technologies — which can be used to validate the estimates from early models as an alternative form of evidence generation.

Generating First Evidence by Eliciting and Updating Prior Distributions

Elicitation of expert opinions can be used to improve early estimates of cost-effectiveness as well as to elicit *a-priori* distributions for clinical trials and VOI analyses. Generally, a number of methodological issues have to be considered for the appropriate elicitation of expert opinions, such as the selection of experts and the number of experts to include; the method of data collection (e.g., face-to-face or telephone interview, email or internet questionnaire); the assessment tool (e.g., visual rating scale, probability wheel); and the method of aggregating opinions of different experts (e.g., behavioral aggregation by Delphi process or statistical aggregation with or without different weights for different experts) (O'Hagan, 2006).

A number of studies have applied methods of expert elicitation (Johnson *et al.*, 2010a; Leal *et al.*, 2007; Grigore *et al.*, 2013). However, the description of methods typically lacks transparency, and much work remains to be done until methods for eliciting expert beliefs are sufficiently reliable, valid, responsive to change, and feasible for wider use in generating early estimates of emerging technologies value (Grigore *et al.*, 2013; Johnson *et al.*, 2010b; Sullivan and Payne, 2011; Haakma *et al.*, 2014).

These priors can be updated on the basis of early clinical trials. An example of how health economic modeling can be integrated into the product life cycle has been provided by Vallejo-Torres for the case of absorbable pins for treating hallux valgus, also known as bunions (Vallejo-Torres *et al.*, 2011).

Managed-Entry Agreements

At a later stage, when a technology is sufficiently developed for use in practice but the evidence barrier about the performance in health care practice is still prohibitively high from the viewpoint of payers, managed-entry agreements (MEA) may provide a valuable context for empirical research to collect further evidence (Adamski *et al.*, 2010). MEAs provide a natural complement to early modeling because they allow for validation of the value propositions established on the basis of early models and complementary preference analyses.

MEAs are contracts between manufacturers or providers and health care payers about the conditional coverage of new health technologies. A large number of MEAs have been reported in the literature (Stafinski *et al.*, 2010; Carlson *et al.*, 2010) and different types and typologies of MEAs exist (e.g., Walker *et al.*, 2012). Some forms of MEA involve the establishment of costly RCTs or medical registries. To minimize the cost of evidence collection, an alternative data source of particular relevance is routine data available from sickness funds (Brandes *et al.*, n.d.; Carlson *et al.*, 2010).

MEAs involve some method of collecting evidence regarding the technology's value — which can involve assessing two components, effectiveness and resource utilization or costs — alongside a technology's use in practice. MEAs that focus on the first component, uncertainty about clinical effectiveness, include (1) provisions covering of the new technology only for research; (2) coverage only alongside evidence development; (3) conditional treatment continuation where coverage is granted for individual patients but under the condition that short-term outcome goals are met; and (4) outcomes-based risk-sharing, where the price paid by health care payers is conditioned on pre-specified outcomes targets. Focusing on the second component, the payer's uncertainty about volume of utilization and costs, MEAs can also include (5) utilization-based risk-sharing where the price paid by the health care payer is linked to the pattern or process of care (e.g., paid for only when an intervention is applied by specialized physicians) and (6) cost-based risk sharing where reimbursed prices can be reduced, for example, if the overall costs or the volume of services exceed a pre-specified amount predicted to be necessary to treat high-need patients (Carlson *et al.*, 2010). The first-mentioned outcomes-based managed-entry schemes are more likely to require the collection of original data, in particular, if outcomes are specified in intermediate endpoints such as tumor progression. The more the schemes are based on utilization and costs, the more likely it is that they can be based on routinely collected data (Brandes *et al.*). For MEAs focusing on uncertainty about the clinical effectiveness of a novel health technology, VOI analysis might provide a helpful contribution to develop the design of the mechanism generating additional evidence on the technology during its use in the health care system.

Evidence regarding the costs and benefits of MEAs is rather limited. This holds particularly for MEAs that attempt to manage uncertainty about health benefits expected from the use of a new technology. It is unknown whether and to what extent these arrangements have kept their promise to reduce health losses — while on the one hand, they can delay the launch of technologies that ultimately prove to be clinically and economically beneficial, on the other hand, they can reduce the waste of scarce financial resources that go toward using technologies that ultimately prove to be ineffective or not cost-effective. Given the almost complete lack of structured *ex post* evaluations of MEAs in the literature, the ISPOR (International Society For Pharmacoeconomics and Outcomes Research) Good Practices for Performance-Based Risk-Sharing Arrangements Task Force has made some recommendations on the standards that should be applied to good practices in the use of MEAs encompassing questions around the desirability, design, implementation, governance, and evaluation of such arrangements (Garrison *et al.*, 2013).

The fundamental rationale for all MEAs is that payers and manufacturers have conflicting interests and, in consequence, potentially different views on the potential value of a novel health technology. Therefore, governance structures and rules assuring the independence of vested interests are essential. Governance must be designed in a way to ensure transparency and accountability, means to mitigate conflicts, independent review of the methods to generate new evidence, and a neutral, independent analysis of this new evidence (Garrison *et al.*, 2013). Given the public debate surrounding the UK multiple sclerosis drugs risk-sharing scheme (MS-RSS), it illustrates the importance of these issues to achieve the aims of the arrangement and avoiding costly failures (Raftery, 2010; Pickin *et al.*, 2009). We will resume this issue of appropriate institutional arrangements in the next section, within the broader context of discussing interaction problems in TM and how to solve them.

Optimizing the Translational Value Chain

Successful TM is highly dependent upon successful societal cooperation — a precondition which can very easily fail. For example, a basic researcher incentivized to increase the scientific output and impact factor may not be interested in dealing with the problems of drop-outs in clinical trials and the side-effects of the newly invented approach in clinical practice. For an entrepreneur or financial investor, the main objective of the further development is to increase sales and maximize profits — regardless of whether applying the technology provides value from a health care system perspective. The analysis of TM from an economic perspective thus includes analyzing the process with a focus on the incentives that may hinder or promote successful and productive cooperation — in order to suggest new institutional designs which overcome interaction problems during the process of TM. In particular, decades of research in new institutional economics which addresses problems of information and incentives have led to a large body of theoretical and empirical literature that may fruitfully be applied to the successful translation of research results into health care practice.

Theoretical considerations about the value of different configurations of translation processes

Following Buchanan's concepts of constitution economics (Buchanan, 1975) and its recent application in economic ethics (Homann and Suchanek, 2000; Luetge, 2005), economics can be understood as the analysis of possibilities and limitations of societal cooperation for mutual advantage (Homann and Suchanek, 2000, p. 5). It analyzes situations of successful and unsuccessful cooperation through concepts such as dilemma structures analogous to the famous game-theory concept of the prisoner's dilemma, wherein because of adverse incentives, two hypothetical prisoners end up in a Pareto-inferior social state. The solution to the dilemma would be an institution that creates stable expectations about each other's commitment to cooperation — in the example of the prisoner's dilemma, an enforceable rule not to defect. Even if such rules limit each individual's freedom, they improve the individual's possibilities of productive cooperation which makes both parties better off and thus leads to a Pareto improvement. New institutional economic theories, such as principal–agent theory, the theory of transaction costs, and the theory of property rights provide insights about how institutional designs can be designed in an incentive-compatible manner that facilitates such societal cooperation.

As mentioned previously, it is not only the characteristics of novel health technologies themselves (their cost-effectiveness, VOI, costs of reversing a positive coverage decision), but also institutional characteristics of coverage decision processes that are relevant for the optimal design of MEAs (Walker *et al.*, 2012). A first framework to assess such coverage decision processes in a formal manner has been recently developed. It combines the decision-analytic framework of net benefit (see the theoretical considerations in the previous section, "*Establishing the value of a potential technology prior to translation*") and the value of information (see the theoretical considerations in the previous section, "*Establishing evidence of value during the translation process*") with the agency theory. In this framework, coverage decision processes can be seen as a value-generating step in TM because uncertainty about whether or not a new technology meets the funding criteria is reduced; furthermore, institutional requirements such as transparency and participation can create incentives to select value-maximizing technologies (and thus overcome moral hazard prior to the final reimbursement decision), and adequate reimbursement and management rules can create incentives for service providers to implement the value-based coverage decisions in clinical practice (Rogowski, 2013).

To our knowledge, little systematic work from an economic perspective has been done on the incentives of the multiple stakeholders involved in the translation process for promoting cost-effective health technologies early on, although there are some global initiatives in place to stimulate this research. For instance, the Center for Translational Molecular Medicine (CTMM) in the Netherlands, the Helmholtz Center Munich in Germany, and Oncotyrol in Austria have a specific interest in health technology assessment during early stages of technology development and scientific discovery.

Generally, different concepts from new institution economics (Milgrom and Roberts, 1992) could be used to analyze problems in translation beyond the decisions about coverage and reimbursement. In particular, the agency theory is likely to be relevant as far as the interests of funding agencies for research and health care may deviate from the interests of researchers or health service providers. As far as the societal objectives of successful translation can be represented by an objective function, decision-analytic frameworks can be used to model the value created or potentially forgone by suboptimal configurations of the translational value chain.

Activities to promote a clear specification of decision criteria for the coverage of new health technologies in the face of scarce resources, which are acceptable to all involved stakeholders, can serve as a basis for information gathering and conflict resolution in the cooperative process of TM. Here, economic theories of value in health care can provide guidance for the discourse among stakeholders. To ensure that the decision frameworks are both implementable and acceptable, it is important that the quantitative economic evaluation methods used to determine value are robust, and also that their normative foundations are well developed, and understood and accepted by decision-makers.

In the practice of research funding, translation is playing an increasingly explicit role. For example, the EU Horizon 2020 program[5] uses implementation of findings as an evaluation criterion and includes a number of calls for proposals explicitly addressing translational medicine. This may be one emerging approach to align the incentives of researchers with the end-users of new medical technology: At least during the phase of grant application which is a necessary aspect of successful scientific careers, researchers increasingly have to consider how their biomedical research results can have an impact on patient benefit. However, much remains to be done to gain a better theoretical understanding of how translation processes can be improved.

---

[5]Horizon 2020 is an EU Research and Innovation program with close to €80 billion of funding available over a time span of 7 years (2014–2020); see http://ec.europa.eu/programmes/horizon2020/en/what-horizon-2020 [accessed 28 January 2015].

Towards empirical approaches

To establish empirical economic methods for optimizing the translational value chain would ideally require, first, a descriptive analysis of translation processes including the relevant problems of information and motivation as well as institutional settings to overcome these; second, it would require structured measurement concepts for collecting quantitative data on these process elements and estimates of their relative performance in solving interaction problems arising during translation; and third, it would require the development of evidence-based, practical tools to measure deficiencies and develop suggestions for improvement in efficiently translating medical discoveries into cost-effective care. Currently, work at all three of these steps is still at a rather early stage, with a focus on descriptive models of translation.

Many descriptive models characterize translation as a process ranging from research to late development stages such as market approval, use in clinical practice or health outcomes; and typically, problems of information are incorporated into existing descriptive frameworks (Sung *et al.*, 2003; Plebani and Marincola, 2006; Westfall *et al.*, 2007; So *et al.*, 2011; Dougherty and Conway, 2008; Simon, 2008). The IOM Clinical research roundtable described the translation process as consisting of two phases (1) from basic science to clinical science and (2) from clinical science to public health impact. This has been further refined as three phases from basic to clinical science ("T1"), to clinical practice ("T2") and further onto health impact ("T3"). Some denotation of three sequential phases of translational medicine (differing in content) can frequently be found in the literature. These characterizations typically incorporate the notion that there are chasms between these phases, and different suggestions have been made about how to bridge them (Drolet and Lorenzi, 2011). Rather than a sequence, translational medicine has also been described as a circle in which entrepreneurial translational researchers identify and bridge the gaps at between different steps (Keramaris *et al.*, 2008). From an economic perspective, with a focus on the translation of valuable technologies, also fourth-hurdle processes need to be integrated into models of translation, i.e., the decision of health care payers about whether or not the new technologies provide value for money (Rogowski *et al.*, 2008).

Furthermore, a large number of players with different perspectives and incentives are involved in TM, supporting the idea that institutional economics could provide a relevant framework for analyzing TM. Identified players include: Basic scientists of different disciplines; manufacturers of health technologies such as drugs and devices; primary care physicians and hospitals; specialized providers, such as laboratories, that provide additional services; patients and patient representatives; citizens, represented by governments; insurers or payers of obligatory or voluntary contribution payments, represented by decision-makers among public and private health care payers; research funding agencies; and further international organizations and independent monitoring agencies (Plebani and Marincola, 2006; Keramaris *et al.*, 2008; Ijzerman and Steuten, 2011).

However, the work on structured methods for measuring different configurations of TM processes or policy options is still limited, although some work has been done. First frameworks have been developed for assessing coverage decision processes (Fischer *et al.*, 2011; Hutton *et al.*, 2006). Existing quantitative empirical studies on coverage decisions have addressed past decisions and attributes of decision processes by partial least square modeling (Fischer *et al.*, 2013b) and regression analysis (Fischer *et al.*, 2013a) and have addressed the impact of process characteristics on decision outcomes.

Also, there is a large and diversified body of empirical literature on a range of topics which are relevant for TM. For example, a number of econometric and other analyses have assessed the process of technology diffusion and different factors associated with increased or delayed diffusion of new technologies (e.g., Berndt *et al.*, 2002; Booth-Clibborn *et al.*, 2000; Greenberg *et al.*, 2005; Hashimoto *et al.*, 2006; Oh *et al.*, 2005, Packer *et al.*, 2006). Translation has also been investigated in a bibliometrical manner, tracing the publications of findings from basic research to publications of experimental studies of health care services (e.g., Contopoulos-Ioannidis *et al.*, 2003). Furthermore, factors that contribute to translation in terms of universities' performance in creating new technology ventures have been investigated (e.g., O'Shea *et al.*, 2005) as well as factors that contribute to the involvement of stakeholders into innovation processes (e.g., Ahmad *et al.*, 2012). However, a synthesis of these findings within a theoretically coherent model of TM from an economic perspective is still lacking.

Regarding frameworks for evaluating translation processes, the descriptive studies frequently incorporate some kind of recommendations about how to improve translation. Here too, first frameworks for assessing translational research processes have been developed (e.g., Rajan *et al.*, 2013). However, again, the development of empirical methods based on theoretical reflection and empirical evidence is still among the tasks that remain to be achieved by THE.

Discussion

This chapter introduces a definition of THE and presents an overview of this emerging area of research. THE is described as a field of research that aims to use economic theories and methods to bridge the gap between the decision to fund and use a new health technology in clinical practice (the back end of translational medicine) and the initial decision to invest in its development (the front end of translational medicine). This goes beyond the traditional concept where health economists primarily provide the results of their economic evaluations to decision-makers responsible for allocating health care funds. THE more closely integrates the development of innovations, and provides links to health care business perspectives and decisions.

This chapter illustrated how health economics can, first, support the analysis of "value" for a potential health technology and the development of a value proposition that is strong enough to justify the initiation of a translation process; second, how health economic methods can be used to generate evidence about an emerging technology's value as early as possible in the translation process; and third, how institutions to overcome barriers of information and motivation in the highly cooperative process of translating new biomedical ideas into value for health care systems and patients can be analyzed from a health economics perspective.

Concepts of particular relevance from a business perspective include the use of early modeling for estimating value-based prices and developing business cases, the use of structured methods for measuring and incorporating user preferences into the development process, and the use of managed entry schemes to facilitate timely market access for innovators.

THE is a new concept, and therefore providing an overview of THE is subject to limitations. In particular, THE is defined by a specific type of problems rather than by a certain methodological approach. Thus, the demarcation line between THE and other areas of health economics is necessarily fuzzy, and it is a difficult topic to cover completely. THE is still a young area of research and this chapter is the first publication which presents an overview of a research field, which is likely to evolve further.

THE promotes a more rational translation of medical technologies toward medical practice in circumstances where they are considered to provide good value for money; however, this process depends on agreement about the criteria of what constitutes value for money in publicly funded health care. Frequently, scarcity of health care resources is handled implicitly rather than explicitly, and evidence of effectiveness is the only consented allocation criterion. Besides numerous questions that still need to be addressed by further research, a lack of clear criteria may provide the most practically relevant limitation to any use of economic methods by decision-makers about initiating translation, managing translation projects, and shaping the translational value chain. From an economic perspective, the decision to initiate a translation process can be seen as an investment decision of scarce public or private resources. The better that value functions are specified by decision-makers (as in the case of NICE in the UK, which specifies the type of health gain as well as willingness to pay), the more precisely can value already assessed during R&D because this provides a value function that can be implemented in early models. Therefore, developing health economic methods is a task not only for research settings but also for normative reflection and input from political deliberation processes that aim to further specify a shared societal understanding of value for money in health care. For this reason, THE also includes theoretical and philosophical reflections of value, evidence of value, and the most appropriate institutional setting in which to generate value in health care.

Research needs in THE associated with the three areas of investigation covered in this chapter include the following: First, regarding the establishment of value for potential health technologies, there are still theoretical and empirical questions about what can be considered "value" in health care. Theoretically, because public payers are typically required to treat the covered population equitably rather than maximizing any unit of outcome such as health (Klonschinski, 2014). Therefore, it needs to be determined how outcome-oriented concepts of efficiency can be applied to health care to anticipate future coverage decisions and which other criteria rather than health gains need to be considered. Empirically, it is unclear how these considerations are to be operationalized and weighted. More work is also needed to determine the appropriate role of preference elicitation and the most valid and reliable methods for this task — different methods arrive at different weights of attributes and subsequent rank orders, therefore more work is needed to determine which can be considered the most valid methods. From a business perspective, more case studies and methodological work is needed to arrive at reliable, easily applicable methods for analyzing and incorporating user preferences into technology development. Finally, more evidence about other technology-related characteristics of translation processes are needed, such as R&D costs and success probabilities for technologies other than drugs in order to arrive at better NPV estimates for translation business cases.

Second, regarding the establishment of evidence about value as early as possible in the process of translation, there are still a number of open questions for the use of VOI analysis, such as how to incorporate structural uncertainty, or which are the appropriate assumptions to make regarding technology life cycles. Furthermore, it is unclear how notions of "value" other than outcome maximization can be accounted for in VOI methods. There is also still a need to compare and validate different approaches for generating evidence early in the translation process. From a business perspective, there is a particular need for further development of technically and legally feasible, smart MEAs that facilitate early market access of valuable innovations. For example, routine data may be a particularly suitable and low-cost data source of MEAs. However, routine data also have limitations and it needs to be explored further under which circumstances they will be able to provide a reliable, valid, and ethically acceptable approach for generating evidence about value alongside a new technology's use in practice.

Finally, further theoretical and empirical research about the optimal translation value chain is needed. Theoretically, it needs to be determined how the institutional economic understanding of value can appropriately be accounted for in value functions used in health economic evaluation. Furthermore, there is a need to further expand the existing theoretical institutional economic work on coverage decisions to earlier stages in the translation process. Finally, there is also a need for further empirical work to assess the effects of different configurations of translation processes and whether institutional changes suggested on the basis of economic theory to improve TM also have the intended effects in practice and empirical investigation.

To conclude, THE is intended to improve translation processes in different ways. In particular, it aims to:

- Increase the chances that inventions are selected for translation that will indeed be used to improve clinical care;
- Reduce the time-span and increase the focus in the overall product development path by making better-informed decisions early on;
- In consequence, increase cost-efficiency of translation as well as the allocative efficiency of resource spending by accounting for the emerging technology's value for money from the beginning of the translation process.

This chapter has provided an overview of current attempts to pursue these aims with health economic methods. It has also illustrated that much work remains to be done to fully exploit the potential of translational medicine, aiming at a thoughtful, logical and financially sustainable allocation of scarce resources and, for those ideas that are found to provide good value for money, to promote the efficient translation of research findings and ideas from bench to clinical practice in a way that is acceptable to all involved stakeholders.

References

Adamski J, Godman B, Ofierska-Sujkowska G, Osinska B, Herholz H, Wendykowska K, Laius O, Jan S, Sermet C, Zara C, Kalaba M, Gustafsson R, Garuoliene K, Haycox A, Garattini S, Gustafsson LL. 2010. Risk sharing arrangements for pharmaceuticals: potential considerations and recommendations for European payers. *BMC Health Services Research* 10: 153.

Ahmad R, Kyratsis Y, Holmes A. 2012. When the user is not the chooser: Learning from stakeholder involvement in technology adoption decisions in infection control. *Journal of Hospital Infection* 81: 163–168.

Allmark P. 2004. Bayes and health care research. *Medicine, Health Care and Philosophy* 7: 321–332.

Assessment, OOT. 1978. *Assessing the Efficacy and Safety of Medical Technologies*. Washington DC, U.S. Government Printing Office.

Banta D. 2003. The development of health technology assessment. *Health Policy* 63: 121–132.

Banta HD, Vondeling H. 1994. Strategies for successful evaluation and policy-making toward health care technology on the move: The case of medical lasers. *Social Science & Medicine* 38: 1663–1674.

Banzi R, Moja L, Pistotti V, Facchini A, Liberati A. 2011. Conceptual frameworks and empirical approaches used to assess the impact of health research: An overview of reviews. *Health Research Policy and Systems* 9: 26.

Bartelmes M, Neumann U, Lühmann D, Schönermark MP, Hagen A. 2009. Methoden zur frühen entwicklungsbegleitenden Bewertung innovativer medizinischer Technologien. *GMS Health Technology Assessment* 94: 1–120.

Belton V, Stewart TJ. 2003. *Multiple Criteria Decision Analysis an Integrated Approach*. Boston, Mass. [u.a.], Kluwer Academic Publishers.

Berndt ER, Bhattacharjya A, Mishol DN, Arcelus A, Lasky T. 2002. An analysis of the diffusion of new antidepressants: variety, quality, and marketing efforts. *Journal of Mental Health Policy and Economics* 5: 3–19.

Birch S, Donaldson C. 2003. Valuing the benefits and costs of health care programmes: where's the 'extra' in extra-welfarism? *Social Science & Medicine* 56: 1121–1133.

Blackorby C, Donaldson D. 1990. A Review Article: The case against the use of the sum of compensating variations in cost–benefit analysis. *Canadian Journal of Economics* 23(3): 471–494.

Bland JM, Altman DG. 1998. Bayesians and frequentists. *British Medical Journal* 317: 1151–1160.

Boadway R, Bruce N. 1984. *Welfare Economics*. Oxford [u.a.], Blackwell.

Booth-Clibborn N, Packer C, Stevens A. 2000. Health technology diffusion rates. Statins, coronary stents, and MRI in England. *International Journal of Technology Assessment in Health Care* 16: 781–786.

Brandes A, Schwarzkopf L, Rogowski WH n.d. Evidence generation in managed entry agreements — When are claims data a suitable source? In press, to be published in *International Journal of Technology Assessment in Health Care.*

Bridges JF, Hauber AB, Marshall D, Lloyd A, Prosser LA, Regier DA, Johnson FR, Mauskopf J. 2011. Conjoint analysis applications in health — A checklist: A report of the ISPOR Good Research Practices for Conjoint Analysis Task Force. *Value Health* 14: 403–413.

Briggs A, Claxton K, Sculpher M. 2006. *Decision Modelling for Health Economic Evaluation*. Oxford u.a. Oxford University Press.

Brouwer WB, Culyer AJ, Van Exel NJ, Rutten FF. 2008. Welfarism vs. extra-welfarism. *Journal of Health Economics* 27: 325–338.

Buchanan JM. 1975. *The Limits of Liberty: Between Anarchy and Leviathan*. Chicago [u.a.], University of Chicago Press.

Butler DF. 2014. *Business Planning for New Ventures a Guide for Start-Ups and New Innovations*. New York, NY u.a., Routledge.

Carlson JJ, Sullivan SD, Garrison LP, Neumann PJ, Veenstra DL. 2010. Linking payment to health outcomes: A taxonomy and examination of performance-based reimbursement schemes between healthcare payers and manufacturers. *Health Policy* 96: 179–190.

Chakma J, Sun GH, Steinberg JD, Sammut SM, Jagsi R. 2014. Asia's ascent — global trends in biomedical R&D expenditures. *New England Journal Medicine* 370: 3–6.

Claxton K. 1999. The irrelevance of inference: A decision-making approach to the stochastic evaluation of health care technologies. *Journal of Health Economics* 18: 341–64.

Claxton K, Ginnelly L, Sculpher M, Philips Z, Palmer S. 2004. A pilot study on the use of decision theory and value of information analysis as part of the NHS Health Technology Assessment programme. *Health Technology Assessment* 8: 1–103.

Claxton K, Sculpher M, Drummond M. 2002. A rational framework for decision making by the National Institute For Clinical Excellence (NICE). *Lancet* 360: 711–715.

Claxton KP, Sculpher MJ. 2006. Using value of information analysis to prioritise health research: Some lessons from recent UK experience. *Pharmacoeconomics* 24: 1055–1068.

Contopoulos-Ioannidis DG, Ntzani E, Ioannidis JP. 2003. Translation of highly promising basic science research into clinical applications. *American Journal of Medicine* 114: 477–484.

Cosh E, Girling A, Lilford R. 2007. Investing in new medical technologies: A decision framework. *Journal of Commercial Biotechnology* 13: 263–271.

Culyer A, Mccabe C, Briggs A, Claxton K, Buxton M, Akehurst R, Sculpher M, Brazier J. 2007. Searching for a threshold, not setting one: The role of the National Institute for Health and Clinical Excellence. *Journal of Health Services Research & Policy* 12: 56–58.

Culyer A, Newhouse JP. 2000. Introduction: The state and scope of health economics. In Culyer A, Newhouse JP. (Eds.). *Handbook of Health Economics*. Elsevier Science B.V.

Cutler DM, Mcclellan M. 2001. Is technological change in medicine worth it? *Health Affairs (Millwood)* 20: 11–29.

DE Bekker-Grob EW, Ryan M, Gerard K. 2012. Discrete choice experiments in health economics: A review of the literature. *Health Economics* 21(2): 145–172.

Devlin N, Sussex J. 2011. *Incorporating multiple criteria in HTA. Methods and processes*, London, Office of Health Economics.

Dougherty D, Conway PH. 2008. The "3T's" road map to transform US health care: The "how" of high-quality care. *Journal of the American Medical Association* 299: 2319–2221.

Drolet BC, Lorenzi NM. 2011. Translational research: Understanding the continuum from bench to bedside. *Translational Research* 157: 1–5.

Fischer KE, Leidl R, Rogowski WH. 2011. A structured tool to analyse coverage decisions: Development and feasibility test in the field of cancer screening and prevention. *Health Policy* 101: 290–299.

Fischer KE, Rogowski WH, Leidl R, Stollenwerk B. 2013a. Transparency vs. closed-door policy: Do process characteristics have an impact on the outcomes of coverage decisions? A statistical analysis. *Health Policy* 112: 187–196.

Fischer KE, Stollenwerk B, Rogowski WH. 2013b. Link between process and appraisal in coverage decisions: An analysis with structural equation modeling. *Medical Decision Making* 33: 1009–1025.

Garber AM. 2004. Cost-effectiveness and evidence evaluation as criteria for coverage policy. *Health Affairs (Millwood),* Suppl Web Exclusives, W4-284-96.

Garrison Jr LP, Towse A, Briggs A, DE Pouvourville G, Grueger J, Mohr PE, Severens JL, Siviero P, Sleeper M. 2013 Performance-based risk-sharing arrangements-good practices for design, implementation, and evaluation: Report of the ISPOR good practices for performance-based risk-sharing arrangements task force. *Value Health* 16: 703–719.

Greenberg D, Peterburg Y, Vekstein D, Pliskin JS. 2005. Decisions to adopt new technologies at the hospital level: Insights from Israeli medical centers. *International Journal of Technology Assessment in Health Care* 21: 219–227.

Gregson N, Sparrowhawk K, Mauskopf J, Paul J. 2005. Pricing medicines: Theory and practice, challenges and opportunities. *Nature Reviews Drug Discovery* 4: 121–130.

Griffin S, Claxton K, Palmer S, Sculpher M. 2007. Dangerous omissions: The consequences of ignoring decision uncertainty. *Medical Decision Making* 27.

Grigore B, Peters J, Hyde C, Stein K. 2013. Methods to elicit probability distributions from experts: A systematic review of reported practice in health technology assessment. *Pharmacoeconomics* 31: 991–1003.

Grossman M. 1972. On the concept of health capital and the demand for health. *Journal of Political Economy* 80(2): 223–255.

Haakma W, Steuten LM, Bojke L, Ijzerman MJ. 2014. Belief elicitation to populate health economic models of medical diagnostic devices in development. *Applied Health Economics and Health Policy* 12: 327–334.

Hartz S, John J. 2008. Contribution of economic evaluation to decision making in early phases of product development: A methodological and empirical review. *International Journal of Technology Assessment in Health Care* 24: 465–472.

Hashimoto H, Noguchi H, Heidenreich P, Saynina O, Moreland A, Miyazaki S, Ikeda S, Kaneko Y, Ikegami N. 2006. The diffusion of medical technology, local conditions, and technology re-invention: A comparative case study on coronary stenting. *Health Policy* 79: 221–230.

Hauschildt J. 2004. *Innovations Management,* 3rd ed., München: Vahlen Verlag.

Hicks J. 1939. The foundation of welfare economics. *Economic Journal* 49: 696–712.

Hilgerink MP, Hummel MJ, Manohar S, Vaartjes SR, Ijzerman MJ. 2011. Assessment of the added value of the Twente Photoacoustic Mammoscope in breast cancer diagnosis. *Medical Devices (Auckland)* 4: 107–115.

Homann K, Suchanek A. 2000. *Ökonomik eine Einführung*. Tübingen, Mohr Siebeck.

Hummel JM, Bridges JF, Ijzerman MJ. 2014. Group decision making with the analytic hierarchy process in benefit–risk assessment: A tutorial. *Patient* 7: 129–140.

Hutton J, Mcgrath C, Frybourg JM, Tremblay M, Bramley-Harker E, Henshall C. 2006. Framework for describing and classifying decision-making systems using technology assessment to determine the reimbursement of health technologies (fourth hurdle systems). *International Journal of Technology Assessment in Health Care* 22: 10–18.

Ijzerman MJ, Steuten LM. 2011. Early assessment of medical technologies to inform product development and market access: A review of methods and applications. *Applied Health Economics and Health Policy* 9: 331–347.

Ishizaka A, Nemery P. 2013. *Multi-Criteria Decision Analysis Methods and Software* s.l. Wiley.

Johnson SR, Tomlinson GA, Hawker GA, Granton JT, Feldman BM. 2010a. Methods to elicit beliefs for Bayesian priors: A systematic review. *Journal of Clinical Epidemiology* 63: 355–369.

Johnson SR, Tomlinson GA, Hawker GA, Granton JT, Grosbein HA, Feldman BM. 2010b. A valid and reliable belief elicitation method for Bayesian priors. *Journal of Clinical Epidemiology* 63: 370–383.

Kaldor N. 1939. Welfare propositions and interpersonal comparisons of utility. *Economic Journal* 49: 549–552.

Keramaris NC, Kanakaris NK, Tzioupis C, Kontakis G, Giannoudis PV. 2008. Translational research: From benchside to bedside. *Injury* 39: 643–650.

Khoury MJ, Gwinn M, Ioannidis JP. 2010. The emergence of translational epidemiology: From scientific discovery to population health impact. *American Journal of Epidemiology* 172: 517–524.

Klonschinski A. 2014. 'Economic Imperialism' in health care resource allocation — How can equity considerations be incorporated into economic evaluation? *Journal of Economic Methodology,* 21(2).

Koerber F, Rolauffs B, Rogowski W. 2013. Early evaluation and value-based pricing of regenerative medicine technologies. *Regeneration Medicine* 8: 747–758.

Leal J, Wordsworth S, Legood R, Blair E. 2007. Eliciting expert opinion for economic models: An applied example. *Value Health* 10: 195–203.

Lichtenberg FR. 2005. The impact of new drug launches on longevity: Evidence from longitudinal, disease-level data from 52 countries, 1982–2001. *International Journal of Health Care Finance Economics* 5: 47–73.

Lichtenberg FR. 2012. Contribution of pharmaceutical innovation to longevity growth in Germany and France, 2001–7. *Pharmacoeconomics* 30: 197–211.

Luetge C. 2005. Economic ethics, business ethics and the idea of mutual advantages. *Business Ethics: A European Review* 14: 108–118.

Macintosh E. 2010. *Applied Methods of Cost–Benefit Analysis in Health Care*. Oxford [u.a.]. Oxford University Press.

Markiewicz K, Van Til JA, Mj IJ. 2014. Medical devices early assessment methods: Systematic literature review. *International Journal of Technology Assessment in Health Care* 30: 137–146.

Mccabe C, Claxton K, Culyer AJ. 2008. The NICE cost-effectiveness threshold: What it is and what that means. *Pharmacoeconomics* 26: 733–744.

Milgrom PR, Roberts J. 1992. *Economics, Organization and Management*. Englewood Cliffs, NJ, Prentice Hall.

Mindell JS, Boltong A, Forde I. 2008. A review of health impact assessment frameworks. *Public Health* 122: 1177–1187.

Morgan S, Grootendorst P, Lexchin J, Cunningham C, Greyson D. 2011. The cost of drug development: A systematic review. *Health Policy* 100: 4–17.

National Institute for Health and Clinical Excellence. 2008. Social value judgements. Principles for the development of NICE guidance. Second Edition. London.

Noorani HZ, Husereau DR, Boudreau R, Skidmore B. 2007. Priority setting for health technology assessments: a systematic review of current practical approaches. *International Journal of Technology Assessment in Health Care* 23: 310–315.

O'hagan A. 2006. *Uncertain Judgements Eliciting Experts' Probabilities*. Chichester u.a., Wiley.

O'shea RP, Allen TJ, Chevalier A, Roche F. 2005. Entrepreneurial Orientation, Technology Transfer and Spinoff Performance of U.S. Universities. *Research Policy* 34: 994–1009.

Ogilvie D, Craig P, Griffin S, Macintyre S, Wareham NJ. 2009. A translational framework for public health research. *BMC Public Health* 9: 116.

Oh Eh, Imanaka Y, Evans E. 2005. Determinants of the diffusion of computed tomography and magnetic resonance imaging. *International Journal of Technology Assessment Health Care* 21: 73–80.

Packer C, Simpson S, Stevens A. 2006. International diffusion of new health technologies: A ten-country analysis of six health technologies. *International Journal of Technology Assessment in Health Care* 22: 419–428.

Paul SM, Mytelka DS, Dunwiddie CT, Persinger CC, Munos BH, Lindborg SR, Schacht AL. 2010. How to improve R&D productivity: the pharmaceutical industry's grand challenge. *Nature Reviews Drug Discovery* 9: 203–214.

Philips Z, Bojke L, Sculpher M, Claxton K, Golder S. 2006. Good practice guidelines for decision-analytic modelling in health technology assessment: A review and consolidation of quality assessment. *Pharmacoeconomics* 24: 355–371.

Philips Z, Claxton K, Palmer S. 2008. The half-life of truth: what are appropriate time horizons for research decisions? *Medical Decision Making* 28: 287–299.

Philipson T, Eber M, Lakdawalla DN, Corral M, Conti R, Goldman DP. 2012. An analysis of whether higher health care spending in the United States versus Europe is 'worth it' in the case of cancer. *Health Affairs (Millwood)* 31: 667–675.

Pickin M, Cooper CL, Chater T, O'hagan A, Abrams KR, Cooper NJ, Boggild M, Palace J, Ebers G, Chilcott JB, Tappenden P, Nicholl J. 2009. The Multiple Sclerosis Risk Sharing Scheme Monitoring Study — early results and lessons for the future. *BMC Neurology* 9: 1.

Plebani M, Marincola FM. 2006. Research translation: a new frontier for clinical laboratories. *Clinical Chemistry and Laboratory Medicine* 44: 1303–1312.

Pluddemann A, Heneghan C, Thompson M, Roberts N, Summerton N, Linden-Phillips L, Packer C, Price CP. 2010. Prioritisation criteria for the selection of new diagnostic technologies for evaluation. *BMC Health Services Research* 10: 109.

Raftery J. 2010. Multiple sclerosis risk sharing scheme: a costly failure. *British Medical Journal* 340: c1672.

Rajan A, Caldas C, Van Luenen H, Saghatchian M, Van Harten WH. 2013. Assessing excellence in translational cancer research: a consensus based framework. *Journal of Translational Medicine* 11: 274.
Reed Johnson F, Lancsar E, Marshall D, Kilambi V, Muhlbacher A, Regier DA, Bresnahan BW, Kanninen B, Bridges JF. 2013. Constructing experimental designs for discrete-choice experiments: Report of the ISPOR Conjoint Analysis Experimental Design Good Research Practices Task Force. *Value Health* 16: 3–13.
Rogowski W, Burch J, Palmer S, Craigs C, Golder S, Woolacott N. 2009a. The effect of different treatment durations of clopidogrel in patients with non-ST-segment elevation acute coronary syndromes: A systematic review and value of information analysis. *Health Technology Assessment* 13: 1–102.
Rogowski WH, Grosse SD, Khoury MJ. 2009b. Challenges of translating genetic tests into clinical and public health practice. *Nature Reviews Genetics* 10: 489–495.
Rogowski WH. 2010. What should public health research focus on? Comments from a decision analytic perspective. *European Journal of Public Health* 20: 484–485.
Rogowski WH. 2013. An economic theory of the fourth hurdle. *Health Economics* 22: 600–610.
Rogowski WH, Grosse SD, Meyer E, John J, Palmer S. 2012. Die Nutzung von Informationswertanalysen in Entscheidungen über angewandte Forschung. Der Fall des genetischen Screenings auf Hämochromatose in Deutschland. *Bundesgesundheitsblatt Gesundheitsforschung Gesundheitsschutz* 55: 700–709.
Rogowski WH, Hartz SC, John JH. 2008. Clearing up the hazy road from bench to bedside: a framework for integrating the fourth hurdle into translational medicine. *BMC Health Services Research* 8: 1–12.
Salter AJ, Martin BR. 2001. The economic benefits of publicly funded basic research: A critical review. *Research Policy* 30: 509–532.
Sanders PM, Ijzerman MJ, Roach MJ, Gustafson KJ. 2011. Patient preferences for next generation neural prostheses to restore bladder function. *Spinal Cord* 49: 113–119.
Schroeder M. 2012. Value Theory. In Edward N. Zalta (ed.). *The Stanford Encyclopedia of Philosophy (Summer 2012 Edition).* Available at http://plato.stanford.edu/archives/sum2012/entries/value-theory/
Sculpher M, Drummond M, Buxton M. 1997. The iterative use of economic evaluation as part of the process of health technology assessment. *Journal of Health Services Research & Policy* 2: 26–30.
Sen A. 1979. The welfare basis of real income comparisons: A survey. *Journal of Economic Literature* 17(1): 1–45.
Sen A. 1999. The possibility of social choice. *The American Economic Review* 89: 349–378.
Severin F, Schmidtke J, Muhlbacher A, Rogowski WH. 2013. Eliciting preferences for priority setting in genetic testing: A pilot study comparing best-worst scaling and discrete-choice experiments. *European Journal of Human Genetics* 21: 1202–1208.
Simon R. 2008. Lost in translation: Problems and pitfalls in translating laboratory observations to clinical utility. *European Journal of Cancer* 44: 2707–2713.

So AD, Gupta N, Brahmachari SK, Chopra I, Munos B, Nathan C, Outterson K, Paccaud, JP, Payne DJ, Peeling RW, Spigelman M, Weigelt J. 2011. Towards new business models for R&D for novel antibiotics. *Drug Resistance Updates* 14: 88–94.

Stafinski T, Mccabe CJ, Menon D. 2010. Funding the unfundable: Mechanisms for managing uncertainty in decisions on the introduction of new and innovative technologies into healthcare systems. *Pharmacoeconomics* 28: 113–142.

Steuten L, Van De Wetering G, Groothuis-Oudshoorn K, Retel V. 2013. A systematic and critical review of the evolving methods and applications of value of information in academia and practice. *Pharmacoeconomics* 31: 25–48.

Sullivan W, Payne K. 2011. The appropriate elicitation of expert opinion in economic models: Making expert data fit for purpose. *Pharmacoeconomics* 29: 455–459.

Sung NS, Crowley WF, Jr, Genel M, Salber P, Sandy L, Sherwood LM, Johnson SB, Catanese V, Tilson H, Getz K, Larson EL, Scheinberg D, Reece EA, Slavkin H, Dobs A, Grebb J, Martinez RA, Korn A, Rimoin D. 2003. Central challenges facing the national clinical research enterprise. *Journal of the American Medical Association* 289: 1278–1287.

Sussex J, Towse A, Devlin N. 2013. Operationalizing value-based pricing of medicines: A taxonomy of approaches. *Pharmacoeconomics* 31: 1–10.

Tuffaha HW, Gordon LG, Scuffham PA. 2014. Value of information analysis in healthcare: A review of principles and applications. *Journal of Medical Economics* 17: 377–383.

Valentin EK. 2015. *Business Planning and Market Strategy*. Los Angeles u.a., Sage Publications Inc.

Vallejo-Torres L, Steuten L, Parkinson B, Girling AJ, Buxton MJ. 2011. Integrating health economics into the product development cycle: A case study of absorbable pins for treating hallux valgus. *Medical Decision Making* 31: 596–610.

Wailoo A, Tsuchiya A, Mccabe C. 2009. Weighting must wait: Incorporating equity concerns into cost-effectiveness analysis may take longer than expected. *Pharmacoeconomics* 27: 983–989.

Walker S, Sculpher M, Claxton K, Palmer S. 2012. Coverage with evidence development, only in research, risk sharing, or patient access scheme? A framework for coverage decisions. *Value Health* 15: 570–579.

Weernink M, Janus S, Van Til J, Raisch D, Ijzerman M. 2014. A systematic review to identify the use of preference elicitation methods in healthcare decision making. *Pharmaceutical Medicine* 28: 175–185.

Weinstein MC, Manning Jr WG 1997. Theoretical issues in cost-effectiveness analysis. *Journal of Health Economics* 16: 121–128.

Westfall JM, Mold J, Fagnan L. 2007. Practice-based research — "Blue Highways" on the NIH roadmap. *Journal of the American Medical Association* 297: 403–406.

Yazdizadeh B, Majdzadeh R, Salmasian H. 2010. Systematic review of methods for evaluating healthcare research economic impact. *Health Research Policy and Systems* 8: 6.

Zweifel P, Breyer FHJ, Kifmann M. 2009. *Health Economics*, s.l. Springer-Verlag.

Index

A
Accelerated Approval, 122–125
Accelerated Development, 120–122
Acceptability, 14–15, 27, 276
Access Reform, 1
Access to Resources, 83
Accessibility, 13–16, 165, 177, 276
Acclimatization with Rural Life, 86
Accommodation, 14–15, 338, 357, 360, 369, 381–382, 393–396
Accountable Care Organizations (*see also* ACOS), 240
Accountants, 56
Accreditation, 7, 28–31, 35, 39, 92
ACE-Inhibitors, 117
Adaptive Licensing, 167
Adaptive Pathways, 126
Affordability, 2, 14, 21, 144, 161–179, 340, 398, 400
Affordable Care Act (*see also* ACA), 239–240
Age and Gender, 76, 215
Age–Gender Composition, 206
Age-Related Sensory and Neurocognitive Changes, 80
Aggregate Income Growth, 206
Aging, 2, 55, 61–63, 78–80, 94
AIDS Treatment, 14
Alcohol Consumption, 109
Alcoholic Drinks, 19
Allocative Efficiency, 8
Allopathic Cadre, 84
Ambulance Drivers, 56
Ambulatory Care Sensitive Conditions (*see also* ACSCs), 252
Angioplasty, 202
Antacids, 117
Antenatal Care (*see also* ANC), 315
Anti-Retroviral (*see also* ARV) Therapy, 69
Appropriateness, 276
Argentina's Plan Nacer, 314
Asia-Pacific Countries, 29
Asthma, 60
Autonomized Units, 36
Autonomy of Professional Labor, 84
Availability of Medicines, 175
Availability of Schools, 86
Ayurvedic and Nursing Cadres, 84

B
Basic Insurance Coverage, 220–224
Behavioral Health Care, 60
Benchmarking Mechanisms, 384–385
Benefits, 2, 16, 30, 39, 56, 64, 72, 81, 108, 126, 144, 190, 198, 250, 327, 360
Beta Blockers, 115–116
'Bianzhi' Nurses, 72–73
Bilateral Agreements, 84
Biosimilars, 121

Blood Pressure, 236, 291, 301
Bottom–Up Costing, 10
Brain Drain, 88, 90
Brain Injury Care, 5
Branded Drugs, 118, 170
Break-Area, 83
Budget Limits, 140
Budgetary Restrictions, 179
Bundled Interventions, 87
Bundling and Private Finance, 353
Burden of Disease, 2, 60, 67, 138
Burnout, 75
Business Consultancies, 175
Business Loans, 88

C
Cancer Drugs, 163
Cancer Treatments, 163
Cancer, 60, 77, 116
Capability, 193, 201, 210, 276
Capital Investment, 198
Capitation Rates, 34
Capitation-Based Components, 236
Capitation-Based Payments, 295
Care Model, 25–26
Career Development Opportunities, 83
Case Complexity, 19
Catering, 356–357, 368, 371, 392, 396
Cause–Effect Relationships, 290
Center for Translational Molecular Medicine (*see also* CTMM), 428
Centers for Medicare & Medicaid Services (*see also* CMS), 316
Central Nervous System (*see also* CNS), 163
Certainty-Enhancing Mechanisms, 180
Certificate of Need Laws, 28
Chronic Diseases, 69, 94, 174, 236, 247, 256, 299, 304, 307
Chronic Illness, 60, 69, 78
Chronic Obstructive Pulmonary Disease (*see also* COPD), 242
Clerical Workers, 56
Clinical Activities, 370
Clinical Benefit, 160
Clinical Efficacy, 272
Clinical Evidence, 198
Clinical Indicators, 312
Clinical Managers, 371
Clinical Officers, 73
Clinical Professionals, 284
Clinical Psychologists, 62
Clinical Service Issues, 398
Clinical Services Cost, 396
Clinical Services Quality, 396
Clinical Training Locations, 65
Clinical Trials, 200
Clinical Value, 146
Clinics and Providers, 341
Co-Insurance, 169
Co-Location with Spouses, 86
Communitarianism, 275
Community Health Workers (*see also* CHW), 74
Comparative Analysis, 40
Competence, 91, 157, 175, 276
Competency-Based Education, 78
Competition, 4, 19–24, 107, 109, 117–119, 121, 139, 171, 248, 297, 392
Conditional Coverage (*see also* CC), 146, 424–425
Conditional Guidance, 289
Conditional Marketing Authorization, 122–123
Constant Returns To Scale (*see also* CRS), 17
Contextual Attributes, 86
Continuity, 276
Contract-Based Nurses, 73
Coronary Artery Bypass Grafts (*see also* CABGs), 210
Coronary Heart Disease (*see also* CHD), 312
Corporatized Units, 36
Cosmetic and Bariatric Surgery, 338, 340

Cost Containment, 149, 152, 155–160, 176, 180, 193
Cost Overruns, 395
Cost Savings, 414
Cost–Benefit Analysis, 137, 376, 386, 391, 401, 411
Cost-Effective Intervention, 86
Cost-Effectiveness, 2, 9, 129, 138, 144, 146, 167, 197, 199, 313, 322, 413–421, 423, 427
Cost-Efficiency, 226
Cost-Plus Pricing, 136
Council for Health Services Accreditation of Southern Africa (*see also* COHSASA), 30
Country Clusters of Health Systems, 221
Country-Level Planning, 94
County-Level HR Officers, 72
Coverage and Access, 191
Coverage with Evidence Development (*see also* CED), 146
Cream Skimming, 248, 372
Cross-Country Data, 203
Cross-Country Variation, 226
Cross-Sectional Analysis, 225

D

Data Availability, 38–39, 176, 193
Data Envelopment Analysis (*see also* DEA), 10, 288
  DEA approach, 17
  DEA results, 13
Decentralization of the Health Care System, 72
Decentralized Control of Health Systems, 222
Decision-Making, 40
Defensive Medicine, 29
Delegation, 223
Delphi Technique, 5
Demand for Health Care, 63, 67–71, 79, 192, 195
Demand Fostering, 372
Demand-Side Intervention, 147
Democratic Republic of Congo (*see also* DRC), 318
Demographic Shifts, 214
Demographics, 66–67, 76, 79, 212
Dengue Fever, 69
Density of Health Services Providers, 58
Density of Physicians, 58
Density of Nurses, 58
Density of Midwives, 58
Dental Assistants, 79
Dental Therapists, 79
Dentists, 73, 79, 339
Design Policies, 94
Diabetes Care, 5
Diabetes, 69–70, 151, 242, 291, 299, 316, 328
Diagnosis-Related Group (*see also* DRG), 23, 192–196, 199, 203, 227, 307, 409
Diet, 109, 299
Differential Pricing and Parallel Trade, 176
Diffusion, 189
Direct Hierarchical Control, 35–36
Disability, 75, 94
Disability-Adjusted Life Years (*see also* DALYs), 9, 277
Discrete-Choice Analysis (*see also* DCE), 418
Disease Burden, 60, 67, 69–70, 73, 85, 94
Diseconomies of Scale and Scope, 16
Dispensers, 127
Diverging Interpretation, 164
Donabedian Model, 5
Donabedian's Framework, 5
Donabedian's Multi-Dimensional Conception of Quality, 7
Donor Organizations, 55, 57, 91, 94
Drug Utilization, 161
Drug-Eluting Stents, 202

E

Early Evaluation, 405, 409, 418, 423
Economic Demand, 65
Economic Efficiency, 8, 168, 362
Economic Incentives, 351
Economic Model of
 health worker labor market, 64
 labor supply and demand, 64
Economies of Scale, 8, 16–17, 30
Education, 4, 31, 61–62, 68–69, 74–81, 86–92, 192, 209, 285–289, 329, 410
Educational Interventions, 86
Efficacy, 81, 117, 120–123, 161, 164, 175
E-Learning Technologies, 78
E-Learning Tools, 61
Emergency Human Resources (*see also* HR) Plan, 72
Empirical Analysis, 201, 203, 224
Employment Policies, 71
Employment Status, 83
Environmental Constraints, 19
Epidemics, 67, 207
Equatorial Guinea, 59, 289
Equity, 1, 13–14, 16, 23, 30, 32, 36, 108, 155, 180, 270–276, 303, 313, 343, 345, 412
Equity Implications of Hospital Performance, 16
Ethnicity, 284, 322
Europe's EUnetHTA Collaboration, 165
European Commission (*see also* EC), 112–113, 122, 150, 158, 178, 352
European Family Health Nursing Project, 77
European Federation of Quality Management (*see also* EFQM) Scale, 4
European Medicines Agency (*see also* EMA), 121–122, 177
European Union (*see also* EU)
 EU Directive on Patient Mobility, 335
 EU Member States, 126, 129–130, 132, 165, 171, 174
 Supplementary Protection Certificate in the EU, 117
Evidence of Corruption and Inaction, 72
Evidence-Based Policy-Making, 109
Exceptional Circumstances, 122–125, 161
Exemption Systems, 15, 32
Exercise, 109
Existence of Monopoly, 117
External Price Referencing (*see also* EPR), 129–130, 134, 156, 180
External Quality Assessment, 29
Externalities, 322–327, 360, 371

F

Facilities Maintenance Staff, 56
Faculty Shortfalls, 65
FADE QI Model, 26
Familiarity, 340
Family Circumstances, 75
Feasibility, 10, 27, 139
Fee Waivers, 33
Fee-For-Service (*see also* FFS), 35, 71, 231, 235, 239, 297, 301, 307, 314, 383
Female Health Workers, 84
Female Nursing, 81
Female Physicians, 81
Finance Remuneration, 94
Financial Burdens, 23, 32
Financial Incentives, 87–88, 108, 114, 128–129, 137, 148–149, 179, 251, 297, 317
Financial Loss of Consumption, 88
Financial Reforms, 72
Financial Risk, 241, 255, 261–262, 273, 297–298, 300
Financial Risk Protection, 270, 273
Financing Mechanism, 39, 107
Financing of Health Employment, 71
Fiscal Management, 380
Fixed Pricing, 156
Formularies, 131–132, 143, 161, 163
France
 France's *Centre HospitalierSud-Francilien* (*see also* CHSF), 364

French Society of Thoracic and Cardiovascular Surgery, 79
temporary authorization for use (*see also* ATU), 126, 172
Full-Service Model, 357–358, 368–369, 398
Funding, 83, 94, 109, 114, 299–300, 323–324, 344, 352–353, 364–367, 394, 400–401, 408–410, 415, 427–428

G
Gabon's Health Worker Density, 59
Gaming, 136, 251, 318, 320–322, 327
Gatekeepers, 222–223, 233, 239, 358
Gate-Keeping, 223
Gender Distribution of Health Care Occupations, 80
Gender of Medicine, 80
General Practitioners (*see also* GPs), 222, 225, 249, 312–313
Generalized Least Squares (*see also* GLS), 209
Generic Competitors, 171–172
Generic Drug Availability, 177
Generic Drugs, 150, 158, 170
Generic Policy, 168, 171
Generic Price Capping, 158
Geographic Boundary, 20
Geographic Disparities, 81
Geographical and Ethnic Affinities, 86
Global Budget, 31, 108, 307, 383
Global Budget Constraints, 222–225
Global Health Policymakers, 55, 57
Global Health Workforce, 55, 57, 73, 95
Global Partners in Anesthesia and Surgery (*see also* GPAS), 78
Good Manufacturing Practice (*see also* GMP), 170
Governance Arrangements for Public Hospitals, 45
Government Agencies, 31, 92, 407
Government Budgets, 192, 225
Governmental Efforts, 71–72
Governmental Organization, 357
Governmental Policies, 71
Gross Domestic Product (*see also* GDP)
GDP per capita, 59, 110, 112, 145, 173
GDP quintiles, 59
Gross National Income (*see also* GNI), 205, 212

H
Harassment, 84
Harvard Global Surgery Workforce Initiative, 60
Health Administration, 281, 392
Health and Development, 269
Health Care Cost Inflation, 28
Health Care Delivery System, 64
Health Care Institutions, 88, 217
Health Care Needs, 56, 60, 62, 67, 71, 73, 79, 91, 231, 248, 393, 412
Health Care Occupations, 65, 78, 80–81
Health Care Policy, 189, 385, 400
Health Care Professionals, 107, 168, 181, 387
Health Care Quadrilemma, 195
Health Care Service Delivery, 356
Health Care Service Providers, 56
Health Care Services, 27, 55–57, 63, 66–79, 92, 110, 279, 300, 313, 327, 387, 400, 430
Health Care Spending Growth, 189, 191, 193, 198, 203–207, 220–225
Health Care System Financing Mechanism, 107
Health Care Systems, 56–57, 93, 127, 138, 280, 408, 414, 431
Health Care Teams, 61–62
Health Care Technologies, 142
Health Care Workers, 56, 60, 66, 71, 74, 76–83, 89, 92, 94, 303, 314
Health Care-Providing Institutions, 2
Health Centers, 2, 62
Health Education Programs, 78, 87
Health Extension Program (*see also* HEP), 81, 92

Health Insurance, 29, 67, 71, 129, 136, 142, 151, 158, 162, 176, 220, 231, 254, 284, 410–411, 414
Health Insurers, 107–109, 127, 136, 139–140, 142, 146, 161, 168, 172, 180
Health Intervention and Technology Assessment Program (*see also* HITAP)
HITAP analyses, 29
HITAP evaluations, 29
Health Management Information System (*see also* HMIS), 312
Health Outcomes, 25, 66–67, 109, 190, 208, 250, 272, 278–279, 283–285, 296–303, 314, 412, 416, 429
Health Policy, 189–210, 214, 220, 225, 243, 269, 327, 355, 410
Health Provider Institutions, 31
Health Results Based Financing, 295
Health Spending Growth, 194, 197, 203–207, 213–218
Health Surveillance Assistants (*see also* HSA), 74
Health System Performance, 78, 269–291, 318
Health System Strengthening and Reform, 269
Health Technology Assessments (*see also* HTA)
HTA agency, 165, 175
HTA bodies, 126, 138, 174
HTA decisions, 165
HTA outcomes, 164–165, 174
HTA procedures and requirements, 175
HTA processes, 164–165, 178
HTA recommendations, 163, 178
Health Tourists, 336
Health Workers, 31, 56–81, 89–94, 318, 320, 334, 343
Health Workforce, 55–65, 69–75, 84, 93–94
Health Workforce Shortages, 66, 69
Healthbasket Research Project, 201
Heart and Orthopedic Surgery, 338
High-Cost Patented Drugs, 166
High-Income Countries, 7, 21, 38, 60–77, 278, 301, 329, 334, 346, 359
Highly-Skilled Workers, 88
HIV/AIDS, 67, 69, 84, 121, 283
Horizontal Differentiation, 117
Hospital Autonomy, 38
Hospital Quality and Performance, 1, 3, 7, 13, 24, 37, 40
Hospital Quality Improvement, 39
Hospital Tuberculosis Care, 5
Hospital Utilization and Access, 15
Hospitalization, 20, 297
Hospitals' Performance Measures, 12
Housing Children's Development, 86
Human Relations Model, 4
Human Resources Capacity, 71
Human Resources for Health (*see also* HRH)
assessment of HRH, 62
employment of HRH, 57
HRH capacity, 77
HRH planning, 55, 57, 93
HRH shortages, 55
HRH units, 94
HRH workers, 55, 57
HRH workforce, 55, 57, 94
remuneration of HRH, 82
Hypertension, 236, 316

I

Impact of Regulatory Intervention, 109, 152
Inappropriate Variation in Clinical Practice, 109
Incentive Policies, 94
Incentives, 8, 16, 30, 88, 92, 108, 114, 128–129, 132, 137–138, 148, 179, 191, 195, 203, 237, 248, 251, 297–303, 314, 316–322, 324–329, 351, 361, 363, 383, 423
Income Workforce Relationship, 59

Income–Technology Interaction Effect, 205, 214–215
Infection Control Measures, 30
Information Management Systems, 94
Infrastructural Model, 357
Infrastructure and Management, 78
Infrastructure Costs, 370, 395
Infrastructure Quality, 395
Innovation, 24, 73, 107, 109, 112–116, 129, 144, 160, 177
Innovation in Management, 393
Innovative Drugs, 156
Innovative Medicines, 116, 137, 145
In-Patent and Off-Patent Generic Products, 127
In-Patent and Off-Patent Pharmaceutical Products, 129
In-Patent Drugs, 117, 119, 153
In-Patent Originators, 153–154
In-Patient Care, 181
Input-Based Components, 235
Input-Based Contracts, 295
In-Service Training, 81, 92
Institution-Based Private Practice, 37
Insurance Agencies, 21, 31
Insurance Coverage, 14–15, 71, 151, 196, 206, 212–219
Intermediate Outcomes, 279, 283, 291, 301
Internal Process Model, 4
Internal Reference Pricing (*see also* IRP), 131, 142–143, 150, 162, 169
International Migration
International Nonproprietary Name (*see also* INN), 121
International Society for Pharmacoeconomics and Outcomes Research (*see also* ISPOR), 426
Intervention Mechanism, 130, 132
Irish Health Service, 63

J

Job Attributes, 75
Job Demand, 83
Job Security, 72, 83, 87
Job Segregation, 80
Joint Commission International (*see also* JCI), 342
Joint Commission on Accreditation of Healthcare, 7

L

Labor Demand, 55
Labor Force Activity, 75
Labor Productivity, 55, 208
Labor Supply, 55, 64, 81, 83
Lagos Teaching Hospital, 6
Language Barriers, 341
Laundry, 356, 368, 370–371, 387, 396
Lean Model, 25–26
Liberalism, 275
Licensing and Credentialing, 91–92
Life Expectancy, 37, 67–69, 80, 116, 277, 280, 286, 289, 405
Life-Threatening Diseases, 84, 121–122
Living Conditions, 84, 86–87
Local Practices, 83
Locality-Specific Recruitment, 88
Long-Run Average Costs (*see also* LRAC), 119
Long-Term Care, 2, 63, 79, 278, 356, 363, 372
Long-Term Supply, 75
Low- and Middle-Income Countries (*see also* LMICs), 1–10, 15–24, 33–44, 59, 302
Lump-Sum Payment, 358, 366, 373

M

Macroeconomic Efficiency, 107–109, 129, 180
Malaria, 9, 69, 74, 79, 311
Maldistribution, 55, 85, 93–94
Managed-Entry Agreements (*see also* MEA), 424
Management and Supervision Practices, 83

Management of Changing Disease Burdens, 60
Mandatory Retirement, 72
Maputo Central Hospital in Mozambique, 16
Market Authorization, 29, 164, 176
Market Conditions, 3
Market Structure and Characteristics, 19, 32
Market Structure and Competition, 117
Marketing and Communication, 336–337
Marketing Authorization, 109, 120, 122, 161, 172, 175
Maternal Care, 14, 63, 359
Maternal Mortality, 34
Measles, 69
Median Density, 59
Medical Devices, 29, 191, 197–199
Medical Doctors (*see also* MDs), 60, 74
Medical Innovation, 189–193, 195–197, 201, 206–207, 211, 214, 218–220, 222, 224–226, 410, 422,
Medical Interventions, 2, 198, 420
Medical Knowledge, 203, 212, 218–219, 227, 363
Medical Migration, 337
Medical Officers, 57, 73
Medical Practice, 2, 86, 210, 431
Medical Price Inflation, 207–209
Medical Research and Development, 192, 197
Medical Technology, 138, 189, 192–198, 202–207, 209–220, 222–226, 406, 409, 411, 414, 428
Medical Tourism, 333–347
Medical Tourists, 333, 336–339, 342–346
Medicare, 189, 196, 199, 240, 252, 253, 315–317, 413
Medication Innovation, 226
Mental Health Conditions, 69
Mental Health Service Providers, 62
Mental Health Services, 69
Mental Health Workers, 65, 70
Mental Illnesses, 69
Mentoring and Supervision, 87
Meta-Analysis, 12, 83, 158, 319–320
Mexican–United States Border, 336
Microeconomic Efficiency, 107, 109, 156
Micro-Economic Efficiency, 168
Middle-Income Countries, 1, 3–4, 7, 10, 15, 20, 24–25, 28, 33, 36, 37–40, 59–61, 69–70, 83, 85, 206, 211, 215, 282
Midwifery Personnel, 81
Midwives, 56–59, 63, 65
Migration, 55, 63, 75, 85, 88–89, 91–92, 94
Millenium Development Goals (*see also* MDGs), 283
Ministries of Health, 35, 60, 77
Ministry of Health and Social Welfare (*see also* MOHSW), 72
Ministry of Health Hospital, 23
Mobilizing Donor Funds, 72
Monitoring and Planning, 93
Monitoring Costs, 303, 322–323, 326–327
Monopolist, 38, 117–119, 136, 158
Monopolistic Competition, 55, 117–119
Monopoly, 19, 117–120, 127, 129, 158
Moral Hazard, 33, 127, 147, 151, 190, 240, 261, 361, 427
Mortality and Morbidity, 67, 124
Motivation, 84, 87, 254, 295, 318–320, 327, 333, 336, 338–339, 340, 359–360, 365, 371, 373, 405, 408, 410, 412, 429, 431
Multi-Criteria Decision Analysis (*see also* MCDA), 417
Multi-Dimensional Value, 417
Multifactorial Approach, 80

N

National Audit Office (*see also* NAO), 357, 387–390, 392, 394–397
National Health Accounts (*see also* NHA), 205

National Health Insurance Scheme, 15
Natural Disasters, 67
NDM1 Bacteria, 342
Need-Based Demand, 65–66
Negotiations, 130, 136, 139, 148, 156–158, 164, 176–178, 351, 364
Neoclassical Welfarism, 411
Nepotism, 72, 93
Net Benefit (*see also* NB), 410, 421–423, 427
Neurocognitive Changes, 80
Non-Budgetary Revenues, 36
Non-Clinical Service Issues, 397
Non-Clinical Services, 356–357, 368, 396–398
Non-Payers, 32
Non-Pecuniary Incentive, 84
Non-Pecuniary Rewards, 83
Novel Health Technology, 413, 425–426
Nurses, 7, 27, 56–59, 62–67, 72–73, 76, 78–85, 87–90, 208
Nurses' Perception of Quality of Care, 22
Nursing Education in Ghana, 78
Nursing Workforce, 72, 86, 93

O

Obstetric Care, 15, 16, 25, 27
Obstetricians, 27, 63
Occupational Injuries, 80
Optimizing Pharmaceutical Regulation, 109
Optimum Resources, 8
Oral Health Services, 73
Organisation for Economic Cooperation and Development (*see also* OECD)
  OECD countries, 63, 69, 80–82, 99, 108, 132, 168–170, 192, 206, 215, 218, 237, 254, 272, 276, 281, 295, 297–298, 304–309, 317, 327–329
  OECD database, 206, 216
  OECD health system survey, 222
  OECD primary care measurements, 308
  OECD primary care payment flow, 309
  OECD Region, 163
  OECD sample, 215–217, 219, 224–225
  OECD survey, 220, 304–306
Organizational Attributes Salary, 86
Organizational Culture, 7, 300, 398
Orphan Drug Act (*see also* ODA), 120
Orphan Drugs, 120, 139, 145, 163–164, 166, 172
Orphan-Designated Products, 122
Outcome Guarantee (*see also* OG), 146–147
Out-Of-Pocket (*see also* OOP)
  OOP responsibility, 215
  OOP share of spending, 213–215, 221
  out-of-pocket expenditure, 23, 288
  out-of-pocket payments, 16, 32, 312, 343
Outpatient and Inpatient Providers, 16
Outpatient and Inpatient Services, 16, 23
Overconsumption, 190

P

Parallel Trade, 118, 175–177
Partial Analysis, 36
Patent Extension Term in the USA, 117
Patent Protection, 117, 120, 141,
Patent-Protected Molecule Level, 118
Patient Advocacy, 30
Patient Care Supplies and Equipment, 83
Patient Centered Medical Home (*see also* PCMH), 240
Patient Characteristics, 4, 38, 251
Patient Experiences, 336, 338
Patient Groups, 126, 284
Patient Referrals, 384
Patient Representatives, 167, 429
Patient Satisfaction, 4, 12–13, 15, 27, 237, 253, 301, 304, 306, 396
Patient's Needs, 14
Patient-Centeredness, 276

Patients' Expectations, 108
Pay-For-Performance (*see also* P4P)
P4P approach, 296–297
P4P designs, 295
P4P effectiveness, 295, 327
P4P evidence, 327
P4P mechanism, 296–297, 328
P4P policy Issues, 328
P4P programs, 250, 295, 299–304, 306–310, 312, 315, 318, 322–324, 327–329
P4P reward payment models, 304
Payment Schemes, 231, 237, 242, 245, 254
Pediatric Care, 5
Perceptions of Workforce, 66
Percutaneous Transluminal Coronary Angioplasty (*see also* PTCA), 210
Perfect Competition, 119, 261
Performance Indicators, 171–172, 276, 280–281, 285, 355, 376, 380, 383
Performance Targets, 306–307
Performance-Based Management (*see also* PBM), 313
Performance-Based Payment, 82–83
Personal Efficacy, 81
Personal Values of Service, 86
Pharmaceutical Companies, 141, 176, 178, 200, 284
Pharmaceutical Costs, 127, 148, 151–152, 168
Pharmaceutical Expenditure, 108–112, 154–156, 168, 172, 178, 180–181
Pharmaceutical Expenditure Trends, 109
Pharmaceutical Innovation, 116
Pharmaceutical Markets, 107–109, 117–120, 127–128, 130, 152
Pharmaceutical Price Differentials, 152
Pharmaceutical Price Regulation, 114, 137–138, 176
Pharmaceutical Price Regulation Scheme (*see also* PPRS), 114, 137
Pharmaceutical Prices, 127–130, 137, 154
Pharmaceutical R&D, 109, 112–114, 200, 218
Pharmaceutical Spending, 107–110, 137, 168
Pharmaceutical Treatments, 177
Pharmacists, 58, 107, 127–128, 147–148, 150–151, 170, 176
Physical Assets, 353
Physician Training, 61
Physicians, 5, 56–94, 127–128, 132–150, 170–179, 191, 225–263, 297–328, 337, 340, 344, 425, 429
Plan–Do–Study–Act (*see also* PDSA) Cycles, 26
Pneumonia, 9
Policy Architects, 33
Policy Objectives, 107–109, 127, 129, 143, 152, 155, 163, 180, 419
Policymakers, 55, 57, 63, 76, 94, 176, 203, 269, 280, 283, 285, 287, 290, 346–347
Policy-Related Research, 38
Polio, 69
Political Governance, 351
Political Ideology, 374
Political Instability, 89
Political Motives, 374, 393
Poor Staffing, 83
Population Demographics, 67
Portfolio Deals, 132, 147
Post Approval Efficacy Studies (*see also* PAES), 122
Prescribers, 119, 127, 132, 168
Prescription-Only Medicines (*see also* POM), 173
Price Fixing, 129, 136, 158, 180
Price Negotiation, 164, 178, 193
Price Variability, 152
Price–Volume Agreements (*see also* PVAs), 130, 136, 165
Price–Volume Deal, 146
Pricing Regulation, 156
Pricing Strategies, 23, 157, 175
Primary Care Center, 354, 358, 363

Primary Care Physicians, 231, 234, 239–340, 250
Primary Care Providers (*see also* PCPs), 231–232, 270
  choice of PCP, 237
  PCP services, 233, 242, 254–255
  PCP shifts costs, 247
  PCPs act as gatekeepers, 233
  PCPs' role in patients' access to primary care, 233
  supply of PCPs, 239
Primary Care Provision, 20
Primary Care Systems, 33, 233, 237
Primary Care Targets, 306
Primary Health Care, 63, 77, 83, 231, 255
Primary Health Organizations (*see also* PHOs), 313
Principal–Agent Contract, 296
Prioritization, 376, 423
Private Companies, 407
Private Finance, 353, 390
Private Hospitals' Pricing Strategies, 23
Private Insurance for Basic Coverage, 221
Private Wards, 16
Privatization, 62, 94
Privatized Units, 36
Procurement, 141, 160
Productivity of Workers, 66
Professional Advancement, 89
Professional and Educational Organizations, 61
Professional Autonomy, 83
Professional Interests, 86
Professional Network, 87
Project Effectiveness, 392
Project Identification, 376
Project Selection, 376, 400–401
Promotion of Industrial Policy, 107
Provider Surplus Extraction, 322–327
Provincial Government Officials, 36
Psychiatrists, 62, 65, 70
Public and Private Ownership, 21, 32
Public Budgets, 192, 198
Public Expectations, 109
Public Health and Prevention, 56
Public Health Budget, 3, 9
Public Health Facilities, 88
Public Integrated System, 221
Public or Private Ownership Status, 3
Public Payers, 32, 199, 417
Public Recognition, 87, 316
Public Sector Comparator, 360, 369, 391, 396, 398
Public Sector Employment, 88
Public Sector Services, 34
Public Service Commission, 34, 72
Public Service Provision, 33
Public Spending, 60, 192, 196, 374, 380
Public-Policy Traps, 373
Public–Private Mix of Health Care, 93
Public–Private Partnerships (*see also* PPPs)
  economic rationale for PPP, 359
  health care PPPs, 385
  hospital PPPs, 355–356, 388, 393, 399
  non-PPP variants, 359
  PPP contract, 351–355, 357–358, 360–362, 364–370, 372, 375–379, 383–384, 386–388, 392–393, 395–396, 399, 401
  PPP efficiency, 386, 394
  PPP management structure, 357
  PPP penalties, 357
  PPP programs, 357, 368, 388
  PPP projects, 361, 364–365, 374, 376, 388, 400
  PPP schemes, 356
Purchaser–Provider Split, 33
Purchasing Power Parity (*see also* PPP), 59, 207

Q

Quality Adjusted Life Year (*see also* QALY), 154, 210, 332, 422

Quality and Outcomes Framework (*see also* QOF), 159, 260, 322
Quality Improvement (*see also* QI) Models, 36
Quality Improvement Programs, 13, 37
Quality of Care, 16–17, 23, 29, 31–39, 46, 117, 139, 159, 190, 230, 247, 251, 260, 288, 307–310, 314, 319, 323, 336, 371
Quality of Health Care, 78, 251, 272, 309, 317, 340
Quality of Life, 89, 108, 164, 198, 200, 405, 412, 416–417
Quality of Work Life, 83, 95

R

Rate-Of-Return (*see also* ROR) Regulation, 128, 130, 137, 157
Recruitment, 62–63, 72, 78, 84, 87–90, 314
Registered Nurses (*see also* RNs), 208
Regression Residual, 209
Regulatory Bodies, 144, 176
Regulatory Policies, 72, 175
Reimbursement Mechanisms, 161
Reimbursement Methods, 160
Reimbursement Negotiations, 139, 176–177
Reimbursement Schemes, 132, 160
Remuneration, 73, 82, 84, 87, 94, 133, 154, 249, 384
Renegotiation, 151, 357, 364, 370–386, 398
Research Funding Agencies, 430
Research Institutions, 407
Residual Claimants, 36
Resource Allocation, 29, 109, 181, 304, 394, 413
Resource Constraints, 109
Responsiveness, 6, 22, 34, 91, 193, 270, 276, 286
Retention, 69, 72, 79, 84–90
Retirement, 72, 75, 79, 91, 93
Returns-To-Scale, 18
Rewards, 76, 81, 83, 89, 132, 148, 251, 302, 318, 327, 383
Rich–Poor Divide, 23
Risk of Violence, 83
Risk Premium Costs, 322–327
Risk Shifting, 297
Risk-Averse Individuals, 240–241
Risk-Averse Provider, 326
Risk-Avoidance, 393
Risks and Regulation, 341
Risk-Sharing, 180, 425–426
Risk-Sharing Agreements (*see also* RSAs), 132, 142, 145–146
RN4CAST Survey, 22
Routine Travel Patterns, 20
Rural Health Issues, 86
Rural Upbringing, 86
Rural–Urban Distribution, 61, 85
Rwandan Ministry of Health, 78

S

Safety Concerns, 89
Sanitary Conditions, 83–84
Scale Efficiency, 9, 13, 17–19
Schizophrenia, 164
Scope of Practice, 72–73, 86
Scottish Medicines Consortium (*see also* SMC), 166
Sectoral Intervention, 3, 28
Service Provision, 2, 16, 33–34, 241–246, 353–355, 360, 371, 385, 399–400, 415
Service Volumes, 38
SERVQUAL Adaptation, 22
SERVQUAL Instrument, 6
Shirking, 303, 317
Short-Term Fluctuations, 67
Six Sigma Model, 25–26
Skilled Health Professionals, 59, 384
Social Determinants of Health, 60, 279
Social Media, 340
Social Workers, 62
Special Purpose Vehicles (*see also* SPVs), 358, 370
Specialized Providers, 357, 429

Staff Safety, 30
Staff Skill Mix, 83
Staffing Models, 83
Dutch Authorities, 160
Step-Down Costing, 10
Stewardship of Public Health Systems, 60
Strategic Management, 384–385
Structural Quality, 12–13
Sub-Saharan Africa, 3, 29, 60, 73
Sunset Clause, 141
Supply-Side Intervention, 129, 139, 141, 156, 158, 160
Supply-Side Rationing, 262

T

Task Shifting, 83–84, 96
Tax Receipts, 98
Taxation Revenues, 31
Taxonomy of Ethical Concepts, 274
Taxpayers, 200, 274, 321, 382
TECH Research Network, 205
Technical Assistance, 94
Technical Efficiency, 8–17, 108, 180
Technical Innovation, 109, 119
Tendering, 131, 139, 141, 158, 160, 351, 376–377, 398
Thoracic, Vascular, and Cardiac Surgeons, 63
Timeliness, 164, 276
Total Health Expenditure, 82, 110, 151, 281
Total Pharmaceutical Expenditure, 110–112
Township–Village Health Centers, 62
Trade in Health Services, 333–334, 347
Training Programs, 65, 75, 81, 86
Translational Health Economics (*see also* THE), 405, 408
Translational Medicine, 405, 408, 428–433
Translational Value Chain, 410, 426, 429, 431
Transparent Value Framework (*see also* TVF), 139
Trauma Care, 6
Treatment of Grievous Illnesses, 116
Tuberculosis, 5, 67, 69, 79, 302, 311
Tumor, 124, 425
Two-Period Theory Model, 246

U

United Kingdom (*see also* UK)
  National Institute of Health and Care Excellence (*see also* NICE), 412
  Private Finance Initiative (*see also* PFI), 355–356
  UK Department of Health (*see also* DH), 137
  UK patients, 335, 344
  UK physicians, 344
  UK residents, 344
United States (*see also* US)
  US Department Of Health And Human Services, 25–26, 190
  US Emergency Plan for AIDS Relief, 79
  US Global Health Initiative (*see also* GHI), 69
  US Institute of Medicine, 7
Universal Access and Equity, 13
Universal Health Care Insurance, 67
Universal Health Coverage (*see also* UHC), 34, 60, 174, 282
Urban–Rural Disparities, 62
Urban–Rural Imbalances, 85
User Fees, 15, 32, 71, 329, 353–354
Utilitarianism, 275
Utilization and Costs, 425

V

Value Assessment, 131, 137–138, 144, 162, 378
Value of Information (*see also* VOI) Analysis, 421, 427
Value-Based Pricing (*see also* VBP), 138, 416
Value-For-Money (*see also* Vfm), 351, 357, 359–360

Variable Returns to Scale (*see also* VRS), 17
Vertical Product Differentiation, 118–119
Voters, 284

W

Wages, 55–56, 64–66, 72, 75–89, 208–209, 343
Waste Management, 370
Web-Based Forums, 337
Welfare Scrounging, 336
Welfarism, 410–412
Whole-Life Costing, 351, 355, 360–363
Work Designs, 83
Work Environment, 84, 87
Workforce Density, 59
Workforce Management Policies, 88
Workforce Supply, 60, 75, 79, 83–84
Working Conditions, 64–65, 81, 83–86, 89–90
Work–Life Balance, 31, 83
Workplace Violence, 84
World Health Organization (*see also* WHO)
  WHO analysts, 277
  WHO database, 214, 216
  WHO dataset, 212–213, 224
  WHO's health worker migration, 89
  WHO Framework for Planning For Human Resources for Health, 91
  WHO Global Code, 90
  WHO Global Surgical Workforce Database, 60
  WHO Guidelines, 27
  WHO sample, 213–216, 225
World Trade Organizations (*see also* WTO)
  General Agreement on Trade in Services (*see also* GATS), 324

Z

Zambia's National Health Strategic Plan, 93
Zimbabwe's Health Results Based Financing (*see also* ZHRBF) Project, 315

World Scientific Handbook of Global Health Economics and Public Policy

❷ Health Determinants and Outcomes

World Scientific Series in Global Health Economics and Public Policy

ISSN: 2010-2089

Series Editor-in-Chief: Richard M Scheffler
University of California, Berkeley, USA

Published:

Vol. 1 Accountability and Responsibility in Health Care: Issues in Addressing an Emerging Global Challenge
edited by Bruce Rosen, Avi Israeli and Stephen Shortell

Vol. 2 The Economics of Social Capital and Health: A Conceptual and Empirical Roadmap
edited by Sherman Folland and Lorenzo Rocco

Vol. 3 World Scientific Handbook of Global Health Economics and Public Policy
edited by Richard M Scheffler

World Scientific Series in Global Health Economics and Public Policy – Vol. 3

World Scientific Handbook of Global Health Economics and Public Policy

❷ Health Determinants and Outcomes

Edited by

Richard M. Scheffler

University of California, Berkeley, USA

World Scientific

NEW JERSEY • LONDON • SINGAPORE • BEIJING • SHANGHAI • HONG KONG • TAIPEI • CHENNAI • TOKYO

Published by

World Scientific Publishing Co. Pte. Ltd.
5 Toh Tuck Link, Singapore 596224
USA office: 27 Warren Street, Suite 401-402, Hackensack, NJ 07601
UK office: 57 Shelton Street, Covent Garden, London WC2H 9HE

Library of Congress Cataloging-in-Publication Data
Names: Scheffler, Richard M., editor.
Title: World Scientific handbook of global health economics and public policy /
[edited by] Richard M. Scheffler.
Other titles: Handbook of global health economics and public policy
Description: New Jersey : World Scientific, 2016. | Includes bibliographical references and index.
Identifiers: LCCN 2015040481| ISBN 9789814612319 (set : alk. paper) |
ISBN 9789814612340 (v. 1 : alk. paper) | ISBN 9789814612357 (v. 2 : alk. paper) |
ISBN 9789814612364 (v. 3 : alk. paper)
Subjects: | MESH: Economics, Medical. | Delivery of Health Care. | Global Health. |
Health Policy. | Quality of Health Care. | Social Determinants of Health.
Classification: LCC RA410.5 | NLM W 74.1 | DDC 338.4/73621--dc23
LC record available at http://lccn.loc.gov/2015040481

British Library Cataloguing-in-Publication Data
A catalogue record for this book is available from the British Library.

In-house Editors: Herbert Moses/Li Hongyan

Typeset by Stallion Press
Email: enquiries@stallionpress.com

Printed in Singapore

Acknowledgment

Jessica Foster was my editorial assistant and partner. She helped me in every way possible. I am very grateful to her. Kati Phillips made the handbook happen. She handled all the details and coordinated all the moving parts without missing a beat. Finally, I would like to thank Zvi Ruder. He worked hard over a long period of time to convince me that the handbook could be done. He was so right.

—Dr. Richard M. Scheffler

Contents

Acknowledgment v

About the Editor ix

List of Contributors xi

Introduction to Volume 2 xxv
Richard M. Scheffler

Mental Health 1
Martin Knapp and Valentina Iemmi

Aging and Long-Term Care 43
Audrey Laporte and Meghan McMahon

Dental Care 83
Marko Vujicic, Eduardo Bernabé, Daniela Garbin Neumann, Carlos Quiñonez, and Elizabeth Mertz

Personalized Medicine: Economic Evaluation and Evidence 123
Kathryn A. Phillips, Katherine Payne, and Ken Redekop

Social Capital and Health 151
Lorenzo Rocco and Eline Aas

Economics of Tobacco Control and Health 191
Ayda Yurekli, Nigar Nargis, Mark Goodchild, Chonlathan Visaruthvong, Sophia Delipalla, Evan Blecher, Anne-Marie Perucic, Teh-Wei Hu, Anita Lee, and Frank Chaloupka

Health Effects of Alcohol Consumption 285
Catherine Lau and Alex Lau

The Health Impacts of Obesity 355
Franco Sassi, Marion Devaux, and Michele Cecchini

The Economics of Women's Health in Low- and Middle-Income Countries: A Life Cycle Approach 397
Marcella Alsan, Afsan Bhadelia, Patricia Foo, Corinna Haberland, and Felicia Knaul

The Role of Policy Making for Investing in Women's and Children's Health 433
Flavia Bustreo, Jennifer Franz-Vasdeki, Shyama Kuruvilla, Blerta Maliqi, and Rachael Hinton

Behavioral Economics: Health Applications in the US 463
Douglas E. Hough

Behavioral Economics: Health Applications in the UK 489
Adam Oliver

Index 511

About the Editor

Richard M. Scheffler (Editor) Richard M. Scheffler is Distinguished Professor of Health Economics and Public Policy at the School of Public Health and the Goldman School of Public Policy at the University of California, Berkeley and holds the endowed Chair in Healthcare Markets and Consumer Welfare. In 2003 Dr. Scheffler served as the elected president of the International Health Economics Association. He has been a visiting professor at a number of universities including the London School of Economics, Charles University in Prague, at the Department of Economics at the University of Pompeu Fabra in Barcelona and at Carlos III University of Madrid, Spain. Dr. Scheffler has been a visiting scholar at the World Bank, the Rockefeller Foundation in Bellagio, and the Institute of Medicine at the National Academy of Sciences. He has been a consultant for the World Bank, the WHO, and the OECD. Professor Scheffler has been a Fulbright Scholar at Pontifica Universidad Catolica de Chile in Santiago, Chile, and at Charles University, Prague, Czech Republic. He was also awarded the Chair of Excellence Award at the Carlos III University of Madrid in 2013. In 2015 Dr. Scheffler was awarded the Gold Medal for Charles University in Prague for his longstanding and continued support of international scientific and educational collaboration. He earned his PhD in economics with honors at New York University.

List of Contributors

(Author bios are arranged as per the Chapter order)

Martin Knapp is a researcher in the areas of health and social care policy and practice. He has been Professor of Social Policy and Director of the Personal Social Services Research Unit at the London School of Economics and Political Science since 1996. Since 2009, Martin has also been Director of the School for Social Care Research funded by the National Institute of Health Research. Martin's research emphases in recent years have primarily been child and adult mental health, dementia, autism and long-term social care, with much of his work having an economic focus. He has published his research widely, including in more than 500 peer-review articles and 15 books, and his work has impacted policy and practice in the UK and elsewhere.

Valentina Iemmi obtained the title of clinical psychologist at the University of Paris (France) in 2006, graduating in health policy, planning and financing at the LSE and the London School of Hygiene & Tropical Medicine in 2009. Since 2006 she has worked in mental health policy for the WHO Collaborating Centre for Research and Training in Mental Health at the King's College London, the LSE Health, the International Centre for Evidence in Disability at the London School of Hygiene & Tropical Medicine, and the National Institute of Health and Medical Research at the University of Paris V. In 2012 she joined the Personal Social Services Research Unit at the LSE, where her work focuses on economic aspects of policy and practice in the mental health and mental disabilities areas.

Audrey Laporte is Associate Professor of Health Economics in the Institute of Health Policy, Management and Evaluation at the University of Toronto and the Director of the Canadian Centre for Health Economics. For over a decade she has served as Chair of the Canadian Health Economics Study Group annual workshop meetings, the leading national meeting of health economists in the country.

Her work has considered a number of issues related to aging and long-term care including, modeling the impact of informal care networks in the form of social capital on health and health care utilization, the impact of caregiving on the health and labor market experiences of informal care providers, factors that influence the use of formal home based health services and their relation to informal care as well as performance evaluation of institutions within the long-term care sector.

Meghan McMahon is Associate Director with the Canadian Institutes of Health Research's Institute of Health Services and Policy Research. She is completing her PhD in the Institute of Health Policy, Management and Evaluation at the University of Toronto and is a Fellow with the Canadian Centre for Health Economics. Meghan previously worked at the UBC Centre for Health Services and Policy Research and completed an internship with the Organization for Economic Cooperation and Development, both in the area of pharmaceutical policy. Meghan has a MSc in Health Services Research from the University of Toronto.

Marko Vujicic is Chief Economist & Vice Presidents, Health Policy Institute at the American Dental Association, responsible for overseeing all of the Association's policy research activities. Previously, he was Senior Economist with The World Bank in Washington DC, directing the global health workforce policy program. He was also Health Economist with the World Health Organization in Geneva, Switzerland. He is the lead author of the book, *Working in Health*, which examines the effect of fiscal policy on the health workforce. He has worked extensively on broader health policy reform in Africa, East Asia, the Caribbean and Eastern Europe. Dr Vujicic obtained his PhD in Economics from the University of British Columbia and a Bachelor's degree in Business from McGill University in Montreal.

Eduardo Bernabé is Senior Lecturer in Dental Public Health and Programme Director for the Master of Science in Dental Public Health at King's College London. He qualified as a dentist in Peru, where he worked as Associate Professor in Universidad Peruana Cayeatano Heredia until 2006. In 2009, he earned his PhD from University College London. He received the Aubrey Sheiham Award for Distinguished Research in Dental Public Health at the IADR in 2015. His primary research interests are on the social determinants of oral health and measuring the burden of oral diseases on individuals and societies.

Dr Bernabé is the co-lead of the Expert Group on Oral Diseases for the Global Burden of Disease Study and work as Associate Editor for BMC Public Health and Health and Quality of Life Outcomes. He has over hundred publications in prestigious medical journals such as The Lancet, American Journal of Public Health and Rheumatology (Oxford) as well as in the top two dental journals, namely the

Journal of Dental Research and the Journal of Clinical Periodontology. He has developed strong collaborations links with research teams from South and North America, East Asia and Europe.

Daniela Garbin Neumann is a dental public health specialist. She concluded her PhD studies at the Federal University of Santa Catarina, Brazil, and as a visiting graduate student at the Faculty of Dentistry, University of Toronto, she developed a strong project in comparative public policy. Her research area includes comparative studies on dental care systems, and public policies for dental care in Brazil.

Carlos Quiñonez is a dental public health specialist and researcher. He is an Associate Professor and the Director of the Specialty Training Program in Dental Public Health at the Faculty of Dentistry, University of Toronto. His research program centers on the politics and economics of dentistry, with a special focus on issues of equity in oral health and oral health care.

Elizabeth Mertz is an assistant professor at the University of California, San Francisco, School of Dentistry where she conducts research on dental health services, workforce, and policy. She has a joint appointment in the School of Nursing's department of Social and Behavioral Sciences, and is affiliate faculty at UCSF's Healthforce Center, the Center to Address Disparities in Children's Oral Health (CANDO) and the Philip R. Lee Institute for Health Policy Studies.

Dr. Mertz's work covers a broad range of health professions workforce issues, primarily focused on dental care, including supply and demand of providers; health care regulation; state and federal workforce policy; delivery system design and finance; access to care; and evolving professional practice models. She has served on numerous of advisory and planning committees for federal & state agencies, and non-profit and philanthropic organizations. Dr. Mertz holds a BA from the University of Southern California, an MA from the University of Minnesota, and a PhD in Medical Sociology from the University of California, San Francisco.

Kathryn A Phillips is Professor of Health Economics and Health Services Research at the University of California, San Francisco and Founder/Director of the UCSF Center for Translational and Policy Research on Personalized Medicine (TRANSPERS), UCSF Department of Clinical Pharmacy, Philip R. Lee Institute for Health Policy Studies, and Helen Diller Family Comprehensive Cancer Center.

Kathryn focuses on the translation of new technologies into improved patient outcomes, particularly personalized/precision medicine and its impact on clinical care, health economics, and health policy. Kathryn has had continuous funding from the NIH as a Principal Investigator for almost 25 years and has published more than 100 peer-reviewed articles in journals, She serves on the editorial board for seven journals, including *Health Affairs,* two scientific advisory boards for GenomeCanada, and has worked with numerous international organizations in Canada, Australia, Spain, UK, Netherlands, and Luxembourg.

Katherine Payne was awarded a personal chair in health economics at The University of Manchester in August 2010 and is based in the Manchester Centre for Health Economics. Katherine is also a registered pharmacist. She holds honorary positions with: the School of Pharmacy, University of Nottingham; PHG Foundation, Cambridge; Central Manchester University Hospitals NHS Foundation Trust; and Nowgen, Manchester. Katherine has an interest in the economics of genomic technologies and services and the application to stratified medicine using model and trial-based methods of economic evaluation and stated preference methods such as discrete choice experiments. Katherine is a member of a National Institute for Health Research funding panel and has also served on panels for funding organisations in Canada, France, The Netherlands, and Luxembourg.

Ken Redekop is an associate professor at the Institute for Medical Technology Assessment, Erasmus University, Rotterdam, The Netherlands. He is a clinical epidemiologist with more than 20 years of experience in observational research, clinical trial analysis, and medical technology assessment and has co-authored over 150 papers in the healthcare field. Recent studies include preclinical cost-effectiveness analyses of medical devices and tests (including personalized therapy), RCT-based economic evaluations, economic evaluations in the Diagnostics Assessment programme of the National Institute for Health and Clinical Excellence (NICE, UK) and studies to assess the real-world effectiveness and cost-effectiveness of expensive medicines.

Lorenzo Rocco attained a PhD in economics at the University of Toulouse I, France, in 2005 before moving back in Italy, where he currently is an Associate Professor of Economics at the University of Padova. An empirical economist, his fields of research include the socio-economic determinants of health, the influence of health on the labor market outcomes and several aspects of the economics of education. His research has been published by The *Economic Journal*, *Health Economics*, *Journal of Public Economics*, *Public Choice* among others. He has also contributed to several reports commissioned by the World Bank, World Health Organization and The European Commission.

Eline Aas is Associate Professor in Health Economics at the Department of Health Management and Health Economics at the University of Oslo, and has an honorary contract with the University of York. Aas' research is related to inequalities in health, social capital on health, estimation of health care costs and economic evaluation.

Ayda Yurekli is a Visiting Senior Research Scientist at University of Illinois, at Chicago. She holds a PhD in economics (1996) from Cornell University, Ithaca, NY. She has nearly 18 years' experience on the economics of tobacco and taxation issues. During her tenure at World Bank and World Health Organization, she initiated and developed multisectoral collaboration with Ministries of Finance (MoF) and Treasuries of about 65 countries worldwide, and has advised MoFs from over 45 countries on tobacco tax policies and administration. She initiated and developed the WHO TaXSiM simulation model that has been used by many MoFs on developing tax policies. She has been collaborating with a number of researchers internationally on areas of economics of tobacco taxation, including the tax burden on poor smokers, excise tax systems and their impacts on public health, government and manufacturers' interest, global illicit trade and its evolvements.

Nigar Nargis is the Director of Economic and Health Policy Research in American Cancer Society. Prior to this position, she served as an Economist in the Tobacco Control Economics Unit, Department of Prevention of Noncommunicable Diseases in the World Health Organization (WHO), Geneva. She also holds the position of an Assistant Professor at the Department of Economics, University of Dhaka, Bangladesh. She obtained her Bachelor's and Master's degree in Economics from the University of Dhaka, Bangladesh, PhD in Economics from Cornell University, USA, and Post Doctorate in Tobacco Control Economics from the University of Waterloo, Canada with fellowship from the Canadian Institutes of Health Research Strategic Training Program on Tobacco Research. She has widely published and serves as a reviewer in various tobacco control research and development economics journals.

Mark Goodchild is a Senior Economist for the Tobacco Control Economics team within the Prevention of Noncommunicable Diseases department of the World Health Organization, Geneva, Switzerland. Mark's primary role is to provide guidance to Ministries of Finance on how to strengthen their tobacco tax policy and administration systems in order to better achieve revenue and public health objectives. In this capacity, Mark has worked closely with over thirty Member States from across Southeast Asia, the Western Pacific, and Eastern Europe. Mark holds an Honors Degree in International and Applied Economics from Massey University of New Zealand.

Chonlathan Visaruthvong is currently a tax economist in Tobacco Control Economics Unit, Prevention of Noncommunicable Diseases in World Health Organization (WHO). Dr Chonlathan is a secondment from Ministry of Finance

Thailand to work with WHO for one year on global tobacco tax policies. She obtained her Masters Degree and PhD in Economics from the University of Chicago and BA in Economics from Thammasat University, Thailand. She has 15 years' experience in studying and implementing excise tax policy and excise tax administration in tobacco taxation. She has provided technical support international organizations, civil society, and a number of governments, including Laos, Cambodia and Vietnam.

Sophia Delipalla is an Associate Professor at the Department of Balkan, Slavic and Oriental Studies, School of Economics and Regional Studies at the University of Macedonia (Thessaloniki, Greece). She is a graduate from the Economics Department at University of Macedonia (1985), with an MA in Economics (1985) and a PhD in Economics (1994) from the University of Essex. Her research interests are Applied Microeconomics, especially Public Economics and Industrial Economics. As her research on commodity taxation (specific versus ad valorem) in oligopolistic markets applies to tobacco taxation, she worked as a senior economist at the TFI at World Health Organization (Geneva), continuing her collaboration today with the Tobacco Control Economics Team at WHO as a consultant. She is a co-author in the forthcoming NCI Monograph on the Economics of Tobacco Control.

Evan Blecher is a Director and Senior Economist in the Health and Economic Policy Research Program at the American Cancer Society and an Affiliate in the Southern Africa Labor and Development Research Unit at the University of Cape Town. Evan is based in South Africa as a visiting academic at the University of Cape Town. He received his bachelor's degree in Economics and Business Strategy from the University of Cape Town, an MA in Economics with Distinction from the University of the West of England, Bristol and a PhD in Economics from the University of Cape Town. Evan was a member of the expert group for the IARC *Handbook on the Effectiveness of Tax and Price Policies for Tobacco Control* and is a co-author for the forthcoming NCI monograph, *Economics of Tobacco Control*. Evan's research focuses on the economics of tobacco control, particularly in low- and middle-income countries, and covers issues including cigarette affordability, tax and price policy, illicit trade, smoke free areas and advertising bans. His research has been an influence on policy globally, providing expert input to parliamentary committees and international forums in several countries.

Anne-Marie Perucic been working since 2001 with WHO on the economics of tobacco control. She works in the department Prevention of Noncommunicable Diseases in the World Health Organization (WHO) in Geneva, Switzerland. Her work focusses on tobacco taxation and she has been providing technical support since 2009 to a number of countries' Ministry of Finance officials in Africa, Asia, Europe and the Middle East in the revision of their tobacco tax policy. She also provided trainings on tobacco taxation in a number of multi-country workshops aimed at Ministry of Health and Finance officials. Additionally, she has been the focal point for the collection and analysis of global price and tax data that are an integral part of the WHO Reports on the Global Tobacco Epidemic (2009, 2011, 2013 and 2015). Ms Perucic holds an M. Sc. in Economics from the University of Montreal with a focus on econometrics as well as an M. Sc. in Public Health from the London School of Hygiene and Tropical Medicine.

Ms Perucic has also gained a deep knowledge of the international regulatory framework of tobacco control through her close involvement in the development and negotiation of the WHO Framework Convention on Tobacco Control. In addition, she has a good understanding of the United Nations system and inter-agency collaboration working between 2001 and 2013 as the focal point for the activities of the United Nations ad hoc Inter-Agency Task Force on Tobacco Control (now integrated into the United Nations Interagency Task Force on the Prevention and Control of NCDs) chaired by WHO.

Teh-wei Hu is a Professor Emeritus of Health Economics. He has served as Associate Dean and Department Chair in the School of Public Health, and Professor in the Graduate School at the University of California, Berkeley. He was the founding president of the North America Chinese Economics Association and has been appointed by the US Government as a member of the Interagency Committee on Smoking and Health.

He served as a consultant in health care reform and tobacco control to the World Bank, the World Health Organization, and Hong Kong and Taiwan governments and was a senior policy advisor to the Ministry of Health in China. Currently, he serves as the Director for International Tobacco Control Policy Research and Evaluation at the Public Health Institute, Oakland, California. In 2010, he was a recipient of the American Public Health Association's Carl Taube Award for his contribution towards mental health services research.

Anita H Lee is Research Scientist at the Center for International Tobacco Control of the Public Health Institute. She has been involved in tobacco control research, doing health promotion research and intervention studies in various provinces in China as well as tobacco economics research in countries including China, Taiwan, Indonesia and a number of African countries.

Frank J Chaloupka is a Distinguished Professor at the University of Illinois at Chicago, where he has been on the faculty since 1988. He is Director of the UIC

Health Policy Center and Director of the WHO Collaborating Centre on the Economics of Tobacco and Tobacco Control. Dr Chaloupka holds appointments in the College of Liberal Arts and Sciences' Department of Economics and the School of Public Health's Division of Health Policy and Administration. He is a Fellow at the University of Illinois' Institute for Government and Public Affairs, and is a Research Associate in the National Bureau of Economic Research's Health Economics Program and Children's Program. Dr Chaloupka is Co-Director of Bridging the Gap: Research Informing Policy and Practice for Healthy Youth Behavior and Director of BTG's ImpacTeen Project. He is also Co-Director of the International Tobacco Evidence Network. Hundreds of publications and presentations have resulted from Dr Chaloupka's research on the effects of economic, policy, and environmental factors on health behavior, including tobacco use, drinking, drug use, diet, physical activity, and related outcomes.

Catherine R. Lau is Assistant Professor of Economics and Finance at Carthage College in Kenosha, WI. She was a Visiting Professor in the Department of Finance at Western Connecticut State University, and has taught at the University of Shanghai for Science and Technology, for the Taiwan Representative Office of Baruch's Zicklin School of Business Executive Education Program, at Hunter College and Pace University. Prior to turning to academia, Cassie held various positions in financial services firms on Wall Street. She was a Vice President at Credit Lyonnais, a Senior Director at Fitch Ratings, and a Managing Director and Group Head at XL Capital Assurance Inc. She also served as a consultant for Paloma Capital, a hedge fund in Greenwich, Connecticut and as a consultant and credit analyst for Deutsche Bank, AG, in New York. Cassie Lau earned her Ph.D. in economics from the City University of New York Graduate Center in June 2012, and holds an M.Phil. in economics from the City University of New York Graduate Center and an M.B.A. in finance from New York University.

Alex Lau is an adjunct professor in the Business Division at Carthage College. He holds an MBA degree in finance and international business from the Stern School of Business at New York University, and a MA-IR degree in international economics and European studies from the School of Advanced International Studies at Johns Hopkins University. His professional career has been primarily in the world of finance in New York, previously working in commercial banking at Citigroup, management consulting at McKinsey and Company, and as a software engineer specializing in applications for trading desks. He worked at Blackstone Alternative Assets Management of the Blackstone Group, where he managed the Event Driven Fund and the Distressed Fund.

Franco Sassi is a senior health economist at the Organization for Economic Co-operation and Development (OECD). He is Head of OECD's Public Health Programme, aimed at supporting public policies to tackle major chronic diseases and associated risk factors, especially poor nutrition, physical inactivity, alcohol and tobacco use. He is the author of numerous publications on economic aspects of prevention, including the book *Obesity and the Economics of Prevention: Fit not Fat*, in 2010, and editor of *Tackling Harmful Alcohol Use: Economics and Public Health Policy*, 2015. Previously, Franco was a senior lecturer in health policy at the London School of Economics and Political Science, and director of the graduate programme in Health Policy, Planning and Financing. Franco obtained his doctorate in health economics from the University of London. He held an adjunct professor position at the Université de Montréal, as well as visiting positions at a number of universities in the United States, including University of California, Berkeley, Harvard University, University of California, San Francisco, Duke University, and the Catholic University of Rome. He was awarded a 2000–2001 Harkness Fellowship in Health Care Policy by the Commonwealth Fund.

Marion Devaux is a Health Policy Analyst and a statistician at the OECD. Over the past seven years, she has worked on the prevention of chronic diseases and their risk-factors as part of the OECD Public Health Programme. In particular, she contributed to the analysis of trends and disparities of various behavioral risk-factors, the relationship between education and obesity, and the social multiplier effects on the spread of obesity, using population-based survey data. She holds a master's degree in statistics from the French National School for Statistics and Information Analysis and a PhD in health economics from Paris Dauphine University. Before joining the OECD, Marion worked on social health inequalities and on intergenerational transmissions of health inequalities at the Institute for Research and Information in Health Economics.

Michele Cecchini is a health economist/policy analyst in the OECD Health Division, working in the Public Health Programme since 2007. His major research interests include priority setting and programme evaluation in the health sector, in particular with regards to the health and economic assessment of policies influencing non-medical determinants of health as, nutrition, physical activity and alcohol consumption. Michele is an adjunct professor in applied health economics at the School of Public Health of the University of Siena and held a visiting position at the Health Services & Systems Research Centre of the Duke-NUS Graduate Medical School in Singapore. After obtaining a degree in Medicine and Surgery at the University of Genoa, Michele completed his specialist training in Public Health at the University of Siena. He holds a master's degree in Health Policy, Planning and Financing from the London School of Economics and Political Science, and the London School of Hygiene & Tropical Medicine.

Marcella Alsan is a physician-economist and Assistant Professor at the Center for Health Policy and Primary Health Outcomes at Stanford University Medical School, board-certified in both internal medicine and infectious disease. Her research concerns the social determinants of health and wellbeing and the influence of infectious disease on child mortality and human capital formation. She completed her graduate training at Harvard University in Economics (PhD) in 2012, her fellowship in Infectious Diseases at Massachusetts General Hospital in 2013, her MPH and MD in 2005 at Harvard and Loyola University, respectively. She currently is on staff as an infectious disease specialist attending at the Palo Alto Veteran's Administration Hospital and an assistant professor of medicine at Stanford University.

Afsan Bhadelia is a Visiting Scientist within the Global Health Systems Cluster in the Department of Global Health and Population at the Harvard T.H. Chan School of Public Health. She conducts health systems analysis on chronic diseases, particularly cancer. She manages the Lancet Commission on Global Access to Pain Control and Palliative Care and co-coordinates the Commission's Scientific Advisory Committee. She is concurrently a PhD Candidate in the health systems program in the Department of International Health at the Johns Hopkins School of Public Health, focusing on bioethics and health economics. She has held various research roles at the Harvard Global Equity Initiative, including Research Director and Research Associate. She previously coordinated the Global Task Force on Expanded Access to Cancer Care and Control.

She has been selected by the Union for International Cancer Control as a Young Leader in 2015 for her on-going contributions to cancer disparities. She is co-editor of the book "Closing the Cancer Divide," distributed by Harvard University Press. She holds a MS from the Friedman School of Nutrition Science and Policy and a BS in Biology and International Relations from Tufts University, as well as a certificate in Humanitarian Studies from the Humanitarian Studies Initiative.

Patricia Foo is an MD-PhD candidate at Stanford University. Her research focuses on incentives, regulation and organizational structure in US health care. She studies how these factors affect each other and how they affect the cost and delivery of medical care. She completed her doctorate in Economics in 2014 and is currently completing her MD degree (expected 2015) at Stanford University

School of Medicine. She received her BA in Biochemical Sciences from Harvard University in 2005 where she graduated summa cum laude.

Corinna Anke Haberland is a Lecturer in the Department of Health Research & Policy at the Stanford University School of Medicine, as well as an Associate of the Stanford Center for Health Policy/Center for Primary Care and Outcomes Research. She received her BA, with honors, in Human Biology at Stanford, and her MD from the University of California, Davis. She then returned to Stanford for a residency in Pediatrics, followed by an extra year as Chief Resident. It was during this time that she became motivated to pursue policy research to improve healthcare on a broader level for her patients. To this end she completed an AHRQ funded post-doctoral fellowship in health policy, and received her MS in Health Research and Policy from Stanford, in 2004. Her research has focused on investigating and improving access and quality of care for pediatric patients. This has included work on pediatric quality measures, and investigations of the impact of deregionalized care on critically ill neonates and patterns of care for pediatric patients presenting with acute illnesses.

Felicia Marie Knaul is Director of the Miami Institute for the Americas and Professor at the Miller School of Medicine at the University of Miami. Previously, she was Associate Professor at Harvard Medical School and Director of the Harvard Global Equity Initiative (HGEI). She is also Honorary Research Professor of Medical Sciences, National Institute of Public Health of Mexico; and, Senior Economist at the Mexican Health Foundation. As a result of her breast cancer experience, in 2008 Dr. Knaul founded Cáncer de Mama: Tómatelo a Pecho, a Mexico-based non-profit agency. She founded and directs the Global Task Force on Expanded Access to Cancer Care and Control. Dr. Knaul is also Chair of the Pan American Health Organization Task Force on Universal Health Coverage and since 2014, of the Lancet Commission on Global Access to Palliative Care and Pain Control. She was a member and lead author of the Lancet Commission on Women and Health. Dr. Knaul has produced over 170 academic and policy publications. Her research is focused on global health, cancer and especially breast cancer in low-and-middle- income countries, women and health, health systems and reform, health financing, and access to pain control and palliative care.

Dr Flavia Bustreo was appointed Assistant Director-General for Family, Women's and Children's Health on 1 October 2010. At WHO, she served as Deputy Director, then Director, of The Partnership for Maternal, Newborn & Child Health from 2006 to 2010. Dr Bustreo's work has focused on policy development concerning child and maternal health, policy implementation and partnership-building with a wide range of stakeholders. In 2015, she led the development of the United Nations Global Strategy for Women's, Children's and Adolescents' Health. Dr Bustreo has worked in several countries, including assignments for WHO country and regional offices in Bangladesh, Brazil, China, Egypt, India, Morocco, Peru, the Philippines, Senegal, Sudan and Uganda. She has also served at the World Bank and as a special advisor to the Norwegian Prime Minister's Initiative for MDGs 4 & 5. She has published numerous academic and popular articles in the field of public health, women's and children's health. Dr Bustreo earned a degree in medicine with honours and a postgraduate qualification in rehabilitation medicine from Padua University, Italy, and later obtained a M.Sc. in Communicable Disease Epidemiology from the London School of Hygiene and Tropical Medicine.

Jennifer Franz-Vasdeki is a consultant for the Partnership for Maternal Newborn & Child Health (PMNCH). She holds a PhD in Economics and has extensive experience in scientific editing, research and writing on a range of subjects, including environmental health and economics, international public health, agriculture and climate change. Her work has primarily focused on communicating and promoting knowledge related to women's and children's health and how it is impacted by social, economic and environmental factors.

Dr Shyama Kuruvilla is Senior Strategic Adviser, Family, Women's and Children's Health, at the World Health Organization. She has over 18 years' experience working on health policy, programmes and research in several countries. In collaboration with governments, United Nations and other organizations, she was the coordinating author for the Global Strategy for Women's, Children's and Adolescents' Health (2016-2030), aligned with the Sustainable Development Goals. She previously worked in academia at the London School of Hygiene and Tropical Medicine, Cornell University and Boston University, and managed a community health and rehabilitation programme at the Christian Medical College and Hospital, Vellore, India. Her PhD. from the London School of Hygiene and Tropical Medicine focused on international health policy, policy science and political philosophy and these areas continue to be a strong focus in her research and work.

Blerta Maliqi is a Senior Technical Officer in the WHO Department of Maternal, Newborn, Child and Adolescent Health in the areas of policy and strategy development, planning and health systems management. She has over fifteen years of experience in leading development and implementation of large public health programmers related to maternal and child survival, HIV, TB and malaria. Her focus is technical assistance to governments and other stakeholders in development and implementation of national health policies, strategies and systems' response to public health concerns. She has worked in different organizational settings from civil society organizations in Central and Eastern Europe, to global technical agencies and funding organizations. Trained as a medical doctor, she holds a PhD in health systems management development and a Master's Degree in health management, planning and policy.

Rachael Hinton is a Technical Officer for the Partnership for Maternal, Newborn & Child health, focusing on bridging the interface between research and policy and practice for women's, children's and adolescent health and rights. In this role she contributes to a range of activities related to policy analyses and implementation for reproductive, maternal, newborn, child and adolescent health (RMNCAH), including the development of the Multisectoral Policy Compendium for RMNCH. She has been involved in knowledge translation work across a range of regions and sectors including supporting the application of culturally appropriate brief interventions for depression and substance misuse among pregnant women and adolescents in Indigenous settings in Australia. She has a PhD in International Health from Curtin University of Technology, Australia and a Masters in Social Sciences (Anthropology) from the University of Waikato, New Zealand.

Douglas E. Hough, Ph.D., is Associate Scientist and Associate Director of the Master in Healthcare Management program in the Department of Health Policy and Management at the Bloomberg School of Public Health, Johns Hopkins University. He teaches in the areas of health economics and strategic planning. His research interests are in the application of the emerging field of behavioral economics to health care issues and in identifying the optimal size and structure of a physician practice. His book, titled, *Irrationality in Health Care: What Behavioral Economics Reveals about What We Do and Why,* was published by Stanford University Press in 2013. Dr. Hough has been a research economist at the American Medical Association, and a consultant in three health care strategy firms. He is a frequent speaker and author on health care issues. Dr. Hough earned his M.S. and Ph.D. in Economics from the University of Wisconsin, and his B.S. in Economics from MIT.

Adam Oliver is a Reader in Social Policy at the London School of Economics and Political Science (LSE). He co-founded the Health Equity Network, the European Health Policy Group and the journal, *Health Economics, Policy and Law*. He has published widely in the areas of health economics, health policy, behavioural economics, and behavioural public policy.

Introduction to Volume 2: Health Determinants and Outcomes

Richard M. Scheffler
Distinguished Professor of Health Economics and Public Policy
Director of the Global Center for Health Economics and Policy Research
University of California, Berkeley

Chapters 1–5 in this volume deal with five of the major inputs in determining health outcomes — the mental health sector, long-term care, dental care, personalized medicine, and social capital. There has been a dramatic increase in mental health problems around the globe. Depression now has the largest number of DALYs lost globally. Mental health problems are especially complex and move over the life-course, affecting not only individuals and families, but communities as well. Chapter 1, *Mental Health*, details the prevalence, mortality, and disability due to mental health problems and their economic implications. It lays out alternative financing strategies and methodologies of evaluating mental health use and spending.

The global aging of the population is one of the most significant trends and has obvious and important implications for the development of long-term care systems, which will be expanding rapidly in the decades ahead. Chapter 2, *Aging and Long Term Care*, looks at the increased demand for formal and informal caregivers, increased spending, and the impact on patients, families, and the health care system. It concludes with an evidence-based review to improve the efficiency of long-term care services. Like mental health and long-term care, oral health needs to be recognized as an input to the overall health of a population. There is evidence that healthy gums are associated with lower risk of heart disease and diabetes. Clearly, one of the most successful public health interventions was the fluoridation of the water supply. Chapter 3, *Dental Care*, discusses the notion that improved oral health can also be linked to increased earnings. The authors also discuss implications of dental care being financed separately from other types of care, which raises issues of coordination. The authors review barriers to dental care across different countries, and the need to improve delivery of dental care across the world. The dramatic and ever increasing growth of genomic technologies — often called personalized medicine — is a rapidly expanding global phenomenon. It requires the understanding of the impact on the health care system. Chapter 4, *Personalized Medicine: Economic Evaluation and Evidence*, summarizes the existing economic evaluation literature on genomic-based medicine; describes how economic evaluation of genomic-based medicine has emerged into practice using case studies of three countries; and describes challenges in defining and measuring the value of genomic-based medicine and synthesizing costs and benefits for use in economic evaluations. It concludes by discussing key challenges in moving and expanding the development of personalized medicine.

A key social determinant of health is social capital, whose role is receiving increased attention in health economics and public policy. There continues to be a debate about the exact definition of social capital, but for the most part, it includes supporting the trust and networks in communities and between individuals, which allows them to improve their health and the overall functioning of the health care system. Chapter 5, *Social Capital and Health*, reviews the debate on how to measure the impact of social and community networks on health, and provides new empirical estimates between social capital and health in 93 countries. Results suggest benefits in social capital and improved health are stronger in developed rather than developing countries.

Globally, tobacco use is the number one preventable cause of death, and is projected to cause over 1 billion deaths in the 21st century with a major impact being on low- and middle-income countries. Chapter 6, *Economics of Tobacco Control and Health*, looks at the emerging issues of tobacco use and methods to control its growth. It reviews evidence on the reduction and harm caused by tobacco and highlights the most successful public policy intervention — the tobacco tax. The authors describe how this tax is implemented, collected, and its economic impact on the health care sector. Other innovative solutions to control the use and spread of tobacco consumption are also evaluated. Another major health care consideration is alcohol. Alcohol has been consumed throughout history in all cultures, countries, and societies and is a major consumption item throughout the globe. Small or moderate use of alcohol has been shown to have positive impacts on health, but large consumption has the opposite effect on health, mental health, and negative economic activity. Chapter 7, *Health Effects of Alcohol Consumption*, reviews the spending on alcohol around the globe, its economic impact, its impact on the health care system, and the health of the population. Chapter 8, *Obesity*, on the obesity epidemic discusses this phenomenon that has been spreading to all countries at all different income levels. It has been generally due to dietary habits and sedentary ways of life, both of which lead to chronic conditions and premature mortality; 1 out of 5 children are overweight or obese in OECD countries. Obesity leads to increased use of medical care and losses in productivity in the economy. The proper role of government and its intervention is discussed, and policy solutions are evaluated with a clear sense that prevention is one of the most cost-effective methods.

Women's health is a particular challenge at every stage in the life course, especially in LMICs. Unfortunately, discrimination against women still exists, leading to ill health and disability across the life span. Chapter 9, *The Economics of Women's Health in Low- and Middle-Income Countries: A Life Cycle Approach*, looks at impacts in infancy and early childhood, including poor access to health care, nutrition, and education. In adolescence, risks for women include: Gender-based violence, early pregnancy, STDs, and early marriages. Challenges include: Obesity, injury, intimate partner violence, and mental health problems. Women have the burden of disease in old age, reflecting a lack of financial security, neglect, and abuse. Although there are still many problems for women's health, there has been much progress in improving the health of women and children in the last 20 years. Chapter 10, *The Role of Policymaking for Investing in Women's and Children's Health,* looks at specific policies, improvements in women's health, and investments and the impact they have had on women and children and the health care system. Specific examples of investments are examined in LMICs, and their successes and failures are examined in a policy framework.

Behavioral economics (U.S.) is a new and important development in health economics. It is used as a framework, which can better explain the behavior of patients and providers in the health care sector than neoclassical economics. Chapter 11, *Behavioral Economics: Health Applications in the US*, lays out some of the most important and fundamental concepts, such as loss aversion, the endowment effect, framing, the power of default, hyperbolic discounting, and System 1 and System 2 theories of thinking. These new tools and concepts are applied to a variety of decision-making and policy objectives in the U.S. including smoking cessation, weight loss, and substance abuse. Behavioral economics is also important in the UK, which has focused on using nudge policy. Chapter 12, *Behavioral Economics: Health Applications in the UK*, describes what nudge policy is, how it is used in the UK, and its concern that nudge policy may not be optimally used by the government. The chapter lays out an alternative use of behavioral economics and policy that will produce and improve results in the development and implementation of health policy.

Mental Health

Martin Knapp and Valentina Iemmi
London School of Economics and Political Science,
Personal Social Services Research Unit
Houghton Street, London WC2A 2AE, UK

Mental health issues can emerge at any age, with incidence particularly common in childhood and young adulthood. The personal and economic consequences can last the life-course, and spillover into family and wider community impacts. Mental health issues are among the most challenging of all illnesses because of the breadth, durability, and complexity of impact.

We describe prevalence, mortality and disability, and discuss challenges arising in the mental health field, each with economic implications. We report expenditure levels, and we discuss issues that arise in financing mental health interventions. Numerous methodological and practical challenges arise when conducting economic evaluation in the mental health field. We describe how evidence from cost-effectiveness and other analyses contribute to better resource utilization decisions.

Throughout the chapter, we argue how most mental health problems are complicated, and have many negative and often distressing consequences for the individuals who are unwell, their families, and the wider society. This complexity often makes them expensive, and the durability and wide sphere of impact add to the economic consequences. Given the pervasive scarcity of resources, decision-makers must think through the economic case for strategies or treatments that might address mental health needs.

Keywords: Mental Health; Mental Illness; Expenditure; Financing; Economic Evaluation; Policy.

Introduction

Mental health issues can emerge at any age, but are particularly likely to become problematic between childhood and young adulthood. They often have highly significant consequences across much of the life-course, not only for the individual, but also for their family and the wider community. Indeed, mental health issues are among the most challenging of all health problems because of the breadth, durability, and indeed complexity of their impacts.

The effects of poor mental health may start even before life begins: Maternal mental illness during pregnancy or in the immediate period after giving birth can negatively affect a child's later emotional, behavioral, and intellectual development. Emotional and behavioral problems that develop in childhood often continue into adolescence and can lead to difficulties that stretch long into adulthood. Similarly, because the most common age of onset of psychoses such as schizophrenia and bipolar disorder is in late adolescence and early adulthood, the long-term consequences of these usually very serious illnesses can be especially marked over much of adult life because so many key investments and decisions are made in the teenage years that shape future careers, personal relationships, and social roles. But mental health problems can also emerge later in life, as a result of traumatic experiences, major losses such as breavement, stresses in the workplace, strained interpersonal relationships, or economic difficulties such as sudden unemployment or unsecured debt. And one of the most challenging of mental health problems is dementia, which in the vast majority of cases does not develop until old age.

We return to some of these topics later — the breadth and durability of impacts, for example — and also discuss associations that may indicate adverse influences that run in the opposite direction. For example, people with mental health problems are more likely to smoke, be overweight, have disrupted education, be unemployed, take time off work for health reasons, fall into poverty, or find themselves in the criminal justice system. It has been shown repeatedly that major mental disorders are associated with premature mortality, and there is of course the link between some mental illnesses, self-harm and suicide.

In Section "Prevalence, Mortality, Disability" of this chapter, we provide introductory information on mental illness, including prevalence, mortality, and disability. In Section "Challenges Associated with Mental Illness," we discuss a series of challenges that arise in the mental health field: For policy formulation, for health care and related practice, and for research to support decisions in these areas. We discuss a series of 'economic opportunities and challenges'. Between them, they reflect the key characteristics of mental illness: Distressing and disabling symptoms that are often chronic if untreated; high rates of comorbidity with other mental health issues and a range of chronic physical health problems; effects on many aspects of individuals' lives, with consequences for a range of public and private budgets; spillover effects on other people, especially family members but also in the wider community; disrupted employment and work-related difficulties; associations with antisocial behavior, substance misuse and crime; links to self-harm and suicide; widespread stigma; discrimination and victimization; and strong associations with socioeconomic disadvantage and inequalities.

In Section "Expenditure and Financing", we discuss how mental health interventions might be financed. Other chapters in this book have already discussed health financing and we do not attempt comprehensive coverage of the topic; rather, we consider the particular issues that arise in the mental health field. We also describe evidence on levels of expenditure on mental health interventions.

We then turn to economic evaluation in Section "Economic Evaluation for Better Mental Health Policies and Treatment", and the methodological questions and practical tasks that arise in the mental health field, particularly those stemming from the challenges in Section "Challenges Associated with Mental Illness". We discuss how economic arguments can support the case for prevention and treatment by describing how evidence from cost-effectiveness and other analyses contributes to better decisions about resource use. In the final section, we make some concluding comments, highlighting the main public policy themes that emerge from our examination of the mental health area.

Prevalence, Mortality, Disability

Prevalence

Mental health problems can be categorized in a number of ways, but the distinction is often made between common mental disorders and more severe mental disorders. The former include illnesses such as depression, generalized anxiety disorder, panic disorder, obsessive–compulsive disorder, and post-traumatic stress disorder. The prevalence of common mental disorders varies slightly between countries, but is in the range 15–20% of the adult population (Substance Abuse and Mental Health Services Administration, 2013; McManus *et al.*, 2009). So-called severe or serious mental health disorders — although, of course, many people with depression and some anxiety disorders would periodically be experiencing serious impairment and distress — include schizophrenia and bipolar disorder (sometimes still referred to as 'manic depression'). The combined prevalence of these severe mental disorders is between 2% and 3%, although again there can be (small) inter-country differences.

Other conditions included within the set of disorders conventionally seen as mental illnesses are alcohol and drug (substance) abuse, suicide and suicidal ideation. The World Health Organization (WHO) additionally includes epilepsy as a mental disorder for the purposes of its monitoring and advisory activities, although this is not a universally accepted convention and we will not discuss epilepsy further in this chapter. We will also say little about developmental disorders such as intellectual disabilities, although many people with these disorders will have comorbid depression or anxiety, and also a greater likelihood of developing dementia.

The classification of mental illnesses is different in childhood, in part because of the difficulty of making a diagnosis and in part because some disorders tend not to emerge until adolescence or early adulthood. Approximately, 6% of children and young people aged under 18 years have behavioral problems adjudged serious enough to be classified as psychiatric disorders (Green *et al.*, 2005). About 4% of children and young people have emotional disorders, but again it is not always straightforward to decide when the problems experienced are 'serious enough' to warrant psychiatric diagnosis. This is obviously not a trivial matter, since diagnosis can be stigmatizing. But it is often the gateway to treatment, and in some countries may trigger family eligibility for free services or income supplements.

In old age new mental health problems may emerge, in particular, the various conditions grouped under the umbrella term 'dementia', the most common being Alzheimer's Disease. Dementia prevalence has a steep gradient with age: Between 1% and 2% for people aged 65–69 years, but 22% for men and 30% for women for those aged 90 and above (Alzheimer's Disease International, 2008). Dementia is, however, not exclusively a problem of old age, since younger adults can develop this devastating disease, although prevalence is very low before age 60. Much policy and public attention is now being focused on dementia because the world's population is aging rapidly, so that there are considerably more people with dementia today than ever before, and the number globally will almost double by 2030 (Prince *et al.*, 2014). There is currently no cure for any of the dementias. Even though there have been indications recently that the age-specific prevalence rate might be slightly slow (Matthews *et al.*, 2013; Langa, 2015), the total number of people with dementia worldwide will still grow rapidly over coming decades unless a disease-modifying treatment is found.

Disability

The consequences of any health problem can be assessed in a number of ways, most obviously by describing the symptoms, the impacts on an individual's ability to lead a 'normal' life (in terms of independence and employment, for instance), and the associated deterioration in quality of life. Symptoms are illness-specific and this makes it hard to make comparisons or conduct aggregations across different illnesses, and so generic metrics for comparison and aggregation have been suggested for disability, health-related quality of life and cost.

The most recent iteration of global burden of disease calculations — couched in disability terms — has been generated by the *Global Burden of Diseases, Injuries, and Risk Factors Study 2010*, and includes figures for 20 mental and substance use disorders (Whiteford *et al.*, 2013). Figures for each disorder are reported in terms of years of life lost (YLLs) to premature mortality, years lived with disability (YLDs), and disability-adjusted life years (DALYs), which are the sum of YLDs and YLLs. Estimates are adjusted for comorbidity.

Globally in 2010, and aggregated over all mental and substance use disorders, the total impact was 184 million DALYs, equivalent to 7.4% of the total burden of disease (i.e., DALYs for all health problems worldwide). Most of this burden came from YLDs (175 million YLDs) — equivalent to 23% of the overall total, and the leading cause of YLDs worldwide — rather than mortality (9 million YLLs; less than 1% of the overall total). Within the total for mental and substance use disorders, depressive disorders made the single largest contribution (41% of DALYs associated with these disorders). The next largest contributors were: Anxiety disorders (15%), illicit drug use disorders (11%), alcohol use disorders (10%), schizophrenia (7%), bipolar disorder (7%), pervasive developmental disorders (mainly autism, 4%), childhood behavioral disorders (3%), and eating disorders (1%). The burden associated with mental and substance use disorders has grown considerably over time: An increase of 38% between 1990 and 2010, mostly driven by population growth and aging, rather than changes in age-specific prevalence rates (Whiteford *et al.*, 2013). Both total and proportional burdens are expected to continue to grow over coming decades, particularly in low- and middle-income countries (LAMICs).

One of the important conclusions to draw from this work — and from similar work conducted on a smaller scale in individual countries — is that the personal and societal impacts of mental health problems cannot be adequately gauged from their effects on mortality, but need to be understood mainly in terms of their deleterious effects on quality of life (broadly interpreted).

This high disease burden obviously follows from the high prevalence and chronic nature of most mental disorders, given that few can currently be cured. Not surprisingly, there are also high associated costs (as we describe in Section "Multiple Needs and Impacts"). But there are also wide gaps between the underlying prevalence and the rate of diagnosis and treatment, especially in LAMICs. A few years ago, the WHO estimated that the proportion of people with serious mental illness who had received no treatment in the previous 12 months was between 76% and 85% in the LAMICs they looked at (World Health Organization, 2008). But even in high-income countries, the proportion not being treated was generally between 35% and 50%. An initiative led by WHO, with buy-in from international donors and clinical and academic communities — the Mental Health Gap Action Program (mhGAP) — is actively encouraging strategic policy-makers across the world to address this major problem of untreated morbidity.

Challenges Associated with Mental Illness

The inherent characteristics of most mental illnesses — many of which would be seen as quite complicated and challenging — have a range of direct and indirect economic implications.

Enduring impacts

Effective treatment of mental health problems will often considerably reduce or perhaps completely remove symptoms. However, chronicity of the underlying condition remains the usual pattern of illness, and given that incidence is often in the formative years of childhood or adolescence, the adverse consequences will often extend long into adult life. Moreover, as noted above, quite high proportions of people with mental health problems do not have their symptoms recognized or adequately treated. The effects of this neglect could obviously include poor health-related quality of life for those individuals, but also antisocial and criminal behavior and substance misuse (often associated with behavioral problems in childhood and perhaps with psychosis), unemployment, poor workplace experiences (and hence absenteeism and presenteeism), poverty and social exclusion.

Each of these consequences could generate high costs over extended periods. For example, Scott *et al.* (2001) looked at follow-up data on a sample of 28-year-old whose behavioral and emotional needs (and many other characteristics) had been studied at age 10. For this London (UK) sample, conduct disorder in childhood (a psychiatric diagnosis; found for the most antisocial 3% of the children in the study) and conduct problems (found for the next 9%) were predictive of considerably higher service-related costs between ages 10 and 28, particularly costs of criminal justice contacts. Costs for the conduct disorder group were almost 10 times higher than those for the group with no mental health problems. Child and adolescent mental health services in the UK in the early 1970s — when this sample were first studied — were under-developed and under-resourced, and so these huge cost differences in early adulthood probably represent what happens when childhood behavioral problems go untreated.

Another London cohort study, which started collecting data on a group of boys a decade later than the group included in the Scott *et al.* study, also found that conduct problems and hyperactivity at age 6–7 years were associated with high service-related costs (again, especially criminal justice costs) 20 years later, but the difference compared to boys without mental health problems was smaller (D'Amico *et al.*, 2014). Given these time trajectories there is clearly the potential for good and timely treatment to confer positive health and economic benefits over many years too (Beecham, 2014).

Childhood mental health problems also commonly lead to employment difficulties in adulthood. Goodman *et al.* (2011) used birth cohort data for over 17,000 children born in Britain in one week in 1958 to show large effects on earnings, labor supply and other sources of family income by age 50 associated with childhood psychological problems. Adulthood economic cost related to childhood mental disorders was much greater than the cost related to physical illnesses: The impacts of poor mental health appeared to occur earlier in adulthood compared to the poor physical health. Broadly similar findings emerged from another British birth cohort: Conduct disorder, attention deficit hyperactivity disorder, and anxiety problems at age 10 were all associated with worse employment-related outcomes at age 30. But there was one important exception: Boys with conduct disorder in childhood had significantly *higher* earnings than boys without conduct disorder, even after adjusting for all relevant covariates (Knapp *et al.*, 2011a).

A long-term American follow-up study charted the impacts of childhood psychological conditions including depression and substance abuse up to 40 years later using data from the US Panel Study of Income Dynamics (PSID) (Smith and Smith, 2010). The authors followed groups of siblings and their parents in an attempt to adjust for some of the covariates that compromise this kind of research; they also adjusted for physical health in childhood. Childhood psychological problems were strongly predictive of poorer educational accomplishments, worse employment patterns, lower family household income and assets, and a lower probability of being married.

Buescher *et al.* (2014) calculated the annual and lifetime costs of autism spectrum disorders (ASD), covering health care, education, social care, special housing, community services, social security benefits, and lost employment (productivity losses) for individuals with ASD and their families. They compared these costs between the UK and USA, finding that the lifetime cost of supporting someone with an ASD who also has intellectual disability (IQ below 70) was \$2.4 million in the US and £1.5 million (\$2.2 million) in the UK. For someone with an ASD but without intellectual disability (e.g., with Asperger's Syndrome) these lifetime costs were \$1.4 million (US) and £0.92 million (UK; \$1.4 million). The similarities in total costs between the two countries were quite striking, although underlying patterns of service support differ.

As noted earlier, the most common age of onset of psychosis is adolescence or early adulthood, which can therefore seriously disrupt education and post-school training, leading to poor educational outcomes and poor long-term employment prospects. The longer the duration of untreated psychosis the worse the health and other outcomes for individuals, including a higher risk of suicide. One systematic review found a completed suicide rate of about 4% in people with schizophrenia, with most of these events occurring early in the course of the illness (Robinson *et al.*, 2010). Health care systems in some high-income countries have invested in early intervention services designed to provide intensive multifaceted support for young people experiencing a first psychotic episode; these services can reduce suicide rates (Melle *et al.*, 2006). More generally, they can reduce symptomatic relapse and improve vocational recovery and quality of life (Killackey *et al.*, 2008), and can substantially reduce short- and long-term health, social care and other service-related costs (Mihalopoulos *et al.*, 2012).

Comorbidities

Two major comorbidity 'themes' are becoming more widely appreciated in this area. One is the high risk of physical morbidity and premature mortality among people with enduring mental health problems, in part linked to the risks that follow from poor health behaviors. The other is the high rate of psychiatric morbidity in people with long-term physical health conditions such as cancer, coronary heart disease and diabetes. In both cases, the comorbidities might considerably impair health and quality of life — the overall impact often being greater than the sum of the parts — which then complicates treatment and adds significantly to health care costs.

Mental and physical health problems often cluster together in childhood, for instance, leading to higher service-related costs (Guevara *et al.*, 2001; Nelson *et al.*, 2013). People with schizophrenia have above-average rates of physical morbidity (particularly cardiovascular disease and type 2 diabetes) and lower life expectancy: Up to 20 years lower compared with the general population (Chang *et al.*, 2011). Indeed, while public health programs have achieved successes in some high-profile areas over recent decades, the relative disadvantage experienced by people with severe mental health problems appears to have widened: A Swedish study found that while deaths from heart disease had decreased in the general population, they *increased* for people with schizophrenia (Osby *et al.*, 2000). Tobacco use is especially high among people with psychosis (Myles *et al.*, 2012) and is above average for people with most mental illnesses (McManus *et al.*, 2010), with obvious long-term health consequences. Treatments might actually exacerbate the situation: Some antipsychotic medications are known to cause rapid weight gain and metabolic complications (Foley and Morley, 2011).

Depression is frequently associated with poor physical health, with diabetes being very common for example, generating difficulties in terms of self-management of health and increasing the likelihood of absenteeism from work (Das Munshi *et al.*, 2007). A calculation for the US suggested that health care costs for individuals with severe depression and diabetes are almost twice those for people with diabetes alone (Simon *et al.*, 2007). The broader economic consequences are also considerable (Molosankwe *et al.*, 2012). However, 'collaborative care' approaches delivered in primary care settings — antidepressant medications, perhaps psychological therapy, and usually with nurse-led case management — have been shown to improve health and to be cost-effective (Katon *et al.*, 2006; Simon *et al.*, 2007). Comorbidity seems to be the rule rather than the exception, and the area of diabetes and depression is one of the few that has been researched and for which interventions have been developed. More attention is now being paid to innovative forms of liaison psychiatry, and the redesigning of payment mechanisms to encourage better integrated working across specialties.

Naylor *et al.* (2012) conservatively estimated that £1 in every £8 of health care expenditure in England on people with long-term (physical) conditions is linked to their (often untreated) poor mental health. The increase in total health care costs was at least 45% for each person with both a long-term condition and a comorbid mental health problem. This evidence review also pointed to complicated patterns of association with other factors: People with comorbid physical and mental health problems were more likely to be living in deprived areas and to have poorer access to economic, social, and health care resources. Associations with inequalities were particularly marked.

One more example can be offered: The interconnections between HIV and mental illness. Two evidence reviews highlight the prevalence of this comorbidity, and the scale of the challenge in Africa. Breuer *et al.* (2011) show how complex this bidirectional interconnection can be, with reported prevalence rates of mental illness among people living with HIV or AIDS being as high as 19% in one study. Brandt (2009) concluded that 'about half of HIV-infected adults sampled had some form of psychiatric disorder, with depression the most common individual problem,' considerably higher than for equivalent people *not* infected with HIV. Antiretroviral treatment was associated with lower rates of psychiatric morbidity. A cohort study in Malawi found that HIV-infected women do not have higher rates of postpartum depression than uninfected women, but depression was higher among women with an HIV-infected child (Dow *et al.*, 2014).

Multiple needs and impacts

Mental health problems that are unrecognized, poorly managed or unresponsive to treatment can have enduring and considerable impacts across many life domains. In turn, there could be needs for intervention from many service or policy sectors, such as social care, housing, employment, criminal justice, income support, and other systems. Consequently, although the direct health care treatment costs will often be substantial — mental health needs account for more than 10% of total health budgets in many high-income countries, for example — the indirect costs can high too.

We discuss employment-related impacts and criminal justice impacts in the forthcoming subsections, but note here that both make substantial contributions to overall costs for many people with mental health problems.

Partly because of the employment difficulties that many individuals with mental health issues face — either in getting a job in the first place, or keeping it, or being able to work full-time — they would benefit from welfare advice, and many are reliant on social security (welfare) payments. Some are caught in a vicious downward spiral: Their mental health problems damage their employment prospects and plunge them into poverty, the stress of which then exacerbates the underlying symptoms. The combined effects of severe and enduring mental illness and persistent poverty can lead to situations where individuals are socially isolated and not able to access appropriate services. Specialist advice around welfare entitlements, debt management, and community resources can be cost-effective (Pleasance and Balmer, 2007; Knapp *et al.*, 2011b).

Another substantial impact of mental health problems outside the health care sector is in the domain of housing. Social and economic disadvantage can generate housing problems. Homelessness is common for people with schizophrenia and other psychotic disorders (Herman *et al.*, 1998). Again there is a vicious circle of mental health problems leading to economic disadvantage, leading in turn to an inability to keep up rental or mortgage payments, which causes more stress and symptomatic relapse. To take just one illustration, patients discharged from psychiatric inpatient settings may relapse if they are not able to move into sufficiently supportive community environments (Rog *et al.*, 2014). Homelessness is itself socially costly, and providing supported housing is also going to need injection of resources from public or charitable sources. Supported housing programs can be effective in improving quality of life and health (Gilmer *et al.*, 2010) and cost-effective in reducing use of emergency room and outpatient services (Gilmer *et al.*, 2010; Russolillo *et al.*, 2014). These successful interventions involve well-coordinated actions across health, housing and other relevant sectors, including help with managing social security benefits and paying bills.

Indeed, a common theme that emerges from much of the evaluative research on interventions in the mental health field is this need for *coordinated action* across sectors, systems and budgets. This helps to avoid gaps through which individuals with complex needs might fall, thereby reducing the occurrence of distressing and costly crises. But a perennial challenge is 'silo-budgeting', where budget-holders are so focused on protecting their own resources and carefully managing their own spending that they shift costs and dump problems onto other budgets. Silo-budgeting is probably more likely in periods when resources are under particular pressure, such as during macroeconomic recession, and yet that is precisely the time when coordinated action is most needed.

Taking a bird's-eye view of these multiple needs and their consequences, we can see from a number of cost-of-illness and similar studies how non-health care costs can stack up relative to health care costs. Charrier *et al.* (2013) for example, reviewed evidence on the cost of schizophrenia in OECD countries, finding substantial productivity losses, high costs to unpaid family carers, and wide-ranging impacts on other service systems. High non-health care costs associated with schizophrenia have also been documented in countries such as Japan (Sado *et al.*, 2013), China (Zhai *et al.*, 2013), and Thailand (Phanthunane *et al.*, 2012). For bipolar disorder, a systematic review found many studies where the non-health care costs dominated health costs (Kleine-Budde *et al.*, 2014), and this pattern is even more marked when looking at depression (Luppa *et al.*, 2007) and anxiety disorders (Konnopka *et al.*, 2009). Indeed, one English study calculated that 90% of the societal cost of depression was due to unemployment and absenteeism from work (Thomas and Morris, 2003). In childhood, there can be high-cost impacts in the education system: Childhood mental health problems in Britain generated costs for frontline education services twelve times greater than costs for specialty mental health services (Snell *et al.*, 2013).

Looking to the future, calculations by Bloom *et al.* (2011) compared expected costs for mental health problems with those for the four non-communicable diseases focused on by a United Nations High-Level Meeting in 2011 (to widespread surprise, the UN excluded mental illness from its list of non-communicable diseases). Bloom found that total lost output from mental health problems over the following 20 years was (on an annual basis) equivalent to about 5% of global GDP in 2010. This impact was greater than that of cardiovascular diseases, and vastly greater than diabetes, chronic respiratory diseases, and cancer.

Impacts on others

There are numerous 'spillover' or 'external' effects of mental health problems on other people, both contemporaneously and over time. Three areas illustrate well these often wide-ranging impacts: Maternal mental illness during the perinatal period, family impacts in schizophrenia, and consequences for health, time and quality of life for unpaid carers of people with dementia. There are also ways in which actions by external parties can have important benefits for people experiencing mental illness.

Perinatal mental health problems can have deleterious consequences for the newly born children as they develop through childhood and adolescence (and also on the mother's partner and other children). There are high risks that the child will have emotional, behavioral or intellectual problems (Murray and Cooper, 1997; Pawlby *et al.*, 2009; Dean *et al.*, 2010; Velders *et al.*, 2011), and also of intergenerational transmission of socio-economic disadvantage (Johnston *et al.*, 2011). Bauer *et al.* (2015) examined the effects and associated costs of perinatal maternal depression on child development up to 16 years of age from a London cohort study. The additional risks that children exposed to perinatal depression would develop emotional, behavioral or cognitive problems ranged from 5% to 21%, and there was a likelihood of 24% of having special educational needs. Discounting costs back to the time of birth, each child exposed to perinatal depression generated public sector costs of £3,030, reduced earnings of £1,400 and health-related quality of life losses valued at £3,760, after adjusting for other covariates. Interventions designed to recognize and treat mental health problems in women during pregnancy or soon after birth, which might already look encouraging in terms of their impacts on mothers and cost-effective (Morrell *et al.*, 2009), might therefore be *further* justified by reference to effects on their offspring. Thus far, however, these wider effects have not been included in evaluative studies.

As with other mental illnesses, the distressing and disabling experiences of people with schizophrenia can have impacts on family members (Smith *et al.*, 2014). If a psychotic episode leads to violence, which can sometimes happen (see Section "Antisocial Behavior and Crime"), then there could be wider external impacts. Families with a member with schizophrenia may incur direct or indirect costs themselves, such as out-of-pocket payments for services or to transport the person with schizophrenia to treatment, or lost earnings if they give up employment or take time off work to provide support. These are largely hidden costs, but they are of importance if a mental health system is heavily reliant on the unpaid inputs of family and other carers. On the other hand, high levels of 'expressed emotion' within a family — high levels of criticism, hostility, emotional over-involvement, and over-exuberant praise — have been known to exacerbate psychotic symptoms. Family-focused therapy can be quite effective in some cases (Pharoah *et al.*, 2010) and also potentially cost-effective (Knapp *et al.*, 2014).

In the dementia area, reliance on unpaid care inputs from spouses and family members is enormous across every country (Wimo and Prince, 2010). Responsibility for caring can take its toll on the health and wellbeing of unpaid carers, with high rates of depression and anxiety, for example (Mahoney *et al.*, 2005). With the right kinds of support, these 'burdens' can often be lessened, and in ways that are cost-effective. A sample of family carers of people with dementia in the UK were given information on where to get emotional support, and taught (personalized) techniques to improve their understanding and manage the behaviors of the person they cared for, change unhelpful thoughts, promote acceptance, improve communication, plan for the future, relax, and engage in meaningful enjoyable activities.

Compared to standard support arrangements, this intervention significantly improved carer health-related quality of life and mental health over a 24-month period, had no effects (negative or positive) on illness severity, neuropsychiatric symptoms or quality of life for the people with dementia, and was no more than costly (Knapp *et al.*, 2013b; Livingston *et al.*, 2014).

Employment

The OECD compiled an excellent, wide-ranging report on the links between mental health and work (Organisation for Economic Co-Operation and Development, 2012). One of its central messages is that the links between mental illness and employment difficulties are many and complex. People with established disorders face greater risks of unemployment and job insecurity, higher rates of absenteeism and presenteeism, lower earnings, and a greater likelihood of early retirement (Kessler *et al.*, 2008; Kawakami *et al.*, 2012).

Another part of this complex set of interconnections is the modal age for incidence of psychotic illnesses (in late adolescence and early adulthood), which can seriously compromise individuals' abilities to build human capital through education and training, and thereby damage their life-long economic potential. Indeed, across a range of psychiatric diagnoses, individuals with disorders have above-average propensities to leave education early (Organisation for Economic Co-Operation and Development, 2012). Employment is the main source of household income for most people, but also influences social status and roles, fosters social participation, and is a source of self-concept. Long-term employment difficulties increase the risk of unmanageable personal debt and poverty, in turn further worsening mental health (Fitch *et al.*, 2011). For the wider society, employment affects community prosperity and national economic growth.

The links between mental illness and employment become especially difficult when an economy is under pressure. A study that looked at the 27 European Union countries demonstrated that people with mental health problems found it harder to get employment during the global macroeconomic recession of recent years than people without such morbidity. Moreover, the relative disadvantage was significantly greater in countries which displayed higher levels of stigmatizing attitudes towards mental illness (Evans-Lacko *et al.*, 2013).

One response to the danger of a damaging, costly downward spiral linking poor mental health and poor employment experiences and outcomes has been to try to create better employment opportunities for people with a history of mental illness, breaking down discriminatory and attitudinal barriers. There is evidence from many countries that supported employment approaches — intensive skilled support both for employees with mental disorders and their employers in 'open employment' settings — are more effective and cost-effective than traditional approaches centered around 'sheltered workshops'. The best known is Individual Placement and Support (IPS) which helps individuals obtain competitive employment as quickly as possible and then provides on-the-job training and support from employment specialists who are usually integrated into clinical teams, with welfare benefits counselling provided through the transition phase into employment. When implemented properly, IPS is cost-effective compared to traditional vocational support approaches (Bond *et al.*, 2012). The six-country EQOLISE study conducted in Europe, for instance, found both lower costs and better employment outcomes for IPS (Knapp *et al.*, 2013a).

There are characteristics of workplaces that can cause mental health problems to emerge or worsen, such as stress and bullying. Consequently, another response to the employment challenge has been the legislation that clarifies and protects rights to employment and to encourage mental disorders to be viewed in the same way as other conditions and disabilities. Most people with mental health problems want to work and can do so when well, deriving therapeutic as well as economic benefits from it, but can become disillusioned and disengaged if their aspirations are repeatedly dashed.

From the perspective of the employer, there are two big issues. One is that someone with a history of mental illness may be perceived to be less productive than someone without such a background. Many individuals therefore choose not to disclose their health histories when seeking employment (Evans-Lacko and Knapp, 2014). Productivity losses that could result if a key employee takes time off work for short or long periods could be tackled by taking appropriate preventive or ameliorative action in the workplace. While not all risk factors for mental disorders are within an employer's control, some of them undoubtedly are, such as the demands made on employees, the opportunities for them to participate in decision-making, prospects for promotion, workplace harassment, and bullying.

Workplace well-being programs and screening for stress can be highly cost-effective, both for the employer and the broader society (Knapp *et al.*, 2011b; Mills *et al.*, 2007; Wang *et al.*, 2006). Among the measures that employers can take to make it easier for individuals with a history of, or currently experiencing mental health problems to remain in work and to remain productive are adjustments to the workplace, such as flexible scheduling or quieter or less stressful working environments, allowing people to work from home, and training managers in better mental health awareness, whilst also helping employees to build up resilience. A number of these workplace-based interventions have been shown to be cost-effective (Hamberg-van Reenen *et al.*, 2012).

Antisocial behavior and crime

There is a widely held view that people who experience or have a history of mental illness are unpredictable and perhaps violent, a view reinforced by inaccurate and irresponsible reporting in some parts of the media. Thornicroft *et al.* (2013) analyzed newspaper reporting of mental health topics by British newspapers, finding that 14% made explicit reference to people with mental health problems being a danger to others and/or using stigmatizing language.

Although the risks are often exaggerated, it is nevertheless correct that some mental illnesses are associated with a greater likelihood of antisocial behavior or crime. We have already alluded to findings that many children with conduct disorder or displaying antisocial behavior will often — without adequate treatment — become adolescent delinquents and adult criminals (Scott *et al.*, 2001). Substance abuse can trigger acquisitive crime, with high costs for the criminal justice system and victims (Healey *et al.*, 2003). It is also known that, for example, 5% of serious violent crime in England and Wales is committed by individuals under the care of specialist mental health services (Flynn *et al.*, 2014), and that a disproportionate number of homicides in Australia are committed by people experiencing their first florid symptoms of psychosis (Nielssen and Large, 2010). A study in the USA found that the risk of violence was highest among individuals with alcohol disorders (25%) and drug disorders (35%), much more than the risk among people with schizophrenia (13%) (Swanson *et al.*, 1990). Not surprisingly, risks are higher for those individuals who are not adhering to their treatment plans (Swartz *et al.*, 1998). Again, the economic consequences can be large.

Societal responses to these patterns can be both inappropriate and appropriate: Stigmatizing and punishing, or constructively responding to needs by offering evidence-based treatment and support. Epidemiological surveys have shown that high proportions of people in prison have previously unrecognized and therefore untreated mental disorders (Wilper *et al.*, 2009). Poor access to mental health services can propel people in the wrong direction: One US study found that when inpatient psychiatric beds availability fell, there was an increase in the risk of imprisonment for minor charges among people with severe mental health problems, linked particularly to substance abuse (Yoon *et al.*, 2013). Legal powers of compulsory treatment exist in most countries, which may be good so long as they are not abused. The systematic murder of huge numbers of mentally ill people by the authoritarian regimes of Hitler's Germany and Stalin's Russia may be at the extreme end of the abuse spectrum, but there are myriad other examples of mistreatment and denial of basic rights across the whole world (van Voren, 2010).

More appropriate responses include a range of criminal justice liaison and diversion services which identify people with mental health problems who come into contact with criminal justice agencies such as police or courts, and then direct them towards more appropriate mental health services. There are suggestions of effectiveness (Scott *et al.*, 2013), but as yet little economic evidence.

It needs to be emphasized that people with a history of mental health problems have an above-average risk of being the *victims* of crime. The risk of being a victim of violence in the previous 12 months is 3 to 10 times greater for people with severe mental illness compared to the general population (Hughes *et al.*, 2012). Analyses of national data for Sweden showed that people with mental health problems were five times more likely to be the victim of homicide than people without such problems (Crump *et al.*, 2013). Experiencing violence is never good, but the consequences can be magnified for people with pre-existing mental illness. Indeed, people who experience violence — whether in childhood or adulthood — are more likely to develop mental health problems later in life (Green *et al.*, 2010).

Although there are policy and practice issues to be addressed, each with an economic dimension, the key message is this, as summarized by Howard *et al.* (2014) in a recent evidence summary: 'Most people with mental illness are not violent, and most people who are violent are not mentally ill'.

Suicide and self-harm

Self-harm, suicide attempts and successful suicides are all relatively rare but obviously very disturbing events. They are closely linked to mental health problems. They are also strongly associated with socioeconomic deprivation, and with the state of the economy. Many studies have now shown that macroeconomic recession — through its effects on unemployment levels and duration, job insecurity, earnings, unsecured debt and so on — is associated with higher suicide rates. Chang *et al.* (2013) examined data for 54 European and American countries, finding that suicide rates increased significantly after the 2008 global economic crisis, more so for men than women, and more noticeably in countries where the recession was deeper (as measured by job losses). In South Korea, income-related inequalities in depression and suicidal behavior widened enormously over a 10-year period following an earlier economic crisis: Poorer groups fared much less (Hong *et al.*, 2011).

Suicide has many distressing impacts. One less distressing but still pertinent impact is the economic cost, including intangible costs such as the value of lost life, lost productivity (both waged and unwaged), police time, and funerals. The cost of a completed suicide for someone of working age in the UK has been estimated to exceed £1.6 million, for example (Platt *et al.*, 2006). Self-harm and non-fatal suicide attempts can also be costly in terms of emergency and other health care, including long-term psychiatric treatment (Sinclair *et al.*, 2011).

Better identification of people at risk of suicide and better responses to self-harm have been shown to be effective, and there is emerging evidence of cost-effectiveness for interventions such as manual-assisted cognitive behavior therapy (CBT) for adults with a history of recurrent deliberate self-harm (Byford *et al.*, 2003), and suicide-awareness training for GPs and other health professionals, followed by CBT (Knapp *et al.*, 2011b).

Stigma and discrimination

The stigma experienced by many people with schizophrenia and psychosis can affect many aspects of their lives, limiting access to employment and housing, harming social relationships, reducing self-esteem and reducing the likelihood that they seek treatment (Thornicroft, 2006; Lauber and Rossler, 2007). Through its impacts on 'employment, income, public views about resource allocation and health care costs' it can also impose sizeable costs (Sharac *et al.*, 2010).

Evans-Lacko *et al.* (2014) systematically mapped European evidence on stigma and social exclusion experienced by people with mental health problems. Although the body of evidence is modest compared to, say, work on clinical trials of interventions, there is now some wide-ranging and high-quality evidence that documents the stigma, discrimination and social exclusion that is so often experienced. But evidence is sadly lacking on interventions that can reduce stigma and promote social inclusion, and there is also a paucity of evidence on interventions that promote resilience or protect against stigma over the life-course. Social marketing campaigns have been suggested 'as a way to reach the public, to modify health or pro-social behaviors and to promote specific health issues' (Evans-Lacko *et al.*, 2013a). These approaches are potentially highly cost-effective (Evans-Lacko *et al.*, 2013b; McCrone *et al.*, 2010).

Poverty and inequalities

Economic 'difficulties' experienced by individuals — such as unemployment, low income, unsecured debt, housing uncertainty, and social deprivation — have all been linked with incidence or exacerbation of health problems, including mental illness and, as we noted earlier, suicide (Stuckler and Basu, 2013). Again as noted above, there is often a vicious circle at work, since having a mental health problem puts an individual at greater risk of employment difficulties, rent arrears, other debt, and poverty (Patel and Kleinman, 2003; Funk *et al.*, 2012).

This has generated two hypotheses about the underlying associations. The *social causation hypothesis* argues that economic disadvantage such as poverty increases the risk of mental illness by augmenting risk factors — such as financial stress, stigma, social exclusion, and malnutrition — and decreasing protective factors such as education and social capital. Mental health problems may worsen if someone is unable to access good treatment. The *social selection or 'drift' hypothesis* argues that people with mental health problems face higher risks of remaining or falling into poverty because of the costs of their treatment (if they have to pay themselves), lost or disrupted employment, lower productivity when at work, and hence reduced earnings. The former explanation may be more relevant for disorders such as depression and anxiety, while the latter might be more relevant for severe mental disorders such as schizophrenia.

The strong but often complex links between poverty and mental disorder support the case for targeted anti-poverty programs to break into the cycle, such as provision of effective treatment and support services that are accessible to all, resilience-building efforts, investment in education and housing, cash transfer and asset-promotion programs, and enforcement of human rights protection (Funk *et al.*, 2012; Lund *et al.*, 2011).

A related question is the impact of inequalities. There are wide and deep-rooted inequalities in incidence and prevalence in relation to mental health needs. Income-related inequalities in mental health are much greater than in physical health (Mangalore *et al.*, 2007). But there are also wide inequalities in access to treatments (and hence to the therapeutic benefits they generate) even in countries like the UK with tax-funded, universal health care provision (Social Exclusion Unit, 2004). Those inequalities are not only income-related but also linked to race, ethnicity, gender, age, language, religion, and place of residence (Alegria *et al.*, 2010).

Expenditure and Financing

Expenditure

Global expenditure on mental health has been estimated to average US$1.63 per person per year (World Health Organization, 2011). This is the median amount, around which there is enormous variation: Expenditure per capita is more than 200 times higher in high-income countries (US$44.84) than in LAMICs (averaging US$0.20 in low-income, US$0.59 in low-middle-income and US$3.76 in upper-middle-income countries). This wide difference is only partly accounted for by the income level: There are also inter-country differences in total health budgets and the priority attached to mental health within them (Ormel *et al.*, 2008). The percentage of the health budget allocated to mental health averages 2.8% (median) across all WHO countries for which data are available. LAMICs spend lower percentages of the health budget on mental health: The averages are 0.53% in low-income countries, and 5.10% averaged across high-income countries.

These expenditures look especially low when compared with the contribution of mental disorders to global burden of disease (DeSilva *et al.*, 2014), and help to explain the wide gap between prevalence and treatment (see Section "Disability"). There is also the problem that quite high proportions of expenditure committed to mental health are tied up in mental hospitals in LAMICs (73%, compared to 54% in high-income countries) (World Health Organization, 2011). Those hospitals can provide treatment only to a small number of people and often what is provided is of dubious quality (Knapp *et al.*, 2006).

Underinvestment in mental health will have unfavorable consequences not only for the mental health and wellbeing of people with or at risk of developing these disorders, but also for economic development (Funk *et al.*, 2012). A study for the World Economic Forum estimated the global cost of mental health problems to be US$2.5 trillion in 2010 (64% of it occurring in high-income countries), projected to rise to US$6.0 trillion by 2030 (Bloom *et al.*, 2011). Two-thirds of the total was accounted for by indirect costs. In the same study, the cumulative global impact of mental disorders in terms of lost economic output was projected to be US$16.3 trillion over the next 20 years (with just over half this amount in high-income countries), estimated to be equivalent to more than 1% of GDP (World Health Organization, 2013). When compared with other non-communicable diseases, mental ill-health ranked alongside cardiovascular disease in terms of its impact on lost economic output, and was substantially greater than cancer, chronic respiratory diseases, and diabetes.

Financing

Financing health care services is complex, with strategic decision-makers — at national, regional or local levels — having to trade-off affordability, targeting, access, equity and efficiency. For most individuals, their risk of needing health care is highly uncertain, but when they are ill, treatment costs and losses in earnings can be huge. This is why all high-income countries rely heavily on pre-payment financing arrangements — through taxation, social health insurance (SHI) or private voluntary health insurance — in order to pool risks and generally redistribute the benefits of health care towards individuals with greater health needs. If pre-payment arrangements are progressive (with poorer individuals paying lower amounts for equivalent health care), then they are also redistributive in this sense too. Both types of redistribution are important in view of the potentially enormous lifetime costs of mental health treatment and the low socioeconomic status of many people with enduring mental health problems.

The chapter in this volume by Preker *et al.* (Forthcoming) comprehensively covers the principles of health care financing; here we briefly discuss the main advantages and disadvantages of different financing mechanisms specifically in relation to *mental health* care.

Taxation-based financing. Taxes can be levied by one or more different tiers of government; some tax revenues might be hypothecated for specific purposes such as health. Taxation-based financing tends to be progressive, with contributions mandatory and linked to income, thus taking an individual's ability to pay into account. It usually offers universal coverage, which is especially important given that mental illness can leave people socially marginalized and economically disadvantaged: Other financing methods may exclude people from coverage if they are not employed or cannot afford insurance premiums (see below). Means-testing can further support redistributive goals, but co-payments may be barriers to utilization for people who are already perhaps reluctant service users, and can therefore undermine pursuit of equity goals.

Although tax-based financing is mainly associated with high-income countries, it is used to resource mental health care in some LAMICs (e.g., Azerbaijan, Kenya, Kyrgyzstan, Zambia) (Dixon *et al.*, 2006), although these countries may also have high levels of out-of-pocket financing such as user charges and co-payments. Health care funding may fluctuate with the state of the national economy: Many countries hit hardest by the recent global economic recession were further hit by governmental austerity measures (Stuckler and Basu, 2013). In low-income countries, government may not be able to raise sufficient tax revenues to pay for a decent health care system, and — as we have seen — mental health may be a low priority compared to other health needs (Saxena *et al.*, 2007). People with mental health problems may find that, although they are covered *in principle*, access is limited and quality is poor. Unhypothecated taxes have been criticized for not being transparent, public sector bureaucracy may be seen as a source of inefficiency, politicians might be seen to be using health care for political purposes, and patients may feel that a tax-based system offers them limited choice.

The efficiency and equity implications of a tax-based system depend somewhat on how funds are allocated from the central collecting body (such as the finance or health ministry) to population subgroups, localities or facilities. In England, fairly sophisticated resource allocation formulae use weightings to capture variations in need linked to age, gender, ethnicity, and indicators of disadvantage. But such an approach is quite data-heavy, and less sophisticated systems may allocate on the basis of historical expenditure patterns, which is unlikely to be efficient or fair, nor will it incentivize innovation or better responsiveness.

Social health insurance. The main alternative to taxation in high-income countries is SHI. It is the dominant financing mechanism in much of Western Europe (e.g., in Czech Republic, France, Germany, Netherlands, Romania), with revenue collected by quasi-public bodies ('sickness funds'). SHI is also increasingly common in Asia (e.g., China, Japan, Korea, Malaysia, Taiwan), South America (although coverage there tends to be confined to urban areas), and many east European and former Soviet Union states (although other financing mechanisms are also used) (Dixon *et al.*, 2006).

SHI systems differ from country to country, but share some common features: Contributions are usually compulsory for all or most of the population, and they are linked to salaries, with employers typically making contributions. People at high risk of mental health problems do not face higher premiums as they would under private voluntary insurance (see below), although if not in employment they may find themselves excluded. If there is no risk-rating, risk-adjustment mechanisms are often used so that no one sickness fund is unduly disadvantaged by the 'risk profile' of the people it covers. Eligibility for benefits is usually standardized for all enrollees. Transfers are often made from general taxation to sickness funds to provide cover for unemployed, retired and other disadvantaged or vulnerable people. In most low-income countries, only those individuals in formal employment tend to be eligible, indeed some SHI schemes are confined to public sector employees in urban areas. This is problematic given that more severe and enduring mental health problems are associated with low employment rates and low income, with the causal connections working in both directions, as we described in Section "Employment." Another concern is that an emerging SHI system in a low-income country could divert resources away from poorer regions or individuals. A more general issue is moral hazard, shared with tax-based financing, when there is no charge at the point of utilization, because individuals may be tempted to over-use health services.

Private (voluntary) health insurance. Private health insurance (or voluntary insurance, as it is sometimes described) shares advantages with tax-based and SHI in that it pools risks across individuals, and allows those individuals to smooth their expected consumption (Preker *et al.*, Forthcoming). A major disadvantage of private insurance is that, because it is often risk-rated (offering lower premiums to lower-risk individuals) and not mandatory, it may not be affordable for people with mental health problems (leaving them uninsured), and can lead to adverse selection, and 'cream-skimming'. In other words, low-risk individuals move out of a scheme if asked to pay more than they consider reasonable, and if they feel they are cross-subsidizing high-risk individuals (such as those with enduring mental health problems). Meanwhile, insurers may try to encourage low-risk individuals by charging lower premiums and using high charges or other means to exclude other groups, again including those with mental health problems. If an insurance plan exempts existing conditions from the benefit packages — which is common — then individuals with a family history of mental health problems or suspected genetic predisposition to mental illness (such as schizophrenia or early-onset dementia) could find premiums to be prohibitively expensive or simply unavailable. As our understanding and use of gene profiling develops, this could become a bigger and bigger issue.

Private health insurance may be the *only* financing mechanism available to large parts of the population other than out-of-pocket payments (as historically in the US, with mental health cover being very limited) (Frank and Glied, 2006a). The failure of this type of financing to provide adequate cover for people with mental health problems led to the Mental Health Parity and Addiction Equity Act (MHPAEA) and the Patient Protection and Affordable Care Act (ACA), both in 2008, which extended health insurance cover to more people and expanded its scope to include mental health and substance abuse benefits (Frank *et al.*, 2014). Private health insurance may fulfill other roles: As a *substitute for SHI* (e.g., in Germany for higher paid workers), as a *complement to public entitlement* (e.g., in France to cover co-payments within the public health system, or in Chile where it is purchased by higher-income groups) or as a *supplement* (e.g., in Ireland to reduce waiting times and improve choice) (Mossialos and Thomson, 2004).

Evidence from many countries clearly shows that private health insurance is inefficient and inequitable when looked at from the perspective of people with mental health needs (Dixon *et al.*, 2006; Frank and Glied, 2006b; de Menil *et al.*, 2014). It may take heavy regulation, generous subsidies or a tax-based or SHI-based safety net to begin to counter some of these disadvantages (Frank *et al.*, 2014; Parameshvara, 2004). Nevertheless, private health insurance has been advocated by the WHO (2000) as better than what might be the only alternative in many LAMICs, which is out-of-pocket payments. There has also been growth in use of private insurance to pay for specialist treatment (e.g., for addictions), or by employers to treat work-related stress.

Out-of-pocket payments. Individuals using services may face user charges or co-payments, one aim being to discourage excessive or inappropriate utilization (where the marginal opportunity cost of delivery exceeds what is seen as the marginal social benefit of treatment). In some contexts, out-of-pocket payments may be considered to be the only feasible way to generate revenue for a mental health system because of a weak tax base, low rates of formal employment, or the very low priority given to mental illness (as in Nepal and Pakistan) (Dixon *et al.*, 2006). Indeed, out-of-pocket payments account for significant proportions of total expenditure on mental health care in most low-income countries, although they tend not to be the dominant financing mechanism.

However, such out-of-pocket payments may deter people from accessing treatment when they need it, with the consequence in some cases that symptoms worsen to the point where expensive, crisis-driven care is needed (Soumerai *et al.*, 1994). The adverse effects of such deterrence are likely to be especially acute in relation to mental health problems, where individuals might already be reluctant to seek treatment because of stigma, fear, impaired cognition, or lack of insight into the state of their health. The efficiency and distributional implications could be dire, especially as many of those in need of mental health treatment will be the least able to pay (de Menil *et al.*, 2014; Tamblyn *et al.*, 2001). Allowing such individuals to be exempted from charges might be one way to address this problem (Nyonator and Kutzin, 1999), but this will add further bureaucracy to what is often already quite a costly system to administer.

International aid. In high-income countries, pre-payment arrangements (various combinations of taxation, SHI and private health insurance) dominate both health care financing in general, and mental health financing in particular. However, in most low-income countries, mental health care is still most likely to be funded directly by users or families through out-of-pocket payments. Even though international non-governmental organizations (NGO) and foreign governments might provide substantial support sometimes for health systems, international aid of this kind very often excludes mental health care. It is also highly variable and unstable as a platform for long-term planning.

Economic Evaluation for Better Mental Health Policies and Treatment

We have already alluded to economic evaluative evidence in the previous section when discussing the main challenges associated with mental health problems. Here we briefly explain what these evaluations look like, and then discuss some methodological issues that can arise in mental health contexts.

Evaluation questions

The central clinical or effectiveness question when evaluating an intervention (such as a service, medication, preventive strategy or wider policy initiative) is whether it reduces or removes symptoms or improves quality of life. The economic question is then whether the resources needed to deliver the intervention are justified by the outcomes achieved. There are different 'types' of economic evaluation, sharing many common features, but differing in how they define and measure outcomes, because they seek to address slightly different questions. When evaluating an intervention targeted on a particular patient group in comparison to another intervention for the same disorder (such as two antidepressant medications), the most relevant outcomes will be specific to the diagnosis (alleviation of depressive symptoms) as well as some more general indicators (such as quality of life and personal functioning). In this case, a cost-effectiveness analysis would be most appropriate, and this is the most commonly conducted type of health economic evaluation. A *cost-effectiveness analysis* tells decision-makers what course of action (i.e., what treatment) best meets clinical needs given available resources (Petrou and Gray, 2011).

Some decisions in health and other systems raise broader questions; for example, should available resources be used to provide treatment for more people with depression or more people with schizophrenia or coronary heart disease? In this case, measuring depressive symptoms will not be enough, because patients with schizophrenia or coronary heart disease may have not have these symptoms, and even if they do, there are other treatment aims to take into account, such as reducing psychotic symptoms or reducing the risk of coronary events. An evaluation would therefore need a common measure of outcome that would allow the decision-maker to make comparisons across these different clinical fields. Economists have developed a generic outcome measure ('utility'), often operationalized in terms of quality-adjusted life years (QALYs), which we describe further below. Another generic measure, used mainly in LAMIC studies, is the DALY. This form of economic evaluation is often called a *cost–utility analysis*: It tells the (strategic) decision-maker where they are likely to get the biggest impact from their resources by deploying them across a range of clinical areas.

An even broader type of economic evaluation is a *cost–benefit analysis*. It is suitable if a decision-maker needs to choose how to allocate resources across quite diverse areas, such as health care, education or housing. The only currently feasible generic outcome measure in these circumstances is a monetary valuation of what is achieved. Cost–benefit analyses are not easy to undertake in mental health contexts, as it is difficult to calculate the societal value of the health and other outcomes of interventions.

Measuring costs and outcomes

We have already seen that the cost impacts of many mental health problems can range broadly over many services and systems. They can also extend over many years. We have also noted the multidimensional implications of poor mental health, which implies that the evaluation of the effectiveness of an intervention should aim to assess what happens in each of those various domains. The breadth of cost and outcome measurement is driven by what health economists call the *perspective* of the study: Is the evaluation intended to help resource allocation within a particular agency (e.g., a community mental health service), or a particular system (e.g., the health care system), or a particular sector (e.g., government), or the whole society? The breadth of perspective will determine the breadth of both cost measurement and, to some extent, the choice of effectiveness or outcome measures.

Costs can be direct and indirect. Direct costs include those associated with treatment of a disorder (e.g., amounts spent on medications and therapy sessions). Indirect costs include the value of lost productivity because of poor mental health, or the (imputed) cost of unpaid care provided by family members. In the mental health field, as we have seen, the indirect costs can often overshadow direct health care costs.

On the outcome side of an economic evaluation, the approach in mental health contexts is the same as in other areas of health, with the most relevant measures when considering treatments for a given disorder being those that assess changes in symptoms, behavior, functioning, and attitudes, and quality of life. QALYs (utilities) or other generic dimensions can also be added as measures to inform more strategic decision-making such as when setting departmental budgets within a hospital, or taking strategic decisions about which needs to prioritize within a national health care system. There has been debate as to whether QALYs can be measured well enough for some mental health diagnoses (see below), but almost every health economic evaluation today — in Europe at least — would include a QALY measure, alongside symptom or similar 'clinical' measures. The most widely used QALY-generating tool is the EQ-5D (EuroQol Group, 1990).

Both costs and outcomes would ideally be measured over a period of some years, given the chronicity of most mental illnesses and the potential for long-term gains from the most effective interventions. However, as with any evaluation, it often proves infeasible or too expensive — or perhaps even ethically inadvisable — to continue to collect data over long periods from the same individuals.

Making trade-offs

The most difficult challenge in interpreting and using findings from an economic evaluation arises when one intervention is found to be more effective than another but also has higher costs. Which of the two interventions would then be seen to represent the best use of scarce resources? There is no simple answer: It depends what value the decision-maker attaches to the greater effectiveness, i.e., on the trade-off better outcomes and lower costs. This boils down to a value judgment.

Health economic evaluations usually illustrate this trade-off by calculating the incremental cost-effectiveness ratio (ICER), defined as the extra cost associated with a new intervention divided by its additional effectiveness. For example, a study of computerized cognitive behavioral therapy (CCBT) for people with depression or anxiety found it to be better in alleviating symptoms and improving work and social functioning compared to treatment as usual (Proudfoot *et al.*, 2004), but it was also found to be more expensive to the health service (McCrone *et al.*, 2004). The cost of achieving an incremental improvement in depressive symptoms (measured by the Beck Depression Inventory) was found to be £21, equivalent to a cost of £2.50 per depression-free day over the study period. The decision-maker must then take a view as to whether this additional cost is worth paying.

In the same study of CCBT, the cost per QALY was £2190. This ICER value is potentially informative because there is a government-funded (but independently managed) body in England and Wales — the National Institute for Health and Care Excellence (NICE) — that was established to help decision-makers in the tax-funded National Health Service (NHS) to weigh up the trade-offs. NICE produces clinical, public health and social care guidelines built on as much evidence as they can find, synthesized into effectiveness and cost-effectiveness conclusions. In helping providers and purchasers to decide whether better outcomes from a particular treatment are 'worth' the higher costs that may be needed to achieve them, they aim to calculate the cost per QALY and compare it with a (widely discussed) threshold value for cost-effectiveness. Currently, a treatment or other intervention that costs more than £30,000 per QALY would generally not be considered 'worth it' (National Institute for Health and Clinical Excellence, 2008). This is because — according to the approach adopted by NICE on behalf of the NHS — the resources (represented by cost) could be better spent elsewhere in the health care system (i.e., on a different treatment, not necessarily for the same illness). The NICE threshold provides guidance rather than a rigid decision-making rule, with the intention of reminding everyone (clinical professionals, purchasers, patients, taxpayers, and politicians) that resources are scarce, so that choices have to made about how they should be used (Appleby *et al.*, 2007). Some other countries have similar processes to guide allocation decisions (McDaid and Cookson, 2003).

Uses of economic evaluative evidence

Results from economic evaluations have many potential uses. Decision-makers in health and related systems across the world are increasingly turning to economics for evidence to inform, shape and support their decisions. More generally, there are many ways in which economic evaluation and other evidence is used. We offer some brief examples here to illustrate how information on costs and cost-effectiveness evidence is being used.

'Cost-of-illness' studies that add up the direct and indirect costs of a particular mental health problem give *lobbyists and advocacy groups* some economic ammunition to argue the case for more attention and resources to improve prevention, treatment and support. Pharmaceutical, medical devices and other companies might also use similar data to draw attention to what they would argue is a neglected or under-resourced area in order to provide a platform for marketing their wares. Those manufacturers might also invest in cost-effectiveness studies to support the case for their products. Indeed, in some countries there may be formal requirements for them to submit information on cost-effectiveness to regulatory or related bodies. Economic evidence can therefore also be used to help shape the local *commissioning* of treatments.

Economic evidence is increasingly being used in the *formulation and monitoring of policy* by public bodies. For example, the Department of Health in England commissioned a study to examine the economic case for mental health promotion and mental illness prevention (Knapp *et al.*, 2011b). Similarly, the WHO has invested in cost-effectiveness evidence within its Choosing Interventions that are Cost Effective Program, collating information for each of the 17 WHO subregions on the costs, impact on population health and cost-effectiveness of different health interventions (Chisholm *et al.*, 2005).

Some high-income countries have *health technology appraisal* (HTA) mechanisms to formally examine the cost-effectiveness of technologies to inform reimbursement and coverage decisions or develop treatment guidelines. NICE in England and Wales is one such body. In evaluating specific technologies and preparing guidelines for clinical practice, NICE makes copious use of economic evidence.

However, even when there is an economic evidence base, it does not necessarily change policy or practice. There could be a number of barriers in the way (Knapp *et al.*, 2006). One of the most challenging is resource insufficiency: There are not enough funds to invest in interventions found to be most cost-effective, perhaps because — even though they are effective — they require a net increase in spending. Another barrier could be that available services are poorly distributed, available at the wrong place or time relative to needs, such as the tendency for specialist psychiatric services to be concentrated in large cities in many LAMICs. Or available services may be inappropriate, not matching what is needed or what would be chosen by individuals; for example, resources could have been sunk in large institutions, whereas best practice would be seen to be community-based. Silo-budgeting is another implementation barrier.

Evaluative challenges

Making an economic case for an intervention does not mean cutting costs but using resources (not just in the health care system, but across the whole economy) to their best effect: That is, ensuring that resources are used so as to achieve the greatest gains in health and quality of life.

The pervasive characteristics of mental health problems and their consequences discussed in Section "Challenges Associated with Mental Illness" have knock-on implications for the design, conduct, interpretation and utilization of cost-effectiveness and other evaluative evidence. One immediate implication stems from the fact that most mental disorders, although primarily defined as 'health problems', have spillover effects in other domains of life, and therefore other domains of public policy. The costs of responding to the needs of children with emotional and behavioral problems, for example, tend to be higher in the education sector than in the health sector. The long-term costs of not adequately responding to childhood behavioral problems are much higher in the criminal justice system than in the health system. The major economic impact of depression is lost productivity because of disrupted employment, rather than treatment or crisis-response costs from health care interventions.

Moreover, many of those spillover impacts are hidden from view. Lost productivity arising through unemployment or absenteeism may be visible and relatively straightforward to measure, but lost productivity through presenteeism is inherently difficult to quantify. Similarly, unpaid support provided by family members or others to someone with a mental illness is almost by its very nature something that is hidden from view, and yet the responsibilities that go with such support can damage a carer's own health, well being and economic position. Economic evaluations therefore need to be at least cognizant of these wider impacts, and better still to include them as measured elements of a study.

We have also emphasized throughout this chapter that most mental health problems are chronic, and whilst effective treatment may alleviate the symptoms, the underlying condition rarely goes away. Indeed, for some people with particularly complicated circumstances or challenging symptoms, there may be no effective treatment. Interventions are usually judged — if only for pragmatic reasons — by their relatively short-term impacts, whether in terms of effectiveness or cost-effectiveness, whereas the true measure of impact ought generally to be assessed over a much longer period.

A related challenge is what could be called '*diagonal accounting*', where the costs of an intervention need to be compared with impacts (economic or otherwise) that are not only in another sector but in another time period. When budgets are tight, it can be hard to persuade decision-makers to spend more, especially if the pay-offs will not be seen immediately and will not even benefit their own service or sector.

Some of the savings from an intervention — whether diagonal, vertical or horizontal — may not anyway be cashable. For example, an intervention that reduces hospital admissions but does not (either immediately or perhaps ever) close inpatient beds might not generate any savings at all. Similarly, reducing the time burden on unpaid family carers does not generally release any resources that are transferable to other uses.

Many people with mental health needs also have other needs. The complex interplay between physical and mental health conditions can make evaluation quite challenging. A linked challenge is the problem of sample attrition in research, usually much higher in mental health studies than in other health economic evaluations. This attrition problem can arise partly because of comorbidities, partly because of the fluctuating nature of some mental illnesses which leave people unable to continue in a study or to participate at certain time-points, and partly because some people live chaotic lives as a result of their illness.

We have mentioned earlier the insights gained by using QALY measures in economic evaluations, linked to the difficult task facing some strategic decision-makers of making comparisons and allocating resources across disease areas or medical specialties. In Europe and many other regions of the world, almost every health economic evaluation includes a QALY (or DALY) measure nowadays, usually alongside symptom and similar 'clinical' outcome measures. But the most widely used QALY-generating tools, such as the EQ-5D, do not always perform well (from a psychometric standpoint) in studies of people with severe mental health problems, or for the youngest or oldest patients (Mulhern *et al.*, 2014). Specific QALY measures have therefore been developed for some conditions, such as dementia (Mulhern *et al.*, 2013).

Benefit measurement — in the evaluative sense of converting outcomes to monetary magnitudes — is even more challenging. It is intrinsically difficult to convert an indicator of symptom or quality of life improvement into a monetary value. In those rare cases where the primary outcome is something such as productivity improvement — as with evaluations of supported employment schemes — it is potentially possible to convert the effectiveness scores into something that can be *directly* compared with costs (Knapp *et al.*, 2013a).

Public Policy Challenges

Some mental health problems are preventable or the risks of their occurrence can be reduced, such as those stemming from traumatic experience, non- or misdiagnosis. An important public policy theme should therefore be to do better at preventing problems from emerging, but when they do emerge, to identify and treat them early. Moreover, as we have emphasized time and again in this chapter, some of these actions — preventive and ameliorative — are needed outside the health sector as conventionally defined.

Relatedly, therefore, early intervention should be, and commonly is, a core policy theme, with good evidence from a number of different diagnostic areas of the effectiveness and cost-effectiveness of early actions to detect and respond to individual needs and preferences.

Suicide is an especially distressing consequence of poor mental health, even if it is relatively rare. Suicide prevention features quite prominently as an objective of many national mental health plans, and has acquired greater urgency in recent years with the realization that economic recession and macroeconomic responses ('austerity policies') are associated with a significantly higher suicide rate.

The roles played by family members in supporting someone with mental health issues are often hidden from view, yet their unpaid, unheralded inputs can often be fundamental to the achievement of a better quality of life. The effects on family members themselves can be considerable, and so an increasingly visible public policy theme is the need to support family carers through information, funding, respite services or family-focused therapies.

Policy needs to address the wide-ranging and durable impacts of many mental health problems, which in turn should imply better co-ordination of local policy and frontline practice responses to ensure that individuals do not 'fall through the net' or get conflicting advice from different agencies. There also needs to be a willingness among policy-makers to invest for the long-term, notwithstanding the almost universal political reluctance to make such commitments.

Another important policy theme is to address the pervasive stigma experienced by people with mental health problems, and how it manifests itself in discrimination in the workplace, education, social relations, citizenship, and participation. Mental health problems are disabilities, and should therefore be treated in a similar way to physical conditions, but they are also different from those conditions in the extent to which people with them are vilified, ostracized and discriminated against. Mental health problems are associated with economic and social disadvantage, with causal connections potentially flowing in both directions. Consequently, public policy in the area of inequalities should pay particular attention to mental health problems, while public policy in the mental health area should pay particular attention to the risk of social and economic marginalization.

Employment is a key element in all of this, given the social and economic benefits that flow from it. Public policy should engage with the challenges that people with mental health problems face in trying to get a job and keeping it; and also encourage employers to pay attention to the well-being and mental health needs of their workforce. This may require economic incentives, particularly in small- and medium-sized enterprises.

Successful population-wide anti-poverty policies will have benefits for people with mental health problems, but there may also be a need for targeted action that recognizes the particular vulnerabilities of people with long-term morbidity. This is another example of the need to take action across a number of conventional sector boundaries, for instance in housing, education, employment, welfare benefits, and taxation policy. Seeing health — and therefore mental health — as part of an anti-poverty strategy has been emphasized by bodies such as the WHO but has generally not yet taken root in many low- or middle-income countries.

Financing mechanisms for mental health vary enormously across the world, with out-of-pocket payments still dominating in low-income countries, even though these are neither efficient nor equitable. In middle-income and high-income countries, pre-payment mechanisms based on taxation, SHI or private health insurance tend to dominate, but can still have their limitations when looking at mental health needs and treatments. This in part explains the wide gap between prevalence and treatment across most of the world, since mental health interventions are funded to highly varying degrees. 'No health without mental health' has become such a common slogan as to have become clichéd, but it reflects the strong view that mental health needs and services have been neglected for too long, especially in most LAMICs.

Discussions of the economic arguments for mental health interventions should mirror discussions in any other health or indeed other field in terms of relevant criteria and methods. However, some of those methods may not be easily applied in the mental health context, with the result that mental health interventions may face disadvantages in trying to get themselves established.

Concluding Comments

As we have demonstrated, most mental health problems are complicated and can have many negative and often distressing consequences for individuals who are unwell, their families, and the wider society. This complexity can make mental illness appear 'expensive', and the durability and wide sphere of impact of many conditions add to the economic consequences. Given the pervasive scarcity of health care and other resources, decision-makers will want to think through the economic case for strategies or treatments that might address mental health needs.

What we have just written in the above paragraph could probably be applied to many health problems, but mental illness tends to be different. What is distinctive is a *troublesome combination of interconnected challenges*: Onset at a key life-stage; chronicity; absence of a cure; widespread personal shame and public stigma; discrimination in many areas of life; impaired capacity during acute phases of illness; close links to suicide and self-harm; associations with dangerous behavior (even if often exaggerated in the media); and restrictions to individual choice and liberty because of assumed or ascribed incapacity or dangerousness.

These features ought to stimulate searches by all affected parties for effective prevention and early intervention, better treatments that are more widely accessible and better coordination of actions, both across different sectors and over the life-course. Paying attention to the economic consequences is obviously essential.

References

Alegria M, Vallas M, Pumariega AJ. 2010. Racial and ethnic disparities in pediatric mental health. *Child and Adolescent Psychiatric Clinics of North America* 19(4): 759–774.

Alzheimer's Disease International. 2008. *The Prevalence of Dementia Worldwide*. Alzheimer's Disease International, London, United Kingdom.

Appleby J, Devlin N, Parkin D. 2007. NICE's cost-effectiveness threshold. *British Medical Journal* 335(7616): 358–359.

Bauer A, Pawlby S, Plant DT, King D, Pariante CM, Knapp M. 2015. Perinatal depression and child development: Exploring the economic consequences from a South London Cohort. *Psychological Medicine* 45(1): 51–61.

Beecham J. 2014. Annual research review: Child and adolescent mental health interventions: A review of progress in economic studies across different disorders. *Journal of Child Psychology and Psychiatry* 55(6): 714–732.

Bloom DE, Cafiero ET, Jané-Llopis E, Abrahams-Gessel S, Bloom LR, Fathima S, Feigl AB, Gaziano T, Mowafi M, Pandya A, Prettner K, Rosenberg L, Seligman B, Stein AZ, Weinstein C. 2011. *The Global Economic Burden of Noncommunicable Diseases*. World Economic Forum, Geneva, Switzerland.

Bond GR, Drake RE, Becker DR. 2012. Generalizability of the Individual Placement and Support (IPS) model of supported employment outside the US. *World Psychiatry* 11(1): 32–39.

Brandt R. 2009. The mental health of people living with HIV/AIDS in Africa: A systematic review. *African Journal of AIDS Research: AJAR* 8(2): 123–133.

Breuer E, Myer L, Struthers H, Joska JA. 2011. HIV/AIDS and mental health research in sub-Saharan Africa: A systematic review. *African Journal of AIDS Research: AJAR* 10(2): 101–122.

Buescher AV, Cidav Z, Knapp M, Mandell DS. 2014. Costs of autism spectrum disorders in the United Kingdom and the United States. *JAMA Pediatrics* 168(8): 721–728.

Byford S, Knapp M, Greenshields J, Ukoumunne OC, Jones V, Thompson S, Tyrer P, Schmidt U, Davidson K. 2003. Cost-effectiveness of brief cognitive behaviour therapy versus treatment as usual in recurrent deliberate self-harm: A decision-making approach. *Psychological Medicine* 33(6): 977–986.

Chang CK, Hayes RD, Perera G, Broadbent MT, Fernandes AC, Lee WE, Hotopf M, Stewart R. 2011. Life expectancy at birth for people with serious mental illness and other major disorders from a secondary mental health care case register in London. *PLoS One* 6(5): e19590.

Chang SS, Stuckler D, Yip P, Gunnell D. 2013. Impact of 2008 global economic crisis on suicide: Time trend study in 54 countries. *British Medical Journal* 347: f5239.

Charrier N, Chevreul K, Durand-Zaleski I. 2013. The cost of schizophrenia: A literature review. *L'Encéphale* 39(Suppl 1): S49–S56.

Chisholm D, van Ommeren M, Ayuso-Mateos JL, Saxena S. 2005. Cost-effectiveness of clinical interventions for reducing the global burden of bipolar disorder. *The British Journal of Psychiatry* 187(6): 559–567.

Crump C, Sundquist K, Winkleby MA, Sundquist J. 2013. Mental disorders and vulnerability to homicidal death: Swedish nationwide cohort study. *British Medical Journal* 346: f557.

D'Amico F, Knapp M, Beecham J, Sandberg S, Taylor E, Sayal K. 2014. Use of services and associated costs for young adults with childhood hyperactivity/conduct problems: 20-year follow-up. *The British Journal of Psychiatry* 204(6): 441–447.

Das Munshi J, Stewart R, Ismail K, Bebbington PE, Jenkins R, Prince MJ. 2007. Diabetes, common mental disorders, and disability: Findings from the UK National Psychiatric Morbidity Survey. *Psychosomatic Medicine* 69(6): 543–550.

de Menil V, Knapp M, McDaid D, Njenga F. 2014. Service use, charge, and access to mental health care in a private Kenyan inpatient setting: The effects of insurance. *PLoS One* 9(3): e90297.

Dean K, Stevens H, Mortensen PB, Murray RM, Walsh E, Pedersen CB. 2010. Full spectrum of psychiatric outcomes among offspring with parental history of mental disorder. *Archives of General Psychiatry* 67(8): 822–829.

DeSilva M, Samele C, Saxena S, Patel V, Darzi A. 2014. Policy actions to achieve integrated community-based mental health services. *Health Affairs (Millwood)* 33(9): 1595–1602.

Dixon A, McDaid AD, Knapp M, Curran C. 2006. Financing mental health: Equity and efficiency concerns for low and middle income countries. *Health Policy and Planning* 21(3): 171–182.

Dow A, Dube Q, Pence BW, Van Rie A. 2014. Postpartum depression and HIV infection among women in Malawi. *Journal of Acquired Immune Deficiency Syndromes* 65(3): 359–365.

EuroQol Group. 1990. EuroQoL: A new facility for the measurement of health-related quality of life. *Health Policy* 16(3): 199–208.

Evans-Lacko S, Courtin E, Fiorillo A, Knapp M, Luciano M, Park AL, Brunn M, Byford S, Chevreul K, Forsman AK, Gulacsi L, Haro JM, Kennelly B, Knappe S, Lai T, Lasalvia A, Miret M, O'Sullivan C, Obradors-Tarrago C, Rusch N, Sartorius N, Svab V, van Weeghel J, Van Audenhove C, Wahlbeck K, Zlati A, McDaid D, Thornicroft G. 2014. The state of the art in European research on reducing social exclusion and stigma related to mental health: A systematic mapping of the literature. *European Psychiatry* 29(6): 381–389.

Evans-Lacko S, Henderson C, Thornicroft G, McCrone P. 2013b. Economic evaluation of the anti-stigma social marketing campaign in England 2009–2011. *The British Journal of Psychiatry Supplement* 55: s95–s101.

Evans-Lacko S, Knapp M, McCrone P, Thornicroft G, Mojtabai R. 2013. The mental health consequences of the recession: Economic hardship and employment of people with mental health problems in 27 European countries. *PLoS One* 8(7): E69792.

Evans-Lacko S, Knapp M. 2014. Importance of social and cultural factors for attitudes, disclosure and time off work for depression: Findings from a seven country European study on depression in the workplace. *PLoS One* 9(3): e91053.

Evans-Lacko S, Malcolm E, West K, Rose D, London J, Rusch N, Little K, Henderson C, Thornicroft G. 2013a. Influence of time to change's social marketing interventions on stigma in England 2009–2011. *The British Journal of Psychiatry Supplement* 55: s77–s88.

Fitch C, Hamilton S, Bassett P, Davey R. 2011. The relationship between personal debt and mental health: A systematic review. *Mental Health Review Journal* 16(4): 153–166.

Flynn S, Rodway C, Appleby L, Shaw J. 2014. Serious violence by people with mental illness: National Clinical Survey. *Journal of Interpersonal Violence* 29(8): 1438–1458.

Foley DL, Morley KI. 2011. Systematic review of early cardiometabolic outcomes of the first treated episode of psychosis, *Archives of General Psychiatry* 68(6): 609–616.

Frank RG, Beronio K, Glied SA. 2014. Behavioral health parity and the affordable care act. *Journal of Social Work in Disability & Rehabilitation* 13(1–2): 31–43.

Frank RG, Glied S. 2006a. Changes in mental health financing since 1971: Implications for policymakers and patients. *Health Affairs (Millwood)* 25(3): 601–613.

Frank RG, Glied S. 2006b. *Better but Not Well: US Mental Health Policy Since 1950*. Johns Hopkins University Press, Baltimore, United States.

Funk M, Drew N, Knapp M. 2012. Mental health, poverty and development. *Journal of Public Mental Health* 11(4): 166–185.

Gilmer TP, Stefancic A, Etter S. 2010. Effect of full-service partnership on homelessness, use and costs of mental health services, and quality of life among adults with serious mental illness. *Archives of General Psychiatry* 66(6): 645–652.

Goodman A, Joyce R, Smith JP. 2011. The long shadow cast by childhood physical and mental problems on adult life. *Proceedings of the National Academy of Sciences of the United States of America* 108(15): 6032–6037.

Green H, McGinnity A, Meltzer H, Ford T, Goodman R. 2005. *Mental Health of Children and Young People in Great Britain, 2004. A Survey Carried Out by the Office for National Statistics on Behalf of the Department of Health and the Scottish Executive.* Palgrave Macmillan, Basingstoke, United Kingdom.

Green JG, McLaughlin KA, Berglund PA, Gruber MJ, Sampson NA, Zaslavsky AM, Kessler RC. 2010. Childhood adversities and adult psychiatric disorders in the national comorbidity survey replication I: Associations with first onset of DSM-IV disorders. *Archives of General Psychiatry* 67(2): 113–123.

Guevara J, Lozano P, Wickizer T, Mell L, Gephart H. 2001. Utilization and cost of health care services for children with attention-deficit/hyperactivity disorder. *Pediatrics* 108(1): 71–78.

Hamberg-van Reenen HH, Proper KI, van den Berg MM. 2012. Worksite mental health interventions: A systematic review of economic evaluations. *Occupational and Environmental Medicine* 69(11): 837–845.

Healey A, Knapp M, Marsden J, Gossop M, Stewart D. 2003. Criminal outcomes and costs of treatment services for injecting and non-injecting heroin users: Evidence from a national prospective cohort survey. *Journal of Health Services Research & Policy* 8(3): 134–141.

Herman DB, Susser ES, Jandorf L, Lavelle J, Bromet EJ. 1998. Homelessness among individuals with psychotic disorders hospitalised for the first time: Findings from the Suffolk County Mental Health Project. *The American Journal of Psychiatry* 155(1): 109–113.

Hong J, Knapp M, McGuire A. 2011. Income-related inequalities in the prevalence of depression and suicidal behaviour: A 10-year trend following economic crisis. *World Psychiatry* 10(1): 40–44.

Howard LM, Shaw J, Oram S, Khalifeh H, Flynn S. 2014. In *Violence and Mental Health*, Davies SC (ed.). *Annual Report of the Chief Medical Officer 2013. Public Mental Health Priorities: Investing in the Evidence*. Department of Health, London, United Kingdom, pp. 227–238.

Hughes K, Bellis MA, Jones L, Wood S, Bates G, Eckley L, McCoy E, Mikton C, Shakespeare T, Officer A. 2012. Prevalence and risk of violence against adults with disabilities: A systematic review and meta-analysis of observational studies. *Lancet* 379(9826): 1621–1629.

Johnston DW, Propper C, Pudney S, Shields MA. 2011. *Child Mental Health and Educational Attainment: Multiple Observers and the Measurement Error Problem*. Institute for the Study of Labor (IZA), Bonn, Germany.

Katon W, Unutzer J, Fan MY, Williams Jr. JW, Schoenbaum M, Lin EH, Hunkeler EM. 2006. Cost-effectiveness and net benefit of enhanced treatment of depression for older adults with diabetes and depression. *Diabetes Care* 29(2): 265–270.

Kawakami N, Abdulghani EA, Alonso J, Bromet EJ, Bruffaerts R, Caldas-de-Almeida JM, Chiu WT, de Girolamo G, de Graaf R, Fayyad J, Ferry F, Florescu S, Gureje O, Hu C, Lakoma MD, Leblanc W, Lee S, Levinson D, Malhotra S, Matschinger H, Medina-Mora ME, Nakamura Y, Oakley Browne MA, Okoliyski M, Posada-Villa J, Sampson NA, Viana MC, Kessler RC. 2012. Early-life mental disorders and adult household income in the World mental health surveys. *Biological Psychiatry* 72(3): 228–237.

Kessler RC, Heeringa S, Lakoma MD, Petukhova M, Rupp AE, Schoenbaum M, Wang PS, Zaslavsky AM. 2008. Individual and societal effects of mental disorders on earnings in the United States: Results from the national comorbidity survey replication. *The American Journal of Psychiatry* 165(6): 703–711.

Killackey E, Jackson HJ, McGorry PD. 2008. Vocational intervention in first-episode psychosis: Individual placement and support v. treatment as usual. *The British Journal of Psychiatry* 193(2): 114–120.

Kleine-Budde K, Touil E, Moock J, Bramesfeld A, Kawohl W, Rossler W. 2014. Cost of illness for bipolar disorder: A systematic review of the economic burden. *Bipolar Disorders* 16(4): 337–353.

Knapp M, Andrew A, McDaid D, Iemmi V, McCrone P, Park A, Parsonage M, Boardman J, Shepherd G. 2014. *Investing in Recovery. Making the Business Case for Effective Interventions for People with Schizophrenia and Psychosis*. Rethink Mental Illness, London, United Kingdom.

Knapp M, Funk M, Curran C, Prince M, Grigg M, McDaid D. 2006. Economic barriers to better mental health practice and policy. *Health Policy and Planning* 21(3): 157–170.

Knapp M, King D, Healey A, Thomas C. 2011a. Economic outcomes in adulthood and their associations with antisocial conduct, attention deficit and anxiety problems in childhood. *The Journal of Mental Health Policy and Economics* 14(3): 137–147.

Knapp M, McDaid D, Parsonage M (eds.). 2011b. *Mental Health Promotion and Mental Illness Prevention: The Economic Case*. Department of Health, London, United Kingdom.

Knapp M, Patel A, Curran C, Latimer E, Catty J, Becker T, Drake RE, Fioritti A, Kilian R, Lauber C, Rossler W, Tomov T, van Busschbach J, Comas-Herrera A, White S, Wiersma D, Burns T. 2013a. Supported employment: Cost-effectiveness across six European sites. *World Psychiatry* 12(1): 60–68.

Knapp M, King D, Romeo R, Schehl B, Barber J, Griffin M, Rapaport P, Livingston D, Mummery C, Walker Z, Hoe J, Sampson EL, Cooper C, Livingston G. 2013b. Cost effectiveness of a manual based coping strategy programme in promoting the mental health of family carers of people with dementia (the START (STrAtegies for RelaTives) study): A pragmatic randomised controlled trial. *British Medical Journal* 347: f6342.

Konnopka A, Leichsenring F, Leibing E, Konig HH. 2009. Cost-of-illness studies and cost-effectiveness analyses in anxiety disorders: A systematic review. *Journal of Affective Disorders* 114(1–3): 14–31.

Langa KM. 2015. Is the risk of Alzheimer's disease and dementia declining? *Alzheimers Research and Theraphy* 7(1): 34.

Lauber C, Rossler W. 2007. Stigma towards people with mental illness in developing countries in Asia. *International Review of Psychiatry* 19(2): 157–178.

Livingston G, Barber J, Rapaport P, Knapp M, Griffin M, King D, Romeo R, Livingston D, Mummery C, Walker Z, Hoe J, Cooper C. 2014. Long-term clinical and cost-effectiveness of psychological intervention for family carers of people with dementia: A single-blind, randomised, controlled trial. *Lancet Psychiatry* 1(7): 537–548.

Lund C, De Silva M, Plagerson S, Cooper S, Chisholm D, Das J, Knapp M, Patel V. 2011. Poverty and mental disorders: Breaking the cycle in low-income and middle-income countries. *Lancet* 378(9801): 1502–1514.

Luppa M, Heinrich S, Angermeyer M, Konig HH, Riedel-Heller S. 2007. Cost-of-illness studies of depression: A systematic review. *Journal of Affective Disorders* 98(1–2): 29–43.

Mahoney R, Regan C, Katona C, Livingston G. 2005. Anxiety and depression in family caregivers of people with Alzheimer disease: The LASER-AD study. *The American Journal of Geriatric Psychiatry* 13(9): 795–801.

Mangalore R, Knapp M, Jenkins R. 2007. Income-related inequality in mental health in Britain: The concentration index approach. *Psychological Medicine* 37(7): 1037–1045.

Matthews FE, Arthur A, Barnes LE, Bond J, Jagger C, Robinson L, Brayne C. 2013. A two-decade comparison of prevalence of dementia in individuals aged 65 years and older from three geographical areas of England: Results of the Cognitive Function and Ageing Study I and II. *Lancet* 382(9902): 1405–1412.

McCrone P, Knapp M, Henri M, McDaid D. 2010. The economic impact of initiatives to reduce stigma: Demonstration of a modelling approach. *Epidemiologia e Psichiatria Sociale* 19(2): 131–139.

McCrone P, Knapp M, Proudfoot J, Ryden C, Cavanagh K, Shapiro DA, Ilson S, Gray JA, Goldberg D, Mann A, Marks I, Everitt B, Tylee A. 2004. Cost-effectiveness of computerised cognitive behavioural therapy for anxiety and depression in primary care: Randomised controlled trial. *The British Journal of Psychiatry* 185: 55–62.

McDaid D, Cookson R. 2003. Evaluating health care interventions in the European Union. *Health Policy* 63(2): 133–139.

McManus S, Meltzer H, Brugha T, Bebbington P, Jenkins R. 2009. *Adult Psychiatric Morbidity in England, 2007*. National Centre for Social Research, London, United Kingdom.

McManus S, Meltzer H, Campion J. 2010. *Cigarette Smoking and Mental Health in England. Data from the Adult Psychiatric Morbidity Survey*. National Centre for Social Research, London, United Kingdom.

Melle I, Johannesen JO, Friis S, Haahr U, Joa I, Larsen TK, Opjordsmoen S, Rund BR, Simonsen E, Vaglum P, McGlashan T. 2006. Early detection of the first episode of schizophrenia and suicidal behavior. *The American Journal of Psychiatry* 163(5): 800–804.

Mihalopoulos C, McCrone P, Knapp M, Johannessen JO, Malla A, McGorry P. 2012. The costs of early intervention in psychosis: Restoring the balance. *The Australian and New Zealand Journal of Psychiatry* 46(9): 808–811.

Mills P, Kessler R, Cooper J, Sullivan S. 2007. Impact of a health promotion program on employee health risks and work productivity. *American Journal of Health Promotion: AJHP* 22(1): 45–53.

Molosankwe I, Patel A, Jose J Gagliardino, Knapp M, McDaid D. 2012. Economic aspects of the association between diabetes and depression: A systematic review. *Journal of Affective Disorders* 142(Suppl): S42–S55.

Morrell CJ, Warner R, Slade P, Dixon S, Walters S, Paley G, Brugha T. 2009. Psychological interventions for postnatal depression: Cluster randomised trial and economic evaluation: The PoNDER trial. *Health Technology Assessment* 13(30): iii–iv, x–xiii, 1–153.

Mossialos E, Thomson S. 2004. *Voluntary Health Insurance in the European Union*. European Observatory on Health Systems and Policies, Brussels, Belgium.

Mulhern B, Mukuria C, Barkham M, Knapp M, Byford S, Brazier J. 2014. Using generic preference based measures in mental health: The psychometric performance of EQ-5D and SF-6D. *The British Journal of Psychiatry* 205(3): 236–243.

Mulhern B, Rowen D, Brazier J, Smith S, Romeo R, Tait R, Watchurst C, Chua KC, Loftus V, Young T, Lamping D, Knapp M, Howard R, Banerjee S. 2013. Development of DEMQOL-U and DEMQOL-PROXY-U: Generation of preference-based indices from DEMQOL and DEMQOL-PROXY for use in economic evaluation. *Health Technology Assessment* 17(5): 1–140.

Murray L, Cooper P. 1997. Effects of postnatal depression on infant development. *Archives of Disease in Childhood* 77(2): 99–101.

Myles N, Newall HD, Curtis J, Nielssen O, Shiers D, Large M. 2012. Tobacco use before, at, and after first-episode psychosis: A systematic meta-analysis. *The Journal of Clinical Psychiatry* 73(4): 468–475.

National Institute for Health and Clinical Excellence. 2008. *Guide to the Methods of Technology Appraisal*. National Institute for Health and Clinical Excellence, London, United Kingdom.

Naylor C, Parsonage M, McDaid D, Knapp M, Fossey M, Galea A. 2012. *Long-Term Conditions and Mental Health: The Cost of Co-Morbidities*. The King's Fund, London, United Kingdom.

Nelson TD, Smith TR, Pick R, Epstein MH, Thompson RW, Tonniges TF. 2013. Psychopathology as a predictor of medical service utilization for youth in residential treatment. *The Journal of Behavioral Health Services & Research* 40(1): 36–45.

Nielssen O, Large M. 2010. Rates of homicide during the first episode of psychosis and after treatment: A systematic review and meta-analysis. *Schizophrenia Bulletin* 36(4): 702–712.

Nyonator F, Kutzin J. 1999. Health for some? The effects of user fees in the Volta Region of Ghana. *Health Policy and Planning* 14(4): 329–341.

Organisation for Economic Co-Operation and Development 2012. *Sick on the Job? Myths and Realities about Mental Health and Work*. OECD Publishing, Paris, France.

Ormel J, Petukhova M, Chatterji S, Aguilar-Gaxiola S, Alonso J, Angermeyer MC, Bromet EJ, Burger H, Demyttenaere K, de Girolamo G, Haro JM, Hwang I, Karam E, Kawakami N, Lepine JP, Medina-Mora ME, Posada-Villa J, Sampson N, Scott K, Ustun TB, Von Korff M, Williams DR, Zhang M, Kessler RC. 2008. Disability and treatment of specific mental and physical disorders across the world: Results from the WHO World Mental Health Surveys. *The British Journal of Psychiatry* 192(5): 368–375.

Osby U, Correia N, Brandt L, Ekbom A, Sparen P. 2000. Time Trends in schizophrenia mortality in Stockholm County, Sweden: Cohort study. *British Medical Journal* 321(7259): 483–484.

Parameshvara DM. 2004. Malaysia mental health country profile. *International Review of Psychiatry* 16(1–2): 167–176.

Patel V, Kleinman A. 2003. Poverty and common mental disorders in developing countries. *Bulletin of the World Health Organization* 81(8): 609–615.

Pawlby S, Hay DF, Sharp D, Waters CS, O'Keane V. 2009. Antenatal depression predicts depression in adolescent offspring: Prospective longitudinal community-based study. *Journal of Affective Disorders* 113(3): 236–243.

Petrou S, Gray A. 2011. Economic evaluation alongside randomised controlled trials: Design, conduct, analysis, and reporting. *British Medical Journal* 342: d1548.

Phanthunane P, Whiteford H, Vos T, Bertram M. 2012. Economic burden of schizophrenia: Empirical analyses from a survey in Thailand. *The Journal of Mental Health Policy and Economics* 15(1): 25–32.

Pharoah F, Mari J, Rathbone J, Wong W. 2010. Family intervention for Schizophrenia. *Cochrane Database of Systematic Reviews* 2010(12): CD000088.

Platt S, McLean J, McCollam A, Blamey A, Mackenzie M, McDaid D, Maxwell M, Halliday E, Woodhouse A. 2006. *Evaluation of the First Phase of Choose Life: The National Strategy and Action Plan to Prevent Suicide in Scotland*. Scottish Executive Social Research, Edinburg, United Kingdom.

Pleasance P, Balmer N. 2007. Changing fortunes: Results from a randomised trial of the offer of debt advice in England and Wales. *Journal of Empirical Legal Studies* 4(3): 465–475.

Preker AS, Glied S, Chernichovsky D, Lapetra MG. Forthcoming. *Economics of Financing Health Care*. In Scheffler R (ed.). *World Scientific Handbook of Global Health Economics and Public Policy*, World Scientific Publishing Co.

Prince M, Albanese E, Guerchet M, Prina M (eds.). 2014. *World Alzheimer Report 2014 Dementia and Risk Reduction. An Analysis of Protective and Modifiable Factors*. Alzheimer's Disease International, London, United Kingdom.

Proudfoot J, Ryden C, Everitt B, Shapiro DA, Goldberg D, Mann A, Tylee A, Marks I, Gray JA. 2004. Clinical efficacy of computerised cognitive-behavioural therapy for anxiety and depression in primary care: Randomised controlled trail. *The British Journal of Psychiatry* 185: 46–54.

Robinson J, Harris MG, Harrigan SM, Henry LP, Farrelly S, Prosser A, Schwartz O, Jackson H, McGorry PD. 2010. Suicide attempt in first-episode psychosis: A 7.4 year follow-up study. *Schizophrenia Research* 116(1): 1–8.

Rog DJ, Marshall T, Dougherty RH, George P, Daniels AS, Ghose SS, Delphin-Rittmon ME. 2014. Permanent supportive housing: Assessing the evidence. *Psychiatric Services: A Journal of the American Psychiatric Association* 65(3): 287–294.

Russolillo A, Patterson M, McCandless L, Moniruzzaman A, Somers J. 2014. Emergency Department utilization among formerly homeless adults with mental disorders after one year of housing first interventions: A randomized controlled trial. *International Journal of Housing Policy* 14(1): 79–97.

Sado M, Inagaki A, Koreki A, Knapp M, Kissane LA, Mimura M, Yoshimura K. 2013. The cost of schizophrenia in Japan. *Neuropsychiatric Disease and Treatment* 9: 787–798.

Saxena S, Thornicroft G, Knapp M, Whiteford H. 2007. Scarcity, inequity and inefficiency of resources: Three major obstacles to better mental health. *Lancet* 370(9590): 878–889.

Scott DA, McGilloway S, Dempster M, Browne F, Donnelly M. 2013. Effectiveness of criminal justice liaison and diversion services for offenders with mental disorders: A review. *Psychiatric Services: A Journal of the American Psychiatric Association* 64(9): 843–849.

Scott S, Knapp M, Henderson J, Maughan B. 2001. Financial cost of social exclusion: Follow up study of antisocial children into adulthood. *British Medical Journal* 323(7306): 191.

Sharac J, McCrone P, Clement S, Thornicroft G. 2010. The economic impact of mental health stigma and discrimination: A systematic review. *Epidemiologia e Psichiatria Sociale* 19(3): 223–232.

Simon GE, Katon W, Lin EHB, Ruter C, Manning WG, Von Korff M, Ciechanowski P, Ludman EJ, Young BA. 2007. Cost effectiveness of systematic depression treatment among people with diabetes mellitus. *Archives of General Psychiatry* 64(1): 65–72.

Sinclair JM, Gray A, Rivero-Arias O, Saunders KE, Hawton K. 2011. Health care and social services resource use and costs of self-harm patients. *Social Psychiatry and Psychiatric Epidemiology* 46(4): 263–271.

Smith JP, Smith GC. 2010. Long-term economic costs of psychological problems during childhood. *Social Science & Medicine* 71(1): 110–115.

Smith L, Onwumere J, Craig T, McManus S, Bebbington P, Kuipers E. 2014. Mental and physical illness in caregivers: Results from an English national survey sample. *The British Journal of Psychiatry* 205(3): 197–203.

Snell T, Knapp M, Healey A, Guglani S, Evans-Lacko S, Fernandez JL, Meltzer H, Ford T. 2013. Economic impact of childhood psychiatric disorder on public sector services in Britain: Estimates from national survey data. *Journal of Child Psychology and Psychiatry* 54(9): 977–985.

Social Exclusion Unit. 2004. *Mental Health and Social Exclusion*. Cabinet Office, London, United Kingdom.

Soumerai SB, McLaughlin TJ, Ross-Degnan D, Casteris CS, Bollini P. 1994. Effects of limiting Medicaid drug-reimbursement benefits on the use of psychotropic agents and acute mental health services by patients with schizophrenia. *The New England Journal of Medicine* 331(10): 650–655.

Stuckler D, Basu S. 2013. *The Body Economic: Why Austerity Kills*. Basic Books, London, United Kingdom.

Substance Abuse and Mental Health Services Administration. 2013. *Results from the 2012 National Survey on Drug Use and Health: Mental Health Findings*. Substance Abuse and Mental Health Services Administration, Rockville, MD.

Swanson JW, Holzer 3rd, CE, Ganju VK, Jono RT. 1990. Violence and psychiatric disorder in the community: Evidence from the Epidemiologic Catchment Area surveys. *Hospital & Community Psychiatry* 41(7): 761–70.

Swartz MS, Swanson JW, Hiday VA, Borum R, Wagner HR, Burns BJ. 1998. Violence and severe mental illness: The effects of substance abuse and nonadherence to medication. *The American Journal of Psychiatry* 155(2): 226–231.

Tamblyn R, Laprise R, Hanley JA, Abrahamowicz M, Scott S, Mayo N, Hurley J, Grad R, Latimer E, Perreault R, McLeod P, Huang A, Larochelle P, Mallet L. 2001. Adverse events associated with prescription drug cost-sharing among poor and elderly persons. *The Journal of the American Medical Association* 285(4): 421–429.

Thomas CM, Morris S. 2003. Cost of depression among adults in England in 2000. *The British Journal of Psychiatry* 183: 514–519.

Thornicroft G. 2006. *Shunned: Discrimination Against People with Mental Illness*. Oxford University Press, Oxford, United Kingdom.

Thornicroft, Goulden R, Shefer G, Rhydderch D, Rose D, Williams P, Thornicroft G, Henderson C. 2013. Newspaper coverage of mental illness in England 2008–2011. *The British Journal of Psychiatry Supplement* 202(s55): s64–s9.

van Voren R. 2010. Political abuse of psychiatry: An historical overview. *Schizophrenia B*ulletin 36(1): 33–35.

Velders FP, Dieleman G, Henrichs J, Jaddoe VW, Hofman A, Verhulst FC, Hudziak JJ, Tiemeier H. 2011. Prenatal and postnatal psychological symptoms of parents and family functioning: The impact on child emotional and behavioural problems. *European Child & Adolescent Psychiatry* 20(7): 341–350.

Wang PS, Patrick A, Avorn J, Azocar F, Ludman E, McCulloch J, Simon G, Kessler R.. 2006. The costs and benefits of enhanced depression care to employers. *Archives of General Psychiatry* 63(12): 1345–1353.

Whiteford HA, Degenhardt L, Rehm J, Baxter AJ, Ferrari AJ, Erskine HE, Charlson FJ, Norman RE, Flaxman AD, Johns N, Burstein R, Murray CJL, Vos T. 2013. Global burden of disease attributable to mental and substance use disorders: Findings from the Global Burden of Disease Study 2010. *Lancet* 382(9904): 1575–1586.

Wilper AP, Woolhandler S, Boyd JW, Lasser KE, McCormick D, Bor DH, Himmelstein DU. 2009. The health and health care of US prisoners: Results of a nationwide survey. *American Journal of Public Health* 99(4): 666–672.

Wimo A, Prince M. 2010. *World Alzheimer Report 2010. The Global Economic Impact of Dementia, Alzheimer's Disease International*. London, United Kingdom.

World Health Organization. 2000. *The World Health Report 2000: Health Systems: Improving Performance*. World Health Organization, Geneva, Switzerland.

World Health Organization. 2008. *Mental Health Gap Action Programme: Scaling Up Care for Mental, Neurological, and Substance Use Disorders*. World Health Organization, Geneva, Switzerland.

World Health Organization. 2013. *Investing in Mental Health: Evidence for Action*. World Health Organization, Geneva, Switzerland.

World Health Organization. 2011. *Mental Health Atlas 2011*. World Health Organization, Geneva, Switzerland.

Yoon J, Domino ME, Norton EC, Cuddeback GS, Morrissey JP. 2013. The impact of changes in psychiatric bed supply on jail use by persons with severe mental illness. *The Journal of Mental Health Policy and Economics* 16(2): 81–92.

Zhai J, Guo X, Chen M, Zhao J, Su Z. 2013. An investigation of economic costs of schizophrenia in two areas of China. *International Journal of Mental Health Systems* 7(1): 26.

Aging and Long-Term Care

Audrey Laporte and Meghan McMahon

Institute of Health Policy, Management and Evaluation
Canadian Centre for Health Economics

Population aging is one of the most important demographic trends facing countries worldwide. This trend is expected to have significant implications for long-term care (LTC) systems, which typically provide health and social services for individuals needing care over a prolonged period of time. Demographic trends are expected to generate increased demand for and spending on LTC services, increased requirements for both formal and informal caregivers, increased affordability concerns for LTC care recipients, and higher expectations from citizens, patients and families about access to and quality of LTC.

This chapter considers the economic and policy implications of an aging population for LTC systems, including the factors that will drive demand for and expenditure on LTC. It draws on international comparative analysis and lessons learned from other country experiences about options for financing, delivering and regulating high-quality, accessible and appropriate LTC. The chapter concludes with evidence-informed reflections on the future of LTC, including policy options to improve the quality, efficiency and value-for-money of an increasingly high-priority sector.

Keywords: Long-Term Care; Aging; Supply and Demand; Financing; Delivering; Regulating.

Introduction

Aging societies and implications for long-term care (LTC)

One of the most important demographic trends facing countries worldwide is the aging of their populations. People aged 80 years and older are the fastest growing population segment in Europe and other countries like Canada and the United States (European Commission, 2012; Canadian Institutes of Health Information,

2011; US Census Bureau, 2014). Whereas in 1950, less than 1% of the global population was aged over 80 years old and in 2010 4% was, by 2050 the share of those aged 80 years and over is expected to more than double, reaching nearly 10% across Organisation for Economic Co-operation and Development (OECD) countries (OECD, 2013). Similarly, the share of the population aged 65 years and over is projected to increase from 17% in 2007 to more than 28% by 2040 in the EU-25 member states alone (Fernández *et al.*, 2009). As discussed below, population aging is an economic, policy and health concern and countries around the world are striving to equip and finance their health and social care systems to deal with the evolving health needs of older adults.

These demographic trends will have significant implications for LTC systems in particular — systems that can be defined as providing care for people needing daily living support over a prolonged period of time — including increased demand for care, increased human resource capacity requirements, increased spending on services, increased affordability concerns for recipients, and higher expectations from citizens, patients and families about access to and quality of care. Moreover, while a significant amount of LTC is currently provided by informal caregivers (mainly family and friends), the pool of potential caregivers is likely to shrink because of labor force trends, including increasing numbers of women working and social policies that no longer support early retirement, which will likely increase capacity demands for formal LTC providers. The share of the working age population is also expected to decline, which has implications for revenue sources for health and pension systems. At the same time, total spending (public and private sector) on LTC, which is currently just over 1% of gross domestic product (GDP) across OECD countries, is projected to double or triple between now and 2050, which has resulted in a number of OECD countries identifying financial sustainability of LTC as their number one policy priority (Colombo *et al.*, 2011; Fernández *et al.*, 2009). Addressing these challenges requires a comprehensive and forward-looking vision of LTC.

Defining LTC

The LTC sector is unique in that it includes traditional medical services as well as social care and often housing services, relies heavily on both formal and informal care providers, and is delivered in home, community and institutional settings. It typically provides care and services for people with reduced functional and health status needing support with activities of daily living (e.g., washing, eating) and instrumental activities of daily living (e.g., preparing meals, shopping) over a prolonged period of time due to chronic illness or physical or mental disability.

LTC systems are complex, often fragmented, and vary by country and region in how they are financed, organized and regulated but they typically comprise multiple services (e.g., medical services, nursing care, social work, personal care services, prevention and rehabilitation, palliative care, domestic help, medical equipments and technologies), delivered by a mix of different providers (nurses, allied health professionals, informal caregivers) in a mix of settings (home, institutional, and community care). This patchwork of fragmented services has been recognized as a challenge for frail older adults as they attempt to navigate multiple types of services paid for multiple types of payers, often resulting in unmet needs and discontinuities in care (Konetzka and Werner, 2010).

Chapter overview

This chapter considers the economic and policy implications of an aging population for LTC, including the factors that will drive demand for and expenditure on LTC as well as options for financing, delivering, and regulating high-quality, accessible and appropriate LTC. Its scope includes both formal and informal LTC and includes data from a number of international comparative analyses (e.g., OECD, European Observatory, European Commission). The chapter concludes with evidence-informed reflections on the future of LTC, including policy options to improve the quality, efficiency and value-for-money of an increasingly high-priority sector.

The Demand and Supply of LTC: An Overview

Who uses LTC and where?

Demand for LTC increases with age, with approximately half of all LTC users aged 80 years or over. As shown in Figures 1(a) and 1(b), most LTC recipients across all age groups and in both homes and institutions are women, likely reflecting higher female than male life expectancy rates. A substantial share of older age LTC recipients suffer from dementia-related problems. Among older adults, health and disability trends are mixed with some countries experiencing declining rates of severe disability while others witness rising rates, though mild disability and chronic disease are generally on the rise (Rechel *et al.*, 2009).

A 2011 OECD Report on LTC (Colombo *et al.*, 2011) illustrated that in the majority of OECD countries, between half and three quarters of all formal LTC is provided in home care settings (Figure 2). While the majority of LTC is received in the home and community, institutional care accounts for the majority of LTC spending, representing 62% of total LTC costs across OECD countries in 2008.

Who provides LTC?

Both formal and informal caregivers are instrumental to the provision of LTC. The formal LTC workforce is comprised mainly of women and includes licensed professionals (e.g., nurses) and unlicensed personal care workers who manage and deliver

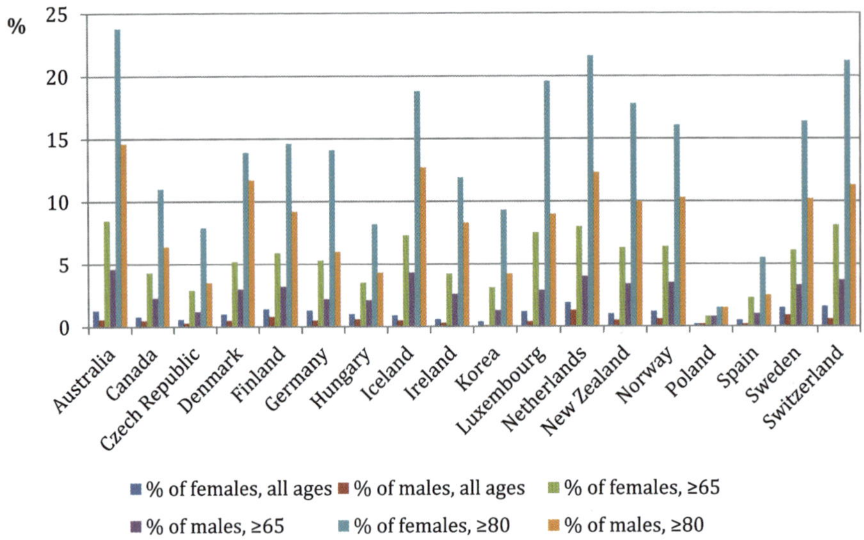

(a)

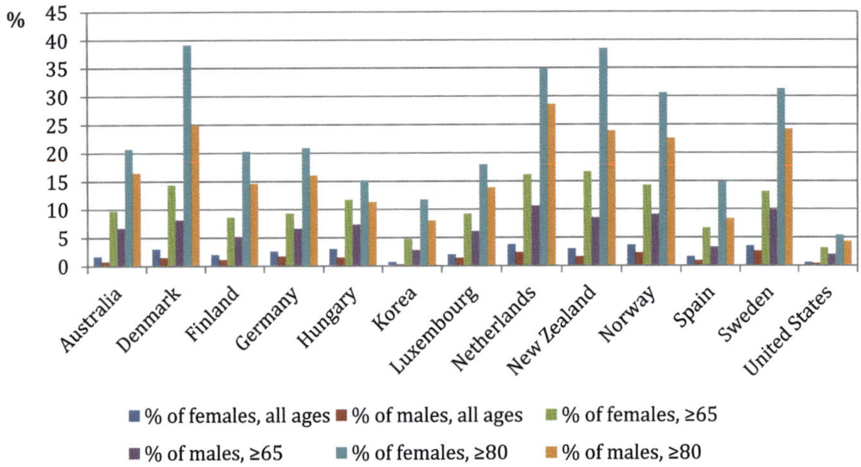

(b)

Figure 1. (a) LTC users (institutional, non-hospital) by age and sex across a subset of OECD countries, 2012. (b) LTC users (home) by age and sex across a subset of OECD countries, 2012

Notes: (a) Data for Denmark and Luxembourg are estimates only. Data for Australia, Canada, Czech Republic and Iceland are for 2009. Data for Australia deviates from OECD definition (OECD, 2014).
(b) Data for Australia deviate from the OECD definition and are from 2011 for "all ages". Data for Luxembourg are estimates only. Data for the United States are from 2007 (OECD Health Statistics, 2014).

LTC services in nursing homes, assisted living facilities, other residential and community-based settings and private residences.

The informal LTC workforce, comprised mainly of families and friends, has been described as the "bedrock" of LTC both because it provides a significant amount of total LTC and because in a fragmented system, where formal care

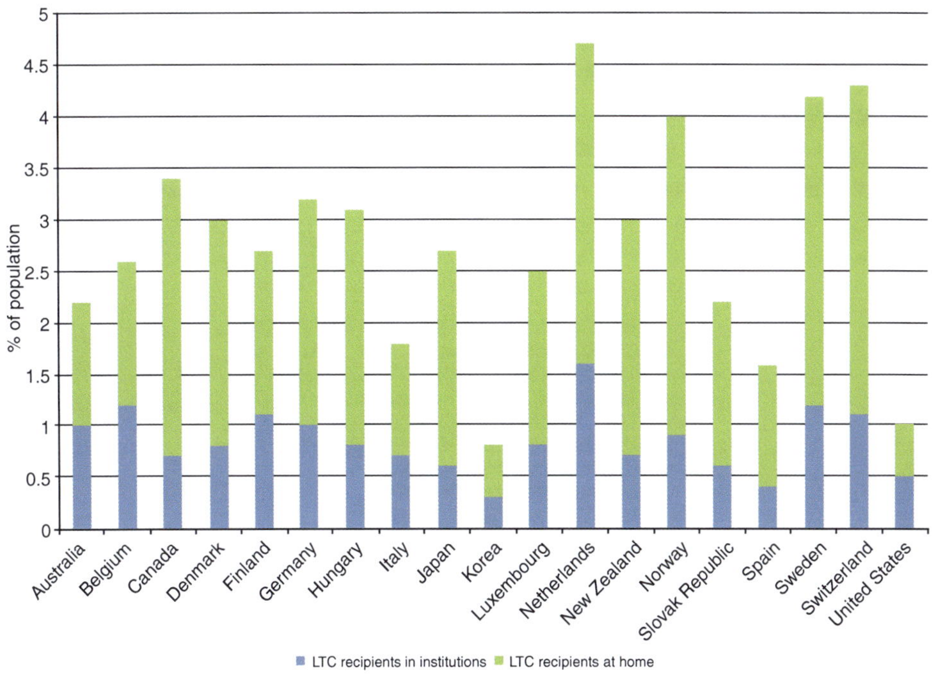

Figure 2. LTC users by setting: Home versus institution, 2012

Notes: Data from Australia are from 2010; Belgium and the United States 2007; and Canada and Japan 2006 (OECD Health Statistics, 2014).

providers change frequently, family caregivers are often the only people who have experienced the entire trajectory of their family member's illness (Levine *et al.*, 2010). Across the OECD, more than one in 10 adults (family and friends) are involved in informal, typically unpaid, caregiving particularly related to activities of daily living (Colombo *et al.*, 2011). When the scope is broadened to include instrumental activities of daily living (i.e., help with shopping or paperwork), closer to one in three adults provide unpaid care.

The supply of informal caregivers is, however, expected to decline over time. Close to two-thirds of informal caregivers are women, and with increased female labor force participation rates and declining fertility rates, the pool of caregivers is projected to shrink. There are also notable differences across countries in perspectives about the role of the family in supporting older adults, and in recent years there has been a decrease in many countries in the willingness to provide informal care (Fernandez *et al.*, 2009). For example, more than half of the EU-27 population believes that older people rely too much on their relatives for support and care, ranging from 42% in Denmark to almost 100% in Bulgaria (Tjadens and Colombo, 2011). These trends in the supply of informal caregivers could have significant implications for the intensity of care that informal caregivers are expected to provide and/or for demand for formal care providers.

Forecasting demand for LTC

Projections surrounding population aging are critical to assist governments in understanding the likely scale of the challenge facing LTC systems and to develop appropriate policies accordingly. OECD data suggest that the percentage of those aged 80 and over is likely to increase from 4% in 2010 to nearly 10% in 2050 in OECD countries, as illustrated in Figure 3.

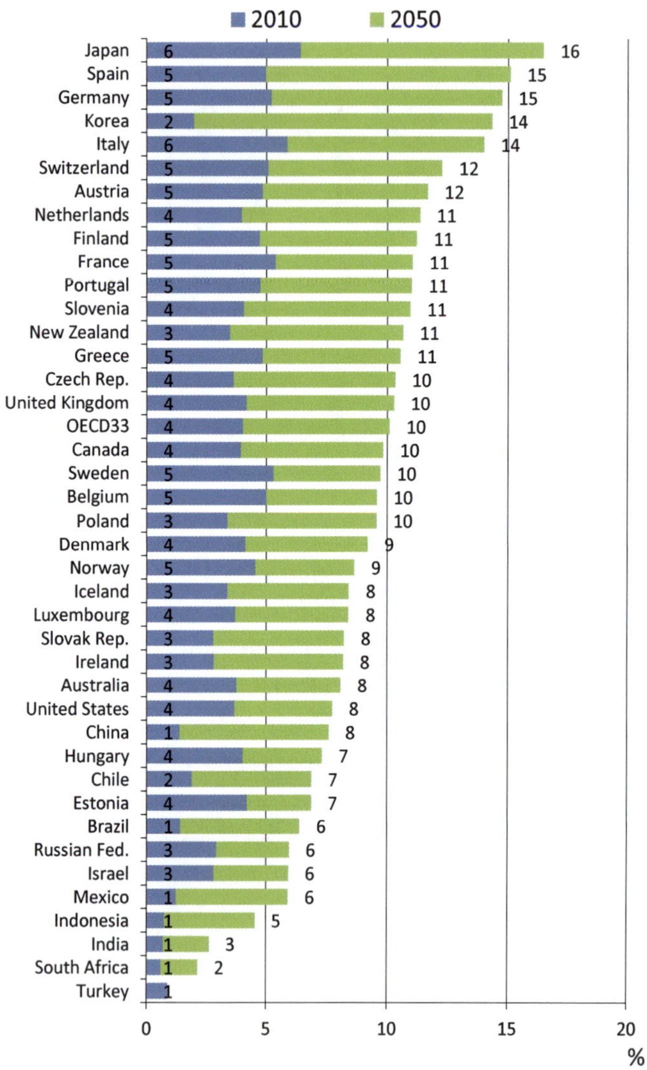

Figure 3. Share of the population aged 80 years and over in OECD countries, 2010 and 2050

Notes: Data are from the OECD Historical Population Data and Projections Database, 2013 (OECD, 2013).
Sources: OECD (2013), *Health at a Glance 2013: OECD Indicators*, OECD Publishing, Paris. http://dx.doi.org/10.1787/health-glance-2013-en.

Equally important for governments to know, however, is whether population aging and increases in life expectancy are accompanied by improvements in healthy life expectancy or, conversely, increases in illness and disability (and therefore increased utilization and demand for LTC). That is, are countries facing a compression or expansion of morbidity? These two scenarios have vastly different implications for countries charged with the task of planning for future LTC demand. Compression of morbidity posits an increase in both absolute lifespan and proportion of the lifespan that is free from disease and disability — that is, greater longevity and more healthy years of life. Expansion of morbidity, conversely, posits that the improvements in health care and prevention made over past decades simply extend the lifespan of individuals with disease and disability — that is, greater longevity and more unhealthy years of life (i.e., more years of life requiring LTC). Evidence from different countries is contradictory, with levels of disability in decline in some countries and on the increase in others (Lafortune and Balestat, 2007; Rechel *et al.*, 2009; Jagger *et al.*, 2011; Payne *et al.*, 2007). While morbidity has been reduced in some countries for all ages, the duration and severity of morbidity increases at older ages which, as Payne *et al.* (2007) explain, implies an aging population may experience more morbidity overall. Recently, it has been suggested that disability projections ought to be based on the occurrence of multimorbidity rather than on single diseases since old age is most frequently characterized by the presence of multiple rather than single diseases, which may provide a more accurate picture of the impact that disability may have on demand for LTC (Jagger *et al.*, 2011). Using a macro-simulation model, Jagger *et al.* (2011) project that, even with assumptions of constant or reduced age-specific disability prevalence over the next 20 years, there will be large increases in the number of individuals requiring LTC.

Despite uncertainties about future trends in disability among older adults, population aging and increasing life expectancy — coupled with other trends related to the supply of informal caregivers and a rise in the number of older adults living alone — are expected to significantly increase demand for formal LTC providers and services. This suggests an urgent need to include prevention, management of chronic disease, and healthy aging strategies in future LTC planning (Comas-Herrera *et al.*, 2011).

Economic consequences of increasing demand for LTC

Population aging creates two potentially major pressures on LTC systems and finances: Increased demand and utilization of health and social services, and decreased revenues (as a declining share of the population is economically active).

The increased demand and utilization of LTC will put upward pressure on public and private LTC expenditure, which is expected to comprise a growing

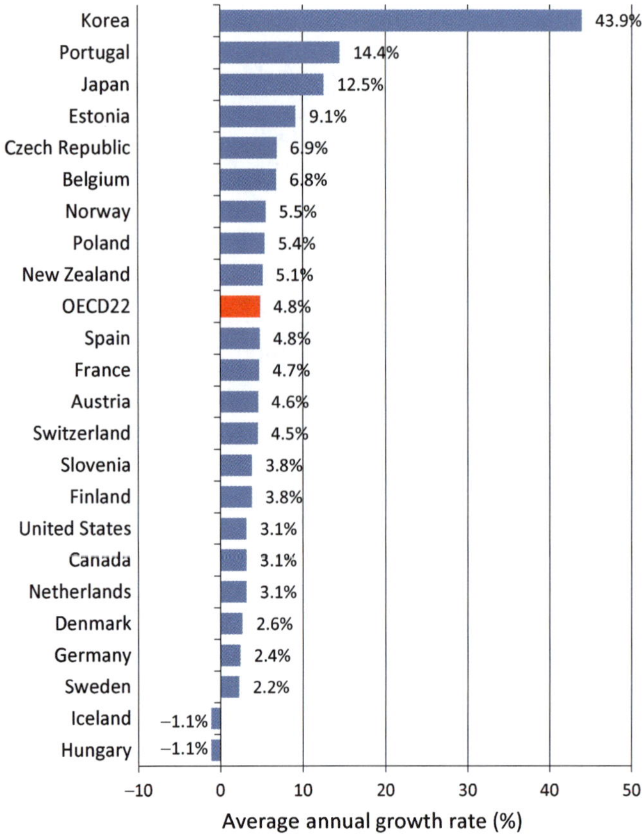

Figure 4. Annual growth rate in public expenditure on LTC across OECD countries, 2005–2011, in real terms

Notes: The OECD average excludes Korea (due to the extremely high growth rate). Information on data for Israel: http://dx.doi.org/10.1787/888932315602 (OECD, 2013).
Source: OECD (2013), *Health at a Glance 2013: OECD Indicators*, OECD Publishing, Paris. http://dx.doi.org/10.1787/health-glance-2013-en.

share of GDP in European countries (European Commission, 2012). OECD data provide a portrait of increasing annual growth in public LTC expenditure over a 6-year period between 2005 and 2011, as shown in Figure 4. Figure 5 illustrates that this growth is observed in both LTC home and institution-based care, though countries differ in where expenditure growth has been most rapid.

Total spending (public and private sector) on LTC, which currently averages just over 1% of GDP across OECD countries, is projected to at least double between now and 2060 to between 2% and 4% of GDP (European Commission, 2012). Colombo and Mercier (2011) caution that these trends will occur concurrently with the growth of other major age-related expenditures like public pensions, with the potential risk of shifting costs to future generations.

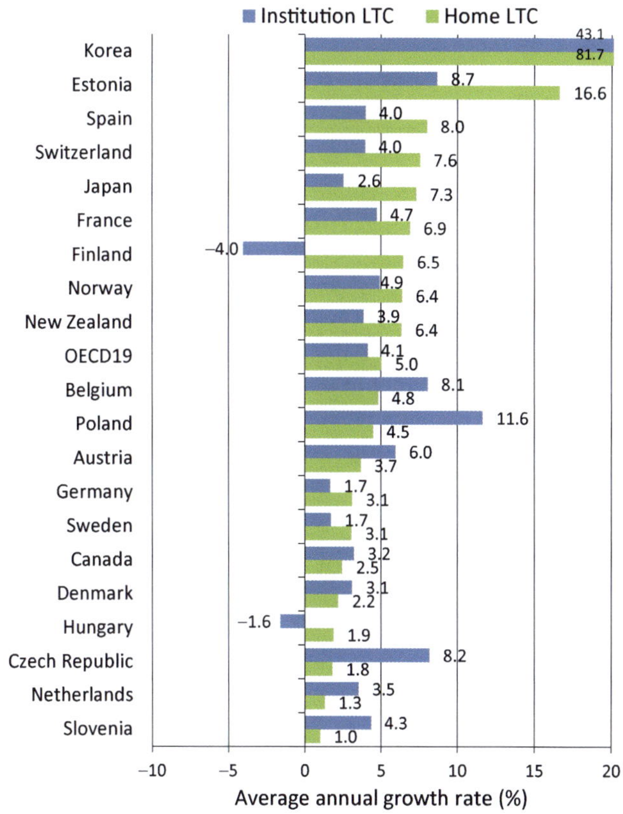

Figure 5. Annual growth rate in public expenditure on LTC institution and at home, in real terms, 2005–2011

Notes: The OECD average excludes Korea (due to the extremely high growth rate). Information on data for Israel: http://dx.doi.org/10.1787/888932315602 (OECD, 2013).

Source: OECD (2013), *Health at a Glance 2013: OECD Indicators*, OECD Publishing, Paris. http://dx.doi.org/10.1787/health-glance-2013-en.

Modeling methodology is increasingly used to predict future LTC demand and expenditures and to examine the potential impact of different LTC policies. Colombo *et al.* (2011) developed five scenarios to predict future LTC expenditures (Table 1) based on country-specific projections from the European Commission 2009 Aging Report for European OECD countries (European Commission, 2009), complemented with projections for the United States, Canada, Australia, New Zealand, and Japan. Table 1 defines the five scenarios (baseline scenario is the pure aging/demographic effect), provides key details and model assumptions, and outlines projection findings. The scenarios are based on a macro-simulation approach that first estimates future demand (volume) of LTC services and then estimates the associated cost. The scenarios assumed demand can be impacted by three key variables,

Table 1. LTC expenditure scenarios

Scenario	Details	Projection
Pure aging/demographic effect (baseline scenario)	Assumes that the number of years with disability will increase in line with future gains in life expectancy. Also assumes the cost of providing LTC will grow in line with wages in the rest of the economy.	Public LTC expenditure is projected to double from around 1.2% to 2.4% for OECD–EU member countries and to about 2.9% of GPD for the selected non-European OECD countries (US, Canada, Australia, New Zealand, Japan) in 2050.
Healthy aging effect	Assumes that gains in life expectancy will lead to a delay in the onset of disability, with half of the increase in lifespan considered to be years with lower dependency. Also assumes the cost of providing LTC will grow inline with wages in the rest of the economy.	Healthy aging mitigates some of the increase in LTC expenditures. Total public LTC spending could decrease by about 5% to 10% by 2050, relative to the baseline scenario.
Productivity gains	Assumes that the cost of providing LTC grows at a slower rate than real GDP per worker due to potential technological efficiency gains.	Public LTC expenditure could decrease by approximately 10%, relative to the baseline scenario.
Wage increases	Assumes the real cost of providing LTC grows at a rate of 1% above real GDP per worker because recruiting and retaining LTC workers in the future could be a challenge that exacerbates pressures on wages.	Public LTC expenditure could increase by approximately 10%, relative to the baseline scenario.
Declining availability of informal care	Assume that the number of individuals able to rely on family will decline at an annual rate of 1% during the first 10 years.	Public LTC expenditure could increase by 5–20%,[a] relative to the baseline scenario.

Notes: [a]Variations mainly reflect differences in the share of the country's dependent population relying on family or no care, as well as their respective average cost of providing care at home or in an institution (Colombo *et al.*, 2011).

including prevalence of disability/dependency by age group, cost of delivering care, and availability of informal care. Overall, Table 1 illustrates that most scenarios point towards increasing LTC expenditures.

Ansah *et al.* (2014) use System Dynamics modeling methodology (which offers a practical approach to examining the impacts of hypothetical policies and scenarios on the behavior of real-world systems over time) to examine the interaction between people with LTC needs and the capacity of the health care system to provide care. They examine four scenarios that differ in how quickly LTC capacity responds and conclude overall that failure to respond proactively to LTC needs (i.e., anticipating the likely demand for LTC in the future, and adjusting LTC capacity accordingly) tends to shift care toward acute care facilities and increase total care needs and therefore total LTC expenditures. Like all simulation models, those developed by Colombo *et al.* 2011 and Ansah *et al.* 2014 are subject to a number of unrealistic assumptions (e.g., that there is no constraint on the supply of health care professionals), but nevertheless provides a basis for discussions around LTC systems planning.

While population aging will contribute to increased health expenditure, a number of analyses have shown that other non-demographic factors, in particular new technologies and devices and physician compensation, are larger contributors to rising health expenditures (Rechel *et al.*, 2009; Canadian Institutes of Health Information, 2013). Evidence is emerging that some of the costs that population aging will bring can be mitigated by prevention and healthy aging initiatives as well as well-coordinated health and social policies (Rechel *et al.*, 2009).

Ability to pay for LTC

Most individuals will require LTC at some point in their lives either through formal or informal care provision. Depending on the intensity and duration of care needed, LTC can be extremely expensive for individuals and societies. Fernández *et al.* (2009) explain that society's capacity to meet the future demand and pay for LTC services depends on its wealth, both in terms of the ability of individuals to pay for their care, and of society's ability to fund a collective care system.

From an individual perspective, LTC is the largest out-of-pocket expenditure risk faced by older adults. Even low levels of LTC need (e.g., <10 hours per week) can consume 60% of a senior's disposable income for those at low and moderate income levels (Colombo *et al.*, 2011). In the United States, annual nursing home costs average more than $75,000 per year (Brown *et al.*, 2012) and while 42% of individuals aged 65 years and older can expect to spend nothing on LTC during their lifetimes, 16% can expect to spend more than $100,000 (Stevenson *et al.*, 2010; Kemper and Alecxih, 2005). This distribution of financial risk points to the role for insurance as a mechanism to spread risk, which will be discussed below.

From a societal perspective, societal wealth is influenced by a number of drivers, including the taxes and/or social insurance contributions of the labor force population since many systems fund LTC on a pay as you go basis — that is the working age population is taxed to pay for services delivered to the current pool of elderly. However, in most OECD countries, the relative (and in some cases absolute) size of the working age population is expected to decrease such that there will be fewer working-age people per retiree. If pay as you go structures are maintained, then unless policies are implemented to push back the legal age for retirement, provide incentives to encourage older adults to remain in the workforce, or broaden the financing base to include older adults, a smaller share of the population will have to finance LTC and likely at a significantly higher contribution rate (Rechel *et al.*, 2009).

Some caution, however, that pushing back the retirement age and encouraging older adults to remain in the workforce may conflict with policies aimed at increasing the level of informal care in the community. Jacobs *et al.* (2014) examined caregiving intensity and retirement status in Canada and found that higher intensity caregiving is associated with being fully retired (relative to working full-time) for retirement-age men and women and their sensitivity analysis suggested that intense caregiving may be an important correlate of early retirement. Their findings lead the authors to caution that a policy context that encourages both later retirement and more informal care in the community may not be fully feasible.

LTC Today: Approaches to Financing, Delivering and Regulating LTC

Financing LTC

With LTC demand and expenditures expected to rise over time, ensuring that sustainable financing systems are in place is of paramount importance to countries around the world. Sustainability refers to the extent to which current revenues equal current expenditures, as well as the extent to which the system is financially equipped to provide care for future older adults.

There are variety of financing mechanisms that can be used to fund LTC as well as a variety of options around the breadth and depth of coverage. Different sources of revenue will generate different incentives and varying degrees of income redistribution. Fernández *et al.* (2009) note that differing national contexts — such as the relative importance placed on the formal LTC sector, societal values, reliance on family care, and resource constraints — will all play a role in determining which financing mechanism is adopted.

The toolkit of financing mechanisms can be broadly organized around those that rely on public contributions (e.g., through taxation or social health insurance), private contributions (e.g., through private health insurance schemes or out-of-pocket payments), or a combination of both. Breadth and depth of coverage can be universal and comprehensive, means-tested, or a mixture of both. Regardless of financing mechanism, there is a strong rationale for pooling the financial risk associated with LTC costs through insurance and for providing basic universal coverage, as individuals face significant uncertainty about future need for LTC and, when needed, expenditure rapidly becomes unaffordable for low and high income individuals alike.

Before delving into the role of public versus private financing systems, it is worth noting that to properly insure against the financial risk of illness needing LTC requires that people begin paying premiums when they are young and the insurer (be it public or private) guarantees that those services will be there should the individual require them when they are older. Having individuals essentially finance their own future care moves us away from the traditional and still most commonly used "pay as you go" approach, which implicitly assumes a constant age distribution. As noted above, this implicit assumption becomes problematic in the context of an aging population since an imbalance emerges between the number of people needing care and the number of people that can be taxed to pay for that care. Japan is an example of a country that has already moved in the pre-payment direction by requiring all individuals aged 40 and over to pay LTC premiums.

OECD data show that the share of public LTC expenditure is substantially higher than that of private LTC expenditure (Figure 6). Indeed, the private LTC insurance

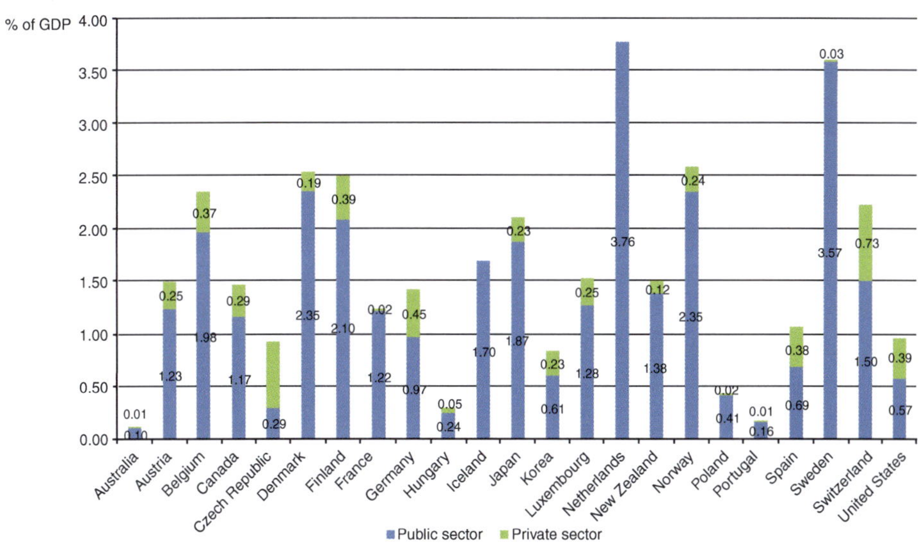

Figure 6. Share of public versus private LTC expenditure in OECD countries as a percentage of GDP, 2011

Note: OECD Health Statistics (2014).

market has remained small for a number of reasons that are discussed below. Overall, countries are moving in the direction of universal, publicly funded LTC systems with targeting of coverage to those in greatest need (Colombo *et al.*, 2011).

Publicly-financed LTC

There is a strong equity rational for public sector LTC financing and a strong efficiency rational for universal coverage. Publicly funded LTC systems can ensure that protection is provided to those in greatest need and help avoid catastrophic costs. Moreover, private sector solutions have failed to provide a sustainable insurance system that can cover a large share of the population, and continued reliance on family support is not possible for many (Fernández *et al.*, 2009).

Public LTC coverage is generally financed through tax-based or social health insurance contributions. Tax-based models are found mainly in the Nordic countries, are typically broad and comprehensive in their coverage of services and people, and tend to result in a relatively large share of GDP spent on LTC — ranging from 2% in Denmark to 3.6% in Sweden (Colombo *et al.*, 2011). LTC recipients typically contribute to the cost of care by way of co-payments. Social health insurance models are found in Germany, Japan, Korea, and the Netherlands and, like tax-based models, tend to provide broad and comprehensive coverage that is supplemented with revenues from co-payments, user charges and/or deductibles. Box 1 provides a short case study of Germany's universal LTC coverage system, which was implemented in 1994 to replace its former means-tested system. Participation in the scheme is typically mandatory for some or all segments of a population (e.g., those employed, or those over a certain age) and predominantly financed through employment-based payroll contributions. As a share of GDP, social health insurance LTC spending is above or around the OECD average of 1.5% (Colombo *et al.*, 2011).

Public LTC coverage can be provided universally to the entire population regardless of income, or targeted to individuals lacking ability to pay. Table 2 provides an overview of different publicly-financed coverage systems, their respective advantages and disadvantages, and the countries in which they are found.

Within the broadly-defined coverage systems featured in Table 2, the comprehensiveness of services can vary according to several dimensions including eligibility rules, level of cost-sharing, and breadth of services included. Services can typically include health and nursing care, domestic care and help with instrumental activities of daily living, and institutional board and lodging costs. There is heterogeneity across countries in which of these services are covered and to what extent. Most LTC schemes do not include coverage for institutional board and lodging except for low-income individuals.

Box 1. A case study of Germany's LTC financing system

In 1994, Germany implemented a statutory coverage system for LTC — *Soziale Pflegeversicherung* — to replace its former means-tested system, which was widely criticized as being at odds with the country's commitment to social solidarity as well as with its universal coverage of acute care (Cuellar and Wiener, 2000). This meant that starting in 1995, all members of statutory SHI sickness funds (including pensioners and the unemployed) as well as all people with full-coverage private health insurance (i.e., who had opted out of the SHI system) were declared mandatory members of the LTC coverage system. In 2013, 69.9 million (87%) were covered by mandatory SHI LTC insurance and about 9.5 million (11.5%) by mandatory private LTC insurance (Busse and Blumel, 2014). Voluntary supplementary private health insurance is also available to cover services not included in the SHI LTC system. In 2009, approximately 1.6 million people (3.5% of the German population aged 40 and over) held this type of LTC coverage (Colombo *et al.*, 2011).

The LTC system provides comprehensive coverage for home and nursing care for people of all ages and regardless of income, based on functional status (i.e., if they require assistance with activities of daily living for a period that is expected to last at least 6 months). Beneficiaries can choose to receive either monetary benefit or professional nursing care at home or in an LTC facility (Garms-Homolova and Busse, 2014).

The SHI LTC system is financed by way of an LTC insurance premium that is uniform and fixed by law at 2.09% of salary as of 2013 (plus an additional 0.25% for people without children), which is shared equally by employers and employees and by retirees and their pension funds (Garms-Homolova and Busse, 2014). It is administered through the country's sickness funds, which are the country's financing mechanism for acute care (quasi-public, quasi-private insurers that are heavily regulated by the national government with mandatory income-related premiums) but with a dedicated and separate budget stream from acute care (Cuellar and Wiener, 2000).

Germany's SHI LTC system is reported to have achieved many of its stated policy goals — shifting the financial burden of LTC off the states and municipalities; expanding home and community-based services and increasing support of informal caregivers; increasing the supply of LTC services; and decreasing reliance on means-tested welfare — without "exploding caseloads or uncontrolled expenditures" (Cuellar and Wiener, 2000). However, because the system is administered by the same sickness funds that administer acute care and because the line between LTC and acute care is oftentimes blurry,

(*Continued*)

Box 1. (*Continued*)

allegations of cost shifting between the two programs are common (Cuellar and Wiener, 2000). Additionally, while having national standards for the provision and financing of LTC services ensures geographic equity, the system has faced criticism for limiting flexibility to tailor programs and benefits to local needs (Cuellar and Wiener, 2000).

While there are many advantages to publicly-financed universal LTC coverage schemes, to maintain cost control it is important to:

- Target benefits to those in greatest need (e.g., via cost-sharing policies and clear definitions of need levels that trigger entitlements);
- Move away from the "pay as you go" model described above and instead move towards forward-looking financing policies that pool finances across generations (e.g., in Japan, individuals aged 40 years and over must pay LTC premiums), include elements of pre-funding, and have a broad source of finances (for example, Japan, the Netherlands, Belgium, and Luxembourg complement payroll contributions with alternative revenues sources and in Germany, retirees are required to contribute to social LTC funds based on their pension) (Colombo *et al.*, 2011);
- Consider developing financial instruments that help with the costs associated with institutional LTC (e.g., home equity release schemes like the Irish Nursing Home Load scheme[1]).

Additionally, Fernández *et al.* (2009) recommend that when determining the parameters of LTC coverage (e.g., universal versus means-tested), consideration for how other related systems like health and housing are financed should be made. For example, the interaction between health systems free at the point of use and means-tested LTC systems could lead to situations where individuals with similar needs are provided with different levels of public coverage depending on whether they are considered to have social or health needs. Incentives and joint budgeting across systems can be used to address this and improve the coordination of health and social care.

Overall, international comparative analyses of LTC financing suggest that the level of public coverage is increasing in low-coverage or highly-targeted countries,

[1]In the Irish Nursing Home Loan scheme, a resident can refer to the time of his or her death while their nursing home contribution is set on the basis of the value of their non-financial assets, such as their home (Colombo and Mercier, 2011).

Table 2. Publicly-financed LTC systems

LTC financing mechanism	Definition	Advantages and Disadvantages	Countries
Safety net/means-tested	Concentrates support on those individuals lacking the financial ability to pay for the cost of services	Can be very effective in controlling state expenditure, but tight restrictions on eligibility can generate significant unmet need, can be costly to administer (i.e., to apply the means testing and user-fees), and can be associated with stigma (i.e., only for the poor).	The United States, the United Kingdom, Southern and eastern European countries
Universal system	Covers the entire population, regardless of income. Co-payments, user charges or deductibles are often required, typically based on income thresholds. Typically financed through taxes or social insurance contributions. Tax-funded universal systems employ expenditure constraints and define eligibility criteria to optimize resource use. Social insurance funded systems tend to be needs driven rather than budget constrained.	Covers the entire population, promoting greater equality (i.e., everyone has access regardless of ability to pay) but at significantly greater cost to government. Health and LTC budgets are often separate, which can impact the continuum of care and lead to cost-shifting incentives between different sectors and providers. Coverage may be universal, but to maintain costs coverage may be limited in breadth and depth of services covered, leaving a significant share of costs to be borne by individuals.	Nordic and northern European countries. Denmark, Sweden, Norway, Finland, Scotland, Germany, Korea, Japan
Progressive universalism (mixed systems)	Combines universal entitlement with a means-tested element	Universal nature of support can increase public support for the system among those who would not qualify for some benefits under the minimum safety benefit system. Because everyone is covered, the stigma attached to the receipt of care in means-tested systems is reduced. As with universal systems, coverage may be universal but limited in breadth and depth of services covered, leaving a significant share of costs to be borne by individuals.	Austria, Belgium, France, Greece, Switzerland, Ireland, Australia

Sources: Fernández *et al.* (2009); Colombo *et al.* (2011).

although there is also greater targeting of public funding in the most comprehensive LTC systems. Colombo *et al.* (2011) conclude from their analysis that overall, the way public LTC systems are financed — through general taxation or social insurance contributions — tends to reflect existing institutional arrangements or political considerations and has little effect on the way LTC benefits are structured. The important policy challenge is how to ensure LTC financing is sustainable over the long-term. Budgeting, pre-funding, tax broadening (or broadening of revenue sources more generally), and public–private partnerships are examples of the various strategies that governments use to balance the sometimes-competing goals of fiscal sustainability and equity of access.

Privately-financed LTC

Views are mixed regarding the merit of private LTC coverage. For some, it is a mechanism to leverage new financial resources towards LTC and alleviate pressure on the public sector. For others, it is a less efficient, less equitable, and more costly way to finance LTC than public coverage. Regardless of perspective, the private LTC insurance sector has remained small in the majority of OECD countries, typically developing around or in complement to a country's public LTC system. Private LTC insurance plays the largest role in the United States and Japan, financing between 5% and 7% of total LTC expenditures and covering between 5% and 15% of the population aged 40 and over. On average across OECD countries, spending on private LTC insurance generally accounts for less than 2% of total LTC spending (Colombo *et al.*, 2011).

Economic theory would suggest that given the significant financial uncertainties in terms of potential need, intensity and duration of LTC, a powerful rationale exists from the LTC user perspective for pooling risk across individuals via private LTC coverage. From an insurer perspective, the rationale for offering coverage is less clear. The literature, mainly from the United States, points to a number of supply- and demand-side factors that help to explain the small size of the private LTC insurance market and are summarized in Table 3 (Stevenson *et al.*, 2010; Brown *et al.*, 2012; Colombo *et al.*, 2011; Barr, 2010). These factors include asymmetric information (e.g., adverse selection and moral hazard), uncertainty about future LTC costs, lack of consumer confidence due to risk of premium volatility, consumer myopia (e.g., consumers' underestimation of future risk or need for LTC), perceived value gap between cost and benefit of LTC insurance, competing financial obligations, and the availability of potential substitutes (e.g., availability of informal care). Table 3 provides brief explanations for each of these factors.

As with public LTC systems, a wide range of private LTC insurance schemes with varying eligibility rules, benefit triggers and benefits paid can be found in

Table 3. Market failures that suggest why the LTC insurance market is small

Factor	Explanation
Asymmetric information: Adverse selection and moral hazard	Risk that only those with high-perceived need will purchase LTC insurance, and that those with coverage will use more than they need, leads insurers to raise premium (affecting demand for coverage) or limit coverage to those without pre-existing conditions (limiting the pool of potential insurees).
Uncertainty about future LTC costs	Insurers face uncertainty about future costs (e.g., onset of dependency, unit costs of care, projected return from accumulated reserves) so charge higher premium to mitigate risk.
Premium volatility/ consumer confidence	To mitigate risk of future market uncertainty (e.g., economic crisis), insurers may include clauses in policies that allow for increases in premium levels if overall risk level shared within a pool of insurees increases. This decreases the predictability of future LTC costs to potential insurees and thus impacts demand for coverage (e.g., some insurees in the U.S. have faced premium rate increases of 15–50%).
Consumer myopia/ underestimating risk	Individuals' perception of the need to plan for the future risk of dependency and LTC costs may be low, especially at younger ages. Individuals may delay purchase of LTC insurance until later ages, when they are more likely to face high premiums or be ineligible due to pre-existing conditions.
Perceived value gap	In the LTC sector, a lower portion of the premium dollar translates into benefits.
Competing financial obligations	Many individuals face competing demands for their financial resources, including child care, education, and housing.
Availability of potential substitutes	The availability and comprehensiveness of potential substitutes for private LTC coverage — including public schemes and informal care — may mitigate demand for private LTC insurance.

Sources: Stevenson *et al.* (2010); Brown *et al.* (2012); Barr (2010); Colombo *et al.* (2011).

OECD countries. Two main products have emerged over time: The reimbursement model, designed inline with private health insurance arrangements; and the indemnity model designed inline with annuity contracts (typically providing eligible recipients with a fixed level of monthly benefits for life, once the insuree meets criteria set in the policy regarding the level of dependency and waiting period). Recent experiences in some OECD countries suggest that the indemnity model is gaining traction, possibly because it appeals to demands for greater consumer choice by way of providing a fixed cash benefit that can be used according to the insuree's preferences.

Governments have employed various strategies to increase the market share and demand for private LTC insurance. For example, tax incentives aim to stimulate demand by reducing the purchase price of a private LTC insurance through deductions or credits based on the level of insurance premium paid. Preferential tax treatment for private LTC insurance exists in the United States, Spain, Mexico, and Austria (Colombo *et al.*, 2011). There is, however, a risk that those who stand to gain the most from tax breaks — namely, high-income groups — are those who would be most likely to purchase LTC insurance regardless of a tax break. Moreover, the costs incurred from providing the tax break or subsidizing the premiums may outweigh the revenues generated from new enrollees (Stevenson *et al.*, 2010). Regulatory interventions are another mechanism used to increase demand for private LTC insurance, including, for example, offering protection of individuals who purchase coverage from canceling coverage or altering premium levels based on change in health status. Public education campaigns to raise public awareness about the importance of understanding the LTC risks they face and plan for the future have also been used to stimulate demand (Stevenson *et al.*, 2010). Finally, mandating the purchase of private LTC insurance among certain population subgroups is another option. For instance in Germany, individuals who have opted out of the social health insurance system must purchase compulsory private LTC insurance. This market provides coverage for about 9% of Germany's population and is highly regulated (Arntz *et al.*, 2007).

To increase demand, expand the range of options available to individuals and meet the needs of diverse populations, countries like the United States, the United Kingdom, Ireland, Australia, Denmark, Sweden, and Singapore have implemented a variety of LTC innovations, including blended life and LTC insurance policies, reverse mortgage/home equity conversion mortgages (e.g., where the loan is payable from the sale of the estate upon death), and closer linkages between the purchase of private LTC insurance and private medical/retirement savings accounts. In Singapore, for example, savings accumulated in a medical savings account can be used to pay for private LTC insurance premiums. However, evidence suggests that thus far, these types of innovations have had little impact on increasing the market or demand for LTC insurance and that the overall market for voluntary private LTC insurance will remain small due in large part to the factors outlined in Table 3 (Zhou-Richter *et al.*, 2010; Colombo *et al.*, 2011).

Summary

Regardless of whether LTC is publicly-financed, privately-financed or financed through a combination of public and private sources, fiscal sustainability is a primary goal worldwide and forward-looking financing policies and strategies are required to achieve it. Such policies include, among others, pre-funding, tax broadening, and intra-generational pooling of resources.

Pre-funding (building up assets to pre-fund future expected LTC-related expenditures) is one strategy suggested to address the fiscal sustainability gap, foster intergenerational equity and ensure a stable set of benefits and services over time. It is more straightforward to apply in practice among countries with dedicated revenue sources for LTC rather than general taxation (e.g., Germany, Japan, Korea, the Netherland), since pre-funding requires that governments sustain a budget surplus over a given time and surpluses are generally subject to competing demands from alternative policy priorities (Colombo *et al.*, 2011). Pre-funding requires a decision on the amount to be pre-funded, and lessons learned from the private insurance industry's experience in premium setting might be useful here.

The concept of intra-generational pooling or funding of LTC noted above is also receiving attention, which would see all individuals of a certain age and older make LTC contributions over the course of their lifespan. Tax broadening — or obtaining LTC revenues beyond those of the working age population, including retirees — is another option. Japan's LTC financing system, for example, includes both intra-generational pooling and tax broadening. Of its total LTC budget, 10% is financed through co-payments and the remaining 90% through taxes and premiums levied on the over 40 population. In Germany, individuals without children have to pay an additional LTC premium of 0.25 percentage points relative to individuals with children based on the assumption that they will use more benefits from social LTC insurance (Colombo et al., 2011). Also in Germany and in other countries including Portugal and France, children are obliged to contribute towards their parent's LTC expenses (mainly board and lodging) and their income and assets are included in the calculation that determines the level of public support their parents will receive.

Delivering LTC: The formal and informal care workforce

- *The formal LTC workforce*

The formal paid LTC workforce is predominantly comprised of (registered) nurses and personal care workers. Women make up the largest share of the workforce.

Many countries face challenges with recruiting and retaining LTC workers and these challenges are exacerbated by the fact that two major recruitment pools are shrinking: Middle-aged women; and inactive women or women with low qualifications (due to increasing labor force participation and education levels). Moreover, the global nursing shortage may have implications for the LTC sector as it is forced to compete with other sectors for nurses, many of which offer higher wages and better working conditions (Tjadens and Colombo, 2011). Indeed, difficult working conditions, low pay and limited professional development opportunities have generated high turnover among LTC providers (Stone and Harahan, 2010).

The literature points to three main policy options for developing an adequate supply of LTC workers:

- *Expand supply*: Improve recruitment of new workers to the field through a variety of mechanisms and incentives including scholarships and loan forgiveness programs as well as targeting high school students through internship opportunities.
- *Improve retention*: Evidence suggests that wages matter and could be increased to be more competitive with wages paid in other health care sectors (Stone and Harahan, 2010), but equally important is the extent to which LTC work and the workforce are valued, as evidenced by attractive benefits packages, safe and rewarding working conditions, and offering (continued) education and career development opportunities.
- *Improve productivity*: Across the OECD, variations in the number of LTC workers per LTC recipient and in skill mix (i.e., the share of nurses relative to the share of lower-skilled LTC workers) suggests that there is scope for enhancing productivity by changing staffing ratios and workers' mix of skills or qualifications (Colombo *et al.*, 2011).

• *The informal LTC workforce*

Families and informal caregivers are widely recognized as the foundation of LTC, as in a fragmented and complex system that can involve multiple providers and care settings they are often the only people who have experienced the entire trajectory of their family member's illness (Levine *et al.*, 2010). Indeed, informal caregivers provide a substantial amount of unpaid LTC related to both activities of daily living (e.g., bathing, toileting) and instrumental activities of daily living (e.g., grocery shopping, preparing meals). OECD estimates suggest that when instrumental activities of daily living are considered, close to one in three adults provides unpaid informal LTC (Colombo *et al.*, 2011). However, there is wide variation across countries in the intensity of care provided (daily versus weekly), as illustrated in Figure 7 where higher rates of daily care are observed in countries with a strong tradition of family caregiving, such as Portugal and Spain, and lower rates in countries like Sweden and Switzerland where LTC is typically provided by formal care providers. Regardless of its intensity, the care that informal caregivers provide has been increasing in complexity over time, due in part to "aging at home" policies that aim to shift care out of institutions and into the home and community, resulting in patients who are discharged from hospital with more complex and ongoing needs.

Most informal care comes from family, friends and neighbors. In terms of the demographic and socioeconomic characteristics of these informal caregivers,

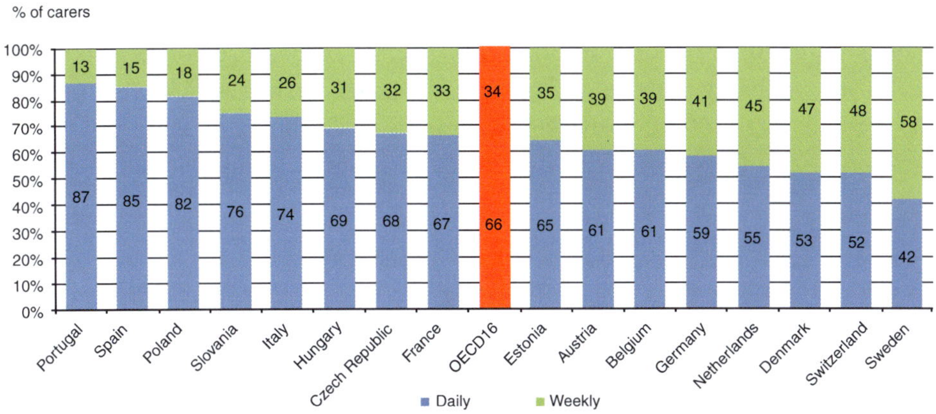

Figure 7. Intensity of care provided by informal caregivers across OECD countries, 2010

Sources: OECD estimates based on 2010 SHARE survey (OECD, 2013). OECD (2013), *Health at a Glance 2013: OECD Indicators*, OECD Publishing, Paris. http://dx.doi.org/10.1787/health-glance-2013-en.

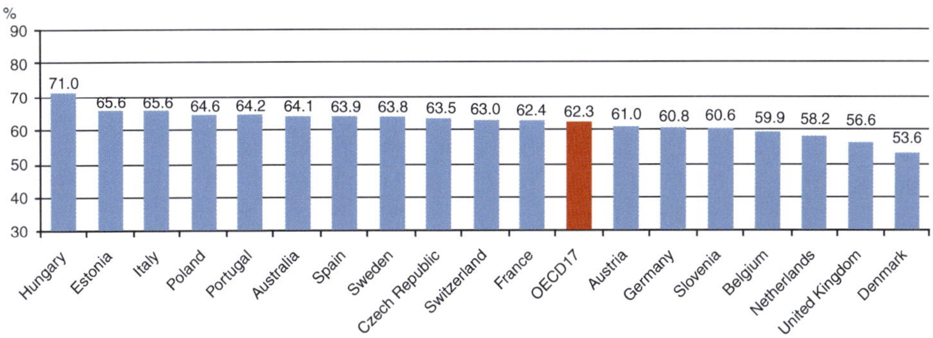

Figure 8. Share of women among all informal caregivers aged 50 and over across OECD countries, 2010

Sources: OECD estimates based on 2011 HILDA survey for Australia, 2009 BHPS survey for the United Kingdom and 2010 SHARE survey for other European countries (OECD, 2013). OECD (2013), *Health at a Glance 2013: OECD Indicators*, OECD Publishing, Paris. http://dx.doi.org/10.1787/health-glance-2013-en.

evidence across a number of countries indicates that they are more likely to be women, as illustrated in Figure 8, but that the gender distribution changes with age with males accounting for a larger proportion of informal caregivers among those aged 75 years and older (Colombo *et al.*, 2011). Overall, the prevalence of caregiving tends to decrease with age. Informal caregivers are less likely to be employed and are more likely than non-caregivers to be home makers (Lilly *et al.*, 2010). Their caregiving tends to be for their spouse or parents.

As with formal LTC providers, the future supply of informal caregivers is a policy concern in many countries. As described above, a number of factors — including the inverted age pyramid, declining family sizes, increased female labor force participation rates, and policies that delay the retirement age — have implications for the future pool of informal caregivers. There is also concern about the health and wellbeing of those who provide informal care, particularly among those who provide high-intensity levels of care (i.e., 15–20 hours or more per week), including risk of psychological distress, strain, overall health deterioration, and poverty.

Informal caregiving has important labor market consequences. Depending on the intensity of care provided, it can be challenging for informal caregivers to balance paid employment with the responsibilities of caregiving. As many informal caregivers are still in their working years, providing care for an elderly parent may have important opportunity costs in terms of labor force participation (Van Houtven *et al.*, 2013; Lilly *et al.*, 2010; Heitmueller, 2007). Indeed, empirical studies find that without support, high-intensity care-giving (generally defined as 15–20 hours or more per week) is associated with reduced hours worked per week in the magnitude of 2 to 10 hours, over-representation in part-time work, wages that are approximately 3% to 6% lower than non-caregivers, and lower levels of overall labor force participation (Jacobs *et al.*, 2013; Van Houtven *et al.*, 2013; Lilly *et al.*, 2010; Colombo *et al.*, 2011; Heitmueller and Inglis, 2007). These effects are mainly observed in women; indeed, Van Houtven *et al.*'s longitudinal analysis examined the effects for men and women separately and found little effect of caregiving on men's hours or wages (2013). In Australia and the United Kingdom where data on the nature of employment are available, caregivers are 30% more likely to hold a temporary job and have a working career that is approximately three years shorter than non-caregivers (Colombo *et al.*, 2011). The association between caregiving and labor force participation is, however, only observed among high-intensity caregivers, even after controlling for potential endogeneity that could arise if, for example, there are unobserved characteristics that make informal caregivers self-select out of the labor force and into informal caregiving or more inclined to enter informal caregiving in the first place (Lilly *et al.*, 2010; Nguyen and Connelly, 2014; Colombo *et al.*, 2011; Heitmueller, 2007). Nevertheless, the reduced labor force participation that high-intensity caregiving is associated with has implications for income tax revenues and social assistance payments that must be weighed against the potential benefit of reduced LTC expenditure.

Jacobs *et al.* (2013) estimated the costs and consequences of various intensities of unpaid caregiving from a government perspective using a cost–benefit analysis based on cross-sectional survey data and a sample of over 23,000 adults aged 45 and over. Overall, they found an overall net benefit to government from low-intensity caregiving and a net cost to government of $641 million from high-intensity caregiving. The factor that had the greatest impact on costs was labor force participation, as high-intensity caregivers were more likely to drop out of the labor force altogether. The authors conclude that government policies that help informal caregivers to balance caregiving responsibilities with paid employment are needed.

Given the impact that caregiving — and in particular high-intensity caregiving — can have on the health, wellbeing and labor force participation of informal caregivers, as well as on costs to government, it is critically important for governments to target policies and economic incentives to support informal caregiving. An analysis of informal caregiving in OECD countries identified a number of examples of such policies and incentives (Colombo *et al.*, 2011), including caregiver allowances (Slovak Republic, Canada); flexible work arrangements; paid care leave (Canada) or unpaid care leave (Germany); support services like respite care, training and counseling for caregivers (the UK); government-paid pension contributions for caregivers (Germany and Austria); government-paid health insurance contributions for caregivers (Austria); and tax credits (Canada). Some countries like the United Kingdom are also targeting informal caregiver training to formal care providers like general practitioners as a mechanism to increase recognition and support for informal caregivers. This is consistent with the recommendation made by Levine *et al.* (2010) that caregiving training and support becomes a core module of professional training and continuing education for providers, and that pay-for-performance and other incentives that include outcome measures be used to encourage broader support for informal caregivers. Evidence on the cost-effectiveness of these and other policies to support informal caregivers is critically needed.

Regulating LTC quality

Providing high-quality LTC is important for a number of reasons. In addition to having responsibility to provide effective and safe care for older adults and protection from abuse, governments are under increasing pressure to improve their accountability and demonstrate that rising LTC expenditures are contributing to high-quality care. How best to ensure the provision of quality of LTC has received significant policy and media attention, stemming in part from the various scandals reported in the media regarding poor treatment of frail elders living in publicly and privately funded LTC facilities (Mor, 2014). Regulation is a policy instrument used by governments to safeguard and control quality, oftentimes in both publicly- and privately-funded facilities, and to identify when intervention may be necessary.

Regulatory measures typically focus on the use of external controls over labor and/or infrastructure inputs, setting minimum acceptable standards, accreditation and certification of providers and organizations, and compliance enforcement (Murakami and Colombo, 2013a), though there is significant heterogeneity across countries in approaches used (Leone *et al.*, 2014).

In most OECD and EU countries, government responsibility for ensuring older adults receives quality and safe care is embedded into legislation (Murakami and Colombo, 2013a). Legislation typically defines the role of providers in ensuring the quality of services and responsibilities like reporting, and the minimum standards expected from providers. Although ultimate responsibility for regulating the quality of LTC generally rests with the central government, a number of countries delegate responsibility for implementing quality control and monitoring compliance to regional levels or arm's length organizations (Leone *et al.*, 2014). Close to one third of OECD countries have decentralized the governance of LTC to state, regional or local-level authorities, including regulating and monitoring LTC quality (Colombo *et al.*, 2011).

Licensing, certifying, and accrediting LTC providers

Most OECD countries regulate labor inputs and require LTC institutions to be officially licensed, registered or certified, although the specified qualifications and skills level vary substantially across countries (Murakami and Colombo, 2013a). Minimum standards are typically used to license, register or certify institutions as a mechanism to mitigate the risk that LTC homes provide unsafe environments or low-quality care. In general, licensure must be met to achieve market entry, while accreditation and certification pertain to quality requirements above and beyond the minimum level required to operate. In many countries, an LTC institution must be accredited or certified in order to be eligible to receive public funding (e.g., England, Spain, Ireland, France, Australia, Germany, Portugal, and the United States). In an OECD analysis of LTC quality improvement in 27 countries, over two-thirds of the countries had accreditation systems in place (Murakami and Colombo, 2013a). The accreditation process typically involves a review of performance against standards set by the accreditation body, self-assessment by the care providers, and ongoing monitoring of performance against the standards. In some countries, recertification or accreditation must be renewed every few years.

Standards to ensure quality care

Partly because self-regulation of quality care does not always work, minimum quality standards are used in a number of countries and are often key elements of evaluation criteria for accreditation or certification. They typically relate to labor and capital inputs, the care process (e.g., quality management systems, medication management, individualized care plans, reporting systems for adverse events and complaints), and expected outputs (e.g., user rights, quality of life) (Murakami and Colombo, 2013a and 2013b).

Examples of common requirements found in a number of OECD countries include staffing structures (e.g., the ratio of registered nurses to personal care workers), the use of quality management systems designed to enhance care processes and outcomes, and setting educational and training requirements of personal care workers. A requirement around the ratio of skilled LTC providers (e.g., nurses and personal care workers) to care recipients is also common, though comparisons across countries and even within countries are difficult as the requirement may be based on the number of staff hours per resident or the total number of full-time staff per resident and, in both cases, the number tends to depend on resident's level of care needs. For example, in LTC facilities across Austria's regions, the number of full-time equivalents (FTE) to residents ranges from 1:10 to 1:24 for those with the lowest level of care needs, and from 1:1 to 1:2 for those with the highest level of care needs (Leichsenring *et al.*, 2014). Conversely in Japan, the nurse to resident ratio must be 1:3 such that a LTC facility with less than 30 residents is required to have one FTE nurse, a facility with 30 to 50 residents is required to have two FTE nurses, and a facility with over 50 residents must have 3 FTE nurses (Ikegami *et al.,* 2014). Murakami and Colombo (2013a) point out that education and qualification requirements of personal care workers varies significantly across countries, ranging from 75 hours in the United States to three years in Japan for similar jobs. Standards and related qualification requirements for LTC providers are generally higher in LTC institutions than for home settings. For example, in the United States, two weeks of training for personal care workers with a high-school diploma is required for home-based care while 75 hours of classroom and practical training is required to work in certified nursing homes. Similarly, in Austria, 400 hours of theoretical and practical instruction is required for home assistants while 1600 hours of practical training is required for those working in a nursing home (Murakami and Colombo, 2013a). Leone *et al.* (2014) note that "homecare remains the most neglected sector from a quality assurance perspective."

Compliance enforcement

Monitoring compliance with standards is primarily performed through surveys and site visit inspections (including unannounced site visit inspections). Some inspections also involve interviews with LTC recipients, their families and facility staff. The frequency with which they are performed varies widely across countries, ranging from one (Germany, Luxembourg, Portugal, and Ontario) to five or seven years (France) or upon request following complaints (Finland, Sweden) (Murakami and Colombo, 2013a). The results of inspections and audits reveal important information about gaps in quality, with common deficiencies including site safety (e.g., infection control), quality of care services and management (e.g., inadequate medication management and records), inadequate staff and training of staff, and lack of re-assessment of recipients' care needs (Murakami and Colombo, 2013a). The consequences of non-compliance are for the most part minimal as most facilities meet the standards and few are sanctioned for non-compliance (Leone *et al.*, 2014; Miller and Mor, 2008; Murakami and Colombo, 2013). This has led some to question the value of compliance enforcement, which is also criticized as being expensive and stifling innovation (Miller and Mor, 2008; Murakami and Colombo, 2013a).

Empirical evidence on the impact of regulation on LTC quality

Empirical evidence on the impact of regulation on quality is limited. The few studies available suggest that stricter control of the LTC industry may improve residents' living conditions, quality of care and quality of life, though these studies are criticized for having methodological limitations including lack of a control group, lack of pre-regulation data, and use of data collected by the LTC facilities themselves (Bravo *et al.*, 2014; Miller and Mor, 2008). A 2014 study in Quebec, Canada empirically examined the impact of a natural experiment involving the government's decision in 2007 to regulate private LTC facilities and found that following the introduction of regulation, quality of care in private facilities improved (Bravo *et al.*, 2014). The authors hypothesize that the observed quality improvements may be attributed in part to the closure of small homes and decrease in resident case-mix complexity that occurred in the private sector following the implementation of regulation. Though the study included a control group (i.e., public facilities, which had been subject to regulation both before and after the introduction of private facility regulation), causation could not be established as cross-sectional data were used.

A recent book on regulating LTC quality using international comparative analysis and in-depth country case studies concluded that "at present there is no consensus as to what constitutes quality LTC nor is there any common framework for measuring it from country to country" (Mor, 2014). Recent calls for "smarter regulation" encourage improvements in data quality, real-time monitoring, and the integration of continuous quality improvement into the oversight process (Miller and Mor, 2008).

The Future of LTC

The importance of prevention, promoting healthy aging, and supportive environments

- *Prevention in LTC*

Population-based interventions to promote health and prevent or postpone disease among older adults are critically important for a number of reasons, including but not limited to improved health and wellbeing, delayed or reduced need for institutional care, and reduced health care utilization and costs (Rechel *et al.*, 2009; Tjadens and Colombo, 2011). When older adults are in good health, studies have shown that they will require fewer health care services and be more likely to remain in the labor force (Rechel *et al.*, 2009). However, questions remain regarding the extent to which prevention is the responsibility of the LTC sector and evidence about the cost-effectiveness of prevention-based interventions is limited given that few have been subject to an economic evaluation.

Japan is recognized as a country that has implemented an innovative prevention-oriented benefit directly within its LTC scheme. In 2006, the Japanese government introduced a community-based prevention benefit within its LTC scheme to improve physical and mental health (e.g., exercise and dementia programs) and quality of life among older adults at risk of needing future care or support (Fukutomi *et al.*, 2013; Tsutsui and Muramatsu, 2007). The underlying goal is to improve the sustainability of the overall LTC insurance scheme, which had attracted higher-than-anticipated uptake when it was introduced in 2000 and, consequently, incurred higher-than-anticipated expenditures (Ishibashi and Ikegami, 2010). Reducing incentives for institutionalization and preventing seniors from becoming dependent by intervening when their care need levels are still low are the key components of the "Prevention of LTC Project," which involves community-based exercise programs, cognitive improvement programs, and malnutrition prevention programs. Some of the preventive services are the same as the traditional LTC services though now framed within the goal of preventing people from becoming dependent (Tsutsui and Muramatsu, 2007). Though widely recognized as an innovative concept, evaluation of the scheme is mixed: Some studies report that there has been a decline in the enrolment and use of LTC services by people with lighter care-need levels, and that savings in LTC insurance have been realized (Campbell *et al.*, 2010; Colombo *et al.*, 2011), while others report that the program did not achieve its intended effect of reducing use of LTC services (Ishibashi and Ikegami, 2010). Further longitudinal analysis of its intended and unintended consequences is needed.

- *Supporting healthy aging and environments in LTC*

As with prevention interventions, policies to support healthy aging and environments for current and future older adults are increasingly recognized as critically important. Several policies fall under the broad umbrella of healthy aging, including increasing community activities to foster social engagement and mitigate risk of cognitive decline and depression; implementing supportive labor and employment policies to enable older adults to remain in paid work; improving lifestyles, health literacy and self-management; providing good quality housing and supportive living environments; better adapting health care systems to the needs of the elderly (Rechel *et al.*, 2009). However, only few countries have integrated specific healthy aging objectives or interventions as part of their LTC insurance systems and uncertainty remains regarding which interventions are most effective and cost-effective (Oxley, 2009; Colombo *et al.*, 2011; Rechel *et al.*, 2009).

Encouraging appropriate use of LTC

LTC is one part of a continuum of health and social care that older adults require. For efficiency, sustainability and appropriateness reasons, it is important to ensure that care is provided in the right setting, that integrated delivery systems are in place encompassing both formal and informal care, and both health and social services, and that transition along the care continuum are as seamless as possible. This can be challenging to achieve for a number of reasons, including the rise in multimorbidity which means that older adults are often seeing a number of different providers of both social and health services (Rechel *et al.*, 2009).

Appropriate utilization can be fostered through a variety of mechanisms such as ensuring adequate supply of services outside hospital and LTC institutions, using payment and coverage systems to incentivize care provision and utilization in appropriate settings, and using multidisciplinary teams and case management to guide users through the continuum of care (Colombo *et al.*, 2011; Johri *et al.*, 2003).

A number of countries have implemented integrated community-based care systems for older adults with varying degrees of success. The On Lok and Program of All-Inclusive Care for the Elderly (PACE) in the United States, the Program of Research to Integrate Services for the Maintenance of Autonomy (PRISMA) and SIPA in Quebec, Canada, and the Darlington model in the United Kingdom are examples that have been relatively well evaluated and analyzed from a comparative perspective. Scoping reviews and comparative analyses of these and other integrated community-based care systems for seniors identify a set of core characteristics that appear to be present in all successful integrated systems, including a multidisciplinary care team with case management, a scope that includes both horizontal and vertical integration, a single point of entry, a person-centered focus and the involvement of caregivers, and financial levers to promote prevention and the downward substation of services (Kodner, 2006; Johri *et al.*, 2003; Williams *et al.*, 2009). Despite heterogeneity in evaluation methodologies, as well as some conflicting results, on the whole the literature suggests that integrated community-based care for older adults can improve access to and use of community services and reduce rates of institutionalization and costs (Johri *et al.*, 2003; Kodner, 2006).

Optimizing LTC quality, efficiency, and value-for-money

Improving quality, efficiency and value-for-money in LTC are goals for most countries, however there are very few empirical assessments or formal evaluations of LTC strategies designed to achieve these policy objectives. Two broad categories of such strategies include public reporting (to inform consumer choice) and provider incentives (to encourage efficiency and quality improvements). Foundational to these market-based incentive strategies is a robust quality measurement system that generates real-time information on LTC quality that can be publicized to inform user choice and incentivize provider behavior.

• *Quality measurement in LTC*

Quality measurement in LTC has been criticized as lagging behind other health care sectors (Murakami and Colombo, 2013b). Only a few OECD countries have robust information systems and indicators for LTC quality and these vary across countries, making cross-country comparisons challenging. Information on LTC quality is derived from a variety of sources, including from standardized assessment instruments like the Resident Assessment Instrument, administrative data, LTC registries, and *ad hoc* surveys of individuals or facilities. While most countries have data on LTC inputs like staffing levels and mix, few countries have data on outputs and outcomes (Murakami and Colombo, 2013b).

Reporting on LTC quality indicators also varies substantially across countries. Quality indicators generally relate to clinical quality (e.g., incidence of falls and fall-related factures, incidence of medication errors, incidence of depression), responsiveness and care coordination (e.g., wait times for LTC admission, avoidable hospital admission for ambulatory care sensitive conditions), and quality of life (primarily based on patient surveys of their experience and/or satisfaction). The challenge with LTC indicators and the instruments used for measurement, particularly with quality of life, is that they can vary widely across countries, making cross-national comparisons challenging (Mor, 2005; Van Malderen *et al.*, 2013). The use of standardized instruments like the Resident Assessment Instrument is believed to hold promise for cross-institution and cross-jurisdictional analyses and for quality improvement outcomes, though a recent systematic review on the use of standardized data for process and quality improvement in LTC suggests more research is needed to understand how to intervene effectively and successfully (Sales *et al.*, 2012).

• *Market-based approaches: Public reporting and provider incentives*

Market-based approaches to improving quality, efficiency and value-for-money in LTC are gaining traction. Pay-for-performance and public reporting, which aim to change the underlying incentive structure facing providers and patients, are two of the dominant approaches used. Both are based on the premise that with the right information provided in the right format, patients will choose the most appropriate settings and types of services given their needs and preferences and, similarly, with the right information, providers will find the most efficient and effective ways to improve quality and outcomes, and thus compete for patients based on quality (Konetzka and Werner, 2010). However, there has been little experimentation and formal evaluation in this arena.

According to recent international comparative analyses (Murakami and Colombo, 2013a and 2013b; Rodrigues *et al.*, 2014), a number of countries monitor LTC quality and performance and publicly report on the results. Public reporting is mandatory in the United States, Japan, England, Germany, Portugal, the Netherlands, and Ontario, Canada. The frequency and level of reporting (e.g., at facility versus provider level), emphasis on process versus outcome indicators, data reporting requirements (e.g., mandatory versus voluntary) and display of information (e.g., star or grade ratings, etc.) vary by country. There is, however, little empirical evidence that public reporting on LTC outcomes leads to improved quality care and where it exists, results are mixed and inconclusive (Mor, 2005; Murakami and Colombo, 2013a and 2013b; Rodrigues *et al.*, 2014). Evidence suggests there is room for improvement in raising public awareness about LTC indicators, in how information is displayed and shared, in the actionability of indicators, and in involving end users in the development of indicators (Rodrigues *et al.*, 2014). It has been recognized that more research is needed to understand if and how consumers use this information to select providers and whether these efforts lead to improvements in care outcomes, and how providers respond to or are activated by the information to change behavior and improve quality (Mor, 2005; Rodrigues *et al.*, 2014). Evidence from the broader field of public reporting in health care suggests that public reporting will have a greater impact on provider behavior than on consumers (Rodrigues *et al.*, 2014).

The issue of how to incentivize LTC providers has received little attention to date but there is growing interest in aligning remuneration mechanisms with LTC system goals. Per diem reimbursement and salaries are typically used in institutional settings, and these come with the standard unintended consequences. Per diem rates that are not risk-adjusted may incentivize cream-skimming, and salary payments that are not aligned with quality or productivity-related goals may incentivize low productivity. Pay-for-performance initiatives — where provider remuneration is based on quality and/or outcomes of care rather than intensity of care — are increasingly common in many health care settings but not yet in LTC and limited to a few examples in the US Medicaid program. There are few formal evaluations of their impacts and the evaluations that do exist point to inconsistent and mixed results, with quality improvements seen in some but not other state

Medicaid nursing homes (Werner *et al.*, 2013). Lack of impact could be attributed to a variety of factors that require further analysis, including incentives that are too small to modify change (i.e., research has shown that the bonus payment should exceed the marginal cost of quality improvement, though with nursing homes in the United States the bonus payments were relatively small), the infrequency of reporting/feedback on performance, and the fact that the incentive or bonus was paid to the nursing home rather than to the individual staff members of the nursing home (Werner *et al.*, 2013).

Research gaps and opportunities for the future

While a number of promising LTC innovations and interventions are taking shape in the LTC sector, a consistent theme throughout this chapter has been the need for better data and more formal evaluations of the impact of these innovations and interventions on widely held health system goals like access, quality, efficiency, sustainability, and health and wellbeing.

With an expected rise in demand for LTC that will put inevitable pressure on limited public funds, developing measures for the economic evaluation (e.g., cost–utility analysis) of LTC interventions will be particularly important. Such measures will need to capture more than health-related quality of life given that improved health outcomes may not be the primary or an appropriate goal of health care services aimed at older adults (Makai *et al.*, 2014; Nieboer *et al.*, 2010). In LTC, for example, interventions may focus primarily on improving non-health aspects of quality of life — such as maintaining independence, dignity, comfort or social interaction — and evaluating such interventions using health-related quality of life instruments may undervalue the non-health benefits (Makai *et al.*, 2014). A systematic review of quality of life and well-being instruments for economic evaluations in LTC for older people identified four promising wellbeing instruments, each with limitations (e.g., health dimensions were only partially captured, preference weights were not available, or the instrument required further validation), and ultimately recommended using the ICECAP-O (the ICEpop CAPability measure for Older people, which is a preference-weighted measure of capability or "wellbeing" in older people) or the ASCOT (the adult social care outcomes toolkit, which is a preference-weighted measure of social care-related quality of life) — both of which have preference-weights but may only partially capture health dimensions and require further validation — alongside the widely utilized and validated EQ-5D or SF-6D instruments (Makai *et al.*, 2014).

Given current emphasis on patient-centered care, understanding user preferences and willingness to pay for various LTC benefits is another area in need of future research attention. Achieving efficient resource allocation decisions that meet user expectations requires knowledge on how individuals place value on particular aspects of LTC. The literature contains a dearth of discrete choice and willingness to pay experiments (Nieboer, 2014).

Conclusions

Population aging is one of the most important demographic trends facing countries worldwide and LTC systems need to be adequately equipped and financed to proactively anticipate and respond to the health needs of older adults. Different LTC systems are at very different stages of development, and much can be learned from the experiences of other countries with respect to the policies, strategies and interventions they are using to prepare their LTC systems for an increasingly aging population.

Key policy issues that are common across a number of countries and that warrant future attention include:

- **Ensuring the fiscal sustainability of LTC systems:** Population aging and increasing life expectancy, coupled with other trends related to the supply of informal caregivers and a rise in the number of older adults living alone, create two potentially major pressures on LTC systems and finances: Increased demand for and utilization of health and social services, and decreased revenues (as a declining share of the population is economically active). Designing LTC financing and delivery systems that are forward-looking, consider long-term fiscal sustainability (and mitigate the potential for inter- and intra-generational inequities), and remain affordable to users is a top priority policy concern. Publicly-financed targeted universal coverage schemes with forward-looking financing systems (e.g., tax broadening, intra-generational pooling of funds, pre-funding) appear to hold promise and, in particular, social insurance schemes where contributions remain earmarked for LTC and are not subject to competition from other demands on public finances as is the case with tax-financed systems. Incorporating prevention and healthy aging strategies within LTC schemes is also garnering increased attention, though robust evaluations of their impact and cost-effectiveness are needed.
- **Ensuring adequate workforce supply to meet demand for care:** Both formal and informal caregivers are essential to meeting rising demand for LTC. Among formal paid care providers (e.g., nurses and personal care workers), difficult working conditions, low pay and limited professional development opportunities have generated high turnover. Improved recruitment and retention strategies are needed, as are mechanism to optimize scopes of practice.

- **Identifying the optimal mix of supports for informal caregivers:** Informal caregivers are an important pillar of LTC but high-intensity caregiving has negative consequences their mental and physical health and paid labor force participation rates. Maintaining their health and wellbeing and thus their continued engagement in providing informal LTC is critical to ensuring adequate supply of current and future caregivers. Countries are experimenting with different supports, incentives and benefits to recognize and value the contributions of informal caregivers, but evidence on the optimal mix of supportive policies is lacking. Additionally, if individuals substitute providing informal care for paid employment due to lack of available formal care alternatives or inflexible work arrangements, supportive policies may help. However, if individuals substitute providing informal care for paid employment because of lack of employability, other types of policies will be needed (i.e., skills training).
- **Reducing fragmentation of LTC services:** This chapter has illustrated that the LTC sector is complex. LTC services are financed by a number of differed payers, provided by a range of different formal and informal caregivers, and delivered in a number of different settings. This complex and oftentimes fragmented system can be challenging for frail older adults to navigate and can result in unmet needs, discontinuities in care, inappropriate utilization and inefficient resource allocation. Policies that promote better integration and improved continuity of care are needed.
- **Fostering innovation, quality, efficiency and value-for-money in LTC:** Much can be learned from the experiences of other health sectors regarding how best to stimulate innovation, improve quality, drive efficiency and achieve value-for-money in LTC. Potential promising practices at this point in time include market-based incentives like pay-for-performance and public reporting. Harnessing the potential of technology to improve productivity is another potential avenue for innovative experimentation (e.g., for patient empowerment, advanced decision support, remote health monitoring and care delivery, population health surveillance and more).
- **Data and evaluation:** Given the magnitude of expenditures the LTC sector is facing and the critical importance of ensuring safe, high-quality and appropriate LTC is provided to an oftentimes vulnerable population, a policy priority for governments around the world should be improving the quality and accessibility of LTC data. The use of common measures and instruments across countries whenever possible will facilitate cross-jurisdictional comparisons and analyses. Encouraging robust evaluations of new LTC policies and interventions should also be top priority.

In summary, this chapter considered the implications of an aging population for LTC, including the factors that are expected to drive demand for and expenditure on LTC, as well as options for financing, delivering, and regulating high-quality, accessible and appropriate LTC. It drew upon data and case studies from a number of international comparative analyses (e.g., OECD, European Observatory, European Commission) to illustrate both differences and commonalities across countries in their LTC systems. The chapter concluded with evidence-informed reflections on the future of LTC, including policy options to improve the quality, efficiency, and value-for-money in an increasingly high-priority sector.

References

Ansah JP, Eberlein RL, Love SR, Bautista MA, Thompson JP, *et al.* 2014. Implications of long-term care capacity response policies for an aging population: A simulation analysis. *Health Policy* 116: 105–113.

Arntz M, Sacchetto R, Spermann A, Steffes S, Widmaier S. 2007. The German Social Long-Term Care Insurance: Structure and Reform Options. *IZA Discussion Paper No. 2625* Bonn, Germany.

Barr N. 2010. Long-term care: A suitable case for social insurance. *Social Policy and Administration* 44(4): 359–374.

Bravo G, Dubois MF, Demersa L, Dubuc N, Blanchette D, *et al.* 2014. Does regulating private long-term care facilities lead to better care? A study from Quebec, Canada. *International Journal for Quality in Health Care* 26(3): 330–336.

Brown JR, Goda GS, McGarry K. 2012. Long-term care insurance demand limited by beliefs about needs, concerns about insurers, and care available from family. *Health Affairs* 31(6): 1294–1302.

Busse R, Blumel M. 2014. Germany: Health system review. *Health Systems in Transition* 16(2):1–296. http://www.euro.who.int/__data/assets/pdf_file/0008/255932/HiT-Germany.pdf?ua=1.

Campbell JN, Ikegami N, Gibson MJ. 2010. Lessons from public long-term care insurance in Germany and Japan. *Health Affairs* 29(1): 87–95.

Canadian Institutes of Health Information. 2011. Health care in Canada 2011: A focus on seniors and aging. https://secure.cihi.ca/free_products/HCIC_2011_seniors_report_en.pdf.

Canadian Institutes of Health Information. 2013. National health expenditure trends: 1975–2013. https://secure.cihi.ca/free_products/NHEXTrendsReport_EN.pdf.

Colombo F, Llena-Nozal A, Mercier J, Tjadens F. 2011. *Help Wanted? Providing and Paying for Long-term Care*. Paris: OECD Publishing.

Colombo F, Mercier J. 2011. Help wanted! Balancing fair protection and financial sustainability in long-term care. *Eurohealth* 17(2–3): 3–6.

Comas-Herrera A, Malley J, Wittenberg R, Hu B, Jagger C. 2011. Disability, dementia and the future costs of long-term care. *Eurohealth* 17(2–3): 10–12.

Cuellar AE, Wiener JM. 2000. Can social insurance for long-term care work? The experience of Germany. *Health Affairs* 19(3): 8–25.

European Commission. 2009. The 2009 aging report: Economic and budgetary projections for the 27 EU member states (2008–2060). *European Commission*, ISBN 978-92-79-11363-9, doi 10.2765/80301. http://ec.europa.eu/economy_finance/publications/publication14992_en.pdf.

European Commission. 2012. The 2012 aging report: economic and budgetary projections for the 27 EU member states (2010–2060). *European Commission*, ISBN 978-92-79-22850-6, doi: 10.2765/19991. http://ec.europa.eu/economy_finance/publications/european_economy/2012/pdf/ee-2012-2_en.pdf.

Fernández JL, Forder J, Trukeschitz B, Rokosová M, McDaid D. 2009. How can European states design efficient, equitable and sustainable funding systems for long-term care for older people? Policy Brief, No. 11, European Observatory on Health Systems and Policies, WHO Regional Office for Europe, Copenhagen.

Fukutomi E, Kimura Y, Wada T, Okumiva K, Matsubayashi K. 2013. Long-term care prevention project in Japan. *Lancet* 381(9861): 116. doi: 10.1016/S0140-6736(13)60049-5.

Garms-Homolova V, Busse R. 2014. Monitoring the quality of long-term care in Germany. In *Regulating Long-Term Care Quality: An International Comparison*. Vincent Mor, Tiziana Leone and Anna Maresso (eds.). Cambridge: Cambridge University Press. ISBN: 9781107323711.

Heitmueller A. 2007. The chicken or the egg? Endogeneity in labour market participation of informal carers in England. *Journal of Health Economics* 26(3): 536–559.

Heitmueller A, Inglis K. 2007. The earnings of informal carers: Wage differentials and opportunity costs. *Journal of Health Economics* 26: 821–841.

Ikegami N, Ishibashi T, Amano T. 2014. Japan's long-term care regulations focused on structure — Rationale and future prospects. In *Regulating Long-Term Care Quality: An International Comparison*, Vincent Mor, Tiziana Leone and Anna Maresso (eds.). Cambridge: Cambridge University Press. ISBN: 9781107323711.

Ishibashi T, Ikegami N. 2010. Should the provision of home help services be contained?: Validation of the new preventive care policy in Japan. *BMC Health Services Research* 2(10): 224. doi: 10.1186/1472-6963-10-224.

Jacobs JC, Laporte A, Van Houtven CH, Coyte PC. 2014. Caregiving intensity and retirement status in Canada. *Social Science & Medicine* 102: 74–82.

Jacobs JC, Lilly MB, Ng C, Coyte PC. 2013. The fiscal impact of informal caregiving to home care recipients in Canada: How the intensity of care influences costs and benefits to government. *Social Science & Medicine* 81: 201–109.

Jagger C, Matthews M, Lindesay J, Brayne C. 2011. The impact of changing patterns of disease on disability and the need for long-term care. *Eurohealth* 17(2–3): 7–9.

Johri M, Beland F, Bergman H. 2003. International experiments in integrated care for the elderly: A synthesis of the evidence. *International Journal of Geriatric Psychiatry* 18: 222–235.

Kemper P, Alecxih L. 2005. Long-term care over an uncertain future: What can current retirees expect? *Inquiry* 42(4): 335–350.

Kodner DL. 2006. Whole-system approaches to health and social care partnerships for the frail elderly: An exploration of North American models and lessons. *Health and Social Care in the Community* 14(5): 384–390.

Konetzka RT, Werner RM. 2010. Applying market-based reforms to long-term care. *Health Affairs(Millwood)* 29(1): 74–80.

Lafortune G, Balestat G. 2007. Trends in severe disability among elderly people: Assessing the evidence in 12 OECD countries and the future implications. *OECD Health Working Paper* No 26. Paris: OECD Publishing, 2007

Leichsenring K, Lamontagne-Godwin F, Schmidt A, Rodrigues R, Ruppe G. 2014. Performance measurement in long-term care in Austria. In *Regulating Long-Term Care Quality: An International Comparison*, Vincent Mor, Tiziana Leone and Anna Maresso (eds.). Cambridge: Cambridge University Press. ISBN: 9781107323711.

Leone T, Maresso A, Mor V. 2014. Regulating quality of long-term care — what have we learned? In *Regulating Long-Term Care Quality: An International Comparison*, Vincent Mor, Tiziana Leone and Anna Maresso (eds.). Cambridge: Cambridge University Press. ISBN: 9781107323711.

Levine C, Halper C, Preist A, Gould DA. 2010. Bridging troubled waters: Family caregivers, transitions, and long-term care. *Health Affairs* 29(1): 116–124.

Lilly MB, Laporte A, Coye PC. 2010. Do they care too much to work? The influence of caregiving intensity on the labour force participation of unpaid caregivers in Canada. *Journal of Health Economics* 29: 895–903.

Makai P, Brouwer WB, Koopmanschap MA, Stolk EA, Nieboer AP. 2014. Quality of life instruments for economic evaluations in health and social care for older people: A systematic review. *Social Science & Medicine* 102: 83–93.

Miller EA, Mor V. 2008. Balancing regulatory controls and incentives: toward smarter and more transparent oversight in long-term care. *Journal of Health Politics, Policy and Law* 33(2): 249–279.

Mor V. 2005. Improving the quality of long-term care with better information. *The Milbank Quarterly* 83(3): 333–364.

Mor V. 2014. A framework for understanding regulation of long-term care quality. In *Regulating Long-Term Care Quality: An International Comparison*, Vincent Mor, Tiziana Leone and Anna Maresso (eds.). Cambridge: Cambridge University Press. ISBN: 9781107323711.

Murakami Y, Colombo F. 2013a. Regulation to improve quality in long-term care. In OECD/European Union, *A Good Life in Old Age?: Monitoring and Improving Quality in Long-term Care.* OECD Publishing.

Murakami Y, Colombo F. 2013b. Measuring quality in long-term care. In OECD/European Union, *A Good Life in Old Age?: Monitoring and Improving Quality in Long-term Care.* OECD Publishing.

Nguyen HT, Connelly LB. 2014. The effect of unpaid caregiving intensity on labour force participation: Results from a multinomial endogenous treatment model. *Social Science & Medicine* 100: 115–122.

Nieboer AP, Koolman X, Stolk EA. 2010. Preferences for long-term care services: Willingness to pay estimates derived from a discrete choice experiment. *Social Science & Medicine* 70(9): 1317–1325. doi: 10.1016/j.

Nieboer P. 2014. Quality of life instruments for economic evaluations in health and social care for older people: A systematic review. *Social Science & Medicine* 102: 83–93.

OECD. 2013. Informal carers. *Health at a Glance 2013: OECD Indicators.* OECD Publishing.

OECD. 2014. OECD health data: Health expenditure and financing: Health expenditure indicators. *OECD Health Statistics* (database). doi: 10.1787/data-00349-en.

Oxley H. 2009. Policies for healthy aging: An overview. *OECD Health Working Papers* No. 42. Paris, OECD.

Payne G, Laporte A, Deber R, Coyte PC. 2007. Counting backward to health care's future: using time-to-death modeling to identify changes in end-of-life morbidity and the impact of aging on health care expenditures. *The Milbank Quarterly* 85(2): 213–257.

Rechel B, Doyle Y, Grundy E, McKee M. 2009. How can health systems respond to population aging? Policy Brief, No. 10, European Observatory on Health Systems and Policies, WHO Regional Office for Europe, Copenhagen.

Rodrigues R, Trigg L, Schmidt AE, Leichsenring K. 2014. The public gets what the public wants: Experiences of public reporting in long-term care in Europe. *Health Policy* 116: 84–94.

Sales AE *et al.* 2012. The use of data for process and quality improvement in long term care and home care: A systematic review of the literature. *Journal of the American Medical Directors Association* 13: 103–113.

Stevenson DG, Cohen MA, Tell EJ, Burwell B. 2010. The complementarity of public and private long-term care coverage. *Health Affairs* 29(1): 96–101.

Stone R, Harahan MF. 2010. Improving the long-term care workforce serving older adults. *Health Affairs* 29(1): 109–115.

Tjadens F, Colombo F. 2011. Long-term care: Valuing care providers. *Eurohealth* 17(2–3): 13–17.

Tsutsui T, Muramatsu N. 2007. Japan's universal long-term care system reform of 2005: Containing costs and realizing a vision. *Journal of the American Geriatrics Society* 55: 1458–1463.

U.S. Census Bureau. 2014. 65+ in the United States: 2010, U.S. Government Printing Office, Washington, DC.

Van Malderen L, Mets T, Gorus E. 2013. Interventions to enhance the quality of life of older people in residential long-term care: A systematic review. *Aging Research Reviews* 12: 141–150.

Van Houtven CH, Coe NB, Skira MM. 2013. The effect of informal care on work and wages. *Journal of Health Economics* 32(1): 240–252.

Werner RM, Konetzka RT, Polsky D. 2013. The effect of pay-for-performance in nursing homes: Evidence from state Medicaid programs. *Health Services Research* 48(4): 1393–1414.

Williams AP, Challis D, Deber R, Watkins J, Kuluski K, Lum JM *et al*. 2009. Balancing institutional and community-based care: why some older persons can age successfully at home while others require residential long-term care. *Healthcare Quarterly* 12: 95–105.

Zhou-Richter T, Browne MJ, Grundi H. 2010. Don't they care? Or, are they just unaware? Risk perception and the demand for long-term care insurance. *Journal of Risk and Insurance* 77(4): 715–747.

Dental Care

Marko Vujicic
Health Policy Institute, American Dental Association
Eduardo Bernabé
Division of Population and Patient Health, King's College London Dental Institute
Daniela Garbin Neumann
CAPES Foundation, Ministry of Education of Brazil
Carlos Quiñonez
Faculty of Dentistry, University of Toronto
Elizabeth Mertz
Preventive and Restorative Dental Sciences, School of Dentistry
University of California

Oral health is closely linked to whole-body health. Healthy gums are associated with a lower risk of heart disease and diabetes, although the exact nature of the links is not fully understood. Routine dental care and other preventive measures in childhood have a significant impact on oral health throughout adulthood. Water fluoridation has been identified as one of the most successful public health interventions of the 20th century. Improved oral health has been linked to enhanced career earnings and other economic benefits as well. Yet in both developed and developing countries, many segments of the population do have adequate access to dental care. In fact, tooth decay is the most prevalent chronic disease for children worldwide. Dental care is often financed and delivered entirely separately from medical care. In this chapter, we analyze select aspects of dental care systems. To begin, we summarize the evidence on the burden of disease for oral conditions and compare oral health across select countries. We then review dental care systems in select countries to illustrate alternative approaches to dental care financing and service delivery. We also analyze the available multi-country data on dental care spending, the supply of dental care providers, dental care utilization, dental insurance, and financial barriers to dental care. Finally, we outline policy options available to address some of the key challenges facing dental care systems and identify critical knowledge gaps that need to be filled in order to help advance policy.

Introduction

The mouth is connected to the body. Thus, not surprisingly, oral health is linked to whole-body health in many ways. For example, although the exact nature of the relationship is not fully understood, healthy gums are associated with a lower risk of heart disease (Lockhart *et al.*, 2012) and diabetes (Simpson *et al.*, 2010). These links are increasingly important given the shifting global burden of disease toward non-communicable conditions. Some cancers and infections that occur in the mouth are also closely linked with those that occur in other parts of the body (Lamster and Eaves, 2011). Dental caries (tooth decay) is the most prevalent chronic disease for children worldwide (World Health Organization (WHO), 2003) and can lead to significant development problems, and indeed even the US Surgeon General has emphasized the importance of the relationship between oral and whole-body health in stating that "you can't be healthy without good oral health" (Department of Health and Human Services (DHHS), 2000). As research advances, new relationships are emerging between oral and whole-body health. In fact, two recent studies have found an association between oral health and cognitive function after controlling for confounding factors (Naorungroj *et al.,* 2013; Stewart *et al.*, 2008).

Aside from the impact on overall health, there is emerging evidence on the economic benefits associated with improved oral health. For example, in the United States, for every 100 children aged 5–17, it is estimated that three days of school per year are missed because of dental symptoms and treatment and for every 100 employees, two days of work per year are lost due to poor oral health. Diminished oral health has also been linked with lower career earnings (Glied and Neidell, 2010). In Thailand, 74% of 35–44-year-olds reported that their state of oral health affected their daily performance, and 46% reported their emotional stability was affected (Adulyanon *et al.*, 1996).

From a broader health systems perspective, there are potential health care cost-savings associated with increased dental care use and improved oral health. A recent analysis showed that treatment of gum disease has been associated with lower overall medical costs among those with diabetes and heart disease and stroke patients (Cigna, 2010). Routine preventive dental care lowers the chance of advanced dental disease in later years and reduces overall dental care treatment costs (Savage *et al.*, 2004). Water fluoridation, due to its significant impact on lowering the rate of dental disease, has been cited as one of the most successful public health interventions of the 20th century (Centers for Disease Control and Prevention (CDC), 1999). It is estimated that one dollar of investment in water fluoridation saves 38 dollars in dental treatment costs (CDC, 2013).

The key drivers of oral health include oral hygiene, nutrition, preventive interventions such as fluoridation, and dental care utilization (CDC, 2006). There is considerable variation across countries in how dental care is delivered and paid for.

In many countries, the dental care system is largely separated from the medical care system, with independent financing, governance, and service delivery arrangements. In some countries, however, there is much more coordination and integration of dental care services with the broader medical care system.

Health economists have observed several important characteristics of the market for dental care, and noted some key distinctions from medical care (Sintonen and Linnosmaa, 2000). There are relatively few dental diseases and their occurrence is more predictable. Patients experience the same dental procedures through the course of their lives and can gain an understanding of the benefits and costs of treatments. In this sense, the potential information asymmetry between patients and providers may be less severe in dentistry than in other medical fields. Dental disease is highly preventable. For example, routine preventive care, fluoride, and a consistent oral health regimen that includes brushing and flossing are very effective ways to prevent dental disease. Finally, dental care is rarely an emergency. These factors help explain why in many settings dental care systems have evolved separately from medical care. However, these peculiarities in the market for dental care do not explain why there is so much variation in dental care systems across countries.

In this chapter, we focus on four objectives. First, we summarize the evidence on the burden of disease for oral conditions and compare oral health across select countries. Second, we review select dental care systems around the world to illustrate alternative approaches to dental care financing and service delivery. As part of this review, we summarize the available data on dental care spending and the supply of dental care providers in various countries. Third, we summarize data on insurance coverage for, utilization of, and financial barriers to dental care for select countries. Fourth, we identify key challenges facing dental care systems in both developed and developing countries and outline policy options available to address some of these challenges. We also identify critical knowledge gaps that need to be filled in order to help advance oral health policy.

(1) Oral health status — burden of disease and oral health outcomes

Two useful indicators determine if a health condition is an important public health problem: Whether the condition is highly prevalent and whether the condition has a significant impact on people and societies. Oral conditions satisfy both criteria. They are widespread and have a significant impact on daily life, thereby placing a major burden on both individuals and the health care system. This statement is supported by findings from the Global Burden of Disease (GBD), 2010 Study (Marcenes *et al.*, 2013) and recent analyses of trends in caries experience among developed and developing countries (Bernabé and Sheiham, 2014a).

Untreated caries, severe periodontitis (gum disease) and total tooth loss were included in the list of 291 conditions evaluated in the GBD 2010 Study (Murray *et al.*, 2012a; Murray *et al.*, 2012b). For this study, a case of untreated caries was defined as having at least one tooth with unmistakable coronal or root cavity at dentin level; a case of severe periodontitis with a Community Periodontal Index score of four; a clinical attachment loss more than 6 mm or a gingival pocket depth more than 5 mm; and a case of total tooth loss resulting in no permanent teeth (Kassebaum *et al.*, 2014; Marcenes *et al.*, 2013).

Untreated caries of permanent teeth was the most prevalent of all 291 conditions in the GBD 2010 Study with a global prevalence of 35% for all ages combined (Table 1). Severe periodontitis, untreated caries of deciduous teeth (baby teeth), and total tooth loss were the 6th, 10th, and 36th most prevalent conditions, affecting 11%, 9%, and 2% of the global population, respectively (Table 1). While the global prevalence and incidence of untreated caries and severe periodontitis have remained fairly stable between 1990 and 2010, a review of the epidemiological data shows significant declines in the global prevalence and incidence of total tooth loss over the same period (Kassebaum *et al.*, 2014).

Dental caries rates in children have declined dramatically in the past 30 years in most industrialized countries (Petersson and Bratthall, 1996). This is evident in Figure 1, which illustrates the decline in dental caries among 12-year-old children living in developed countries. It was assumed by policymakers in many settings that this decline would translate to older age cohorts and lead to declining dental disease across all ages. This assumption, however, was not based on a rigorous analysis of the relative influences of age, period, or cohort effects on caries trends. A synthetic cohort analysis of data from four series of nationally representative cross-sectional surveys conducted over the past 50 years in England and Wales, the United States, Japan, and Sweden suggests that caries levels increase with age and continue to be a major problem in adults. This was observed despite recent declines in caries among children in these four developed countries, some

Table 1. Prevalence of health conditions, including oral conditions, in the world

Rank	Condition	in (millions)	(%)
1	Untreated caries of permanent teeth	2,432	35
2	Tension-type headache	1,431	21
3	Migraine	1,012	15
4	Fungal skin diseases	985	14
5	Other skin and subcutaneous diseases	804	12
6	Severe chronic periodontitis	743	11
7	Mild hearing loss	725	11
8	Acne vulgaris	646	9
9	Low back pain	632	9
10	Untreated caries of deciduous teeth	622	9
36	Total tooth loss	158	2

Source: Marcenes *et al.*, 2013.

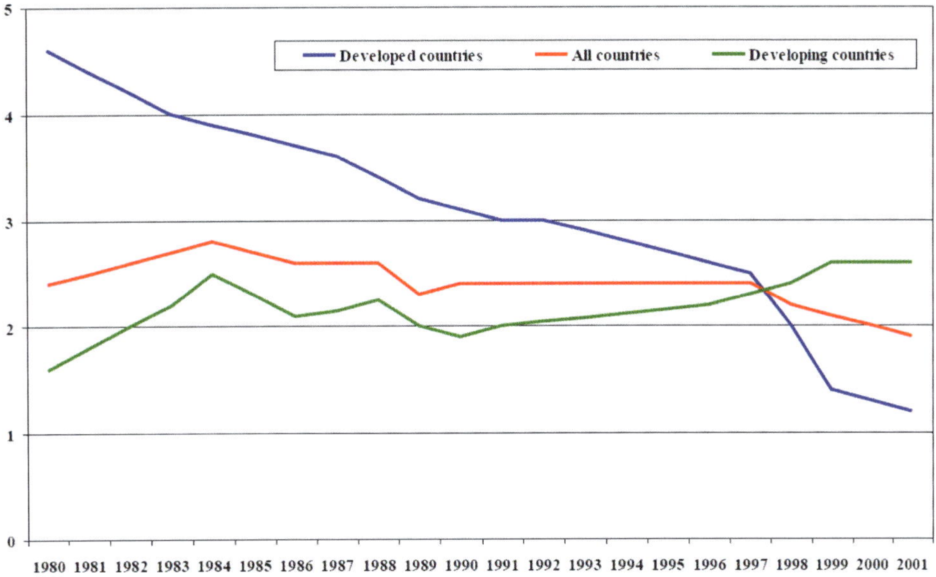

Figure 1. Dental caries (DMFT) trends in 12-year-olds, developed and developing countries

Source: Petersen PE, WHO. Oral health information systems, Figure 7.

with well-organized dental prevention programs directed at children and high utilization of fluoride toothpastes (Bernabe and Sheiham, 2014a). In the best longitudinal study of dental caries to date — the Dunedin Multidisciplinary Health and Development Study in New Zealand, which involved several oral examinations through the first half of life and high participation rates — dental caries levels increased as participants transitioned from childhood to adult life, despite widespread free access to dental care and caries preventive measures in childhood and adolescence (Broadbent *et al.*, 2006; Broadbent *et al.*, 2008; Broadbent *et al.*, 2013).

Newer evidence suggests that the same age-increasing trend in caries experience is occurring in other developed countries and in the developing world. A key measure of caries experience in dental epidemiology is the decayed, missing and filled teeth (DMFT) index, which represents the number of decayed (D), missing due to caries (M), and filled (F) teeth (T). There are no well-established and universally accepted measures of oral health status (Glick and Meyer, 2014) and the DMFT index has its limitations (Baelum *et al.*, 2007; Broadbent and Thomson, 2005). Still, it has been used for more than 75 years and is routinely included in epidemiological surveys to monitor population oral health trends.

In 23 out of 26 countries examined by Bernabe and Sheiham (Bernabe and Sheiham, 2014b), there was a five-fold difference in the number of DMFT between 12-year-olds and 35–44-year-olds. In 7 countries there was at least a ten-fold difference and in 10 of the 26 countries, the relative difference between children and adults was at least ten-fold, irrespective of the DMFT levels in the 12-year-olds (Bernabe and Sheiham, 2014b). Adults are indeed a caries-active group, with incidence rates at least as great as those of children and adolescents (Broadbent *et al.*, 2006; Glass *et al.*, 1987; Griffin *et al.*, 2005; Mejare *et al.*, 2004; Thomson, 2004).

The GBD 2010 Study is unique because it quantifies the comparable magnitude of health loss due to various diseases, injuries, and risk factors for years 1990, 2005, and 2010 for 21 regions covering the entire globe. Comparing the effects of different health outcomes, including those from fatal and non-fatal conditions, as well as injuries, is not a straightforward task. A single standardized summary measure of health loss was used across all the conditions evaluated in the study; that measure is called disability-adjusted life-years (DALYs) and is the sum of years of life lost (YLLs) due to premature mortality and years of life lived in less than ideal health or years lived with disability (YLDs). The implicit inclusion of YLDs in the calculation of DALYs emphasizes that health is about more than avoiding death. Individuals, households, and health care systems around the world devote enormous resources to the treatment, prevention, and amelioration of non-fatal complications of diseases and injuries. Some form of periodic accounting about the burden of non-fatal illness in populations, and how it is changing, should therefore be available for policymaking and planning (Murray *et al.*, 2012a; Murray *et al.*, 2012b). Since death as a direct result of oral conditions is rare, YLLs due to oral conditions are assumed to be zero, leading to all DALYs due to tooth loss to be equal to YLDs (Marcenes *et al.*, 2013).

In 2010, untreated caries, severe periodontitis and total tooth loss were among the top 35 causes of YLDs globally. The three conditions combined accounted for 15 million YLDs globally; representing 1.9% of all YLDs and 0.6% of all DALYs in the world (Marcenes *et al.*, 2013; Vos *et al.*, 2012). Among non-fatal outcomes, oral conditions ranked comparably with many non-communicable diseases, including maternal conditions, hypertensive heart disease, schizophrenia, and diseases of the blood. Furthermore, oral conditions accounted for more YLDs than 25 of 28 categories of cancer; only stomach, liver and trachea, and bronchus and lung cancers ranked higher than oral conditions (Vos *et al.*, 2012). As DALYs for oral conditions were identical to YLDs, oral conditions dropped down in the DALYs ranking when compared with conditions that led to significant YLLs, but were still among the top 100 causes of DALYs (Marcenes *et al.*, 2013; Murray *et al.*, 2012b).

Furthermore, DALYs due to oral conditions have been on the rise in recent years. There was a 21% increase in DALYs due to oral conditions in the past 20 years — from 12 million in 1990 to 15 million in 2010 — mainly driven by increases in population size and life expectancy despite changes in age-and sex-specific disease rates.

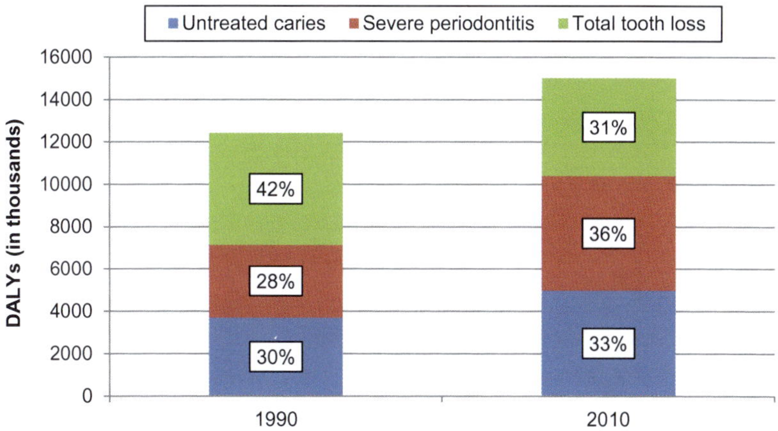

Figure 2. Disability-adjusted life years (DALYs) due to oral conditions in 1990 and 2010
Source: Marcenes *et al.* (2013).

In addition, the global burden of oral conditions has shifted from total tooth loss toward severe periodontitis and untreated caries (Figure 2). In 2010, untreated caries, severe periodontitis and total tooth loss each accounted for a third of DALYs due to oral conditions worldwide (Marcenes *et al.*, 2013).

A comparison of the burden of oral conditions by economic development status in 2010, using the World Bank's classification of income, shows that DALYs due to oral conditions were higher in middle-income countries than in high- and low-income countries (Figure 3). As explained earlier, population growth and aging as a result of increased life expectancies are the main drivers behind the growing number of DALYs. China and India, the two countries with the world's largest populations, were classified respectively as upper- and lower-middle-income countries in 2010, therefore accounting for a significant proportion of DALYs in those income groups. Increased population and longevity may also explain why there were more DALYs in high-income and middle-income than in low-income countries (Marcenes *et al.*, 2013).

DALYs are affected by population size, which means that when comparing two countries with similar levels of disease, the burden will be higher in the country with more individuals, simply because total DALYs are the sum of all DALYs for the entire population. An alternative way to express burden of disease is DALYs per capita, which accounts for changes in population size and demographic profile (distribution by sex and age). The GBD 2010 Study produced estimates for total DALYs and DALYs per capita by region, with the globe divided into 21 regions according to the mean age of death (Murray *et al.*, 2012b; Wang *et al.*, 2012). There were large geographical variations in total DALYs due to oral conditions, with the biggest burden seen in South Asia and

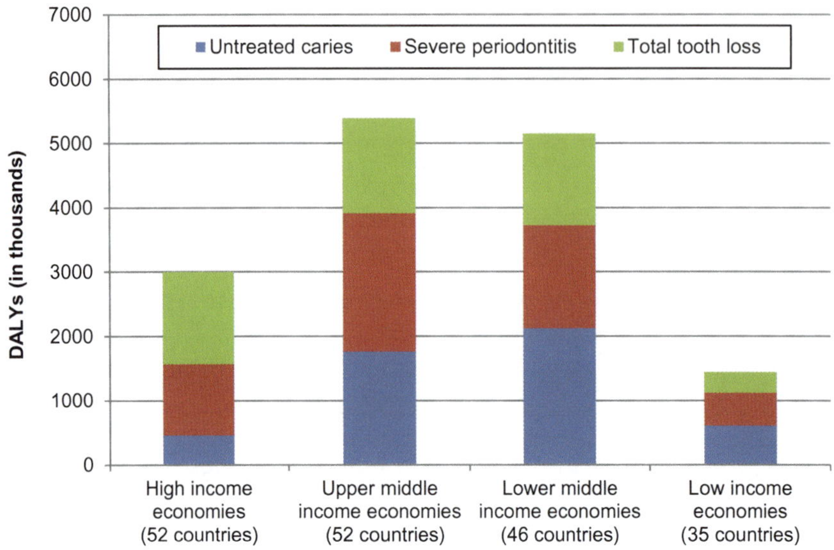

Figure 3. Disability-adjusted life years (DALYs) due to oral conditions in World Bank-designated high-, middle- and low-income economies

Source: Marcenes *et al.*, 2013.

East Asia, which is not surprising due to the fact that the two are the most populous regions in the world. Severe periodontitis was the leading cause of DALYs due to oral conditions in Australasia, East Sub-Saharan Africa, Central, East and Southeast Asia, and Southern, Central, Tropical and Andean Latin America. Untreated caries was the leading cause of DALYs due to oral conditions in Oceania, South Asia, North Africa/Middle East, and West, Central and Southern Sub-Saharan Africa. And severe tooth loss was the leading cause of DALYs due to oral conditions in High-Income North America, Western Europe, High-Income Asia Pacific, Eastern and Central Europe, and the Caribbean (Marcenes *et al.*, 2013).

A different picture emerges when looking at DALYs per capita. In Figure 4, world regions are presented in descending order according to mean age of death. The mean-age-of-death measure reflects both the population's age structure and age-specific death rates, and ordering countries in this way provides a simple summary measure of where regions are in the demographic (i.e., shift from high fertility and mortality to low fertility and mortality) and epidemiological (i.e., shift from communicable to non-communicable diseases) transition (Murray *et al.*, 2012b; Wang *et al.*, 2012).

The per capita burden of the three oral conditions is highest in regions such as Eastern and Central Europe, and Southern Latin America, which are going through a demographic transition from high fertility and mortality to low fertility and

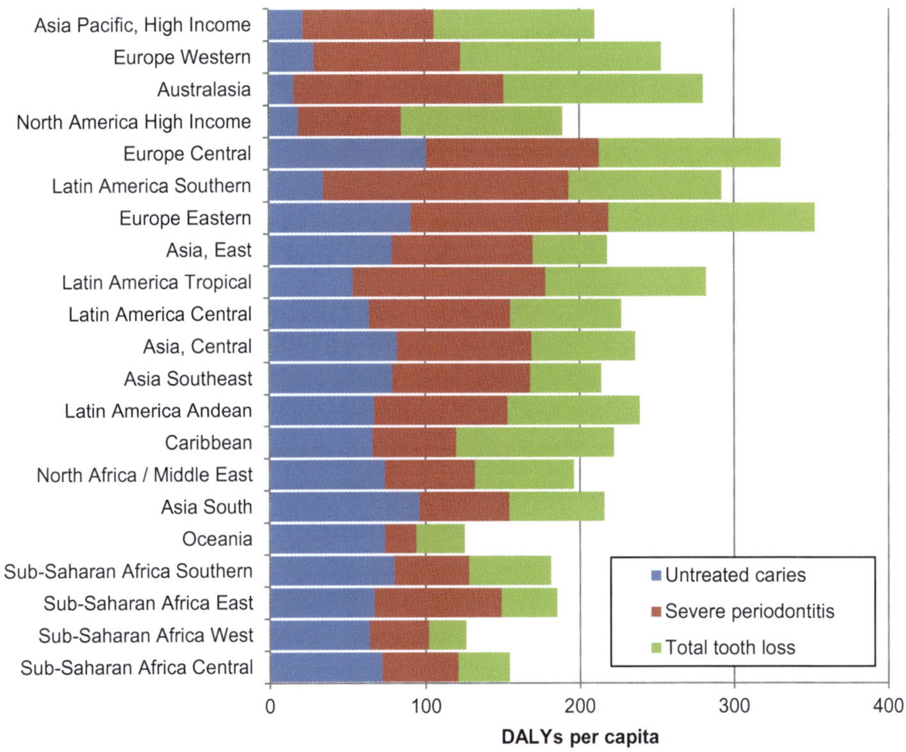

Figure 4. DALYs per capita (per 100,000 people) due to oral conditions for 21 geographical regions. Regions are sorted in descending ordered by mean age of death

Source: Marcenes *et al.*, 2013.

mortality. This demographic shift is typically accompanied by an epidemiological transition from communicable to non-communicable diseases. The oral conditions graphed in Figure 4 were lowest in regions such as Sub-Saharan Africa and Oceania, which have not yet experienced these transitions.

DALYs per capita also show that the burden of untreated caries decreases while the burden of severe periodontitis and total tooth loss increases as regions experience these transitions. As severe periodontitis and total tooth loss are age related, increases in longevity will be accompanied by greater prevalence of severe periodontitis and persistent disability caused by total tooth loss compared to regions where life expectancy is shorter. These trends have already been seen in more developed regions. The lower burden of untreated caries in more developed regions could be explained by the effectiveness and greater use of caries preventive measures.

In summary, oral conditions are highly prevalent and account for a significant burden of disease globally. The burden of oral conditions has increased in the past 20 years, but not evenly across regions of the world.

Table 2. DMFT index for children aged 12, select OECD countries

	1990	1995	2000	2005	Average annual % reduction
Australia	1.4	1.0	0.9	1.1	1.4
Austria	4.2	2.4	1.4	1.2	4.8
Belgium	2.7	1.8	1.4	1.0	4.2
Canada	3.7	—	—	—	—
Chile	3.5	3.5	2.7	2.7	1.6
Czech Rep.	—	3.2	3.1	2.8	1.1
Denmark	1.3	1.2	1.0	0.8	2.6
Estonia	4.1	3.4	—	—	3.4
Finland	1.2	1.2	1.2	1.0	1.4
France	3.0	2.0	1.6	1.6	3.2
Germany	4.1	2.3	1.2	0.7	5.5
Greece	—	2.5	2.4	2.1	1.6

Note: Average annual percent reduction is calculated for varying timeframes for different countries based on data availability.
Source: OECD Health at a Glance, 2013. Available at http://www.oecd-ilibrary.org/social-issues-migration-health/health-at-a-glance-2013_health_glance-2013-en.

As Table 2 shows, all 12 Organisation for Economic Cooperation and Development (OECD) countries for which data are available experienced a significant decline between 1990 and 2005 in the DMFT index for 12-year-old children. These gains in oral health status are not universal across different income and racial sub-groups in particular countries (Dye *et al.*, 2007). Nevertheless, these data show that significant progress has occurred over time in reducing dental disease among children. Similar multi-country data for adults are not available.

(2) Dental care systems around the world
Current knowledge of the world's dental care systems varies considerably. Researchers have studied some countries' dental care systems in depth and others not at all. Nevertheless, sufficient data exist to make some meaningful comparisons, especially among OECD nations, where data are more readily available.

Table 3 summarizes dental care spending, dental care use, and the supply of dentists in select OECD countries. It provides a snapshot of quantitative data available from OECD Health Data 2013 that relates to dental care in addition to the DMFT data presented in Table 2. Table 3 demonstrates the significant variation across countries in resources devoted to dental care. For example, per capita dental spending adjusted for purchasing power parity (PPP) varies from $51 in Hungary to $348 in the United States. This nearly seven-fold difference is slightly higher than the difference in total health spending for the same set of countries.

The US is an outlier among the OECD countries when it comes to total health spending. While the US also has the highest level of dental care spending with the OECD, the difference between the next two countries, Switzerland and Canada, is

Table 3. Select data on dental care systems in OECD countries

	Per capita GDP, $2011 PPP	Per capita health expenditure, $2011 PPP	% of health spending from private sources	Per capita dental expenditure, $2011 PPP	% of dental spending from private sources	Dental spending as % of total health spending	Mean number of dentist visits per person per year	Dentists per 1,000 population
Australia	$44,023	$3,800	31.7%	$223	77.6%	5.9%		0.55
Austria	$42,888	$4,546	22.7%	$213	51.5%	4.7%	1.2	—
Belgium	$39,840	$4,061	24.3%	$145	43.2%	3.6%	2.5	—
Canada	$41,163	$4,522	29.9%	$313	94.7%	6.9%	—	0.60
Czech Rep.	$27,047	$1,966	16.1%	$109	46.4%	5.5%	1.9	—
Denmark	$41,831	$4,448	15.3%	$251	65.8%	5.6%	0.9	0.83
Estonia	$23,310	$1,303	19.5%	$78	66.7%	6.0%	1.3	—
Finland	$38,618	$3,374	25.7%	$112	71.6%	3.3%	1.2	0.86
France	$36,381	$4,118	22.3%	$176	66.1%	4.3%	1.7	0.67
Germany	$40,980	$4,495	23.0%	$278	36.1%	6.2%	—	0.83
Greece	$27,046	$2,361	31.6%	$186	98.8%	7.9%	—	1.30
Hungary	$22,413	$1,689	36.8%	$51	68.8%	3.0%	0.7	—
Iceland	$38,216	$3,305	19.6%	$204	85.4%	6.2%	—	0.94
Japan	$34,321	$3,213	17.6%	$185	23.4%	5.8%	3.1	0.78
Korea	$29,035	$2,199	43.2%	$161	84.7%	7.3%	1.6	—
Luxemburg	$88,848	$4,246	15.7%	$234	51.7%	5.5%	0.6	—
Netherlands	$43,148	$5,099	14.3%	$214	72.6%	4.2%	2.3	0.50
New Zealand	$31,720	$3,182	17.3%	$107	63.5%	3.4%	—	0.45
Norway	$61,896	$5,669	15.2%	$274	73.7%	5.1%	—	0.99
Poland	$21,748	$1,452	29.1%	$63	85.7%	4.3%	0.8	0.35
Slovak Rep.	$25,128	$1,915	26.2%	$83	48.6%	4.3%	1.2	0.49
Slovenia	$28,156	$2,421	26.7%	$85	56.4%	3.5%	—	0.63
Spain	$31,732	$3,072	27.1%	$162	98.9%	5.3%	1.6	—
Sweden	$41,763	$3,925	18.4%	$248	65.1%	6.3%	—	0.85
Switzerland	$51,302	$5,643	34.6%	$338	93.6%	6.0%	2.1	—
U.S.	$49,854	$8,508	51.5%	$348	90.3%	4.1%	0.9	0.61
OECD average	$38,554	$3,636	25.2%	$186	68.5%	5.2%	1.5	0.72

Source: OECD Health at a Glance, 2013. Available at http://www.oecd-ilibrary.org/social-issues-migration-health/health-at-a-glance-2013_health_glance-2013-en.

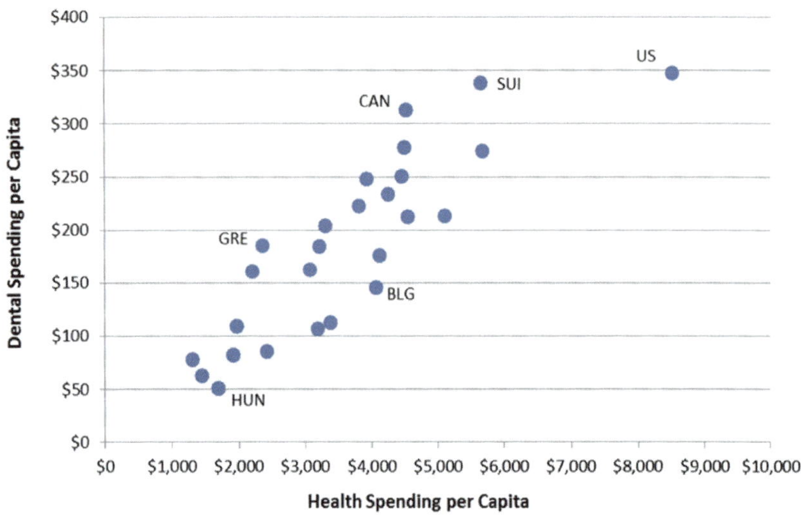

Figure 5. Per capita health and dental care spending in OECD countries

Source: OECD Health at a Glance, 2013. Available at http://www.oecd-ilibrary.org/social-issues-migration-health/health-at-a-glance-2013_health_glance-2013-en.

only a few dollars (Figure 5). Belgium and Canada have very similar levels of health spending but dental care spending in Canada is more than twice the level in Belgium. There has not been a thorough quantitative analysis that explores why dental care spending levels vary so widely across OECD countries and what impact these variations have on dental care utilization and oral health outcomes.

Dental care is financed differently than overall health care. Unlike overall health care, dental care in almost all OECD countries is financed primarily through private insurance and out-of-pocket spending. Only Japan and the Slovak Republic have the majority of dental spending coming from public sources. In the US, dental care is privately financed to a much larger extent than medical care.

There is considerable variation in the share of total health spending devoted to dental care, with a low of 3.0% in Hungary to a high of 7.9% in Greece. Despite having the highest per capita dental spending level, dental care in the US accounts for a lower-than-average share of total health spending compared to other OECD countries. On average, dental spending accounts for 5.2% of total health spending across OECD countries.

A strong empirical finding in the global health economics literature is that higher income countries spend more on health care, both in per capita terms and as a share of gross domestic product (GDP). For an overview of the literature in this area, see *The Determinants of Health Expenditure: A Country-Level Panel Data Analysis* (Xu *et al.*, 2011).

To the best of our knowledge, there has been little empirical analysis of multi-country variations in dental spending. Figure 6 demonstrates that, as with health

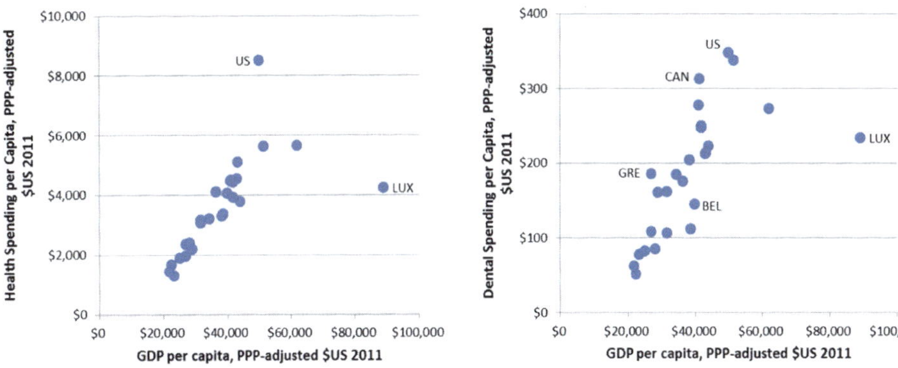

Figure 6. Health spending, dental spending, and GDP

Source: OECD Health at a Glance, 2013. Available at http://www.oecd-ilibrary.org/social-issues-migration-health/health-at-a-glance-2013_health_glance-2013-en.

care spending, dental care spending at the national level is tied to per capita GDP, although the relationship is not as strong. Dental spending varies as much as three foldamong several countries with roughly the same level of income. Analysis of the relationship using dental spending as a share of GDP reveals a similar pattern. While the data suggest that dental care spending behaves similarly to overall health care spending with respect to GDP levels, more research is needed to study key drivers of dental expenditure at the country level.

As Table 3 shows, the supply of dentists varies significantly across OECD countries. On average, there are 0.7 dentists per 1,000 population in OECD countries, compared to 3.3 physicians per 1,000 population. Poland has the fewest dentists per capita, at 0.35 per 1,000 population, while Greece has nearly four times as many, at 1.3 per 1,000 population.

As with many other health care occupations, issues such as shortages, geographic distribution, and international migration (Parkash *et al.*, 2006) are relevant in the dental care sector in both developed and developing countries (Yamalik, *et al.*, 2014). For example, the average density of dentists to population in Africa is 1–150,000 and in Ethiopia, the lack of access is even more dramatic with a density of only 1 dentist per 1.3 million people. Even in countries with fast growing populations of dentists, unequal access to dental care is a major obstacle to optimal oral health. India registers some 20,000 new dental graduates each year, yet there are still not enough dentists to adequately deal with the population's needs. Brazil has a high proportion of dentists but they tend to remain in urban areas, leaving vast rural areas without enough qualified dental practitioners to meet the needs of the population (WHO, 2012).

Figure 7 shows the supply of dental personnel averaged across countries of similar by per capita income levels. The analysis is based on a total of 40 countries where comparable data are available. The data are from WHO's Global Health

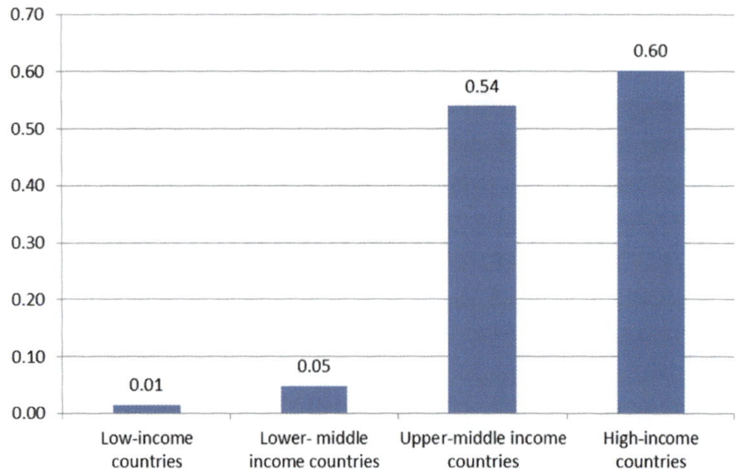

Figure 7. Dental personnel per 10,000 population by country income level

Note: Based on data from 40 countries. Countries are grouped based on World Bank income classifications.
Source: WHO Global Health Observatory Data Repository. Available at http://apps.who.int/gho/data/node.main.A1444?lang=en.

Observatory and cover a very broad definition of dental personnel including dentists, dental surgeons, dental hygienists, dental assistants, dental technicians, dental therapists (DTs), dental auxiliaries, dental nurses, or dental specialists. Thus, these data are not based on a standardized definition of the dental care workforce.

There are startling global disparities in the availability of dental personnel across the globe. There is more than a 60-fold difference between low-income and high-income countries. This is far greater a disparity than for any other type of health care provider for which the WHO tracks data and clearly illustrates the severe lack of dental personnel in low-income settings relative to the disease burden.

To help shed light on the variation in dental spending, dental care use and other data summarized in Table 3, it is useful to review some illustrative examples of how dental care is financed and delivered in different countries. Here, we focus only on a small set of countries that illustrate some of the different approaches.

The United States (US)

The US health care system is mainly characterized by its high cost and fragmentation. Different people obtain health care through different means, and not all Americans are automatically covered by health insurance. Consequently, there are wide gaps in coverage across the population. In 2011, most of the US population received health care coverage from private health insurers. Public programs (namely Medicare, an insurance program primarily serving people age 65 and older, and Medicaid, an assistance program for low-income people of all ages) covered about 32% of the population, and 15.7% of US residents — almost 49 million people — were uninsured (Thomson *et al.*, 2012; DeNavas-Walt *et al.*, 2012). Under the recent health care reform law, the Affordable Care Act, dental care for children is considered one of 10 essential health benefits mandated by the law, but dental care for adults is not.

Dental insurance coverage is less prevalent than medical insurance coverage. According to the most recent data, 56% of US adults have private dental insurance. More than 34% have no form of dental insurance (Nasseh and Vujicic, 2014a). Among adults with low incomes, Medicaid is the primary vehicle for oral health care, but while Medicaid programs are required to cover comprehensive dental services for children, states have flexibility to determine what dental benefits to provide to adult enrollees. Thus, the largest source of financing for oral health care is private health insurance, followed by out-of-pocket payments (Wall *et al.*, 2014a).

Independent private practitioners deliver most oral health care in the US. Individual states are the final authority on dentists' licensure requirements. Dental hygienists, dental assistants, dental laboratory technicians are also recognized as dental providers. Some states also recognize DTs, which are widely used outside the US, denturists, and community dental health coordinators, a relatively new provider type unique to the US. State practice acts determine the level of supervision dental allied providers require to deliver services within their scope of practice.

In 2012, 35.4% of the US adults and 47.6% visited a dentist (Nasseh and Vujicic, 2014b). About 1 in 10 Americans reported an unmet dental need due to cost in the past year (Wall *et al.*, 2014b). However, there is a six-fold difference between low-income and high-income adults in the likelihood of facing financial barriers to dental care. Large differences in affordability also exist by insurance status, further highlighting important social inequalities in access to oral health care (Dye *et al.*, 2007; Bloom *et al.*, 2012; Manski and Brown, 2012).

The United Kingdom (UK)

The UK's National Health Service (NHS) was established in 1948. As part of a postwar government plan, it provides preventive medicine, primary care and hospital services largely free at the point of use to all who are "ordinarily resident" in the UK. Public sources account for almost 83% of all health care expenditure, with the remainder funded privately, either through private insurance or out-of-pocket payments (Boyle, 2011).

Oral health services are delivered in acute and some single-specialty hospitals (secondary and tertiary services), community settings (screening of schoolchildren, oral health promotion and services for patients with special needs), and small independent practices (ambulatory services to meet most oral health needs). There are more than 33,000 practicing dentists (0.54 per 1,000 population), and roughly 27,000 of them are working within the NHS (Kravitz and Treasure, 2009; Blackburn, 2011; Boyle, 2011).

Since 1951, copayments have applied to oral health care, although oral health services provided in hospitals and community settings remain free at the point of use. Therefore, individuals in the UK are entitled to immediate access to urgent oral health care when required and also have the right — subject to a set of co-payments — to all clinically necessary treatments. Although individuals have these treatment entitlements under the NHS, many choose to receive a mix of private and NHS treatment, with nearly 12% of the population purchasing supplemental private dental plans. Because many services are not covered by public and private dental insurance, out-of-pocket payment accounts for 54% of UK dental spending (Blackburn, 2011; Boyle, 2011; Office of Fair Trading (OFT), 2012).

The majority of the UK population visited a dentist within the past year. The NHS remains the dominant provider of oral health services in the UK, as 71% of the population had used the NHS for their last course of treatment. Only 3% of people who felt they needed oral health services in the previous 12 months were unable to receive them, with minimal differences across income groups. This is among the lowest rates of financial barriers to dental care among European countries (Rooney *et al.*, 2010; European Commission, 2010; OECD, 2012).

Sweden

The Swedish health care system is a socially focused system with a commitment to ensure health care for all citizens. There is a mix of publicly and privately owned health care facilities, but they are generally publicly funded. Thus, the public sector accounts for more than 81% of all health care expenditure and the remainder is paid almost entirely out-of-pocket (Anell *et al.*, 2012).

Oral health care is part of the national social insurance system, and coverage is universal. No user fees apply for people under 20 years old. Adults are eligible for two types of subsidies for clinically necessary dental services: (1) A fixed general annual subsidy for preventive care and general examinations, and (2) a separate high-cost insurance policy that reimburses up to 85% of costs for other dental care services. Nevertheless, the majority of oral health care is still financed through out-of-pocket payments since the coverage is not extensive for many types of oral care services (Anell *et al.*, 2012; OECD, 2013; 2014).

The Public Dental Service (PDS) is the main provider of oral health care for children. Adults and elderly people can get subsidized dental care from the PDS or from dentists in private practice. There are almost 8,000 professionally active dentists, or 0.85 per 1,000 population (Kravitz and Treasure, 2009; OECD, 2014).

In 2009, about two-thirds of the adult population had visited a dentist for a regular check-up during the previous 12 months. Although only 8.5% of individuals had an unmet need for oral health care, differences among socioeconomic groups are present, as this number increases to 15.1% in the lower income quintile (European Commission, 2010; OECD, 2012; 2014).

France

The French health care system is a mix of public and private providers and insurers. Public insurance, the Statutory Health Insurance (SHI), is compulsory and is financed by both employee and employer contributions. All those legally residing in France are entitled to oral health care under the SHI, which has reached almost universal coverage.

Although generous in terms of services covered, SHI requires coinsurance for most dental treatments. These payments can be fully reimbursed by Complementary Health Insurance (CHI), which is supplemental voluntary private health insurance that covers 95% of the population. Public expenditure accounts for about 77% of total health care expenditure (Chevreul *et al.*, 2010, OECD, 2011; Durand-Zaleski, 2012).

Self-employed practitioners are the main providers of oral health care, representing 91% of the roughly 42,000 active practitioners. Licensing is granted by *Ordre National des Chirugiens-Dentistes* (the national dentists association).The only recognized auxiliary personnel are dental assistants and dental technicians (Kravitz and Treasure, 2009; OECD, 2014).

A considerable part of oral health care expenditure is financed by out-of-pocket payments. As a result, inequalities in access to and utilization of oral health services have developed. On average, 8.4% of individuals who felt they needed oral health care services did not receive them. This number decreases to 4.3% among high-income people and reaches 15.5% among low-income people (Union Francaise de Santé Bucco-Dentaire (UFSBD), 2006; European Commission, 2010; OECD, 2012; 2014).

Canada

The Canadian health care system is predominantly publicly financed and is highly decentralized in terms of governance, organization, and service delivery. Medically necessary hospital, diagnostic, and physician services are free at the point of service for all residents. More than 70% of health care is publicly financed (Table 3) and private insurance is complementary, that is, it covers services excluded from or only partially covered by public insurance. Oral health care is, in general not part of the publicly financed coverage, as only select surgical-dental services delivered in hospital are included in Medicare, the universal national health insurance program, with almost all dental care being privately financed and delivered (CIHI, 2005; Quiñonez *et al.*, 2008; Marchildon, 2013).

Private dental insurance covers 62.6% of Canadians, generally by way of employment-based benefit plans. Only 5.5% of Canadians are covered by public policies, mostly targeted to children, seniors, eligible aboriginal individuals and the disabled, and the remainder of the population is uninsured. Consequently, the private sector makes up the largest component of oral health care spending in Canada, with private insurers contributing 52.1% of total oral health care expenditure (Health Canada, 2010; CIHI, 2011; OECD, 2014).

Independent practitioners deliver almost all of the oral health care in Canada. The country currently has more than 20,000 dentists, and the dentist-to-population ratio is 0.6:1000 (Table 3). Provincial organizations are responsible for licensing and regulating professionals, and in select jurisdictions, dental hygienists, DTs, and denturists have legislated practice and offer services autonomously (CIHI, 2013; Marchildon, 2013).

National estimates show that 74.5% of the population made a dental visit within the last 12 months. At the same time, 17% of the population has avoided visiting a dentist because of cost, and this percentage is higher among uninsured, lower-income adults (Health Canada, 2010).

Brazil

Brazil has developed a dynamic and complex health system, known as the *Sistema Único de Saúde* (SUS) or Unified Health System. The SUS aims to provide universal health care services that are "free at the point of delivery." The public sector has generally been responsible for 47% of total health care expenditure, with the remaining spending coming from private sources (WHO, 2010; Paim *et al.*, 2011).

The 2004 Brazilian Oral Health Policy, "Smiling Brazil," has increased dental insurance coverage for oral care from 15.2% to 37% of the population between 2002 and 2012. Still, most dental care is financed through private dental insurance and out-of-pocket payment (Pucca-Junior, 2009; Instituto Brasileiro de Geografia e Estatística (IBGE), 2010; Agência Nacional de Saúde Suplementar (ANS), 2012; Brasil, 2013).

Publicly financed oral health care is usually provided in local community settings. There are about 257,000 registered dentists in Brazil and a dentist/population ratio of 1.14 per 1,000. Almost 27% are working in the public sector, with significant differences in provider availability between the more and less developed regions. Most oral health care is delivered in independent private dental offices, where dentists can earn their living entirely through fees paid by their patients and/or by dental plans (Morita *et al.*, 2010; Victora *et al.*, 2011; CFO, 2013).

(3) Dental insurance coverage, dental care use, financial barriers to dental care
Table 3 reveals considerable variation in the share of health spending devoted to dental care, with a low of 3.0% in Hungary to a high of 7.9% in Greece. Despite having the highest per capita dental spending level, dental care in the US accounts for a lower-than-average share of health spending compared to other OECD countries. On average, dental spending accounts for 5.2% of health spending across OECD countries.

Unlike medical care, dental care in almost all OECD countries is financed primarily through private insurance and out of pocket spending. Only Japan and the Slovak Republic have the majority of dental spending coming from public sources. In the US, dental care is privately financed to a much larger extent than medical care.

Dental insurance coverage

According to a recent OECD survey on health system characteristics, basic primary health coverage is available to the vast majority of residents of OECD countries. Dental care is typically covered at a lower level than other types of health care services, and coverage is much more limited for adults than it is for children (Paris *et al.*, 2010). Beyond these two observations, it is difficult to draw broad conclusions about dental insurance globally. We could not find a reliable source of multi-country data on dental insurance coverage rates that uses a consistent methodology. Neither WHO nor the OECD routinely collects this information. As a result, in this section we review dental insurance policies and arrangements in a select group of countries. Our selection of countries is not meant to be representative of any particular region or of the global picture. Rather, we aim to illustrate the wide variety of arrangements across the globe.

In Austria, compulsory health insurance provides health coverage to around 99% of the population. The cost of basic restorative and conserving dental treatments are generally covered by the insurance, although benefits vary. Crowns and bridges, implants, fixed orthodontic appliances, and other complex or cosmetic treatments are not covered and have to be paid for by patients. Children are covered by the same insurance as their parents. About 5% of the population also purchases private insurance to help meet additional dental care costs (Kravitz and Treasure, 2009).

Denmark has a NHS, which is funded through general taxation. Children up to the age of 18 receive free dental care through their school, including free orthodontics. Private dental care for children is also available, but 35% of the cost of such private dental services is met by the patient. Generally, there is no free dental care for adults. Instead, a system of subsidies operates whereby around 80% of the cost of privately provided dental care is met by the patient, with the state meeting the balance. Around 30% of the adult population has private health insurance. Some disadvantaged groups — the disabled, the elderly and those on low incomes — have their dental care costs met by the state (Kravitz and Treasure, 2009).

In Finland, health care is financed through general taxation. Although it is centrally planned, delivery of state-funded services (including dental services) is via municipal authorities. Dental services are delivered either through a network of public health centers or by private dentists, denturists (a type of dental technician) and dental laboratories. Public health centers are relatively autonomous and each determines who can access their subsidized public dental services, although children and special groups are usually given priority. Copayments often apply. Overall, the cost of dental services in Finland is broadly shared between individuals (around 56% of the cost), the state (around 36%), and the national social insurance scheme (around 7%). Around half of the adult population also has private health insurance (Kravitz and Treasure, 2009).

Germany has a statutory health insurance system, in which some 87.5% of Germans belong to not-for-profit 'sick funds', which must provide a legally sanctioned package of health care. Premiums for membership of these funds are shared between employees and employers. Membership in a sick fund entitles the member to a package of free basic dental care, with advanced treatment options such as crowns, bridges and orthodontics sometimes requiring significant patient copayments. Those not entitled to sick fund membership (the self-employed and those on high incomes) can opt to join a private health insurance fund. Supplementing these arrangements is a public dental service, but the type of care provided is restricted to examination, diagnosis and prevention (Kravitz and Treasure, 2009).

In Greece, health care is provided by a mixture of private practitioners, social security organizations and, since 1983, a basic state-funded NHS. Dental care is nominally offered free by NHS clinics to all, but services are generally targeted toward children and prevention. Most other patients contribute to the cost of dental care, which is also subsidized to varying amounts by social security organizations that have contracts with dentists and clinics. However, one-third of total private health care spending in Greece is spent on dental health services. Very few people use private health insurance to cover dental costs (Kravitz and Treasure, 2009).

In Italy, most health care is publicly funded through general taxation, although small copayments may apply. Comprehensive dental care is meant to be provided through NHS, although dental implants are excluded. However, in practice, the comprehensiveness of the service depends on local priorities and thus varies considerably even within a region. In many areas, only emergency dental treatment is provided by the NHS. As a consequence, publicly provided dental treatment mainly comprises extractions and rarely, restorations. Waiting lists are often long. Consequently, most people seek treatment in the private sector. Although some private health insurance is available, comprehensive dental coverage is often excluded from such plans (Kravitz and Treasure, 2009).

Since 2003, the Polish health care system has been financed through a common health insurance fund, the Narodowy Fundusz Zdrowia (NFZ). Citizens pay an obligatory premium of 9% of their income to finance the NFZ. As well as paying for their health services, membership in the NFZ entitles citizens to a limited range of dental services from either publicly funded clinics or dentists under contract to the NFZ. At a minimum, this includes a once-a-year dental check-up, but children under 18 and pregnant women are able to obtain a wider range of services more frequently. Not all dentists work in the state system; around two-thirds work outside the public system in private practice, although some provide dental services under contract to NFZ. Basic services provided under NFZ are free, although some services also require a copayment and the availability of services is limited. The cost of dental services provided in private practice is met by the patient (Kravitz and Treasure, 2009).

Spain provides universal access to health care for all citizens, however, some services such as dentistry are not comprehensively covered. Health services provided by the government (or the regions) are funded mainly through compulsory social security deductions from income, supplemented by other sources. These deductions are aggregated into a national social security pool. Although most dental care is provided by private practitioners and is paid for by patients, each regional health care organization operates a small public dental service. Generally, these dental services are delivered through clinics, which provide free emergency care or antibiotic treatment. Some of these are also able to offer supplementary services, such as free pediatric dentistry (including fillings, extractions, and cleanings) and prevention services (Kravitz and Treasure, 2009).

The US provides an interesting case study of alternative approaches to dental insurance coverage for adults compared to children. Only 13% of children lack some form of dental insurance, compared to 34% of adults (Nasseh and Vujicic, 2014b). The major reason for this difference is that within the main public insurance programs for children, Medicaid and the Children's Health Insurance Program, dental insurance is compulsory. In contrast, within Medicaid, adult dental insurance is optional and most states provide limited coverage. The expansion of public dental insurance coverage for children in recent years has been a major driver of expanded access to dental care for children (Vujicic and Nasseh, 2014) while the reduction in dental coverage for adults has led to, among other things, increased emergency room visits for dental conditions (Wall *et al.,* 2014c).

Dental care utilization

Figure 8 summarizes dental care utilization rates, as measured by the average number of dental visits per capita per year. Figure 7 plots these data alongside physician visits for comparison. When the data are presented this way, they provide insight into differences in dental care utilization across countries as well as dental care utilization relative to general health care utilization.

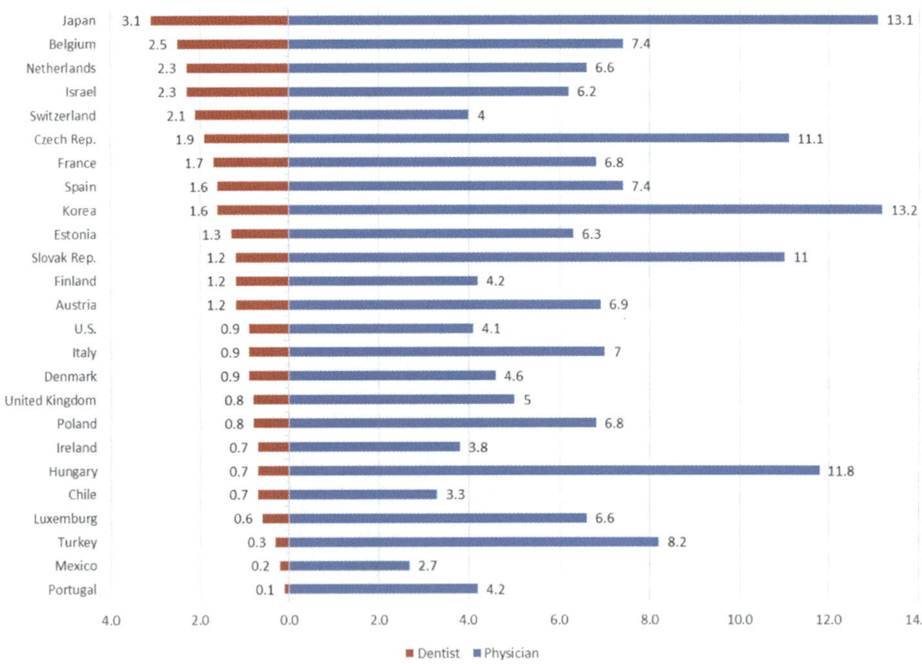

Figure 8. Average number of dentist and physician visits per person per year, select OECD countries

Source: OECD Health at a Glance, 2013. Available at http://www.oecd-ilibrary.org/social-issues-migration-health/health-at-a-glance-2013_health_glance-2013-en.

Japan has the highest utilization rate for both dentist and physician visits. Switzerland has the smallest difference between dental care and medical care utilization, while Portugal has the largest difference. In our view, two key policy questions emerge from Figure 8 related to dental care utilization. What is driving the significant differences in dental care utilization across countries, and, does increased dental care utilization translate to improved oral health outcomes? These questions have not been sufficiently addressed in the literature and are important areas for future research. Based on the data in Figure 8, there is little correlation between dental care use and both the supply of dentists and dental spending. Other factors such as household income levels, disease patterns, and population preferences, therefore, could explain at least part of the variation in dental care use.

Financial barriers to dental care

Another key aspect of access to dental care is affordability. The evidence suggests strongly that, at least in developed countries, affordability is an important factor that potentially limits access to and utilization of dental care (Wall *et al.*, 2014d).

There are numerous measures that could be used to assess affordability of dental care, including prices of dental care services, average out-of-pocket payments for dental visits, and self-reported measures. For example, one insightful indicator is the share of the population who indicate they have delayed or skipped needed dental care due to cost.

Another method of identifying the relative importance of financial barriers to care is to examine the main reasons people do not visit a dental care provider. For example, recent data from a large survey in the United States shows that the most common reasons adults cite for not visiting the dentist relate to cost (Wall *et al.*, 2014d). Financial barriers to dental care are most acute among young adults and have increased substantially over time in the US. In fact, affordability issues, in turn driven by declining dental insurance rates and household incomes, are a key factor explaining declining dental care use among US adults.

Data from the Commonwealth Fund, an independent think tank in the US, sheds light on the importance of financial barriers to both medical and dental care in select OECD countries (Schoen *et al.*, 2010). Figure 9 shows the percentage of adults in 11 countries within the OECD that report not being able to obtain the medical or dental care they need because of cost. These data provide several important insights. First, the US has the highest level of financial barriers for both medical and dental care. On the medical side, this is not a new finding and is consistent with extensive empirical evidence showing the US health care system provides poor financial protection to the population relative to other OECD countries (Schoen *et al.*, 2010). Second, in most countries the financial barriers to

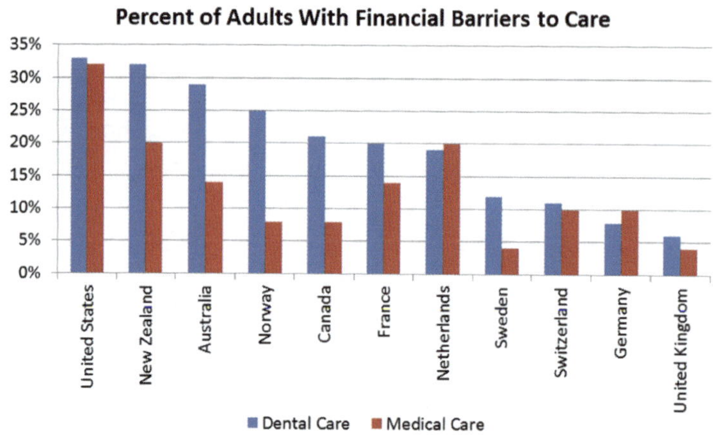

Figure 9. Financial barriers to medical and dental care in select OECD countries

Note: Data are based on percent of respondents indicating they did not see doctor when sick or did not get recommended care because of cost in the past year and the percent of respondents indicating they skipped dental care or checkups because of cost in the past year.

Source: 2013 Commonwealth Fund International Health Policy Survey. Available at http://www.commonwealthfund.org.

dental care are much higher than for medical care. The notable exceptions are the US, the Netherlands, Switzerland, and Germany. Germany and Switzerland have a relatively low rate, with only about 10% of adults reporting financial barriers to dental and medical care. In the US, the level is much higher — about one out of three adults — but is still surpassed by financial barriers to medical care. Third, the United Kingdom has the lowest level of financial barriers for both medical and dental care of any of the countries.

These multi-country differences in financial barriers to dental care and differences between medical and dental care within a country can be explained, in part, by variations in how dental care is financed. In Canada, for example, medical coverage is universal and care is paid for primarily through a single-payer system. However, dental coverage for adults is not included in the essential benefits and is financed primarily through private (employer-provided) dental insurance and out-of-pocket payments. This could explain the stark difference between the level of financial barriers to medical and dental care in Canada (Quiñonez and Grootendorst, 2011). Of all 11 countries in Figure 9, the UK goes furthest in limiting out-of-pocket spending and the financial burden of health care. The NHS requires little or no cost sharing for a very comprehensive set of benefits, which include dental care. In the Netherlands and Switzerland, medical coverage is provided mainly through private insurance that must cover core benefits through a tightly regulated marketplace.

Where data are available, they tend to strongly indicate that financial barriers to dental care are lowest among children and highest among working age adults.

For example, reports indicate that only 5.8% of US children delay or skip needed dental care because of financial reasons, compared to 14.8% of young adults aged 19 to 34 (Nasseh and Vujicic, 2014c). An analysis of adult dental care use in 24 European countries revealed a strong correlation between socioeconomic inequalities and the non-use of dental care among adults both within and across countries. A survey conducted in the United Kingdom found that 43% of adults reported avoiding the dentist due to cost. Of those adults, 26% reported suffering long-term tooth decay, and 13% reported suffering a periodontal abscess as a result (Simpson *et al.*, 2010). A national sample of Canadian adults demonstrated that 30% reported avoiding or delaying dental visits, and 32.2% reported not being able to receive all the treatment that was recommended due to cost (Locker *et al.*, 2011).

Low financial barriers to dental care among children reflect the fact that dental care financing is organized differently for children compared to adults in many OECD countries. For example, in the US, the Medicaid program, which is the main source of health insurance coverage for the low-income population, mandates that all states provide dental benefits to eligible children. But adult dental benefits are optional, and many states provide very limited coverage (Vujicic, 2014).

Affordability of dental care for older populations is an issue in many developed countries (Petersen *et al.*, 2010). As developed countries experience population aging, access to dental care for seniors is likely to become an increasingly important issue to heath care policymakers.

(4) Policy issues in dental care systems

The OECD data in Table 3 and the descriptions we have gathered of select dental care systems raise several important policy questions. Chief among them, how do different dental care financing and delivery arrangements impact access to dental care and, ultimately, oral health?

There have been several studies that help in answering this question. For example, the European Union publishes a manual of dental practice describing how oral health care fits within the health system of each European nation. There are also several studies that contribute important empirical evidence to the study of dental care systems. One study of seven OECD countries applies the ‘production function’ framework to compare the efficiency of dental care systems (Parkin and Devlin, 2003). One part of the study found that the French dental care system is more productive than the Irish and Dutch, but the underlying factors explaining the differences were not identifiable. Another part of the study, using a different econometric approach, found that the lower the ratio of population to dentists, the higher the average age of dentists, the more preventively oriented the fee structure and the lower the patient out-of-pocket costs, the greater the output of the system in terms of oral health achievements. The authors stated clearly that their results should be treated with caution because of the very small sample size and a host of other factors. Their objective was to illustrate the value of a production function approach and the need to expand the analysis to include many more countries.

Another study describes and analyzes dental care delivery systems in nine settings across six countries, comparing oral health outcomes, e.g., DMFT and periodontal disease rates (Chen *et al.,* 1997). The limited sample size, as well as other data constraints limit both the generalizability of the findings as well as the inferences that can be drawn regarding the impact of alternative dental care delivery systems and oral health outcomes.

In our view, the global evidence on how alternative dental care financing and delivery systems affect outcomes such as access to care, affordability, dental care utilization, and oral health is very limited. While several studies describe alternative dental care systems around the world (Widström and Eaton, 2004), few have attempted such a comparative analysis using a health systems framework (WHO, 2000). In our view, one major factor constraining such an analysis is the lack of agreement within the global oral health community on how oral health should be defined and measured (Glick and Meyer, 2014). Earlier in this chapter, for example, we have outlined the shortcomings of the very commonly used DMFT index. A multi-country comparative analysis that focuses on a large set of countries (e.g., the OECD), focuses on more recent experiences, and adopts an analytic approach that identifies how alternative dental care financing and delivery arrangements impact key outcomes would be an enormous contribution to the global health policy knowledge base and would, ultimately, help advance oral health.

Nevertheless, our review of the global evidence has identified several common dental care system challenges in both developed and developing countries. One challenge relates to provider adequacy relative to both the need for dental care, a clinical concept determined mainly by disease burden, and the demand for dental care, an economic concept determined by various other factors (Vujicic, 2014). Many countries regularly estimate current and future 'shortages' of dental care providers based on measures such as population to provider ratios that are meant to capture the need for dental care.

As noted in earlier sections on the chapter, another major challenge is affordability of dental care, or financial protection for dental care, or cost barriers to care. In some countries, like the US, there is considerable inequality in 'financial access' to dental care. A major driver of affordability is dental insurance coverage. However, as the experience of the UK, US, Sweden, France, Canada, and Brazil show, dental coverage is not the only factor driving affordability.

A third challenge is coordinating dental care with other health care services. The degree to which dental care is financed and delivered separately from the rest of the health care system varies across countries. However, in most OECD settings dental care is largely separate. This is an important issue, particularly in ageing societies, since evidence is emerging that oral and systemic health are linked, particularly among populations with high chronic disease burdens (Lockhart *et al.*, 2012; Simpson *et al.*, 2010).

A fourth challenge is that oral health is generally a neglected area of global health and has traditionally ranked low on the radar of national policymakers. The reasons for this situation are complex and varied. In many countries, oral health is not included in national health surveys. Moreover, if data are actually collected, they are usually isolated from the context of general health. Furthermore, in some cultures, oral health is neglected because teeth are seen as expendable. In addition, because poor oral health affects morbidity more than mortality, governments have viewed oral conditions as less important than other, more life-threatening diseases (Moysés, 2012).

A fifth challenge, most relevant in developing countries, is scaling up effective prevention strategies. For example, water fluoridation is considered one of the most significant public health achievements in history due to its effect on dental disease (CDC, 1999). However, weaknesses in infrastructure in developing countries make it extremely challenging to fluoridate drinking water. Even in developed countries, recent efforts are calling into question the need to fluoridate community water supplies (Kliff, 2013).

What policies can be considered to address some of these challenges?

Prevention

The WHO has identified several priority action areas for countries to consider when initiating or strengthening national oral health programs (Petersen *et al.,* 2005): effective use of fluorides for prevention of dental caries; oral health and prevention of oral disease through a healthy diet; control of tobacco-related oral disease by involving oral health professionals in tobacco cessation and preventing children and youth from adopting the tobacco habit; oral health promotion in schools; oral health improvement among the elderly through health promotion and older adult-friendly primary health care; integration of oral health into national and community health programs; development of oral health systems and orientation of services towards prevention and health promotion; strengthening the prevention of Human Immunodeficiency Virus/Acquired Immunodeficiency Syndrome (HIV/AIDS)-related oral disease, particularly in developing countries; development of oral health information systems; and research for oral health, oriented toward bridging the research gaps between developed and developing countries.

In the area of prevention, the use of fluoride is a cost-effective, evidence-based approach to reducing dental decay. Water or salt fluoridation is a possible population-wide approach but its implementation depends on the development and infrastructure of the country, as well as political will and community acceptance. Policies that address the risk factors for oral diseases, such as intake of sugars and tobacco use, can also be implemented, especially because these moves help reduce chronic diseases. Oral diseases and chronic diseases, such as cardiovascular diseases, cancer, chronic respiratory diseases, and diabetes, share many common risk factors. In 2007, a World Health Assembly resolution called for oral health to be integrated into chronic disease prevention programs (WHO, 2007).

The Dental Care Workforce

Expanding the dental work force can be achieved through increased enrollment in dental training programs (e.g., dentist and hygienist training programs), increased in-migration of providers, or task-shifting (e.g., altering scope of practice policies and practices).

Dental school capacity in developing countries is generally very low. In many developed countries, the supply of dental care providers is increasing, often motivated by the belief that a lack of providers is constraining access to care among vulnerable groups and an increased supply of dentists will address the issue. For example, several new dental schools have recently opened and existing dental schools are expanding enrolment in both the US and Canada. In fact, 12 new dental schools have opened since 2000 in the US and the number of graduates now exceeds 5,000 annually (American Dental Education Association (ADEA), 2013). Many of these new US dental schools have an explicit goal of educating dentists to serve in rural areas or to treat segments of the population that have difficulty affording dental care. It is too early to tell whether expanded dental school enrolment is increasing access to dental care. However, the global experience suggests that simply increasing the supply of providers without considering important labor market dynamics is an ineffective strategy for improving access to care for vulnerable groups (Vujicic, 2014).

An alternative approach to expand capacity is to consider task-shifting among existing providers or to introduce new types of dental care providers. A recent analysis in the US found that task-shifting certain types of dental care services to hygienists through less restrictive scope of practice regulations can reduce the cost of dental care (Marier and Wing, 2012) and increase dental care use among underserved populations (Buchmueller *et al.*, 2013). Teledentistry, the use of distance technologies that allow providers to collaborate in the care of a patient without being collocated, also provides an opportunity to increase provider capacity (Daniel and Kumar, 2014; Daniel *et al.,* 2013).

Over the past 20 years, there has been an increase in the types and scope of practice of many dental care providers in the US in response to the country's struggles to address problems with access to dental care. A 2003 Surgeon General's report explicitly called for increasing the capacity, diversity and flexibility of the dental workforce (DHHS, 2003). By 2014, workforce innovation had become a central oral health policy issue in the US (Mertz and Finocchio, 2010). These new workforce models rely on new roles for existing providers or new types of providers. Researchers will continue to evaluate the effectiveness of new workforce models and the roles each of these providers play in promoting oral health. Here is what we know today.

Dental assistant roles have changed over time, primarily with regard to their scope of practice. As dentistry has become more technologically advanced and complicated, dental assistants have moved from being helpers with on-the-job training to individuals who are licensed or registered based on academic qualifications at various levels (Dental Assisting National Board (DANB), 2014). While each state is different, California provides a good example of how this workforce has diversified. There are now five categories of dental assisting in California that create a career ladder within the field. The US Bureau of Labor Statistics (BLS) notes that dental assisting is one of the higher growth occupations (BLS, 2014).

Dental hygienists' professional roots are in public health but they have solidified their role as a critical member of the dental team in the private practice of dentistry. Over the past 20 years, hygienists have seen their role expanded in some states through changing laws on the supervision and employment regulations for dental hygiene work (American Dental Hygiene Association (ADHA), 2012). In some states independent practice policies that allow dental hygienists to practice independently have been initiated, although in all cases except Colorado (Astroth and Cross-Poline, 1998), this entails a collaborative practice agreement with a dentist (Mertz and Glassman, 2011). A recent analysis found that task-specific occupational regulations that limit hygienist scope of practice increase dental care prices by about 12%. Moreover, there are direct effects of such regulations on the utilization of basic dental services. When insurers are permitted to directly reimburse hygienists for their work dental care utilization increases by 3 to 4%age points (Marier and Wing, 2012; Petersen *et al.*, 2005).

Primary care providers such as family physicians, pediatricians, nurse practitioners (NPs), and physician assistants (PAs) can also play an important role in oral health care. Provision of oral health education and prevention services by these providers did not require a scope of practice change, but in some states it did require reimbursement systems to accommodate dental billing by medical providers. Several studies in the US show that engaging medical providers in oral care services expands access to dental care and can lower costs (Pahel *et al.*, 2011; Stearns *et al.*, 2012; Rozier *et al.*, 2003; Kranz *et al.*, 2014).

Community Dental Health Coordinator is a new type of community health worker with an oral health focus, part of a pilot program adopted by seven states in the US (American Dental Association (ADA), 2014a). The coordinator provides education about oral health disease and prevention with the goal of helping underserved communities better manage their own oral health and access the formal dental care system. Originally intended as a program to provide oral health knowledge to community health workers, the program has attracted many dental hygienists and therefore has refocused on providing hygienists with community health worker skills. Evaluations are currently underway that examine the impact of this type of provider on access to care but early results are very promising (ADA, 2014b).

DT is a provider with a larger scope of practice than a hygienist, typically able to perform some restorative procedures. DTs are widespread, with 54 countries having this type of provider. A comprehensive analysis of DTs worldwide was conducted and found that they offer safe, effective dental care (Will Keith Kellogg Foundation (WKKF), 2012). DTs were introduced in the US as part of a strategy to expand access to primary dental care, particularly with underserved populations. To date, four different kinds of DTs have been codified into practice, and each has been evaluated differently, but primarily in terms of clinical technical performance (Bader *et al.*, 2011). In the US, evaluations are currently underway that examine the effect of DTs on access to care. Initial evaluations have focused on the educational programs, technical efficiency, impact on disease rates (Wright *et al.*, 2013), and quality issues (Wetterhall *et al.*, 2010). Case studies have examined economic feasibility issues, including whether additional revenues from employing DTs exceed employment costs (Kim, 2013).

Affordability and Financial Protection

Dental insurance coverage is an important driver of access to dental care, affordability, and dental care use (Vujicic and Nasseh, 2014). Developed countries have wide variation in the extent of dental insurance coverage and how that coverage is provided (Biggs and Parliament of Australia Department of Parliamentary Services, 2012), e.g., as part of a universal health insurance program or purchased separately from a private insurance company.

It is evident from the analysis that most developed countries have adopted 'two divides' when it comes to dental insurance coverage. The first divide is that children have much more extensive dental insurance coverage than adults. This is true in both public and private dental insurance programs. The second divide is that dental insurance is usually provided separately from medical insurance. In essence, when it comes to health care financing policy, the mouth is largely disconnected from the body, and the status of the mouth changes when one enters adulthood. The divide in dental insurance coverage between children and adults in the US has led to considerable differences in access to care between adults and children, particularly in lower income groups (Vujicic, 2014c). Less is known about the implications of the divide between medical care and dental care financing, although it is extremely likely that this separation inhibits the coordination of dental care with overall medical care.

Conclusion

Oral health is an important component of overall health. Not only do oral conditions contribute significantly to the burden of disease in both developed and developing countries, but a healthier mouth can contribute to reduced health care costs, improved overall health status, and even increased earnings. The link between oral health and non-communicable diseases is particularly important for middle- and high-income countries with aging populations. At the same time, a significant share of the world's population, especially in developing countries, simply does not have sufficient access to dental care services, which are an important driver of oral health. Dental care ranks near the top among all health care services when it comes to difficulty accessing and paying for care.

Our analysis demonstrates that there are multiple approaches across countries to financing and delivering dental care. In some countries basic dental care is included in national health insurance systems while in others it is financed almost exclusively through private funding, including private dental insurance and out-of-pocket payments. In every country for which we had data, however, the share of spending from public sources was significantly lower for dental care compared to medical care. In developed countries, dental care is delivered primarily by dentists and other personnel working under the supervision of dentists. In developing countries a broader cadre mix is used due, in part, to a severe lack of dentists.

We summarized the numerous dental care system challenges faced by policy makers and highlighted some of the alternative approaches to addressing these challenges. In our view, the available evidence on the effectiveness of these alternative approaches needs to be strengthened. More fundamentally, we feel that the evidence base linking alternative dental care financing and care delivery arrangements with key outcomes such as dental care utilization, affordability of dental care, and oral health is extremely weak. There have been very few empirically sound, data-driven, cross-country analyses of dental care systems around the world. Part of the reason is data availability, especially outside of the OECD, and part is a lack of consensus on a definition of oral health and what indicators can be used to measure it. We feel there is a significant need to increase the evidence base on how various approaches to financing and delivering dental care impact key outcomes. This would include, as one of the first steps, gaining some international consensus on how oral health ought to be measured. It would also include an up-to-date, data-driven comparative analysis of a large set of countries. There are significant lessons to be learned from the global experience and policy makers — and ultimately the public — would benefit greatly from a synthesis of this experience.

References

Adulyanon S, Vourapukjaru J, Sheiham A. 1996. Oral impacts affecting daily performance in a low disease Thai population. *Community Dentistry and Oral Epidemiology* 24: 385–389.

Agência Nacional de Saúde Suplementar (ANS). 2012. *Caderno de Informação da Saúde Suplementar: beneficiários, operadoras e planos.* ANS: Rio de Janeiro.

American Dental Association (ADA). 2014a. About Community Dental Health Coordinators. Available at http://www.ada.org/en/public-programs/action-for-dental-health/community-dental-health-coordinators.

American Dental Association (ADA). 2014b. Impact of CDHPs. Available at http://www.ada.org/en/public-programs/action-for-dental-health/community-dental-health-coordinators/impact-of-cdhcs.

American Dental Education Association (ADEA). 2013. Washington, DC.

American Dental Hygiene Association website (ADHA). 2012. Available at http://www.adha.org/scope-of-practice.

Anell A, Glenngård AH, Merkur S. 2012. Sweden: health system review. *Health Systems in Transition* 14(5): 1–159.

Astroth DB, Cross-Poline GN. 1998. Pilot study of six Colorado dental hygiene independent practices. *Journal of Dental Hygiene* 72(1): 13–22.

Bader JD, Lee JY, Shugars DA, Burrus BB, Wetterhall S. 2011. Clinical technical performance of dental therapists in Alaska. *Journal of the American Dental Association* 142(3): 322–326.

Baelum V, Van Palenstein Helderman W, Hugoson A, Yee R, Fejerskov O. 2007. A global perspective on changes in the burden of caries and periodontitis: Implications for dentistry. *Journal of Oral Rehabilitation* 34: 872–906.

Bernabe E, Sheiham A. 2014a. Extent of differences in dental caries in permanent teeth between childhood and adulthood in 26 countries. *International Dental Journal* 64(5): 241–245.

Bernabe E, Sheiham A. 2014b. Age, period and cohort trends in caries of permanent teeth in four developed countries. *American Journal of Public Health* 104(7): e115–e121.

Biggs A, Parliament of Australia Department of Parliamentary Services. 2012. Dental Reform: An Overview of Universal Dental Schemes. Available at http://www.aph.gov.

au/About_Parliament/Parliamentary_Departments/Parliamentary_Library/pubs/BN/2011-2012/DentalSchemes#_ftn20.

Blackburn P. 2011. *Dentistry: UK Market Report* 2011. Laing & Buisson: London.

Bloom B, Simile CM, Adams PF, Cohen RA. 2012. Oral health status and access to oral health care for US adults aged 18–64: National Health Interview Survey, 2008. National Center for Health Statistics. *Vital Health Stat* 10(253): 1–22.

Boyle S. 2011. United Kingdom (England): health system review. *Health Systems in Transition* 13(1):1–486.

Brasil. 2013. Ministério da saúde.*Sala de Apoio à Aestão Estratégica*. Available at http://189.28.128.178/sage/ [5 March 2013].

Broadbent JM, Thomson WM. 2005. For debate: problems with the DMF index pertinent to dental caries data analysis. *Community Dentistry and Oral Epidemiology* 33(6): 400–409.

Broadbent JM, Thomson WM, Poulton R. 2006. Progression of dental caries and tooth loss between the third and fourth decades of life: A birth cohort study. *Caries Research* 40(6): 459–465.

Broadbent JM, Thomson WM, Poulton R. 2008. Trajectory patterns of dental caries experience in the permanent dentition to the fourth decade of life. *Journal of Dental Research* 87(1): 69–72.

Broadbent JM, Foster Page LA, Thomson WM, Poulton R. 2013. Permanent dentition caries through the first half of life. *British Dental Journal* 215(7): E12.

Buchmueller TC, Orzoi S, Shore-Sheppard LD. 2013. The effect of medicaid payment rates on access to dental care among children. *NBER Working Paper* No. 19218.

Centers for Disease Control and Prevention (CDC). 1999. Achievements in Public Health, 1900–1999: Fluoridation of Drinking Water to Prevent Dental Caries. *Morbidity and Mortality Weekly Report.* http://www.cdc.gov/mmwr/preview/mmwrhtml/mm4841a1.htm [19 October 2014].

Centers for Disease Control and Prevention (CDC). 2006. Oral Health for Adults. Available at http://www.cdc.gov/oralhealth/publications/factsheets/adult_oral_health/adults.htm.

Centers for Disease Control and Prevention (CDC). 2013. Cost Savings of Community Water Fluoridation. Available at http://www.cdc.gov/fluoridation/factsheets/cost.htm.

Chen M, Andersen RM, Barmes DE, Leclerq MH, Lyttle CS. 1997. *Comparing Oral Health Care Systems: A Second International Collaborative Study*. World Health Organization: Geneva.

Chevreul K, Durand-Zaleski I, Bahrami S, Hernández-Quevedo C, Mladovsky P. 2010. France: Health system review. *Health Systems in Transition* 12(6): 1–291.

Cigna. 2010. *Improved Health and Lower Medical Costs: Why Good Dental Care is Important, A White Paper*. [8 January 2014]. Available at: http://www.cigna.com/assets/docs/life-wall-library/Whygooddentalcareisimportant_whitepaper.pdf.

Canadian Institute for Health Information (CIHI). 2005. *Exploring the* 70/30 *Split: How Canada's Health Care System is Financed.* Canadian Institute for Health Information: Ottawa.

Canadian Institute for Health Information (CIHI). 2011. *National Health Expenditure Trends*, 1975 *to* 2012. Canadian Institute for Health Information: Ottawa.

Canadian Institute for Health Information (CIHI). 2013. *Canada's Health Care Providers*, 1997 *to* 2011 *— A Reference Guide*: *Overview and Methodological Notes.* Canadian Institute for Health Information: Ottawa.

Daniel SJ, Wu L, Kumar, S. 2013. Teledentistry: a systematic review of clinical outcomes, utilization and costs. *Journal of Dental Hygiene* 87(6): 345–352.

Daniel SJ, Kumar, S. 2014. Teledentistry: a key component in access to care. *Journal of Evidence-Based Dental Practice* 14(Suppl): 201–208.

DeNavas-Walt C, Proctor BD, Smith JC. 2012. Income, Poverty, and Health Insurance Coverage in the United States: 2011. US Census Bureau, *Current Population Reports* P60–243.

Dental Assisting National Board, Inc. website (DANB). 2014. Available at http://www.danb.org/Meet-State-Requirements/State-Specific-Information.aspx.

Durand-Zaleski I. 2012. The French Health Care System, in Thomson S, Osborn R, Squires D, Jun M (eds.). *International Profiles of Health Care Systems*. 2012. The Commonwealth Fund. Available at http://www.commonwealthfund.org/~/media/Files/Publications/Fund%20Report/2012/Nov/1645_Squires_intl_profiles_hlt_care_systems_2012.pdf. [25 February 2013].

Dye BA, Tan S, Smith V, Lewis BG, Barker LK, Thornton-Evans G *et al.* 2007. Trends in oral health status: United States, 1988–1994 and 1999–2004. National Center for Health Statistics. *Vital and Health Statistics* 11(248): 1–92.

European Commission. 2010. *Special Euro barometer 330 — Oral Health*. Available at http://ec.europa.eu/public_opinion/archives/ebs/ebs_330_en.pdf.

Glass RL, Alman JE, Chauncey HH. 1987. A 10-year longitudinal study of caries incidence rates in a sample of male adults in the USA. *Caries Research* 21(4): 360–367.

Glick M, Meyer DM. 2014. Defining oral health: A prerequisite for any health policy. *Journal of the American Dental Association* 145(6): 519–520.

Glied S, Neidell M. 2010. The economic value of teeth. *Journal of Human Resources* 45(2): 468–496.

Griffin SO, Griffin PM, Swann JL, Zlobin N. 2005. New coronal caries in older adults: Implications for prevention. *Journal of Dental Research* 84(8): 715–720.

Health Canada. 2010. *Report on the findings of the oral health component of the Canadian Health Measures Survey* 2007–2009. Publications Health Canada: Ottawa. Available at http://www.fptdwg.ca/assets/PDF/CHMS/CHMS-E-summ.pdf.

Instituto Brasileiro de Geografia e Estatística (IBGE). 2010. *Pesquisa de Orçamentos Familiares* 2008–2009: *Despesas, Rendimentos e Condições de Vida.* Instituto Brasileiro de Geografia e Estatística: Rio de Janeiro. Available at http://www.ibge.gov.br/home/estatistica/populacao/condicaodevida/pof/2008_2009/POFpublicacao.pdf.

International Collaborative Study on Oral Health Care Systems and WHO Oral Health Programme. 1997. Also listed as authors on Chen paper at this URL http://apps.who.int/iris/handle/10665/41976.

Kassebaum NJ, Bernabe E, Dahiya M, Bhandari B *et al.* 2014. Global Burden of Severe Tooth Loss: A Systematic Review and Meta-analysis. *Journal of Dental Research* 93(7 suppl): 20S–28S.

Kim F. 2013. *Economic Vialbility of Dental Therapists.* Prepared for Community Catalyst. Available at http://www.wkkf.org/resource-directory/resource/2013/05/economic-viability-of-dental-therapists.

Kliff S. 2013. A brief history of America's fluoride wars. *The Washington Post Wonkblog.* Available at http://www.washingtonpost.com/blogs/wonkblog/wp/2013/05/21/a-brief-history-of-americas-fluoride-wars/.

Kranz AM, Rozier RG, Preisser JS, Stearns SC *et al.* 2014. Examining continuity of care for Medicaid-enrolled children receiving oral health services in medical offices. *Maternal and Child Health Journal* 19(1): 196–203.

Kravitz A, Treasure E. 2009. *Manual of Dental Practice.* The Council of European Dentists. Available at http://www.eudental.eu/library/eu-manual.html. [17 April 2013].

Lamster IB, Eaves K. 2011. A model for dental practice in the 21st century. *American Journal of Public Health* 101(10): 1825–1830.

Locker D, Maggirias J, Quiñonez C. 2011. Income, dental insurance coverage, and financial barriers to dental care among Canadian adults. *Journal of Public Health Dentistry* 71(4): 327–334.

Lockhart PB, Bolger AF, Papapanou PN, Osinbowale O *et al.* 2012. Periodontal disease and atherosclerotic vascular disease: does the evidence support an independent association? A scientific statement from the American Heart Association. *Circulation* 125: 2520–2544.

Manski RJ, Brown E. 2010. *Dental coverage of adults ages 21–64, United States*, 1997 *and* 2007. Agency for Healthcare Research and Quality: Rockville. Available at http://www.meps.ahrq.gov/mepsweb/data_files/publications/st295/stat295.pdf. [3 May 2013].

Marchildon GP. 2013. Canada: Health system review. *Health Systems in Transition* 15(1): 1–179.

Marcenes W, Kassebaum NJ, Bernabe E, Flaxman A *et al.* 2013. Global burden of oral conditions in 1990–2010: Asystematic analysis. *Journal of Dental Research* 92(7): 592–597.

Marier A, Wing C. 2012. Effects of Occupational Regulations On The Cost Of Dental Services: Evidence From Dental Insurance Claims. Available at http://chess.bsd.uchicago.edu/events/documents/DentalRegsFeb12012.pdf.

Mejare I, Stenlund H, Zelezny-Holmlund C. 2004. Caries incidence and lesion progression from adolescence to young Adulthood: a prospective 15-year cohort study in Sweden. *Caries Research* 38(2): 130–141.

Mertz EA, Finocchio L. 2010. Improving oral healthcare delivery systems through workforce innovations: an introduction. *Journal of Public Health Dent*istry 70(Suppl 1): S1–S5.

Mertz E, Glassman P. 2011. Alternative practice dental hygiene in California: past, present, and future. *Journal of the California Dental Association* 39(1): 37–46.

Morita MC, Haddad AE, Araújo ME. 2010. *Perfil Atual e Tendências do Cirurgião-Dentista Brasileiro.* Dental Press: Maringá.

Moysés SJ. 2012. Inequalities in oral health and oral health promotion. *Brazilian Oral Research* 26(Supplement 1): 86–93.

Murray CJL, Ezzati M, Flaxman AD, Lim S *et al.* 2012a. GBD 2010: design, definitions, and metrics. *The Lancet* 380(9859): 2063–2066.

Murray CJL, Vos T, Lozano R, Naghavi M *et al.* 2012b. Disability-adjusted life years (DALYs) for 291 diseases and injuries in 21 regions, 1990–2010: A systematic analysis for the Global Burden of Disease Study 2010. *The Lancet* 380(9859): 2197–2223.

Naorungroj S, Schoenbach VJ, Beck J, Mosley TH *et al.* 2013. Cross-sectional associations of oral health measures with cognitive function in late middle-aged adults: A community-based study. *Journal of the American Dental Association* 144(12): 1362–1371.

Nasseh K, Vujicic M. 2014a. *Dental Benefits Expanded for Children, Young Adults in* 2012. American Dental Association Health Policy Institute. Available from: http://www.ada.org/~/media/ADA/Science%20and%20Research/HPI/Files/HPIBrief_1014_5.ashx.

Nasseh K, Vujicic M. 2014b. *Dental Care Utilization Rate Highest Ever Among Children, Continues to Decline Among Working-Age Adults.* American Dental Association Health Policy Institute. Available from: http://www.ada.org/~/media/ADA/Science%20and%20Research/HPI/Files/HPIBrief_1014_4.ashx.

Office of Fair Trading (OFT). 2012. *Dentistry: an OFT market study.* Office of Fair Trading: London. Available at http://www.oft.gov.uk/shared_oft/market-studies/Dentistry/OFT1414.pdf. [15 April 2013].

Organisation for Economic Cooperation and Development (OECD). 2011. *Health at a Glance* 2011: *OECD Indicators.* OECD Publishing. Available at http://dx.doi.org/10.1787/health_glance-2011-en. [27 February 2013].

Organisation for Economic Cooperation and Development (OECD). 2012. *Health at a Glance*: *Europe* 2012, OECD Publishing. Available at http://dx.doi.org/10.1787/9789264183896-en. [17 April 2013].

Organisation for Economic Cooperation and Development (OECD). 2013. *Health at a Glance 2013*: *OECD Indicators*, OECD Publishing. Available at http://dx.doi.org/10.1787/health_glance-2013-en. [22 June 2014].

Organisation for Economic Cooperation and Development (OECD). 2014. OECD. StatExtracts Database. Available at http://stats.oecd.org/. [24 June 2014].

Pahel BT, Rozier RG, Stearns SC, Quiñonez RB. 2011. Effectiveness of preventive dental treatments by physicians for young Medicaid enrollees. *Pediatrics* 127(3): e682–e689.

Paim J, Travassos C, Almeida C, Bahia L, Macinko J. 2011. The Brazilian health system: history, advances, and challenges. *Lancet* 377: 1778–1797.

Paris V, Devaux M, Wei L. 2010. Health Systems Institutional Characteristics: A Survey of 29 OECD Countries. *OECD Health Working Paper No. 50.* OECD Publishing. Available at http://dx.doi.org/10.1787/5kmfxfq9qbnr-en.

Parkash H, Mathur VP, Duggal R, Jhuraney B. 2006. *Journal of Dental Education* 11(suppl): 22–26.

Parkin D, Devlin N. 2003. Measuring Efficiency in Dental Care. In: Scott, A *et al.* (eds.). *Advances in Health Economics.* Wiley: Chichester. doi: 10.1002/0470867922.ch8.

Petersen PE, World Health Organization. 1997. Oral Health Information Systems, Figure 7. Available at http://www.who.int/oral_health/media/en/orh_figure7.pdf?ua=1.

Petersen PE, Saskia Estupinan-Day S, Ndiaye C. 2005. WHO's action for continuous improvement in oral health. *Bulletin of the World Health Organization* 83(9): 641–620. Available at http://www.who.int/bulletin/volumes/83/9/editorial10905html/en/.

Petersen PE, Kandelman D, Arpin S, Ogawa H. 2010. Global oral health of older people — Call for public health action. *Community Dental Health* 27(2): 257–268.

Petersson GH, Bratthall D. 1996. The caries decline: a review of reviews. *European Journal of Oral Sciences* 104(4): 436–443.

Pucca-Junior GA, Costa JFR, Chagas LD, Silvestre RM. 2009. Oral health policies in Brazil. *Brazilian Oral Research* 23(Suppl): 9–16.

Quiñonez C, Grootendorst P. 2011. Equity in dental care among Canadian households. *International Journal for Equity in Health.* Available at http://www.biomedcentral.com/content/pdf/1475-9276-10-14.pdf. Accessed 2011.

Quiñonez CR, Locker D, Sherret L, Grootendorst P *et al.* 2008. *An environmental scan of public dental programs in Canada.* Community Dental Health Services Research Unit and the Office of the Chief Dental Officer: Health Canada.

Rooney E, Davies G, Neville J, Robinson M, Perkins C, Bellis MA. 2010. *Oral Health Survey of 12-year-old Children* 2008/2009: *summary of caries prevalence and severity results.* NHS Dental Epidemiology Programme for England. Available at http://www.nwph.net/dentalhealth/reports/Report_NHS_DEP_for_England_OH_Survey_12yr_2008-09.pdf. [17April 2013].

Rozier RG, Sutton BK, Bawden JW, Haupt K *et al.* 2003. Prevention of early childhood caries in North Carolina medical practices: Implications for research and practice. *Journal of Dental Education* 67(8): 876–885.

Savage MF, Lee JY, Kotch JB *et al.* 2004. Early preventive dental visits: Effects on subsequent utilization and cost. *Pediatrics* [online] 114(4): e418-e423. Available at http://pediatrics.aappublications.org/content/114/4/e418.short. [5 November 2013].

Schoen C, Osborn R, Squires D, Dotty MM *et al.* 2010. How health insurance design affects access to care and costs, by income, in eleven countries. *Health Affairs* 29(12): 2323–2334.

Simpson TC, Needleman I, Wild SH, Moles DR, Mills EJ. 2010. Treatment of periodontal disease for glycemic control in people with diabetes. *Cochrane Database of Systematic Reviews* 5: CD004714.

Sintonen H, Linnosmaa I. 2000. Economics of Dental Services. In: Culyer AJ, Newhouse JP, (eds.). *Handbook of Health Economics,* Vol. 1. Elsevier: Amsterdam, pp. 1251–1296.

Stearns SC, Rozier RG, Kranz AM, Pahel BT, Quiñonez RB. 2012. Cost-effectiveness of preventive oral health care in medical offices for young Medicaid enrollees. *Archive of Pediatric and Adolescent Medicine* 166(10): 945–951.

Stewart R, Sabbah W, Tsakos G, D'Aiuto F, Watt RG. 2008. Oral health and cognitive function in the Third National Health and Nutrition Examination Survey (NHANES III). Psychosomatic Medicine 70(8): 936–941.

Thomson S, Osborn R, Squires D, Jun M (eds.). 2012. *International Profiles of Health Care Systems*. The Commonwealth Fund. Available at http://www.commonwealthfund.org/~/media/Files/Publications/Fund%20Report/2012/Nov/1645_Squires_intl_profiles_hlt_care_systems_2012.pdf. [25 February 2013].

Thomson WM. 2004. Dental caries experience in older people over time: What can the large cohort studies tell us? *British Dental Journal* 196(2): 89–92.

Union Francaise de Santé Bucco-Dentaire (UFSBD). 2006. *La Santé Bucco-Dentaire Des Enfants de 6 et 12 Ans en France, en 2006*. Available at http://www.sante.gouv.fr/IMG/pdf/La_sante_bucco-dentaire_des_enfants_de_6_et_12_ans_en_France_en_2006.pdf. [23 April 2013].

US Bureau of Labor Statistics (BLS). Occupational Outlook Handbook. Available at http://www.bls.gov/ooh/healthcare/dental-assistants.htm.

US Department of Health and Human Services (DHHS). 2000. *Oral Health in America: A Report of the Surgeon General*. US Department of Health and Human Services. National Institute of Dental and Craniofacial Research, National Institutes of Health: Rockville. Available at http://silk.nih.gov/public/hck1ocv.@www.surgeon.fullrpt.pdf.

US Department of Health and Human Services (DHHS). 2003. *National Call to Action to Promote Oral Health*. US Department of Health and Human Services, National Institute of Dental and Craniofacial Research, National Institutes of Health: Rockville, MD: Available at http://www.ncbi.nlm.nih.gov/books/NBK47472/.

Victora CG, Barreto ML, Leal MC *et al*. 2011. Health conditions and health-policy innovations in Brazil: the way forward. *Lancet* 377: 2042–2053.

Vos T, Flaxman AD, Naghavi M, Lozano R *et al.* 2012. Years lived with disability (YLDs) for 1160 sequelae of 289 diseases and injuries 1990–2010: A systematic analysis for the Global Burden of Disease Study 2010. *The Lancet* 380(9859): 2163–2196.

Vujicic M. 2014. Health Labor Markets in Developing Countries. In: Culyer AJ, ed. *Handbook of Health Economics,* Vol. 1. Elsevier: San Diego, pp. 111–407.

Vujicic M, Nasseh K. 2014. A decade in dental care utilization among adults and children (2001–2010). *Health Services Research* 49(2): 460–480.

Wall T, Nasseh K, Vujicic M. 2014a. *US Dental Spending Remained Flat Through 2012.* American Dental Association Health Policy Institute. Available from: http://www.ada.org/~/media/ADA/Science%20and%20Research/Files/HPRCBrief_0114_1.ashx.

Wall T, Nasseh K, Vujicic M. 2014b. *Majority of Dental-Related Emergency Department Visits Lack Urgency and Can Be Diverted to Dental Offices.* American Dental Association Health Policy Institute. Available from: http://www.ada.org/~/media/ADA/Science%20and%20Research/HPI/Files/HPIBrief_0814_1.ashx.

Wall T, Nasseh K, Vujicic M. 2014c. *Fewer Americans Forgoing Dental Care Due to Cost.* American Dental Association Health Policy Institute. Available from: http://www.ada.org/~/media/ADA/Science%20and%20Research/HPI/Files/HPIBrief_1014_6.ashx.

Wall T, Nasseh K, Vujicic M. 2014d. *Most Important Barriers to Dental Care are Financial, Not Supply Related.* American Dental Association Health Policy Institute. Available from: http://www.ada.org/~/media/ADA/Science%20and%20Research/HPI/Files/HPIBrief_1014_2.ashx.

Wang H, Dwyer-Lindgren L, Lofgren KT, Rajaratnam JK *et al.* 2012. Age-specific and sex-specific mortality in 187 countries, 1970–2010: A systematic analysis for the Global Burden of Disease Study 2010. *The Lancet* 380(9859): 2071–2094.

Wetterhall S, Bader JD, Burrus BB, Lee JY, Shugars DA. 2010. Evaluation of the Dental Health Aide Therapist Workforce Model in Alaska. Final Report. RTI International: Research Triangle Park. Available at https://www.rti.org/pubs/alaskadhatprogram evaluationfinal102510.pdf.

Widström E, Eaton KA. 2004. Oral healthcare systems in the extended European union. *Oral Health & Preventive Dentistry* 2(3): 155–194.

W.K. Kellogg Foundation (WKKF). 2012. A Review of the Global Literature on Dental Therapists. Available at http://www.wkkf.org/resource-directory/resource/2012/04/nash-dental-therapist-literature-review.

World Health Organization (WHO). 2003. Dental Diseases and Oral Health. Available at http://www.who.int/oral_health/publications/en/orh_fact_sheet.pdf.

World Health Organization (WHO). 2007. Resolution WHA60.17. Available at http://apps.who.int/gb/ebwha/pdf_files/WHASSA_WHA60-Rec1/E/reso-60-en.pdf.

World Health Organization (WHO). 2010. Global Health Expenditure Database. http://apps.who.int/nha/database/StandardReport.aspx?ID=REPORT_2_WHS. [6 March 2013].

World Health Organization (WHO). 2012. Statistics Database. Available at http://knoema.com/WHOSDB2012/world-health-organization-statistics-database-2012?tsId=1115640.

Wright JT, Graham F, Hayes C, Ismail AI *et al.* 2013. A systematic review of oral health outcomes produced by dental teams incorporating midlevel providers. *Journal of the American Dental Association* 144(1): 75–91.

Xu K, Saksenaa P, Holly A. 2011. The Determinants of Health Expenditure: A Country-Level Panel Data Analysis. Available at http://www.who.int/health_financing/documents/report_en_11_deter-he.pdf.

Yamalik N, Ensaldo-Carrasco E, Cavalle E, Kell K. 2014. Oral health workforce planning part 2: Figures, determinants and trends in a sample of World Dental Federation member countries. *International Dental Journal* 64(3): 117–126.

Personalized Medicine: Economic Evaluation and Evidence

Kathryn A. Phillips
University of California at San Francisco
Center for Translational and Policy Research
on Personalized Medicine (TRANSPERS)
Department of Clinical Pharmacy;
UCSF Philip R. Lee Institute for Health Policy;
and UCSF Helen Diller Family Comprehensive Cancer Center
3333 California St, Room 420, Box 0613
San Francisco, CA 94143

Katherine Payne
Manchester Centre for Health Economics
The University of Manchester
Oxford Road, Manchester M139PL, UK

Ken Redekop
Institute of Health Policy and Management
Erasmus University Rotterdam
PO Box 1738, 3000 DR Rotterdam
The Netherlands

There is a recent expansion in the development and application of genomic technologies, often called "personalized medicine" (PM). This growth in technological capability requires consideration of the potential impact on constrained health care budgets before it moves into clinical practice. There is a need for robust evaluative frameworks to provide decision-makers allocating scarce health care resources with robust evidence of the relative costs and benefits of applications of genomic-based medicine. This chapter: summarizes the existing economic evaluation literature on genomic-based medicine; describes how economic evaluation of genomic-based medicine has emerged into practice using case studies of three countries; and describes challenges in defining and measuring the value of genomic-based medicine and synthesizing costs and benefits for use in economic evaluations. The chapter concludes by looking at the (near) future and describes some key challenges associated with evaluating the economic impact of introducing new 'sequencing' technologies into clinical practice. Health economists have two key challenges in the context of genomics and PM. The first is to continue to apply robust methods of economic evaluation. The second is to tackle the methodological and practical issues to generate a sufficient evidence base to inform resource allocation decisions.

Keywords: Personalized Medicine; Economic(s); Value; United States (US); United Kingdom (UK); The Netherlands.

Introduction

Genomics has now firmly embedded itself as a real concept in the practice of medicine. Genomics is distinguished from genetics, that focuses on the function of single genes, as it 'addresses all genes and their inter-relationships in order to identify their combined influence on the growth and development of the organism'(*WHO Definitions of Genetics and Genomics*, 2004). There is a recent expansion in the development and application of genomic technologies, often called "personalized medicine." This expansion is likely to continue as new techniques are developed with increasing clinical applications. Application of genomics in health care offers an extensive array of technologies that enable different degrees of targeting and personalization of screening strategies, diagnostics and treatments. In terms of screening and diagnostic technologies, we are no longer reliant on Sanger sequencing methods[1] that, although accurate and reliable, only identified single mutations in single genes (*Sanger Institute*, 2012). The advent of next generation sequencing and whole exome or genome sequencing (hereafter termed 'sequencing' as shorthand) means that it is now feasible to test for panels of genes at one time and, in theory, sequence the whole human genome. This expansion in technological capability has resulted in the introduction of genomic-based diagnostics in new areas of medicine, and in some instances, may completely replace existing services, such as cytogenetics.[2] This expansion in technical capability can effectively move genomic testing to the front of the diagnostic care pathway. There are also examples of genomics moving from just being the remit of specialist clinical genetics services into mainstream health care. The prime examples are applications of genomics in clinical oncology in which genomic-based targeted medicines are frequently used in current practice. The early examples of

[1] Sanger Sequencing is a method of DNA sequencing based on the selective incorporation of chain-terminating dideoxynucleotides by DNA polymerase during *in vitro* DNA replication.

[2] Cytogenetics involves preparing a sample of a patient's chromosomes, staining them and looking for structural changes using a microscope. The advent of new genomic technologies can potentially replace this manual process by identifying structural changes.

genomic-based targeted medicines in oncology being the monoclonal antibody trastuzumab, which is approved for the treatment of HER2-positive breast cancer and the tyrosine kinase inhibitor imatinib, which is licensed for the treatment of BCR–ABL translocation-driven chronic myeloid leukemia (Yap and Workman, 2012). There is likely to be a continued expansion in the future to other areas in mainstream health care such as cardiology and treatment of rheumatoid arthritis. This continued expansion in genomic-based technologies must, however, be viewed within the context of constrained health care budgets. Therefore, there is a need for robust evaluative frameworks to be used to provide decision-makers allocating scarce health care resources with robust evidence of the relative costs and benefits of applications of genomic-based medicine.

The specific objectives of this chapter are to:

- Summarize the existing literature on economic evaluation in the context of genomic-based medicine;
- describe how economic evaluation of genomic-based medicine has emerged into practice using case studies of three countries;
- describe challenges in defining and measuring the value of genomic-based medicine; and
- describe challenges in collating and synthesizing costs and benefits for use in economic evaluations and illustrate these challenges with case studies.

The chapter will end by taking a look at the (near) future and describing some key challenges associated with evaluating the economic impact of incorporating sequencing into clinical practice.

Why is Economics Relevant to Genomics?

The development of genomic technologies has introduced the concept of personalized medicine (PM), which is now ubiquitous. However, there is little consistency in how PM is either defined or used in clinical practice. Various authors have attempted to bring together the different definitions of PM (see, for example, Redekop and Mladsi, 2013; Schleidgen *et al.*, 2013). Redekop and Mladsi (2013) offer this useful working definition of PM:

> "the use of combined knowledge (genetic or otherwise) about a person to predict disease susceptibility, disease prognosis, or treatment response and thereby improve that person's health."

This is the definition adopted in this chapter because it facilitates discussion of broad implications when considering the economics of PM, rather than adopting the narrower focus on using genomics to target medicines.

Irrespective of how PM is defined, decision-makers charged with allocating finite health care budgets require robust and timely evidence to support the cost-effectiveness of technologies used to 'personalize' the diagnosis, prevention or treatment of diseases. Health economics provides evaluative frameworks that can be used to design studies to provide evidence on how to best spend finite health care resources. The underlying premise is that choices have to be made because health care resources are limited and some systems are set up with a finite, and generally annual, budget specifically allocated to provide health care services, treatments and interventions. The objective of health care providers then becomes how to spend resources to achieve maximum benefits to patient populations. Evidence suitable for informing decision-making can be generated from a range of methods, each underpinned by different economic theories that guide the resulting evaluative framework. Economic evaluation, which provides a framework to enable the assessment of an intervention's incremental benefits and costs over existing treatments, is one method available to health economists who want to generate evidence to inform decision-making. In this chapter, we focus on the use of economic evaluation methods, such as cost-effectiveness or cost–utility analysis, drawing on model-based and trial-based evaluations and their application to genomic-based technologies.

What is Already Known About the Economics of PM

A common perception is that PM will save health care costs by better targeting medications and interventions to patient groups that are most likely to benefit. This assumption is conceptually appealing, but evidence is needed to show whether it is borne out in actual practice. The need to understand this evidence base has been the stimulus for the extensive number of published systematic reviews that have identified and summarized published economic evaluations of PMs (Carlson *et al.*, 2005; Giacomini *et al.*, 2003; Hatz *et al.*, 2014; Jarrett and Mugford, 2006; Phillips *et al.*, 2013b; 2014; Phillips and Van Bebber, 2004; Vegter *et al.*, 2008; 2010; Wong *et al.*, 2010). The findings from these reviews cannot be compared directly because different definitions of PM, different search strategies and inconsistent study inclusion criteria have been used. However, a common finding from all of the published systematic reviews is that the economic evidence base is both increasing in volume and improving in quality, but some key methodological challenges remain for the design and conduct of cost-effectiveness analyses (CEAs) of PM. A key challenge for all systematic reviews was the lack of a common nomenclature in PM, which resulted in heterogeneous search strategies in an attempt to identify all the published economic evaluations. Economic evaluations have, however, only been conducted on a fraction of the available genomic tests and potential applications in health care, with most of the cost-utility analyses focusing on more common conditions such as breast cancer (Phillips *et al.*, 2014). The focus has been on using cost-effectiveness and cost-utility analysis rather than cost–benefit analysis. In general, studies to date suggest that applications of PM have similar incremental cost-effectiveness ratios (ICERs) as pharmaceuticals. The majority of studies suggested that PM is relatively more cost-effective than alternative strategies, with a minority of PM interventions shown to be cost-saving.

The series of systematic reviews has shown significant growth in the evidence base over time. The first review, published by Phillips and Van Bebber (2004) aimed to identify all published cost-effectiveness analyses (CEAs) and cost–utility analyses (CUAs) of pharmacogenomics interventions and found just 11 studies. More recent examples include reviews which focused on identifying the current economic evidence base supporting the use of genomic-based strategies to diagnose and target treatments, respectively (Hatz *et al.*, 2014; Phillips *et al.*, 2014). Hatz *et al.* (2014), conducted a systematic review of cost-effectiveness and cost-utility analyses published in English or German and located 84 studies, most of which were from the US, were CUAs, and were published since 2005. The median value of CUAs was found to be around US$22,000 per QALY gained, similar to the median found in another review of CUAs of pharmaceuticals (Neumann *et al.*, 2009). These authors concluded that:

> "individualized medicine neither seems to display superior cost-effectiveness than other types of medical interventions nor to be economically inferior. Instead, rather than 'whether' health care was individualized, the question of 'how' it was individualized was of economic relevance."

In 2013, Phillips and colleagues also assessed the quantity and quality of evidence on the economic value of PM tests and identified the gaps in the evidence base. They did so by creating a unique evidence base using data on published CUAs from the Tufts Cost-Effectiveness Analysis Registry (CEAR) (Phillips *et al.*, 2014). The CEAR is a comprehensive database that abstracts and aggregates information on over 3,000 original, English-language, health-related CUAs published between 1976 and 2011 and indexed in PubMed (Neumann *et al.*, 2005). A total of 59 CUA studies were identified that examined personalized medicine tests (1998–2011). A majority (72%) of the cost per QALY gained ratios indicated that testing provides better health although at higher cost than the relevant alternative. Still, almost half of the ratios were under the threshold of $50,000 per QALY gained, indicating they can be considered a cost-effective use of health care resources (Grosse, 2008). One-fifth of the results indicated that tests may save money while improving health. The key conclusion was that many PM tests have been found to be relatively cost-effective although fewer have been found to be cost-saving and many available or emerging medicine tests have not been evaluated. In summary, there has been a growth in the quantity and quality of economic evidence available supporting the use of PM but more evidence on the potential added value will be needed to inform decision-making and assessment of genomic priorities. The development of this economic evidence base also needs to take account of key methodological and practical challenges in the design and conduct of economic evaluations of PM.

What is Known about the Economics of PM by Country?

This section starts by comparing the existing evidence base for CUA of PM across countries. This is a new analysis of the studies identified by Phillips *et al.* (2014). The section then continues by providing descriptive case studies reporting the economics of PM in three exemplar countries: The US, the UK, and The Netherlands.

The 59 CUAs identified and summarized in Phillips *et al.* (2014) were used to provide a comparison between studies based in the US ($n = 30$) and non-US countries ($n = 29$). The country codes from the Tufts CEAR (reflecting the relevant country population) were linked with the 59 identified CUAs and used to group studies into these two categories. In some instances, the analyses reported multiple results as cost per QALY gained, therefore, the weighted QALYs across the reported ratios for each study ($n = 139$ ratios) was calculated. Looking at the combined data for US-based and non-US-based studies, the majority (72%) of the ICERs indicated that the PM interventions provide better health although at higher cost. Around half of the ICERs were above a threshold of $50,000 per QALY gained and some 20% were higher than a threshold of $100,000 per QALY gained (Phillips *et al.*, 2014).[10] The distribution of the ICERs was marginally different between US and non-US studies ($p = 0.07$) (see Figure 1). The US-based studies reported generally lower ICERs compared with the non-US-based studies. This analysis and data do not allow us to determine why cost-effectiveness may differ between countries, but some speculative reasons are: Specific type of test under investigation; the choice of comparator (e.g., treat all, treat none); impact of unit drug costs; or the impact of downstream treatment options.

The next three sections of this chapter draw on three case studies in the US, UK, and the Netherlands to explore how economic evidence is used in the context of PM. The existence of published economic evaluations is a necessary but insufficient condition for the use of economic evidence to inform decision-making in the context of PM. To understand if, and how, economic evidence is, or could be,

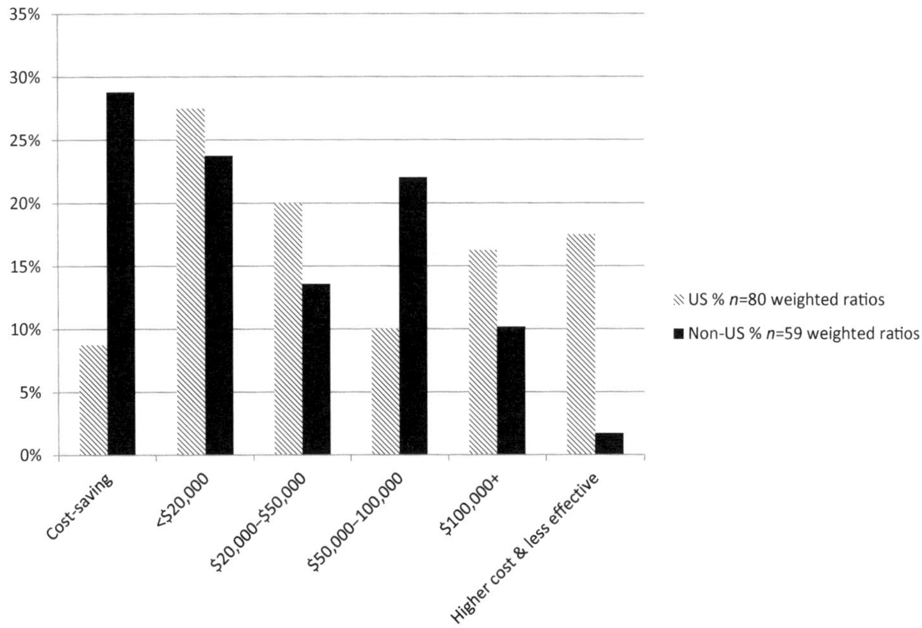

Figure 1. Distribution of ICERs from cost–utility analyses of interventions to personalize medicine tests comparing US-based and non-US-based studies (Phillips *et al.*, 2014)

used to inform resource allocation decisions for PM, it is also necessary to consider the context in which such decisions are made at the country level. Given the substantial differences between funding mechanisms and health service provision across countries, it is also necessary to take account of country-specific differences in how economic evaluation is used to inform resource allocation decisions for PM.

PM and economics in the United States (US)

The unique features of the US health care system compared with other systems are well-known. The US system can be described as a patchwork of public and private providers and insurers in a competitive system that is less regulated than in other countries. Thus, not surprisingly, there is a wide range of approaches to assessing PM and economics in the US. We highlight below some key initiatives and organizations.

- *National Institutes of Health (NIH)*

The NIH is the principal federal agency for health research in the US, funding about $30 billion in research annually (*National Institutes of Health Budget*, 2014). NIH is a major funder of research on PM throughout its 27 institutes. In 1989, the NIH established a center focusing specifically on genomics research — now called the National Human Genome Research Institute (NHGRI). Historically, NIH has funded primarily basic research in genomics (and other areas) with little emphasis on economics or other applied research. However, the legislation creating NHGRI stipulated that 5% of its extramural research funding be allocated to ELSI related grants (Ethical, Legal, and Social Implications). Although the definition of ELSI research does not explicitly include the term "economics," in recent years NHGRI has become more interested in funding economic and other related research. For example, the senior author of this chapter (Kathryn A. Phillips) was funded by NHGRI to conduct a 4-year study of the benefit–risk tradeoffs of whole genome sequencing, including an analysis of its economic value (described further below).

The NIH has also recently funded several grants focusing specifically on the economics of PM through its Common Fund. The NIH Common Fund was enacted in 2006 to support high-impact, trans-NIH programs. NIH Common Fund programs are intended to be transformative, catalytic, synergistic, cross-cutting, and unique. The Common Fund's Health Economics Program aims to support theoretical and applied research to understand how innovations in treatments, diagnosis, and preventive strategies can be most effectively deployed to improve health and well-being. In 2013, the NIH Common Fund Health Economics Working Group partnered with the editors of the Forum for Health Economics & Policy to publish a special issue on the economics of personalized health care and prevention. In addition, the Health Economics Program funded four studies in 2013 to conduct economic research on the determinants and consequences of personalization in health care and prevention (Tufts Medical Center, Georgetown University, Vanderbilt University Medical Center, and University of Washington).

- *Institute of Medicine (IOM)*

The IOM, which is the health arm of the National Academy of Sciences, is an independent, nonprofit organization that works outside of government to provide unbiased and authoritative advice to decision-makers and the public. As with the NIH, genomics and economics is a frequent topic across different areas of medicine, for example, oncology. Of particular relevance is the IOM Roundtable on Translating Genomic-Based Research for Health, which brings together leaders from academia, industry, government, foundations and associations who have a mutual interest in addressing the issues surrounding the translation of genomic-based research. The mission of the Roundtable is to advance the field of genomics and improve the translation of research findings to health care, education, and policy. In 2012, the Roundtable held a workshop on "Assessing the Economics of Genomic Medicine," which assessed the potential economic impact that the advent of genomic medicine may have on clinical practice and research (Feero *et al.*,

2013). The authors concluded that genome-scale information challenges traditional economic assessment much as it challenges approaches of traditional health care delivery. Four overarching points became apparent during the meeting. First, genomic researchers, health care practitioners, payers, and economists are not comfortable in each other's domains. Second, the evidence base demonstrating that genomic data improve health outcomes is critically underdeveloped, and commonly accepted evidence thresholds for clinical utility and value for money do not exist. Third, traditional methods for economic assessment are not readily scalable to the pace of genomic discovery in terms of turnaround time and expense. Fourth, there is a need to develop a formal approach for dealing with what has come to be known as "personal utility", e.g., the value to the individual beyond clinical utility, and its role in assessing the value of sequencing.

- *Centers for Disease Control and Prevention (CDC)*

The CDC is the major public health and health protection organization in the US. Of particular relevance is the Office of Public Health Genomics (OPHG), which provides timely and credible information for the effective and responsible translation of genomics research into population health benefits. One activity sponsored by OPHG is the EGAPP Working Group (Evaluation of Genomic Applications in Practice and Prevention), which was established in 2005 to support the development of a systematic process for assessing the available evidence regarding the validity and utility of rapidly emerging genetic tests for clinical practice. This independent, multidisciplinary panel prioritizes and selects tests, reviews CDC-commissioned evidence reports and other contextual factors, highlights critical knowledge gaps, and provides guidance on appropriate use of genetic tests in specific clinical scenarios. Although most of the work conducted by OPGH and EGAPP is not directly focused on assessing economics of PM, economic value is one of the issues it tracks and considers as relevant.

- *Health Technology Assessment (HTA) Organizations*

In a previous study (Trosman *et al.*, 2011), we identified seven US-based organizations that conduct HTA, which are used to inform private payer coverage decisions related to PM: Blue Cross Blue Shield Technology Evaluation Center (BCBS TEC); Emergency Care Research Institute (ECRI); Evaluation of Genomic Applications in Practice and Prevention (EGAPP); Hayes; Institute for Clinical and Economic Research (ICER); United States Preventive Services Task Force (USPSTF); and UpToDate. We found that these organizations had varying characteristics and addressed different research questions. The seven HTA organizations included two private companies, two independent panels developed by the government, and three nonprofit organizations. Several of the organizations charge a fee for access to their HTAs. Few of the reviews focused on cost-effectiveness, which was seen as a shortcoming by a large majority of the private payers that were interviewed. Of particular interest was that, although all interviewed payers reported using at least one external HTA organization in their coverage-decision making related to personalized medicine, the number of HTA organizations used by individual payers ranged from one to all seven.

To provide an illustration of one specific center that includes a focus on PM and economics, we now summarize some of the key research and findings conducted by the *University of California, San Francisco Center for Translational and Policy Research on Personalized Medicine* (TRANSPERS). Launched in 2008, TRANSPERS is a research center dedicated to developing evidence-based information to objectively assess how personalized medicine can be most beneficial and efficient in improving health outcomes. The Center has three key foci: (i) Access, utilization, and preferences; (ii) Coverage and reimbursement; (iii) Economic value.

In a recent article (Phillips *et al.*, 2013b), we reviewed the Center's work since its inception and reached the following conclusions about key findings:

(1) There is a lack of evidence on how PM is implemented in actual practice and thus its value in "real world" settings.
(2) It is unclear whether PM will be cost-saving or more cost-effective than other alternatives.
(3) Analyses of targeted testing need to consider the method of targeting in order to appropriately assess the value of PM.
(4) Behavior of family members is a key factor in determining the value of PM for inherited mutations.
(5) Patient and provider preferences may affect the cost-effectiveness of PM.
(6) Payers struggle with how to assess the value of PM for making coverage and reimbursement decisions.
(7) Diffusion of PM appears to lag for certain subgroups such as the underserved, with implications for utilization and cost-effectiveness.

These findings now help set the stage for a future research agenda, not only in the US but also in other countries.

PM and economics in England

As is well known, the UK has a publicly funded health care system called the National Health Service (NHS). A minority of the British public also purchase private health care insurance, but most people access health care services that are free at the point of use. The budget for health care provision is set each year. Funding of the NHS together with service commissioning decisions are both now devolved to the constituent members of the UK: England, Scotland, Wales, and Northern Ireland. The devolved nature of service commissioning has led to differences in decision-making bodies charged with allocating health care resources across the UK constituent countries.

In the UK, once a medicine has a product license, based on safety, efficacy and quality data, then it is eligible for prescribing by NHS clinicians. Similarly, diagnostics can gain regulatory approval but there are also examples of laboratory-developed tests that are used in the NHS. Following regulatory approval some medicines and diagnostics can be subsequently appraised by the National Institute for Health and Care Excellence (NICE) using a structured health technology assessment based on a combination of a systematic review of the available clinical evidence and a model-based cost effectiveness analysis. Below, we describe the main national research funding and decision-making bodies that have an impact on developing economic evidence to support the use of PM in England.

The NHS is a complex and ever-changing system and it is within this context that PM has to move from research into clinical practice, ideally supported by robust clinical and economic evidence. This evidence base can be produced by academics, industry, health technology assessment bodies and clinicians, and others working at the provider level. Funding is clearly required to support the development of a robust evidence base. There has been a national funding strategy for generating an evidence base to develop PM at the basic bioscience level and to inform how best to translate the basic science into clinical practice (*Realising the Potential of Stratified Medicine*, 2013). Stratified Medicine focused initiatives have been established by national funding bodies such as the Medical Research Council (*Medical Research Council*, 2014) and the Technology Strategy Board (*Stratified Medicine Innovation Platform*, 2011) to focus on generating the basic science and clinical evidence. Alongside this, the National Institute for Health Research (NIHR) has commissioned Biomedical Research Centres (*Biomedical Research Centres*, 2014) and Experimental Cancer Medicine Centres (*Experimental Cancer Medicine Centres*, 2014) to support the development of innovative genomic-based technologies. To supplement these initiatives, Diagnostic Evidence Co-Operatives (*Diagnostic Evidence Co-Operatives,* 2014) have been established to generate evidence of clinical utility and cost-effectiveness of diagnostics, including genomic-based technologies. These funding streams are also supplemented by funding for specific projects that has been commissioned under the remit of The NIHR Evaluation, Trials and Studies Coordinating Centre (NETSCC), which was established in April 2008 and has five core streams: Efficacy and Mechanism Evaluation

Programme; Health Services and Delivery Research Programme; Health Technology Assessment Programme; Public Health Research Programme and the Systematic Reviews Programme. It is the NETSCC that supports the development of the evidence base for decision-making bodies such as the National Institute for Health and Care Excellence (NICE) that leads the appraisal and assessment of health care technologies, diagnostics, and public health interventions and programmes.

A national funding strategy is a necessary but not sufficient requirement to support the introduction of PM. It is also necessary to have clear processes for the evaluation and appraisal of the evidence base to inform if, and how, to introduce new genomic-technologies into clinical practice. In England specifically, three systems have emerged as potentially relevant to genomics and PM: The NICE technology appraisal process; the NICE Diagnostics Assessment Programme and the United Kingdom Genetic Testing Network (UKGTN). The UKGTN also has a remit in Scotland, Wales, and Northern Ireland. However, NICE is primarily relevant to England only.

The process used by NICE to inform resource allocation decisions is transparent, well-structured and now has over 10 years of practical experience in the appraisal of the clinical and cost effectiveness of pharmaceuticals. The technology appraisal process set up by NICE has become the gold standard for using evidence of clinical and cost effectiveness to inform national guidelines, which are subsequently used by decision-makers choosing how best to spend the NHS budget at a regional level. NICE is now also attempting to deal with the challenge of evaluating products that do not have like-for-like regulatory evidence requirements, such as companion diagnostics, and diagnostics more generally (Payne, 2009).

There is a distinction made in terms of how NICE views companion diagnostics-medicine combinations compared with other genomic-based diagnostics as part of these appraisal processes. If the genomic-based diagnostic is clearly linked with a specific new medicine and is by definition a companion diagnostic-medicine combination, then this type of technology will generally feed into the NICE Technology Appraisal (TA) Programme. However, if the genomic diagnostic has the potential to inform the selection of more than one medicine, or if more than one version of the test is available, and the diagnostic is likely to add to an existing care pathway, then the technology will generally be appraised as part of the Diagnostics Assessment Programme (DAP) (*Diagnostics Assessment Programme*, 2014). The Medical Technical Appraisal Committee (MTAC) within NICE makes the final decision as to which programme the technology is most suitable to be assessed within. The distinct TA and DAP processes mean that different committees and different methods are used for companion genomic diagnostics and genomic diagnostics with multiple applications. However, despite different methods guides being used for the two processes, only subtle differences in the actual assessment processes apply. Both processes state a clear preference for the need for robust CEA to be used in decision-making and for evidence of the benefit of the technology or diagnostic test to be based on the QALY outcome.

The UKGTN was established before NICE implemented the Diagnostics Assessment Programme. The UKGTN now liaises closely with NICE to ensure no overlap or duplication of work and has a specific remit to act as an advisory organization to provide commissioning support on genetic tests to the NHS and the Department of Health for NHS patients (*UK Genetic Testing Network,* 2014). The main purpose of the UKGTN is to promote equity of access to genetic testing for rare conditions, and it does not specifically focus on companion diagnostics to target medicines. The UKGTN developed and introduced Gene Dossiers, a system for the evaluation of new genetic tests that aims to inform the commissioning of services in the NHS. Gene Dossiers are a voluntary system of control for laboratories providing genetic testing in which evidence about the disease condition to be tested, the test's clinical validity and utility together with the proposed cost of the test is submitted. Gene Dossiers consider budget impact but not relative cost effectiveness per se. Genetic tests can be provided on a national basis upon successful submission of a Gene Dossier and subsequent approval by the Specialist Commissioning Group who report to local service commissioners. Genetic tests without a dossier can only be offered on a regional basis. This is the more common route for a genetic test to move from the research laboratory environment directly into clinical service. The Dossier process shares a similar remit to NICE making recommendations to commissioners but differs considerably in the source and type of evidence submitted. The evidence submitted by the NHS laboratory who wants to provide the test will include a summary of the literature and in-house validation studies of test sensitivity and specificity with a budget impact assessment. To date, evidence from trials or economic models has not formed part of the evidence submitted. A tariff-setting exercise found large variability in pricing between laboratories and the process does not work on a national price list of genetic tests. This lack of a nationally agreed price list has a direct implication, for instance, if a genetic test was to be considered by NICE. In its current appraisal mechanisms NICE uses publicly available unit costs for the technologies, therefore, it will be necessary to contact laboratory providers directly to determine the unit cost of a genomic-based diagnostic in the absence of a national price list.

To summarize, a substantial national budget has been diverted to developing and evaluating new genomic-based technologies. In addition, NICE and the UKGTN have processes in place to provide support for decision-makers deciding how to allocate the finite NHS budgets. However, some clear gaps remain in the evidence produced and appraised at a national level, which means that decision-makers working at a regional level and within health service provider organizations still have to judge if, and how, to introduce PM into practice using their own initiative. It is how to close this evidence gap that remains an enduring challenge for research funding and health technology assessment organizations in England and constituent members of the UK.

PM and economics in The Netherlands

The Netherlands has a health care system characterized by mandatory universal coverage in combination with competing private health plans. When it comes to acute medical care, all private health insurance companies are obliged to reimburse a defined set of insured treatments (a so-called basic package); expenditures through this insurance accounted for approximately 40% of all health care expenses in 2012 (*Zorgrekeningen; uitgaven (in lopende en constante prijzen) en financiering*, 2014). Advice regarding the contents of the basic health care package is provided the National Health Care Institute (Zorginstituut Nederland, until recently known as CVZ, the name which is therefore used in this chapter), a government organization, to the Minister of Public Health, Welfare and Sport, who makes final decisions. This section describes aspects of the system in order to highlight how PM is assessed in The Netherlands.

Le Polain *et al.* (2010) provide an in-depth, albeit dated in parts, description of the Dutch drug reimbursement process. Historically, advice about the reimbursement of outpatient medicines was provided by the CFH (*Commissie Farmaceutische Hulp*, meaning Pharmaceutical Care Committee), a committee operating as part of CVZ. The CFH based the reimbursement eligibility of a medicine on its therapeutic value, efficacy, and economic impact. Advice from CFH and CVZ was then provided to the Minister, who could add drugs to one of two so-called "positive lists" (Schedules 1A and 1B). Schedule 1A consisted of clusters of similar medications with a reimbursement limit for each of these clusters while Schedule 1B consisted of "dissimilar" medications, for which no price limit is set. If the chance of inappropriate use of a medicine (e.g., off-label use) was high, conditions could be placed on its reimbursement and the medicine was added to a so-called Schedule 2 list.

The CVZ applies a variety of assessment and appraisal criteria: Medical need, (added) therapeutic value (including effectiveness and safety), cost-effectiveness, feasibility, necessity to insure, budget impact, disease severity, rarity of the disease, individual responsibility, accessibility, social affordability, and public health benefit.

While this approach to reimbursement seems very rational, there have been indications that the system does not work as well as one might expect. For example, it was found that conditions placed by CVZ on the use and reimbursement of in-patent statins were rarely followed by clinicians; in practice, clinicians' decisions about statin use were more often in line with the recommendations found in clinical practice guidelines (Niezen *et al.*, 2007). Interestingly, policymakers indicated that they were aware of the problem but viewed the conditions as a way to communicate to health insurers and doctors that they should exercise restraint when prescribing and reimbursing statins.

In the Netherlands, specialist medicines (or "inpatient drugs") are reimbursed only after they have been reviewed by CVZ; once approved, they will be included in the basic insurance package. In addition, they may be financed through a policy for conditional access ("*Voorwaardelijke toelating/financiering van zorg*"). If certain conditions are met, such as a high national budget impact, then add-on financing can be requested by a health care provider or health insurer on behalf of all hospitals. The provision of conditional access is linked with the obligation to examine the degree of appropriate drug use and incremental cost-effectiveness in daily practice over a 4-year period. At the end of this period, a report of reassessment (including an updated estimate of the cost-effectiveness of the drug), will be assessed by CVZ, who will then decide whether or not additional financing will continue. A favorable (or low) cost-effectiveness ratio is expected to increase the likelihood of continued reimbursement, while an unfavorable (or high) ratio would likely reduce the likelihood.

The roots of this additional financing are worth examining since they have a relevant connection with PM. In 2003, both patients and clinicians indicated that trastuzumab for the treatment of HER2-positive metastasized breast cancer was not being used sufficiently in practice. In response to these concerns, the Dutch Breast Cancer Association conducted a study in 2004 to determine the extent to which patients with HER2-positive metastatic breast cancer were treated with trastuzumab (*Availability of trastuzumab for breast cancer patients with HER2-positive tumors [report, in Dutch]*, 2007). This study revealed that only 39% of the patients eligible for treatment with trastuzumab actually received it; the underlying reasons for the low percentage of use could not be ascertained since this study relied on a database of treatments provided to patients. Moreover, the percentage of trastuzumab use varied greatly between provinces. The Dutch Breast Cancer Association found this "postal code medicine" unacceptable and insisted that the government, insurers, hospital administrators, and physicians should ensure compliance with national clinical guidelines and provide adequate funding. The concerns expressed by various parties about postal code medicine eventually culminated in a new policy to provide partial government financing of expensive inpatient drugs. This was unique, since the drugs administered in a hospital were normally not reimbursed separately from other hospital activities; very expensive drugs therefore represented an exception to that rule. The explicit purpose of this policy was to ensure that hospitals using these medicines were sufficiently reimbursed and thereby avoid any postal code medicine. In 2012, the policy was replaced with a rule which allows hospitals to declare these drugs in a separate DBC (Diagnosis-Related Group (DRG)-like system), a so-called add-on DRG.

The new policy to partially reimburse expensive in-hospital drugs was presented as a means to prevent postal code medicine as well as ensure timely access to promising new drugs. However, it also came with strings attached. It was, in fact, what could be called a coverage with evidence development policy, meaning that these drugs would be reimbursed for a limited period of time to enable clinicians, researchers and reimbursement authorities to ascertain if the drugs are being used as expected ('appropriate use,' assessed based on aspects like patient characteristics, dosages, and dose modifications) and if their so-called 'real-world' effectiveness and cost-effectiveness were acceptable. During this limited period of reimbursement, these criteria are not used to make reimbursement decisions. However, this system requires that evidence has to be provided twice: Once at the time of the initial reimbursement application and again during a reassessment based on the drug's use in daily practice and its real-life effectiveness and cost-effectiveness. As one might expect, implementation of this policy brings with it a myriad of methodological challenges (Franken *et al.*, 2013). One of the major concerns has been the lack of a randomized controlled setting, which results in problems with internal validity. Other challenges include the role of data synthesis and modeling, the use of existing data sources, the applicability of outcome measures commonly used in clinical trials, timeliness of evidence, and generalizability of the results. A recent paper described the issues that arose when the pilot studies were conducted (Franken *et al.*, 2014). In brief, although coverage with evidence development policies and outcomes research seem to be an attractive policy option, many unanswered questions remain regarding their actual value and feasibility. In the Netherlands, the policy of coverage with evidence generation combined with outcomes research requirements was first introduced for expensive inpatient drugs in 2006. Since 2013, this policy has been extended to cover specific groups of outpatient drugs; the impact of this extension will only be clear in a few years.

The exemplars of PM described above primarily relate to targeted medicines. In other cases, the focus is more on the test and less on the medicine. Examples of such applications include Oncotype Dx® and Mammaprint®, two diagnostic tests which help to determine whether chemotherapy will improve the prognosis of a woman with breast cancer. As in England, the decision-making process regarding these types of applications is different from the process seen with drugs. In order to help the health care minister make reimbursement decisions, CVZ gathers input from various sources throughout the various phases of its evaluation. This approach essentially has two aims: To ensure that the advice given to the minister is based on correct and complete knowledge and to ensure, wherever possible, that all stakeholders will support its final advice. The second aim is arguably an example of the Dutch consensus-based 'polder model,' where cooperation is sought amongst stakeholders despite their differences (*Polder Model*, 2014). In Dutch law, four different principles are applied when making reimbursement decisions about the addition of a technology: Necessity (medical and financial), effectiveness (including safety), cost-effectiveness, and feasibility. Financial necessity relates to the issue of whether or not an individual can be expected to pay for the care; factors here include the predictability of the need to receive that care and ability to pay. Medical necessity focuses on disease severity and the proportion of future health that a patient may lose due to illness (proportional shortfall) (Stolk *et al.*, 2004). Considerations about effectiveness relate to the state of both the clinical science and medical practice, which essentially means an examination of not only the evidence of effectiveness found in the literature but also what is used in daily clinical practice, particularly in The Netherlands. The opinions of medical specialists, including the contents of Dutch clinical practice guidelines can play a role here. The principle of cost-effectiveness focuses on the methods and techniques used worldwide and does not differ that much from the principles used by NICE. The fourth and final principle of feasibility relates to the issue of whether the technology being evaluated can be provided to all eligible patients in The Netherlands. This principle relates to the aim of fairness to all; important doubts about whether the technology will be available country-wide will mean a delay in positive advice about reimbursement.

The case of MammaPrint® for breast cancer provides a useful example of how CVZ operates. MammaPrint® is a prognostic test used to guide adjuvant treatment decisions in patients with node-negative breast cancer. It has been claimed that categorizing patients into a high-risk or a low-risk group based on the MammaPrint® is a more accurate method than the standard risk estimates in use and that its use could reduce overtreatment with chemotherapy. An example of this claim can be found in Retel *et al.* (2010), which compared its use with two alternative approaches (Sankt Gallen guidelines, Adjuvant Online Software) to determine its relative impact on survival, quality of life and costs (Retel *et al.*, 2010). They used a Markov model to simulate the 20-year costs and health outcomes in a hypothetical cohort of node-negative, estrogen receptor positive breast cancer patients in the Netherlands. Prognostic accuracy (sensitivity and specificity) of the approaches was based on analyses of tumor samples from three different validation studies. It was shown that the MammaPrint test resulted in the highest degree of quality-adjusted survival and had the highest probability of being cost-effective at willingness-to-pay levels beyond €12,000. During its assessment of the MammaPrint test, CVZ noted that the available results regarding the predictive value and clinical utility of the MammaPrint® test were based only on retrospective research (*Background Report on Assessing Whether the Gene Expression Test MammaPrint® in the Treatment of Breast Cancer Complies with Established Medical Science and Medical Practice,* 2010). It pointed out that prospective studies were both feasible and necessary to demonstrate the added value of the MammaPrint® test and concluded that the clinical utility of the MammaPrint® had not yet been demonstrated and that it did not fulfill the criterion of 'established medical science and medical practice'. Perhaps not coincidentally, CVZ was aware of an ongoing prospective, randomized, multicentre study (MINDACT) to compare MammaPrint® with standard clinical risk estimates. One can only speculate what the CVZ would have concluded if no such study was taking place or was being planned.

The Netherlands requires all health insurers to reimburse all of the technologies included in the basic reimbursement package; the contents of this package are determined by the minister. Since the minister, based on advice by CVZ, decided not to reimburse MammaPrint, health insurers were not obliged to reimburse it. However, it appears that most health insurers have opted to reimburse it nevertheless. In their explanations for their decision, they indicate a willingness to ensure that patients have access to PM even though clinical trials are still underway; this attitude is not unique to PM and can potentially be seen with other innovative therapies. It will be interesting to see how many other promising PM applications are also voluntarily reimbursed by health insurers in the future.

This concludes the description of examples of current funding and evaluation mechanisms that have included evidence on the economics of PM in three different countries. The experiences in these countries reveal the variety of developments that have taken place, both at the basic science and at the policy level. If we look into the future, we can see a number of common global issues that will need to be addressed. The next section examines these issues in more detail.

Challenges in Defining and Measuring Value of PM

In general, the design and conduct of cost-effectiveness analyses to show the added value of interventions to PM is no different than the evaluation of any other health care intervention. In particular, there are close analogies that can be drawn with the evaluation of diagnostics. However, there are some specific technical and practical challenges when conducting a CEA of a personalized medicine. A number of commentators have published papers on the specific issues for the design of CEAs of PM (Annemans *et al.*, 2013; Buchanan *et al.*, 2013; Conti *et al.*, 2010; Faulkner *et al.*, 2012). Generally, these papers have focused on issues for the economic evaluation of technologies concerned with identifying a single gene to stratify patient populations into sub-groups more likely to respond safely and effectively to a targeted treatment. In 2002, Danzon and Towse explored some specific issues related to the economics of gene therapy, concluding that such extreme examples of the 'personalization of medicines,' down to the individual patient level, are likely to be prohibitively expensive given the relative size of the benefits to patient populations (Danzon and Towse, 2002).

Buchanan *et al.* (2013) described some key methodological challenges for conducting economic evaluations of genomic-based diagnostic or prognostic tests, including those used to target treatment strategies (Buchanan *et al.*, 2013). The methodological challenges described related to how to define the relevant comparator, study perspective and time horizon for the analysis. The authors also described challenges associated with identifying and quantifying resource use and effectiveness data in an environment in which there are limited trials of the interventions being evaluated and there is limited evidence on patient and clinician behavior in terms of if/how they use genomic information in practice. Finally, the authors outlined the challenge of how to quantify the benefits to patients from genomic technologies because sometimes the use of health status, as valued in a cost-effectiveness or cost–utility analysis, may not capture all the relevant outcomes of interest. This methodological challenge arises because many of the potential clinical applications of sequencing are used as tests to diagnose conditions for which there are no available treatment options. This means that simply measuring change in health status would not be possible and it may be necessary to go beyond health and include some non-health outcomes such as the inherent value of diagnostic information (Grosse *et al.*, 2008). Work is ongoing in the US, for example, (*Center for Translational and Policy Research on Personalized Medicine*, 2014) and in the UK (*The University of Manchester — Katherine Payne*, 2013) to define how to measure the economic value of genomic-based diagnostics, which can be related to aspects such as empowerment linked to the capability to make an informed decision.

More recently, Annemans *et al.* (2013) used a more focused definition of PM and described 10 methodological challenges for generating estimates of cost-effectiveness using model-based economic evaluations of strategies used to stratify patient populations into groups of safe and effective responders to screening or treatment options (Annemans *et al.*, 2014). Some key issues described mirrored points raised by Buchanan *et al.* (2013), including the correct framing of the research question, data collection challenges and how to measure the value of tests (Buchanan *et al.*, 2013). Additional points described were specific to designing model-based evaluations of complex interventions that require a link to be made between if and how tests are used, the process of obtaining a diagnosis and interpretation of test results and informing a subsequent treatment decision to which patients adhere. Furthermore, Annemans *et al.* (2014) and Buchanan *et al.* (2013) described how the analysis can even become very complex if different tests are combined or sequentially used as there is a need to calculate the combined sensitivities and specificities of the tests (Annemans *et al.*, 2014; Buchanan *et al.*, 2013). Each of these issues leads to a higher degree of uncertainty in economic models designed to identify and quantify the incremental costs and benefits of personalized medicine compared with their simple pharmaceutical counterparts.

A key practical challenge that generally arises in the context of PM is the lack of a sufficient clinical evidence base to support the population of model-based economic evaluations. This practical challenge of producing an economic model populated with sufficiently robust data is exemplified using two published HTAs of an example companion diagnostic medicine technology, a pharmacogenetic test called *CYP2D6*. Two HTA reports looking at applications of *CYP2D6* testing for two pharmaceutical treatments, antipsychotics for people with schizophrenia (Fleeman *et al.*, 2010) and tamoxifen for women with breast cancer, (Fleeman *et al.*, 2011) respectively. In both HTAs, the most startling conclusion was that of the impact of the limited clinical evidence base to inform an economic model and the difficulty in differentiating between evidence of no effectiveness rather than no evidence of effectiveness of *CYP2D6* testing in these applications. This lack of evidence of clinical utility and cost effectiveness remains the enduring challenge for national centralized decisions to support the use of personalized medicines in clinical practice.

It is also important to have a clear understanding about the extent of adherence to the recommendations of the diagnostic test to target a medicine and to quantify the impact of the recommendations on prescribing behavior. In general, however, there is a paucity of evidence to support if, and how, clinicians use the results of companion diagnostics and how the test results affect subsequent prescribing and medicine-taking behavior. The importance of considering the impact of evidence about this level of decision-making can be illustrated using the findings from a prospective pragmatic randomized controlled trial of a pharmacogenetic test, the thiopurine methyltransferase test (*TMPT*), to predict the risk of neutropenia (a profound depletion in the number of white blood cells, that are used to fight infections) from the azathioprine used to treat autoimmune conditions (The TARGET study). This trial was pragmatic in design in that the intervention involved providing the *TPMT* genotype result and associated advice (regarding the appropriate azathioprine prescription) in the form of a clinical report to clinicians, and the comparator was current prescribing practice for each participating clinician (Newman *et al.*, 2011). It was anticipated, before the trial, that using the *TPMT* test would encourage clinicians to confidently start azathioprine at a treatment dose earlier in the patient's treatment plan rather than the current practice of slowly titrating up from a low start dose with frequent monitoring of blood results to reduce the risk of adverse effects like neutropaenia (Newman *et al.*, 2011). In the *TPMT* testing arm, the trial attempted to establish whether genotyping altered clinicians' prescribing behavior, and found that the clinicians were initiating treatment at a lower dose for *TPMT* heterozygotes as advised by the genotype result. However, overall there was no difference between the prescribing dose patterns of azathioprine between initiation and at 4 months between the two arms of the RCT which indicated that clinicians were not following the recommendations in the clinical test report. In a subsequent paper, the impact of the *TPMT* test compared with current practice was measured using a generic measure of health status (the EQ-5D) (Thompson *et al.*, 2014; *WHAT IS EQ-5D?*, 2014). A small negative difference in health status in the genotype arm compared with the no test arm was observed.

The causal reason for this observation cannot be known but may have been a reflection of the lack of adherence to test recommendations that subsequently manifest as a small detrimental effect on health benefit from testing (Thompson *et al.*, 2014). The TARGET study was underpowered and therefore unable to yield a statistical difference in health status between the two arms, but a positive change in health would have been predicted for the *TPMT* test arm. Several observations can be made from this study. It was apparent that clinicians were not changing their prescribing behavior, which might have been a consequence of a perceived lack of confidence in using the *TPMT* test. Clinicians, like decision-makers working at a policy level, require robust evidence of potential effect of using a companion diagnostic test before modifying their current prescribing behavior.

Furthermore, this trial was one of very few prospective randomized studies of a pharmacogenetic test, which resulted in moderate evidence of a modest effect of using TPMT to inform prescribing behavior and reduce the risk of neutropaenia. The trial required extensive expense, time and effort to conduct and yet still resulted in a smaller sample size than planned which meant the robustness of the findings were minimal. However, there is a continued demand for prospective trials to support the introduction of personalized medicines at national, local and the individual patient level. The feasibility of meeting this demand for RCT evidence is questionable given available funding resources and research effort.

Economics of New Genomic Sequencing Technologies: The Next Frontier in PM

Until recently, genetic-based testing was performed using technologies that identified known, specific, single-gene variants, such as analysis of the *HER2* gene for making decisions about treatment for breast cancer or the *BRCA1/2* genes for determining breast and ovarian cancer risk (Phillips *et al.*, 2013a). The advent of genomic-based testing and new sequencing technologies which rapidly analyze multiple genes in parallel (referred to as "next generation", "high throughput", or "massively parallel" sequencing, herein shortened to "sequencing"), has dramatically reduced the unit cost per gene and time associated with examining human genetic variations across the entire genome. Such sequencing technologies are now being used in research settings and are rapidly moving into clinical care (Faruki, 2013; Johansen Taber *et al.*, 2013). These emerging technologies can be used to examine gene panels, the entire coding portion of the genome which makes proteins (known as "whole exome sequencing"), or the whole genome including non-coding regions (known as "whole genome sequencing"). Several private companies in the US are offering gene panels based on sequencing technologies for clinical use, particularly for cancer treatment. In the UK, sequencing has some clinical applications in the NHS such as next generation sequencing for *BRCA1/2* (*Northern Genetics Service: Next Generation Sequencing*, 2014). To date, there are no clinical applications of whole exome or whole genome sequencing, but these technologies are currently being developed in research settings. These research-based applications of new sequencing technologies potentially allow genetic service providers to deliver an increased capacity (throughput) of genomic-based diagnostic tests to a wider population of patients; test results in a timely manner to inform subsequent management pathways information about multiple genes in one test rather than performing sequential single-gene tests; and genomic-based diagnostic testing at the front of the diagnostic pathway rather than the current situation in which a sequence of pre-tests focusing on clinical signs and symptoms (or 'work-up' tests) are used to suggest the need for subsequent genetic-based diagnosis.

Assessing the economic value of clinical applications of such new sequencing technologies is complex because the diagnostic can provide a multitude of results that include:

- Clinically actionable findings — findings where there is expert consensus that the results can be used for treatment or prevention.
- Findings that are not directly clinically actionable — findings that may have some usefulness but with unclear treatment or prevention implications.
- Findings of unknown significance — findings that currently have no known usefulness.

Figure 2 illustrates the relevant pathway of events that would need to be captured in an economic model. There is currently a lack of consensus about to what extent all findings should be returned to patients because of concerns that providing information that does not have any known clinical utility could be harmful if there

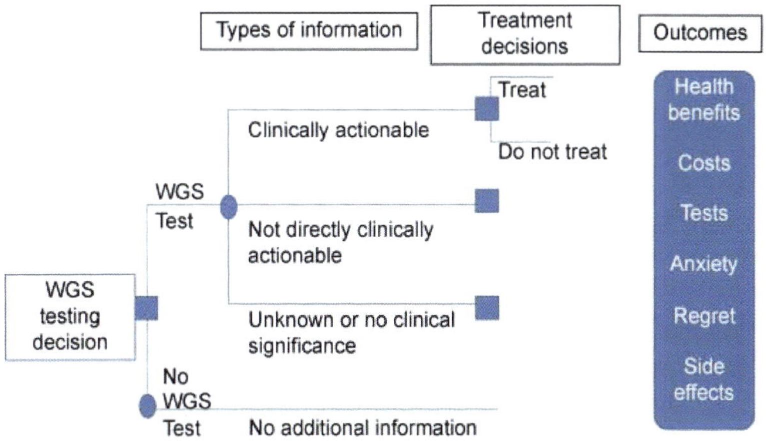

Figure 2. Example of pathways and outcomes for sequencing technologies
Source: Modified from Phillips *et al.* [2013b].

are no available or acceptable treatments or if the information leads to confusion or unwarranted health care.

Although studies are beginning to collect data on the costs associated with examples of sequencing, (Dewey *et al.*, 2014) to our knowledge there have not been any published economic evaluation studies. Furthermore, it is probably not feasible to produce reliable, fully specified cost-effectiveness analyses of new sequencing technologies because the clinical application has not yet been clearly specified. This evaluation challenge is further compounded by the potential for the sequencing technologies to test for multiple genes that makes the definition of what the intervention and its relevant comparators complex. A practical challenge is that there is too limited clinical evidence based on the intervention resulting in extensive uncertainty. The case study of genetic testing for hereditary breast cancer (*BRCA1/2*) can be used to illustrate some potential evaluation challenges when evaluating new sequencing technologies. This clinical area has a well-established clinical service offered using Sanger sequencing. In the UK, due to capacity constraints related to the current turnaround time for genetic testing, it is common practice to offer the test only to women deemed at high risk. For example, in the UK, the decision to offer a test is based upon a decision rule whereby women must be deemed to be at high-risk and a ≥20% risk of having a *BRCA1* or *BRCA2* mutation before qualifying for a genetic test (Sullivan *et al.*, 2012). The use of new sequencing technologies to test for *BRCA1/2* mutations facilitates a faster turnaround time and removes the need to use a 'risk' threshold before testing, and this means that more women can be offered testing. This implies there is the potential for new sequencing technologies to increase the capacity to provide testing to a greater proportion of individuals who otherwise would not have been offered the test in current practice. This situation introduces a key economic question to address and thus inform whether the potential for increased capacity provides added value to the health care system and patients.

Concluding Remarks

The rapid technological advances in PM threaten to outpace our ability to use these interventions effectively in clinical practice and to address the associated health policy issues. Whether genome-based sequencing technologies can achieve their potential to improve patient outcomes will depend on how patients and providers value the information provided, whether it will be covered by payers and recommended in guidelines, and whether the economic value to the health care delivery system outweighs the costs. The challenge for health economists is to continue to apply robust methods of economic evaluation and also tackle the methodological and practical issues that need to be addressed to generate a sufficient evidence base to inform resource allocation decisions in the context of genomics and PM.

References

Annemans L, Brignone M, Druais S, De Pauw A, Gauthier A, Demyttenaere K. 2014. Cost-effectiveness analysis of pharmaceutical treatment options in the first-line management of major depressive disorder in belgium. *Pharmacoeconomics* 32: 479–493.

Annemans L, Redekop K, Payne K. 2013. Current methodological issues in the economic assessment of personalized medicine. *Value Health* 16: S20–S26.

Availability of trastuzumab for Breast Cancer Patients with HER2-positive Tumors [Report, in Dutch] [Online]. 2007. Dutch Breast Cancer Association. Available: www.borstkanker.nl/php/bibliotheek_ext/download.php?id=366&bestand=HerceptinRapport2007_DEFINIT.pdf [Accessed 8 October 2014].

Background Report on Assessing Whether the Gene Expression Test MammaPrint® in the Treatment of Breast Cancer Complies with Established Medical Science and Medical Practice [Online]. 2010. Dutch National Health Care Institute. Available: http://www.zorginstituutnederland.nl/binaries/content/documents/zinl-www/documenten/publicaties/publications-in-english/2010/1010-background-report-on-assessing-whether-the-gene-expression-test-mammaprint-in-the-treatment-of-breast-cancer-complies-with-established-medical-science-and-medical-practice/1010-background-report-on-assessing-whether-the-gene-expression-test-mammaprint-in-the-treatment-of-breast-cancer-complies-with-established-medical-science-and-medical-practice/Background+report+on+assessing+whether+the+gene+expression+test+Mammaprin t+in+the+treatment+of+breast+cancer+complies+with+established+medical+science +and+medical+practice.pdf [Accessed 16 October 2014].

Biomedical Research Centres [Online]. Available: http://www.nihr.ac.uk/about/biomedical-research-centres.htm [Accessed 8 October 2014].

Buchanan J, Wordsworth S, Schuh A. 2013. Issues surrounding the health economic evaluation of genomic technologies. *Pharmacogenomics* 14: 1833–1847.

Carlson JJ, Henrikson NB, Veenstra DL, Ramsey SD. 2005. Economic analyses of human genetics services: A systematic review. *Genetics in Medicine* 7: 519–523.

Center for Translational and Policy Research on Personalized Medicine [Online]. 2014. Available: http://clinicalpharmacy.ucsf.edu/transpers/ [Accessed 16 January 2014].

Conti R, Veenstra DL, Armstrong K, Lesko LJ, Grosse SD. 2010. Personalized medicine and genomics: challenges and opportunities in assessing effectiveness, cost-effectiveness, and future research priorities. *Medical Decision Making* 30: 328–340.

Danzon, P, Towse, A. 2002. The economics of gene therapy and of pharmacogenetics. *Value Health* 5: 5–13.

Dewey FE, Grove ME, Pan C, Goldstein BA, Bernstein JA, Chaib H, Merker JD, Goldfeder RL, Enns GM, David SP, Pakdaman N, Ormond KE, Caleshu C, Kingham K, Klein TE, Whirl-Carrillo M, Sakamoto K, Wheeler MT, Butte AJ, Ford JM, Boxer L, Ioannidis JP, Yeung AC, Altman RB, Assimes TL, Snyder M, Ashley EA, Quertermous T. 2014. Clinical interpretation and implications of whole-genome sequencing. *The Journal of the American Medical Association* 311: 1035–1045.

Diagnostic Evidence Co-Operatives [Online]. Available: http://www.nihr.ac.uk/about/diagnostic-evidence-co-operatives.htm [Accessed 8 October 2014].

Diagnostics Assessment Programme (DAP) [Online]. Available: http://www.nice.org.uk/About/What-we-do/Our-Programmes/NICE-guidance/NICE-diagnostics-guidance [Accessed 8 October 2014].

Experimental Cancer Medicine Centres [Online]. Available: http://www.nihr.ac.uk/about/experimental-cancer-medicine-centres.htm [Accessed 8 October 2014].

Faruki H. 2013. Genomic testing: The clinical laboratory perspective. *Clinical Pharmacology and Therapeutics* 94: 190–192.

Faulkner E, Annemans L, Garrison L, Helfand M, Holtorf AP, Hornberger J, Hughes D, Li T, Malone D, Payne K, Siebert U, Towse A, Veenstra D, Watkins J, Personalized Medicine D, Reimbursement Working G. 2012. Challenges in the development and reimbursement of personalized medicine-payer and manufacturer perspectives and implications for health economics and outcomes research: A report of the ISPOR personalized medicine special interest group. *Value Health* 15: 1162–1171.

Feero WG, Wicklund C, Veenstra DL. 2013. The economics of genomic medicine: Insights from the IOM Roundtable on translating genomic-based research for health. *The Journal of the American Medical Association* 309: 1235–1236.

Fleeman N, Martin Saborido C, Payne K, Boland A, Dickson R, Dundar Y, Fernandez Santander A, Howell S, Newman W, Oyee J, Walley T. 2011. The clinical effectiveness and cost-effectiveness of genotyping for CYP2D6 for the management of women with breast cancer treated with tamoxifen: A systematic review. *Health Technology Assessment* 15: 1–102.

Fleeman N, Mcleod C, Bagust A, Beale S, Boland A, Dundar Y, Jorgensen A, Payne K, Pirmohamed M, Pushpakom S, Walley T, De Warren-Penny P, Dickson R. 2010. The clinical effectiveness and cost-effectiveness of testing for cytochrome P450 polymorphisms in patients with schizophrenia treated with antipsychotics: A systematic review and economic evaluation. *Health Technology Assessment* 14: 1–157.

Franken MG, Gaultney JG, Blommestein HM, Huijgens PC, Sonneveld P, Redekop WK, Uyl-De Groot CA. 2014. Policymaker, please consider your needs carefully: Does outcomes research in relapsed or refractory multiple myeloma reduce policymaker uncertainty regarding value for money of bortezomib? *Value Health* 17: 245–253.

Franken MG, Van Gils CW, Gaultney JG, Delwel GO, Goettsch W, Huijgens PC, Steenhoek A, Punt CJ, Koopman M, Redekop WK, Uyl-De Groot CA. 2013. Practical feasibility of outcomes research in oncology: Lessons learned in assessing drug use and cost-effectiveness in The Netherlands. *European Journal of Cancer* 49: 8–16.

Giacomini M, Miller F, O'Brien BJ. 2003. Economic considerations for health insurance coverage of emerging genetic tests. *Community Genetics* 6: 61–73.

Grosse SD. 2008. Assessing cost-effectiveness in health care: History of the $50,000 per QALY threshold. *Expert Review of Pharmacoeconomics & Outcomes Research* 8: 165–178.

Grosse SD, Wordsworth S, Payne K. 2008. Economic methods for valuing the outcomes of genetic testing: Beyond cost-effectiveness analysis. *Genetics in Medicine* 10: 648–54.

Hatz MH, Schremser K, Rogowski WH. 2014. Is individualized medicine more cost-effective? A systematic review. *Pharmacoeconomics* 32: 443–455.

Jarrett J, Mugford M. 2006. Genetic health technology and economic evaluation: A critical review. *Applied Health Economics and Health Policy* 5: 27–35.

Johansen Taber KA, Dickinson BD, Wilson M. 2014. The promise and challenges of next-generation genome sequencing for clinical care. *JAMA Internal Medicine* 174(2): 275–280.

Le Polain M, Franken M, Koopmanschap MA, Cleemput I. 2010. Drug reimbursement systems: International comparison and policy recommendations: KCE Reports 147C. Belgian Health Care Knowledge Centre.

Medical Research Council [Online]. 2014. Available: http://www.mrc.ac.uk/research/initiatives/stratified-medicine/funding/ [Accessed 11 June 2014].

National Institutes of Health Budget [Online]. 2014. National Insitutes of Health. Available: http://www.nih.gov/about/budget.htm [Accessed 17 October 2014].

Neumann PJ, Fang CH, Cohen JT. 2009. 30 years of pharmaceutical cost–utility analyses: Growth, diversity and methodological improvement. *Pharmacoeconomics* 27: 861–872.

Neumann PJ, Greenberg D, Olchanski NV, Stone PW, Rosen AB. 2005. Growth and quality of the cost-utility literature, 1976–2001. *Value Health* 8: 3–9.

Newman WG, Payne K, Tricker K, Roberts SA, Fargher E, Pushpakom S, Alder JE, Sidgwick GP, Payne D, Elliott RA, Heise M, Elles R, Ramsden SC, Andrews J, Houston JB, Qasim F, Shaffer J, Griffiths CE, Ray DW, Bruce I, Ollier WE. 2011.

A pragmatic randomized controlled trial of thiopurine methyltransferase genotyping prior to azathioprine treatment: The Target study. *Pharmacogenomics* 12: 815–826.

Niezen M, De Bont A, Stolk E, Eyck A, Niessen L, Stoevelaar H. 2007. Conditional reimbursement within the Dutch drug policy. *Health Policy* 84: 39–50.

Northern Genetics Service: Next Generation Sequencing [Online]. 2014. Available: http://www.newcastle-hospitals.org.uk/services/northern-genetics_new-technology_next-generation-sequencing.aspx [Accessed 10 June 2014].

Payne K. 2009. Fish and chips all round? Regulation of DNA-based genetic diagnostics. *Health Economics* 18: 1233–1236.

Phillips KA, Ann Sakowski J, Trosman J, Douglas MP, Liang SY, Neumann P. 2014. The economic value of personalized medicine tests: What we know and what we need to know. *Genetics in Medicine* 16: 251–257.

Phillips KA, Milne RL, Rookus MA, Daly MB, Antoniou AC, Peock S, Frost D, Easton DF, Ellis S, Friedlander ML, Buys SS, Andrieu N, Nogues C, Stoppa-Lyonnet D, Bonadona V, Pujol P, Mclachlan SA, John EM, Hooning MJ, Seynaeve C, Tollenaar RA, Goldgar DE, Terry MB, Caldes T, Weideman PC, Andrulis IL, Singer CF, Birch K, Simard J, Southey MC, Olsson HL, Jakubowska A, Olah E, Gerdes AM, Foretova L, Hopper JL. 2013a. Tamoxifen and risk of contralateral breast cancer for BRCA1 and BRCA2 mutation carriers. *Journal of Clinical Oncology* 31: 3091–3099.

Phillips KA, Sakowski JA, Liang S, Ponce NA. 2013b. Economic Perspectives on personalized health care and prevention. *Forum for Health Economics and Policy* 16: 57–86.

Phillips KA, Van Bebber SL. 2004. A systematic review of cost-effectiveness analyses of pharmacogenomic interventions. *Pharmacogenomics* 5: 1139–1149.

Polder Model [Online]. 2014. *Wikipedia*. Available: http://en.wikipedia.org/wiki/Polder_model [Accessed 10 May 2014].

Realising the Potential of Stratified Medicine [Online]. 2013. The Academy of Medical Sciences. Available: http://www.acmedsci.ac.uk/viewFile/51e915f9f09fb.pdf [Accessed 10 June 2014].

Redekop WK, Mladsi D. 2013. The faces of personalized medicine: A framework for understanding its meaning and scope. *Value Health* 16: S4–S9.

Retel VP, Joore MA, Knauer M, Linn SC, Hauptmann M, Harten WH. 2010. Cost-effectiveness of the 70-gene signature versus St. Gallen guidelines and Adjuvant Online for early breast cancer. *European Journal of Cancer.* 46: 1382–1391.

Sanger Institute [Online]. 2012. Available: https://www.sanger.ac.uk/resources/technologies/sequencing.html [Accessed 17 October 2014].

Schleidgen S, Klingler C, Bertram T, Rogowski WH, Marckmann G. 2013. What is personalized medicine: Sharpening a vague term based on a systematic literature review. *BMC Medical Ethics* 14: 55.

Stolk EA, Van Donselaar G, Brouwer WB, Busschbach JJ. 2004. Reconciliation of economic concerns and health policy: Illustration of an equity adjustment procedure using proportional shortfall. *Pharmacoeconomics* 22: 1097–1107.

Stratified Medicine Innovation Platform [Online]. 2011. Available: https://connect.innovateuk.org/web/stratified-medicines-innovation-platform [Accessed 10 June 2014].

Sullivan W, Evans DG, Newman WG, Ramsden SC, Scheffer H, Payne K. 2012. Developing national guidance on genetic testing for breast cancer predisposition: the role of economic evidence? *Genetic Testing and Molecular Biomarkers* 16: 580–591.

Thompson AJ, Newman WG, Elliott RA, Roberts SA, Tricker K, Payne K. 2014. The cost-effectiveness of a pharmacogenetic test: A trial-based evaluation of TPMT genotyping for azathioprine. *Value Health* 17: 22–33.

Trosman JR, Van Bebber SL, Phillips KA. 2011. Health technology assessment and private payers' coverage of personalized medicine. *Journal of Oncology Practice* 7: 18s–24s.

UK Genetic Testing Network [Online]. 2014. Available: http://ukgtn.nhs.uk/ [Accessed 10 June 2014].

University of Manchester — Population Health — Katherine Payne [Online]. 2013. Available: http://www.population-health.manchester.ac.uk/staff/19433/ [Accessed 10 June 2014].

Vegter S, Boersma C, Rozenbaum M, Wilffert B, Navis G, Postma MJ. 2008. Pharmacoeconomic evaluations of pharmacogenetic and genomic screening programmes: A systematic review on content and adherence to guidelines. *Pharmacoeconomics* 26: 569–587.

Vegter S, Rozenbaum MH, Postema R, Tolley K, Postma MJ. 2010. Review of regulatory recommendations for orphan drug submissions in the Netherlands and Scotland: Focus on the underlying pharmacoeconomic evaluations. *Clinical Therapeutics* 32: 1651–1661.

What is EQ-5D? [Online]. 2014. Available: http://www.euroqol.org/ [Accessed 17 October 2014].

WHO Definitions of Genetics and Genomics [Online]. 2004. World Health Organization. Available: http://www.who.int/genomics/geneticsVSgenomics/en/ [Accessed 17 October 2014].

Wong WB, Carlson JJ, Thariani R, Veenstra DL. 2010. Cost effectiveness of pharmacogenomics: A critical and systematic review. *Pharmacoeconomics* 28: 1001–1013.

Yap TA, Workman P. 2012. Exploiting the cancer genome: Strategies for the discovery and clinical development of targeted molecular therapeutics. *Annual Review of Pharmacology and Toxicology* 52: 549–573.

Zorgrekeningen; uitgaven (in lopende en constante prijzen) en financiering [Online]. 2014. Available: http://statline.cbs.nl/StatWeb/publication/?DM=SLNL&PA=71914ned&D1=37-43&D2=a&HDR=G1&STB=T&VW=T [Accessed 10 June 2014].

Social Capital and Health

Lorenzo Rocco
University of Padova
Eline Aas
University of Oslo

Among the social determinants of health, social capital is gaining increasing attention in health economics and health policy. Although the boundaries of the concept of social capital are still under debate, the essence of social capital is that of favoring and supporting cooperation within communities, allowing them to supply a range of services which are beneficial to individual health. This chapter, after a brief overview of the debate about the conceptualization of social capital, discusses in some detail the mechanisms which relate social capital to health and offers a review of the recent empirical literature, focusing, although not exclusively, on developing countries. In the second part, this chapter contributes to the empirical literature by estimating the association between individual social capital and health in a cross-country setting including 93 countries, the largest ever used in this literature. Results confirm the beneficial role that social capital has in individual health and unveil a pattern so far rather overlooked, that the influence of social capital seems to be stronger in developed than developing countries. The third part of the chapter focuses on policy interventions and recommendations. It provides a broad taxonomy of policies, motivated by theoretical models of investment in social capital. Next, it discusses a number of academic papers describing and evaluating interventions aimed at creating social capital, and concludes by describing a few interventions realized by two organizations whose purpose is to help communities accumulate social capital.

Keywords: Social Determinants; Social Capital; Developing Countries; Generalized Trust; World Values Survey; Beliefs; Values; Willingness to Cooperate; Informal Health Care; Informal Assistance; Compliance; Collaboration; Community; Causal Effects.

Introduction

Is social capital a determinant of individual health? This chapter reviews what health economists and public health scientists have discovered, mainly in the last decade, as regards the relationship between social capital and health and makes a step forward, by providing further evidence derived from the largest cross-country empirical analysis carried out so far.

To begin with, it is important to clarify what is meant by social capital. In the first part of this chapter, we will summarize the long debate on the definition of social capital, which stems from the fact that social capital is a concept difficult to enclose in precise boundaries because it is multi-faceted and overlaps multiple disciplines, primarily sociology and economics. The second step will be to clarify the reasons that suggest that, *a priori*, social capital can plausibly play a role in individual health. The literature has indeed hypothesized multiple possible pathways or mechanisms. To complete the background, we will present a review of a number of empirical studies on social capital and health, selected to cover different countries and continents and give a global perspective. The large majority of the studies suggest that there exists a positive influence of social capital on individual health, regardless of the empirical method adopted or the health outcome considered. This is especially the case when social capital is measured by the indicator of self-reported generalized trust (i.e., how much an individual reports to trust other people). Remarkably, generalized trust has been suggested to be the indicator fitting best with the recent conceptualization of social capital.

In the second part of the chapter, the association between generalized trust and self-reported general health has been estimated using a large dataset derived from World Values Survey, which includes individuals residing in 93 countries over about 20 years. The purpose of the exercise is to analyze how the association varies across countries. We have grouped countries into three sets: High-income, upper-middle income and, taken together, lower-middle and low-income. The estimates indicate that the influence of social capital on individual health increases with national income, although absolute differences are not large. Indeed, in high-income countries, people rich in social capital are 7% more likely to report being in good health compared to the social capital poor, while the corresponding figure is 5.9% in upper-middle income countries and 5% in lower-middle and low-income countries.

In the third part of the chapter, we focus on policy interventions and recommendations. We start by providing a broad taxonomy of policies, motivated by theoretical models of investment in social capital. Next, we review a number of academic papers describing and evaluating interventions aimed at creating social capital, particularly in developing countries. Finally, we describe a few examples of interventions realized by two organizations whose purpose is precisely that of helping communities to develop and accumulate social capital.

What is Social Capital?

Social capital is a multi-faceted concept with unclear boundaries. Intuitively, it has been defined by the World Bank as the glue of a society, the ingredient that favors cooperation and coordination among individuals. Higher degrees of cooperation and coordination enhance social and individual welfare because they facilitate market and non-market transactions (LaPorta *et al.*, 1997).

The term social capital is often traced back to the work of the sociologist Bourdieu (1977), but it became popular in the 1990s, mostly owing to Coleman (1990) and Putnam (1993), and has gained wide acceptance in social sciences and, more recently, in economics, where it has been used to explain economic growth (Knack and Keefer, 1997), size of firms (La Porta *et al.*, 1997), institutions' design and performance (Djankov *et al.*, 2003), financial development (Guiso *et al.*, 2004; 2008b), crime (Glaeser *et al.*, 1995), the power of the family (Alesina and Giuliano, 2007), innovation (Fountain, 1997), and the spread of secondary education (Goldin and Katz, 2001).

Several possible empirical indicators exist and have been adopted in the literature: Trust towards other people, membership in social organizations, social network density, voting turnout, and blood and organ donation among others.

Though widely used, the concept of social capital is contested at both the conceptual and the measurement level. Indeed, a key limitation relates to the ambiguity of its definition (Durlauf and Fafchamps, 2005). On the one hand, social capital has been conceptualized as a group attribute, i.e., as a property of an organization or community as opposed to a characteristic of the individual members. Sociological and political science definitions have tended — though by no means exclusively — to emphasize the aggregate level perspective. Putnam referred to social capital as those "features of social organization, such as trust, norms, and networks that can improve the efficiency of society by facilitating coordinated actions" (Putnam, 1993: 167). On the other hand, there is a so-called "network school" which defines social capital as both an individual attribute and a property of the social network. By contrast, economists have commonly expressed a preference for a more individualistic notion. Glaeser *et al.* (2002) emphasize the individual-level perspective by defining social capital as an individual's social characteristics that enable private returns via interaction with others. They also point out that it is only if social capital is an individual concept that we can hope to rationalize it and discuss its accumulation and its production by applying the economic framework of utility maximization.

Recently, Guiso *et al.* (2008a; 2011) have defined social capital as "good" culture, i.e., a set of individual beliefs and values that facilitate cooperation among members of a community. In essence, according to Guiso *et al.* individual social capital can be summarized as an individual belief about others' willingness to cooperate, a conceptualization of social capital that convincingly answers to the Solow's critique (Solow, 1995).[1] Indeed, beliefs are individual and vary across people; they can change when new information is acquired by means of social interactions (accumulation or decumulation of social capital) and can be transmitted from parents to children (transfer of social capital). Moreover, beliefs can be represented by probabilities and thus they have well defined and undisputed metric.[2] Last but not least, defining social capital as a belief helps to avoid the common confusion between social capital and some of its outcomes such as the quantity or quality of social relationships or involvement in social organizations, and makes social capital clearly distinct from human capital[3] because its returns are contingent on the norms and beliefs of other community members.

The Pathways between Social Capital and Health

Among the socioeconomic determinants of health, growing attention is being devoted to the role of social capital. Many analyses have found a strong positive association between social capital and individual health, and the discussion about the pathways through which this relationship manifests itself has been mounting in recent years (Folland *et al.*, 2012).

Health economics and public health literature suggest several potential pathways for the influence of social capital on health. First, social capital, by favoring the set-up of many and more frequent social interactions, may expand the informational resources available to individuals, allowing for faster and more intense circulation of health-relevant information (Berkmann and Glass, 2000; Scheffler and Brown, 2008). Second, social capital favors the formation of informal networks and safety nets which provide mutual insurance to its members in case of health shocks (Murgai *et al.*, 2002). Social capital may facilitate the provision of informal health care and/or psychological support. Financial support may be required to cover the out-of-pocket costs of health care. The market or the public health care system is usually unable to provide such services. Therefore, people agree on mechanisms of informal assistance between neighbors or friends. Such support tends to arise only in a context of reciprocal trust, as there is no

---

[1] Solow (1995) argues that the term capital is inappropriate: By definition, a capital can be accumulated and decumulated, it can be transferred between individuals and it yields a return to its owner. Solow urges explaining how these characteristics apply to social capital.

[2] One's belief about whether other people are cooperative or uncooperative is representable as a probability ranging from zero to one.

[3] In economics, human capital is an individual's endowment of skills, competencies, know-how and capabilities, which are accumulated by schooling, training and experience.

enforceable contract guaranteeing obligations. Third, social capital may increase a community's political weight, making it easier to obtain more and better public goods and social welfare programs — in other words, social capital may facilitate people's lobbying efforts and coordination to obtain health-enhancing goods and services (Kawachi *et al.,* 1997; Mellor and Milyo, 2005). Fourth, in a dynamic context where the probability of survival depends on an individual's health, social capital, could discourage unhealthy behaviors, such as smoking, drinking or unhealthy eating, by increasing the utility the individuals can enjoy if survive (Folland, 2006). Fifth, social capital might increase individual compliance with public health regulations (such as smoking bans in public places), as individuals rich in social capital tend to account for the positive externalities that such regulations often imply (Rocco and d'Hombres, 2014). Sixth, social capital increases collaboration between doctors, health personnel and patients and contributes to improve health care quality and patients' compliance (Thom *et al.*, 2004). Seventh, by strengthening the feeling of being part of a community, of not being isolated, social capital shields individuals against stress and uncertainty reduces the risks of depression (Wilkinson, 1996). All pathways are motivated by the fundamental characteristic of social capital, favoring cooperation between individuals.

However, it should also be noted that more intense social relationships may also help spread bad health (e.g., through increased susceptibility to infectious diseases or relationships that encourage the adoption of unhealthy behaviors), by means of stronger peer effects (Kawachi and Berkman, 2001).

The relationship between social capital and health in developing countries

The relative importance of the individual pathways by which social capital affects health may differ between developing and developed countries because there are relevant cultural, historical and institutional differences, as well as differences in disease prevalence and burden (Anchorena *et al.*, 2014).

Social capital particularly affects the amount of health information to which one has access in developing countries. Individuals who are better connected in a community may have access to more sources of health information, and individuals in denser networks may be more likely to share the same health norms and health information. Since health information may be less readily accessible in low- and middle-income countries contexts, social capital may play a particularly important role in the health information one receives in these countries. Edgeworth and Collins (2006) observe that households with weaker social and human capital tended to be excluded from information on appropriate self-care treatments for diarrhea in Bangladesh. Thiede (2005) argues that trust, by influencing the credibility of information to the recipient, determines to what extent information induces individuals to access and use health care services.

Social capital may also affect the amount and type of care people seek. Trusting patients are more likely to access care at earlier phases of illness or injury, while mistrusting patients may not seek health care or may seek care only when conditions deteriorate (Goepp, 2006). In Sri Lanka, Russell (2005) finds that poor interpersonal relationships with public health care providers act as an access barrier that pushes many people to utilize the private sector. In Cambodia, Ozawa *et al.* (2011) report that trust is an important determinant of provider choice, especially for people seeking care from private providers. Once the relationship between patient and health care provider is set, more trustful patients may be more willing to disclose sensitive information to physicians, allowing the physicians to provide more appropriate care and make fewer unnecessary referrals or diagnostic tests (Thom *et al.*, 2004). Social capital may also improve the therapeutic response through better adherence to treatment, as Ware *et al.* (2009) observe in HIV/AIDS patients' adherence to antiretroviral therapy in Sub-Saharan Africa.

Typically, developing countries have underdeveloped health insurance programs, and those that do exist tend to be voluntary. Zhang *et al.* (2006) find that social capital is positively associated with the probability of that farmers will be willing to join community-based health insurance programs in rural China. Social capital is also crucial in the formation of informal safety nets in traditional societies in Eritrea, where voluntary mutual-aid community associations and health insurance programs are built on existing social networks (Habtom and Ruys, 2007).

Literature Review

Empirical economic and public health literature have almost unanimously found a positive influence of social capital on individual general health or particular health outcomes. While most of the earlier literature look for associations between several measures of social capital and health indicators, more recently the focus has moved in the direction of identification of causal effects. Causal effects are more interesting than associations because the latter might be misleading, as they include the role played by confounding factors which act on health in parallel to social capital and the feedback effect from health to social capital. Elicitation of causal effect requires more sophisticated statistical analysis, such as instrumental variables (IVs) estimators or techniques which exploit quasi-experimental settings. Nonetheless, these methods rest on relatively strong assumptions which may sometimes be controversial.[4] For this reason, the search for associations remains important, at least as a source of preliminary evidence about the existence of possible causal relationships. In this section, we separately review a number of selected studies which belong to both the associations and causal effects approaches.

Associations

The large majority of the literature published so far has sought associations between social capital indicators and *general* health. A smaller number of studies considered other, more specific health outcomes or behaviors. We initially discuss of the influence of social capital on general health and then we move to studies examining more specific health indicators. The typical empirical strategy in this literature involves multi-level models that account for the hierarchical structure of the data (individuals — communities — regions — country). A few papers adopt a cross-country perspective. Poortinga (2006) uses the first round of the European Social Survey, which covers 22 countries, to analyze whether two social capital measures — an index of social trust (related to generalized trust) and an index of social participation — benefit self-reported general health. By means of a two-level model including both individual and community social capital, defined as the average individual social capital in the community, he finds that both measures of individual social capital are strongly associated with health while the community-level social capital is not. However, the author also finds that the association between individual social capital and health is stronger when community social capital is larger. These results suggest that social capital matters to individual health only when the individual is personally connected to the community and participates to community social life. Instead, *per se* a lively community is ineffective in the absence of individual involvement. Similarly, Olsen and Dahl (2007), by using the same data and a similar methodology, find that individual social capital, defined as intensity of relationships with friends, relatives, and colleagues, is always significantly associated with general health. Mansyur *et al.* (2008) again adopts an approach similar to Poortinga's but covers the 45 countries surveyed in the first and second wave of the World Values Survey. In this larger set of countries, he confirms the pattern of results found by Poortinga (2006).

In the US, Kim and Kawachi (2006) estimate a two-level model, including both individual and community social capital, and find that there is a modest (positive) association between each of three community social capital indices

[4] Details on methods and assumptions necessary to identify causal effects are available in Rocco and Fumagalli (2014).

(individual social attitudes, social participation, and political participation) and self-rated health while most individual-level social capital measures are strongly protective of health. In the UK, Snelgrove *et al.* (2009) find that both individual and community social capital (measured by generalized trust and participation in voluntary organizations) are positively and significantly associated with individual general health. Petrou and Kupek (2008) include in their model only individual social capital indicators and find that high stocks of social capital across the domains of trust and reciprocity, perceived social support, and civic participation are significantly associated with better health status. Giordano and Lindstrom (2010) exploit the longitudinal dimension provided by the British Household Panel Data and estimate a dynamic model where lagged social capital are related to current individual health, finding positive and significant associations between generalized trust and general health.

Considering Scandinavian countries, Islam *et al.* (2006) find that in Sweden, voting participation is positively associated with general health among males but not among females. A similar result is also found by Iversen (2008) in Norway.

In France, Jusot *et al.* (2008) suggest that membership in social organizations and social support are positively associated with general health, while, surprisingly, trust is not. In the Netherlands, Mohnen *et al.* (2011) find a positive association between neighborhood social capital and individual health and note that residents in urban neighborhoods particularly benefit from their neighborhood social capital.

Using a rich dataset from Russia, Rose (2000) shows that some measures of social capital (i.e., trust and the presence of someone to rely on when one is ill) are positively associated with better physical and emotional health, but those who rely on friends for information have worse physical and emotional health. Ferlander and Ma'Kinen (2009) obtain weaker results in a study of Moscovites, showing that the association between self-reported health and social capital, measured by frequency of visits to relatives and friends and by participation in civic associations, is significant for men but not for women. Rojas and Carlson (2006) use a survey of individuals in Taganrog, Russia, and find that being a member of an organization (which they separate into trade unions or political organizations and "any other organization") is positively related to self-reported health. When they interact, these variables with the level of education, a subtler picture appears: Participating in trade unions or political organizations is beneficial for less-educated individuals, while participating in other types of organizations is beneficial for highly educated individuals.

Outside of Europe, Baron-Epel *et al.* (2008) study whether a battery of social capital indicators, including social trust and social support, are associated with self-reported health with different intensities between Israeli Jewish respondents and

Israeli Arab respondents. They find that Jewish respondents with higher social capital report better health, while among Arabs, only social support is significantly associated with health. However, the association is also statistically weaker among the Arabs than among Jews. In China, in three rural counties of the Shandong Province, Yip *et al.* (2007) estimate a two-level model (individual, village) and conclude that social capital (measured by membership in party organizations, membership in voluntary organizations, and trust) is positively associated with general health, psychological health, and overall well-being, with the trust index exhibiting the most consistently positive associations with all three outcome indicators. Wang *et al.* (2009) examine self-reported health and social capital as measured by interpersonal trust and mistrust in rural China, observing that only when personal trust levels reach a certain point does social capital begin to be associated with health. Mistrust effects are generally more pronounced at the individual level, while trust effects are more pronounced at the village level. In Japan, Fujisawa *et al.* (2009) find that perceived helpfulness of the neighborhood, kindness and greeting exchange, considered as indicators of social cohesion at the local level in Japan, are positively and significantly associated with an index of perceived general health. Miller *et al.* (2006) look at the association between community-level social capital and general health in Indonesia. Community social capital is captured by the number of types of community-level organizations. Ordinary Least Squares estimates indicate that social capital is positively associated with good health and that there is mixed evidence for the existence of interactions between social capital and human capital. Hurtado *et al.* (2011) report the estimates of a two-level model in Colombia and find that generalized trust is significantly associated with health after controlling for socio-demographic characteristics. Browne-Yung *et al.* (2013) find a strong positive association between social network participation and general health among the Aboriginal Australians residing in urban areas.

A smaller number of studies analyze specific health outcomes or behaviors, such as smoking or specific diseases. Brown *et al.* (2006) find that the supply of nonprofit organization with a religious origin, a measure of community social capital, is associated with less smoking incidence and intensity in the US. They do not observe effects associated with other kinds of nonprofit organizations. Kim *et al.* (2007) relate indicators that capture attitudes and social, civic and political participation to obesity and physical activity during leisure time. This is one of the very few cases where the association between social capital and health outcomes is weak and not statistically significant. Scheffler *et al.* (2008) find that in Northern California, community social capital reduces the recurrence of acute coronary syndrome mainly for those living in poorer areas, i.e., those people who have less access to the health care system. Nauenberg *et al.* (2011) study how social capital influences use of health care services (GP visits) in Canada. Their results depend on the size of the community: Community social capital is negatively associated with GP visits in large urban areas only, suggesting that social capital can act as a substitute for formal health services. Individual social support is also negatively associated with GP visits in large urban areas, while religious attendance and affiliation are positively associated with GP visits in smaller communities. Also in Canada, recently Devlin and Rudolph-Zbarsky (2014) have found a positive, significant association between social support (mainly sense of belonging) and the probability of having a family doctor. Hyyppa *et al.* (2007) report that in Finland an index of social trust is negatively associated with mortality (distinguishing between all causes and CVD mortality). Giordano and Lindstrom (2012) exploit longitudinal data from the UK and find a strong positive association between social capital and psychological health by means of a dynamic model, where lagged psychological health is directly controlled for as well as social capital, socio-economic characteristics and other measures of social support (such as marriage).

Causal effects

Several more recent studies have attempted to identify the causal effects of social capital. Several empirical strategies have been followed, the most common of which uses IVs.

IV techniques require using exogenous-to-the-model sources of variation to achieve identification of the causal effect. Unfortunately, finding appropriate instruments is far from trivial. Besides the relatively easy requirement of relevance — that is, a strong correlation between the instrument and the supposed endogenous social capital variables — instruments must be exogenous, that is, uncorrelated with the error term, conditional on the remaining exogenous regressors. One implication of exogeneity is the so-called exclusion restriction, which requires that instruments must have no direct effect on the dependent variable (health) beyond the effect mediated by social capital (see for instance Angrist and Pischke (2009), for an ampler discussion and technical details).

Brown *et al.* (2011) use as an IV community social capital, measured by the Petris Index, with weather characteristics and ethnic heterogeneity at the county level, and they find that social capital significantly reduces smoking in California. Folland (2007), by exploiting variation among states in the US, use geographical latitude and state contributions to college education as instruments. Social capital has the expected and significant sign for most but not all indicators of health.[5] Deri (2005) analyzes Canadian data and instruments community social capital with a

[5] Social capital significantly reduces total mortality, cancer mortality, accident mortality, and the suicide rate.

measure of social capital in a larger area. He finds that social network intensity increases the probability of the first contact with the health care system. d'Hombres *et al.* (2010) consider data from eight former Soviet Union Republics and use indices of community heterogeneity in terms of income, education, and religion and the average of community social capital indicators as instruments for individual social capital. They find that trust and social isolation are statistically significant determinants of health while there is no effect of membership to informal social organizations. Ronconi *et al.* (2010) studies Argentina and instrument individual social capital with the presence or lack of public transportation in the neighborhood and with an indicator reporting whether transportation is an important problem in the respondent's life. Significant effect of social capital on health result for both men and women. Kim *et al.* (2011) apply an IV strategy to the cross sectional data collected by the European and World Values Survey. They analyze the role of contextual social capital (i.e., individual social capital averaged at the national level) on individual health, after controlling for individual social capital, and instrumenting contextual social capital with country corruption, population density and religious fractionalization.[6] The estimated effect of contextual social capital on health is positive and results double in size under IV than under OLS.

Two papers, Sirven and Debrand (2011) and Rocco *et al.* (2014), recognize that social capital influences health and that people in better health could accumulate more social capital. Therefore, the relationship between the two variables is circular. Both papers make use of a cross-country dataset, define two-equation models and find that social capital and health are indeed part of a circular relationship.[7] Rocco *et al.* (2014) show that this result is robust to alternative definitions of community (reference groups) and to the possibility that individuals misreport social capital (measured by generalized trust in this study). According to Sirven and Debrand (2011),

[6] Also in this paper social capital is captured by generalized trust.

[7] Sirven and Debrand (2011) exploit longitudinal information and relate current health with lagged social capital and current social capital with lagged health, so the equations are not properly simultaneous; simultaneity derives instead from the assumed correlation between the error terms of the two equations. Individual heterogeneity is explicitly parameterized by exploiting retrospective information referring to individual childhood. The model is estimated by a maximum likelihood bi-variate probit estimator. Rocco *et al.* (2014), on the other hand, explicitly model the simultaneous circular relationship between social capital and health. As in standard simultaneous equation models, identification of the structural parameters is achieved by means of exclusion restrictions. In particular, having been victim of a burglary or an assault is an explanatory variable included in the social capital equation but excluded from the health equation. Symmetrically, measures of health care supply are included in the health equations but are excluded from the social capital equation. The plausibility of the exclusion restrictions depends on a long battery of controls included in both equations. As both social capital and health are categorical variables, a two-step ordered probit estimator is employed, as derived in Stern (1989).

who use an index of participation in social organizations as a measure of social capital and who focus on individuals over age 49, the feedback effect from health to social capital is stronger than the direct effect from social capital to health.

By taking quite a different approach, in order to control for unobserved individual family backgrounds, early health conditions, and genetic endowment, Fujiwara and Kawachi (2008) compare pairs of monozygotic (MZ) and dizygotic (DZ) twins. By first differencing social capital (measured by social trust), self-reported health, and other controls between twin pairs, they remove common unobservables and make it possible to show that the association between social capital and health does not depend on common experiences in the twins' early lives or their common genetic endowment. Actually, the estimates obtained separately from the sample of MZ twins (common genetic endowment) and DZ twins (partially different genetic endowment) are not significantly different, suggesting that genetic endowment does not play a central role. However, as Diez Roux (2008) point out, twin fixed effects cannot control for the life-course and adult experiences, which are likely to differ.

Rocco and d'Hombres (2014), exploiting a quasi-experimental setting related to the introduction of smoking bans in public places in Germany, found that individuals rich in social capital (the more trustful) respond more to the bans by reducing incidence and intensity of smoking.

Evidence from the World Values Survey

The World Values Survey (WVS) is a global research project that explores people's values and beliefs, their stability or evolution over time, and their impact on the social and political development of societies in different countries of the world.

The WVS is a repeated cross-section including six waves from 1981 to 2014. Representative national samples of individuals are interviewed, using a standardized questionnaire. WVS recently finished collecting the 6th wave of survey (2010–2014). This wave is the largest, covering nearly 60 countries, and was released in April 2014.

In this chapter, we have pooled all WVS waves where information on generalized trust, our indicator of social capital, and general self-reported health, education, income, and household characteristics are available. For lack of complete data, the first wave and a few participating countries have been excluded. We have eventually retained 93 countries, which makes ours the broadest cross-country analysis carried out so far in the literature on social capital and health. Most of the retained countries participated in more than one wave of the WVS. Overall, the sample we use in this chapter includes 246,000 observations.

Individual health is measured by means of a self-reported evaluation of own health, coded between 1 and 5, from poor to very good. Given the distribution of this variable, which is concentrated on level 4 (good health) and has relatively few individuals reporting less than good health, we have dichotomized the original indicator by defining a dummy variable, *goodhealth*, which takes 1 if reported health is good or very good (the original levels 4 or 5) and 0 otherwise. In the sample, *goodhealth* takes 1 for about 65% of the observations. No other measures of health are available in the data.

Measuring social capital is perhaps the biggest challenge to applied researchers because social capital has many complementary dimensions. In the literature social capital has been measured by trust toward other people, membership in social organizations, social network density, voting turnout, blood and organ donation among others. The recent theory suggests considering indicators related to individual beliefs and values, as Guiso *et al.* (2008; 2011) convincingly argue. Accordingly, this chapter adopts the indicator that most closely fits with this definition, i.e., generalized trust, which quite naturally captures individual beliefs about others' willingness to cooperate.[8] In so doing, we follow an extensive practice in the social capital literature (Borgonovi, 2010; d'Hombres *et al.*, 2010; Giordano and Lingstrom, 2010; Hurtado *et al.*, 2011; Mansyur *et al.*, 2008; Petrou and Kubek, 2008; Portinga, 2006b; Rostila, 2007; Snelgove *et al.*, 2009). Generalized trust has been shown to have predictive validity for a number of other objective social capital indicators, e.g., the share of wallets returned in wallet drop experiments from capitals around the world (Zak and Knack, 2001), and with indicators of corruption and violent crime (Uslaner, 2002). In addition, studies find a close correlation between generalized trust in surveys and actual behavior as observed in experiments (e.g., Glaeser *et al.*, 2000; Fehr and Fischbacher, 2003).

Generalized trust is coded as a dummy, *trust*, which takes 1 if the respondent reports that "most people can be trusted" and 0 if the respondent reports that "you can't be too careful in dealing with others." In the sample, about 27% report of being trustful (*trust* = 1). Other possible indicators of social capital are included in the WVS, such as membership to voluntary and informal social organizations or voting turnout. Besides the doubtful appropriateness of these social capital indicators, they are available only for some waves or for some countries. For these reasons, we have preferred to focus on generalized trust only.

The selected control variables are age and gender, household composition (marital status and the number of children), education level (coded according to

[8]This approach has the advantage of simplifying the analysis and the interpretation of the results, since the object of interest is much more focused. Of course, the cost is that of losing results' richness and variety compared to an analysis dealing with a multi-faceted concept.

ISCED classification) and income. The latter is reported country-by-country on a scale from 1 (lowest) to 10 (highest) and should therefore be interpreted as relative to the prevailing country and time specific economic conditions.

The model

Given that the dependent variable, *goodhealth*, is a dummy, we estimate a linear probability model where individual health is regressed on generalized trust plus controls. Specifically, our model is

$$goodhealth_{ict} = a\ trust_{ict} + X_{ict}b + \theta_{ct} + \theta\varepsilon_{ict} \quad (1)$$

where X stands for the vector of controls (demographic variables, household characteristics, education, and income) and θ_{ct} is a country-by-year fixed effect which captures in a flexible way all determinants of individual health which varies by country, time of the survey, and jointly by country and time, such as culture, climate and geographical conditions, total expenditure in health care, the economic cycle and so on. Estimated standard errors are robust to heteroskedasticity and observations are weighted in order to make national samples representative of national populations.

In Table 1, we report estimates based on the full sample where all countries have been pooled by adding, in turn, additional controls. In all specifications, country-by-time fixed effects are included. The addition of demographic characteristics contributes substantially to the goodness-of-fit of the model (Column 2) but has a little impact of the estimated association between *trust* and *goodhealth*,

Table 1. The association between social capital and health

Variables	(1) goodhealth	(2) goodhealth	(3) goodhealth	(4) goodhealth
Trust	0.070***	0.072***	0.071***	0.062***
	(0.002)	(0.002)	(0.002)	(0.002)
Observations	245,747	245,747	245,747	245,747
R-squared	0.092	0.164	0.167	0.185
Country-by-year FE	YES	YES	YES	YES
Demographic controls	NO	YES	YES	YES
Family controls	NO	NO	YES	YES
Education and income controls	NO	NO	NO	YES
Mean health	0.652	0.652	0.652	0.652
Mean trust	0.267	0.267	0.267	0.267

Notes: Robust standard errors in parentheses. ***$p < 0.01$, **$p < 0.05$, *$p < 0.1$.

while household characteristics (column 3) and education and income (column 4) play a marginal role in explaining the total variation in *goodhealth* but are important confounder factors of *trust,* as the change in the estimated parameter of *trust* reveals.

Results in Table 1 indicate that trustful individuals are about 6% more likely to report that they are in good health. This is not a causal effect but as an association, which can hide spurious correlations with omitted and unobservable variables, such as individual attitudes, preferences, how optimistic or pessimistic they are in evaluating and reporting their current and future conditions. Nonetheless, the sign and the magnitude are coherent with the results in the literature that aim to uncover causal effects.

The association between social capital and health likely varies across countries and over time. The estimates reported in Table 1 are an average of the associations existing at the country level and over time, so it may mask important heterogeneities. To explore such heterogeneity more in depth, we first separate the pool of countries into three groups, high-income, upper-middle income, and lower-middle and low-income, according to the 2013 World Bank classification, and we estimate Model (1) separately by group.

Group estimates are reported in Table 2. For all groups, the more complete specification of Model (1) has been adopted. Results indicate that the magnitude of the association between social capital and health grows with income. In high-income countries, trustful individuals are 7% more likely to report being in good health than the non-trustful. This figure compares to the 5.9% in upper-middle income countries and the 5% in lower-middle and low-income countries. However,

Table 2. The association between social capital and health by country income

Variables	**(1) Low- and lower-middle income**	**(2) Upper-middle income**	**(3) High-income**
Trust	0.050***	0.059***	0.070***
	(0.005)	(0.004)	(0.003)
Observations	71,186	90,318	84,243
R-squared	0.180	0.163	0.205
Country-by-year FE	YES	YES	YES
Demographic controls	YES	YES	YES
Family controls	YES	YES	YES
Education and income controls	YES	YES	YES
Mean health	0.634	0.656	0.703
Mean trust	0.215	0.211	0.331

Notes: Robust standard errors in parentheses. ***$p < 0.01$, **$p < 0.05$, *$p < 0.1$.

differences among country groups are sizeable but not dramatic. Regardless of the national level of income, the association is always positive and statistically significant.

To explore whether the association changes over time, in Table 3 we have further refined the analysis by estimating Model (1) by group of countries and wave of the WVS. To save space, we have left wave 2 out and focused only on wave 3, collected between 1995 and 1998, wave 4, collected between 1999 and 2004, wave 5, collected between 2005 and 2009, and wave 6, collected between 2010 and 2014. There appear quite marked variations from wave to wave, the third and the fifth systematically revealing a stronger association compared to the fourth and sixth. This pattern is unrelated to the dynamic of the average level of health and social capital (reported at the bottom of Table 3): The former is increasing in all three country groups while the latter is stable or slightly declining in all country groups. Rather, we speculate that, at least to some extent, the time pattern seems to be related with the world economy cycle. Years between 1999 and 2004 (fourth wave) are those of the burst of the internet economy bubble, and the crisis followed to September 11th attack while the years between 2010 and 2014 span over the worst years of the big economic crisis which is still affecting especially continental Europe.

Finally, in Figure 1 we have mapped the estimated association between social capital and health, together with their 90% confidence intervals, on a country-by-country base. Countries are ranked by the magnitude of the association. In only 6 countries out of 93 the point estimate turns out to be negative but never statistically significantly so. In about one quarter of the sample, the association is non-significantly different from zero and with few exceptions these are low- and lower-middle income countries. In the remaining three quarters, the estimated association is positive and statistically significant ranging from 4 to 11%, with few outliers (Ethiopia, Slovenia, Serbia, and Latvia) at the right-most margin of Figure 1, where the magnitude is between 11% and 15%. Detailed figures of these estimates are reported in Table A1 in Appendix.

Discussion

Our results indicate that the association between social capital, measured by trust, and health is stronger in richer countries, a pattern consistent with that recently observed by Anchorena *et al.* (2014) on a smaller set of countries. This pattern holds in spite of a relatively marked time variation.

A priori one could expect that social capital played a larger role in the less developed countries where the informal economy is large and where many services (insurance, credit, caring) are provided to a large extent by informal social organizations, especially in rural areas. In this context, cooperation among

Table 3. The association between social capital and health by income group and wave

	High-income countries				**Upper-middle income countries**				**Lower-middle and low-income countries**			
Variables	**Wave 3**	**Wave 4**	**Wave 5**	**Wave 6**	**Wave 3**	**Wave 4**	**Wave 5**	**Wave 6**	**Wave 3**	**Wave 4**	**Wave 5**	**Wave 6**
Trust	0.062***	0.051***	0.085***	0.067***	0.061***	0.053***	0.073***	0.048***	0.082***	0.032***	0.063***	0.036***
	(0.007)	(0.009)	(0.006)	(0.006)	(0.009)	(0.008)	(0.008)	(0.008)	(0.011)	(0.009)	(0.009)	(0.009)
Observations	20,985	9,023	26,730	26,824	22,365	20,828	19,003	23,282	12,605	17,438	20,295	18,348
R-squared	0.250	0.128	0.183	0.190	0.152	0.140	0.192	0.176	0.186	0.135	0.169	0.213
Country-by-year FE	YES	YES	YES	YES	YES	YES	YES	YES	YES	YES	YES	YES
Demographic controls	YES	YES	YES	YES	YES	YES	YES	YES	YES	YES	YES	YES
Family controls	YES	YES	YES	YES	YES	YES	YES	YES	YES	YES	YES	YES
Education and income controls	YES	YES	YES	YES	YES	YES	YES	YES	YES	YES	YES	YES
Mean health	0.628	0.759	0.716	0.732	0.605	0.661	0.677	0.691	0.518	0.634	0.621	0.702
Mean trust	0.329	0.345	0.338	0.318	0.228	0.250	0.208	0.181	0.227	0.250	0.207	0.178

Notes: Robust standard errors in parentheses. ***$p < 0.01$, **$p < 0.05$, *$p < 0.1$.

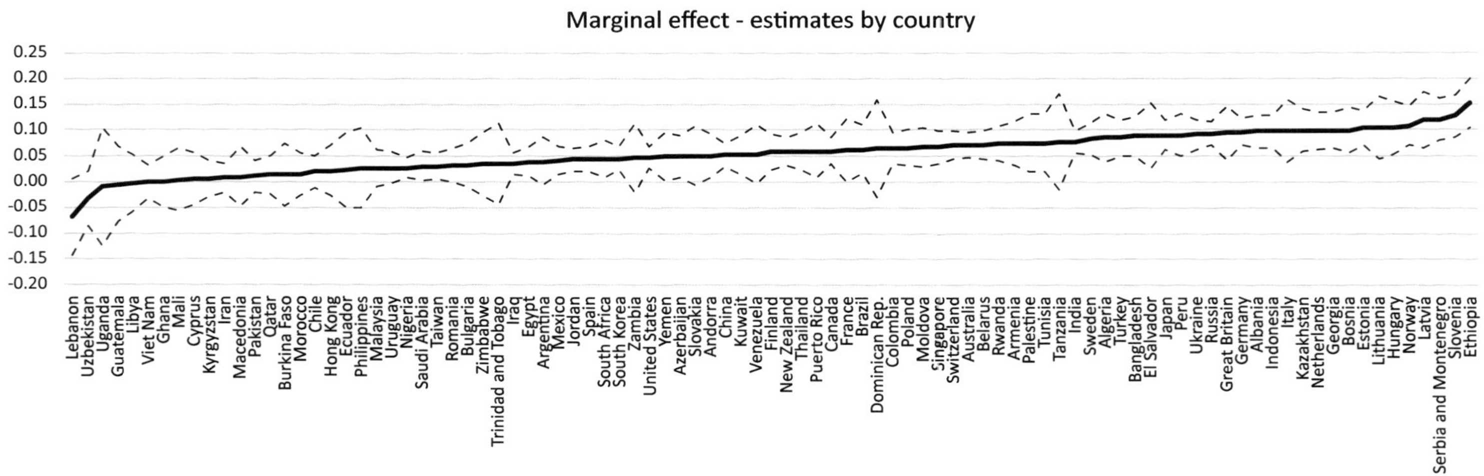

Figure 1. The association between social capital and health by country with the 90% confidence interval

Note: Estimates based on the most comprehensive specification of model (1).

individuals based on trust and reciprocity cannot be substituted by formal legally enforced contracts. Hence, it seems reasonable to expect that social capital is essential to enable a number of transactions directly or indirectly relevant to individual health much more than it is in developed countries generally, where there are effective legal protections.

However, other factors should be taken into account. Trusting individuals benefit from their collaborative attitude only when they interact with other people willing to collaborate. Indeed, when two or more trusting individuals interact, social connections establish favoring the circulation of information, the creation of informal systems of support, insurance and caring. When, instead, trusting individuals happen to interact with less collaborative individuals, collaboration does not occur, or occurs to a lesser extent. As a result, the "return" to *trust* is higher the higher the probability of interacting with other trusting individuals, a probability that we observe to be much larger in high-income countries. In fact, the proportion of trusting people is about 33% in high-income countries and only about 21% in middle and low-income countries.[9]

Another possible explanation depends on the relatively larger prevalence of mental health problems compared to physical health problems in developed countries. If trust reduces stress and, as a result, mental health problems, then trust should have a larger effect on general (i.e., total) health in those countries where mental illness is more prevalent.

Further research is needed to better rationalize these findings, possibly by distinguishing physical from mental health and, even more importantly, by adopting more objective, medically diagnosed, health indicators. Indeed, although self-reported health has been widely used and has been proved to be highly correlated with mortality and morbidity, it is nonetheless affected by reporting heterogeneity both across individuals and across countries. Two individuals with the same health conditions, when objectively measured, could report differently simply because they adopt different evaluation scales or different ways of reporting their condition.

Building Social Capital

Given that the very definition of social capital has yet to be universally agreed upon and accepted, it is not easy to observe programs aimed at building social capital in a community. Many potentially relevant interventions have been carried out all over the world, but for very few of them have the purpose been explicitly that of building social capital.

---

[9] We recognize, however, that this gap might be in part due to reporting heterogeneity across countries.

In this section, we initially propose taxonomy of potentially effective policies that could be derived from the literature, but which remain at a general and abstract level, although concrete examples are provided whenever possible. Next, we review a set of academic papers which analyze and evaluate interventions aimed at building social capital. Finally, we briefly present two organizations whose purpose is that of building social capital, the Asset-Based Community Development Institute (ABCD — http://www.abcdinstitute.org/) and Home-Start Worldwide (http://homestartworldwide.org/).

A taxonomy of policy measures

Effective policy measures for building social capital should encourage both the individual's willingness to invest in social capital and communities' accumulation of social capital. As social capital is an important factor for progress and achievement in several areas, including health, sustaining social capital is not only important from a governmental point of view, but also for the individual and for institutions and communities.

The models of social capital creation and accumulation presented by Tabellini (2008), Guiso *et al.* (2004; 2008) and Aghion *et al.* (2008), all explain transmission of values, like trust, within families. However, they could also be applied to communities, even though the ties may not be as strong as within families. Based on the theoretical models, four categories of policies can be distinguished: (1) Financials incentives, (2) Regulations, (3) Information campaigns at the community or the national level, and (4) Facilitating organizations, communities or services (Aas, 2014).

Financial incentives

A possible financial measure is that of subsidizing organizations to increase or extend the number of groups in a community, such as AAA groups or support groups for people living with cancer or cardiovascular diseases, in order to increase the number and density of social ties. Larger availability of groups would reduce the physical distance to access social networks, which in Gleaser *et al.* (2002) is suggested to be an important barrier for investment in social capital.

For parents, free access to health care centers for newborns can be an instrument to observe the health of the child, and in addition gives the opportunity to establish groups of parents with children born almost at the same time and living in the same area. Such groups could result in an accumulation of social capital over time for both parents and children. In these groups, parents could share information that could result in positive health gains. Such policy measures are implemented in several countries (UK, Sweden, Norway, etc.).

Similarly, the simultaneous increase of health deprivation and the need for health care as ones age implies that a substantial value should be attached to the accumulation of social capital among the elderly and their relatives. Financial incentives could be applied to foster investment in social capital. For instance, membership fees to social organizations could be partly or fully subsidized, by either reducing the price or by allowing for a tax deduction. Using a direct subsidy might be the most effective measure, as transaction costs would be lower. Another alternative is that of subsidizing the costs related to social activities, like travel costs, by allocating free taxi rides.

The family is an important source of social capital. Financial incentives to alleviate the burden of the elderly to their relatives could be a substitute for other types of social interventions. Welfare arrangements that give relatives an opportunity for days off from work to care for their parents could be a possible cost-effective measure. In a recent study, Fevang *et al.* (2012) study the labor supply among relatives of lone parents. They find that labor supply reduces significantly during the terminal stage of the lone parents' lives (and in some cases, reduction lasts after parents' death).

Mobility is predicted to have a negative effect on the accumulation of social capital. Indeed, securing stable living conditions by using financial incentives to encourage homeownership has the potential of accumulating social capital. Measures like zero taxes on savings earmarked for investments in properties and tax deductions for interest rates on loans are relevant to achieve a higher rate of homeownership (Norwegian Ministry of Finance, 2012).

Several of the above measures are already integrated in policy, but few, if any, have been evaluated as regards their ability to build social capital. Later in this section, evidence from research on microfinance as a financial measure to build social capital will be presented.

Regulations

To induce members of a community to participate in activities that are important for a society to sustain and grow, regulation could be an effective tool. For activities like jury duty, civil preparedness, or participation in the Red Cross or caring groups, labor market regulation that legislates the opportunity to participate in these activities could ensure job security. Further, financial compensation to either employers or employees could also be considered to reduce the burden.

The strong relationship between mistrust and level of regulation is discussed in Aghion *et al.* (2008). Regulations are needed to adjust for externalities in communities with a low level of civic capital, for instance, communities with high levels of tax evasion. It is also suggested in Guiso *et al.* (2010), that education is an important measure to increase civic engagement. In school, children are not only dependent on transmission of values and beliefs from their parents, but they could also accumulate it during their schooling. Ensuring the right to education could therefore increase civic engagement.

Campaigns: Campaigns could be used to increase the flow of knowledge and subsequently encourage social interaction, voting and civic engagement. For instance, campaigns could be used to inform individuals in a community about positive trends in the crime rate in their neighborhood. The awareness of living in a safe neighborhood likely reduces the barriers for social interaction given that reciprocal trust increases. Campaigns could also be used to inform people about legislated regulations, for instance legislation that ensures no risk of losing one's job when participating in civil preparedness activities.

One important effect of social capital is that of improving access to information. Since the health care sector is characterized by strong asymmetric information between the doctor and the patient, a larger network could reduce such asymmetry by allowing people to share information on medication, diagnostics and former experiences with hospitals and doctors. Campaigns in the media, over the internet, or through the working place or other institutions, could reinforce and complement the information-spreading effect of social capital and help individuals learn about their opportunities and rights, and about the quality of health care institutions.

Facilitating actions: The government could arrange logistics and facilities for organizations to be evenly distributed in a community in order to bring organizations closer to the user. The government could also coordinate locations for similar or complementary organizations. For instance, clustering health-related organizations (training groups or support groups) in the same place, possibly close to the general practitioner office, the nursing home or the physiotherapist, could be an effective measure to increase social capital in the community. An example of this is shown in a study by Hicks *et al.* (2011), who demonstrate that the elderly participate in their weekly physical training only if they are at a walking distance from the training place.

Health care is often informal (Bolin *et al.*, 2008; Bonsang, 2009; van Houtven and Norton, 2004; 2008). To receive and give informal care, for instance care for children or help at home, an extensive social network is required, especially for those unable to purchase even the more fundamental services from the formal health care system. To compensate for lack of social capital or the ability to pay charges, the government could support the construction of voluntary organizations where the aim is to have a large group of people exchanging services both between organization members, but also providing services to individuals not able to exchange. In the absence of government intervention, such organizations would be totally dependent on the level of trust in the community.

In the next section, we report findings from some studies where the objective of the intervention (mainly or partly) was to build social capital. The interventions are concentrated along two measures, financial incentives and facilitating actions.

Review of studies on building social capital

Most of the published literature on building social capital refers to studies in developing countries or poor areas, or areas experiencing unstable periods (such as disasters and war, or related to HIV/AIDS). We have searched for papers that evaluate the effect of interventions on social capital building, regardless of their effects on health.

One financial measure that has been applied to build social capital, although not necessarily as the primary outcome, is microfinance. The purpose of microfinance is to reduce poverty by supporting individuals and entrepreneurs with microloans. This form of banking is based on relationships, through regular meetings and discussion of projects. In their review, Schrieder and Sharma (1999) argue that microfinance has a direct effect on community development because microfinance creates new *ad hoc* networks. Moreover, microfinance has an indirect effect because it enables and facilitates community development as an externality of its primary purpose, that of supporting entrepreneurship and economic development. According to the Schrieder *et al.* (1999), findings about the effect of microfinance on social capital are mixed in Berger (1989), Khandker (1998), Nguyen and Osmani (1998), Schrieder and Pfaff (1997), and Zaman (1998). Microfinance did, however, have a positive effect on women's empowerment in one study (Schuler *et al.*, 1997) and increased participants' capability to design, develop and manage community projects in another study (Srinivas and Pallen, 1998).

Feigenberg *et al.* (2010), carry out an experiment among women in India aimed at identifying the effect of group lending on social capital and especially the formation of new networks. A "Grameen Bank" style microfinance program is tested in this study. The Grameen Bank was established in 1983 and specialized in financial support for the poor, defining poor as owing less than half an acre of land. Social capital is created within the Grameen Bank system by forming horizontal (among equal agents of similar relation and power in a hierarchy) and vertical networks (among unequal agents in unequal relation and power in a hierarchy), establishing new norms and fostering a new level of social trust to solve collective action problems of accessing capital (Dowla, 2006). Based on these principles, Feigenberg *et al.* (2010) focused on the effect of different meeting schedules in the microfinance institution (MFI), hypothesizing that more frequent mandatory meetings between first-time borrowers would generate more social capital. The total sample consisted of 1026 clients, randomized either to an MFI group with either weekly (30 groups with 307 clients) or monthly (70 groups with 721 clients) group meetings. Further, a lottery combining expected return with a ticket-giving decision was tested to identify reciprocal behavior among the ticket recipient. In the initial lottery, each client had a 1 to 11 chance of winning, and then the client was given the opportunity to give out additional lottery tickets to the MFI group. Given away tickets reduced the client's probability of winning, but increased the overall likelihood of winning in the MFI group. The client would only increase the expected payoff if the group member decided to share the winnings. Giving away tickets indicated that the client considered the "resource potential" in the group. Two levels of prize were tested, one voucher and four vouchers. At the time of the lottery, additional loan cycles were initiated among a sub-sample that was re-randomized into weekly or monthly repayment schedules. This additional intervention enabled the authors to study interaction among new and old group members.

Feigenberg *et al.* (2010) find that weekly meetings generated persistent increases in social contact with group members in their homes and the number of events and visits to others outside the MFI group. These gains were mainly among clients who did not know each other well before the trial. Findings from the lottery show that a client was 67% more likely to give away a lottery ticket to a group member if the voucher was divisible. Further, based on the re-randomization, it is also found that individuals in regular weekly group meetings gave away more lottery tickets (increasing the resource potential). The authors conclude that the latter effect implies that more frequent group meetings help sustaining cooperation by reducing the costs and increasing the benefits of coordination actions.

In a social experiment in Nicaragua, building social capital by facilitating community development was tested in post-conflict communities (Brune and Bossert, 2009). In the study, three communities (Pantasma, Waslala and Cinco Pinos) with 200 households were included, all with low levels of social capital. In two communities, a program to develop management and leadership (M&L) was implemented with the purpose of strengthening the community's organization and self-management capabilities, encourage development through higher participation in community activities, and increase trust both among citizens and between citizens and public organizations. The M&L was implemented on a wide scale, through providing technical assistance information from formal organizations; leadership training of leaders in the community as well as teachers and others; an information and educational campaign to reach all citizens in the community using radio; and, finally, systematic outreach to people in the community to increase participation.

Social capital was measured along several dimensions: Participation, meetings per month, contribution to the community (money, goods, material and/or labor), general trust (*Do you trust most people?*), solidarity (*Do you think that most people in this village are willing to help if you need it?*) and social interaction (*In the last month, have you met with people in a public place to talk or to eat/drink?*). For further details, see Brune and Bossert (2009). In addition, the study included questions related to civic participation and empowerment. Separate analyses of the effect of social capital on several health outcomes were also presented.

Results from this small study indicate that M&L had an effect on several social capital components, especially attitudes of trust in the community and civic participation. In addition, they found that social capital had an effect on health behavior, such as the use of modern medicine and treatment of children's respiratory illnesses. There are several methodological issues with the study by Brune and Bossert (2009), such as the sample size and biased groups, implying that we should be cautious with the interpretation of the findings.

In a study from Brazil, building social capital through intergenerational interaction was tested to find its effect on health (de Souza and Grundy, 2007). The randomized control trial was carried out in Ceilândia, one of the satellite cities of Brasilia. This area is an area predisposed to poor levels of social cohesion, hence relevant for interventions aiming at improving social integration. Students in 11 classes in seventh and eighth grade in one school were included in the trial. Improved social integration was measured along several dimensions, such as trust, honesty, helpfulness, selfishness and family relationship. One class was included in the pre-study pilot, and five of the remaining 10 classes randomized to the intervention. The study contained 253 adolescents (age 12 to 18 years). In the same catchment area, 266 elders (age 60 years and over) where included in the study. The intervention included two-hour sessions once a week during school hours over a 14-week period. The teachers facilitated the activities by initiating topics for conversation, using triggers such as interviews, photos or old objects. The teachers had 20 hours of training ahead of the trial. Of the 149 elders included in the intervention group, only 32 participated in the intervention activities. The results with regard to social capital and health were ambiguous. In the experimental group, the proportion of adolescents reporting that people are selfish increased during the study period, and also the proportion reporting improved family relationship and quality of family relationship increased. The elders in the intervention group, however, were more likely to report an increase during the study period on helpfulness of neighbors, judging most people to be good and reporting family relationships as good. Even though this study is based on a randomized trial, baseline characteristics identify that the experimental group was not equal with the control group on all dimensions. Further, it is problematic interpreting the findings when only one fourth of the elders actually participated. More studies are needed to provide policy recommendations both on how intergenerational interactions could be built and whether social capital increases as a consequence of such interactions.

According to the literature, social capital seems to be an important measure in prevention and treatment of HIV/AIDS (see Kennedy *et al.*, 2014, for an overview). In a study by Pronyk *et al.* (2008) the effect of microfinance and a two phase training program were evaluated in villages in rural South Africa (Limpopo). Based on cluster randomization, the poorest women from eight of the villages with no prior access to microfinance were included and matched with women from comparable villages. The women were allocated to a loan centers, and joined one of eight groups of five women, all loan recipients, who met every two weeks. In addition to accessing microfinance, the women participated in a two-phase training program. The first phase contained a 12-month HIV training program, called Sisters-For-Life, covering topics like gender roles, women's work, gender and HIV, domestic violence, knowledge is power, and empowering change. In the second phase, the main objective was to encourage community mobilization. Social capital was measured by structural components, defined by intensity of membership (distinguishing between being a member, active member and a leader) and cognitive social capital, measured by perceived reciprocity and community support, solidarity and participation in collective action. The study included 419 women with a 90% and 84% follow-up rate in the intervention group and the control group, respectively. Both structural and cognitive social capital turned out to be higher in the intervention group. Women in the intervention groups increased their participation in social groups and reported higher perceived levels of community solidarity and collective action.

Contrary to the studies above, one study examined the possibility of destroying social capital. Olken (2009) estimates the effect of accessibility of television and radio on social capital in Indonesia. Two exogenous shocks are used to achieve identification, variation in signal reception and differential introduction of private television. Olken (2009) finds that social capital, measured by participation in social organizations and self-reported trust was reduced with improved reception, implying more hours allocated to watching television or listening to radio. Local governance, measured by the ability to carry out a road building project, was not affected by reception.

Two actors building social capital

The Asset-Based Community Development Institute (ABCD) is a center that builds on the skills of local residents, the power of local associations, and the supportive functions of local institutions and draws upon existing community strengths to build stronger, more sustainable communities for the future. ABCD developed a methodology to build social capital that rests on social assets, the gifts and talents of individuals, social networks that are important for local communities and informal networks. The ABCD methodology consists of collecting information about successful stories in a community that could reveal capacities, defining a group to be in charge of putting the process forward, mapping the capacities in the community, building relationships among local assets for mutual benefit, mobilizing all available assets for improving economic development, ensuring that plans for community development have sufficient support, and finally, exploring and leveraging activities, investments and resources outside the community. The ABCD approach has been applied to projects all over the world. Here are some examples.

*The **Mercado Central** is a retail business cooperative that was developed by the Latino immigrant community in Minneapolis, Minnesota. The Mercado Central (Cooperative Mercado Central) is the result of the creativity and hard work of members of this community, who joined forces with a faith-based organizing group and numerous community organizations to build a traditional marketplace in their inner-city neighborhood. Currently home to 44 businesses, the Mercado Central has transformed the lives of people in this community by recognizing their capacity to build their own local economy in a manner that reflected their traditions.*

(http://www.abcdinstitute.org/about/)

***Our Town Rocks.** The S2AY Rural Health Network, a regional health agency, set out on a long-term project to help residents of rural Yates County, New York, kick-start their community. The agency brought residents together and helped them discover their own strengths, and Our Town RoCKS, short for "Raising our Community, especially our Kids, to be Strong," was born.*

(http://www.abcdinstitute.org/abcd09/)

In Ethiopia, ABCD's approach was applied to develop local communities (Peters *et al.*, 2011). The research design included 400 people from seven communities. In this project, two types of mapping were carried out: (1) Based on interviews among participants their social ties were identified by listing informal and voluntary associations in the community and discussing their relative importance and roles, and (2) physical assets were mapped, such as number of acres, houses and livestock, to identify resources. A "Leaky Bucket"[10] tool was used to

[10]The "leaky bucket" is a popular education tool that helps people at the grassroots better understand their local economy. It enables them to identify and quantify the main flows of money coming into

help participants learn more about which resources already exist in the community and which resources are needed but not available in the community. If the assets in the community increase, the wealth increases. The "Leaky Bucket" is also a useful tool to identify changes in conditions, such as prices on fuel, and how these changes influence the opportunities. Through group meetings and interviews, an action plan was developed for future changes that included a detailed description of which community assets could be used and the assets that would be required from others. In this project, several changes were identified with regard to social capital through increased organizational capacity within the community.

Pan *et al.* (2005) put forward several arguments for the appropriateness of the ABCD method in pediatrics. The main components of the discussion are social relationships, social capital and health. Two steps were suggested: First, mapping the pediatrician's assets, and next mapping the community's assets. The pediatrician's assets consist of their professional skills and knowledge as a pediatrician, their passion for children and their clinical position (often as a leader in a clinical or hospital setting). In a community setting, a pediatrician is an asset in the development of care for children in the community. Second, community assets would need to be mapped through detailed discussions and interviews with parents, teachers, leaders and other stakeholders in the community. Based on the discussions and interviews, available resources in the community would identified as well as how the community could develop by prioritizing measures to improve children's health.

Another type of organization aimed at building social capital is Home-Start Worldwide, an organization that consists of volunteers in 22 countries around the world helping parents with young children through difficult periods. The main purpose is for volunteers to build parents' confidence by encouraging them to do independent activities and to sustain and/or build networks. One important measure to achieve this goal is to ensure continuity, as the volunteers visit the family regularly until the youngest child starts school or until the parents feel confident standing on their own two feet.

Home-Start has been evaluated in two studies in the Netherlands (Asscher *et al.*, 2008; Hermanns *et al.*, 2013;). In Asscher *et al.* (2008) the introduction of Home-Start was evaluated among 54 families and compared with families in areas where Home-Start was not yet implemented. One of the main activities for the Home-Start volunteer to help enlarge the parents' social networks. Asscher *et al.* (2008) found that Home-Start had an effect on perceived parenting competence,

and out of their community. In turn, this process often leads to revealing economic opportunities, which may help community members to improve their community and household well-being, see http://www.coady.stfx.ca/tinroom/assets/file/op9.pdf.

parental consistency and observed sensitivity. In Hermanns *et al.* (2013), Home-Start was evaluated in a randomized community sample. Initially, 59 families were allocated to the intervention group and 56 to the comparison group. After three years, only 33 and 45 families were in the sample. Based on a three-year follow-up, the authors found that Home-Start had a positive effect on parental wellbeing, competence and behavior. Further, the Home-Start group showed more responsiveness and less oppositional defiant behavior. The authors concluded that the findings were promising, but that more research is needed.

Discussion

The effect of social capital on health is analyzed and documented in several studies, but less is known about what measures are effective in building social capital. Based on taxonomy of policies, we suggest a number of possible interventions including financial incentives, regulations, information campaigns and facilitating actions. In one example, we discussed the use of free access to clinics for parents with newborns and its effect on enabling the formation of informal parent groups who share information about child health issues, as well as contributing to the accumulation of social capital over time for both parents and children. Such policy measures are implemented in several countries (UK, Sweden, and Norway). Most of the examples in this section are based on well-functioning communities where regulations and financial measures could easily be implemented. Measures building social capital in developing countries might be different, since in these countries communities have less formal structure. Further, as trust is lower among low-income countries (see the results from WVS), the fact that most evidence for building social capital is from low-income countries is not surprising. In the future, it would be both interesting and highly relevant to evaluate the effect of some of the suggested interventions to see if their introduction actually results in an accumulation of social capital and, consequently, better health. Such analyses would allow the identification of the most cost-effective policy measures. For the informal parent groups, we know that the additional cost of bringing the parents together is almost zero as they are already at the clinic; hence the challenge is whether these informal groups are really able to build stable social networks and improve health.

The review of studies building social capital has identified a limited number of relevant papers. Some refer to microfinance. Building social capital via microfinance is related to how microfinance is organized in the community through both vertical and horizontal networks. One well-designed experiment uses microfinance to build social capital, and results suggest that it is possible to build social capital by increasing meeting frequency (weekly compared to monthly). Other studies also indicate an effect of microfinance on social capital, such as in the prevention and follow-up of HIV/AIDS. Two papers describing a management and learning program and intergenerational activities indicate ways to potentially increase social capital, although both of these studies have methodological limitations. One paper finds that higher accessibility to television and radio can destroy social capital. Generally, too few studies have been designed to properly identify the effect of interventions on social capital. There is a need for evaluations that include a higher number of individuals and communities and a well-defined control group (via experiments or randomized control trials).

Worldwide organizations like ABCD and Home-Start are large players involving a lot of volunteers. ABCD in particular has set social capital accumulation as one of its main purposes and has acknowledged the effect of social capital on other outcomes. It would be an important contribution to social capital research if such organizations, with clear identities and distinctive methodologies, could facilitate proper evaluations of their interventions. For Home-Start, there are some examples of research on the effects of their programs, which show it is possible to design interventions while taking into account the needs of a subsequent evaluation.

Conclusions

We conclude by answering the question posed at the beginning of this chapter: Social capital can be considered a socio-economic determinant of health. The empirical evidence, also the most recent aiming at identifying causation, almost unanimously supports this conclusion in spite of ongoing debate surrounding the ways in which social capital and health influence one another. The influence of social capital on health might vary depending on the social capital indicator and the health outcome being studied and depending on the particular context where the analysis is carried out. In particular, we have observed that social capital plays a larger role in developed countries than in developing countries. However, the difference is not that large, a result which reinforces the claim that social capital could be a lever to achieve better health everywhere. In these years of increasing concerns about the sustainability of the health care systems, threatened by continuously mounting costs, developing social capital could reveal to be a cost-effective alternative to more traditional health policies. Its importance, however, has yet to be fully acknowledged by policymakers. To convince them and to demonstrate the effects of social capital building, much effort will have to be spent to design interventions able to increase social capital both at the individual and at the community level. We have provided a number of examples and ideas in this regard, but a ready-to-use policy is still to be defined.

References

Aas 2014. Policy implications. In Folland S. and Rocco L. (eds.). *The Economics of Social Capital and Health. A Conceptual and Empirical Roadmap*. World Scientific Publishing.

Aghion, Philippe, Yann Algan, Pierre Caluc, Andrei Shleifer. 2008. Regulation and Distrust, National Bureau of Economic Research, *Working Paper* 14648.

Alesina A, Giuliano P. 2007. *The Power of the Family*. Working Paper, Harvard University.

Anchorena J, Ronconi L, Ozawa S. 2014. Social Capital and Health in Low- and Middle-Income Countries. In Folland S, Rocco L (eds.). *The Economics of Social Capital and Health. A Conceptual and Empirical Roadmap*. World Scientific Publishing.

Angrist JD, Pischke JS. 2009. *Mostly Harmless Econometrics: An Empiricist's Companion*. Princeton University Press.

Asscher JJ, Hermanns JMA, Dekovic M. 2008. Effectiveness of the Home-Start parenting Support Program: Behavioral Outcomes for Parents and Children. *Infant Mental Health Journal* 29: 95–113.

Baron-Epel O, Weinstein R, Haviv-Mesika A, Garty-Sandalon N, Green MS. 2008. Individual-level analysis of social capital and health: A comparison of Arab and Jewish Israelis. *Social Science & Medicine* 66(4): 900–910.

Berger M. 1989. Given women credit: The strengths and limitations of credit as a tool for alleviating poverty. *World Development* 17(7): 1017–1032.

Berkman LF, Glass T. 2000. Social integration, social networks, social support, and health. In Berkman LF, Kawachi I. (eds.). *Social Epidemiology* (pp. 137–173). New York: Oxford University Press.

Bolin K, Lindgren B, Lundborg P. 2008. Informal and formal care among single-living elderly in Europe. *Health Economics* 17(3): 393–409.

Bonsang E. 2009. Does informal care from children to their elderly parents substitute for formal care in Europe? *Journal of Health Economics* 28(1): 143–154.

Borgonovi F. 2010. A life-cycle approach to the analysis of the relationship between social capital and health in Britain. *Social Science & Medicine* 71(11): 1927–1934.

Bourdieu P. 1977. *Outline of a Theory of Practice*. Cambridge University Press: Cambridge.

Brown TT, Colla CH, Scheffler RM. 2011. Does community-level social capital affect smoking behavior? an instrumental variables approach, working paper presented at the 3rd Workshop of the Global Network on Social Capital and Health (Oslo, September 2010).

Brown TT, Scheffler RM, Seo S, Reed M. 2006. The empirical relationship between community social capital and the demand for cigarettes. *Health Economics* 15(11): 1159–1172.

Browne-Yung K, Ziersch A, Baum F, Gallaher G. 2013. Aboriginal Australians' experience of social capital and its relevance to health and wellbeing in urban settings. *Social Science & Medicine* 97: 20–28.

Brune NE, Bossert T. 2009. Building social capital in post-conflicting communities: Evidence from Nicaragua. *Social Science & Medicine* 68: 885–893.

Coleman JS. 1990. *Foundations of Social Theory*. Cambridge, MA: Harvard University Press.

de Souza EM, Grundy E. 2007. Intergenerational interaction, social capital and health: Results from a randomized controlled trial in Brazil. *Social Science & Medicine* (65): 1397–1409.

Deri C. 2005. Social networks and health service utilization. *Journal of Health Economics* 24(6): 1076–1107.

Devlin RA, Rudolph-Zbarsky J. 2014. Social networks and the probability of having a regular family doctor. *Social Science & Medicine* 115: 21–28.

d'Hombres B, Rocco L, Suhrcke M, McKee M. 2010. Does social capital determine health? Evidence from eight transition countries. *Health Economics* 19(1): 56–74.

Diez Roux AV. 2008. The effects of social capital on health. What twin studies can tell us. *American Journal of Preventive Medicine* 35(2): 182–183.

Dowla A. 2006. In credit we trust: Building social capital by Grameen Bank in Bangladesh. *The Journal of Socio-Economics* 35: 102–122.

Durlauf S, Fafchamps M. 2005. Social capital. In Durlauf S, Aghion P. (eds). *Handbook of Economic Growth*, 1B, North Holland: Amsterdam. pp. 1639–1699.

Edgeworth R, Collins A. 2006. Self-care as a response to diarrhoea in rural Bangladesh: Empowered choice or enforced adoption? *Social Science & Medicine* 63: 2686–2697.

Fehr E, Fischbacher U. 2003. The nature of human altruism. *Nature* 425: 785–791.

Feigenberg B, Field EM, Pande R. 2010. Building social capital through microfinancing. *NBER Working Papers 16018.*

Ferlander S, Mäkinen IH. 2009. Social capital, gender and self-rated health evidence from the Moscow Health Survey 2004. *Social Science & Medicine* 69(9): 1323–1332.

Fevang E, Kverndokk S, Røed K. 2012. Labor Supply in the Terminal Stages of Lone Parents' Lives. *Journal of Population Economics*, forthcoming.

Folland S. 2006. Value of life and behavior toward health risks: An interpretation of social capital. *Health Economics* 15: 159–171.

Folland S. 2007. Does 'community social capital' contribute to population health? *Social Science & Medicine* 64(11): 2342–2354.

Folland S, Islam MK, Kaarbøe OM. 2012. Social Capital and Types of Illness: A Look at How Its Results Are Achieved, Mimeo, Presented at the IV workshop of the Global Network on Social Capital and Health, Padova (Italy) October 4–5, 2012.

Fountain JE. 1997. Social Capital: A Key Enabler of Innovation in Science and Technology, In Branscomb LM, Keller J. (eds.). *Investing Innovation: Toward a Consensus Strategy for Federal Technology Policy*. MIT Press.

Fujisawa Y, Hamano T, Takegawa S. 2009. Social capital and perceived health in Japan: An ecological and multilevel analysis. *Social Science & Medicine* 69(4): 500–505.

Fujiwara T, Kawachi I. 2008. Social capital and health: A study of adult twins in the US. *American Journal of Preventive Medicine* 35(2): 139–144.

Giordano GN, Lindstrom M. 2010. The impact of changes in different aspects of social capital and material conditions on self-rated health over time: A longitudinal cohort study. *Social Science & Medicine* 70(5): 700–710.

Giordano GN, Lindstrom M. 2012. Social capital and change in psychological health over time. *Social Science & Medicine* 72: 1219–1227.

Glaeser E, Laibson D, Sacerdote B. 2002. An economic approach to social capital. *The Economic Journal* 112(483): 437–458.

Glaeser E, Laibson DI, Scheinkman JA, Soutter CL. 2000. Measuring Trust. *The Quarterly Journal of Economics* 115(3): 811–846.

Glaeser E, Sacerdote B, Scheinkman JA. 1995. Crime and social interactions. *The Quarterly Journal of Economics* 111: 507–548.

Goepp JG. 2006. Reflections on trust and health services utilization. *Preventive Medicine* 42: 81–82.

Goldin C, Katz L. 2001. Human capital and social capital: The rise of secondary schooling in America, 1910–1940. In Rotberg R. (ed.). *Patterns of Social Capital*. Cambridge University Press.

Guiso L, Sapienza P, Zingales L. 2011. *Civic Capital As The Missing Link*. In Benhabib J, Bisin A, Matthew Jackson (eds.). *The Handbook of Social Economics*. North Holland.

Guiso L, Sapienza P, Zingales L. 2004. The role of social capital in financial development. *American Economic Review* 94(3): 526–556.

Guiso L, Sapienza P, Zingales L. 2008a. Alfred Marshall lecture social capital as good culture. *Journal of the European Economic Association* 6(2–3): 295–320.

Guiso L, Sapienza P, Zingales L. 2008b. Trusting the stock market. *Journal of Finance* 63(6): 2557–2600.

Habtom GK, Ruys P. 2007. Traditional risk-sharing arrangements and informal social insurance in Eritrea. *Health Policy* 80(1): 218–235.

Hermanns JMA, Asscher JJ, Zijlstra BJH, Hoffenaar PJ, Dekovic M. 2013. Long-term changes in parenting and child behavior after the Home-Start family support program. *Children and Youth Services Review* 35: 678–684.

Hicks GE, Benvenuti F, Fiaschi V, Lombardi B, Segenni L, Stuart M, Pretzer-Aboff I, Gianfranco G, Macchi C. 2011. Adherence to a community-based exercise program is a strong predictor of improved back pain status in older adults: An observational study. *The Clinical Journal of Pain* 28(3): 195–203.

Hurtado D, Kawachi I, Sudarsky J. 2011. Social capital and self-rated health in Colombia: The good, the bad and the ugly. *Social Science & Medicine* 72(4): 584–590.

Hyyppa MT, Maki J, Impivaara O, Aromaa A. 2007. Individual-level measures of social capital as predictors of all-cause and cardiovascular mortality: A population-based prospective study of men and women in Finland. *European Journal of Epidemiology* 22(9): 589–597.

Islam MK, Merlo J, Kawachi I, Lindstrom M, Burstrom K, Gerdtham UG. 2006. Does it really matter where you live? A panel data multilevel analysis of Swedish municipality-level social capital on individual health-related quality of life. *Health Economics, Policy, and Law* 1(3): 209–235.

Iversen T. 2008. An exploratory study of associations between social capital and self-assessed health in Norway. *Health Economics, Policy, and Law* 3(4): 349–364.

Jusot F, Grignon M, Dourgnon P. 2008. Access to psycho-social resources and health: Exploratory findings from a survey of the French population. *Health Economics, Policy, and Law* 3(4): 365–391.

Kawachi I, Kennedy BP, Lochner K, Prothrow-Stith D. 1997. Social capital, income inequality, and mortality. *American Journal of Public Health* 87: 1491–1498.

Kawachi I, Berkman L. 2001. Social ties and mental health. *Journal of Urban Health Bulletin of the New York Academy of Medicine* 78(3): 458–467.

Kennedy CE, Fonner VA, O'Reilly KR, Sweat MD. 2014. A systematic review of income generation interventions, including microfinance and vocational skills training, for HIV prevention. *AIDS Care* 26: 659–673.

Khandker M. 1998. Socio-economic and psychological dynamics of empowerment of Grameen Bank and BRAC borrowers, *PRUS Working Paper* No. 3. Workshop proceedings Recent research on micro-finance: Implication for policy. In Matin I, Sinha S, with Alexamdner P. (eds.). Brighton, Sussex, UK: University of Sussex, Poverty Research Unit at Sussex (PRUS) pp. 43–56.

Kim D, Kawachi I. 2006. A multilevel analysis of key forms of community- and individual-level social capital as predictors of self-rated health in the United States. *Journal of Urban Health: Bulletin of the New York Academy of Medicine* 83(5): 813–826.

Kim D, Baum CF, Ganz ML, Subramanian SV, Kawachi I. 2011. The contextual effects of social capital on health: A cross-national instrumental variable analysis. *Social Science & Medicine* 73: 1689–1697.

Kim D, Subramanian SV, Gortmaker SL, Kawachi I. 2007. US state- and county-level social capital in relation to obesity and physical inactivity: A multilevel, multivariable analysis. *Social Science & Medicine* 63(4): 1045–1059.

Knack S, Keefer P. 1997. Does social capital have an economic impact? A cross-country investigation. *Quarterly Journal of Economics* 112(4): 1252–1288.

La Porta R, Lopez de Silanes F, Shleifer A, Vishny R. 1997. Trust in large organizations. *American Economic Review* 87(2): 333–338.

Mansyur C, Amick BC, Harrist RB, Franzini L. 2008. Social capital, income inequality, and self-rated health in 45 countries. *Social Science & Medicine* 66(10): 43–56.

Mellor J, Milyo J. 2005. State social capital and individual health status. *Journal of Health Politics, Policy and Law* 30(6): 1101–1130.

Miller DL, Scheffler R, Lam S, Rosenberg R, Rupp A. 2006. Social capital and health in Indonesia. *World Development* 34(6): 1084–1098.

Mohnen SM, Groenewegen PP, Völker B, Flap H. 2011. Neighborhood social capital and individual health. *Social Science & Medicine* 72: 660–667.

Murgai R, Winters P, Sadoulet E, de Janvry A. 2002. Localized and incomplete mutual insurance. *Journal of Development Economics* 67: 245–274.

Nauenberg E, Laporte A, Shen L. 2011. Social capital, community size and utilization of health services: A lagged analysis. *Health Policy* 103(1): 38–46.

Nguyen, TDPG. 1998. Food insecurity and the evolution of indigenous risk-sharing institutions in the Sahel. Ph.D. Thesis. Columbus, OH, USA: The Ohio State University (OSU), Department of Agricultural Economics.

Norwegian Ministry of Finance. 2012. For budsjettåret 2013. Skatter, avigifter og toll 2013 (Budget, Taxes, fees and custom 2013). Prop. 1LS2012–2013.

Olken BA. 2009. Do television and radio destroy social capital? Evidence from Indonesian villages. *American Economic Journal: Applied Economics* 1(4): 1–33.

Olsen KM, Dahl S. 2007. Health differences between European countries. *Social Science & Medicine* 64(8): 1665–1678.

Osmani LNK. 1998. Credit and Relative Well-being of Women: The Experience of Grameen Bank, Bangladesh. *PRUS Working Paper* No. 3. Workshop Proceedings Recent Research on Micro-financc: Implication for Policy. 21–28, In Matin I, Sinha S, with Alexamdner P. (eds.). Brighton, Sussex, UK: University of Sussex, Poverty Research Unit at Sussex (PRUS).

Ozawa, Sachiko, Walker, Damian. 2011. Comparison of trust in public vs. private health care providers in rural Cambodia. *Health Policy and Planning* 26: i20–i29.

Pan RJ, Littlefield D, Valladolid SG, Tapping PJ, West DC. 2005. Building healthier communities for children and families: Applying asset-based community development to community pediatrics. *Pediatrics* 115: 1185–1187.

Peters B, Gonsamo M, Molla S. 2011. Capturing unpredictable and intangible change: Evaluating an asset-based community development (ABCD) approach in Ethiopia. Occasional Papers Series No. 10, Coady International Insititute.

Petrou S, Kupek E. 2008. Social capital and its relationship with measures of health status: Evidence from the health survey for England 2003. *Health Economics* 17(1):127–143.

Poortinga W. 2006. Social capital: An individual or collective resource for health? *Social Science & Medicine* 62(2): 292–302.

Pronyk PM, Harpham T, Busza J, Phetla G, Morison LA, Hargreaves JR, Kim JC, Watts CH, Porter JD. 2008. Can social capital be intentionally generated? A randomized trial from rural South Africa. *Social Science & Medicine* 67: 1559–1570.

Putnam RD, Leonardi R, Nanenetti R. 1993. *Making Democracy Work: Civic Traditions in Modern Italy*. Princeton University Press: Princeton, NJ.

Rocco L, d'Hombres B. 2014. Social capital and smoking behavior. *Eastern Economic Journal* 40(2): 202–225.

Rocco L, Fumagalli E. 2014. The empirics of social capital and health. In Folland S, Rocco L. (eds.). *The Economics of Social Capital and Health. A Conceptual and Empirical Roadmap*. World Scientific Publishing.

Rocco L, Fumagalli E, Suhrcke M. 2014. From social capital to health — and back. *Health Economics* 23(5): 586–605.

Rojas Y, Carlson P. 2006. The stratification of social capital and its consequences for self-rated health in Taganrog, Russia. *Social Science & Medicine* 62(11): 2732–2741.

Ronconi L, Brown TT, Scheffler RM. 2010. Social capital and self-rated health in Argentina. *Health Economics* 21(2): 201–208.

Rose, Richard. 2000. How much does social capital add to individual health? A survey study of Russians. *Social Science & Medicine* 51(9): 1421–1435.

Rostila M. 2007. Social capital and health in European welfare regimes: A multilevel approach. *Journal of European Social Policy* 17(3): 223.

Russell S. 2005. Treatment-seeking behavior in urban Sri Lanka: Trusting the state, trusting private providers. *Social Science & Medicine* 61: 1396–1407.

Scheffler RM, Brown TT. 2008. Social capital, economics, and health: New evidence. *Health Economics Policy Law* 3(4): 321–31.

Scheffler RM, Brown TT, Syme L, Kawachi I, Tolstykh I, Iribarren, C. 2008. Community-level social capital and recurrence of acute coronary syndrome. *Social Science & Medicine* 66(7): 1603–1613.

Schrieder G, Pfaff K. 1997. Mise en place d'un réseau de caisses d'épargne villageoises au Niger. *Working Paper* 28. Stuttgart, Germany: University of Hohenheim, Development Theory and Policy (490a).

Schrieder G, Sharma M. 1999. Impact of finance on poverty reduction and social capital formation: A review and synthesis of empirical evidence. *Savings and Development* (1): 67–93.

Schuler SR, Hashemi SM, Riley AP. 1997. The influence of women's changing roles and status in Bangladesh's fertility transition: Evidence from a study of credit programs and contraceptive use. *World Development* 25(4): 563–575.

Snelgrove JW, Pikhart H, Stafford M. 2009. A multilevel analysis of social capital and self-rated health: Evidence from the British Household Panel Survey. *Social Science & Medicine* 68(11): 1993–2001.

Solow R. 1995. Trust: The Social Virtues and the Creation of Prosperity (Book Review). *The New Republic* 213: 36–40.

Srinivas H, Pallen D. 1998. The environmental colors of microfinance. http://soc.titech.ac.jp/icm/environ/environ.html.

Stern S. 1989. Measuring the effect of disability on labor force participation. *Journal of Human Resources* 24(3): 361–395.

Tabellini G. 2008. The scope of cooperation: Values and incentives. *Quarterly Journal of Economics* 3: 905–950.

Thiede M. 2005. Information and access to health care: Is there a role for trust? *Social Science & Medicine* 61: 1452–1462.

Thom DH, Hall MA, Pawlson LG. 2004. Measuring patients' trust in physicians when assessing quality of care. *Health Affairs* 23(4): 124–132.

Uslaner EM. 2002. *The Moral Foundations of Trust*. Cambridge University Press.

van Houtven CH, Norton EC. 2004. Informal care and health care use of older adults. *Journal of Health Economics* 23(6): 1159–1180.

van Houtven CH, Norton EC. 2008. Informal care and Medicare expenditures: Testing for heterogeneous treatment effects. *Journal of Health Economics* 27(1): 134–156.

Wang Hongmei Schlesinger M, Wang H, Hsiao W. 2009. The flip-side of social capital: The distinctive influences of trust and mistrust on health in rural China. *Social Science & Medicine* 68: 133–142.

Ware N, Idoko J, Kaaya S, Biraro I, Wyatt M, Agbaji O, Chalamilla G, Bangsberg D. 2009. Explaining adherence success in Sub-Saharan Africa: An ethnographic study. *PLoS Medicine* 6(1): e1000011.

Wilkinson RG. *Unhealthy Societies: The Afflictions of Inequality*. London: Routledge, 1996.

Yip W, Subramanian SV, Mitchell AD, Lee DT, Wang J, Kawachi I. 2007. Does social capital enhance health and well-being? Evidence from rural China. *Social Science & Medicine* 64(1): 35–49.

Zak PJ, Knack S. 2001. Trust and Growth. *The Economic Journal* 111(470): 295–321.

Zaman H. 1998. BRAC's impact on poverty and empowerment: A summary of findings from Matlab. *PRUS Working Paper* No. 3. 13–20. In Matin I, Sinha S, Alexamdner P. (eds.). Workshop Proceedings Recent research on micro-finance: Implication for Policy. Brighton, Sussex, UK: University of Sussex, Poverty Research Unit at Sussex (PRUS).

Zhang L, Wang H, Wang L, Hsiao W. 2006. Social capital and farmer's willingness-to-join a newly established community-based health insurance in rural China. *Health Policy* 76(2): 233–242.

Appendix

Table A1. The association between social capital and health by country

Country	Marginal effect	Std error	Observations	R^2	Share of respondents in good health	Share of trustful respondents
Albania	0.0969***	(0.0187)	1,815	0.265	0.742	0.256
Algeria	0.0848***	(0.0282)	2,042	0.116	0.563	0.150
Andorra	0.0511**	(0.0258)	943	0.153	0.848	0.207
Argentina	0.0391	(0.0280)	2,098	0.055	0.637	0.163
Armenia	0.0741***	(0.0246)	2,850	0.176	0.448	0.174
Australia	0.0721***	(0.0143)	4,032	0.077	0.784	0.467
Azerbaijan	0.0495**	(0.0246)	2,608	0.139	0.628	0.177
Bangladesh	0.0883***	(0.0227)	2,814	0.054	0.538	0.216
Belarus	0.0724***	(0.0165)	3,267	0.198	0.309	0.295
Bosnia	0.0992***	(0.0258)	1,849	0.151	0.625	0.210
Brazil	0.0635**	(0.0276)	3,107	0.134	0.720	0.0810
Bulgaria	0.0327	(0.0244)	1,553	0.303	0.566	0.256
Burkina Faso	0.0142	(0.0370)	1,187	0.057	0.723	0.141
Canada	0.0607***	(0.0159)	3,432	0.075	0.823	0.415
Chile	0.0205	(0.0189)	3,832	0.167	0.658	0.176
China	0.0525***	(0.0137)	5,782	0.085	0.663	0.560
Colombia	0.0666***	(0.0182)	4,440	0.163	0.761	0.0771
Cyprus	0.00563	(0.0309)	1,985	0.141	0.765	0.0894
Dominican Rep.	0.0641	(0.0562)	311	0.173	0.711	0.264
Ecuador	0.0228	(0.0446)	1,198	0.157	0.742	0.0718
Egypt	0.0388**	(0.0171)	7,217	0.110	0.640	0.257
El Salvador	0.0890**	(0.0378)	1,016	0.196	0.682	0.151
Estonia	0.104***	(0.0204)	2,440	0.272	0.438	0.307
Ethiopia	0.152***	(0.0286)	1,279	0.072	0.657	0.240
Finland	0.0580***	(0.0204)	1,792	0.222	0.696	0.537
France	0.0611*	(0.0367)	878	0.145	0.719	0.192
Georgia	0.0991***	(0.0205)	3,275	0.208	0.448	0.185
Germany	0.0963***	(0.0154)	5,230	0.186	0.644	0.377
Ghana	0.000696	(0.0303)	2,971	0.089	0.839	0.0685
Great Britain	0.0943***	(0.0312)	785	0.133	0.743	0.327
Guatemala	−0.00462	(0.0440)	941	0.102	0.620	0.152
Hong Kong	0.0216	(0.0297)	1,044	0.101	0.629	0.424

(Continued)

Table A1 (*Continued*)

Country	Marginal effect	Std error	Observations	R^2	Share of respondents in good health	Share of trustful respondents
Hungary	0.105***	(0.0309)	950	0.349	0.585	0.296
India	0.0772***	(0.0119)	6,562	0.097	0.638	0.345
Indonesia	0.0971***	(0.0187)	2,366	0.052	0.756	0.477
Iran	0.00786	(0.0169)	4,096	0.065	0.718	0.327
Iraq	0.0355***	(0.0122)	5,686	0.152	0.701	0.405
Italy	0.0980***	(0.0363)	622	0.155	0.728	0.328
Japan	0.0894***	(0.0172)	3,778	0.052	0.545	0.411
Jordan	0.0436***	(0.0139)	3,448	0.166	0.835	0.234
Kazakhstan	0.0990***	(0.0239)	1,500	0.203	0.616	0.383
Kuwait	0.0525**	(0.0225)	1,053	0.089	0.855	0.305
Kyrgyzstan	0.00602	(0.0213)	2,392	0.099	0.678	0.273
Latvia	0.119***	(0.0317)	1,116	0.160	0.361	0.247
Lebanon	−0.0698	(0.0450)	1,057	0.068	0.746	0.110
Libya	−0.00390	(0.0343)	1,891	0.048	0.855	0.106
Lithuania	0.104***	(0.0360)	892	0.243	0.439	0.224
Macedonia	0.00918	(0.0350)	1,576	0.093	0.715	0.110
Malaysia	0.0271	(0.0219)	2,494	0.065	0.879	0.0858
Mali	0.00422	(0.0377)	918	0.129	0.663	0.181
Mexico	0.0419***	(0.0155)	6,350	0.142	0.630	0.223
Moldova	0.0677***	(0.0222)	2,807	0.188	0.392	0.183
Morocco	0.0144	(0.0249)	2,778	0.154	0.710	0.156
Netherlands	0.0990***	(0.0215)	2,303	0.097	0.735	0.577
New Zealand	0.0596***	(0.0159)	2,439	0.080	0.819	0.543
Nigeria	0.0278**	(0.0122)	6,033	0.064	0.841	0.207
Norway	0.108***	(0.0223)	1,967	0.146	0.795	0.716
Pakistan	0.0108	(0.0187)	3,557	0.187	0.694	0.250
Palestine	0.0746**	(0.0334)	881	0.218	0.757	0.175
Peru	0.0902***	(0.0244)	4,973	0.106	0.508	0.0775
Philippines	0.0270	(0.0476)	2,370	0.048	0.569	0.0572
Poland	0.0668***	(0.0203)	2,835	0.334	0.529	0.201
Puerto Rico	0.0599*	(0.0314)	1,699	0.176	0.708	0.148
Qatar	0.0134	(0.0223)	1,042	0.101	0.885	0.213
Romania	0.0318	(0.0201)	4,079	0.233	0.574	0.151
Russia	0.0928***	(0.0136)	5,637	0.229	0.355	0.264

(*Continued*)

Table A1 (*Continued*)

Country	**Marginal effect**	**Std error**	**Observations**	R^2	**Share of respondents in good health**	**Share of trustful respondents**
Rwanda	0.0737***	(0.0200)	2,929	0.348	0.591	0.111
Saudi Arabia	0.0304*	(0.0173)	1,296	0.034	0.888	0.540
Serbia and Montenegro	0.120***	(0.0238)	4,115	0.180	0.524	0.246
Singapore	0.0680***	(0.0191)	1,918	0.072	0.806	0.371
Slovakia	0.0510	(0.0344)	861	0.243	0.524	0.271
Slovenia	0.127***	(0.0247)	1,949	0.194	0.609	0.191
South Africa	0.0456**	(0.0216)	7,128	0.126	0.719	0.177
South Korea	0.0456***	(0.0139)	4,725	0.065	0.794	0.284
Spain	0.0449***	(0.0144)	3,770	0.217	0.748	0.247
Sweden	0.0828***	(0.0184)	2,884	0.094	0.768	0.638
Switzerland	0.0711***	(0.0155)	2,609	0.099	0.839	0.479
Taiwan	0.0308*	(0.0158)	2,368	0.089	0.870	0.276
Tanzania	0.0771	(0.0556)	969	0.065	0.637	0.0826
Thailand	0.0596***	(0.0221)	1,462	0.128	0.763	0.410
Trinidad and Tobago	0.0354	(0.0478)	1,948	0.125	0.737	0.0353
Tunisia	0.0751**	(0.0329)	1,121	0.186	0.710	0.161
Turkey	0.0849***	(0.0208)	8,179	0.060	0.638	0.102
Uganda	−0.0102	(0.0696)	544	0.153	0.757	0.0764
Ukraine	0.0913***	(0.0174)	4,351	0.223	0.374	0.278
United States	0.0481***	(0.0124)	4,592	0.093	0.819	0.358
Uruguay	0.0276	(0.0190)	2,597	0.161	0.785	0.217
Uzbekistan	−0.0329	(0.0326)	1,437	0.185	0.738	0.141
Venezuela	0.0536	(0.0344)	1,093	0.132	0.757	0.132
Viet Nam	−0.000476	(0.0200)	2,352	0.099	0.595	0.469
Yemen	0.0491*	(0.0287)	924	0.154	0.711	0.402
Zambia	0.0467	(0.0408)	1,145	0.107	0.728	0.106
Zimbabwe	0.0349	(0.0367)	2,321	0.164	0.716	0.103

Notes: Estimates based on the most comprehensive specification of model (1).

Economics of Tobacco Control and Health

Ayda Yurekli
University of Illinois, Chicago
Nigar Nargis
American Cancer Society
Mark Goodchild
World Health Organization
Chonlathan Visaruthvong
Ministry of Finance, Thailand
Sophia Delipalla
University of Macedonia
Evan Blecher
World Health Organization
Anne-Marie Perucic
World Health Organization
Teh-Wei Hu
University of California, Berkeley
Anita Lee
Center for International Tobacco Control, Public Health Institute
Frank Chaloupka
University of Illinois, Chicago

Tobacco use remains the world's leading cause of preventable death, and is projected to cause over 1 billion deaths in the 21st century, with a disproportionate impact on low- and middle-income countries. This chapter reviews current and emerging evidence on tobacco use and tobacco control efforts worldwide. The chapter explores tobacco prevalence and consumption levels around the globe, trends in tobacco production and international trade, the health and economic consequences of tobacco use among different populations, illicit trade patterns, and the fundamental economic relationship between tobacco taxation, final price and consumer demand.

There is a sound evidence base and experience throughout the world that tobacco control measures are effective in reducing the harm caused by tobacco use. Tobacco taxation has proven to be one of the most cost-effective and efficient tobacco demand reduction measures available. Combined with other tobacco control measures such as those recommended in the WHO Framework Convention on Tobacco Control, there is growing optimism that the tobacco epidemic can be reversed and prevented throughout the world. However, tobacco control measures still face challenges from the tobacco industry that require innovative solutions, collaboration and political commitment on the part of governments.[1]

Keywords: Non-communicable Diseases (NCDs); Excise Taxes; RIP; Illicit Trade.

Introduction

The tobacco epidemic currently represents the world's largest cause of preventable death. It is estimated that tobacco currently causes over 5 million deaths per year, and the death toll from tobacco in the 21st century is predicted to exceed 1 billion deaths per year (Eriksen *et al.*, 2012).

At the same time, tobacco is a relatively recent phenomenon in the context of human history. Its widespread worldwide use dates back little more than a century, with the advent of affordable mass-produced cigarettes. Combined with a relative lack of health knowledge, smoking became a cultural norm in many countries, with prevalence among men exceeding 50% in many countries at its peak (WHO, 2013a). It has only been in recent decades that evidence-based science has begun to emerge on tobacco control and public health.

This chapter will review the current state of tobacco and tobacco control as of 2014, including areas such as prevalence and consumption, health impacts and demand as well as tobacco control areas and policy issues such as taxation and pricing, affordability of tobacco products, smuggling and illicit trade, and supply-side interventions for farmers. It reviews current science in these areas, and summarizes key trends in understanding and resolving the current crisis of tobacco use.

Global Tobacco Market

The manufacture and consumption of cigarettes was close to 6 trillion in 2008, a 13% increase over the previous decade (Eriksen *et al.*, 2012). A disproportionate amount of this consumption now takes place in low- and middle-income countries, where there is still nascent growth of smoking in general, particularly among

[1]The authors alone are responsible for the views expressed in this article and they do not necessarily represent the views, decisions or policies of the institutions with which they are affiliated.

groups such as women and youth, and resources are more limited for both tobacco control efforts and to address the health consequences of smoking. For example China, where the largest growth in tobacco use has taken place this century, alone consumes more than 2 trillion cigarettes per year (Euromonitor, 2014).

The market for manufactured cigarettes far dominates the use of tobacco. However, other tobacco products are more popular in specific cultures, such as bidis in India (700 billion pieces per year) and clove-flavored kretek in Indonesia (200 billion pieces per year, and over 90% of the local tobacco market) (Barber *et al.*, 2008). Smokeless tobacco products are also in use in many countries, with higher rates of prevalence in specific cultures and countries such as India. Nonetheless, the vast majority of today's tobacco market revolves around the use of manufactured cigarettes, and tobacco control today is largely synonymous with efforts to eradicate cigarette smoking.

Tobacco consumption

Tobacco is consumed worldwide in the form of combusted or non-combusted products. Combusted products include white cigarettes that contain tobacco; kreteks[2] that contain both tobacco and cloves; bidis[3] that are wrapped in tendu leaves (used for example in India); biris that are hand-rolled in cigarette paper (Bangladesh); and loose tobacco rolled in papers called roll your own (RYO) or smoked in devices such as a pipe or nargile[4] (water pipe). Non-combusted products include different types of snuff and chewing tobacco products.

Globally, manufactured cigarettes account for approximately 90% of smoked tobacco products (Table 1) and are thought to account for more than 80% of total tobacco leaf production (IARC, 2011).

- *Cigarettes*

Almost 5.8 trillion cigarettes were sold in 2012, with roughly 80% of consumption (sales) occurring in low- and middle-income countries. China led this consumption accounting for more than 40% of global sales alone. Between 2000 and 2012,

---

[2]Kreteks are also known as clove cigarettes, as they typically contain 40% cloves and 60% tobacco.

[3]Bidis/biris are small hand-rolled cigarettes that tend to be smaller than conventional cigarettes and are exotically flavored with ingredients promoted as natural and healthy. They typically contain a few hundred milligrams of tobacco wrapped in a tendu or temburni leaf.

[4]Pipe tobacco is loose tobacco that is usually smoked in smoking pipes or water pipe devices. Water pipes (also called shisha or nargile) are products in which tobacco smoke is passed through water ("bubbled") before inhalation.

Table 1. Volume and market share of combusted tobacco products 2012

Sales of combusted tobacco products 2012	Measure (billion)	Volume	Global market share (%)
Cigarettes*	Sticks	5,718.9	91.4
Smoking tobacco**	Grams	236.6	3.8
Pipe tobacco	*Grams*	133.1	2.1
RYO	*Grams*	103.5	1.7
Bidis/biris***	Sticks	300.0	4.8
Total	Sticks	6,255.5	100.0

Notes: *Cigarettes include kreteks cigarettes. **Smoking tobacco includes pipe and roll-your-own (RYO) cigarettes and we assume that 1 gram of smoking tobacco is equivalent to one stick. ***The tobacco content of bidis/biris varies from 0.20 to 0.30 gram per stick.
Source: Numbers are compiled by authors using historical statistical sales data from EuroMonitor, 2014.

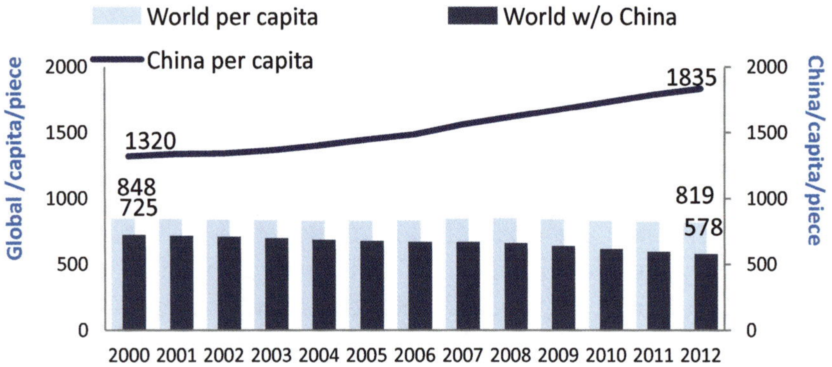

Figure 1. Global cigarette consumption, number of pieces per capita, 2000–2012
Source: Figure constructed by authors' calculations using sales data from Euromonitor, population by the World Bank HNP database from 2000 to 2012.

however, global per capita cigarette consumption decreased by 8%, from 848 pieces to 810 pieces per capita. When China is excluded, global cigarette consumption in fact has experienced a 24% decrease, from 725 pieces to 578 pieces per capita during the same period (see Figure 1 and Table 2).

Looking at trends in consumption between 1997 and 2012 (Figure 2), data shows that unlike in developed (high-income) countries where consumption has tapered, consumption has been steadily increasing in developing countries.

Regionally, the European (EUR) and American (AMR) regions have experienced reductions in sales, while a steady and marked increase has been seen in the Western Pacific Region (WPR), driven particularly by large increases in consumption in

Table 2. Summary of total sales breakdown by income groups and WHO regions

	Cigarette sales (Billion sticks)	Percentage of total sales (%)	Per capita (PC) adult consumption (sales) (number of sticks)
High Income (HI)	1,156.3	20.0	1,299.6
Upper Middle-Income (UMI)	3,550.7	61.6	1,761.5
Low Middle-Income (LMI)	923.0	16.0	525.6
Low Income (LI)	137.9	2.4	291.4
World	5,767.8		1,123.8
Africa Region (AFR)	126.0	2.2	262.7
Americas Region (AMR)	558.0	9.7	771.3
East Mediterranean Region (EMR)	345.7	6.0	868.7
European Region (EUR)	1,270.3	22.0	1,702.9
South-East Asia Region (SEAR)	449.2	7.8	354.1
West Pacific Region (WPR)	3,018.6	52.3	2,045.2

Sources: Table constructed by authors' calculations using sales data from Euromonitor, income group classification of the World Bank in 2012 and UN World Population Prospects 2012.

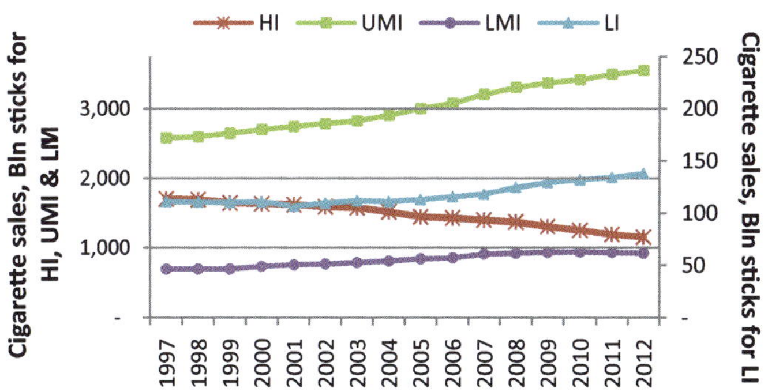

Figure 2. Trends in sales by income group (1997–2012)

Source: Figure constructed by authors' calculations using sales data from Euromonitor and income group classification of the World Bank in 2012.

China (57% between 1997 and 2012), the Philippines (48%) and Vietnam (135%). The South-East Asia (SEAR) and Eastern Mediterranean (EMR) regions have also seen regular increases in sales, particularly in Bangladesh and Indonesia (50% increase for each) in SEAR and Iran, Jordan, Kuwait, Lebanon and Qatar (more than 200% increase each) in EMR. The African region (AFR) shows a steady but conservative increase over time (Figure 3).

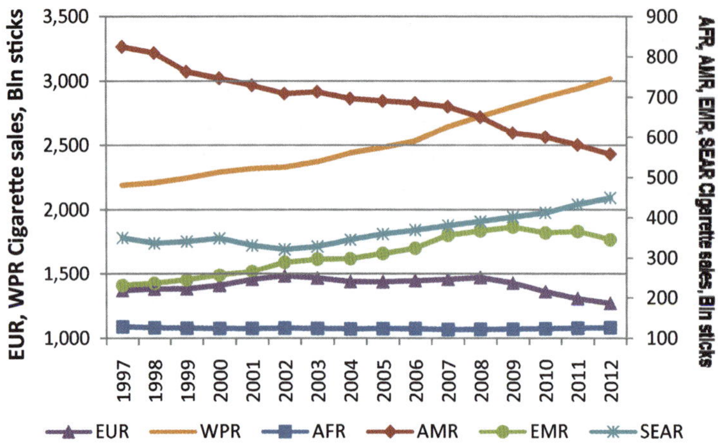

Figure 3. Trends in cigarette sales, by WHO regions (1987–2012)

Source: Figure constructed by authors' calculations using sales data from Euromonitor and WHO regional groupings.

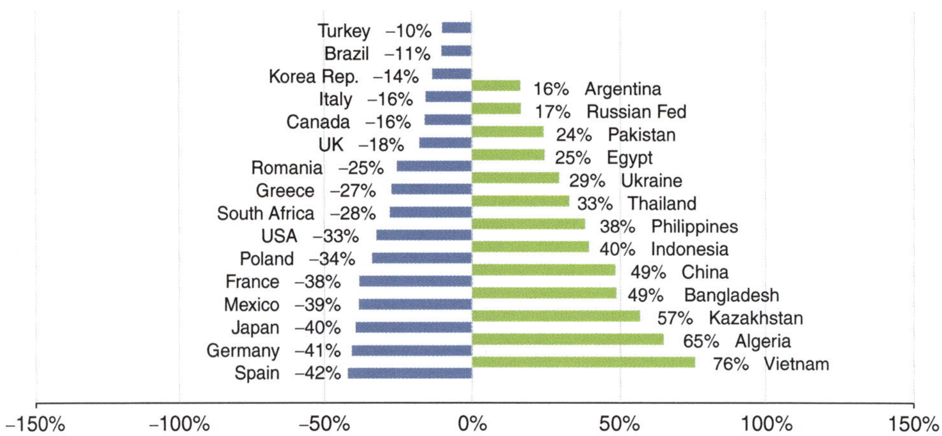

Figure 4. Percentage change of total cigarette sales 2000–2012 among top cigarette consuming countries

Source: Authors' estimates using historical statistical sales data from 2000 to 2012 by Euromonitor 2014.

However, among many of the top cigarette-consuming countries, total cigarette sales fell considerably between 2000 and 2012, ranging from a 42% decline in Spain to a 10% decline in Turkey. At the same time, sales increased in a number of the most populated developing countries, including Vietnam, Bangladesh, China, Indonesia, Philippines, Egypt, Pakistan and the Russian Federation (Figure 4).

- *Other tobacco products*

Tobacco use also shows considerable variation across different geographic locations. For example, bidi/biris are consumed mainly in South-East Asia. Kreteks are used in some countries in the Western Pacific Region (e.g., Indonesia, Malaysia). Water pipes are a common form of pipe tobacco use in North Africa and the Middle East that is also becoming common in other parts of the world.

All of these products have a relatively limited market compared to cigarettes, but their share can be considerable in certain countries. For example, biris are smoked mainly in Bangladesh where their tax-paid sales were around 48–50 billion sticks[5] or about 47% of the total Bangladeshi cigarette market (white + biris) in 2012 (WHO, MOF/NBR Bangladash 2012). Bidis, on the other hand, are popular in India, Sri Lanka and a few other South Asian countries, but India is the largest consuming country with an estimated 295 billion sticks or 72% of the smoked tobacco market in India in 2012.[6] Roll-your-own (RYO) cigarettes also show a similar pattern to bidis. Their share in the global smoking market is only 2% (based on data from 121 countries), but they have a significant market share exceeding 40% in a number of countries including Luxembourg, Belgium and the Netherlands. Their use is also relatively substantial among large cigarette consuming countries such as Germany (with a 24% market share), France (14%), UK (12%) and Spain (11%). Between 2007 and 2012, total sales of RYO increased by 19% globally, with significant increases occurring in large cigarette-consuming countries, including Italy (307%), Japan (169%), and South Africa (160%) (WHO, 2014a; Euromonitor, 2014) (Figure 5).

Pipe tobacco consumption is the highest in EMR countries, as it is used mainly in water pipes. However, it is now becoming popular in other parts of the world including the US, Bolivia, Georgia, Belarus, Chile and the Caribbean Islands (Figure 6).

Smokeless tobacco is the most-widely used non-combustible tobacco product, with 84% of the global market consumed in India in 2012, followed by the US at 12%. Nonetheless, between 2007 and 2012, smokeless tobacco sales declined by 17% from 589 thousand tons to 487 thousand tons, mainly because of a 21% market reduction in India during that period (Figure 7).

[5]Estimates of bidi consumption in Bangladesh come from different sources: (1) The ITC Bangladesh Survey in 2012 estimates the amount to be 48 billion sticks, (2) The Ministry of Finance, Bangladesh provides a number amounting to 51 billion sticks (excise paid in 2012), (3) Estimates from the Global Adult Survey for Bangladesh GATS in 2009 estimates a consumption of 50 billion sticks.

[6]Data provided to WHO by the Ministry of Finance, India, 2014.

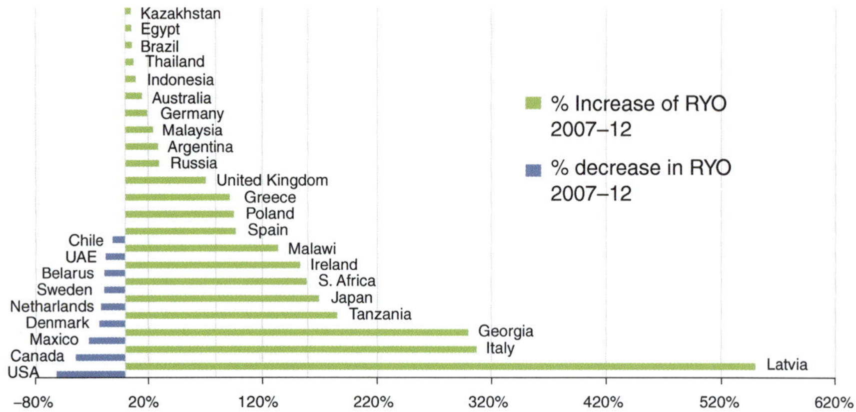

Figure 5. Highest changes in RYO sales by country in 2012

Source: Graph constructed by authors using Euromonitor data 2014.

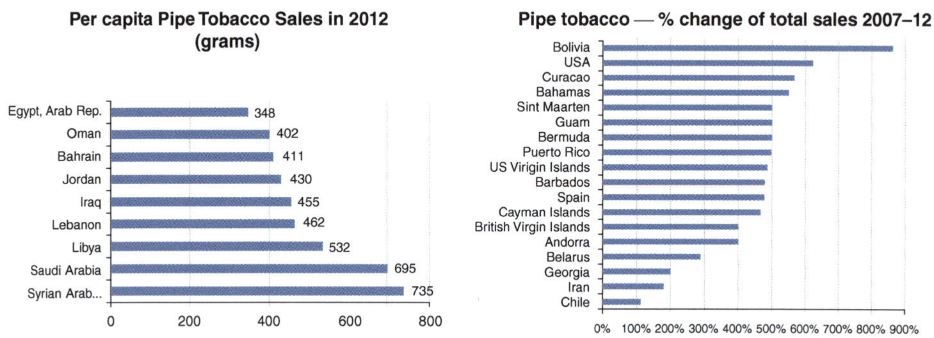

Figure 6. Pipe tobacco sales in 2012 and changes between 2007 and 2012

Source: Graphs are constructed by authors using Euromonitor data 2014.

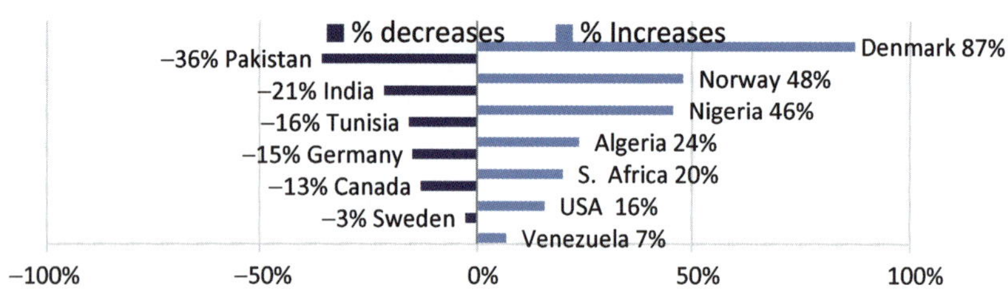

Figure 7. Percentage change in smokeless tobacco sales 2007–2012

Source: Graph is constructed by authors by using Euromonitor data from 2007 to 2014.

Prevalence of tobacco use

Cigarettes have the most global reach, being available in most countries, including non-filter variations common to Eastern Europe. Cigarette use has therefore been studied more extensively around the world than other tobacco products.

- *Prevalence of cigarette use*

The WHO has calculated cigarette use throughout the world based on nationally representative surveys of smoking prevalence (WHO, 2010a). In 2012, WHO estimated that there were 1 billion adult cigarette smokers, accounting for as much as 20% of the total global adult population. The prevalence rate of smoking tends to increase with country income, a pattern that is heavily influenced by the greater uptake of smoking among women as incomes increase, discussed later in this section (Table 3). Similarly, the global pattern is influenced by China and India with their large populations. As expected, almost half of adult cigarette smokers globally live in upper middle-income (UMI) countries, primarily because of China.

By WHO Region, smoking prevalence is highest in Europe followed by the Western Pacific Region (e.g., China, Philippines, and Vietnam) and the Americas (Table 4). Africa records the lowest rate of smoking, with half of all countries recording prevalence rates of less than 10% of the adult population. Daily cigarette consumption is the highest in the WPR Region and the lowest in the AFR Region. Table 3 provides complete details on the adult prevalence and consumption of cigarette smoking by income group in 2012 whereas Table 4 elaborates adult prevalence and consumption of cigarette smoking by WHO region in 2012, respectively.

Table 3. Prevalence of cigarette smoking by income group in 2012

	Adult rate of current cigarette smoking	**Number of adult cigarette smokers**	**Daily cigarette consumption**
	(% of population aged 15+)	**(Million adults)**	**(Sticks per day, per adult smoker)**
	Total	Total	
High Income (HI)	25	220	14.3
Upper Middle-Income (UMI)	25	499	19.4
Lower Middle (LMI)	14	235	10.6
Low Income (LI)	13	56	5.9
World	20	1,011	15.5

Source: World Health Organization 2013 Report on Global Tobacco Epidemic and Euromonitor 2013.

Table 4. Prevalence of cigarette smoking by WHO region in 2012

	Adult rate of current cigarette smoking	**Number of adult cigarette smokers**	**Daily cigarette consumption**
	(% of population aged 15+)	***(Million adults)***	***(Sticks per day, per adult smoker)***
	Total	Total	
Africa (AFR)	8	35	8.8
Americas (AMR)	20	136	10.9
Eastern Med. (EMR)	15	57	16.6
Europe (EUR)	31	227	15.2
South-East Asia (SEAR)	14	174	7.0
Western Pacific (WPR)	26	382	21.7
World	20	1,011	15.5

Source: WHO 2013 Report on Global Tobacco Epidemic, Euromonitor 2013.

- *Prevalence of other tobacco products*

Existing evidence shows that for a number of countries, the use of products such as bidis, kreteks, water pipe, or smokeless tobacco is much more common than cigarettes. In India, for example, 25.9% of adults use smokeless tobacco compared to 14% that use smoking tobacco product and among those, only 5.3% smoke cigarettes and rest smoke bidis (GATS Factsheet India, 2009–2010). This is also the case for Bangladesh, where the prevalence of smokeless tobacco (27.2%) is higher than that for tobacco smoking (23%) (GATS Factsheet Bangladesh, 2009). In Indonesia, kreteks are the most widely used tobacco product, in contrast to common cigarettes (usually called white cigarettes). The overall 36.1% prevalence rate for tobacco use in Indonesia is mainly driven by kretek use, with a 31.5% prevalence rate in 2001 (GATS Factsheet Indonesia, 2011). The prevalence of current smokeless tobacco, white cigarettes and hand-rolled cigarettes use in Indonesia is much smaller with overall rates of 1.7, 2.2, and 4.7% respectively.

Most smokers worldwide consume manufactured cigarettes. In a number of countries, cigarettes are also rolled by hand to smoke, either in the context of a cottage industry, like in India or Indonesia, or by tobacco users themselves who purchase shredded tobacco for their own consumption such as in Thailand. These are commonly called Roll Your Own (RYO) in Europe and the United States.

The data reveal that the use of RYO cigarettes among tobacco smokers is significant, nearly reaching levels of (manufactured) cigarette smoking in some countries. This is the case in Thailand, where prevalence of manufactured cigarettes and RYO were 15.2% and 14.4% respectively in 2001 (GATS Factsheet Thailand,

Table 5. Prevalence of cigarettes and RYO among current smokers, 2008*

	Exclusive factory-made	**Predominant RYO**	**Some RYO use**
Australia	78.2%	15.4%	6.4%
Canada	87.9%	8.8%	3.3%
United Kingdom	32.0%	31.5%	6.6%
US	89.1%	5.7%	5.2%
	Exclusive factory-made	Exclusive RYO	Both
New Zealand	47.5%	38.2%	14.3%

Note: *Results are from surveys undertaken by the International Tobacco Control Policy Evaluation Project (the ITC Project).
Source: Young *et al.* (2010; 2012).

Table 6. Smoking prevalence of cigarettes and pipe tobacco

	Current tobacco smoking	**Current cigarette smoking**	**Current water pipe smoking**
Egypt (2009)	19.4%	16.3%	3.3%
Qatar (2013)	12.1%	10.2%	3.4%

Source: Global Adult Tobacco Survey (GATS). Factsheet: Egypt, 2009 and Qatar, 2013.

2011). This is also the case in the UK and New Zealand (Young *et al.,* 2010; 2012) as shown in Table 5.

Based on available information from GATS in Egypt and Qatar, prevalence rates for water pipe tobacco may look low, but they are not insignificant relative to cigarettes smoking as demonstrated in Table 6. Qatar, for example, had a cigarette-smoking prevalence of 10.2% compared to a water pipe-smoking prevalence of 3.4% in 2013.

• *Prevalence by socioeconomic groups*

Gender and youth: In many low- and middle-income countries, social and cultural norms have historically prevented women from smoking. As a result, the prevalence of smoking is much higher among adult males than females (WHO 2010a). Table 7 illustrates the prevalence of cigarette smoking for each gender by income group and by region, showing that the highest prevalence of cigarette smoking among women occurs in developed countries (19%) and the rate decreases concurrently with decreases in income groups.

Table 7. Current cigarette prevalence for each gender by income group and region in 2012

	Adult rate of current cigarette smoking (% of population aged 15+)		Number of adult cigarette smokers (*Million adults*)	
	Males	**Females**	**Males**	**Females**
High Income (HI)	31	19	135	85
Upper Middle Income (UMI)	43	7	426	73
Lower Middle Income (LMI)	24	3	213	22
Low Income (LI)	25	2	51	5
Africa (AFR)	14	1	32	3
Americas (AMR)	25	15	84	52
Eastern Med. (EMR)	27	2	53	4
Europe (EUR)	41	22	143	85
South-East Asia (SEAR)	24	2	159	15
Western Pacific (WPR)	47	4	355	27
World	33	7	825	185

Source: WHO 2013 Report on Global Tobacco Epidemic.

Table 8. Overall prevalence of tobacco use and smoking cigarettes by gender

	India — 2009–2010		Thailand — 2011		Indonesia — 2011	
	Current tobacco use (%)	**Current cigarette smoking (%)**	**Current tobacco use (%)**	**Current cigarette smoking** (%)**	**Current tobacco use (%)**	**Current tobacco smk* (%)**
Males	47.9	10.3	47.2	30.1	67.4	67.0
Females	20.3	0.8	7.6	1.1	4.5	2.7
Overall	34.6	5.7	26.9	15.2	36.1	34.8

Notes: *White and kretek cigarettes, **manufactured.
Source: Ministry of Health and Family Welfare, Government of India. Global Adult Tobacco Survey (GATS) Factsheet: India 2009–2010. GATS Factsheet: Thailand, 2011.

As further evidence on types of tobacco use by gender become available, the prevalence rate for tobacco use among women is turning out to actually be higher than previously thought. Data from three of the most populated and highest tobacco prevalence countries demonstrates this fact in Table 8.

High prevalence rates of smokeless tobacco use among women, especially in India (18.4%) and Thailand (5.3%), are responsible for higher prevalence of rates of tobacco use among women in those countries. Similarly, with respect to water pipe use, its use among women is as high as cigarette smoking as illustrated in Table 9.

Table 9. Smoking prevalence of cigarettes and pipe tobacco in Egypt and Qatar

		Current cigarette smoking (%)	Current water pipe smoking (%)
Egypt (2009)	Males	31.8	6.2
	Females	0.2	0.3
Qatar (2013)	Males	17.9	4.9
	Females	1.8	1.6

Source: Global Adult Tobacco Survey (GATS). Factsheet: Egypt, 2009 and Qatar, 2013.

Table 10. Evolution of prevalence and number of smokers over time

	Prevalence %		Number of daily smokers (million adults)	
	1980	2012	1980	2012
Men	41.2	31.1	571.7	807.3
	(40.0–42.6)	(30.2–32.0)	(552.7–591.3)	(783.9–829.4)
Women	10.6	6.2	149.0	160.0
	(10.2–11.1)	(6.0–6.4)	(143.1–155.7)	(155.5–164.8)
Both	25.9	18.7	720.7	967.3
	(25.1–26.6)	(18.2–19.1)	(700.2–742.0)	(943.8–989.1)

Note: Numbers between brackets indicate 95% confidence interval.
Source: Ng *et al.* (2014).

A recent publication by Ng *et al.* (2014), looking at trends in smoking prevalence for 187 countries from 1980 to 2012, showed global reductions in smoking prevalence among both men and women but also increases in the number of smokers because of population increases. Ng *et al.* show that the rate of decrease in prevalence has slowed since 2006 with an apparent increase in smoking prevalence for men since 2010. This was partly due to increases in the number of smokers in large countries like Bangladesh, China, Indonesia and Russia. Table 10 provides a brief summary of the changes between 1980 and 2012.

With regards to prevalence rates among the youth, analysis of data from the Global Youth Tobacco Use Survey (GYTS)[7] undertaken by US Centers for Disease

[7]The GYTS is a school-based survey that collects data on students aged 13–15 years using a standardized methodology for constructing the sample frame, selecting schools and classes, and processing data. GYTS has been conducted for all income group of countries but developing countries represent the majority. http://www.cdc.gov/tobacco/global/.

Table 11. Prevalence of youth aged 13–15 who used tobacco, selected countries, GYTS 1999–2001

	Currently use any tobacco product (%)	Currently smoke cigarettes (%)	Currently use other tobacco products (%)
Ghana (2000)	16.8	4.2	14.5
Nigeria (Cross River State 2001)	18.1	7.0	14.0
Bahamas (2000)	16.2	7.1	11.8
Dominica (2000)	19.3	11.6	10.7
Jordan (1999)	20.6	16.6	11.2
Sri Lanka (1999)	9.9	4.0	7.2
India (Bihar 2000)	59.9	13.9	46.7
Philippines (2000)	23.3	18.2	11.1

Source: Global Youth Tobacco Survey Collaborative Group (2002).

Control in collaboration with the World Health Organization in 1999 and 2001 shows that the overall median rate of current smoking globally was 13.9%, ranging from 39.6% to less than 1% among students 13 to 15 years old in some countries (CDC OSH, 2002). Using more recent GYTS data from between 2000 and 2011, we estimate that on average 15% of youth (1.3 million out of 8.8 million youth aged 13–15 years old) among 24 high-income countries and 7% of youth (22.4 million out of 330 million youth aged 13–15 years) among 130 developing countries[8] are identified as current smokers (meaning that they smoked at least one cigarette during the last 30 days prior to survey). GYTS data reveals that, among those students who smoke, nearly 25% said that they had their first cigarette before the age of 10 years (CDC OSH, 2002). Furthermore, GYTS data reveal that youth are not only using cigarettes but also other tobacco products that equal or surpass by far their use of cigarettes (Table 11).

These numbers are alarming in terms of future public health outcomes, meaning premature mortality and morbidity, private and public health care costs, lost productivity and hence negative outcome on the development process — as it will be discussed in Health and Economic Consequences of smoking and tobacco control section of this chapter — especially, for developing countries, since they have a relatively higher share of youth population compared to that of developed countries. Indeed, developing countries are home to 71% of the global youth (0–14 age group) population — more than 1.5 billion persons (United Nations Secretariat, 2012). In some countries the share of young population reaches as high as 34% of total population (World Bank HNP Population Data, 2014).

[8] We gathered the data from CDC GYTS database. We eliminated a number of small islands due to unavailability of youth data.

National surveys of smoking among youth populations (aged 13–15) also often show that young women report higher rates of cigarette use than adult women and have similar rates of use to their young male counterparts. This pattern could be a reflection of aggressive tobacco industry marketing to young women, and is very concerning because it suggests substantial increases in adult women smoking in the near future. The number of female smokers has been forecasted to double between 2003 and 2025 (Mackay and Amos, 2003).

With regards to socio-economic status, cigarette smoking and tobacco product prevalence tends to be higher among the poor or people from lower socio-economic status levels (usually defined in terms of individual or household income level, expenditure level or educational level of individuals) (IARC, 2011). Recent evidence from 13 low- and middle-income countries shows that higher SES is associated with a lower probability of smoking (Kostova *et al.*, 2013).

A more comprehensive study by Bobak *et al.* (2000) examined the relationship between smoking and socioeconomic status in 74 studies and developed a ratio of the smoking prevalence rate of the lowest to the highest socioeconomic groups. This study shows that smoking prevalence is higher among the lowest socioeconomic groups in almost all countries including both developed to developing countries, except for a few countries such as Bolivia, Japan and Thailand where smoking prevalence is higher among the highest socioeconomic groups. We see similar results in Turkey, where a Turkish expenditure survey in 2003 shows that smoking prevalence is higher in rich households compared with the poor households (Table 12). These varying results are attributed to the different stages of where these countries stand in the tobacco epidemic.[9] For example, if a country is at a relatively early stage of the tobacco epidemic, when the prevalence of smoking is increasing, then lower prevalence rates are observed among lower socioeconomic groups. This is not surprising, as we will discuss below in detail; the affordability of tobacco products has been increasing over the years, as per capita income increases at a higher rate than the increases in retail prices of tobacco products. As their per capita income and education level increases, smokers in higher socioeconomic groups are more likely to internalize the health risks associated with smoking at a faster pace than less educated, lower-income groups.

[9]Four stages outline the evolution of the global tobacco epidemic. The first stage sees smoking initiation among men and a slow rise in prevalence, while prevalence in women is almost nil. During the second stage, smoking increases markedly among men to reach very large proportions (prevalence above 60%) and deaths among men start to be observed. At the same time, women start taking up the habit but proportions are still low. In the third stage, prevalence in men reaches a maximum and starts to decrease but deaths among men continue to increase substantially. Prevalence in women continues to increase and deaths among women are observed and on the rise. During the fourth stage, prevalence in men continues to decrease and deaths in men reach a maximum and start to decrease. Women's prevalence also starts to go down but deaths are on the rise.

Table 12. Smoking prevalence among households in Turkey, 2003

Expenditure tertiles	Smoking prevalence by households (%)	Average number of packs smoked per month
The poor	54.1	31.5
Middle	59.1	32.7
Rich	59.5	33.1
Total	57.6	32.5

Source: Turkish household expenditure survey 2003 (Önder and Yürekli, 2014).

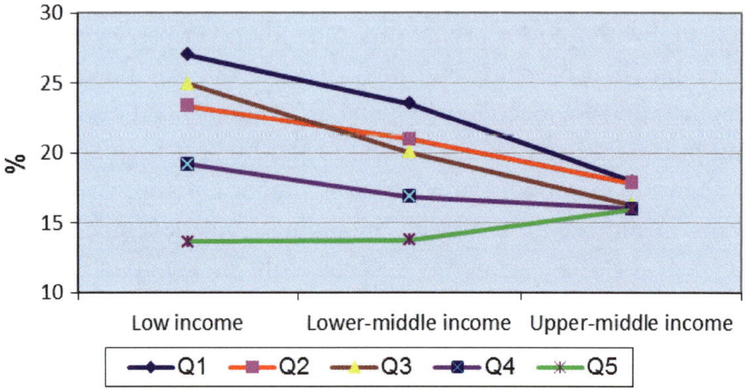

Figure 8. Prevalence of daily tobacco smoking by income group and income quintile, 2004

Notes:

1. Q1–Q5 indicate income quintiles, Q1 being the lowest income group and Q5 the highest income group.
2. The graph was made using average prevalence figures from 44 countries. Prevalence levels for China and India were removed from these averages to avoid skewed results from their large population weights.

Source: David *et al.* (2010).

Using prevalence data from the World Health Survey for 44 countries, David *et al.* (2010) showed that the gap in prevalence in daily smoking tobacco between different socioeconomic groups was larger in lower income countries in 2004. This gap narrowed as the income level of countries increased. A similar trend was seen within country-level income groups, with prevalence higher in lower-income households and decreasing as the income of the household increased (see Figure 8).

Globalization of the tobacco market

Over the past three decades, the global landscape for the tobacco market has witnessed dramatic changes with respect to: (i) Ownership status of producers of tobacco products including flow of trade and trade agreements (ii) strength of tobacco control policies, and (iii) changing consumers' demand for tobacco products and product differentiation.

- *Ownership status of producers*

Many developed and developing countries that have long traditions of state involvement and production of tobacco products joined the global privatization movement, especially in the 1990s, and privatized their state-owned tobacco processing and manufacturing facilities. These mainly involved multinational tobacco companies (MTCs) including British American Tobacco (BAT), Philip Morris International (PMI) and Atria (US affiliation of PMI), Imperial Tobacco (IT), and Japan Tobacco International (JTI). By 2010, the global tobacco industry became a highly consolidated industry with a few large players dominating global tobacco product production, especially for cigarettes (Figure 9).

By 2012, only a handful of governments have kept significant ownership in national cigarette manufacturing companies. For example, Japan and Egypt still have 49% and 52% ownership in state-owned firms respectively, as the rest of ownership has changed to local private hands. Other countries including Algeria, Belarus, China, Ethiopia, Lebanon, Moldova, Thailand, Tunis, and Vietnam still have 100% ownership. However, based on available data, the market share of state-owned tobacco companies' brands have declined dramatically to 70% in Thailand, 66% in Tunis, 64% in Egypt, 60% in Belarus, 56.6% in Algeria and 44% in Vietnam in 2012. Only China and Ethiopia keep their market share above 90% of the domestic market. Figure 9 shows global cigarette market concentration and the shares of the largest cigarette producers in global cigarette market, respectively.

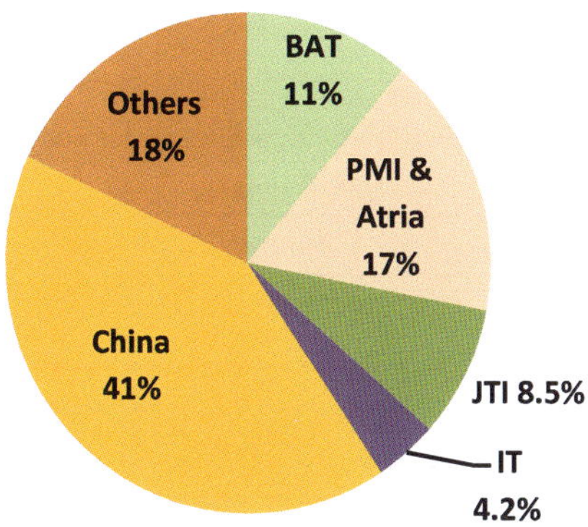

Figure 9. Market concentration and global market share 2012

Notes: BAT: British American Tobacco, PMI & Atria: Philipp Morris International and Atria, JTI: Japan Tobacco, IT: Imperial Tobacco.

Source: Graph is constructed by authors using Euromonitor data 2014.

- *Global tobacco production and trade*

Between 1980 and 2012, global tobacco leaf production increased by 73% from 6.2 million tons to 10.7 million tons, and the land devoted for tobacco leaf production increased by 11% from 3.9 million hectares to 4.3 million hectares, respectively. Yield per hectare increased as well, especially in the developing countries (FAO database, 2014).

Cigarette production has increased globally by about 12% from 5.3 trillion pieces to 5.9 trillion pieces between 2000 and 2012 (Figure 10). Over the years, as developed countries decreased their production of manufactured and unmanufactured tobacco, developing countries have taken the lead in tobacco production (Table 13).

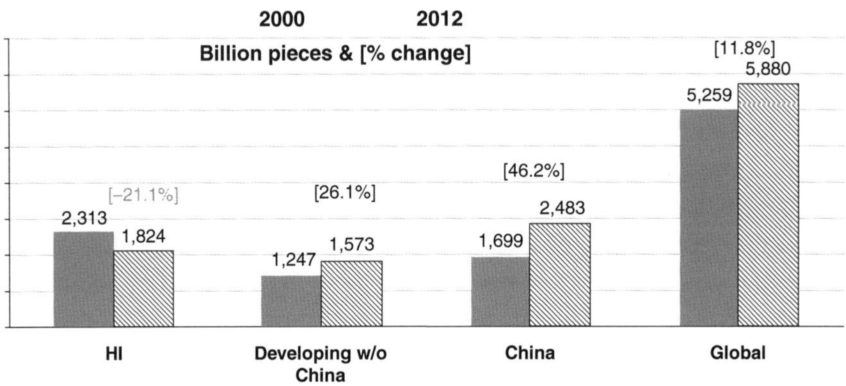

Figure 10. Cigarette Production and percentage change in production level between 2000 and 2012

Notes: Columns represents the production level by billion pieces, % change in production level is given in the brackets.

Source: FAO for unmanufactured tobacco data, Euromonitor for cigarettes, Bangladesh and Pakistan by MoF of respective countries.

Table 13. Unmanufactured tobacco production HI and LMIC (developing)

	(Million tons)			% change	
Unmanufactured tobacco	**1980**	**2000**	**2012**	**1980–2012**	**2000–2012**
Developed (HI Countries)	1.8	1.1	0.7	−64	−39
Developing Countries	4.4	8.2	10.0	130	22
Developing Countries, excluding China	3.5	5.7	6.8	98	21
China	0.9	2.6	3.2	256	25
Global	6.2	9.3	10.7	73	15

Source: FAO for unmanufactured tobacco data, Euromonitor for cigarettes, Bangladesh and Pakistan by MoF of respective countries.

Tobacco Trade: As globalization has proceeded, many countries have established bilateral trade agreements and have become members of regional economic/monetary or customs unions as well as the World Trade Organization. One purpose of trade agreements has been to reduce traditional protectionist policies through reducing or eliminating import duties between members and impose a common external tariff for imports from non-member countries. In consequence, between 2000 and 2012 alone, global tobacco export value increased by 80% and rose from US$21 billion in 2000 to US$38.4 billion in 2012. About 53% of this export value was generated by cigarettes in 2012, followed by unmanufactured tobacco with 29%.

The export value of unmanufactured tobacco more than doubled between 2000 and 2012, and reached US$11.3 billion in 2012 compared with US$5.4 billion in 2000 (Figure 11). Developing countries generated 70% of this export value (See Tables A.1 and A.2).

As developed (HI) countries have reduced their tobacco production, they have also became net importers of tobacco and run into trade deficits on unmanufactured and manufactured (cigarette) trade (Figure 12). In fact, the tobacco trade deficit has widened from US$−0.5 billion in 2000 to US$−6.6 billion in 2012. Developing countries, on the other hand, have turned their trade deficit from US$−4.09 billion in 2000 to a positive trade balance of US$3.22 billion in 2012 (Details by income group in Tables A.1 and A.2).

In 2012, there are only three countries around the globe with a significantly high positive trade balance, Brazil (one of the major tobacco leaf producers), the Netherlands and Germany, the latter two of which are top cigarette producing

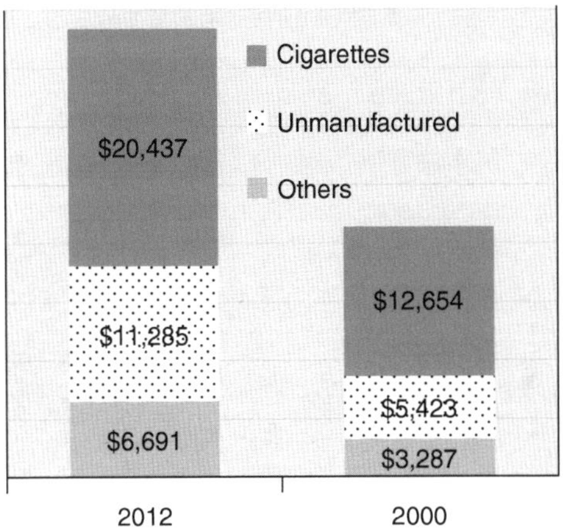

Figure 11. Global tobacco exports in 2000–2012 (Billion US$)

Note: *Unmanufactured tobacco and cigarettes.

Source: Figure constructed by authors' using estimation from UN COMTRADE database 2014.

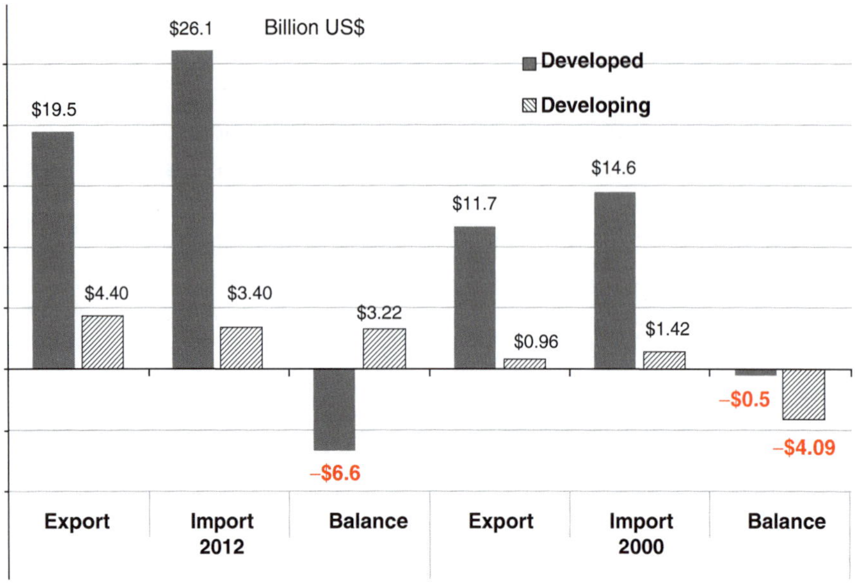

Figure 12. Tobacco *trade value and balance (billion US$) 2000–2012

Note: *Unmanufactured tobacco and cigarettes.
Source: WHO estimation from UN COMTRADE database 2014.

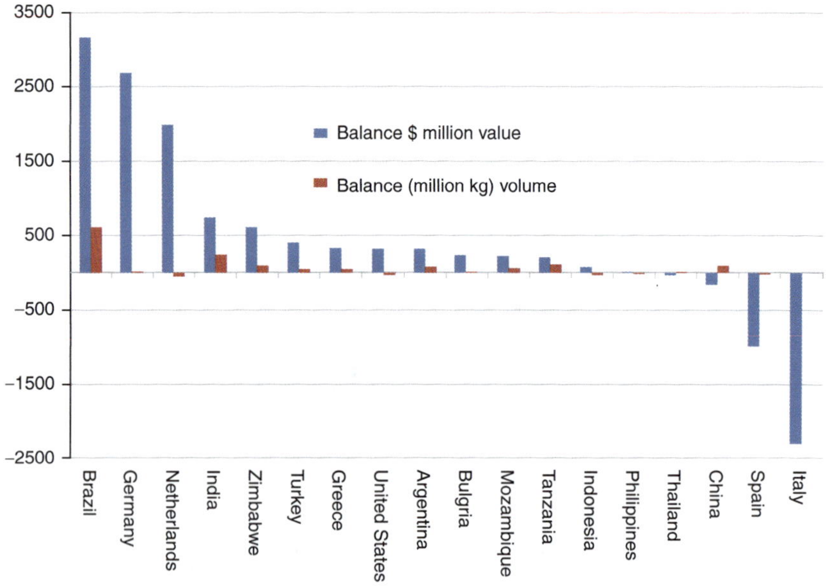

Figure 13. Tobacco (cigarette and tobacco leaf) trade balance in volume and value by highest producers, 2012

Source: UN COMTRADE database 2014.

countries (Figure 13). Interestingly, some top tobacco leaf and/or cigarette-producing countries such as China, Spain, and Italy have trade deficits by value.

Market development and emerging trends

- *Product differentiation and consumers' perception*

Implementation of strong and comprehensive tobacco control measures such as warning people about the dangers of tobacco use[10], banning tobacco advertisement and promotion[11], protecting people from tobacco use, offering help to those who wish to quit smoking, and raising tobacco taxes as discussed in detail later in the chapter, is one of the many factors that has more likely increased mass populations' awareness of the harmful effects of using tobacco products and their smoking behavior (details of Member States' implementation status can be found in WHO 2013a). Global Adult Tobacco Survey (GATS) from most populated countries with high smoking prevalence show that 80% or more of populations are aware that smoking causes serious illness, except China with only 22% believing this (Figure 14) (GATS, 2008–2012).

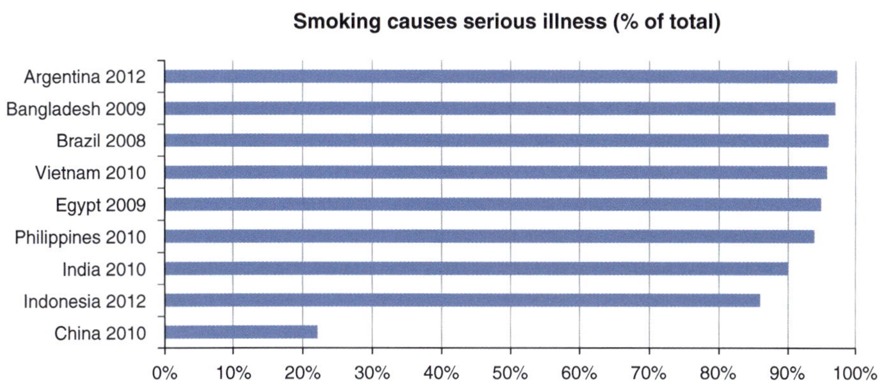

Figure 14. People's awareness about harmful use of tobacco 2009–2012

Source: GATS Country Reports. http://nccd.cdc.gov/gtssdata/Ancillary/DataReports.aspx?CAID=3. Last accessed 8 May, 2014.

---

[10]Not all tobacco users fully understand the risks associated with smoking. Large and clear health warnings describing tobacco-attributable illnesses placed on both sides of tobacco packages have an impact on smokers. Use of graphic images demonstrating the harm of tobacco use are proved to be more effective than worlds alone in convincing users to quit (WHO, 2013a).

[11]A complete total ban applying to all direct and indirect advertising and marketing categories, promotion and sponsorship are found to be effective in substantially reducing tobacco consumption and protecting people especially from industry marketing tactics.

Increasing awareness supported by strong tobacco control measures, especially for cigarettes may explain part of the decrease in global demand for cigarettes (Figure 1) and perhaps the increase in popularity of other tobacco products. For example, the increase in water pipe tobacco's popularity, particularly in the East Mediterranean Region and especially among youth and women, is largely due to the misperception that it is less harmful to health than cigarette smoking (WHO 2006). In addition, in order to retain health-cautious smokers in the market and to attract potential smokers, manufacturers have altered traditional smoking products and deceived smokers by promoting them as less harmful, such as low tar cigarettes or charcoal filtered cigarettes.

Government reactions towards product differentiation vary. By 2012, many governments (101 out of 194) have banned descriptors such as "light, ultra-light and mild" on tobacco products, as they misled consumers as being "safer" alternatives to traditional cigarettes (WHO NCI Ongoing Monograph 19, WHO, 2012). The EU has also banned the sales of menthol and chocolate cigarettes as well as those designed like lipstick.

Some government legislation requires companies to comply with tobacco control policies and also in some cases require companies to alter the content of their products. For example, some governments, such as the UK, Australia, Brazil, China, Malaysia and some Gulf countries (e.g., Saudi Arabia, UAE) require companies to reduce the tar and nicotine levels of cigarettes, or to use charcoal filters instead (Ongoing WHO NCI Monograph No. 19). However, evidence shows that although charcoal added cellulose acetate filters can reduce selected vapor phase of smoke constituents (e.g., aldehydes and benzene), they have little impact on the other potentially hazardous particulate phase constitutes such as tar and nicotine levels inhaled (WHO NCI Ongoing Monograph 19, Sarkar *et al.*, 2008). Despite these facts, smokers may still perceive charcoal filter cigarettes as a safer alternative, especially in developing countries (Table 14). Although charcoal filtered cigarettes represented only 8% of the global cigarette market in 2012[12], in some countries, their market share has increased to quite high levels, such as 97% in Venezuela, 93% in South Korea, 70% in Japan and 42% in Turkey. Our analysis shows a positive and significant relationship between the percentage change in total cigarette sales and the percentage change in the market share of charcoal filter cigarettes. This indicates that the higher the increases in total cigarettes sales, the higher the percentage change in the market share of charcoal filtered cigarettes (Figure 15).

Similarly, the market share of low and ultra-low tar cigarettes increased by 1% globally, from 20% to 21% of total sales between 2007 and 2012. In China, where

[12] Data exist only for 77 countries.

Table 14. Charcoal filter cigarette sales 2007–2012 (billion pieces) and percentage change by income group

Income Groups	2007	2012	% change
HI	1.4	1.2	−18
UMI	3.2	3.5	11
LMI	0.8	0.8	2
LI	0.05	0.06	25
Total	5.4	5.5	2

Notes: HI = 34, UMI = 28, LMI = 15 and LI = 1 countries.
Source: Euromonitor 2014.

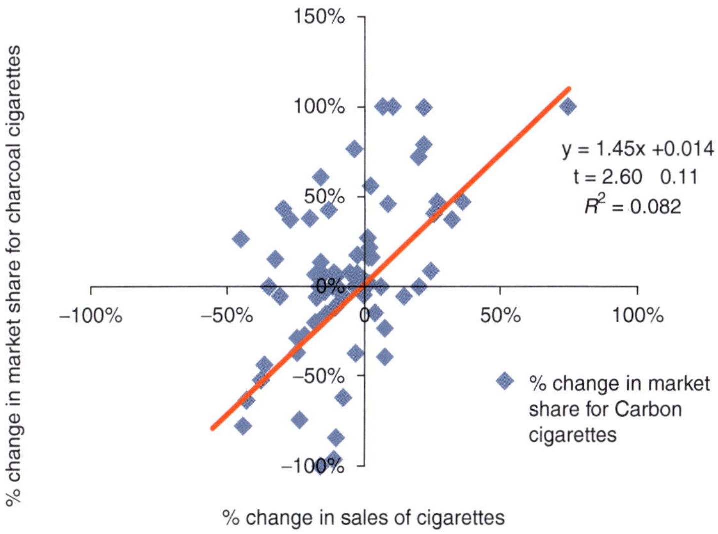

Figure 15. Relationship between percentage changing total cigarette and charcoal filter cigarette sales
Source: Graphs are constructed by WHO by using Euromonitor data 2014.

high-tar cigarettes dominated the market with a 95 % market share, mid- and-low-tar cigarette sales increased by 257% and 658% during the period between 2007 and 2012, presumably due to anincreasing number of female smokers who prefer lower tar content (Figure 16).

At the global level, we also find a statistically significant and positive relationship between the female prevalence rate and the market share of low tar cigarettes, based on 2012 data from 78 countries (Figure 17).

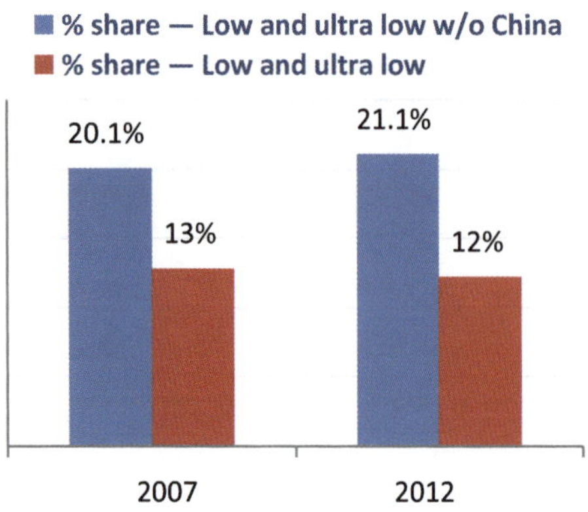

Figure 16. Share of low and ultra-low tar cigarette market in 2007–2012

Source: Graphs are constructed by authors by using Euromonitor Data 2014 and WHO 2013 Report on Global Tobacco Epidemic.

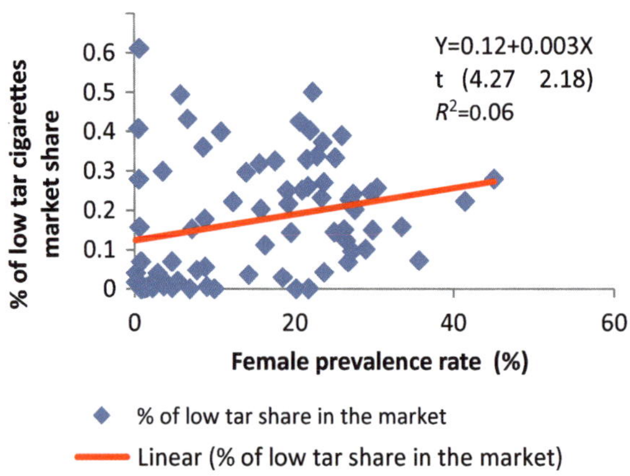

Figure 17. Low tar cigarettes and female prevalence of smoking in 2012

Source: Graphs are constructed by authors by using Euromonitor Data 2014 and WHO 2013 Report on Global Tobacco Epidemic.

Health and Economic Consequences of Smoking and Tobacco Control

The health impact of tobacco use

Smoking is a major cause of premature death and morbidity (Table 15). Epidemiological studies over the past 50 years have shown that tobacco kills one-third to one-half of all people who use it (Peto *et al.*, 2003; Doll *et al.*, 2004). Smoking is responsible for up to 90% of lung cancers and is a significant risk

Table 15. Smoking-attributable deaths by WHO region in 2004

	Smoking-attributable deaths (000s, aged >30 years)			Percent of adult deaths (% of all adult deaths)		
	Males	**Females**	**Total**	**Males**	**Females**	**Total**
Africa	124	21	145	5	1	3
Americas	473	385	858	17	15	16
Eastern Med.	169	18	186	12	2	7
Europe	1,143	328	1,472	25	7	16
South-East Asia	815	222	1,037	14	5	10
Western Pacific	850	555	1,405	14	11	13
World	3,574	1,529	5,103	16	7	12

Source: WHO Global Report: Mortality Attributable to Tobacco (2012).

factor for other non-communicable disease (NCDs) such as strokes and heart attacks as well as tuberculosis and other respiratory infections (WHO, 2002; 2012b). Smokeless tobacco causes cancer of the head and neck, esophagus and pancreas, as well as many oral diseases (Boffetta *et al.*, 2005). Furthermore, users are not the only ones affected by tobacco use as second-hand smoke indirectly causes death and disease among non-smokers.

The WHO estimates that about 5 million adults globally die each year from tobacco use (WHO, 2012b). A further 600,000 people worldwide are estimated to die each year from second-hand smoke (Öberg *et al.*, 2011). The greatest number of smoking-attributable deaths occurs in the European Region followed by the Western Pacific Region which includes China (Table 15). Smoking is responsible for 16% of deaths among adult males and 7% of deaths among adult females. Its pattern of mortality generally reflects underlying prevalence rates of smoking with Europe and the Americas showing the highest proportion of adult deaths from smoking-related diseases.

Overall, tobacco use is responsible for approximately 12% of all adult deaths globally. The proportion of adult deaths caused by tobacco tends to be highest in developed countries compared to developing countries reflecting higher prevalence rates of smoking and greater intensity of use in these countries generally, as well as relatively high mortality rates from communicable diseases in many developing countries (Figure 18). This pattern in which rates of smoking and smoking-attributable deaths tend to increase with the level of development also highlights the potential risk profile for many low- and middle-income countries. This risk profile is especially the case if smoking is taken up by young women in these countries as their economies develop and liberalize.

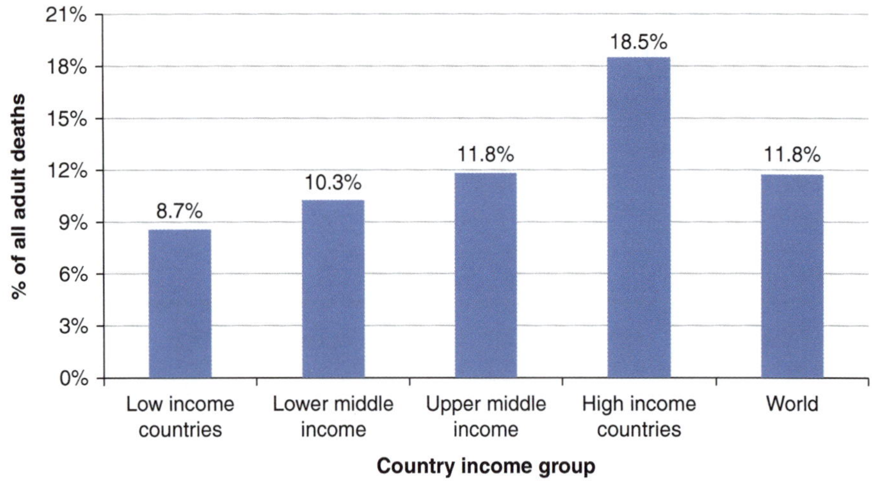

Figure 18. Smoking-attributable deaths as a % share of all adult deaths in 2004

Source: Authors calculations from WHO Global Report: Mortality Attributable to tobacco 2012 and World Bank Income Classification in 2012.

As the risks of smoking are usually associated with prolonged use or exposure, it is often mistakenly believed that smoking-attributable diseases afflict only the elderly. In fact, smoking is responsible for 10% of male deaths in the 30–44 age cohort and close to 20% of male deaths in the 45–59 age cohort globally. Overall, almost 30% of all deaths from smoking occur in men and women under the age of 60 years, and on average smokers fatally afflicted by smoking-related diseases lose 15 years of normal life expectancy (WHO, 2012b; World Bank, 1999). This highlights that smoking has a significant detrimental impact not just on the elderly but also on the middle-aged and economically active populations of society.

- *Expected tobacco-attributable deaths*

The impact of tobacco use on the health status of populations can be assessed in different ways. Aside from retrospective studies, forward-looking analyses quantify the expected impact of tobacco use on health outcomes in the future. As part of World No Tobacco Day 2014, WHO developed a model of the global cigarette market in order to demonstrate the potential for tobacco taxation to generate extra revenue while also improving public health. In this study, the potential public health impact of tobacco use was measured in terms of the expected number of smoking-attributable deaths amongst the current population alive in 2012. This single cohort approach has been used extensively in studies to quantify the potential impact of tobacco and tobacco taxation both globally (World Bank, 1999; Levy *et al.*, 2013) as well as nationally (e.g., Ross *et al.*, 2008; John *et al.*, 2010;

Table 16. Expected number of smoking-attributable deaths by WHO region

	2012 Population (millions)		Smoking prevalence	Smokers (millions)			Smoking attributable-deaths (millions)		
	Adults	Youth	(% adults)	Current	Future	Total	Current	Future	Total
Africa	467	344	8	34	24	58	12	8	20
Americas	674	212	20	136	42	178	45	14	59
Eastern Med.	379	180	15	43	22	65	15	7	22
Europe	734	153	31	227	46	273	76	15	91
South-East Asia	1,283	524	14	173	70	243	58	24	82
Western Pacific	1,486	351	26	382	90	472	127	30	157
World	**5,022**	**1,765**	**20**	**996**	**294**	**1,290**	**332**	**98**	**430**

Source: Authors' Calculation (WHO, 2014b).

Waters *et al.*, 2010). A limitation of this approach though, is that it does not incorporate dynamic aspects of changes in demographics and smoking rates.

WHO crude age-adjusted rates of current adult cigarette smoking by gender were used to calculate the number of current smokers globally. This gave a total of close to 1 billion current adult smokers in 2012. Epidemiological studies over the past 50 years have shown that tobacco kills one-third to one-half of all people who use it (Peto *et al.*, 2006; Doll *et al.*, 2004). Taking a low-range mortality rate of 33%, this suggests that 332 million adult smokers alive in 2012 will die early from smoking-attributable diseases (Table 16).

In addition, if today's youth population (aged 15 years and under) take up smoking at a similar rate as their parents when they themselves become adults, there will be some 294 million future smokers from among the population in 2012. Around 98 million of these future smokers (33% of 294 million) would also be at risk of dying from smoking-attributable diseases, bringing the potential death toll from smoking among the current population in 2012 to around 430 million.

Economic consequences of smoking by development perspective

Government policymakers and health professionals would like to know the importance of smoking beyond the epidemiological focus of morbidity and mortality. The economic costs of smoking consist of two components: Direct costs and indirect costs. Direct costs include all health care expenditures for treating smoking-related illnesses, such as outpatient visits, inpatient hospitalization, and self-medication. Indirect costs represent losses for which there is no monetary exchange in the market place, but nonetheless involves a loss of productivity caused by smoking-related illnesses, including disability, absence from work and premature death. It also includes the value of time spent by caregivers and their foregone productivity.

The economic impact of smoking has been studied most extensively in the US and other high-income countries. These studies tend to find that smoking-attributable diseases account for 6–15% of national health expenditures (World Bank, 1999). A recent study of 27 European Union (EU) Member States found that smoking-attributable diseases accounted for an average of 6% of public health expenditures in the EU ranging from 3.6% in Cyprus to 11.9% in Hungary (GHK, 2009). Within these 27 countries, the share of public health expenditure accounted for by smoking-attributable diseases was closely correlated with the death rate from smoking (Figure 19).

The impact of smoking on health spending in low- and middle-income countries has been less commonly documented. Available evidence suggests that smoking accounts for a lower share of health expenditures in these countries, possibly because the tobacco epidemic is at an earlier stage of development or due to more limited access to medical care in these countries (Ross *et al.*, 2007). During the early 2000s, a number of studies in Asia bear this out with smoking accounting for 3 to 5% of health expenditures in China, India and Vietnam (Sung *et al.*, 2006; John, 2008a; Ross *et al.*, 2007). Bangladesh records the highest share among these studies at around 7% of health spending (WHO, 2005).

The full economic cost of smoking also includes the loss in productivity associated with early death and disability from smoking-attributable diseases. Smoking-related disability has a subtle effect on productivity, with studies confirming that

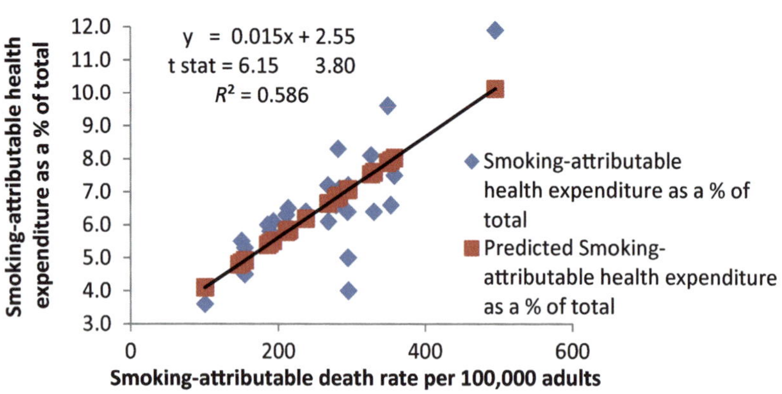

Figure 19. Smoking-attributable death rate per 100,000 adults and smoking-attributable health expenditure as % of total, European Countries, 2009

Sources: GHK (2009); WHO (2012b).

smokers have excess rates of workplace absenteeism over non-smokers (Berman *et al.*, 2013). Furthermore, absenteeism due to smoking is not evenly distributed. For example, the average EU smoker suffering from cancer, COPD or cardiovascular disease loses 92, 122 and 136 workforce days to ill health, respectively (Suhrcke *et al.*, 2008). Such high rates of absenteeism surely impact the earnings potential of those suffering from such chronic diseases, while other smokers facing prolonged illnesses may need to withdraw from the labor force altogether.

A review article by Lightwood *et al.* (2000) assessed the full economic cost of smoking including the productivity losses from smoking-attributable mortality. They concluded that the total economic costs of smoking represent a significant loss for the wider economy, reaching 2.1–3.4% of GDP in Australia, 1.3–2.2% of GDP in Canada, and 1.4–1.6% of GDP in the US. Similarly, a more recent study of 27 Member States of the EU found that the total cost of smoking-attributable diseases amounts to about 3.4% of the EU's GDP (GHK, 2009).

In addition to the negative effect of smoking on health and productivity, smoking also has an impoverishing impact on many families both by diverting household income to tobacco use and by leading to household expenditures on medical care associated with the treatment of tobacco-attributable diseases. The impact of smoking on poverty was estimated in a study that used the 1998 China National Health Services Survey. The results indicated that the excess medical spending attributable to smoking in 1998 have caused the poverty rate to increase by 1.5% for the urban population and by 0.7% for the rural population (Liu *et al.*, 2006).

In 2009, Eriksen *et al.* (2012) estimated the direct private and public medical costs of treating tobacco-attributable diseases for select countries based on available data. The cost is determined by the number of people being treated and the costs of treatments for these tobacco-attributable diseases. The results reveal that many countries, including both developed and developing ones, already face high costs[13] (Figure 20). For example, the share of tobacco-attributable diseases in total health care expenditures varies from 2% in China, Canada and Germany to 3.5% in the USA, 6% in France, 9% in Mexico and Malaysia, and 10% in the Philippines.

The full economic cost of tobacco use in low- and middle-incomes countries has rarely been fully documented. However, studies within countries confirm that the economic effect of tobacco use on the poor is greater than that for higher-income groups. Taking education as a proxy for income, data from countries around the world suggest that poor people consume more tobacco products than those in higher income groups. In the UK, the least educated group of people smoke three times more than the highest-educated group, and this difference is up

[13] Indirect costs such as losses in labor productivity, cigarette butt littering, fire damage, environmental harm from destructive farming practices, and the intangible suffering of the victims and their families are not included.

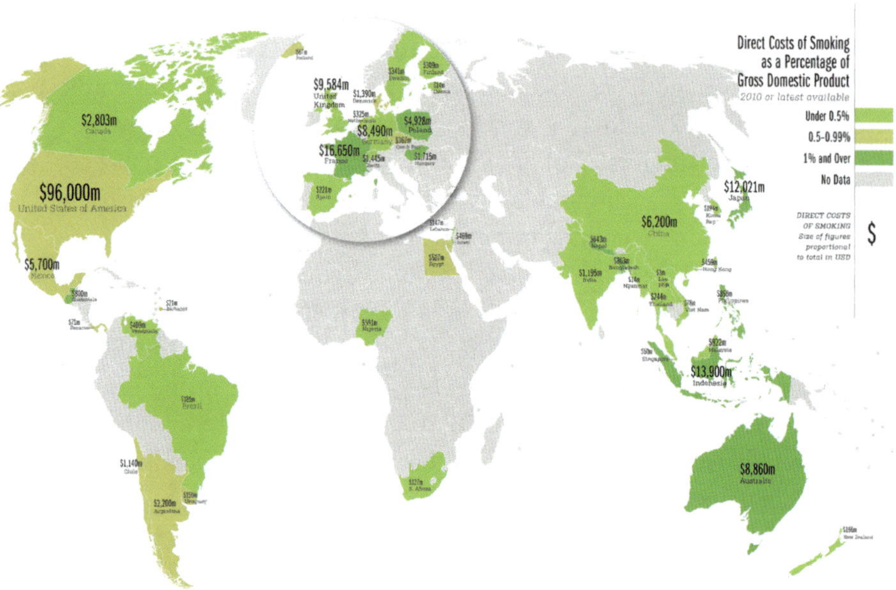

Figure 20. Direct costs of smoking as a percentage of gross domestic product
Source: Eriksen *et al.* (2012).

to seven times more in some developing countries. The risk of death from tobacco use is also related to income (World Bank, 1999). One study in Canada found the risk of death from smoking to be 5% for high-income earners, rising to 15% for the poorest population group.

Tobacco control, health and development

- *Tobacco control*

Since 2005, the global landscape on tobacco control has been changing, and the WHO Framework Convention for Tobacco Control (FCTC) has become the first international treaty on tobacco control that includes very comprehensive tobacco control measures for governments to adopt. By January 2014, 177 countries made commitments to implement these measures by ratifying the Convention treaty. In 2008, a package of six evidence-based tobacco-use prevention and control measures that have been proven to reduce tobacco use and improve public health outcomes were put together in WHO MPOWER package. MPOWER stands for (1) Monitor tobacco use and prevention policies, (2) Protect people from tobacco smoke, (3) Offer help to quit tobacco use, (4) Warn about the dangers of tobacco, (5) Enforce bans on tobacco advertising, promotion and sponsorship, and (6) Raise taxes on tobacco.

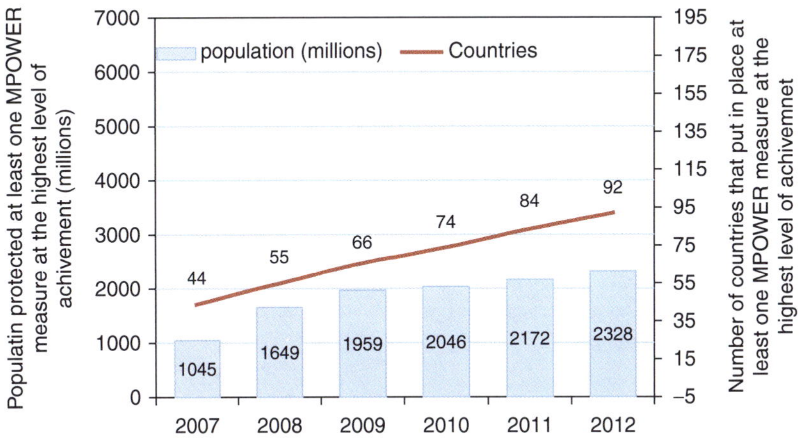

Figure 21. Five years of progress in select tobacco control measures 2007–2012

Notes: 2009 and 2011 data include some estimation where the year of complete O and R policies was not known. Data on Monitoring of tobacco use and Mass media campaigns are not included.
Source: WHO 2013 Report on Global Tobacco Epidemic.

In 2007, about 1 billion people in 44 countries implemented at least one of the MPOWER measures which has reached to more than 2.3 billion people living in 92 countries in 2012 (WHO, 2013a) (Figure 21). WHO reports that almost all progress made in implementing MPOWER measures during 2007 and 2012 have been achieved in low- and middle-income countries. This is an important development as the tobacco epidemic has already shifted to LMICs (WHO 2013).

Between 2007 and 2012, 32 countries (including 26 LMICs) adopted complete smoking bans[14], resulting in 1.1 billion people or 16% of world's population, being protected from the dangers of second-hand smoke. Similarly, in the past 5 years, the number of people are exposed to strong, graphic health warning labels on

[14]Countries are assessed into four groupings based on the following health warnings' information about the characteristics of cigarette pack warnings. These groupings include countries that have: (1) No warning or small warnings (average of front and back of package is less than 30%), (2) medium size warnings (average of front and back of package is between 30% and 49%) missing some (one or more) appropriate characteristics OR large warnings (average of front and back of the package is at least 50%) missing one or more appropriate characteristics, (3) medium size warnings with all appropriate characteristics OR large warnings missing one or more appropriate characteristics, (4) large warnings with all appropriate characteristics. Appropriate characteristics include the following criteria: (i) Specific health warnings mandated, (ii) appearing on individual packages as well as on any outside packaging and labelling used in retail sale, (iii) describing specific harmful effects of tobacco use on health, (iv) are large clear, visible and legible (e.g., specific colors and front style and sizes are mandated), (v) rotate, (vi) include pictures or pictograms; written in (all) the principal language(s) of the country (WHO GTCR 2013 Technical Note 1).

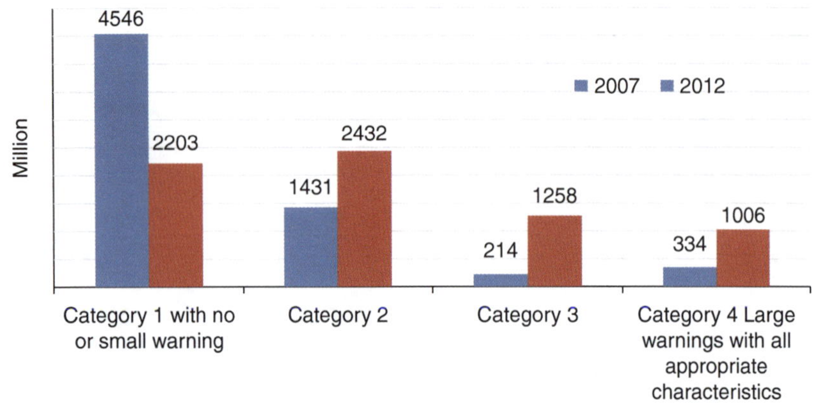

Figure 22a. Warning people of the dangers of smoking: Number of people who are exposed to the strength of health warnings on cigarette packs in 2007 and 2012

Notes: Total 194 countries data are compiled. Total global population is estimated as 6,525 million in 2007 and 6,900 million in 2007. In 2007, group 1 has 115 countries, and among those countries 72 stay in the same group in 2012 while 20, 14 and 9 countries move to groups 2, 3 and 4, respectively. In 2007, group 2 has 62 countries. As 37 countries stay in the same group, 17 and 8 countries move to groups 3 and 4, respectively. There are only 7 countries in group 3 in 2007, and 3 countries move to group 4, the rest stay in the same group in 2012. Number of countries in group 4 has increased from 10 in 2007 to 30 in 2012.
Source: Authors' estimation by WHO 2013 Report on Global Tobacco Epidemic.

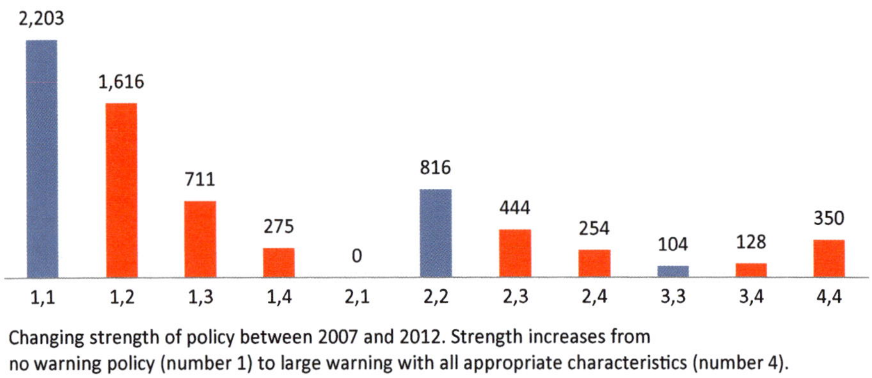

Figure 22b. Global population covered by the changing strengths of cigarette pack health warnings 2007–2012

Notes: People (million) who are covered by the strength of health warnings on cigarette packages: From no warning or small warning (1) To large warning with all appropriate characteristics (4) between 2007 and 2012.
Source: Authors' estimation by WHO 2013 Report on Global Tobacco Epidemic.

cigarette packs has nearly tripled from 356 million people in 10 countries in 2007 to more than 1 billion people in 30 countries in 2012 (Figure 22a).

An increasing number of countries improved the information on characteristics of health warnings on cigarette packs during these 5 years with total 3.4 billion people seeing the characteristics of cigarette pack health warnings improve between 2007 and 2012 (Figure 22b).

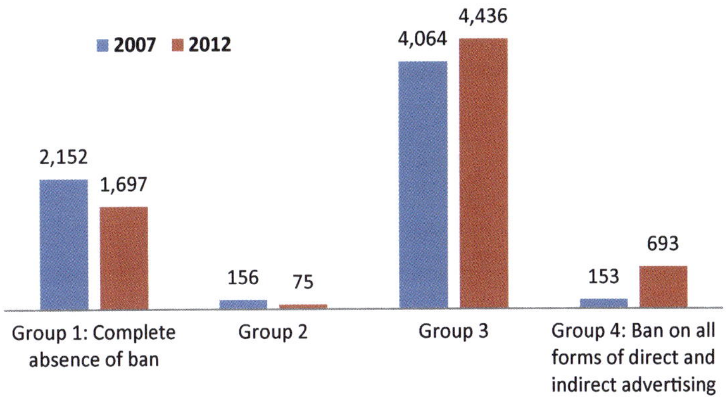

Figure 23a. Ban on tobacco advertising, promotion and sponsorship policies 2007–2012

Notes: People (Million) covered by the strength of banning tobacco advertising, promotion and sponsorship policy-from no ban policy (1) to complete ban policy (4) between 2007 and 2012.
Source: Authors' estimation by WHO 2008 and 2013 Reports on Global Tobacco Epidemic.

Finally, by 2012, 694 million people in 24 countries were protected by complete ban on all forms of direct and indirect tobacco advertising, promotion and sponsorship policy[15], compared to 170 million people in 8 countries in 2007 (Figure 23a).

Progress has been made by many countries (meaning countries moved from their existing grouping to higher grouping number (1, 2, 3 to 2, 3, 4, respectively), to the extent that about 1.23 billion people see improved policy and stayed in the best policy (group 4) between 2007 and 2012. By 2012, 71% of total population — 5.1 billion out of 7.0 billion — live in countries with better (group 3) or best (group 4) policies on banning tobacco advertising, promotion and sponsorship (Figure 23b).

[15]Countries are assessed into four groupings based on the following bans on advertising, promotion, and sponsorship indicators. (1) Complete absence of ban, or ban that does not cover national television (TV), radio and print media, (2) ban on national TV, radio and print media only, (3) ban on national TV, radio and print media as well as on some (but not all) other forms of direct and/or indirect advertisement, (4) ban on all forms of direct and indirect advertising. Direct advertising bans include: (i) national TV and radio, (ii) local magazines and newspapers, (iii) billboards and outdoor advertising, and (iv) point of sale. Indirect advertising bans include: (i) free distribution of tobacco products in the mail or through other means; (ii) promotional discounts; (iii) non-tobacco products identified with tobacco brand names (brand stretching), (iv) brand names of non-tobacco products used for tobacco products (brand sharing), (v) appearance and tobacco brands or products in TV and/or films (product placement) OR, appearance of tobacco products in TV and/or films, (vi) sponsored events, including corporate social responsibility programs (see Corporate social Responsibility Activities in GTCR 2013, Appendix VI).

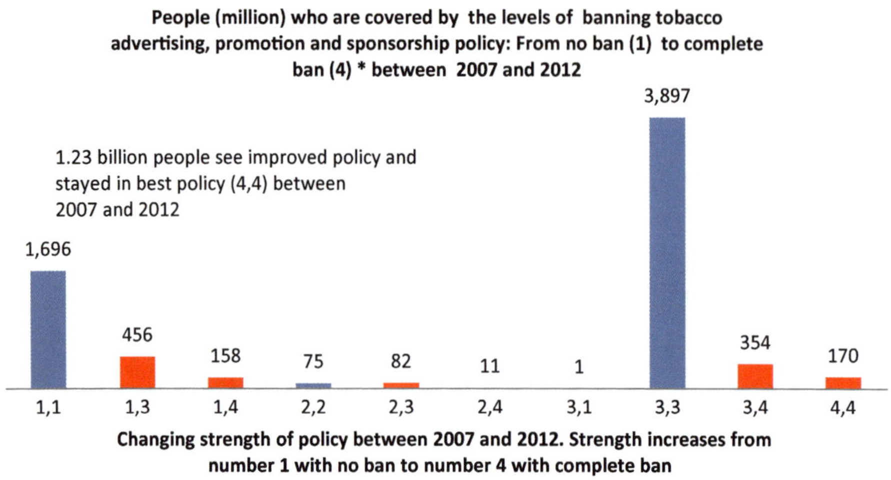

Figure 23b. Achievements in banning tobacco advertising, promotion and sponsorship policies 2007–2012

Notes: Total number of countries are 193. In group 1, there are 96 countries in 2007. In 2012, 65 countries stay in group 1, 25 countries move to group 3 and 7 countries to group 4. In 2007, there are 3 countries in group 2 and by 2012 only 1 country stays in group 2 while other two countries move to group 3 and 4. In 2007, there are 86 countries in group 3 and the number increased to 103 countries in 2012. In this group, as 77 countries kept their status in group 3, 8 countries move from group 3 to group 4 between 2007 and 2012. Only one country fell from group 3 to group 1 during that period. Finally, the number of countries in group 4 increased from 8 to 24 between 2007 and 2012, respectively. Eight countries kept their status in group 4.
Source: Authors' estimation by WHO 2008 and 2013 Reports on Global Tobacco Epidemic.

- *Health and economic impacts of tobacco control*

Models that assess the prospective impact of tobacco control measures on global cigarette demand date back to the 1980s (Levy *et al.* 2006; Hanewinkel and Isensee, 2010a, b). Ranson *et al.* (2000) completed one of the earliest studies of tobacco control at the global level and found that non-price measures together (warning labels, bans on smoking in public places, etc.) would cause 23 million smokers to quit and prevent some 5 million smoking-attributable deaths. They also found that a 10% increase in the real or inflation-adjusted price of cigarettes worldwide would cause 42 million smokers to quit and prevent 10 million smoking-attributable diseases.

Prospective models tend to conclude that the introduction of non-price interventions will reduce smoking prevalence by around 15% in the short term. For example, based on country-level evidence Asaria *et al.* (2007) assumed that smoke-free policies, health warnings, media campaigns against smoking and bans on cigarette advertising would reduce smoking prevalence by 4%, 2%, 7% and 2% respectively. Similarly, the SimSmoke Model of tobacco control measures adopts parameters based on expert panels and published literature

Table 17. Global impact of fully implemented MPOWER policies in period from 2007 to 2010

Policy	Smokers in countries meeting policies (000s)	Reduction of smokers due to policy (000s)	Reduction in deaths from smoking (000s)
Protect air	84,445	5,033	2,516
Cessation treatments	29,847	759	380
Warnings on packages	100,633	1,380	690
Enforced marketing bans	9,334	613	306
Raise taxes	62,416	7,056	3,528
Total	286,675	14,840	7,420

Source: Levy *et al.* (2013).

reviews (Levy *et al.*, 2013) to conclude that smoke-free policies, health warnings, and bans on advertising would reduce prevalence by around 6%, 1% and 5% respectively. In addition, cessation services could further reduce prevalence by 1–3%.

A recent study assessed the impact of WHO's recommended set of MPOWER policies over the first three years of implementation from 2007 to 2010 (Levy *et al.*, 2013). The authors restricted their analysis to countries that had fully implemented at least one MPOWER measure between 2007 and 2010, and found that these actions will result in 14.8 million fewer smokers compared to the 2007 baseline and prevent 7.4 million smoking-attributable deaths (Table 17). The authors concluded that tobacco control measures have enormous potential to reduce deaths and disease from smoking, but cautioned that those measures with the greatest impact (i.e., smoke-free air laws and taxation) remain alarmingly under-adopted in many countries.

Tax, Price and Demand for Tobacco Products

Theoretical framework

Classical models of demand assume that consumers are fully rational and sovereign in their decision-making. Within this framework, tobacco is considered to be a good just like any other and a chosen behavior is *a priori* assumed to be optimal because a person has rationally chosen it. However, if a product is addictive, the assumption of consumer sovereignty no longer applies. The addictiveness of the product 'forces' a consumer to buy a good that they might not otherwise have been bought. Economic models of addiction can be divided into three basic groups: Models of myopic addictive behavior, models of rational addictive behavior and models of imperfectly rational addictive behavior (Chaloupka and Warner, 2000).

Addictive behavior was initially modelled through myopic demand models in which only previous consumption and price levels influence current consumption. A myopically addicted person does not consider the future in determining current consumption. As such, the future is discounted at an infinitely high rate. This approach can be traced back to the irreversible demand models of the late 1940s. Houthakker and Taylor (1966) pioneered empirical applications of the model during the 1960s by formally modelling demand as a function of a 'stock of habits' representing the depreciated sum of all past consumption.

The forward-looking rational addiction models emerged during the late 1980s. Under this framework, a rationally addicted person's current consumption is determined not only by past consumption and past prices, but also by future prices. For example, if an addicted consumer predicts that the price of the addictive product will increase in the future, that knowledge will cause his/her current consumption of the product to decrease. Importantly, the full price of the product includes not only the monetary price of the product but also the negative health effects associated with consumption.

Empirical applications of the rational addiction model have largely been underpinned by the theoretical framework formally introduced by Becker and Murphy (1988). The essence of the rational addiction model is that people with stable preferences may rationally decide to engage in an addictive behavior since this maximizes their lifetime utility.

Chaloupka (1991) used data from the Second National Health and Nutrition Examination Survey conducted in the late 1970s in one of the earliest empirical applications of the rational addiction model. He found consistent evidence that cigarette smoking was an addictive behavior and that smokers did not behave myopically.

However, the rational addiction framework has been severely criticized, particularly with respect to the assumption of perfect foresight. Akerlof (1991) noted that individuals who become addicted in the rational addiction model do not regret their past decisions, since they are assumed to be fully aware of the consequences of their consumption. Yet this assumption is unrealistic. For example, surveys often show that adult smokers want to quit and regret having taken up smoking (Fong *et al.*, 2004; Chol *et al.*, 2011; Licht *et al.*, 2011).

Orphanides and Zervos (1995) addressed this issue by introducing uncertainty into their model of addiction, by assuming inexperienced users are not fully aware of the potential harm associated with consuming an addictive substance. Instead, an individual's knowledge comes from the observed effects of the addictive good on others as well as through personal experimentation. Interestingly, this extension of the theoretical framework helps to explain youth experimentation and the importance of peer influences.

Gruber and Kozsegi (2004) made a significant contribution by arguing that consumer preferences may not be stable over time. Preferences are time-inconsistent if a person when asked on different occasions displays different relative preferences. This raises the possibility of 'hyperbolic discounting' in which people make relatively far-sighted decisions taking into account all costs and benefits, but take relatively short-sighted action based on some immediate costs or benefits. This framework is supported by results from laboratory and psychological research, which suggest that consumers can be time-inconsistent and exhibit self-control problems. In short, many smokers may want to quit, but the immediate gratification from nicotine dominates the desire to quit.

Income and demand for tobacco — upward shifting for quality

Econometric studies show that there is a positive relationship between a country's income and its demand for cigarettes, which will be discussed in more detail in Section "Tobacco taxes".

As income increases, the demand for tobacco products increases. Based on the United Nations Conference on Trade and Development (UNCTAD) database, real GDP per capita increased in all income groups of countries between 2000 and 2012, where the highest percentage increase was observed in the middle-income groups — real GDP per capita increased by 43% in lower middle income countries and by 41% in upper-middle income countries (UMICs) followed by 31% in low-income countries (LICs), and 12% in high-income countries (HICs). Contrary to the expectation that higher income will bring in higher consumption of tobacco products with income growth, per capita cigarette consumption has decreased at a global level. In effect, the impact of income growth has been reflected in growing demand for higher price brands. This trend has been observed especially in middle-income countries, where between 2007 and 2012, the market shares of mid-price and premium cigarettes have increased and the market share of economy brands decreased (Figure 24a and b).

Our analysis that examines the relationship between income and demand for premium cigarettes by using data from 78 countries between 2007 and 2012 shows a positive and significant relationship between the level of per capita income and the relative demand for premium cigarette brands (Figure 25).

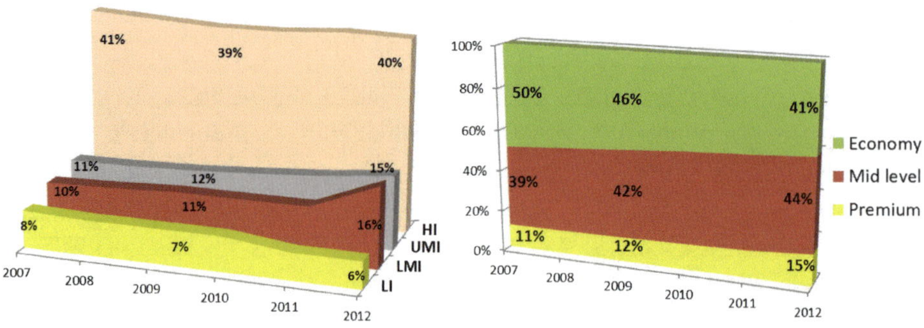

(a) Premium brand market share by income group countries

(b) Market share of price band in middle-income group of countries 2007–2012

Figure 24. Changing market share of cigarette price band (economy, mid-priced and premium brands) by income group 2007–2012

Source: Graphs are constructed by authors' estimtation by using Euromonitor data 2014 and IMF World Economic Outlook database 2014.

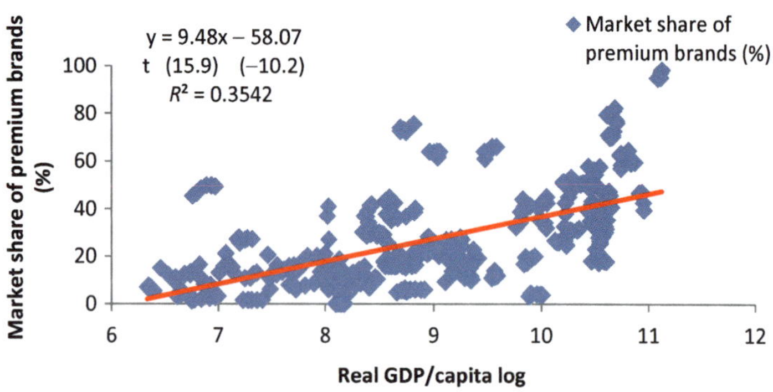

Figure 25. Country income and demand for premium brand cigarettes 2007–2012

Source: Author's estimation by using Euromonitor data on market share of premium cigarette brands and, IMF World Economic Outlook 2014 database for real GDP/capita.

Price and demand for tobacco

Price is an important determinant of the demand for products. Since the classical era of the Marshallian Law of demand, it has been recognized that consumers reduce their demand for products in response to price increases. Tobacco products are no exception to this law. The relationship between price and tobacco consumption is found to be negative in most cases. Moreover, the fact that tobacco is addictive may make its consumption less price sensitive (price elasticity is usually less than one).

When governments raise tobacco excise taxes, it raises costs to producers and/or importers. These producers and/or importers, in general, raise the retail price of tobacco products by the same amount as the tax increase, or sometimes even more than the tax increase, to push some or all of the tax burden onto the consumers and gain more revenue. Therefore, tax and price generally have a positive relationship — the higher the taxes, generally the higher the prices for tobacco products.

However, under rare circumstances, the industry may act differently by adjusting other components of retail prices and absorbing the cost of the tax burden by reducing industry profit, reducing distribution margin or even cutting other costs to keep the retail price the same or even lower. For example, in China in 2011, when the Chinese government raised cigarette taxes, the State Tobacco Monopoly Administration (STMA) maintained the same wholesale prices and retail prices nationwide. The STMA absorbed the increased tax burden itself. The tax increase, therefore, had no impact on cigarette retail prices (Gao *et al.*, 2012).

There are several types of taxes that governments can levy on tobacco products such as import and/or export duties, excise taxes, value added taxes (VAT), general sales taxes (GST), and other special taxes. All of these taxes positively affect the prices of tobacco products and generate revenue for governments. However, there is a basic difference between excise and general types of sales taxes. While excise taxes are meant for specific products to raise their price relative to other products and discourage their consumption, general sales tax or value added tax are applied generally to all products and do not affect the relative price. As such, excise taxes are the most important in achieving the public health objectives of tobacco taxation, given that excise taxes apply uniquely to tobacco products and increase the price of these products relative to other goods and services. Globally, about 90% of countries levy excise taxes on tobacco products.

The excise tobacco tax is a specific consumption tax that are collected at the producers' or importers' level and passed on to consumers. Governments generally levy excise taxes on the producers and/or importers of tobacco products, which raises their costs. Taxes are a significant component of the retail price along with other components including cost of production, industry profit and wholesale and retail distribution margins. The higher the proportion of tax as a component of retail price, the more important these taxes will be in determining the retail price. The generic breakdown of the tax and other components of retail prices for domestic and imported tobacco products are shown in Figure 26. Note that the proportions do not represent the real data from any particular country and may vary from one country to another.

Evolution of empirical studies on tobacco demand

The empirical evidence on the effect of price on tobacco demand has evolved in a number of waves since the 1940s. In a review done by a group of more than

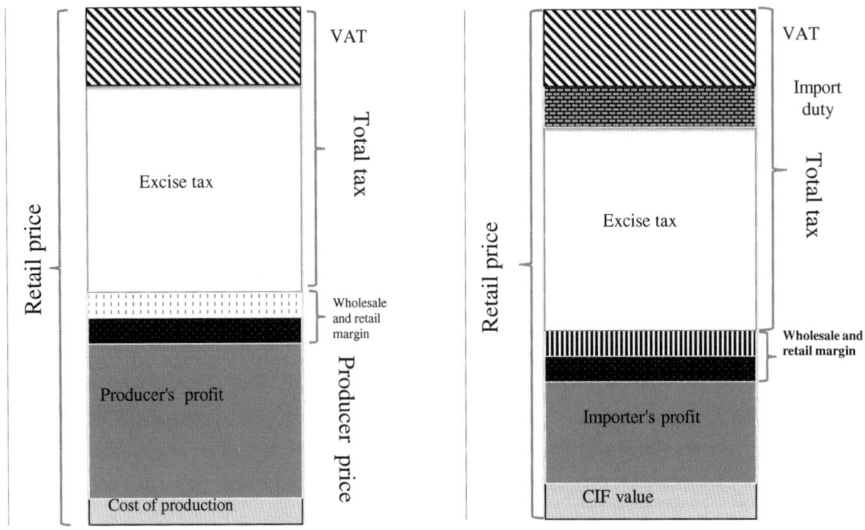

Figure 26. Tax as a component of retail prices for tobacco products
Source: WHO Manual on Tobacco Tax Administration 2010.

20 experts at the International Agency for Research on Cancer IARC (2011), three waves were identified with respect to the evolution of the empirical literature on tobacco demand. In this chapter, we also discuss a fourth wave that came in the aftermath of the WHO Framework Convention on Tobacco Control (FCTC) studying the effectiveness of tobacco control policies in general, and of tobacco taxation in particular, in reducing tobacco demand. These waves are delineated in Box 1 with reference to the timeline and the focus of evidence base.

Box 1. Waves of empirical literature on tobacco demand

Wave 1: 1930s–1960s. During the 1930s through the early 1960s, a few studies investigated demand for cigarettes as a part of the developing literature on the demand for household goods. This was primarily during the era prior to the documentation of the adverse health consequences of smoking in the US Surgeon General Report 1964 (USDHEW, 1964). Hence, public health implications were absent from the analyses in these studies.

Wave 2: 1970–1990. The second wave of empirical research on tobacco demand emerged with the recognition of the public health implications of tobacco use. The focus shifted away from the scholarly estimation of price and income elasticities to policy analytic studies based on the impact of advertising expenditures,

(*Continued*)

Box 1. (***Continued***)

controls on advertising, restrictions on the right to smoke, and health awareness and health warnings, in addition to price and income effects. This trend was set forth by Bass (1969), followed by a number of studies in the 1970s and 1980s. These studies observed that anti-smoking publicity reduced the demand for cigarettes, but found no consensus on the impact of advertising expenditure on the demand for cigarettes.

Wave 3: 1990–2000. The first two waves of empirical work in tobacco demand examined the impacts only in developed countries (e.g., USA, UK, Australia, West Germany, Austria, Greece, New Zealand) and this empirical work continued in the 1990s and 2000s. Studies on developing countries, on the other hand, started to appear in the 1990s beginning with the publication of price elasticity estimates for Papua New Guinea (Chapman and Richardson, 1990). Studies on both developed and developing countries focused on the estimation of the price sensitivity of tobacco consumption. This trend was sparked by the growing concern about the gradual shift in the burden of tobacco use from developed to developing countries in the 21st century.

Wave 4: 2000 onwards. The turn of the 21st century was marked by the consolidation of the tobacco control efforts around the globe into one landmark international treaty known as the Framework Convention on Tobacco Control (FCTC) that came into force in 2003 and was signed and subsequently ratified by the Member States of the World Health Organization. Parties that signed onto this treaty are committed to fight against the tobacco epidemic through the implementation of FCTC measures including tobacco taxation. As countries have made progress with the ratification and implementation of the FCTC, a body of literature has flourished to evaluate the efficiency and effectiveness of tobacco control measures in these countries. Hu and Mao (2002), for example, showed that with estimated price elasticity at −0.54, a 10% increase in cigarette tax per pack would significantly increase central government revenue that would twice exceed total losses in industry revenue, tobacco farmers' income and local tax revenue. Moreover, this tax increase is estimated to save between 1.44 and 2.16 million lives.

In 2009–2010, more than 20 tobacco control experts invited by the International Agency for Research on Cancer (IARC) evaluated the effectiveness of tax and price policies on tobacco demand based on available scientific evidence. The expert group found strong evidence of the effectiveness of increased tobacco excise taxes and price in reducing tobacco consumption and improving public health (Chaloupka *et al.*, 2011; IARC, 2011).

The current wave of literature also dwells on the effectiveness of different tax systems and tax administration in serving both public health and the revenue goals of governments. The underlying principle is that the efficiency and effectiveness of tax systems and tax administration and the market characteristics influence the transmission of tax increases into price increases. Additionally, this literature examines tax evasion and avoidance behavior of both producers and consumers, which in turn determines the effectiveness of tax and price policy to reduce tobacco demand. A simple tax structure has been well recognized as a best practice for tobacco tax policy (WHO, 2010b). In a cross-country study, Chaloupka *et al.* (2014) observed that more complex tax structures give rise to greater variability of price and scope for downward switching (meaning that consumers purchase lower-price products), undermining the quitting behavior normally resulting from tax and price increases. Two other country-level studies have looked at the consequences of complex tax structures for tax avoidance and public health in India (Jha *et al.*, 2011; Joseph and Chaloupka, 2014) and Bangladesh (Nargis *et al.*, 2014b) for example.

A parallel line of research looks at the compensatory behavior of smokers that can potentially undermine the effectiveness of tax and price increases to reduce overall tobacco consumption. These studies investigate the adjustments in the behavior of tobacco users to counteract cost increases due to higher taxes and prices of tobacco products, such as switching to higher nicotine cigarettes (Evans and Farrelly, 1998), substituting cheaper tobacco products (Haewinkel and Isensee, 2007a; 2007b; Ramos, 2009; Young *et al.*, 2006; Laxminarayan and Deolalikar, 2004; Oshfeldt and Boyle, 1994; 1997; Oshfeldt *et al.*, 1998; Thompson and McLeod, 1976; Pekurinen, 1989; 1991), purchasing cigarettes from cheaper or untaxed sources (Guindon *et al.*, 2014; Fix *et al.*, 2014; Yao *et al.*, 2014), cross-border purchasing (Nagelhout *et al.*, 2013; Cornellius *et al.*, 2014; Nargis *et al.*, 2014a; White *et al.*, 2014), or bulk purchases in cartoons (Huang *et al.*, 2014).

Estimation of the impact of price on tobacco demand

The empirical strategy of identifying the impact of price on tobacco demand involves the estimation of a demand equation that specifies quantity consumed or sold as a function of price controlling for income, prices of substitutes and/or complements, and other socio-economic, demographic and environmental factors including tobacco control policy variables.

- *Aggregate level studies*

Beginning in 1945 up to the year 2011, IARC (2011) found 66 cigarette demand studies — half of which are from the US — that used aggregate data from different high-income countries. In contrast, the empirical literature on cigarette demand in LMICs started off in 1990. By 2011, only 31 studies were published for these countries. A few cross-country studies have also been done for 22 OECD countries, 52 European countries and 51 countries including 30 LMICs.

Using either time series or panel data, these studies estimated price elasticity of demand and some studies reported income elasticity of demand as well. The aggregate level time series data reported observations on a particular country or region (e.g., state, province) in specified intervals of time (e.g., month, quarter, year). Panel data consisted of pooled time series data on countries or regions. There was wide variation in the theoretical models and the econometric methods applied to these data.

Prior to the 1990s, some of the aggregate level studies included past consumption level as an explanatory variable to account for habit persistence in the model and were used to differentiate between the short-run and long-run price elasticity of demand. The long-run price elasticity of demand was expected to be larger than the short-run price elasticity, implying that people are allowed more time to adjust their behavior in the long-run. The rational addiction models, on the other hand, focused on future price or consumption as the explanatory variable to allow for future considerations in the decision to smoke.

Since the 1990s, the time-series econometric techniques used in aggregate level studies made a remarkable shift to address the non-stationarity of time-series data that causes spurious correlation between variables from long-run upward or downward trends. These studies have used co-integration or vector autoregression techniques to deal with the non-stationarity problem.

All of these studies provide evidence for a strong negative relationship between aggregate tobacco consumption and price. Their price elasticity estimates clustered between −0.20 and −0.60 for high-income countries and between −0.20 and −0.80 in LMICs. It appears that demand for tobacco products in LMICs is at least as responsive, and often more responsive, to price than it is in high-income countries (Chaloupka *et al.*, 2012).

- *Micro-level studies*

The availability of individual-level or household-level data collected through large-scale national or regional surveys gave way to micro-level studies beginning in the 1980s in the US and other high-income countries, and in the 2000s and onwards for LMICs.

There is a wide variation in the econometric methods applied to these micro-level studies. Most of these studies used the two-part model of demand developed by Cragg (1971) that explains tobacco consumption behavior in two stages — the first, to decide to smoke, and the second, how much to consume once the decision to smoke is made. The first part is estimated by the limited dependent variable techniques (logit or probit) and the second part is estimated by the ordinary least squares (OLS) technique. The price elasticity estimated from the first step — deciding to smoke — is called price elasticity of prevalence and the one estimated from the second step — deciding how much to smoke — is called price elasticity of intensity. The total price elasticity of demand is given by the sum of the price elasticities of prevalence and intensity.

Both the prevalence and the amount of tobacco consumed are negatively influenced by taxes and prices. Estimates from high-income countries show that about half of the overall impact of price increase on tobacco use comes from the reduction in prevalence and the other half from reduction in consumption or intensity by continuing users (IARC, 2011). The estimates from LMICs, however, show considerable variation in the relative impact on prevalence and consumption (IARC, 2011).

The impact of taxes and prices on prevalence reflects the effect of price increases in inducing successful quit attempts and cessation, which seem to play a more important role in reduction in tobacco use in high-income countries where cessation aids are more readily available compared to low- and middle-income countries. However, recent evidence from Global Adult Tobacco Surveys (GATS) in Eastern Europe (Poland, Russia and Ukraine) shows that a 10% increase in cigarette taxes during the post-transitional period of 1990s and 2000s increased the probability of smoking cessation among smokers by 1.6% to 2.3%. Further evidence from the GATS in 14 LMICs shows that higher cigarette prices are associated with higher probability of quit attempts, and higher bidi prices are associated with higher probabilities of both quitting and quit attempts in Southeast Asian countries where bidi use is common (Shang *et al.,* 2014).

Tax and youth smoking: Higher taxes and prices are particularly effective among youth in preventing the initiation of regular smoking behavior among those with occasional or experimental cigarette use. While these findings are globally evident, recent studies using data from the Global Youth Tobacco Surveys (GYTS) have shown that youth in LMICs are more price sensitive than in high-income countries (Nikaj and Chaloupka, 2014; Sweis and Chaloupka, 2013). The effectiveness of higher taxes and prices in deterring tobacco use among youth has been also proven across different tobacco products such as cigarettes, bidis and smokeless tobacco in India (Joseph and Chaloupka, 2014).

Tax and smoking by gender: The evidence on the price sensitivity of tobacco use by gender is mixed. While some studies observe women to be relatively unresponsive to price (Sweis and Chaloupka, 2013) and men to be more likely than women to have quit or tried to quit due to price increase (Shang *et al.*, 2014), other studies observe girls being more price sensitive than boys (Joseph and Chaloupka, 2014). Although smoking prevalence is lower among women than men, the number of female smokers is expected to increase, as mentioned in Section "Prevalence by socioeconomic groups". The issue of price sensitivity among women is therefore important from the perspective of effective tobacco control.

Tax and smoking by socio-economic group: In high-income countries, tobacco use among people of lower socioeconomic status (SES) is found to be more responsive to tax and price changes than tobacco use among people with higher SES. The evidence on the relationship between price sensitivity and SES in LMICs, however, is relatively limited. Studies conducted up to 2010 from LMICs show mixed evidence — while some countries found a negative gradient of price elasticity by SES, others did not find any significant difference in price elasticity across SES groups (IARC, 2011).

Tobacco Taxes

Purpose of taxation of tobacco products — health and economic justification

Taxation of tobacco products can be justified on two grounds. First, tobacco consumption creates a negative externality, a cost on others who choose not to consume the tobacco product. A corrective tax is imposed to internalize this cost that is otherwise not taken into account by the price mechanism (Pigou, 1932). The external cost of tobacco consumption includes not only the direct externalities experienced by non-smokers, such as second-hand smoke, but also the resource costs borne by society, such as the cost of the medical treatment for smoking-related diseases when this cost is publicly funded.

Second, tobacco consumption creates an internality that is harmful to the person who chooses to consume the product. Tobacco consumers act against their own interest because they do not understand fully the cost of their present decision to smoke or do not anticipate correctly the full effects of the addictive nature of the tobacco product they choose to consume. That is, their current action creates an externality to their future self (see, e.g., Gruber, 2003; Viscusi, 1995). The tax is imposed to reflect this cost but also to help consumers change their behavior. It is, however, difficult to measure the externalities and internalities associated with the consumption of tobacco products. The external and internal costs of consuming a particular product may also differ across different groups in society.

According to the economic approach, tobacco products are a good candidate for higher taxation as they are price-inelastic. According to Optimal Tax Theory, and more specifically, according to "the inverse elasticity rule" products with a low price elasticity of demand are an efficient source of revenue. However, with respect to revenue-raising efficiency, the Corlett–Hague Rule suggests that we should tax more heavily goods that complement leisure, rather than substitute for it. Whether cigarette consumption is a complement with leisure or not is not clear *a priori*: Some smokers consume the product in their leisure, while others may use it to cope with work-related stress. There is no sufficient evidence to support one argument or the other (see e.g., Parry, 2003; Crawford *et al.*, 2010).

Types of taxes levied on tobacco products

Tobacco products, as already mentioned in Section "Price and demand for tobacco", are subject to a variety of taxes, the most common types including excise taxes, value-added taxes (VAT) or sales taxes, custom/import duties and other taxes (e.g., statistical/administrative fees, levies for regional blocs, environmental taxes).

Excise taxes: Both domestic and imported products are subject to excise taxes. The World Trade Organization (WTO) recommends that the domestic and imported tobacco products should be treated with an equal excise tax rates. However, it is the sovereign right of every country to determine the excise tax system and tax rates as set out in Article 6.2 of WHO FCTC.

Value added tax (VAT)/sales tax: VAT is a type of consumption tax that is placed on a product whenever value is added at a stage of production and at final sale. It is a "multi-stage" tax that a country may choose to impose *on all consumer goods and services* applied proportionally to the price the consumer pays for a product. Although manufacturers and wholesalers also participate in the administration and payment of the tax along the manufacturing/distribution chain, they are all reimbursed through a tax credit system, so that the only entity who pays in the end is the final consumer. The amount of VAT that the user pays is thus the cost of the product, less any of the costs of materials used in the product that have already been taxed. Some countries, however, impose sales taxes instead. Unlike the VAT, sales taxes are only levied at the point of retail on the total value of goods and services purchased.

As a general tax, the VAT/sales tax leaves the relative price of one product in relation to another unaffected, and as such has great practical appeal for revenue generation. However since VAT is usually applied on all consumed products, increasing this tax for tobacco control purposes is not an effective approach because this will lead to increases in prices across all products, not just tobacco, therefore raising the issue of inflation. Additionally, raising VAT will not raise the relative price of tobacco products and may therefore be effective in making them less affordable compared to other products.

Import duties: In general, import duties are collected by the customs authority of the government from the importing companies at the point of entry into the country. The main objective of such duties is to protect domestic production and raise a country's revenue. Their lower administration cost is especially attractive to countries with limited resources to devote to tax administration, a lack of qualified personnel, and limited accounting sophistication by taxpayers.

Almost all countries levy a tariff on imported cigarettes. However, import duties do not apply under free trade agreements that usually require participating countries to gradually phase them out. For example, Uganda imports most of its locally consumed cigarettes from Kenya without paying any import duty, as Uganda and Kenya are both member states of the East African Community, forming a customs union. If the country is a WTO member, its import duty may be bound, that is, subject to a maximum rate. As import duties are gradually phased out, governments lose the revenues they generated and need to impose or raise other taxes to compensate for the loss.

Most governments levy excise taxes and other taxes on tobacco products and apply duties to imported tobacco products. Based on available data, about 90% of countries impose tobacco excise taxes, almost as many apply a VAT or sales tax to tobacco products, and nearly all impose import duties.

Countries that do not levy tobacco excises include those in the Gulf Cooperation Council, some Pacific Island and Caribbean Island countries, and a few others; in many of these countries, there is little or no domestic tobacco production and governments generate tobacco revenues through duties on imported tobacco products.

VAT rates vary widely, ranging from 2% to 20% in those countries that apply a VAT on tobacco products. Similarly, import duties on tobacco products vary widely, with rates of more than 100% of importers' declared CIF (cost, insurance, freight) value in some countries.

Excise taxes on tobacco products

Excise taxes are meant for some specific commodities, the consumption of which are undesirable from the society's point of view and hence need to be discouraged. Excise taxes on tobacco products are targeted to reduce tobacco consumption in order to avoid its undesirable public health consequences of deaths and disabilities. Hence, excise taxes are discussed in more detail in this section.

There are three types of excise taxes that may be imposed on tobacco products:

(1) **Specific excise:** A specific excise tax is a monetary value per quantity (e.g., pack, weight, piece, and carton) of tobacco products.
(2) **Ad-Valorem excise:** An ad valorem excise is levied as a percentage of the value of the products (retail price, producer price, wholesale price, cost, insurance, freight value, etc.).
(3) **Hybrid/mixed excise:** Both specific and *ad-valorem* excise are combined in a mixed excise system.

Among the 187 countries covered by the WHO Report on the Global Tobacco Epidemic 2013, 59 countries apply specific excises on cigarettes, 52 countries apply *ad valorem* excises, 57 countries have a mixed system and 19 countries do not have any excise tax on cigarettes. The excise rate can be uniform or differential (tiered) based on different product characteristics (e.g., retail price, length, producer price, volume of production, packaging characteristics, etc.). Globally, 20 countries apply tiered specific excises on cigarettes, six countries apply tiered ad valorem excises, and seven countries have tiered mixed systems.

Governments around the world use varying approaches to the taxation of other tobacco products. In the United States, for example, all states apply uniform specific taxes on cigarettes, but most states apply *ad valorem* taxes on other tobacco products, with the excise taxes on these products typically accounting for a much lower share of retail prices than is accounted for by the cigarette tax in cigarette prices. In India, manufactured bidis are taxed at a rate of 26 rupees per 1,000 sticks, while handmade bidis are taxed at 14 rupees per 1,000, well below the lowest cigarette excise tax of 669 rupees per 1000 sticks.

In the EU, while it is compulsory for sellers to apply a mixed system of excise taxes on cigarettes, the regulation on the types of taxes for other tobacco products is not as restrictive. The difference is striking when comparing cigarettes with fine cut tobacco used in RYO cigarettes as shown in in Figure 27. The lower tax burden for fine cut tobacco encourages substitution of RYO for cigarettes and discourages quitting because RYO is a common substitute for cigarettes in a number of EU countries.

As a result of the discriminatory rates of tax, between 2002 and 2013, the total sale of cigarettes went down while that of RYO went up (Figure 28).

Which is the right type and level of tobacco tax?

If tobacco taxation is imposed to "internalize" to some extent the negative externality caused by smoking, then quantity and not price is the right criteria for specifying the

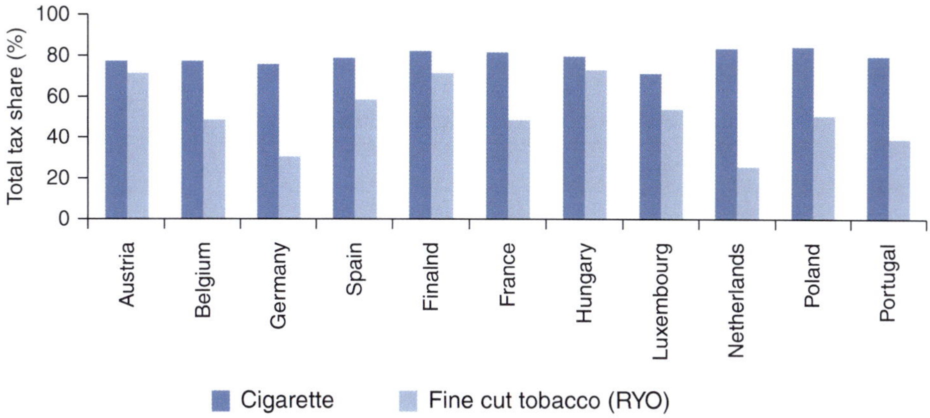

Figure 27. Total tax as a proportion of price for different tobacco products in the EU, July 2014

Source: Excise Duty Tables, European Commission, January 2014.

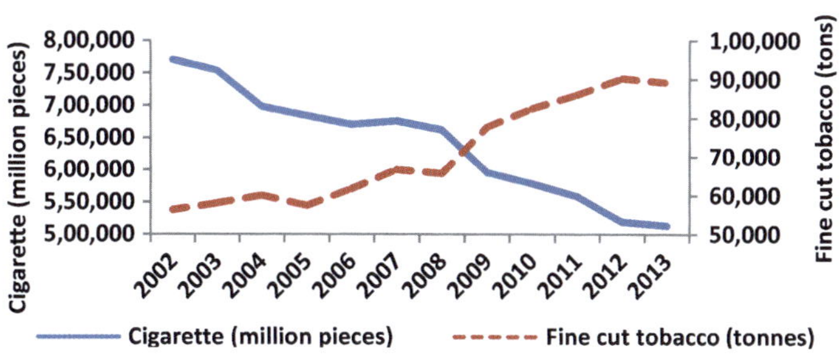

Figure 28. Sales of cigarettes and fine cut tobacco in the European Union 2002–2013

Notes:

1. Total EU covers all EU member countries except Romania (27 countries).
2. Cigarette equivalent calculation assumes each cigarette contains one gram of tobacco.

Sources: European Commission Releases for Cigarettes and Fine Cut Tobacco Consumption Database 2014; European Union (2013).

tax base. If tobacco taxation is imposed to raise price and discourage consumption, reducing the "internality" specific taxation is preferred again. It is well documented in the theoretical literature that, in imperfectly competitive markets, for a given level of tax revenue, specific taxation leads to a higher price than ad valorem taxation (see the survey by Keen (1998) and references therein). It is also evident in Table 18, which provides a weighted (by number of current cigarette smokers) average of the price and excise tax levels of countries based on the type of excise they apply on cigarettes. Countries that rely on specific excise only or those that apply a mixed system but rely more on the specific component of their excise tend to have higher price and excise tax levels. Countries that do not apply an excise tend to have prices lower than all others countries.

Table 18. Weighted average price and excise tax in purchasing power parity dollars (PPP$) by excise structure, 2012

Excise tax structure	Average price PPP$	Average excise PPP$
Specific only	3.73	1.57
Ad valorem only	2.50	1.28
Mix system	2.86	1.32
Relying more on specific	3.84	1.67
Relying more on ad valorem	2.29	1.11
No excise	1.70	—

Source: WHO 2013 Report on the Global Tobacco Epidemic.

Specific taxation, however, raises market power and increases industry profitability, because it allows the manufacturers to maneuver the price while the tax liability does not vary. In markets with monopoly power and little product differentiation, concerns about market dominance would make ad valorem taxation a more attractive option. This, however, would lead to a relatively lower price, a practice not consistent with the correcting purpose of tobacco taxation.

Most tobacco markets are characterized by both horizontal and vertical product differentiation. *Ad valorem* taxes, due to a 'multiplier effect' (meaning that a change in producer price has a larger impact on consumer price), tend to discourage costly improvement in product specifications, while specific taxation encourages it. *Ad valorem* taxation, however, promotes more intense price competition between producers and results in lower average price compared to specific excise tax, which is not desirable from public health point of view. Governments with distributional concerns might prefer *ad valorem* taxation to preserve the low price variants of the tobacco products. This, of course, is not the right approach, as the distributional objective of this approach conflicts with the public health objective. There are more appropriate instruments to deal with distributional concerns.

Calculating and implementing the optimal tax is not so straightforward. It requires information about market structure and the degree to which the tax is passed on to consumers, as well as data on demand elasticities. Calculating the right tax to internalize the externality is not easy either, especially as this is not the only distortion in the market. Tobacco markets are characterized by market power as well as externalities. This makes the calculation of the right tax more complex. Moreover, feasible rates depend on other economic aspects, such as industry regulation, administration, compliance and enforcement, tax avoidance and evasion opportunities, as well as political dimensions, such as concerns over jobs or apparent tax regressivity. Much of the tax rate differentiation, especially in low-income countries, is driven by distributional considerations, such as favoring lower income consumers by charging lower tax rates on lower-priced brands or protecting domestic industry from competition with importing companies. Setting differing tax rates for different variants of tobacco products introduces costly complexity, unintended inefficiencies, and scope for lobbying as well as health inequities.

Overview of cigarette prices and taxes at global and regional levels

From a public health perspective, the importance of excise taxation is based on the share of excise tax in the final retail price of tobacco products. It indicates to what extent price increases can be induced from a given tax increase. According to the WHO Report on the Global Tobacco Epidemic 2013 Database, the global average price of a pack of 20 cigarettes of the most sold brand in each country as of July 2012 is PPP$3.00 per pack and the average share of excise tax in retail price (weighted by estimated number of smokers in each country) is 45.35%. The global average is far below the WHO recommended share of 70%. As shown in Figure 29, the average price and excise tax share are the highest in the European region (EUR) and the lowest in the Western Pacific Region (WPR). A closer look at the country profiles in relation to the global and regional averages reveal considerable variation in prices and excise tax shares across countries and regions. In the

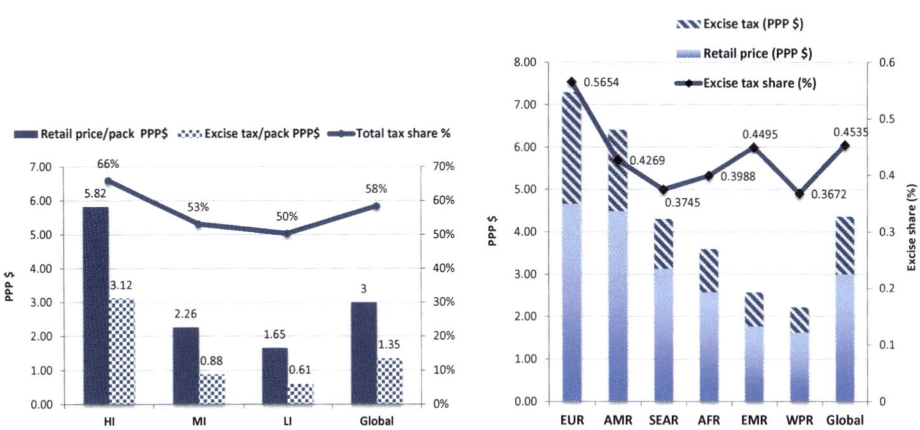

Figure 29. Average price, excise tax per pack and the share of excise and total tax on average price by country income groups and World Health Organization regions, 2012

Notes:

1. Retail price is the most popular brand's price.
2. HI = High-income; MI = Middle-income; LI = Low-income.
3. EUR = European Region; AMR = American Region; SEAR = South-East Asia Region; AFR = African Region; EMR = Eastern Mediterranean Region; WPR = Western Pacific Region.

Source: WHO Report on the Global Tobacco Epidemic, 2013a. WHO regions are, African region (AFR) Americas Region (AMR), Eastern Mediterranean region (EMR), European region (EUR), South East Asia region (SEAR), and Western Pacific region (WPR).

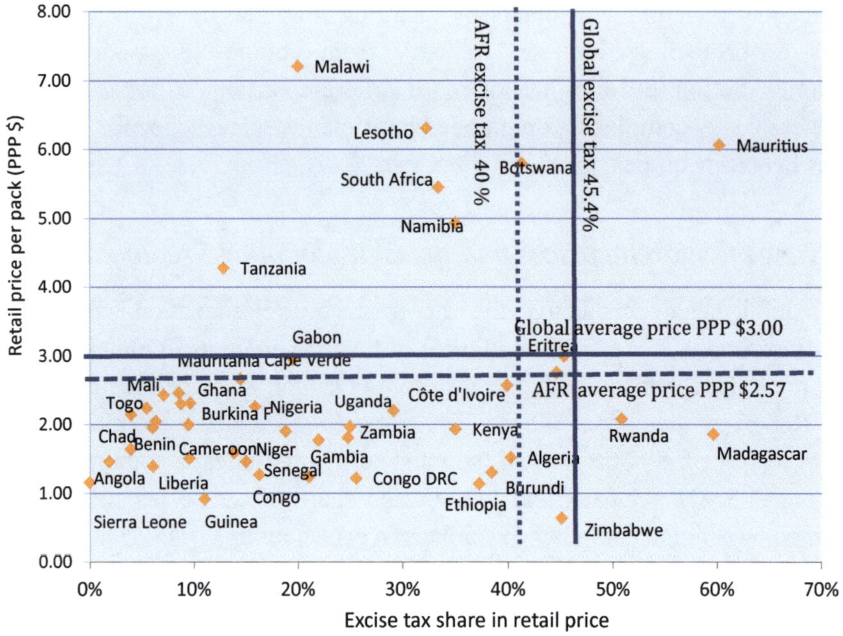

Figure 30. African Region (AFR) cigarette excise tax rates, retail price sand countries' status in relation to the global and regional averages, 2012

Source: WHO 2013a, Report on the Global Tobacco Epidemic.

African Region (AFR), the average price of cigarettes (PPP$2.57) and excise tax share (39.9%) are below the global averages (Figure 30). These countries are at high risk of expanding their markets for cigarettes, particularly among youth, and are in great need of higher taxes and prices in order to avoid wider cigarette use. Only two countries in this region, Mauritius and Seychelles, are above the global average price and tax shares of the most sold brands. In Botswana, Lesotho, Malawi and the United Republic of Tanzania, prices are higher than the global average; however excise tax shares are lower than the global average, implying that the tax has an insignificant role in determining the price. Madagascar and Rwanda on the other hand, have lower than global average prices and higher than global average excise tax shares, indicating that taxes need to be increased further to raise the price level. Thus, to make progress in pricing-related tobacco control, countries would benefit from moving towards the North-East direction of the graph, which will shift the global and regional average prices and excise tax shares in that direction as well.

In the Americas (AMR), the average regional price of cigarettes (PPP$4.49) is higher than the global average, driven up by a number of countries such as Barbados, Canada, Jamaica, Panama, the US, and Venezuela (Figure 31). The excise tax share for many countries in this region is, however, lower than the global average, making

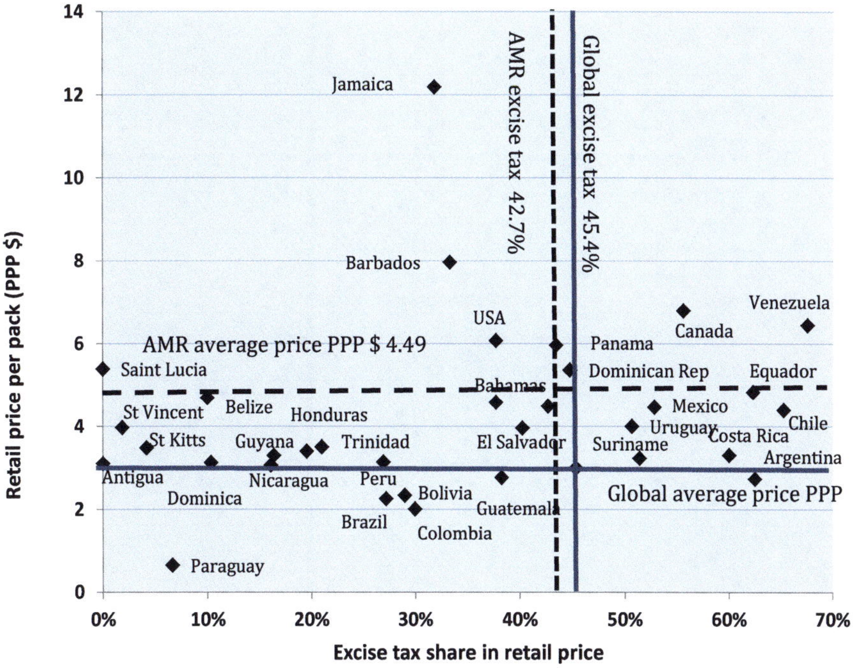

Figure 31. American Region (AMR) cigarette excise tax rates, retail prices and countries' status in relation to the global and regional averages, 2012.

Source: WHO 2013a Report on the Global Tobacco Epidemic.

the regional average excise tax share for AMR just 42.69%. Countries such as Bolivia, Brazil, Colombia, and Paraguay are in need of raising both the taxes and prices to catch up with the global average.

In the Eastern Mediterranean Region (EMR), the regional average price of cigarettes (PPP$1.77) is well below the global average (Figure 32). While the average excise tax share (44.95%) is close to the global average, a number of countries in this region do not have any excise tax on cigarettes and are in need of introducing one.

The average price of cigarettes (PPP$4.66) and excise tax share (56.54%) in the European Region (EUR) are both higher than the global averages (Figure 33). While countries such as Ireland and United Kingdom have price and excise tax shares well above the EUR averages, a number of former Soviet Republic countries are on the opposite side of the graph below the global average and from a tobacco control standpoint are in need of raising taxes and prices.

In the South-East Asia Region (SEAR), the average price of cigarettes (PPP$3.13) is slightly above the global average, although the average excise tax share (37.45%) is significantly below the global average (Figure 34). Sri Lanka outperforms all the SEAR countries in respect to price and tax share. Maldives is the only SEAR country that does not apply any excise tax on cigarettes. Bangladesh and Myanmar have prices below the regional average, India and Timor-Leste have

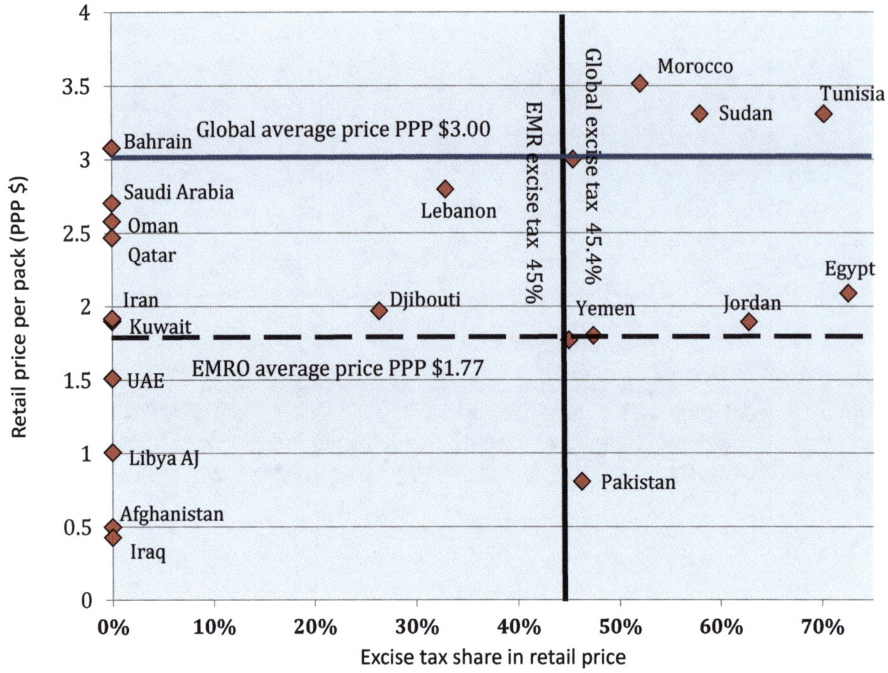

Figure 32. Eastern Mediterranean Region (EMR) cigarette excise tax rates, retail prices and countries' status in relation to the global and regional averages, 2012.

Source: WHO 2013a Report on the Global Tobacco Epidemic.

excise tax shares below the regional average and Nepal has both price and excise tax share below the regional averages.

In the Western Pacific Region (WPR), a number of countries have price and excise tax shares above the global averages (Figure 35). However, their regional averages are brought down below the global average due to low prices and taxes in Cambodia, China, Lao People's Democratic Republic, Mongolia, the Philippines, and Vietnam. Some countries, such as Fiji, Papua New Guinea, Solomon Islands, and Tuvalu have prices higher than global averages, although the excise tax shares are low in these countries. All these countries are in need of raising their taxes and prices to reach regional and global averages.

Tobacco taxes and the poor

Governments and others often raise concerns about the negative impact of excise tax increases on poor smokers: As taxes increase, the poor will spend a higher percentage of their limited incomes on tobacco; the income inequity between the poor and the rich will widen; and the poor will disproportionately pay higher taxes as a share of income compared to that of the rich. Following these arguments, tobacco taxes are labelled "regressive." Evidence shows that low-income

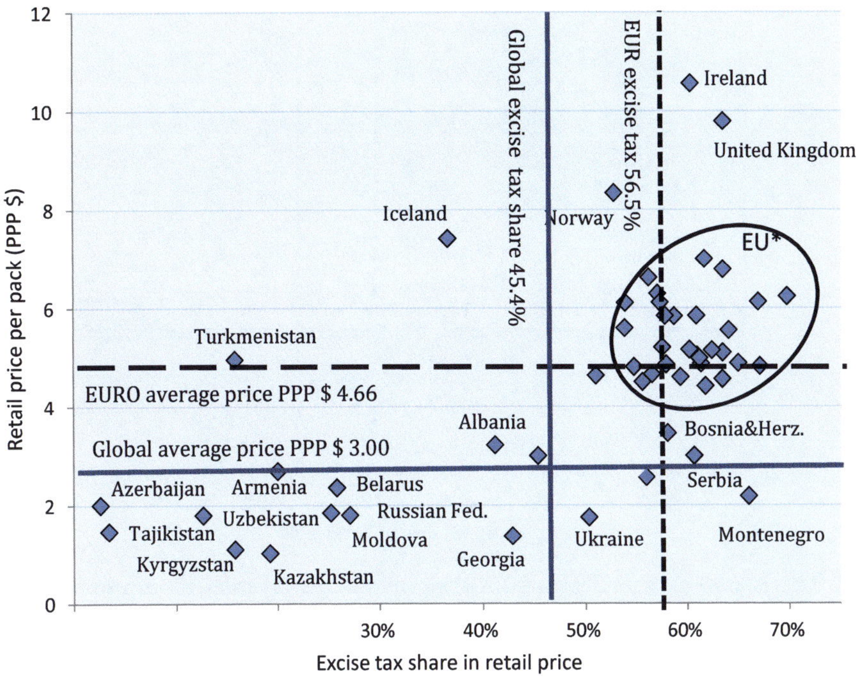

Figure 33. European Region (EUR) cigarette excise tax rates, retail prices and countries' status in relation to the global and regional averages, 2012

Sources: WHO 2013a Report on the Global Tobacco Epidemic. EU*= Austria, Bulgaria, Belgium, Croatia, Cyprus, Czech Republic, Denmark, Estonia, Finland, France, Germany, Greece, Hungary, Israel, Italy, Latvia, Luxembourg, Lithuania, FYR of Macedonia, Netherlands, Malta, Poland, Romania, Portugal, Slovakia, Slovenia, Spain, Sweden, Switzerland, Turkey.

households in LMICs already spend a relatively higher share of their household income on tobacco, ranging from 4.25 to 7.2%, compared to 1.65 to 3% in high-income households (Önder, 2002; Karki *et al.*, 2003; Arunatilake and Opatha, 2003; Adioetomo *et al.*, 2005).

In general, there are two schools of thoughts when it comes to the impact of tobacco taxes on the poor. The first school evaluates tax increases from traditional and welfare perspectives. The traditional view of incidence analysis compares the share of cigarette taxes as a proportion of household expenditures, and calculates the tax burden by income or expenditure groups.

From a welfare perspective, the first school also claims that even if the poor quit smoking due to higher taxes, they will still be worse off because they give up on something providing positive utility (Remler, 2004). The second school of thought evaluates the higher taxes from a broader perspective and argues that with equal consumption patterns assumed, a tobacco tax increase will account for a greater *burden of income* for the poor than for the rich. Evidence, however, clearly shows that the poor are more sensitive to higher prices than the rich. In LMICs, the price

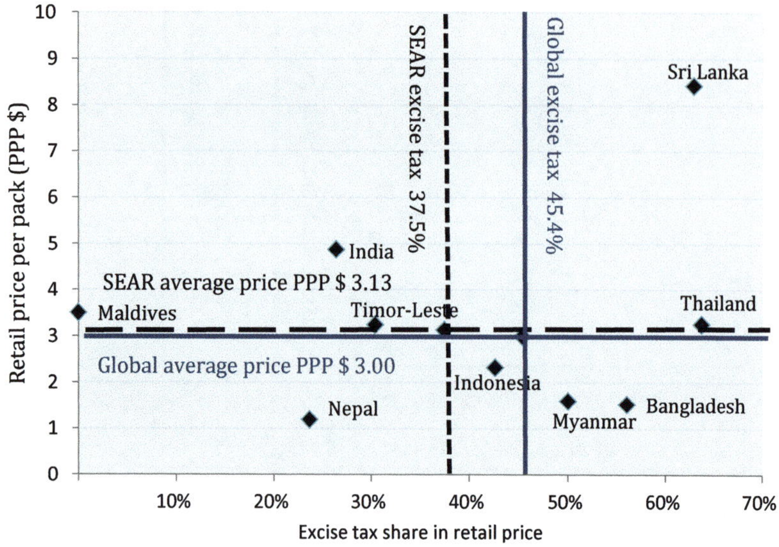

Figure 34. South-East Asia Region (SEAR) cigarette excise tax rates, retail prices and countries' status in relation to the global and regional averages, 2012.

Source: WHO 2013a Report on the Global Tobacco Epidemic.

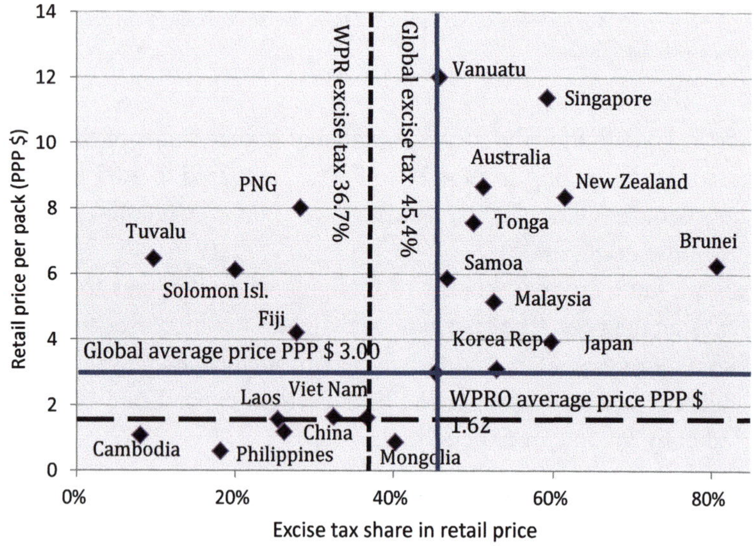

Figure 35. Western Pacific Region (WPR) cigarette excise tax rates, retail prices and countries' status in relation to the global and regional averages, 2012

Source: WHO 2013a Report on the Global Tobacco Epidemic.

elasticity of tobacco demand ranges from −1.9 to −0.15 among poor and −1.48 to +0.51 among the rich (see IARC (2011).

Therefore, when the higher price sensitivity of the poor is taken into account, their consumption pattern cannot be assumed to be equal, as they are more likely to quit or reduce their tobacco consumption as the tobacco tax increases. In consequence, tax increases may not be regressive if the poor reduce consumption more than the rich, and furthermore, tax-induced behavioral change to encourage quitting benefit the poor in at least two ways. First, smokers' health will improve and their productivity will increase, which could break the vicious cycle of consumption–sickness–premature death–low productivity and loss of income–poverty. Second, the opportunity costs of tobacco spending will be reduced so that they can allocate more money on other goods and services (Chaloupka and Warner, 2000).

Indeed, evidence from low-income countries show that smoking has an immediate negative impact on living standards by diverting scarce household resources away from essential expenditures. For example, a 2002 survey in China, examined expenditures among 2,400 households across Southwest China (Hu *et al.,* 2005). Expenditures on cigarettes constituted 7.7% of family expenditures in poor or near-poor urban smoking households and 11.1% of family expenditures in poor or near-poor rural smoking households. The study reveals that smoking households' spending on other household necessities, such as food, housing, and education, were lower than that of non-smoking households. Wang *et al.* (2006) estimated the impact of tobacco spending on other household expenditures and found a negative and significant relationship between tobacco and other goods including food, education and medical care. A study in Bangladesh showed that cigarette expenditures can reduce the nutritional status of low-income households by displacing expenditures on food and estimated that 10 million people who are currently malnourished could have an adequate diet if money spent on tobacco were spent on food instead (Efroymson *et al.*, 2001). John (2008) found similar results in India as he compared tobacco using and non-using households' expenditures. The results show that on one hand, the budget share of food, education and entertainment falls as tobacco expenditure increases. On the other hand, the budget share for health care expenditures increases.

Economic evidence on the tax burden experience by the poor when excise taxes increase is mixed. For example, in earlier literature, Townsend *et al.* (1994) found that the absolute value of price elasticity was inversely related to social class in the UK for men in 1987, and both genders in 1994. She argued that the lowest social class was more likely to alter their smoking behavior as taxes increased and was therefore able to reduce the burden of tax increases. Borren and Sutton (1992), on the other hand, argue otherwise by showing that men in the lowest social class pay over eight times more in increased tax than men in highest social class. Research from Gruber and Koszegi (2004) indicates that higher taxes can work as a commitment mechanism for the smokers to quit smoking, who cannot commit otherwise. They argue that this self-control function benefits lower income groups more, as they are more sensitive to higher prices. They conclude that incidence of cigarette taxes is much less than previously assumed and are even progressive for a wide variety of parameter values. However, their results appear to be sensitive to the parameter values and the assumptions made. (For more evidence, see Chapter 7 of IARC 2011 for the existing literature.)

Higher prevalence rates of smoking among lower-income groups can be attributed to the fact that poor smokers may value the utility they get from smoking and their sense of well being at the current time at a higher degree than higher income groups, and they may discount the harmful consequences of tobacco use in the future (IARC, 2011; Becker and Murphy, 1988; Becker *et al.*, 1994). Given their higher sensitivity to price, any tax or and price increase would impose a greater cost on the poor, especially those who cannot quit or reduce their smoking levels. However as the tax increases, given their level of price sensitivity, total consumption will be reduced by poor and the low-income groups, which will then reduce their share of excise tax payment as a portion of total excise tax revenue for tobacco (IARC, 2011). Önder and Yürekli (2014) examine the share of excise revenue paid by different expenditure tertiles in 2003 in Turkey, and the simulation results show that as the excise tax per pack increases, the share of total tobacco excise tax revenue that is paid by the poor households is reduced (Table 19).

Existing evidence consistently suggests that increasing taxes and prices to make tobacco products less affordable would help the poor relatively more than the rich. Especially in the long run, tax-induced reductions in consumption will improve health outcomes and economic welfare, which would increase the quality of life. Moreover, studies suggest that excise taxes on tobacco be increased for both revenue and health gains (Stotsky and Woldemariam, 2002; Owen *et al.*, 2001).

Table 19. Simulation of the estimated share of total cigarette excise tax revenue that would be paid by poor, middle-income and rich households in the presence of excise tax increases in Turkey 2003

	Portion of tobacco tax revenue paid by expenditure tertiles		
	Poor (%)	**Middle (%)**	**Rich (%)**
Base 2003 Case	23.8	33.9	42.2
10% excise/pack increases	23.1	34.2	42.7
25% excise increase	21.8	34.6	43.6
50% excise increase	18.9	35.5	45.6
75% excise increase	14.6	36.9	48.5

Source: Önder and Yürekli (2014).

The revenue gain from higher excise taxes is expected primarily due to the fact that the demand for tobacco products is price inelastic so that consumption reduces less than proportionately when there is price increase. Even if demand is price elastic, revenue may increase when the share of tax in price is very low. Revenues generated by higher taxes can be spent progressively for social programs that the poor would benefit from, such as on national health insurance programs. This has been done by a number of countries including the Philippines, where both tobacco and alcohol excise taxes increased substantially in 2012 and 85% of excise tax revenues are allocated for national health insurance (MoF Philippines, 2012).

Tobacco taxes and public health

Tobacco taxation is widely recognized to be one of the most effective measures for reducing the demand for tobacco products. Tax increases raise the consumer price of tobacco products, thereby reducing their affordability and leading some users to quit, while many others will reduce their level of consumption. The evidence also finds that about half of the overall drop in tobacco consumption results from reductions in the number of tobacco users (CDC, 2004; World Bank, 1999; IARC, 2011) and, that poor and youth populations are the most sensitive to price increases. Reductions in use among young people due to price increases are on average two-to-three times greater than those that occur among adults (IARC, 2011).

A number of retrospective studies have quantified the link between higher taxes and public health outcomes. Moore (1996) used US data from 1954–1988 to examine the effect of tobacco excise taxes on changes in mortality. After controlling for state, year, socioeconomic variables and alcohol taxes, Moore found that variations in tobacco taxes were inversely related to smoking-attributable mortality and concluded that a 10% increase in tobacco taxation would save 6,000 lives per year. Another study in Switzerland using time series data from 1965–1994 found that tobacco taxes were inversely related to the male standardized suicide rate (Yamasaki *et al.*, 2005). France increased its taxes substantially between the early 1990s and 2005 leading to cigarette prices tripling in inflation-adjusted terms. The health impact of these increases were seen just a few years later with lung cancer deaths rates for young men falling by 50% over the same period (Jha and Peto, 2014; Hill, 2013).

Several studies from California have identified a clear association between tobacco taxation and mortality at the sub-national level. In 1989, California increased tobacco taxation and earmarked part of the revenue to go to its tobacco control program. Based on data collected between 1980 and 1995, a regression model showed that, California's tobacco control program was able to reduce deaths by about 12,000 per year by preventing cardiovascular and stroke deaths (Lightwood and Glanz, 1997). Another study compared per capita cigarette consumption and the death rate from heart disease for California to that of the other 49 states in the US (Fichtenberg and Glanz, 2000). The regression results showed that California had 33,000 fewer deaths from heart disease between 1989 and 1992 than would have been expected had the tobacco control program not been implemented. A major limitation of these studies is that the program included measures other than just taxation. Although it is difficult to separate the net effect of taxation alone, it is the key feature of the tobacco control program in California and thus much of the overall effect can likely be attributed to taxes.

- *Expected lives saved by higher tobacco taxes*

The theme for World No Tobacco Day 2014 was tobacco taxation, and as part of this event, the WHO developed a model of the global cigarette market in order to demonstrate the potential for tobacco taxation to generate extra revenue while also improving public health. The model found that if all countries increased the amount of excise tax on cigarettes by 50%, then the retail price of cigarettes would increase on average by 26.5% globally (Table 20). Prevalence elasticities of demand ranging from −0.25 in low-income countries to −0.15 in high-income countries were applied to each country in the model to determine how smoking prevalence would respond to these higher retail prices. Overall, smoking prevalence would decrease by 3.8% globally reflecting 49 million fewer smokers from among the 2012 population as described in Section "Expected tobacco-attributable deaths".

The impact on public health outcomes can also be measured in terms of reduced smoking-related mortality among those who are expected to

Table 20. Impact of increasing the amount of cigarette excise tax by 50% by WHO Region

	Increase in cigarette retail prices (%)	**Decrease in smoking prevalence (%)**	**Decrease in total number of smokers (millions)**	**Smoking attributable deaths averted (millions)**
Africa	19.7	−2.8	−1.6	0.4
Americas	25.0	−3.9	−6.9	1.5
Eastern Med.	32.7	−5.5	−3.5	0.8
Europe	32.4	−4.8	−13.0	2.9
South-East Asia	26.8	−4.0	−9.8	2.2
Western Pacific	22.6	−3.0	−13.9	3.1
World	**26.5**	**−3.8**	**−48.8**	**10.8**

Source: Authors calculation (WHO, 2014b).

quit smoking. The benefits of cessation are many and occur early for a number of serious diseases. After one year of cessation, the risk of coronary heart diseases is about half that of a smoker. The risk of stroke is reduced to that of a non-smoker in 5–15 years after quitting. After 10 years of cessation, the risk of lung cancer falls to about half that of a smoker. Overall, adults who quit before middle age avoid almost all the excess hazards of smoking (Doll *et al.*, 2004). However, not all smokers can avoid early death from smoking because of the accumulated effects of their use. Studies that assess the economics of tobacco and tobacco taxation typically use a mortality adjustment of 67% to allow for this (Ranson *et al.*, 2000; John *et al.*, 2010; Waters *et al.*, 2010). This means that among those smokers who quit, 67% of those who would have died early from a disease caused by their smoking will avoid early death by quitting.

Table 20 shows the number of smoking-attributable deaths averted under the scenario described above in which 49 million smokers quit in response to the higher cigarette taxes and prices. The number of smoking attributable deaths in the future from among the world's population in 2012 (refer to Table 16) would decrease by 10.8 million (49 million quitters multiplied by expected mortality of 33% and the 67% adjustment factor).

Studies also confirm that tobacco control measures are cost-effective. The 2002 World Health Report (WHO, 2002) examined the cost-effectiveness of priority interventions and found taxation to be the most cost-effective tobacco control measure available in addition to having the greatest potential impact on public health. The World Health Report highlighted that taxes together with bans on advertising and information dissemination campaigns would be affordable and cost-effect in the majority of countries. A subsequent study by Jha *et al.* (2006) found that the Cost per Disability-Adjusted Life Year (DALY) saved from a 33% increase in cigarette prices through higher taxation ranged from US$13–US$195 per DALY saved, making it a highly cost-effective public health measure. The cost of non-price tobacco control measures ranged from US$233–US$2,916 per DALY saved, also reflecting good value for the investment compared to many other potential health interventions in low- and-middle income countries.

In 2011, a United Nations high-level meeting on non-communicable disease (NCD) prevention also highlighted the importance of tobacco control to the global NCD agenda. This event was only the second time in UN history that the General Assembly met to discuss a health issue (the last issue was AIDS). WHO research leading up to the Assembly highlighted tobacco taxation, smoke-free policies, health warnings and bans on advertising as "best buy" interventions that are not only highly cost effective, but also feasible to implement within the constraints of LMIC health systems (WHO, 2011).

Concerns and Evidence on the Impact of Higher Taxes

Illicit trade in tobacco products

Illicit trade in all its forms is perhaps the most widely used argument against raising tobacco taxes worldwide. Governments are keenly concerned about the revenue loss and criminality that this activity entails. Illicit trade is a concern for public health since it undermines the impact of tobacco control measures including taxation, warning labels and restrictions to sales of minors (IARC, 2011).

The illicit market is a highly complex and diverse set of illegal activities, including grey areas relating to abuses of legal duty-free sales and cross-border shopping. The diverse and complex nature of illicit trade makes it difficult to quantify. A recent study by Joossens *et al.* (2010), however, found that the illicit market accounted for 12% of global cigarette consumption in 2007. The market share of illicit trade varied from an average of 17% in low-income countries to an average of 10% in high-income countries.

Figure 36 shows the breakdown of illicit trade in tobacco by the main types of illicit activity in 2012, as estimated by Euromonitor (2012). Although the narrative on illicit trade often focuses on the incentives for bootlegging or internet shopping by individuals, studies suggest that these forms of circumvention are comparatively small, especially internet purchases (IARC, 2011). Evidence shows that large-scale smuggling by organized networks is the prominent channel responsible for around 72% of global illicit trade as indicated in Figure 36.

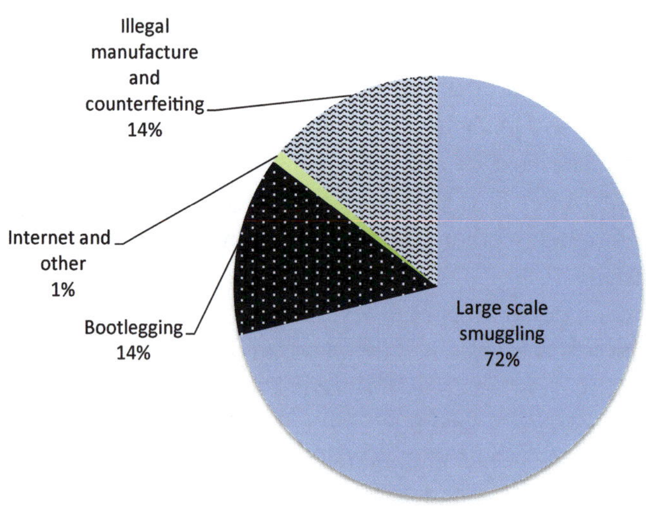

Figure 36. Illicit trade in tobacco by type of illicit activity, 2012

Source: Euromonitor (2014).

The illicit cigarette market is comprised of two main activities — production and trade. In either case, the aim is to evade taxes in one or several markets. Illicit cigarettes can be produced by legal or illegal manufacturers. Illegal production facilities are completely outside the tax net and so can be difficult to trace. In India, for example, illegal manufacturing is often undertaken by small 'mobile' production facilities that can easily relocate if they are at risk of being caught by the authorities.

Legal manufacturers can also engage in illicit activity by producing contraband original or unknown brands that do not pay all applicable taxes. Brazil has perhaps the best-known case of illicit production by legal manufacturing companies. In 2007, after electronic monitoring system for cigarette producers is implemented in 2007, the Brazilian Government found that three legitimate cigarette companies had been producing illicit cigarettes leading to tax revenue losses in the order of US$280 million per year. The three companies were not able to meet their resulting overdue tax liabilities and were consequently shut down (MoF Brazil, 2009). Many other countries including Bangladesh and Pakistan have similar experiences with local producers (MoF, NBR, Bangladesh 2010, MoF, FBR, Pakistan 2009).

Illicit trade can also involve the direction of trade flows. Smuggling occurs when authorities in the destination market have not been informed of the product's arrival and consequently the product evades destination market taxes. Smuggled cigarettes can be original brands (contraband), fake original brands (counterfeit) or unknown brands (WCO, 2012; OCTA, 2011; European Commission, 2013). Smuggling can also occur in the form of bootlegging by individuals taking advantage of duty-free or cross-border shopping opportunities, or in the form of large-scale smuggling by organized networks. Paraguay is an example of the latter, where locally produced cigarettes are directly brought by criminal networks from factories without any taxes being paid, then shipped illegally for sale in neighboring Brazil as well as other countries throughout the world (CIET, 2009).

The second variant with respect to trade is the emergence of 'cheap white' cigarettes. These are cigarettes that have been legally produced typically in low-tax jurisdictions, where they likely pay the local taxes, however, the quantities are vastly surplus to legitimate demand in that jurisdiction and thus destined to be smuggled-out. Cheap whites have been identified as a major concern by international agencies such as the World Customs Organization and by regional institutions particularly in the European Union (EU).

Measurement of illicit trade

Due to its complex and interwoven nature, it can be difficult to quantify the level and extent of illicit trade in tobacco. However, a number of methodologies have

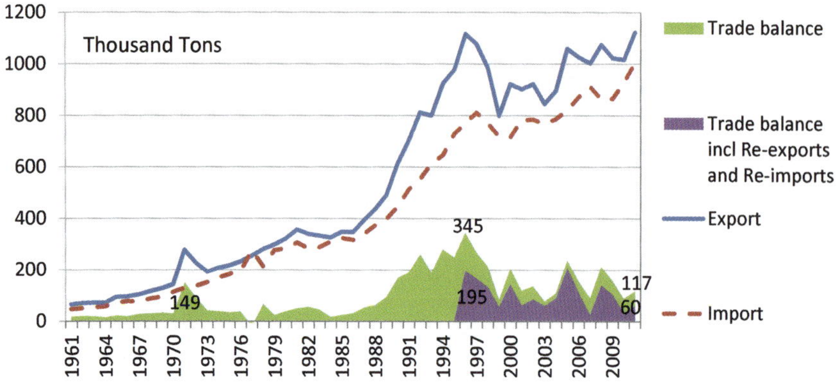

Figure 37a. Global Export and Import of Cigarettes and the Trade Discrepancy, 1960–2011
Source: Constructed by authors by using FAO and COMTRADE databases.

Table 21. Illicit cigarette trade volume and customs seizures 2010

2010	Illicit trade volume* (million sticks)	Customs seizures** (million sticks)	Seizure as % of illicit trade (% total sticks)
Asia and the Pacific	300,974	281	0.1
Europe	106,040	2,502	2.4
Americas	78,601	42	0.1
Middle East and Africa	55,504	354	0.6
World	**541,118**	**3,180**	**0.6**

Notes: *Euromonitor estimates. **World Customs Annual Report 2011–2012.
Source: Euromonitor (2014) and World Customs Annual Report 2011–2012.

been developed to shed light on this activity. This includes the use of trade statistics to quantify trade discrepancies between cigarette export and import volumes (Figure 37a), customs seizures (Table 21), expert opinion, and market or consumer surveys. Each methodology comes with its own shortcomings.

Customs seizures are another source of country-level information. However, seizures provide only a very partial picture of the illicit market since it can also reflect the strength or lack thereof in the customs administrations of different jurisdictions. In addition, seizures account for only a small fraction of the overall illicit market in most countries and regions. For example, EU law enforcement agencies are reported to have seized 4.7 billion illicit cigarettes in 2009 (European Commission, 2013). Given that the total EU cigarette market as around 650 billion sticks annually, these seizures represent less than 0.05% of the market and thus understate the true extent of illicit market. As discussed below, studies estimated

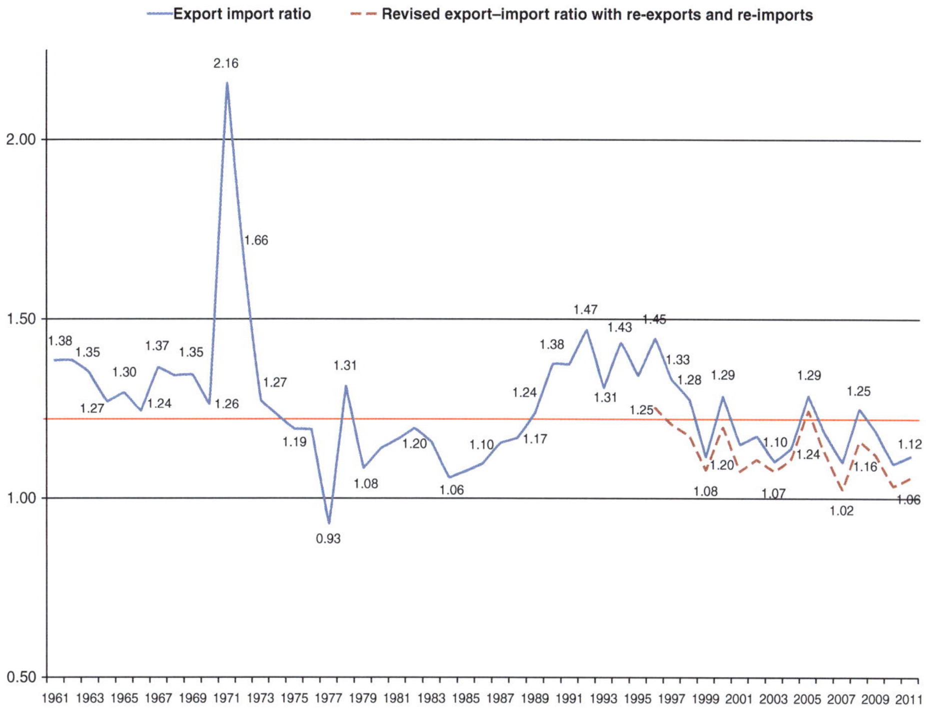

Figure 37b. Global trade discrepancy (export–import ratio) of cigarettes 1960–2011

Source: Constructed by authors by using FAO and COMTRADE databases.

that illicit cigarette market in EU is between 8% and 11% (KPMG, 2005; 2012; Joossens *et al.*, 2010a). Similarly, the World Customs Organization (WCO) (2012) reports that almost 3.2 billion and 1.9 billion pieces of cigarettes respectively were captured in 2010 and 2011 by the customs agencies of 64 countries. Based on Euromonitor estimates of the illicit cigarette market globally, these seizures represent less than 1% of the total illicit trade of 541 billion pieces annually.

In our illustration of the trade balance between 1960 and 2011 (Figure 37), we also estimate the export–import ratio (trade discrepancy) for cigarettes from 1960 to 2011 (Figure 37b). We find that the average global ratio between 1960 and 2011 is 1.23, meaning that global reports of cigarette export volume is 1.23 times higher than global reports of cigarette import volume. As illustrated in Figure 37b, the periods between 1960 and the mid-1970s (ratio varies between 1.24 and 1.37) and also between 1990 and 1998 (ratio varies from 1.31 to 1.47), the trade discrepancy is much higher than the global average. Relatively high ratios before the mid-1970s could be due to poor data reporting by the countries. For example the highest and the lowest trade discrepancies are estimated as 2.16 in 1971 and 0.98 in 1977. Since early 1980s, the data reveals two interesting points. First, from the early 1970s until the late 1980s, and after the late 1990s until 2011, the trade discrepancy (export–import ratio) fluctuates below global average in most years. Second, trade discrepancy between 1990 and 1997 stands out with its consistently higher import–export ratio between minimum 1.31 to maximum 1.47 throughout 1960 and 2011 period. During the 1990s, illicit trade for cigarettes is one of the most discussed and analyzed issue, as will be discussed later on. Trade discrepancy does not indicate the level of illicit trade due to the fact that there are many reasons for such discrepancies, including quality and quantity of data reporting and recording that includes all trade activities including re-exports and re-imports. As the re-export and re-import data starts becoming available with 14 countries in 1996 to 35 countries in 2005 and 25 countries in 2012, we revise the export–import ratio starting 1996 by including available limited re-exports and re-imports data into estimation. Although the revised ratio (trade discrepancy) is relatively lower than the ratio that does not take into re-exports and re-imports volumes, the discrepancies of trade balances still persist in 1996 and 2011. Trade is a very lucrative business and it is very likely that many more countries engage in re-exports and re-imports but only few probably report the data. Therefore, it is important to conduct careful analysis to determine what percentage of export–import ratio is illicit trade. Merriman (2010) applied the trade discrepancy technique to data between the mid-1970s and the mid-1990s and concluded that approximately 6% of total tobacco products sold in 1995 were smuggled through the diversion of untaxed exports from legal to illegal channels.

Experts' opinion tends to be the most widely used method of quantifying illicit cigarette trade, especially in the case of LMICs where data are less widely available. Experts are those who due to their profession or position have particular insight, information or knowledge about the illicit market (IARC, 2011). However, this approach has shortcomings since opinions are subjective by definition, and can be biased for many reasons including the interests of the institutions they represent.

A number of survey techniques have been developed by academics and others in recent years in order to make the estimation of illicit trade more analytically robust. For example, Lakhdar (2008) used survey and tax paid retail sales data for 2005 and 2006 to estimate that illicit cross-border shopping accounted for 15% of cigarette consumption in France. In the United States, Stehr (2005) compared per capita consumption and the tax paid sales in 2001. Based on the difference between these two datasets, he reported that 13% of cigarettes did not have taxes paid from their home state. In the UK Her Majesty (HM) Customs and Excise, and HM Treasury compared consumption data gathered from a national survey to official customs clearance data to conclude the 18% of the UK's cigarette market was illicit in 2000 (HMRC, 2000), and decreased to 13% in 2005 and 2006 (HMRC, 2006).

In recent years, collecting cigarette packs from wastebaskets has become another common methodology for measuring the size of the illicit market. For example, Merriman (2010) collected littered cigarette packs around Chicago and found that about 75% of packs collected did not have a Chicago tax stamp. However, this does not necessarily correspond to the level of tax avoidance, since a majority of the population commutes to Chicago from neighboring jurisdictions. In addition, Chicago has high tourism levels. Therefore, it is likely that their finding will have overstated the actual level of tax avoidance. In Poland, a marketing consulting firm Almares funded by the National Tobacco Industry Association collected 10,500 packs in 63 cities across five regions in three consecutive years from 2001–2003. The study found that the share of cigarettes from among the collected packs that were not duty paid in Poland averaged 15.2% (Ciecierski, 2007). A similar technique was used by Ciecierski *et al.* (2009), who collected packs from 30 districts across Warsaw and concluded that nearly 13% of cigarette packs had foreign tax stamps.

KPMG examined illicit trade in 25 EU Member States by combining two methodologies — collecting empty cigarette packs and conducting consumer surveys (KPMG, 2005; 2012). The study found that illicit cigarettes accounted for 8.3% and 11.1% of the EU market in 2005 and 2012, respectively.

In 2010, the Pricing Policies and Control of Tobacco in Europe (PPACTE) project that used computer assisted personal interviews among adults 15 years old and older in 18 select European countries revealed that, a significant number of respondents in Latvia (26%), Bulgaria (12%), Czech Republic (11%), and Poland (11%) said that they had purchased smuggled cigarettes in the preceding month (Joossens *et al.*, 2010a). By comparison, the International Tobacco Control Policy Evaluation Project (ITC) Surveys (Hyland *et al.*, 2006), which have detailed questions to detect untaxed or lower-tax purchases show that individual tax avoidance[16] is relatively low at around 1.1% in Australia, less than 4% in Canada, and range between 5% and 6.1% in the US between 2002 and 2003.

Causes of illicit trade

- *Tax and price differences*

Differences in tobacco taxes and prices between countries or jurisdictions are most commonly identified as the cause of illicit trade. Researchers have measured the impact of cigarette taxes and prices on illicit trade with different results. Several studies find that higher cigarette prices are the primary motivation for cross-border

[16]These surveys include questions on cross-border, duty-free, Native American reservation, Internet, and other direct purchases, and other options that potentially reflect untaxed or lower-tax purchases.

shopping and bootlegging (Baltagi and Levin, 1986; 1992; Tsai *et al.*, 2003; Taal *et al.*, 2004; Lakhdar, 2008; Goel, 2008; DeCicca *et al.*, 2010; Merriman, 2010). A number of these studies have examined the relationship between price and illicit trade among neighboring US states with different tax rates. These studies found that a 10% increase in the price of cigarettes in a neighboring state would increase cigarette sales by up to 30.1% (DeCicca *et al.*, 2010).

Tsai *et al.* (2003), examine the Taiwan market by using survey data from 2000. They found that the likelihood of purchasing smuggled cigarettes increases at least 2.6 times for every 1% increase in cigarette prices. In Europe, Taal *et al.* (2004) estimated legal and illegal cigarette purchases by Estonians and by foreign visitors to Estonia between 1993 and 2000. They found that purchases by foreign visitors, especially by Finnish tourists constituted up to 50% of the total Estonian market, as the prices in Estonia are up to four times lower than its neighbors. In the UK, the HM Treasury stated that the illicit market reached to 18% in 2000, due in part to a 25%% increase in cigarette prices between 1997 and 2000 (HMRC, 2000).

While the evidence shows that price and tax differences can motivate bootlegging by individuals, especially in border or transit areas, this finding does not necessarily translate into other forms of illicit trade, particularly large-scale smuggling by organized networks. This is important because large-scale smuggling is the source of illicit activity that dominates globally and thus has the greatest threat to government tax bases and to public health. Furthermore, unlike bootlegging, the reasons behind organized-large-scale smuggling are not only price and tax differences. Other factors, such as corruption in a country, people's perception (positive or negative) of counterfeit cigarettes, lack of communication between and among customs and also involvement of tobacco manufacturers may play more important roles than the price/tax differences (World Bank, 1999; Yürekli and Saygınsoy,

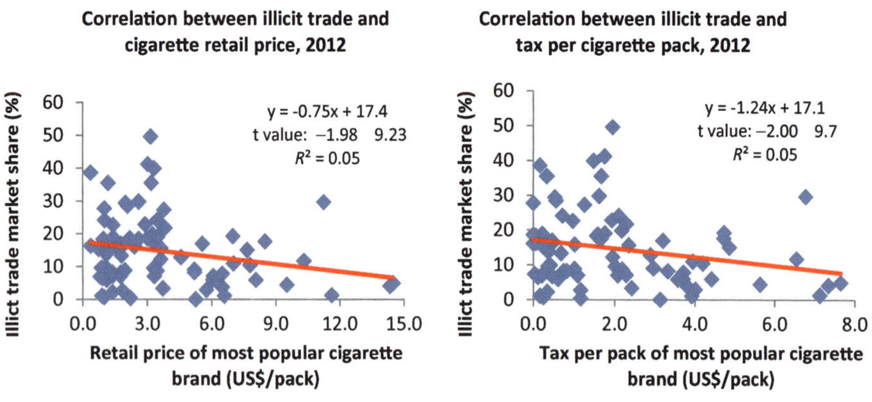

Figure 38. Correlation between illicit trade, cigarette price and excise tax per pack 2012
Source: Euromonitor for illicit market share, WHO 2013 Report on Global Tobacco Epidemic for price and tax data.

2008; Joossens *et al.*, 2010). We examine the relationships between illicit market (share of illicit-counterfeit cigarettes in total cigarettes, sold in a market), and the most popular brand prices as well as excise taxes per pack by 77 countries in 2012 by using 2 × 2 analysis (Figure 38). Results show a negative and significant relationship between the level of illicit market and the price-tax level per pack, suggesting that other factors may have a larger impact on the level of illicit cigarette market than the tax-price differences alone. This could explain the reason that researchers do not find a simple, positive cross-country correlation between cigarette taxes or prices and the market share of illicit trade.

For example, a recent study by Joossens *et al.* (2012) also confirms that no statistically significant relationship exists between cigarette prices and tax evasion (illicit trade). This led the authors to conclude that factors other than price influence illicit trade. The authors identified the ease and cost of operating in a country, industry participation, criminal networks and corruption levels as among the key factors. Other studies have used tobacco industry behavior to shed doubt on the simple link between higher cigarette prices and illicit trade. For example, Gilmore and Reed (2014) examined the cigarette industry's pricing behavior in the UK. They concluded that if the industry was genuinely concerned that price increases would fuel illicit tobacco use, it would surely not have increased prices to the extent it has. Their findings are consistent with evidence from Ireland which showed that between 2000 and 2010, 36% of the price increases in cigarettes were imposed by the industry, despite its claims every budget that tax (and thus price) increases would lead to smuggling.

- *Other non-price enabling factors*

Non-price factors may be as important to the illicit tobacco market as price differences, since they encompass disincentives such as the probability and cost of being caught. Such non-price considerations include weaknesses in supply chain monitoring and control, where manufacturers and exporters have no legal obligation to monitor the movement of their products throughout the supply chain, and consequently customs and tax administrators are unable to properly trace the movement or final destination of products.

Another common factor is that customs and tax administrators often have inadequate human resources and technologies to detect illicit activities. Technology such as specialized equipment to identify product origin, scanners, sniff dogs, and appropriate IT systems can enable risk analysis for the supply movement at the borders. Customs and tax administrations can also have inadequate communication and coordination mechanisms in place both within and between countries. Lenient and ambiguous legislation that creates grey areas for smuggling, imposes low penalties, gives inadequate authority to customs,

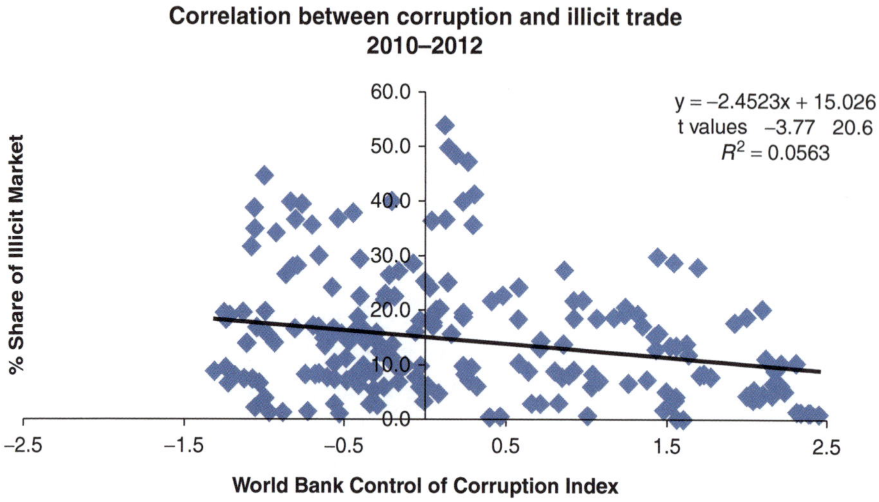

Figure 39. Illicit trade market and corruption

Source: Authors' estimation by using database by World Bank and Euromonitor.

and entails lengthy prosecution factor into play (European Commission, 2013; OCTA, 2011; CIET, 2009).

Customs officials can also face personal security concerns, especially in remote areas. In many developing countries with vast and/or inhibited border areas, agents may face retaliation by smugglers that jeopardize their safety (MoF Pakistan, 2009). Lastly, corruption can infiltrate all levels of administration, especially where internal control is weak, administrators have inadequate salaries, or there is infrequent rotation and a lack of appropriate training of agents (European Commission, 2013; OCTA, 2011).

Figure 39 shows the correlation between corruption and illicit trade during 2010–2012. From this figure, We examine the relationship between corruption level and the market share of illicit cigarette trade by using the World Bank corruption index and Euromonitor data respectively from 70 countries for 3 years between 2010 and 2012. The corruption level is indexed between −2.5 (the most corrupt) and +2.5 (the least corrupt). Our simple 2 by 2 analysis shows a negative relationship, indicating that higher the corruption level, the higher the share of illicit market for cigarettes.

- *Impact on government revenues*

The primary purpose of levying higher excise taxes from the Ministry of Finance perspective is to generate more revenues. However, their concern is that higher taxes and prices will increase smuggling activity. As tax-induced smuggling increases, demand for legal cigarettes is expected to fall, which will then lead to

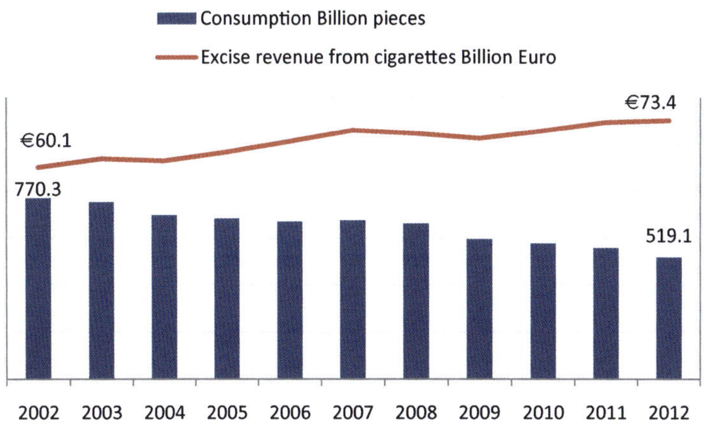

Figure 40. Consumption and excise tax revenues of cigarettes in EU 2002–2012

Source: European Commission July 2013. EU Excise duty tables, tax receipts-manufactured tobacco and release for consumption of cigarettes. http://ec.europa.eu/taxation/index. 2002 consumption data excludes Romania.

lower expected revenues. However, these concerns have typically proven to be unfounded. For example, the EU provides clear evidence to the contrary. Figure 40 shows the correlation between cigarette consumption and excise tax revenues from cigarettes in EU 2002–2012. From this figure, it is known that the EU has among the highest taxes and prices as a region globally and faces illicit trade from neighboring areas, particularly Eastern Europe. Yet even as cigarette consumption has declined, and even smuggling is present revenues from cigarette excise taxes have increased, regardless of the level of smuggling the EU countries face. Two factors played important roles on this trend. First, the EU has implemented strong tobacco control measures as discussed below and those countries that face large illicit trade have reduced the market share of illicit cigarettes dramatically. Second, the level of tax increase has been high enough that it accounts for the loss in consumption and smuggling.

• *Responses to illicit trade*

Many countries have successfully implemented measures to protect tax revenues from both the risk and reality of illicit trade. For example, Brazil and Turkey have been among the most innovative, having implemented automated systems for monitoring cigarette production in the late 2000s. In the case of Brazil, the Ministry of Finance estimates that this measure reduced the amount of evasion by US$100 million in 2008. In 2011, Kenya piloted an electronic cargo tracking system to ensure cigarette exports actually exit Kenya. An evaluation of this pilot project found that tax-paid sales increased by up to 30% in some Western border areas, presumably reflecting a decline in smuggling. The EU and its Member

States have also implemented a broad range of measures to tackle illicit trade including through increased customs corporation among member states. The UK in particular has developed and reviewed sector-wide strategies specifically aimed at addressing illicit trade in tobacco. Indeed, according to Eurmonitor data, illicit cigarette share in the total cigarette market reached almost 27% in 2002 and by 2012, it fell to 12.6% of the total cigarette market. Similar successes have been seen in Italy and Spain, where illicit cigarette shares of the total cigarette market reached 15% to 21% in the mid-1990s, and reduced to 2% to 1% in 2008, respectively (Euromonitor, 2014). At a global level, the Protocol to Eliminate Illicit Trade in Tobacco Products was the first protocol adopted by the Conference of Parties to the WHO Framework Convention on Tobacco Control (WHO FCTC). The Protocol took 4 years to negotiate and was finally adopted by the 5th Conference of Parties in Seoul on 12 November 2012. As of 2014, it is currently open for ratification by the Parties of the WHO FCTC. The Protocol aims to eliminate all forms of illicit trade in tobacco products by requiring Parties to implement a package of national measures to monitor and control supply chain and through the promotion of international cooperation. Supply chain control measure is considered to be the "heart" of the Protocol. The "Tracking and Tracing" provision within the supply chain control measure requires Parties to establish a national or regional tracking and tracing system for all tobacco products that are manufactured or imported into its territory, with the cost of these systems to be borne by the cigarette manufacturers. Other provisions include (i) due diligence (Article 7) requires all natural and legal persons engaged in the supply chain of tobacco, tobacco products and manufacturing equipment to know their customers, that includes monitoring their sales, identifying their intention of use and marketing products, and taking all necessary measures to ensure compliance; (ii) record keeping (Article 9); (iii) security and preventive measures (Article 10); (iv) sales by internet (Article 11); (v) duty free sales (Article 13); and (vi) implementing control measures in free zones and international transit (Article 12) by the Member States (WHO, 2013b).

Affordability of cigarettes

Consumers' decisions to buy cigarettes are influenced by their income and the prices of cigarettes. The combination of income and price determines the affordability of cigarettes. The affordability concept is relevant to tobacco control only when assessed over time in order to compare the changes in consumers' demand for tobacco products within the same population, as opposed to a snapshot across countries. For example, there has been a concern that cigarettes have become more affordable over time in developing countries.

Affordability refers to the amount of resources (not exclusively monetary) or cost required to be able to purchase a certain product (in this case tobacco products). The affordability concept simultaneously considers the net outcome from both the price effect and income effect on tobacco consumption. It holds that the quantity demand of tobacco decreases when the prices of tobacco increase and the quantity demand of tobacco increases when incomes increase. If both tobacco prices and incomes increase, the quantity of demand of tobacco will respond to these simultaneous changes. The net outcome of income and price changes will influence whether cigarettes become more affordable (e.g., when income increases faster than price increases) or less affordable (e.g., when income increases more slowly than price increases).

Conventional studies consider the effect of price and income separately. A limited number of studies have investigated the affordability of cigarettes. Guindon *et al.* (2002) and Kan (2007) defined affordability as the time worked to purchase a pack of cigarettes. Guindon *et al.* (2002) found that cigarettes became less affordable in most countries between 1990 and 2000. Blecher and van Walbeek (2004; 2009) defined the Relative Income Price (RIP) as a broad measure of affordability. The RIP is the percentage of annual per capita Gross Domestic Product required to purchase 100 packs of the cheapest cigarettes. Blecher (2010) used the concept of affordability to assess the risks of aggressive economic growth on tobacco consumption by using a case study of South Africa. He proposed that cigarette taxation should link to the change in affordability (increases in tax should be indexed to inflation and per capita increases simultaneously) rather than targeting the price increases alone (e.g., increases in price could be levelled off by the increases in inflation and/or per capita income) or excise tax incidence alone (e.g., increases in the share of excise — let's say from 30% to 40% of price (such as of producer price, wholesale price or retail price) does not necessarily increase the tax and hence the retail price level if the initial base price is low to start with).

There are various affordability measurements used in the literature, such as the percentage of per capita GDP required to purchase 100 packs of the cheapest cigarettes or RIP (Blecher and van Walbeek, 2004; 2009), the percentage of daily income required to buy a pack of cigarettes (Kan, 2007), the minutes of labor required to purchase the cheapest pack of cigarettes (Guindon *et al.*, 2002), the ratio of GDP per capita to consumer price index of tobacco (Guindon *et al.*, 2010), and the percentage of disposable income per capita required to buy a pack of cigarettes (Hu *et al.*, 2008).

Using price data from the Economist Intelligence Unit and income data from the World Bank we calculate the RIP for as many as 90 countries between 1990 and 2012. Figure 41 shows the average annual change in RIP since 1990.

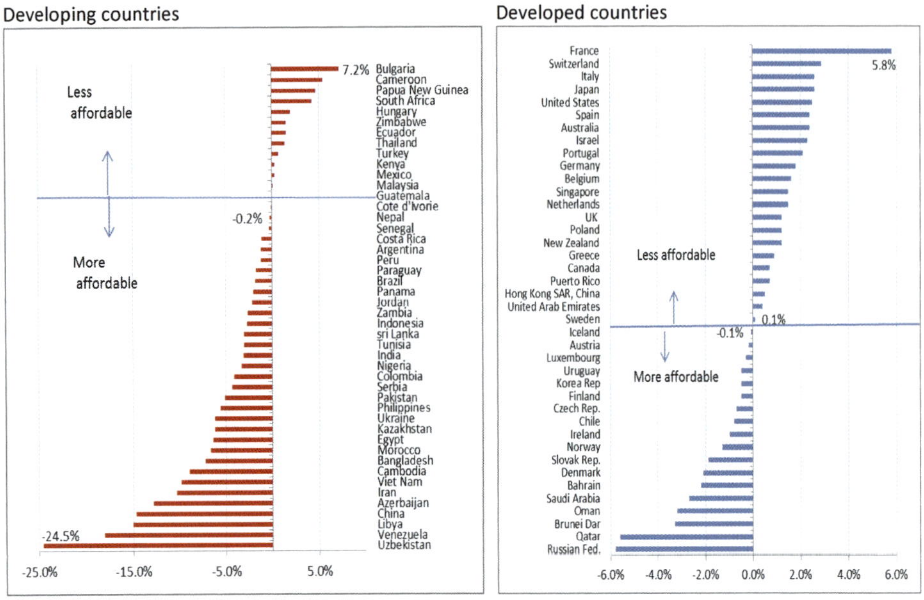

Figure 41. Average annual percentage change in Relative Income Price of cigarettes (1990–2012)

Source: Authors' estimation by EIU database (2013).

A positive value means that cigarettes have, on average, become less affordable in the country. Countries are sorted first by development status (developed vs. developing) and then by the average annual change in affordability.

Cleary, cigarettes have become more affordable in 33 LMICs, and less affordable in only 13, mainly due to the fact that tax-induced retail price increases could not keep pace with the income increases. This is not an encouraging result from a tobacco control perspective. The trend in high-income countries is more encouraging where cigarettes have become less affordable in 22 countries and more affordable in only 18 countries. From a policy perspective it is important to understand what is driving the changes in affordability. For example, cigarettes becoming more affordable in a country could be driven by either declines in real cigarette prices or increases in real income, or because increases in real incomes are greater than increases in real prices. (Please see Figure A.1 for the decomposition of the average annual percentage change of RIP).

South Africa is one of the most well-known cases of the use of tax increases as a tobacco control tool in the developing world. Between 1990 and 2012, real excise taxes rose by 552% leading to an increase in real prices of 217% (Figure 42). The impact of price increases lead to increases in the RIP from 2.0% to 3.8% (Figure 43).

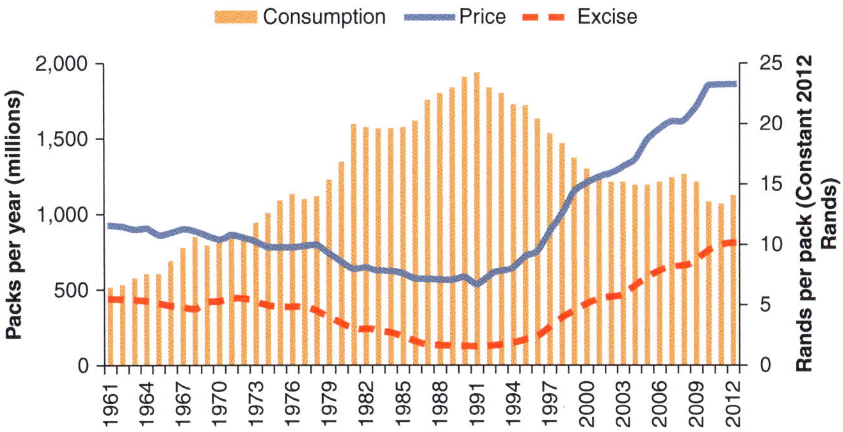

Figure 42. Taxes, prices and cigarette consumption in South Africa 1961–2012
Source: Authors' estimation from data gathered by Ministry of Finance South Africa.

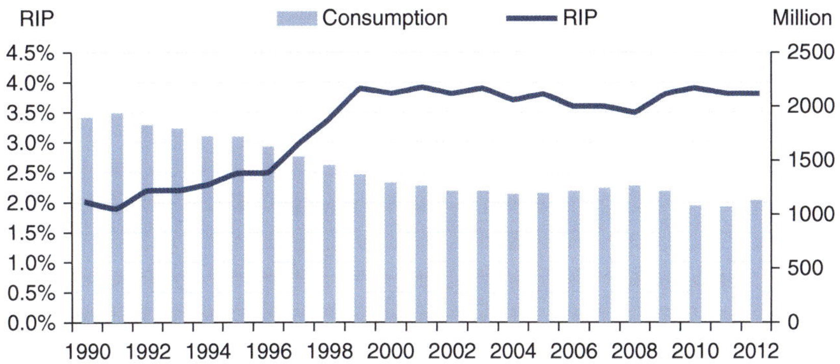

Figure 43. Affordability and cigarette consumption in South Africa 1990–2012
Source: Authors' estimation from data gathered by MoF South Africa and EIU.

Price increases reduced the affordability of cigarettes, and hence led to a reduction in total and per capita cigarette consumption by 41% and 66% respectively. This coincided with a decline in adult smoking prevalence from 32.6% to 20.1% between 1993 and 2012. A notable artifact from the analysis in South Africa is that while excise taxes and prices rose consistently between 1990 and 2012, it did not result in cigarettes becoming consistently less affordable. While cigarettes became less affordable at a rapid rate between 1990 and 1999, stronger economic conditions from 2000 onwards resulted in the RIP becoming more stable. This changes in affordability also coincided with patterns in consumption. When cigarettes were becoming rapidly less affordable the declines in consumption were most rapid. When the affordability measure flattened, the decline in consumption also slowed.

Estimations of RIP income Price over the more recent period from 2008 to 2012 shows more cause for optimism. Data reveal that at a global level and among all income groups, cigarettes are becoming less affordable. The highest decrease in affordability is estimated in low-income countries within 5 years, followed by middle-income countries (Figure 44). Affordability appears to decrease the least in high-income countries, despite higher increases in the average price of cigarettes. That is because increases in GDP/capita is relatively higher than the increases in price, and consequently increases in GDP/capita offset the impact of price increases on affordability (Figure 45).

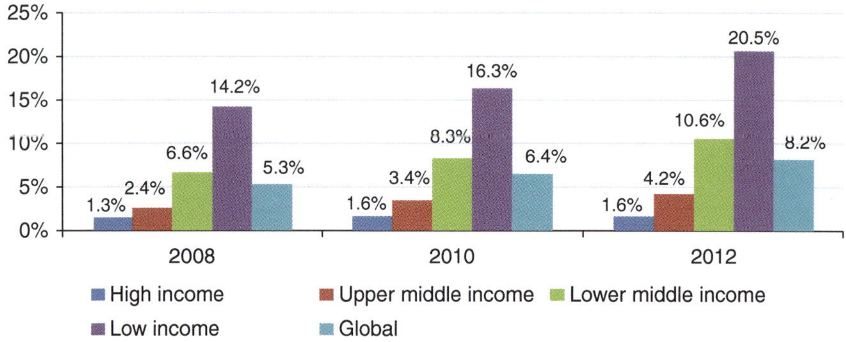

Figure 44. RIP* of cigarettes 2008–2012 by country income

Notes: (*) % GDP per capita to buy 100 packs of most sold brand cigarettes.

Source: Authors' estimation by using prices of most sold brand cigarettes in WHO 2013 Report on Global Tobacco Epidemic.

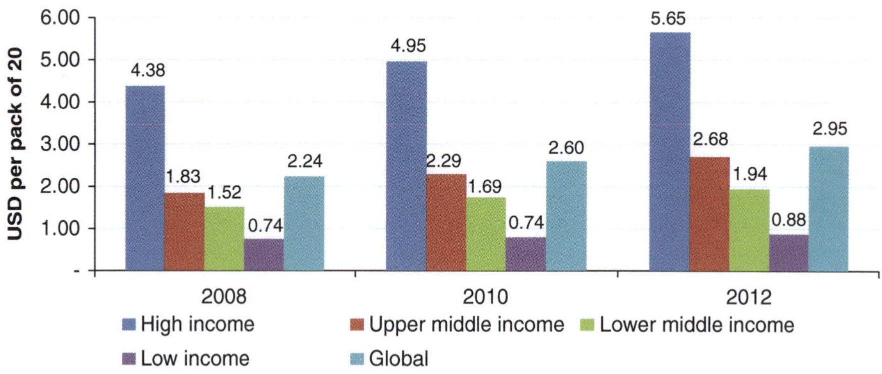

Figure 45. Average price per pack of most sold brand cigarettes, USD in 2008, 2010, 2012

Note: Data from 170 countries, WHO GTCR database.

Source: Authors' estimation by WHO 2009, 2011 and 2013 Reports on Global Tobacco Epidemic, and based on 2012 World Bank income category.

To evaluate the effectiveness of tobacco tax interventions, governments should focus on a comparison of the affordability trend of a country over time. Therefore, to effectively reduce tobacco consumption, governments should raise the taxes and prices of tobacco productions by taking into consideration both inflation rate and the increases in per capita income simultaneously so that they are less affordable over time.

Employment and Farmers

Changing technologies and capitalization with respect to ownerships

A common concern raised against tobacco taxation is that it reduces final demand for tobacco products and thus upstream employment in tobacco growing, manufacturing and distribution. Although tobacco-related employment has been falling over time, this pattern was not driven by tobacco control measures. Global consumption of tobacco products has not fallen nearly enough to reduce employment in the tobacco sector to the extent experienced in many countries. The two main factors that have reduced employment are the introduction of new labor-saving technologies and the privatization of state-owned enterprises (Yürekli *et al.*, 2010).

Moreover, employment tends to be expanding more rapidly in other sectors of the economy such as the service industries. This means that tobacco sector employment can be broadly stable in absolute terms but declining as a share of total employment. This is the case in Indonesia for example, where employment in the tobacco sector has increased in absolute terms from 132,000 in 1970 to 230,676 in 1995 but fallen from 38% to 5.6% as a share of manufacturing employment (de Beyer and Yürekli, 2000). Overall, employment in manufacturing has been increasing much faster than employment in the tobacco industry, as Indonesia's economy has grown and diversified, and greatly reduced its reliance on tobacco for employment.

Another consideration is the part-time and temporary nature of employment in tobacco growing, which contributes to significant underemployment in terms of both hours and income. In Bangladesh, the National Board of Revenue (NBR) undertook a comprehensive enumeration of employment in bidi cigarette manufacturing sector in 2012. In the 198 operating bidi factories, a total of 32,180 persons were found working on factory premises and 134,927 persons were working from home on a contractual basis. The full-time equivalent employment of these two types of workers was estimated at 76,706 persons or 49% of total number of heads employed by bidi industry (WHO, MoF/NBR Bangladesh, 2012).

From a broader macro-economic perspective, the impact on employment from any decrease in final demand for tobacco products from higher taxes will be offset by increased government expenditure and thus upstream employment in other sectors of the economy (Warner *et al.*, 1996; IARC, 2011). Similarly, individuals who quit or reduce their tobacco use can shift their spending to other household goods and services. Most retailers except for specialized tobacconists will be left largely unaffected in aggregate terms. However, aggregate employment may in fact increase as final demand is shifted from the relatively capital-intensive nature of tobacco production to the more labor-intensive production of other goods and services. Nonetheless, tobacco farming is perceived by many developing countries as a means to alleviate poverty, providing employment and cash income to poor farmers.

- *Tobacco farming and crop substitution*

It has been argued that increasing tobacco tax could lead to a reduction in cigarette consumption in the long run, leading to a reduction in demand for tobacco leaf.

It is recognized that successful tobacco control policies should ultimately lead to a reduction in demand for tobacco as a farm or intermediate product. For this reason, Articles 17 and 18 of the WHO Framework Convention on Tobacco Control (FCTC) mandate that signatory countries provide tobacco farmers with viable alternative crops to reduce the amount of land cultivated for tobacco leaf and to enable tobacco farmers to switch to an alternative livelihood. In the 10 years since the WHO FCTC, however, not much progress has been reported in this area by the signatory countries. Individual crop substitution programs exist, and have shown success. But major national efforts to implement these two articles of the FCTC have not been apparent.

Part of the problem lies in the use of informal labor — the use of women and children in tobacco cultivation is common in countries such as Brazil, Indonesia and the African tobacco growing countries. The labor-intensive processes of planting, watering, weeding, harvesting, stringing and hanging the leaves for curing are often done by women and children. In Malawi, for example, it is reported that 30% of the tobacco labor force are children, some as young as 5 years old (Lecours *et al.*, 2012). Farmers can also effectively become bonded or indebted to the industry as it is common practice in many countries for tobacco companies or their affiliates to provide loans or otherwise subsidized inputs for leaf production. However, the real return to farmers once these loans or subsidies are accounted for are low and tends to perpetuate the cycle of poverty and reliance on the tobacco industry.

The economic return of growing tobacco can also be less attractive than other cash crops, as studies have shown (Keyser, 2007), yet tobacco farmers continue in their livelihood. Another important contributing factor is the lack of knowledge and technical support to substitute other cash crops. Coupled with the lack of marketing channels and skills and the possible loss of employment and income, tobacco farmers face numerous hurdles to switch to other crops.

This is an area where government action, as well as assistance from non-government organizations and other civil society organizations, may play an important role. Research to show which crops are suitable substitutes, pilot programs and technical assistance to show the way, loans to farmers to kick-start the initiative, and advocacy for government policies that can promote such crop substitution and protect employment, are all needed if tobacco crop substitution is to have a chance to succeed.

Inflation

Governments are often concerned about the inflationary impact of raising tobacco taxes, especially if they index government spending such as wages, social security and pension payments to inflation. Two key factors can determine the extent to which higher tobacco taxes filter through to measures of inflation. The first is the extent to which higher tax rates will translate into higher cigarettes prices. This differs by country, depending on the share of excise in the final retail price of cigarettes and the size of the increase in the excise tax. The second factor is the weight that is given to tobacco products in the overall basket of goods and services used to measure inflation.

In 2011, for example, the government of Turkey had planned to increase the excise tax on cigarettes from 63% to 69% of retail price, however this tax increase would have raised the inflation rate by 2.5 percentage points. Instead, the government decided to increase the rate to 65% of the retail price to lessen the impact on inflation (Personal communication with MoF Turkey). The weight of cigarettes in the consumer price index was 5.3% and an increase of excise from 63% to 69% of retail price would have led to a 50% increase in the average retail price. In turn, that would have raised the inflation rate by approximately 2.5 percentage points (50% price increases multiplied by 5.3% weight). Although this may not sound high, given Turkey's history battling high inflation, the government's action on excise tax is understandable.

WHO technical manual on tobacco tax administration (2010) has illustrated the inflationary impact of excise tax increases under various combinations of the share of excise tax as percentage of retail price and the weight of cigarettes or tobacco products in the consumer price index, as shown in Table 22.

As illustrated in Section "Tax, Price and Demand for Tobacco Products", Figure 26, at a global average level the share of excise tax as a percentage of retail

Table 22. Inflationary impact of tobacco tax increases

% Share of excise on retail price			Tobacco weight in price index			Inflationary impact		
Low (<40%)	**Medium (40–70%)**	**High (>70%)**	**Low (<2%)**	**Medium (2–4%)**	**High (4–8%)**	**Low (<1.0%)**	**Medium (1.0–2.5%)**	**High (>2.5%)**
×			×			×		
	×		×			×		
		×	×			×		
×				×		×		
	×			×			×	
		×		×			×	
×					×		×	
	×				×		×	
		×			×			×

Note: Midpoints of ranges for tax and tobacco weight are used for computing inflationary impact.
Source: WHO Tax Manual 2010.

price is 45% due to the low share of excise in most developing countries. As a result, the inflationary impact of excise tax increases on cigarettes is expected to be relatively small. Furthermore, for those countries where cigarettes have a higher weight in consumer price indices, as excise tax increases, reduced consumption levels would reduce cigarettes' weight in the CPI and the inflationary impact would be less than expected.

From a public health perspective (Alchin, 1995), and for alleviating the inflationary impact of excise tax increases, one alternative would be excluding tobacco products from the basket of goods used in computing the price index for government spending, as is already done in several countries. For example, tobacco was excluded from price indices used for adjusting minimum wages in France (1992), as well as for services that are linked to wage scale in Belgium (1994) and Luxembourg (1991). In addition, the EU has recommended that its member states exclude tobacco from price indices (Baille, 1998).

Conclusion

While tobacco use has declined in many countries, particularly in most high-income countries, tobacco remains the world's largest source of preventable death, and forms a particular burden for LMICs. The vast majority of the world's current 1 billion smokers worldwide are in LMICs, as well as the majority of annual preventable deaths. The growth of tobacco use in LMICs, particularly among youth and women, remain a major public health concern. As a result, the projected 1 billion deaths in the 21st century is approximately 10 times that of the previous century, with concomitant economic, labor and health care consequences (Eriksen, 2012).

The most important key development in recent years has been the implementation of the first ever global public health treaty, the WHO Framework Convention for Tobacco Control (WHO FCTC) (WHO, 2003). First implemented in 2005, and now ratified by 177 countries, this treaty mandates tobacco use prevention and control policies and programs that have been demonstrated to be effective in reducing tobacco use and its health and economic consequences. This treaty, with the force of law behind it, is a tangible example of using scientifically valid data collection and analysis to help curb the tobacco epidemic and create a more smoke-free society. By 2012, nearly 1 billion people living in 39 countries are covered by two or more of the MPOWER measures at the highest level (e.g., implementation level as discussed in 3.1.1 of the Tobacco Control Section, where the complete/comprehensive implementation of TC laws are given scores of 4 or 5), and the most progress has been made in low-and middle-income countries (WHO, 2013a).

More research remains to be done, particularly on the impact of tobacco use and tobacco control in LMICs, however a clear consensus is starting to emerge on how best to reduce and ultimately end the worldwide tobacco epidemic. While tobacco use remains a multi-dimensional problem with aspects ranging from tax policy to smuggling, we now have the tools to substantially change the current course of public health outcomes. It has become clear that policy interventions, particularly taxation, have now become the most important tools alongside other areas such as education and cessation to reduce the use of tobacco in society. In response to one of the greatest public health crises in human history, we have now developed a strong evidence base and a growing plan of action for countering this problem, with a long road of implementation and research still ahead of us.

Annex

Tobacco Trade

Among developing countries, the middle income groups (Upper Middle and Lower Middle) have both exported and imported significant amount of unmanufactured tobacco, but only the Upper Middle Income group (Table A.1) generated a positive trade balance, and the Lower Middle Income group ended up with a trade deficit by 2012. Low-income countries became the net exporters of unmanufactured tobacco in 2012 and turned the negative (US\$−4.3 billion) trade deficit of 2000 to a positive trade balance by 2012.

Table A 1. Unmanufactured trade value and balance by income group of countries 2000–2012

2012	2012 (Billion $)			2000 (Billion $)			% change 2000–2012	
	Export	Import	Balance	Export	Import	Balance	Export	Import
HI	$3.5	$7.5	−$4.0	$2.4	$5.2	−$2.8	47	45
UMI	$5.4	$3.2	$2.2	$1.8	$1.0	$0.7	204	203
UMI w/o China	$4.7	$2.0	$2.8	$1.6	$0.88	$0.74	192	123
LMI	$1.1	$2.2	−$1.1	$0.4	$0.4	−$0.04	212	437
LI	$1.3	$0.21	$1.1	$0.9	$5.2	−$4.3	39	–96
China	$0.66	$1.2	−$0.54	$0.2	$0.16	−$0.013	334	629

Source: WHO estimation from UN COMTRADE database 2014, and 2012 WB income group categories.

Table A.2. Cigarette trade balance

	2012 (Billion $)			2000 (Billion $)			% change 2012–2000	
	Export	Import	Balance	Export	Import	Balance	Export	Import
HI	$16.0	$18.6	−$2.6	$11.70	$9.40	$2.3	37	97
UMI	$2.6	$1.9	$0.64	$0.70	$0.50	$0.20	266	285
UMI w/o China	$2.1	$1.9	$0.27	$0.58	$0.46	$0.12	267	301
LMI	$1.7	$1.1	$0.67	$0.21	$0.77	−$0.56	720	39
LI	$0.1	$0.4	−$0.29	$0.05	$0.15	−$0.094	97	166
China	$0.5	$0.08	$0.37	$0.16	$0.04	$0.087	259	93

Source: WHO estimation from UN COMTRADE database 2014, and 2012 WB income group categories.

The trade data also reveal another interesting result in China. China is the largest tobacco leaf and cigarette producer in the world. Despite having a negative trade balance for unmanufactured tobacco, China has experienced a positive trade balance on cigarettes.

Affordability

Figure A.1 decomposes the average annual change in Relative Income Prices for cigarettes into price and income components. The countries are ordered on cigarette

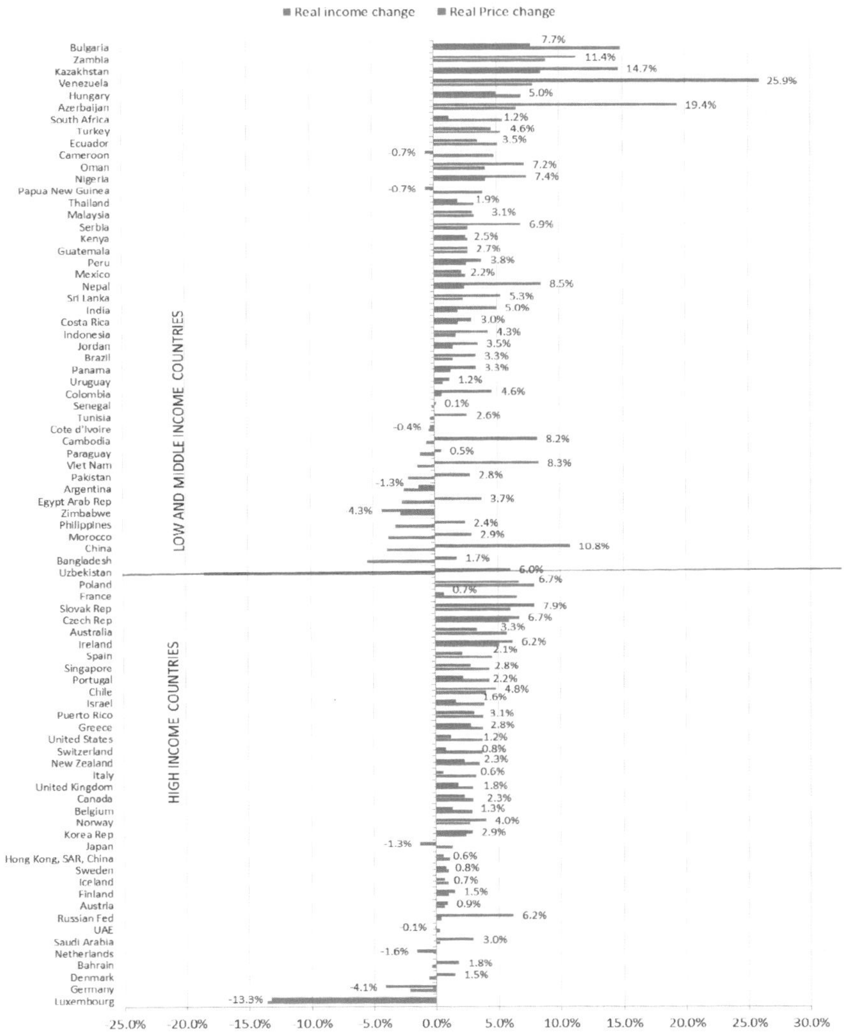

Figure A.1. Decomposition of average annual percentage change in Relative Income Price (1990–2012)

Note: High-income status is based on 2012 World Bank classification.
Source: Authors' estimation from IMF World Economic Outlook and EIU databases.

affordability from those that became less affordable most rapidly from the top to those that have become more affordable most rapidly at the bottom. Data show that 46 countries saw cigarettes, on average, become more affordable, 29 countries saw real prices, on average, increase, and 43 countries saw real incomes increase. On the other hand, 35 countries saw cigarettes become less affordable, of which 32 countries saw real prices increase.

References

Adioetomo S, Djutaharta T, Hendratno. 2005. Cigarette Consumption, Taxation, and Household Income: Indonesia Case Study. *HNP Discussion Paper* — Economics of Tobacco Control Paper, No. 26. Washington DC: The World Bank.

Alchin TM. 1995. A note on tobacco product prices in the Australian CPI. *Applied Economic Letters* 2: 473–477.

Akerlof G. 1991. Procrastination and obedience. *American Economic Review* 81: 1–19.

Arunatilake N, Opatha M. 2003. The Economics of Tobacco in Sri Lanka. *HNP Discussion Paper*, Economics of Tobacco Control Paper, No. 12. Washington DC: World Bank.

Asaria P, Chisholm C, Mathers C, Ezzati M, Beaglehole R. 2007. Chronic disease prevention: Health effects and financial costs of strategies to reduce salt intake and control tobacco use. *The Lancet* 370(9604): 2044–2053.

Baille J. 1998. Baille, L'Union Européenne et la tabac. Thése de Docteur en Médecine. Faculté de médecine de Marseille, Université de la Méditerranée Aix-Marseille II.

Baltagi B, Levin D. 1986. Estimating dynamic demand for cigarettes using panel data: The effects of bootlegging, taxation and advertising reconsidered. *The Review of Economics and Statistics* 68(1): 148–155.

Barber S, Adioetomo SM, Ahsan A, Setyonaluri D. 2008. Tobacco Economics in Indonesia. Paris: International Union Against Tuberculosis and Lung Disease.

Bass F. 1969. A simultaneous equation regression study of advertising and sales of cigarettes. *Journal of Marketing Research* 6: 291–300.

Becker G, Murphy K. 1988. A theory of national addiction. *Journal of Political Economy*, 96: 675–700.

Becker G, Grossman M, Murphy K. 1994. An empirical analysis of cigarette addition. *The American Economic Review* 84(3): 396–418.

Berman M, Crane R, Seiber E, Munur M. 2013. Estimating the cost of a smoking employee. *Tobacco Control* 23(5): 428–433.

Blecher EH. 2010. Targeting the affordability of cigarettes: A new benchmark for taxation policy in low-income and middle-income countries. *Tobacco Control* 19: 325–330.

Blecher EH, van Walbeek CP. 2004. An international analysis of cigarette price affordability. *Tobacco Control* 13: 339–346.

Blecher EH, van Walbeek CP. 2009. Cigarette affordability and trends: An up-date and some methodological comments. *Tobacco Control* 18: 167–175.

Bobak M, Jarvis M, Skodova Z, Marmot M. 2000. Smoke intake among smokers is higher in lower socioeconomic groups. *Tobacco Control* 9(3): 310–312.

Boffetta P, Aagnes B, Weiderpass E, Andersen A. 2005. Smokeless tobacco use and risk of cancer of the pancreas and other organs. *International Journal of Cancer* 114(6): 992–995.

Borren P, Sutton M. 1992. Are increases in cigarette taxation regressive. *Health Economics* 1(4): 245–253.

Centers for Disease Control and Prevention (CDC). 2002. Office on Smoking and Health (OSH). 2002. Tobacco use among youth: A cross country comparison. The Global Youth Tobacco Survey Collaborative Group. *Tobacco Control* 11: 252–270.

Centers for Disease Control and Prevention (CDC). 2004. The health consequences of smoking: a report of the Surgeon General. Washington DC. Department of Health and Human Services, Centers for Diseases Control and Prevention, National Center for Chronic Disease Prevention and Health Promotion, Office on Smoking and Health.

Chaloupka F, Warner KE. 2000. The economics of smoking. In Newhouse J, Culyer A. (eds.). *The Handbook of Health Economics* 1, Part B: 1539–1627.

Chaloupka FJ. 1991. Rational addictive behavior and cigarette smoking. *Journal of Political Economy* 99(4): 722–742.

Chaloupka FJ, Straif K, Leon ME. 2011. Working Group International Agency for Research on Cancer. Effectiveness of tax and price policies in tobacco control. *Tobacco Control* 20(3): 235–238.

Chaloupka FJ, Yürekli AA, Fong G. 2012. Tobacco taxes as a tobacco control strategy. *Tobacco Control* 21: 172–180.

Chaloupka FJ, Kostova D, Shang C. 2014. On behalf of the GATS collaborative group. Cigarette excise tax structure and cigarette prices: Evidence from the Global Adult Tobacco Survey and the US National Adult Tobacco Survey. *Nicotine & Tobacco Research* 16(Suppl 1): S3–S9.

Chapman S, Richardson J. 1990. Tobacco excise and declining tobacco consumption: The case of Papua New Guinea. *American Journal of Public Health* 80(5): 537–540.

Ciecierski C. 2007. The market for legal and illegal cigarettes in Poland: A closer look at demand and supply-side characteristics. *IDRC Working Paper Series*. http://www.idrc.ca/tobacco/ev-84071-201-1-DO_TOPIC.html.

Ciercieski D, Merriman D, Stoklosa M. 2009. Cigarette tax avoidance: Evidence from littered cigarette packs in Warsaw, Poland. (Working paper).

CIET. 2009. *Illegal Trade in Tobacco in MERCOSUR Countries*. Uruguay.

Choi K, Hennrikus D, Forster J, *et al.* 2012. Use of price-minimizing strategies by smokers and their effects on subsequent smoking behaviors. *Nicotine & Tobacco Research* 14(7): 864–870.

Cornelius ME, Driezen P, Fong GT, *et al.* 2014. Trends in the use of premium and discount cigarette brands: Findings from the ITC US surveys (2002–2011). *Tobacco Control* 23: i48–i53.

Cragg JG. 1971. Some statistical models for limited dependent variables with application to the demand for durable goods. *Econometrica* 39(5): 829–844.

Crawford I, Keen M, Smith S. 2010. Value added tax and excises. In Mirrlees J, Adam S, Besley T, Blundell R, Bond S, Chote R, Gammie M, Johnson P, Myles G, Poterba J (eds.). *Dimensions of Tax Design: The Mirrlees Review.* Oxford University Press for Institute for Fiscal Studies.

David A, Esson K, Perucic AM, Fitzpatrick C. 2010. Tobacco use: Equity and social determinants. In: Blas E, Sivasankara Kurup A (eds.). *Equity, Social Determinants and Public Health Programmes*. World Health Organization.

de Beyer J, Yürekli AA. 2000. Curbing the tobacco epidemic in Indonesia. Watching Brief. East Asia and the Pacific Region. World Bank 6.

DeCicca P, Kenkel D, Liu F. 2010. Excise tax avoidance: The case of state cigarette taxes. *National Bureau of Economic Research, Inc, NBER Working Papers*.

Doll R, Peto R, Boreham J, Sutherland I. 2004. Mortality in relation to smoking: 50 years' observations on male British doctors. *British Medical Journal* 328(7455): 1519.

Efroymson D, Ahmed S, Townsend J, Alam SM, Dey AR, Saha R, Dhar B, Sujon AI, Ahmed KU, Rahman O. 2001. Hungry for tobacco: An analysis of the economic impact of tobacco consumption on the poor in Bangladesh. *Tobacco Control* 10(3): 212–217.

Eriksen M, MacKay J, Ross H. 2012. *Tobacco Atlas, 4th Edition* American Cancer Society and World Lung Foundation.

Euromonitor 2012. Illicit trade in tobacco products: Will the new protocol prove effective? *Euromonitor International.*

Euromonitor 2014. Types of tobacco sales and production data from 2007–2012. *Euromonitor International.*

European Commission. 2013. Communication from the Commission to the council and the European Parliament. Stepping up the fight against cigarette smuggling and other forms of illicit trade in tobacco products. A comprehensive EU strategy. European Union, Brussels.

Evans WM, Farrelly MC. 1998. The compensating behavior of smokers: Taxes, tar, and nicotine. *RAND Journal of Economics* 29: 578–595.

FAO. 2014. FAOSTAT. Food and Agricultural Commodities Production. Accessed 17 March 2014. Available from: http://faostat.fao.org/site/339/default.aspx.

FAO. 2014. FAOSTAT. Food and Agricultural Trade. Accessed 17 March 2014. Available from: http://faostat.fao.org/site/342/default.aspx.

Fichtenberg CM, Glantz SA. 2000. Association of the California Tobacco Control Program with declines in cigarette consumption and mortality from heart disease. *The New England Journal of Medicine* 343(24): 1772–1777.

Fix BV, Hyland A, O'Connor RJ, *et al.* 2014. A novel approach to estimating the prevalence of untaxed cigarettes in the USA: Findings from the 2009 and 2010 international tobacco control surveys. *Tobacco Control* 23: i61–i66.

Fong GT, Hammond D, Laux FL, Zanna MP, Cummings KM, Borland R, Ross H. 2004. The near-universal experience of regret among smokers in four countries: Findings from the International Tobacco Control Policy Evaluation Survey. *Nicotine and Tobacco Research* 6(Suppl 3): S341–S351.

Gao S, Zheng R, Hu T-W. 2012. Can increases in cigarette tax rate be linked to cigarette retail prices? Solving mysteries related to the cigarette pricing mechanism in China. *Tobacco Control* 21(6): 560–562. Doi:10.1136/tobaccocontrol-2011-050027.

GATS 2008–2014. Global Adult Tobacco Survey. Global Tobacco Surveillance System Data. Centers for Disease Control, Office on Smoking and Health.

GATS Factsheet Bangladesh. 2009. Global Adult Tobacco Survey (GATS).

GATS Factsheet Egypt. 2009. WHO Global Adult Tobacco Survey (GATS).

GATS Factsheet India. 2009–2010. WHO Global Adult Tobacco Survey (GATS).

GATS Factsheet Indonesia. 2011. WHO Global Adult Tobacco Survey (GATS).

GATS Factsheet Qatar. 2013. WHO Global Adult Tobacco Survey (GATS).

GATS Factsheet Thailand. 2011. WHO Global Adult Tobacco Survey (GATS).

GHK. 2009. A study on liability and the health costs of smoking: Final report. DG SANCO of European Commission (2008/C6/046).

Gilmore AB, Reed H. 2014. The truth about cigarette price increases in Britain. *Tobacco Control* 23:(e15–e16). Doi:10.1136/tobaccocontrol-2013-051048.

Goel RK. 2008. Regulatory bottlenecks, transaction costs and corruption: A cross-country investigation. *BOFIT Discussion Papers 10/2008, Bank of Finland, Institute for Economies in Transition 10.*

Guindon GE, Nguyen TTH, Hoang VK, McGirr E, Trung DV, Nguyen LT. 2010. Tobacco taxation in Vietnam. *International Union Against Tuberculosis and Lung Disease. Paris, France.*

Guindon Ge S, Tobin S, Yach DD. 2002. Trends and affordability of cigarette prices: ample room for tax increases and related health gains. *Tobacco Control* 11(1): 35–43.

Guindon GE, Driezen P, Chaloupka FJ, *et al.* 2014. Cigarette tax avoidance and evasion: Findings from the International Tobacco Control Policy Evaluation Project. *Tobacco Control* 23: i13–i22.

Gruber J. 2003. Smoking's internalities. *Regulation*: 52–57.

Gruber J, Köszegi BB. 2004. Tax incidence when individuals are time inconsistent> the case of cigarette excise taxes. *Journal of Public Economics* 88(9–10): 1959–1988.

Global Youth Tobacco Survey Collaborative Group (GYTS). 2002. *Tobacco Control* 11(3): 252–270.

Hill C. 2013. Cancer prevention and screening. *Bulletin du Cancer* 100(96): 547–554.

Hanewinkel R, Isensee B. 2007a. Access to cheaper cross-border cigarettes may decrease smoking cessation intentions in Germany. *Tobacco Control* 16: 70–1.

Hanewinkel R, Isensee B. 2007b. Five in a row — reactions of smokers to tobacco tax increases: Population-based cross-sectional studies in Germany 2001–2006. *Tobacco Control* 16: 34–37.

Houthakker HS, Taylor LD. 1970. *Consumer Demand in the United States 1929–1970: Analyses and Projections*. Harvard University Press, Cambridge.

Hu TW, Mao Z. 2002. Effects of cigarette tax on cigarette consumption and the Chinese economy. *Tobacco Control* 11: 105–108.

Hu T-w, Mao Z, Liu Y, de Beyer J, Ong M. 2005. Smoking, standard of living, and poverty in China. *Tobacco Control* 14: 247–250.

Hu T-w, Moa Z, Shi J, *et al.* 2008. *Tobacco taxation and its potential impact in China.* International Union Against Tuberculosis and Lung Disease (The Union), Paris–France.

Her majesty's Revenues and Customs. (HRMC). 2000. *Tackling Tobacco Smuggling London, March 2000.* available at http://www.hmce.gov.uk.

Her Majesty's Revenue and Customs. 2006. *New responses to new challenges: Reinforcing the Tracking Tobacco Smuggling Strategy.* London.

Huang J, Zheng R, Chaloupka FJ, *et al.* 2014. Chinese smokers' cigarette purchase behaviors, cigarette prices and consumption: Findings from the ITC China Survey. *Tobacco Control* 23: i67–i72.

Hyland A, Laux FL C. Higbee C, Hastings G, Ross H, *et al.* 2006. Cigarette purchase patters in four countries and the relationship with cessation: findings from the International Tobacco Control (ITC) Four Country Survey. *Tobacco Control* 15 (Suppl 3): iii59–iii64.

International Agency for Research on Cancer (IARC) 2011. *IARC Handbooks of Cancer Prevention, Tobacco Control.* Volume 14: Effectiveness of tax and price policies in tobacco control. Lyon, France.

Jha P, Chaloupka FJ, Moore J, Gajalakshmi V, Gupta PC, Peck R, Asma A, Zatonski W. 2006. Tobacco Addiction. In Jamison D, *et al.* (eds.). *Disease Control Priorities in Developing Countries. 2nd Edition.* Washington (DC): World Bank.

Jha P, Guindon E, Joseph R, Nandi A, John RM, Rao K, Chaloupka FJ, Kaur J, Gupta CG, Rao MG. 2011. *Economic and Political Weekly* 46(42): 44–51.

Jha P, Peto R. 2014. Global effects of smoking, quitting and of taxing tobacco. *New England Journal of Medicine* 370(1): 60–68 doi: 10.1056/NEJMra1308383.

John RM. 2008. Crowding out effect of tobacco expenditure and its implications on household resource allocation in India. *Social Science & Medicine* 66(6): 1356–1367.

John, RM, Sung H-Y, Max W. 2008a. The economic cost of tobacco use in India, 2004. *Tobacco Control* 18: 138–143.

John, RM, Rao RK, Rao MG, *et al.* 2010. *The Economics of Tobacco and Tobacco Taxation in India.* Paris, International Union Against Tuberculosis and Lung Disease.

Joseph RA, Chaloupka FJ. 2014. The influence of prices on youth tobacco use in India. *Nicotine & Tobacco Research* (Suppl 1): 24–29.

Joossens l, Merriman D, Ross H, Raw M. 2010. The impact of eliminating the global illicit cigarette trade on health revenue. *Addiction* 105: 1640–1695.

Joossens L, Gilmore A, Gallus S. 2010a. PPACTE — WP2 European Survey: Pricing Policies and Control of Tobacco in Europe (PPACTE), www.ppacte.eu.

Joossens L, LugoA, Vecchia C, Gilmore A, Clancy L, Gallus S. 2012. Illicit cigarettes and hand rolled tobacco in 18 European countries: A cross-section survey. *Tobacco Control.* Doi 10.1136/tobaccocontrol-2012-050644.

Kan MY. 2007. Investigating cigarette affordability in 60 cities using the cigarette price-daily income ratio. *Tobacco Control* 16(6): 429–432.

Karki Y, Pant K, Pande P. 2003. A study on the economics of tobacco in Nepal, *HNP Discussion Paper Series. Economics of Tobacco Control Paper No. 13,* Washington DC, The World Bank.

Keen M. 1998. The balance between specific and ad valorem taxation. *Fiscal Studies* 19 (1): 1–37.

Keyser J. 2007. Crop substitution and alternative crops for tobacco. A technical document for the first meeting of the *Ad Hoc* Study Group on Alternative Crops established by the Conference of the Parties to the WHO Framework Convention for Tobacco Control.

Kostova D, Tesche J, Perucic AM, Yurekli AA, Asma A. 2013. Exploring the relationship between cigarette prices and smoking among adults: A cross-country study of low-and-middle-income nations. *Nicotine and tobacco research* 16(1): S10–S15.

KPMG, Study on the collection and interpretation of data concerning the release for consumption of cigarettes and fine-cut tobacco for rolling of cigarettes. Brussels: KPMG Belgium (2005, 2012).

Lakhdar CB. 2008. Quantiative and qualitative estimates of cross-border tobacco shopping and tobacco smuggling in France. *Tobacco Control* 17: 12–16. Doi:10.1136/tc.2007.020891.

Laxminarayan R, Deolalikar A. 2004. Tobacco initiation, cessation, and change: Evidence from Vietnam. *Health Economics* 13: 1191–1201.

Lecours N, Almeida GEG, Abdallah JM, Novotny TE. 2012. Environmental health impacts of tobacco farming: A review of the literature. *Tobacco Control* 21: 191–196 doi: 10.1136/tc-2011-050318.

Levy DT, Bauer JE, Lee HR. 2006. Simulation modelling and tobacco control: Creating more robust public health policies. *American Journal of Public Health* 96(3): 494–498.

Levy DT, Ellis JA, Mays D, Huang AT. 2013. Smoking-related deaths averted due to three years of policy progress. *Bulletin of the World Health Organization* 91: 509–518.

Licht AS, Hyland AJ, O'Connor RJ, *et al.* 2011. How do price minimizing behaviors impact smoking cessation? Findings from the International Tobacco Control (ITC) Four Country Survey. *International Journal of Environment Research and Public Health* 8: 1671–1691.

Lightwood JM, Glantz SA. 1997. Short-term economic and health benefits of smoking cessaiotn. Myocardial infarction and stroke. *Circulation* 96: 1089–1096. doi:10.1161/01.CIR.96.4.1089.

Lightwood JM, Collins D, Lapsley H, Novotny TE. 2000. Estimating the costs of tobacco use. In: Jha P, Chaloupka FJ. (eds.). *Tobacco Control in Developing Countries*. Oxford: Oxford University Press.

Liu Y, Rao K, Hu T-W, Sun Q, Mao Zhenzhong. 2006. Cigarette smoking and poverty in China. *Social Science & Medicine* 63: 2784–2790.

Mackay J, Amos A. 2003. Women and tobacco. *Respirology (Carlton, Vic.)* 8: 123–130.

Merriman D. 2010. The micro-geography of tax avoidance: Evidence from littered cigarette packs in Chicago. *American Economic Journal: Economic Policy* 2(2): 61–84(24).

MoF, NBR Bangladesh 2010. A joint internal document on excise tax system and the consequences to Bangladesh economy, prepared in collaboration with WHO and National Board of Revenue.

MoF Brazil 2009. Federal Revenue Secretariat, Production Control, Track and Trace System, Presentation at WHO Geneva.

MoF, FBR, Pakistan–WHO, 2009. Federal Board of Revenue (FBR), Ministry of Finance. Excise Duty Assessment on Cigarettes in Pakistan — An analysis by Baloch AA, Khoso MA, Kamboh GN. (Internal MoF document).

MoF Philippines 2012: MoF, Department of Finance (DoF) and WHO collaborative work and internal document on Philippines excise tax system and a way forward, prepared jointly by WHO and DoF/MoF.

Moore M. 1996. Death and tobacco taxes. *RAND Journal of Economics* 27(2): 415–428.

Nagelhout GE, van den Putte B, Allwright S, *et al.* 2014. Socioeconomic and country variations in cross-border cigarette purchasing as tobacco tax avoidance strategy. Findings from the ITC Europe Surveys. *Tobacco Control* 23: i30–i38.

Nargis N, Fong GT, Chaloupka FJ, *et al.* 2014a. The choice of discount brand cigarettes: A comparative analysis of International Tobacco Control surveys in Canada and the USA (2002–2005). *Tobacco Control* 23: i86–i96.

Nargis N, Ruthbah UH, Ghulam Hussain AKM, Fong G, Huq I, Ashiquzzaman. 2014b. The price sensitivity of cigarette consumption in Bangladesh: Evidence from the

International Tobacco Control (ITC) Bangladesh wave 1 (2009) and wave 2 (2010) surveys. *Tobacco Control* 23(01): i139–147. Doi:10.1136/tc-2012-050835.

Ng M, Freeman MK, Fleeming TD, Robinson M, Dwyer-Lindgren L, Thomson B, Wollum A, Sanman E, Wulf S, Lopez AD, Murray CJL, Gakidou E. 2014. Smoking prevalence and cigarette consumption in 187 countries, 1980–2012. *The Journal of the American Medical Association* 311(2): 183–192. Doi:10.1001/jama.2013.284692.

Nikaj S, Chaloupka FJ. 2014. The effect of prices on cigarette use among youths in the Global Youth Tobacco Survey. *Nicotine & Tobacco Research* (suppl 1): S16–S23.

Öberg M, Jaakkola MS, Woodward A, Peruga A, Prüss-Ustün A. 2011. Worldwide burden of disease from exposure to second-hand smoke: A retrospective analysis of data from 192 countries. *Lancet* 377(9760): 139–146. Doi:10.1016/S0140-6736(10)61388-8.

OCTA. 2011. EU Organized Crime threat Assessment. Europol. *02-Analysis & Knowledge.* The Hague, 28/04/11. File no. 2530-274.

Önder Z. 2002. The economics of tobacco in Turkey: New evidence and demand estimates. *HNP Discussion Paper Series*, Economics of Tobacco Control Paper No. 2, Washington DC, World Bank.

Önder Z, Yürekli AA. 2014. Who pays the most cigarette excise tax in Turkey? *Tobacco Control* doi:10.1136/tobaccocontrol-2014-051639.

Orphanides A, Zervos D 1995. Rational addiction with learning and regret. *Journal of Political Economy* 103(4): 739–758.

Oshfeldt RL, Boyle RG. 1994. Tobacco excise taxes and rates of smokeless tobacco use in the US: An exploratory ecological analysis. *Tobacco Control* 3: 316–323.

Ohsfeldt RL, Boyle RG, Capilouto EI. 1997. Effects of tobacco excise taxes on the use of smokeless tobacco products. *Health Economics* 6: 525–532.

Ohsfeldt RL, Boyle RG, Capilouto EI. 1998. Tobacco taxes, smoking restrictions, and tobacco use. *NBER Working Paper No. 6486*, National Bureau of Economic Research.

Owen D, Bassett S, Lane C, Mumssen C, Weisfeld H, Fassina S, Ishikawa S. 2001. Georgia: Recent Economic Developments and Selected Issues. IMF Country Reports, No. 211.

Parry I. 2003. On the costs of excise taxes and income taxes in UK. *International Tax and Public Finance* 10: 281–304.

Pekurinen MJ. 1989. The demand for tobacco products in Finland. *British Journal of Addiction* 84: 1183–1192.

Pekurinen MJ. 1991. Economic Aspects of Smoking: Is There a Case for Government Intervention in Finland? National Agency for welfare and Health. Research reports 16. Helsinki: Vapk-Publishing.

Peto R, Lopez A, Boreham J, Thun M. 2006. Mortality from smoking in developed countries 1950–2000. 2nd ed. International Union Against Cancer. Geneva, Switzerland.

Pigou AC. 1932. The economics of welfare. (Macmillan and Company, London. 4th edition.

Ramos A. 2009. Illegal trade in tobacco in MERCOSUR countries. *Centro de Investigacion de la epidemia de tabaquismo (CIET-Uruguay). Working Paper.* http://www.fctc.org/dmdocuments/INB3_report_illegal_trade_in_MERCOSUR.pdf.

Ranson K, Jha P, Chaloupka FJ, Son N. 2000. The effectiveness and cost-effectiveness of price and other tobacco control policies. In: Jha P, Chaloupka F. (eds.). *Tobacco Control in Developing Countries*. Oxford, Oxford University Press.

Remler DK. 2004. Poor smokers, poor quitters and cigarette tax regressivity. *American Journal of Public Health* 94(2): 225–229.

Ross H, Trung DV, Phu VX. 2007. The costs of smoking in Viet Nam: The case of inpatient care. *Tobacco Control* 16(6): 405–409.

Ross H, Shariff S, Gilmore A. 2008. The economics of tobacco and tobacco taxation in Russia. Paris, International Union Against Tuberculosis and Lung Disease.

Sarkar M, Kapur S, Frost-Pineda K, Feng S, Wang J, Liang Q, Roethig H. 2008. Evaluation of biomarkers of exposure to selected cigarette smoke constituents in adult smokers switched to carbon-filtered cigarettes in short-term and long-term clinical studies. *Nicotine & Tobacco Research* 10(12): 1761–1772.

Shang C, Chaloupka FJ, Kostova D. 2014, Who quits? An overview of quitters in low- and middle-income countries. *Nicotine & Tobacco Research* 16(Suppl 1): S44–S55.

Stehr M. 2005. Cigarette tax avoidance and evasion. *Journal of Health Economics* 24: 277–297.

Stotsky J, Woldemariam. 2002. A Central American tax reform: Trends and possibilities. *IMF Working Paper Series*, No: 02/227.

Suhrcke M, Arce RS, McKee M, Rocco L. 2008. Economic costs of ill health in the European Region. In: Figueras J, McKee M (eds.). *Health Systems, Health, Wealth and Societal Well-Being: Assessing the Case for Investing in Health Systems*. WHO Regional Office for Europe and European Observatory on Health Systems and Policies.

Sung H, Wang L, Jin S, Hu T-W, Jian Y. 2006. Economic burden of smoking in China. *Tobacco Control* 15(Suppl 1): i5–i11. doi:10.1136/tc.2005.015412.

Sweis N, Chaloupka FJ. 2013. The economics of tobacco use in Jordan. *Nicotine and Tobacco Research* 15(Suppl 1): S30–S36.

Taal A, Kiivet R, Hu T-W. 2004. The economics of tobacco in Estonia. World Bank Economics of Tobacco Control Paper No. 19. Washington DC: World Bank.

Thompson ME, McLeod I. 1976. The effects of economic variables upon the demand for cigarettes in Canada. *Math Sci* 1: 121–132.

Townsend J, Roderick P, Cooper J. 1994. Cigarette smoking by socioeconomic group, sex, and age: effects of price, income, and health publicity. *British Medical Journal* 309(6959): 923–927.

Tsai Y, Sung H, Yang C, Shih S. 2003. The behavior of purchasing smuggled cigarettes in Taiwan. *Tobacco Control* 12(1): 28–33.

Warner K, Fulton G, Nicolas P, Grimes D. 1996. Employment implications of declining tobacco product sales for the regional economies of the United States. *The Journal of the American Medical Association* 275(16): 1241–1246.

Waters H, Saenz de Miera, Ross H, *et al.* 2010. *The economics of tobacco and tobacco taxation in Mexico*. Paris, International Union Against Tuberculosis and Lung Disease.

White JS, Li J, Hu TW, *et al.* 2014. The effect of cigarette prices on brand-switching in China: A longitudinal analysis of data from the ITC China survey. *Tobacco Control* 23: i54–i60.

USDHEW, *Smoking and Health: Report of the Advisory Committee to the Surgeon General of the Public Health Service.* Washington, United States Department of Health, Education and Welfare (1964).

United Nations Secretariat 2012. *Population Division of the Department of Economic and Social Affairs of the United Nations Secretariat, World Population Prospects: the 2012 Revision.* New York, United Nations.

Viscusi W. 1995. Cigarette taxation and the social consequences of smoking. *Tax Policy and the Economy* 9: 51–102.

Wang H, Sindelar J, Busch S. 2006. The impact of tobacco expenditure on household consumption patterns in rural China. *Social Science & Medicine* 62(6): 1414–1426.

World Bank 1999. *Curbing the Epidemic. Governments and the Economics of Tobacco Control* In Jha P, Chaloupka FJ. (eds.). Washington DC, World Bank.

World Bank. 2014. Health Nutrition and Population Statistics Database. http://data.worldbank.org/data-catalog/health-nutrition-and-population-statistics.

WCO. 2012. Annual Report 2011–12. World Customs Organization. 2012. www.wcoomd.org.

WHO 2002. Reducing risks, promoting healthy life. *World Health Report 2002.* World Health Organization, Geneva, Switzerland.

WHO. 2003. *Framework Convention on Tobacco Control.* World Health Organization 2003. Geneva Switzerland.

WHO. 2005. *Impact of Tobacco-Related Illnesses in Bangladesh.* In Zaman MM, Nargis N. (eds.). Dhaka, Bangladesh, World Health Organization 2005.

WHO 2006. *World No Tobacco Day Brochure: Tobacco: Deadly in Any Form or Disguise*, World Health Organization 2006. Geneva, Switzerland.

WHO. 2008. The MPOWER Package. *WHO Report on the Global Tobacco Epidemic: World Health Organization, 2008. Geneva, Switzerland.*

WHO. 2010a. *Gender, Women and the Tobacco Epidemic.* In Samet J, Young SY. (eds.). World Health Organization, 2010 Geneva, Switzerland.

WHO. 2010b, *WHO Technical Manual on Tobacco Tax Administration*, In Yürekli AA, Delipalla S, Chaloupka FJ, Perucic AM. (eds.). World Health Organization 2010. Geneva, Switzerland.

WHO. 2012. Warning about the dangers of tobacco. *WHO Report on the Global Tobacco Epidemic.* World Health Organization 2012, Geneva Switzerland.

WHO, MoF/NBR Bangladesh 2012. Biris employment in Bangladesh In Nargis N, Huq MS, Z aman MM, Ahmed N, and Ministry of Finance/National Bureau of Revenue (eds.). World Health Organization 2012.

WHO. 2012b. *WHO Global Report: Mortality Attributable to Tobacco.* World Health Organization 2012 Geneva, Switzerland.

WHO. 2013a. Enforcing Bans on Tobacco Advertising, Promotion and Sponsorship. *WHO Report on the Global Tobacco Epidemic.* World Health Organization 2013, Geneva, Switzerland.

WHO 2013b. Protocol to eliminate illicit trade in tobacco products. WHO Framework Convention on Tobacco Control (FCTC). Geneva, Switzerland.

WHO. 2014a. *WHO Tobacco Tax Training Material*. World Health Organization 2014, Geneva, Switzerland.

WHO 2014b. *Tobacco Taxes and Saving Lives*. World Health Organization 2014, Geneva, Switzerland.

Yamasaki A, Chinami M, Suzuki M, Kaneko Y, Fujita D, Shirakawa T. 2005. Tobacco and alcohol tax relationships with suicide in Switzerland. *Psychological Reports* 97(1): 213–216.

Yao T, Huang J, Sung H-Y, *et al.* 2014. Who purchases cigarettes from cheaper sources in China? Findings from the ITC China Survey. *Tobacco Control* 23: i97–i101.

Young D, Borland R, Hammond D, *et al.* 2006. Prevalence and attributes of roll-your-own smokers in the International Tobacco Control (ITC) Four Country Survey. *Tobacco Control* 15(Suppl. III); iii: 76–82.

Young D, Yong HH, Borland R, Shahab L, Hammond D, Cummings KM, Wilson N. 2012. Trends in roll-your own smoking: Findings from the ITC Four-Country Survey (2002–2008). *Journal of Environmental and Public Health*. Vol no. 2012, Article ID 406283. http://dx.doi.org/10.1155/2012/406283.

Young D, Wilson N, Borland R, Edwards R, Weerasekera D. 2010. Prevalence, correlates of, and reasons for using roll-your-own tobacco in a high RYO use country: Findings from the ITC New Zealand survey. *Nicotine and Tobacco Research* 12(11): 1089–1098.

Yürekli A, Saygınsoy Ö. 2008. Worldwide organized cigarette smuggling: An empirical analysis. *Applied Economics* 42(5): 545–561.

Yürekli AA, Önder Z, Elibol M, Erk N, Cabuk A, Fisunoğlu M, Erk S, Chaloupka FJ. 2010. The economics of tobacco and tobacco taxation in Turkey. International Union against Tuberculosis and Lung Disease Paris, France.

Health Effects of Alcohol Consumption

Catherine Lau and Alex Lau
Carthage College

Humans have consumed alcohol for centuries for social, religious, and medicinal reasons. Production and sale of alcoholic beverages are important contributors to GDP for many countries around the globe. Since alcohol is a normal good, consumption increases as income increases. Empirical evidence supports this positive relationship between consumption and income on both a micro and macroeconomic level, which means that economic growth fosters greater use of alcohol. In moderate amounts, alcohol can have a positive effect on physical and mental health, but over-imbibing has serious health and societal effects and imposes a significant economic toll on society. Various policies have been formulated by governmental agencies to combat the negative effects of alcohol consumption: This chapter analyzes the costs and benefits of the main policies employed globally.

Keywords: Alcohol Consumption; Binge Drinking; Moderate Consumption; Public Health Perspective; Direct Costs; Indirect Costs; Health Benefits.

Introduction

The World Health Organization (WHO) defines alcohol as a "psychoactive substance with dependence-producing properties" (WHO, 2014), while *The Economist* (2001) reports that beer may be the foundation of western civilization. Immediately, we see there is a dichotomy in views on alcohol and its place in society, which makes formulating and implementing policies to control its consumption difficult.

From a public health perspective, alcohol consumption contributed to almost 6% of all deaths globally (3.3 million), and just over 5% of the global burden of disease and injury could be attributed to alcohol consumption in 2012. The harm caused is determined by the amount of alcohol consumed, the pattern of drinking, and to a lesser extent, the quality of the alcohol consumed. Consumption of alcohol is linked to over 200 diseases and injury conditions, the foremost being alcohol dependence, cirrhosis of the liver, cancers and injury (WHO, 2014).

Besides these direct negative effects of alcohol, there are a multitude of indirect costs to society, which include loss of productivity, higher unemployment, and reduced earnings potential. There are also intangible costs to excessive alcohol use, such as lower quality of life for both the alcohol-dependent person and their family. The full cost to society is substantial, estimated to vary from between 1.3% for the lowest country measured (Thailand) to 3.3% of gross domestic product for the country with the highest cost (WHO, 2014) (Rehm *et al.*, 2009).

It is clear that alcohol has been consumed throughout history, and has been praised for its medicinal qualities. A primary reason for the domestication of cereal crops may have been to produce beer. Wine was mixed with water by the Romans both to provide a thirst quencher and to make the water safe to drink. It is a source of nutrients/calories, has analgesic and antiseptic properties, and is used as medicine. It is also seen as a social lubricant, a relaxer, an enhancement to food. Some believe that "it has always been misused by a minority of drinkers, [but] it has proved to be beneficial to most" (Hanson, 1995). However, this notion is open for debate.

In Europe, alcohol is viewed as an accompaniment to meals and can symbolize the importance of an event or the division between work and leisure (Anderson and Baumberg, 2006). This pattern of drinking is important when we look at alcohol in a public health context: Moderate drinking with food has been found to lower coronary heart disease (CHD) and blood pressure and have a positive effect on lipids, and drinking with food may reduce alcohol absorption while speeding alcohol elimination from the body (Rehm *et al.*, 2003)

Since alcohol consumption has such strong roots in human culture and its first uses supposedly had positive health benefits, parsing out the overall health effects of alcohol consumption and recommending public policies that will curtail the negative effects without eliminating the positive attributes is a complicated process.

Public opinion of alcohol consumption has evolved over the centuries and has directly impacted policy implementation. The ambivalence toward alcohol's harms is highlighted by Room, who points out that the indices of three prominent epidemiology texts have 42 references to cigarette smoking yet only three for alcohol (Room, 1984). Efforts taken to since 1980 in OECD countries, including restrictions on alcohol advertising and sales as well as taxes, have had mixed results, with overall consumption down but increases in the UK, Ireland, and Nordic countries, and perhaps more troublesome, increases in heavy episodic and binge drinking (OECD, 2011).

Alcohol is an imbedded part of most cultures around the globe today and accounts for significant portions of GDP in most regions, which makes the task of controlling its harm seem Sisyphean. In this chapter, we will attempt to give a balanced view of the topic, highlighting the benefits of light to moderate alcohol consumption for a portion of the population and the harms of certain consumption patterns and any consumption for certain people, and we will incorporate the most recent and relevant empirical findings to make policy suggestions, being mindful of cultural differences around the globe.

Drinking Levels Definitions

Since the effects of alcohol consumption are closely linked to the amount of alcohol consumed, it is important to begin by defining the more commonly used terminology for various consumption levels.

The National Institute on Alcohol Abuse and Alcoholism (NIAAA) in the United States specifies three categories: Moderate alcohol consumption, binge drinking, and heavy drinking. Moderate drinking is up to 1 drink per day for women and up to 2 drinks per day for men. Binge drinking brings blood alcohol concentration (BAC) levels to 0.08 g/dL in about two hours, which is typically after 4 drinks for women and 5 drinks for men. Heavy drinking is drinking 5 or more drinks on the same occasion on each of 5 or more days in the past 30 days.

Global Alcohol Market: An Overview

The global alcohol consumption data reported in this chapter are taken from the Global Status Report on Alcohol and Health, 2014 Edition, published by the World Health Organization (WHO).[1] This WHO Report provides historical data as well as projections on various alcohol consumption metrics for each of its member countries. It also provides aggregate data for different WHO regions and World Bank (WB) country income groups. For aggregate data, the WHO report uses population reports from the United Nations (UN) to calculate population-weighted averages.

When presenting data in this chapter, in some cases, data directly from the WHO report will be used. In other instances, alcohol consumption data from the Global Information System on Alcohol and Health (GISAH) and UN population data will be used to perform calculations to arrive at information that is relevant for the chapter. In both cases, the sources of data will be clearly identified. The UN population data come from the UN Department of Economic and Social Affairs, Population Division (2013), World Population Prospects: The 2012 Revision, DVD Edition.

---

[1]The English version of this report may be downloaded from the WHO website at this link: http://www.who.int/substance_abuse/publications/global_alcohol_report/en/. The underlying data for the report may be obtained from the WHO Global Information System on Alcohol and Health (GISAH), in Microsoft Excel, HTML, and other electronic formats at this link: http://apps.who.int/gho/data/node.main.GISAH?lang=en.

Alcohol consumption levels are presented using the same indicator used by the WHO report — alcohol per capita consumption (APC). The WHO defines APC as the per capita amount of alcohol consumed in liters of pure alcohol in a given population (WHO Report, p. 28). Most of the available alcohol consumption data have been collected and compiled for individuals aged 15 years and older (15+). However, for 2010, separate alcohol consumption data are available for those aged between 15 and 19 years. This presents interesting opportunities to further analyze alcohol consumption levels and patterns in this adolescent group, as well as the ability to perform similar analyses only on individuals aged 20 years and older.

The WHO also makes the distinction between recorded and unrecorded alcohol. The WHO defines unrecorded alcohol as "alcohol that is not taxed in the country where it is consumed because it is usually produced, distributed and sold outside the formal channels under government control.[2]

With regard to the electronic database which we constructed using data from GISAH and the UN, we were able to replicate the data in the published WHO report for each member country's 2010 profile, specifically each country's population and percentage of alcohol consumption by type of alcoholic beverages. Corrections to a country's World Bank income group designation was made wherever necessary to match the designation as published in the WHO report. Aggregate summary data presented in this chapter, unless otherwise specifically noted, are those calculated using our own database.

Total and per capita alcohol consumption, 2010

In 2010, globally, over 32.3 billion liters of pure alcohol were consumed by just over 5 billion individuals aged 15+. Of that total, 24.5 billion liters were recorded alcohol, while 7.8 billion liters (24% of the total) were unrecorded alcohol.

Following table shows the WHO region codes and their respective region names:

WHO Region Code	WHO Region Name
AFR	African Region
AMR	Region of the Americas
EMR	Eastern Mediterranean Region
EUR	European Region
SEAR	South-East Asia Region
WPR	Western Pacific Region

[2]See WHO Report, p. 30, Box 13, for more detailed explanation of unrecorded alcohol.

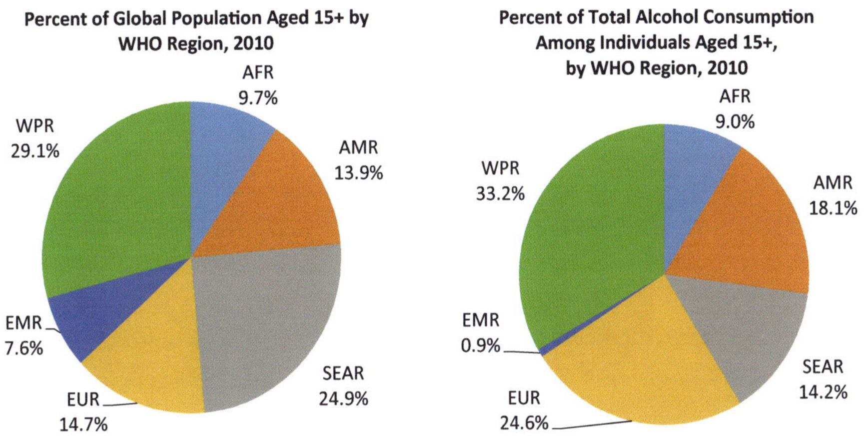

Figure 1. Percent of global population and percent of total alcohol consumption by WHO Region, 2010

Sources: WHO GISAH and UN Department of Economic and Social Affairs, Population Division (2013), World Population Prospects: The 2012 Revision, DVD Edition.

WPR accounted for about 33% of total alcohol consumption worldwide in 2010 (see Figure 1). This is not surprising at this level of analysis because China, which is in this region, accounted for over 22% of the world's 15+ population, and almost 26% of the world's total alcohol consumption in 2010. The EUR region, with the second highest total volume consumption among WHO regions, had the highest alcohol consuming level relative to its population size, with 14.7% of the world's 15+ population, and 24.6% of the world's total alcohol consumption. The EMR region consumed the least amount of alcohol among all WHO regions in 2010. This is consistent with historical trends, both in terms of total consumption and per capita consumption. As noted in the WHO Report, differences in alcohol consumption levels and patterns among the WHO regions are manifestations of differences in many social, economic, demographic and cultural factors.

Figure 2 shows the actual total number of liters (in billions) of pure alcohol consumed in each WHO region in 2010. It shows a different perspective of total alcohol consumption from the pie charts in percentage terms in Figure 1. It also provides a convenient visual transition to our next chart, in Figure 3, where we show the breakdown of total alcohol consumption between recorded and unrecorded alcohol in 2010 among the WHO regions.

It is noteworthy that the EMR region's unrecorded alcohol consumption was slightly higher than its recorded alcohol consumption (i.e., unrecorded alcohol consumption was 51.7% of total alcohol consumption), and that in the SEAR Region, unrecorded alcohol consumption in 2010 was 45.3% of total alcohol consumption, almost the same amount in total liters of pure alcohol as recorded alcohol

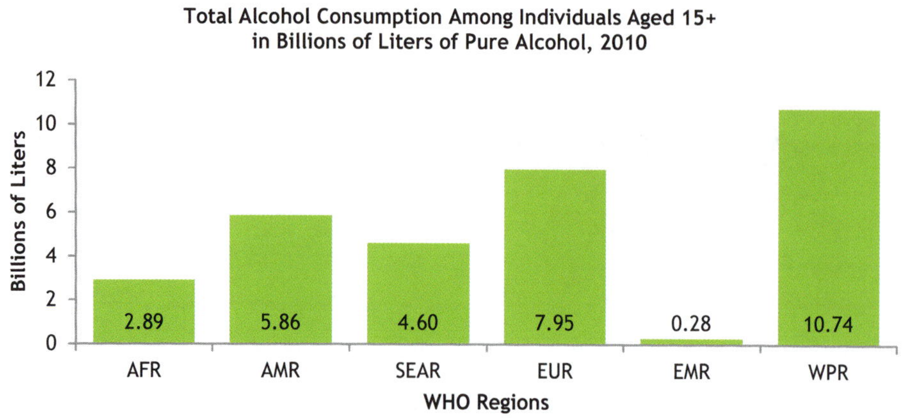

Figure 2. Total alcohol consumption by WHO Region, 2010

Sources: WHO GISAH and UN Department of Economic and Social Affairs, Population Division (2013), World Population Prospects: The 2012 Revision, DVD Edition.

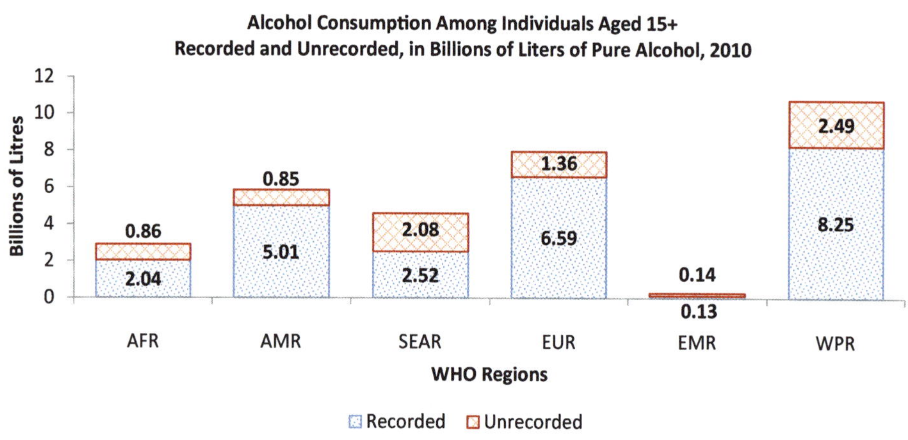

Figure 3. Recorded and unrecorded alcohol consumption by WHO Region, 2010

Sources: WHO GISAH and UN Department of Economic and Social Affairs, Population Division (2013), World Population Prospects: The 2012 Revision, DVD Edition.

consumption. The WHO report attributes this large proportion of unrecorded alcohol relative to total alcohol consumption to the facts that: (1) In many low-income and lower-middle-income countries in the SEAR region, home-made alcohol consumption is a significant portion of total alcohol consumption, and that (2) in some countries where alcohol is officially banned, as is the case in some Islamic states in the EMR Region, unrecorded alcohol consumption is often 100%, or close to 100%, of total alcohol consumption.

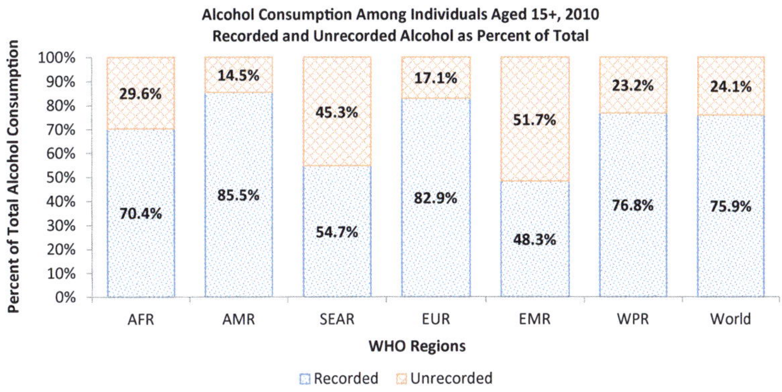

Figure 4. Recorded and unrecorded alcohol consumption as percent of total alcohol consumption, by WHO Region, 2010

Sources: WHO GISAH and UN Department of Economic and Social Affairs, Population Division (2013), World Population Prospects: The 2012 Revision, DVD Edition.

In the AMR and the EUR regions, unrecorded alcohol consumption in 2010 accounted for only 14.5% and 17.1% of total alcohol consumption, respectively (see Figure 4). Alcohol consumption by country income level will be examined later in this section. It is worth noting here, however, that in the AMR and EUR regions, about 90% of the aged 15+ populations live in high-income or upper-middle-income countries.

On a per capita basis, globally, individuals aged 15 years and older consumed on average 6.4 liters of pure alcohol in 2010. This population-weighted average is derived from total (i.e., the sum of recorded and unrecorded) alcohol per capita (APC) consumption data from each of the WHO member countries and UN population data for those countries. As can be expected, the total APC in the different WHO regions vary widely from the global 6.4 liter average. Figure 5 shows each WHO region's total APC and the world's total APC for 2010, while Figure 6 presents the same data with the respective breakdowns between recorded and unrecorded alcohol.

In contrast to Figures 2 and 3, which showed the WPR region with the highest total alcohol consumption level, followed by the EUR Region in second place, Figures 5 and 6 show that, on a per capita basis, the EUR Region had the highest total APC consumption in 2010, followed by the AMR Region. This again suggests that populations in higher-income countries tend to consume more alcohol.

We now turn our attention to alcohol consumption by World Bank (WB) country income group, and explore how total alcohol consumption breaks down

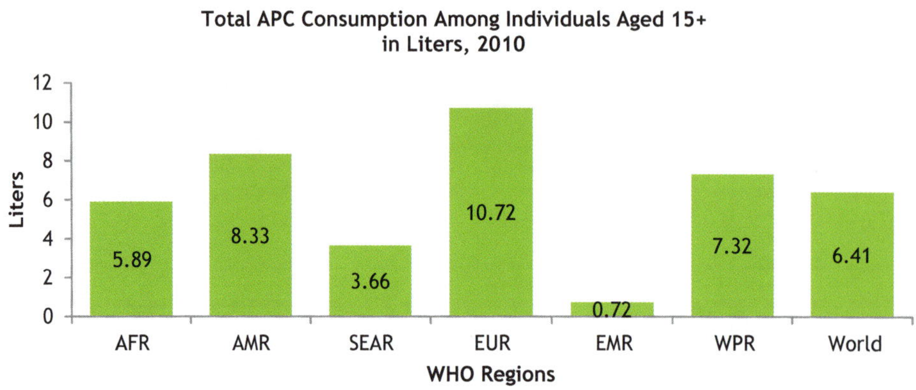

Figure 5. Total APC consumption by WHO Region, 2010

Sources: WHO GISAH and UN Department of Economic and Social Affairs, Population Division (2013), World Population Prospects: The 2012 Revision, DVD Edition.

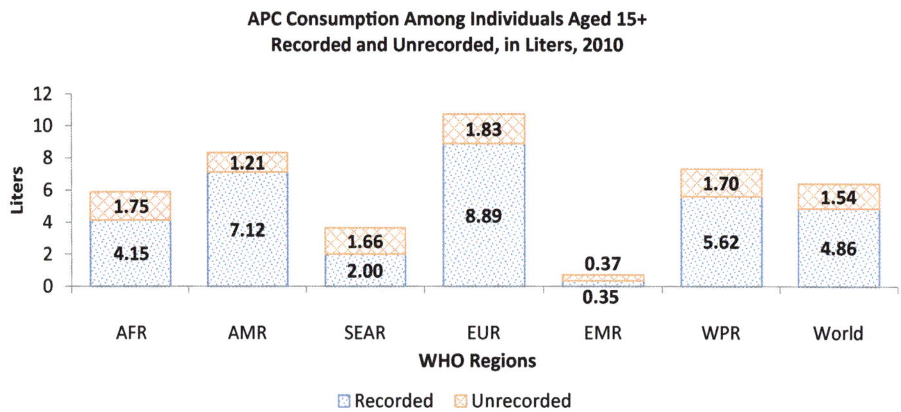

Figure 6. Recorded and unrecorded APC consumption by WHO Region, 2010

Sources: WHO GISAH and UN Department of Economic and Social Affairs, Population Division (2013), World Population Prospects: The 2012 Revision, DVD Edition.

among those income groups. Following table shows the WB country income group codes and their respective names:

WB Income Group Code	WB Income Group Name
LI	Low-Income
LMI	Lower-Middle-Income
UMI	Upper-Middle-Income
HI	High-Income

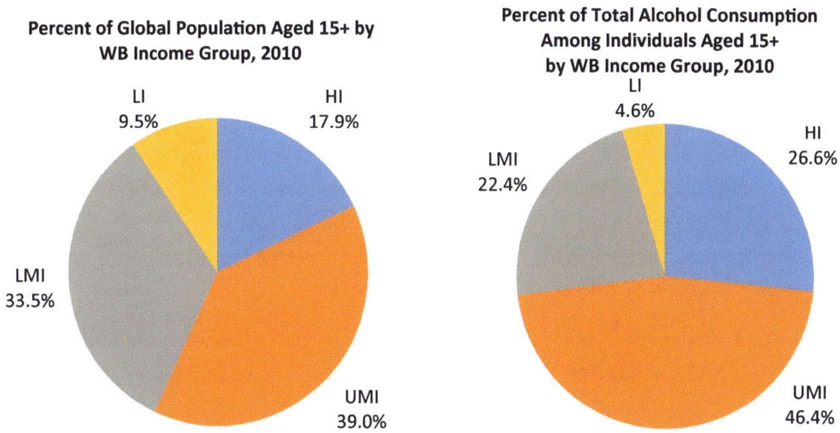

Figure 7. Percent of global population and percent of total alcohol consumption by WB Income Group, 2010

Sources: WHO GISAH and UN Department of Economic and Social Affairs, Population Division (2013), World Population Prospects: The 2012 Revision, DVD Edition.

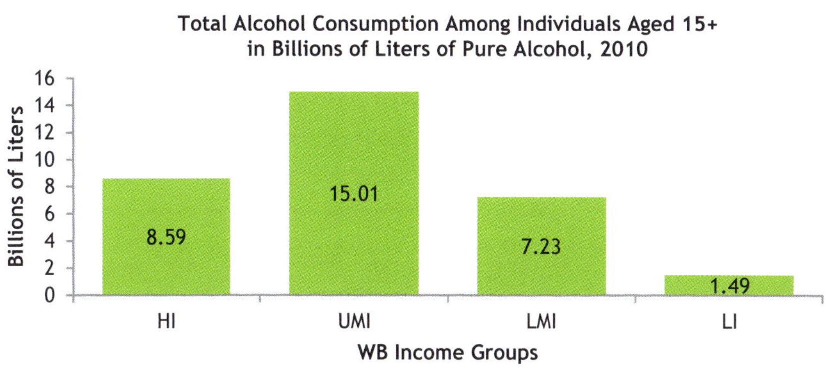

Figure 8. Total alcohol consumption by WB Income Group, 2010

Sources: WHO GISAH and UN Department of Economic and Social Affairs, Population Division (2013), World Population Prospects: The 2012 Revision, DVD Edition.

The pie charts in Figure 7 confirm that, at least globally, countries in the two higher income groups (i.e., the HI and UMI groups) did consume disproportionately more alcohol in 2010 than countries in the two lower income groups. Figure 8 shows the actual total number of liters (in billions) of pure alcohol consumed in each WB income group in 2010, which confirms what we saw in the pie charts in Figure 7, from a different perspective.

Figure 9 shows the same consumption totals broken down into recorded and unrecorded alcohol components. Of interest in this chart is the information that not

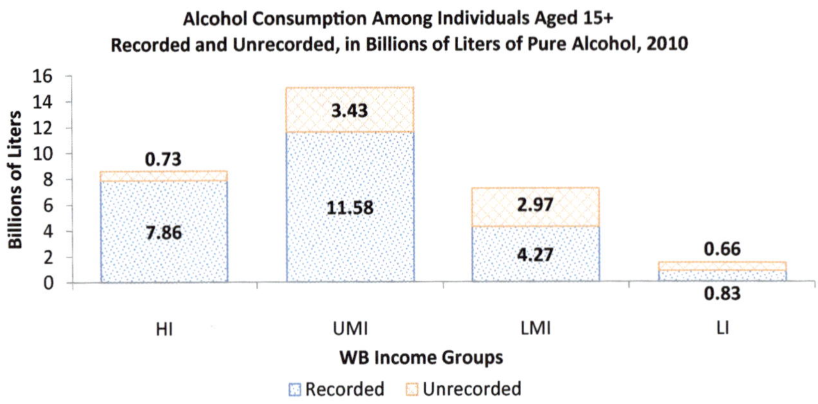

Figure 9. Recorded and unrecorded alcohol consumption by WB Income Group, 2010

Sources: WHO GISAH and UN Department of Economic and Social Affairs, Population Division (2013), World Population Prospects: The 2012 Revision, DVD Edition.

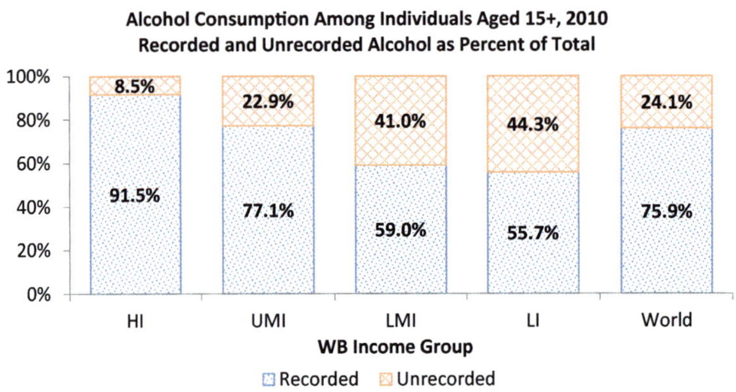

Figure 10. Recorded and unrecorded as percent of total alcohol consumption, by WB Income Group, 2010

Sources: WHO GISAH and UN Department of Economic and Social Affairs, Population Division (2013), World Population Prospects: The 2012 Revision, DVD Edition.

only did HI and UMI countries consume more alcohol than the LMI and LI countries, the HI and UMI countries together consumed both recorded and unrecorded alcohol in greater quantities than the LMI and LI countries combined.

However, within WB income groups, unrecorded alcohol consumption in both LMI and LI exceeded over 40% of their respective total consumption (see Figure 10). In contrast, the HI countries consumed only 8.5% of their alcohol in the form of unrecorded alcohol, and UMI countries had just under 23% of their alcohol consumption in the form of unrecorded alcohol.

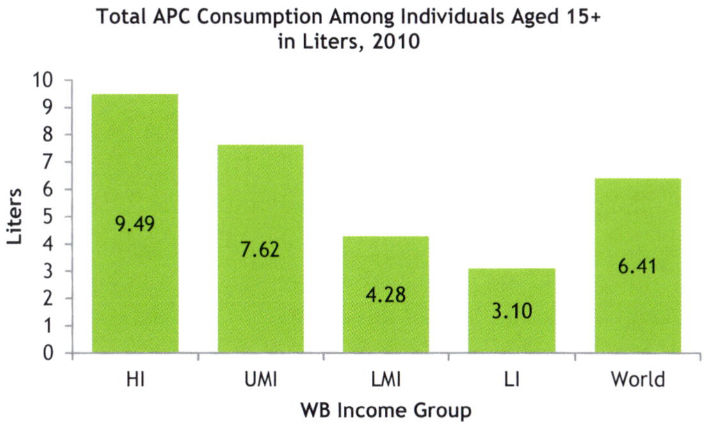

Figure 11. Total alcohol per capita (APC) consumption by WB Income Group, 2010

Sources: WHO GISAH and UN Department of Economic and Social Affairs, Population Division (2013), World Population Prospects: The 2012 Revision, DVD Edition.

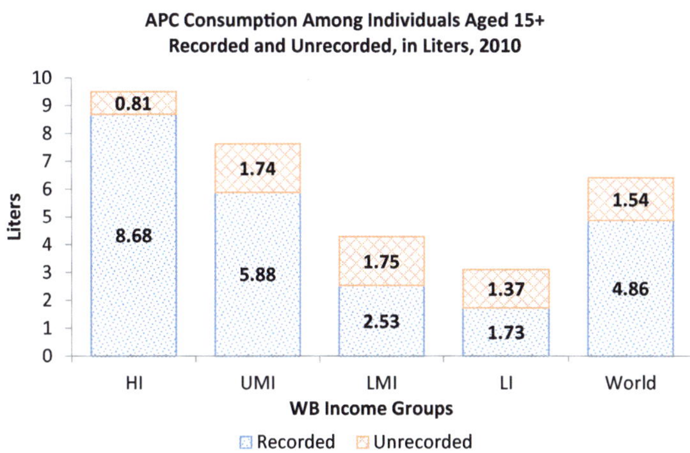

Figure 12. Recorded and unrecorded alcohol per capita (APC) consumption by WB Income Group, 2010

Sources: WHO GISAH and UN Department of Economic and Social Affairs, Population Division (2013), World Population Prospects: The 2012 Revision, DVD Edition.

The correlation between income level and level of alcohol consumption is best highlighted in Figure 11, which shows the APC consumption by WB income group in 2010. Higher income countries did not just consume more alcohol in terms to total quantities; they also consumed more alcohol per capita.

With regard to per capita consumption of recorded relative to unrecorded alcohol, Figure 12 shows that higher income countries consumed more recorded alcohol in 2010 relative to other income groups, generally consistent with the direct correlation exhibited in Figure 11 on total APC consumption. For unrecorded alcohol, however, the UMI and LMI groups consumed about the same number of liters per capita, while those in the LI group slightly less. Those in the HI income group consumed less than 50% of unrecorded APC consumption of the UMI and LMI groups. Note that Figure 9 above showed that the HI group consumed 0.73 billion liters of pure alcohol in 2010. That represented only about 20% and 25% of total unrecorded alcohol consumption in the UMI and LMI groups in 2010, respectively. The numbers in Figure 12 are consistent with those shown in Figure 9 because the HI group made up only about 18% of the world's 15+ population in 2010, while the UMI and LMI groups each made up over 30% of that world population.

Total and per capita alcohol consumption, change from 2005 to 2010

in 2005, globally, over 27.5 billion liters of pure alcohol were consumed by about 4.7 billion individuals aged 15+. Of that total, 19.3 billion liters were recorded alcohol, while 8.2 billion liters (30% of the total) were unrecorded alcohol. Going from 2005 to 2010, the world saw an 8.1% increase in its aged 15+ population, and a 17.5% increase in total alcohol consumption.

Figure 13 shows the percentage of the world's population in each WHO region and the percentage of total alcohol consumption in 2005. Comparing this pair of pie charts to those in Figure 1, which shows the same data for 2010, we can see that while the world's population increased from 2005 to 2010, each region's share of the world's population remained relatively stable. The share of the world's total alcohol consumption, however, saw some notable changes.

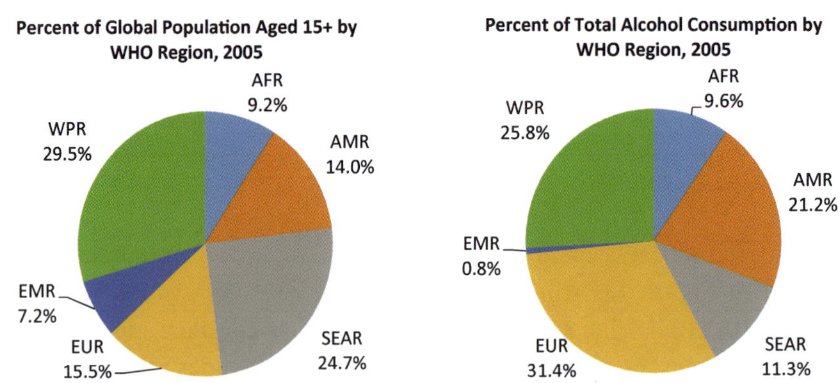

Figure 13. Percent of global population and percent of total alcohol consumption by WHO Region, 2005

Sources: WHO GISAH and UN Department of Economic and Social Affairs, Population Division (2013), World Population Prospects: The 2012 Revision, DVD Edition.

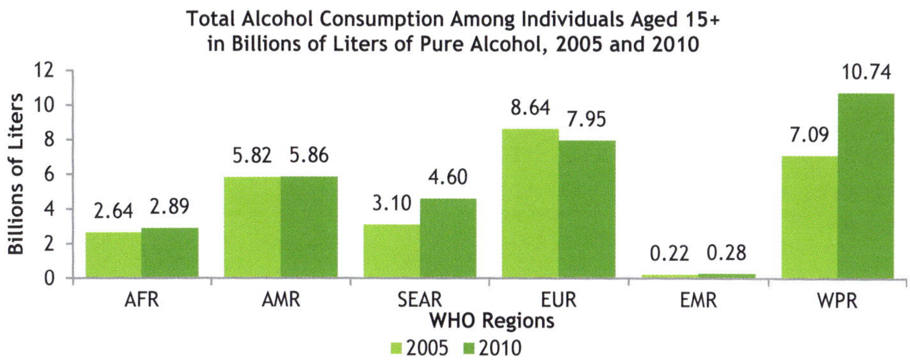

Figure 14. Total alcohol consumption, by WHO Region, 2005 and 2010

Sources: WHO GISAH and UN Department of Economic and Social Affairs, Population Division (2013), World Population Prospects: The 2012 Revision, DVD Edition.

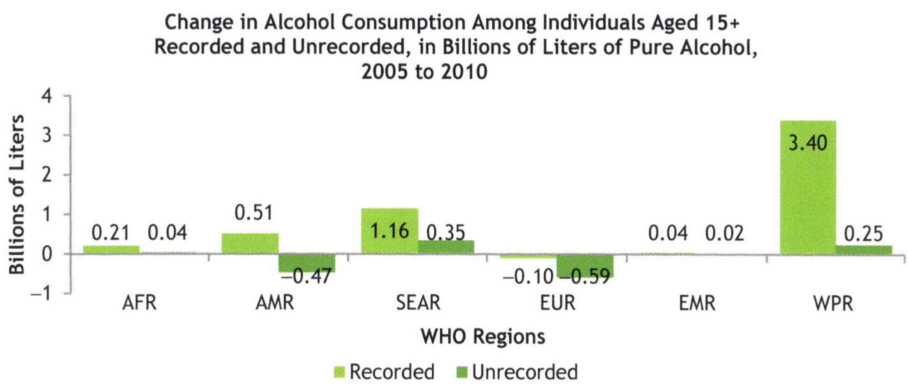

Figure 15. Change in recorded and unrecorded alcohol consumption by WHO Region, 2005 to 2010

Sources: WHO GISAH and UN Department of Economic and Social Affairs, Population Division (2013), World Population Prospects: The 2012 Revision, DVD Edition.

The SEAR region's share of total alcohol consumption went from 11.3% in 2005 to 14.2% in 2010, while that of the WPR region increased from 25.8% to 33.2% during that same period. Those percentage share gains evidently were made at the expense of the EUR (from 31.4% down to 24.6% of the world's total alcohol consumption) and AMR (from 21.2% down to 18.1%) regions. From Figure 14, however, we can see that much of those gains were due to significant increases in total alcohol consumption in the SEAR and WPR regions. The EUR region did experience a decline in the actual quantity of alcohol consumed from 2005 to 2010, while the AFR, AMR and EMR regions all showed modest increases in total consumption during that same period. Specifically, as shown in Figure 15,

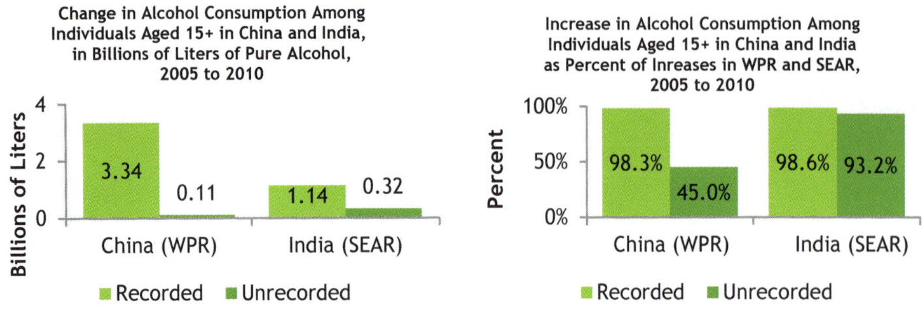

Figure 16. Change in recorded and unrecorded alcohol consumption in China and India, 2005 to 2010

Sources: WHO GISAH and UN Department of Economic and Social Affairs, Population Division (2013), World Population Prospects: The 2012 Revision, DVD Edition.

EUR saw a decline of 690 million liters of pure alcohol consumption between 2005 and 2010, of which about 590 million liters were unrecorded alcohol. The AMR region also saw a significant drop in unrecorded alcohol consumption, though that was offset by an increase in recorded alcohol consumption.

While fair warning should be noted about using data from individual countries, especially on unrecorded alcohol consumption, it is important when citing the dramatic increases in alcohol consumption between 2005 and 2010 in the WPR and in the SEAR regions to point out that China (in WPR) and India (in SEAR) accounted for most of the increases in those two regions.

Figure 16 shows that between 2005 and 2010, China's consumption of recorded alcohol increased by 3.34 billion liters of pure alcohol, which accounted for 98.3% of the WPR region's increase. China also accounted for 45% of the WPR region's increase in unrecorded alcohol consumption in the same period. In the case of India, its increase in recorded and unrecorded alcohol consumption between 2005 and 2010 accounted for 98.6% and 93.2% of the SEAR region's increase in that period. In no other region of the world did any one country dominate its region's change in alcohol consumption to the same extent as China and India did in their respective regions.

With regard to the changes in alcohol consumption among the WHO regions on a per capita basis, it is useful to see the actual population sizes in each region in 2005 and 2010, to help maintain proper perspective on the APC data. It would also help our understanding of the changes in APC consumption to see the percentages changes of total populations and total alcohol consumption in the WHO regions over that time period. Changes in APC consumption are affected by both the changes in quantities of alcohol consumed and changes in the 15+ population. Figure 17 shows that every WHO Region experienced population increase from

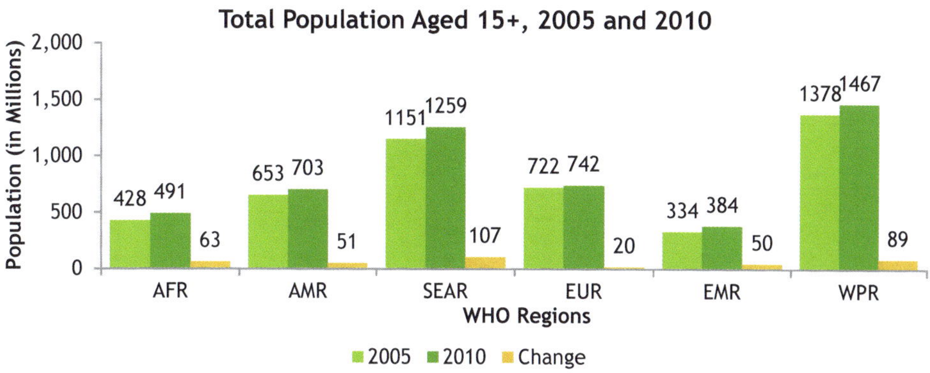

Figure 17. Total population aged 15+ by WHO Region, 2005 and 2010

Sources: WHO GISAH and UN Department of Economic and Social Affairs, Population Division (2013), World Population Prospects: The 2012 Revision, DVD Edition.

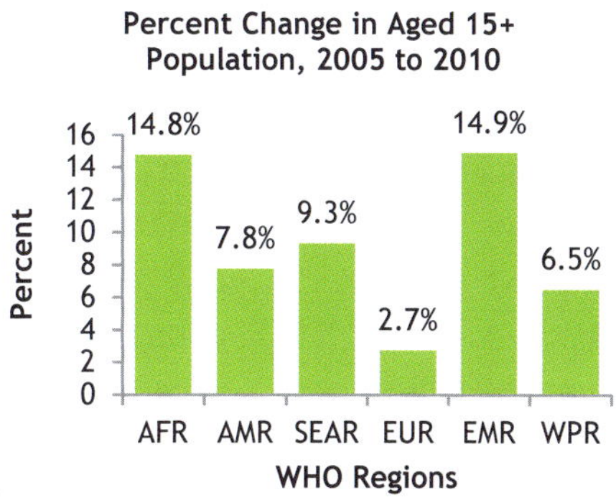

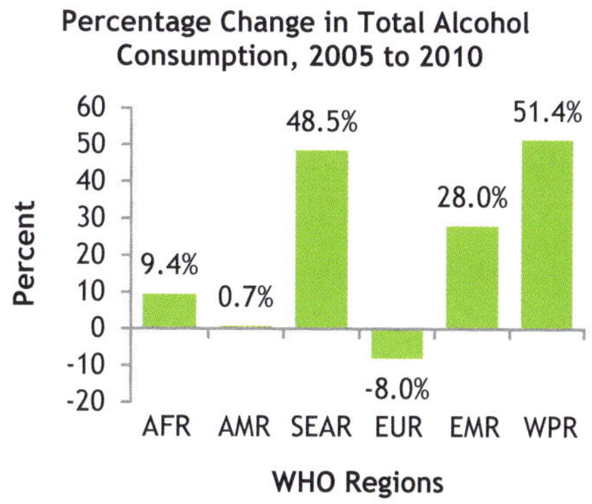

Figure 18. Percent change in aged 15+ population and percent change in total alcohol consumption, by WHO Region, 2005 to 2010

Sources: WHO GISAH and UN Department of Economic and Social Affairs, Population Division (2013), World Population Prospects: The 2012 Revision, DVD Edition.

2005 to 2010 in the 15+ age group, with the largest changes in headcount in the SEAR and WPR regions.

Figure 18 shows the percentage increases in the 15+ population by WHO region from 2005 to 2010, with the two regions with the smallest populations, AFR and EMR, showing the largest percentage increases (14.8% and 14.9%, respectively). The chart also shows the percentage increase in total alcohol consumption in each region over that same time period. The juxtaposition of the two charts helps us make sense of the changes in APC alcohol consumption, which is shown in Figure 19.

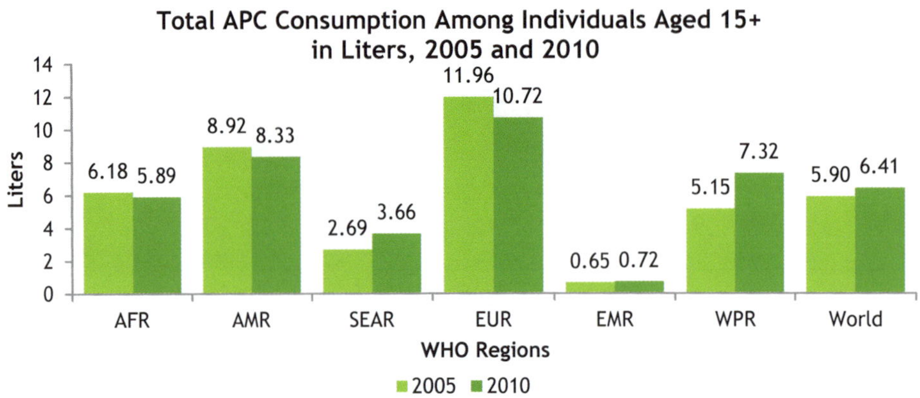

Figure 19. Total APC consumption by WHO Region, 2005 and 2010

Sources: WHO GISAH and UN Department of Economic and Social Affairs, Population Division (2013), World Population Prospects: The 2012 Revision, DVD Edition.

On a per capita basis, the SEAR region's APC consumption increased from 2.69 to 3.66 liters of pure alcohol, an increase of 35.8%, from 2005 to 2010. The WPR region's increase, from 5.15 to 7.32 liters, was 42.2% in that same period. The EMR region's increase was 11.4%, though the overall consumption level in that region remained very low. APC consumption in the AFR, AMR and EUR regions all declined from 2005 to 2010. In the AFR and AMR countries, this decline occurred because population growth among those aged 15+ simply outpaced the increase in total alcohol consumption in those regions. Only in the EUR region was there an actual decline in total alcohol consumption.

Figure 20 shows the breakdown of the changes in APC alcohol consumption by WHO region from 2005 to 2010, into the recorded and unrecorded components. Both AMR and EUR regions showed significant decrease in per capita consumption of unrecorded alcohol. In the SEAR and WPR regions, the dramatic APC increases are primarily due to increased alcohol consumption in India and China, respectively, as shown in Figure 16.

How did the changes in total alcohol consumption between 2005 and 2010 manifest themselves among WB income groups?

Similar to the case in WHO regions, the share of the world's 15+ population among WB income groups remained stable. The HI group's share of the world's total alcohol consumption, however, decreased from 32.8% in 2005 (see Figure 21) to 26.6% in 2010 (see Figure 7). That 6.2% share drop was picked up mostly by the UMI group, which gained 3.6% share, and the LMI group, which gained 2.5% share. The LI group picked up the remaining 0.1% share.

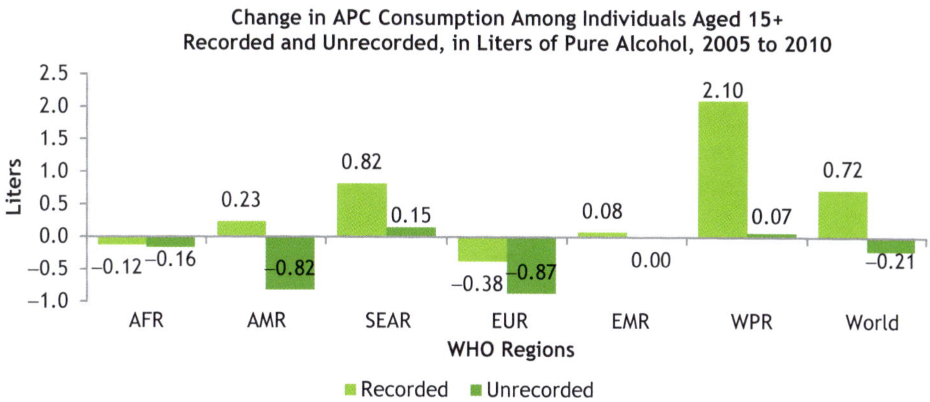

Figure 20. Change in recorded and unrecorded APC consumption by WHO Region, 2005 to 2010

Sources: WHO GISAH and UN Department of Economic and Social Affairs, Population Division (2013), World Population Prospects: The 2012 Revision, DVD Edition.

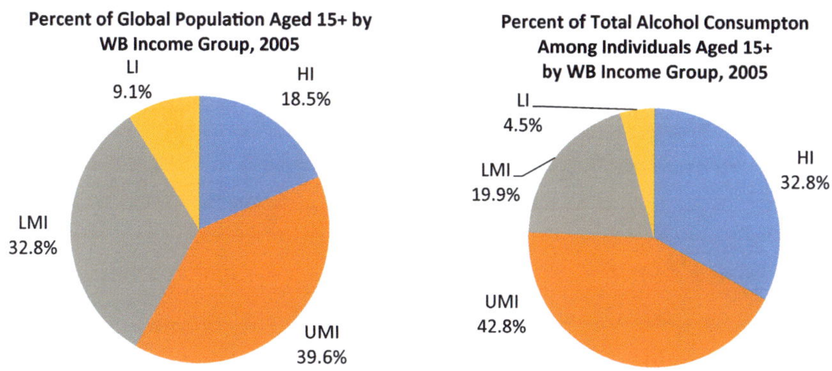

Figure 21. Percent of global population and percent of total alcohol consumption by WB Income Group, 2005

Sources: WHO GISAH and UN Department of Economic and Social Affairs, Population Division (2013), World Population Prospects: The 2012 Revision, DVD Edition.

In Figure 22, we see the actual changes in total alcohol consumption among the WB income groups from 2005 to 2010. The UMI's increase was due primarily to the presence of China in that group, while the same is true of the LMI group with India as one of its members. The HI group is the only group which saw an actual decrease in total alcohol consumption. This is consistent with our previous observations that in the EUR region there was an actual decrease in alcohol consumption during this period, and there was only a very modest increase in alcohol

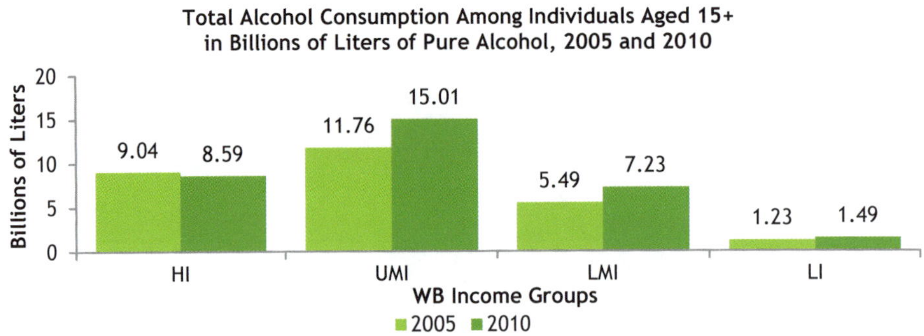

Figure 22. Total alcohol consumption and percentage change, by WB Income Group, 2005 and 2010

Sources: WHO GISAH and UN Department of Economic and Social Affairs, Population Division (2013), World Population Prospects: The 2012 Revision, DVD Edition.

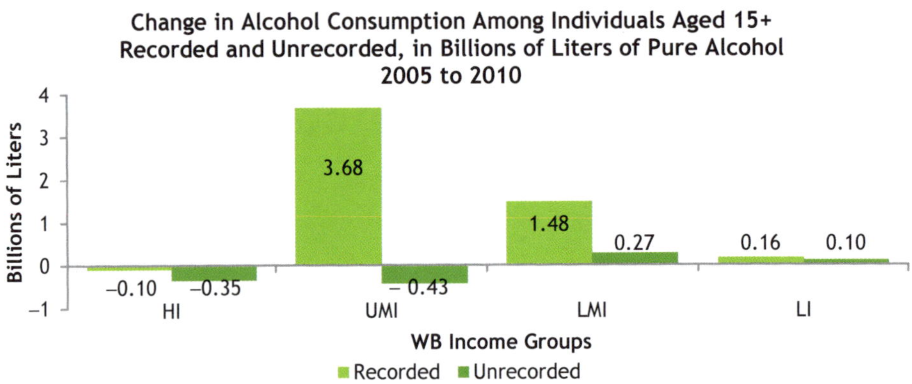

Figure 23. Change in recorded and unrecorded alcohol consumption by WB Income Group, 2005 to 2010

Sources: WHO GISAH and UN Department of Economic and Social Affairs, Population Division (2013), World Population Prospects: The 2012 Revision, DVD Edition.

consumption in the AMR region. EUR is home to over 45% of high-income countries, while over 30% of high-income countries belong to the AMR Region.

In Figure 23, which shows changes in recorded and unrecorded alcohol consumption by WB income group, the UMI group showed a decrease in unrecorded pure alcohol consumption of 430 million liters between 2005 and 2010, despite the presence of China in that group. A closer look at the data shows that while China registered an increase of 110 million liters of unrecorded alcohol consumption in that period, that increase was more than offset by decreases from other UMI countries, most notably Russia in the EUR region, the United States, Mexico and Brazil

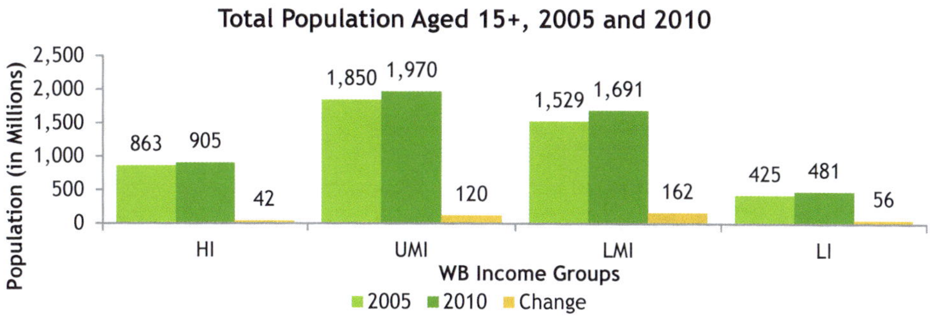

Figure 24. Total population aged 15+ by WB Income Group, 2005 and 2010

Sources: WHO GISAH and UN Department of Economic and Social Affairs, Population Division (2013), World Population Prospects: The 2012 Revision, DVD Edition.

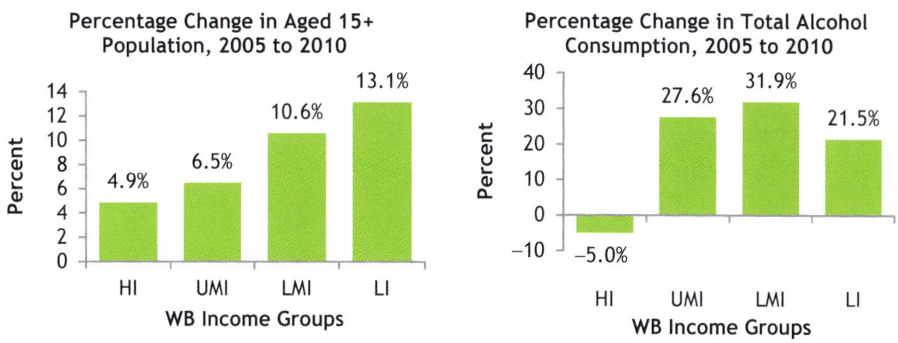

Figure 25. Percent change in aged 15+ population and percent change in total alcohol consumption, by WB Income Group, 2005 to 2010

Sources: WHO GISAH and UN Department of Economic and Social Affairs, Population Division (2013), World Population Prospects: The 2012 Revision, DVD Edition.

in the AMR region, and Nigeria in the AFR region. The increases in recorded alcohol consumption in the UMI and ULI groups are, again, primarily due to the presence of China and India in those respective income groups.

Figure 24 shows that every WB income group show similar information as in Figures 17 and 18, except that the information is presented by WB income group instead of by WHO Region. The charts are to help us better understand the per capita data by WB income group. Figure 24 shows that every WB income group showed an increase in its 15+ population from 2005 to 2010. The largest head-count increases were in the UMI and LMI countries.

The LI group, with the world's smallest population among the four income groups, showed the largest percentage increase in its 15+ population between 2005 and 2010 (see Figure 25). Figure 25 also shows that alcohol consumption increases

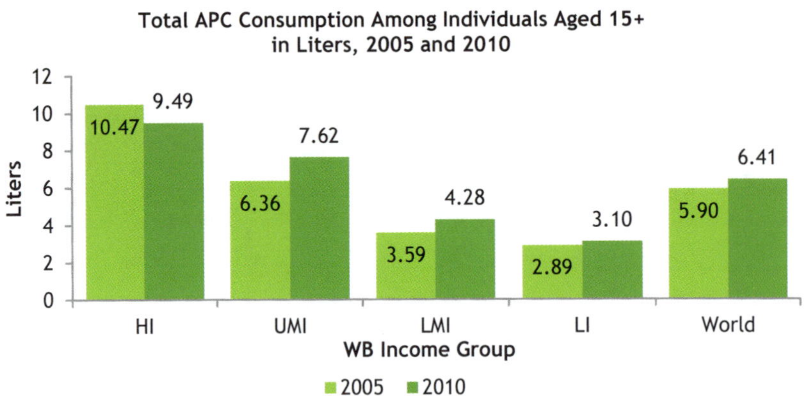

Figure 26. Total APC consumption by WB Income Group, 2005 and 2010

Sources: WHO GISAH and UN Department of Economic and Social Affairs, Population Division (2013), World Population Prospects: The 2012 Revision, DVD Edition.

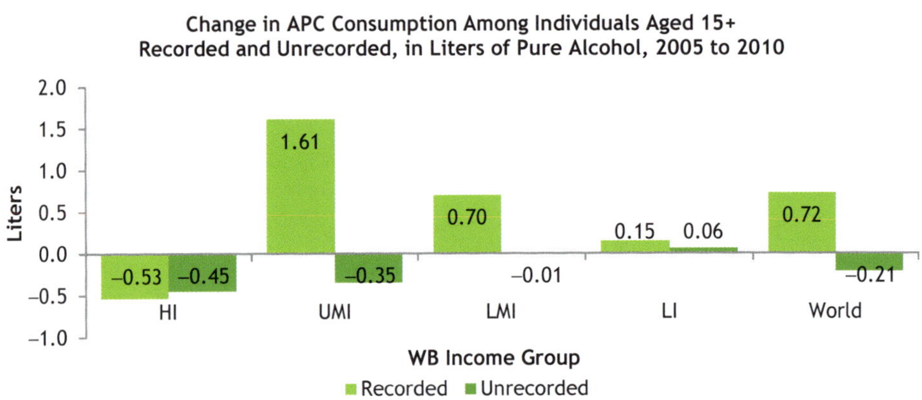

Figure 27. Change in recorded and unrecorded APC consumption by WB Income Group, 2005 to 2010

Sources: WHO GISAH and UN Department of Economic and Social Affairs, Population Division (2013), World Population Prospects: The 2012 Revision, DVD Edition.

in every income group except HI far outpaced the increase in their respective 15+ population in that period.

It logically follows, then, as shown in Figure 26, that the HI countries as a group saw a decline in APC consumption from 2005 to 2010, with its increase in its 15+ population and decrease in total alcohol consumption. APC consumption in all other income groups increased in that same period, as expected.

The final chart in this section (see Figure 27) shows the changes in recorded and unrecorded APC consumption from 2005 to 2010 by WB income group. The HI group experienced declines in APC in both recorded and unrecorded alcohol consumption, as it saw declines in total consumption in both those categories.

The UMI and LMI groups saw dramatic increases in per capita recorded alcohol consumption in this period. It should be noted that while the data show APC consumption declines for the HI group from 2005 to 2010, countries in that group still consumed the most alcohol on a per capita basis in 2010 (see Figures 11 and 12).

Total and per capita recorded alcohol consumption by type of alcohol product, 2010

The WHO 2014 report provides alcohol consumption data by the following product categories — spirits, beer, wine, and other alcoholic beverages. The "Other" category includes fortified wines, rice wine or other fermented beverages made of sorghum, millet or maize. This information, however, is only available for recorded alcohol consumption. This section presents this recorded alcohol consumption data by product type for each WHO Region and for each WB Income Group, in each case in terms of total consumption and APC (per capita) consumption. As was the case in the preceding sections, alcohol consumption volume refers to liters of pure alcohol.

While analysis of this data may yield useful insights on preferences as to type of alcoholic beverages consumed, and changes in such preferences over time, it must be noted that no assumption can be made from this recorded alcohol consumption data about unrecorded alcohol consumption. Countries in different regions and income groups may consume recorded alcohol and unrecorded alcohol in vastly different proportions.

Before we delve into the alcohol consumption data by product type, we revisit a familiar pair of pie charts in Figure 28. The charts shows the percent of global

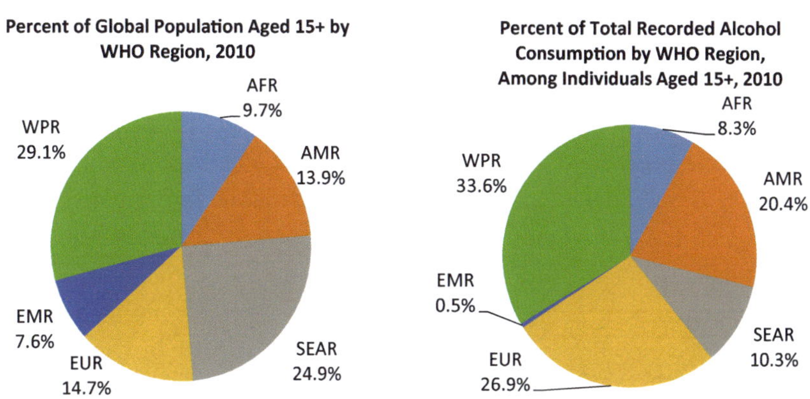

Figure 28. Percent of global population and percent of total recorded alcohol consumption by WHO Region, among individuals aged 15+, 2010

Sources: WHO GISAH and UN Department of Economic and Social Affairs, Population Division (2013), World Population Prospects: The 2012 Revision, DVD Edition.

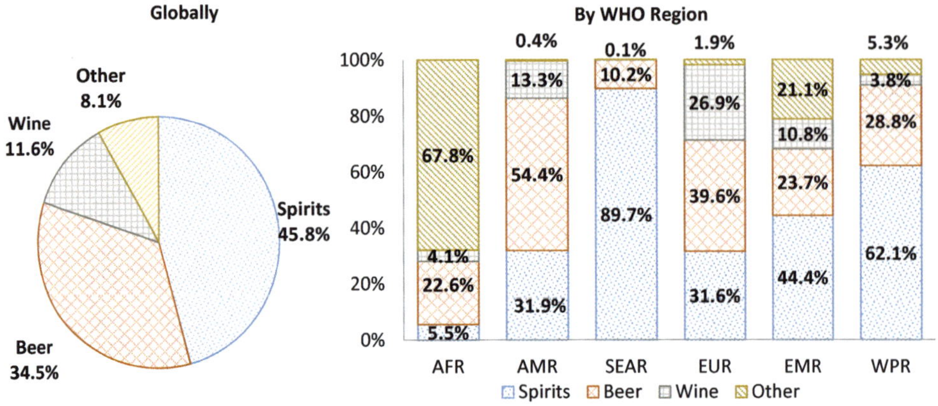

Figure 29. Recorded alcohol consumption by product type, among individuals aged 15+, percent of total consumption, globally and by WHO Region, 2010

Sources: WHO GISAH and UN Department of Economic and Social Affairs, Population Division (2013), World Population Prospects: The 2012 Revision, DVD Edition.

population aged 15 and older by WHO region in 2010, and the percent of total recorded alcohol consumption by those individuals in each WHO region. Figure 1 presented a similar picture, except in that chart the pie chart on the right showed percent of total — i.e., recorded plus unrecorded — alcohol consumption in 2010. While Figure 28 shows no alarming divergence from Figure 1, the information will prove useful as we look next into recorded alcohol consumption by product type.

Figure 29 shows that in 2010, globally, 45.8% of all recorded alcohol consumption by individuals aged 15 and older was in the form of spirits, with beer in second place at 34.5%, wine at 11.6%, and other alcoholic beverages making up the rest, at 8.1%.

Among the WHO regions, however, the distribution of total consumption among beverage types vary widely. In the AFR region, for example, over two-thirds of recorded alcohol consumption in 2010 was in the form of other alcoholic beverages, while beer came in a distant second at 22.6%. In contrast, in the WPR region, 62.1% of recorded alcohol consumption was in the form of spirits in 2010. Spirits was also the overwhelming alcoholic beverage of choice in the SEAR, at 89.7% of total alcohol consumption, with beer in second place at 10.2%. The SEAR registered no meaningful consumption of other alcoholic beverages in 2010, and showed only 0.1% of total consumption in the form of wine. In both the EUR and the AMR regions, beer was the most popular alcoholic beverage, followed by spirits, wine, and others, in that order.

While it is interesting to note the vast differences in proportions of recorded alcohol consumption by product type among the WHO regions, we need to take into account the actual volume of recorded alcohol consumption by product type, to come to an accurate picture of the relative significance of those regional differences. Figure 28 shows that EUR, home to 14.7% of the world's population aged 15 and older in 2010, accounted for 26.9% of the world's recorded alcohol consumption that year. From Figure 29, we see that of those 26.9% of total world consumption, 31.6% was in the form of spirits, 39.6% in the form of beer, 26.9% in the form of wine, and the remaining 1.9% as other alcohol beverages. In contrast, while Figure 29 shows that in the EMR Region, 44.4% of its recorded alcohol consumption was in the form of spirits, that region, as shown in Figure 28, accounted for only 0.5% of global recorded alcohol consumption in 2010.

Figure 30 shows the total volume of recorded alcohol consumption in each WHO Region in 2010, in billions of liters of pure alcohol, and those totals broken down into the product types. The chart on right with the product type break-downs shows only a few data labels, to avoid clutter. Figure 30 highlights the relative significance of each region's consumption relative to global consumption, both in terms of total consumption and consumption by product type. One can see visually that in 2010, the WPR Region consumed the most recorded alcohol, with EUR in second place and AMR in close third. The EMR Region consumed the least amount of recorded alcohol by a wide margin. One can also see that the EUR Region accounted for a large share of global wine consumption, while the WPR Region held that distinction on spirits consumption, and the AFR region accounted for most of the recorded consumption of other alcohol.

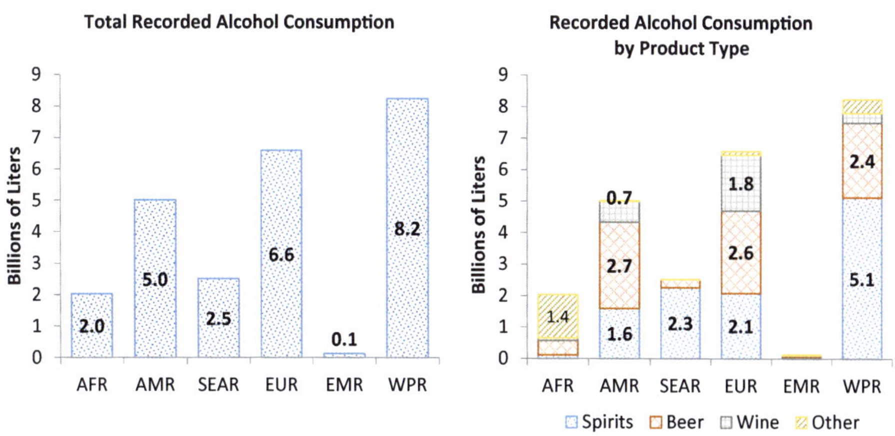

Figure 30. Recorded alcohol consumption by WHO Region and product type, among individuals aged 15+, 2010

Sources: WHO GISAH and UN Department of Economic and Social Affairs, Population Division (2013), World Population Prospects: The 2012 Revision, DVD Edition.

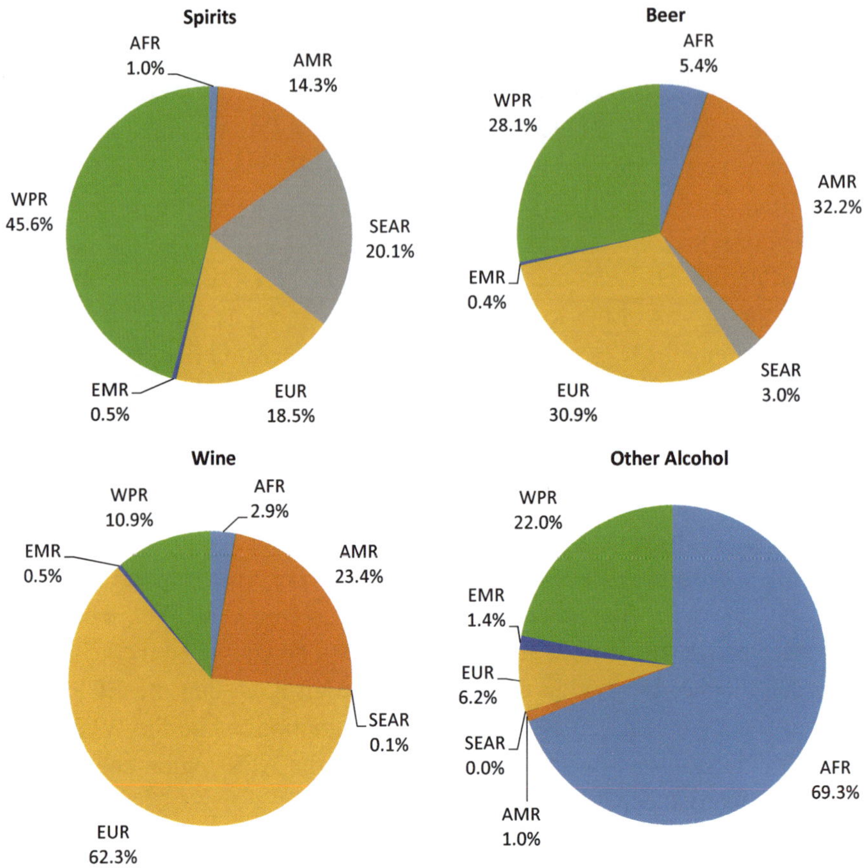

Figure 31. Percent of recorded alcohol consumption by product type and by WHO Region, among individuals aged 15+, 2010

Sources: WHO GISAH and UN Department of Economic and Social Affairs, Population Division (2013), World Population Prospects: The 2012 Revision, DVD Edition.

That visual intuition is confirmed in Figure 31, which shows the percent of recorded alcohol consumption in each WHO Region, by product type. In 2010, 45.6% of all global recorded spirits consumption took place in the WPR Region. EUR accounted for 62.3% of global recorded wine consumption, while AFR accounted for 69.3% of global recorded consumption of other alcohol. Beer, for its part, enjoyed a relatively even distribution among the three regions with the highest volume of recorded alcohol consumption — 32.2% of global recorded beer consumption in 2010 took place in the AMR region, while 30.9% and 28.1% were consumed in the EUR and WPR regions, respectively.

On a per capita basis, we see from Figure 32 that globally, individuals aged 15 and older each consumed 4.86 liters of recorded pure alcohol in 2010. Of that 4.86

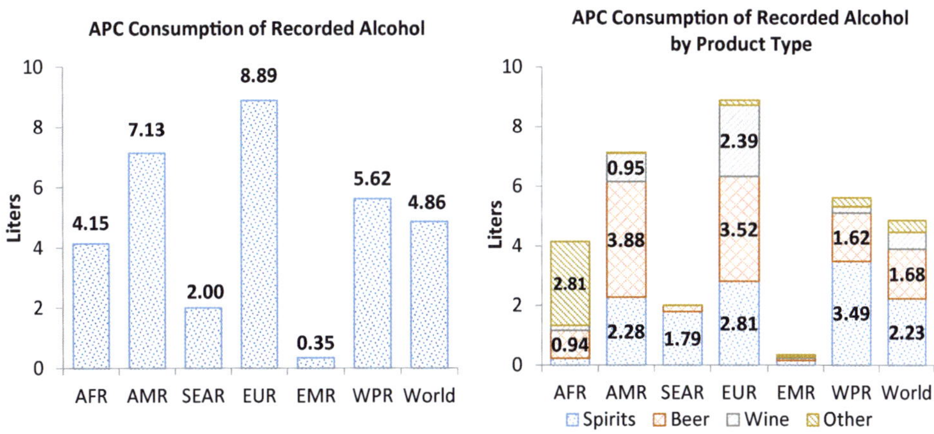

Figure 32. APC consumption of recorded alcohol by WHO Region and product type, among individuals aged 15+, in liters, 2010

Sources: WHO GISAH and UN Department of Economic and Social Affairs, Population Division (2013), World Population Prospects: The 2012 Revision, DVD Edition.

total, 2.23 liters were consumed in the form of spirits, and 1.68 liters were in the form of beer. The charts in Figure 32 also show APC consumption of recorded alcohol in each WHO Region, and within each region, the APC amount for each product type. In the EUR Region, which registered the highest APC recorded alcohol consumption in 2010, the most popular form of APC alcohol consumption was in the form the beer, followed by spirits, then wine. However, EUR's APC wine consumption, similar to what we saw in Figures 30 and 31, accounted for a majority of APC wine consumption worldwide in 2010. Note that while the chart in Figure 32 showing APC recorded alcohol consumption by product type does not show all data labels, to avoid clutter on that chart, the information is shown on the charts in Figure 33.

Figure 33 shows APC consumption of recorded alcohol by individuals aged 15 and older by each type of alcohol, within each WHO region. For spirits, the WPR region consumed the most in 2010, over 50% more than the global average of 2.23 liters of pure alcohol per capita. The EUR and AMR regions also registered APC spirits consumption levels above the global average. For beer APC consumption, both the AMR and EUR regions consumed more than twice the global average in 2010. Wine APC consumption, as noted before and shown in Figure 33 again, was led by the EUR Region by a wide margin. APC consumption of other alcohol products were done mostly in the AFR region in 2010. In the SEAR Region, most of the APC alcohol consumption in 2010 was in the form of spirits, with beer in distant second place, and insignificant amounts of consumption in the forms of wine and other alcohol. In the EMR Region, APC recorded alcohol consumption in 2010 showed a fairly even

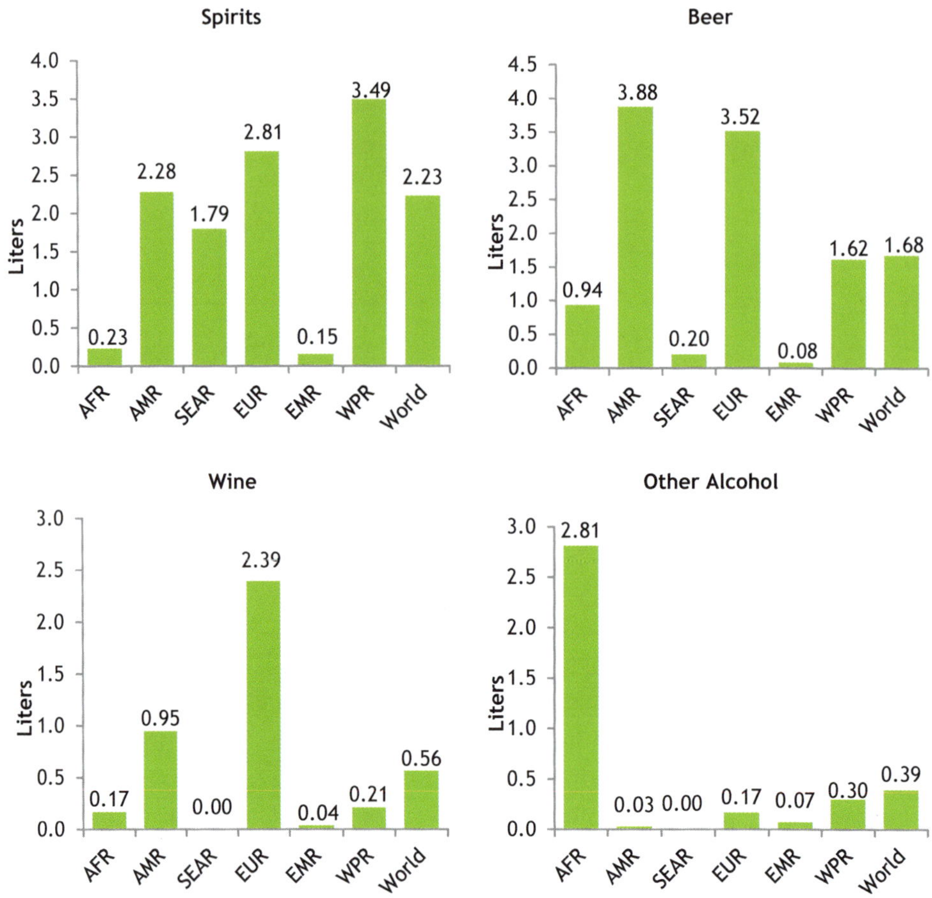

Figure 33. APC consumption of recorded alcohol by type of alcohol beverage and by WHO Region, among individuals aged 15+, 2010

Sources: WHO GISAH and UN Department of Economic and Social Affairs, Population Division (2013), World Population Prospects: The 2012 Revision, DVD Edition.

distribution among the four product types, though the actual volume of alcohol consumption was very low, at 0.35 liters per capita (see Figure 32).

In Figures 34–39, we show recorded alcohol consumption by WB income group. Figure 34 shows the percent of the global population aged 15 years and older by WB income group in 2010, and the percent of recorded alcohol consumption by each group. The HI income group accounted for 17.9% of global population aged 15 and older in 2010, and consumed a disproportionate 32% of global consumption of recorded alcohol. The UMI income group, with 39% of the world's population aged 15 and older, consumed 47.2% of global consumption of recorded alcohol. The LI and LMI groups combined, home to 43% of the global population aged 15 and older, accounted for 20.8% of global recorded alcohol consumption in 2010.

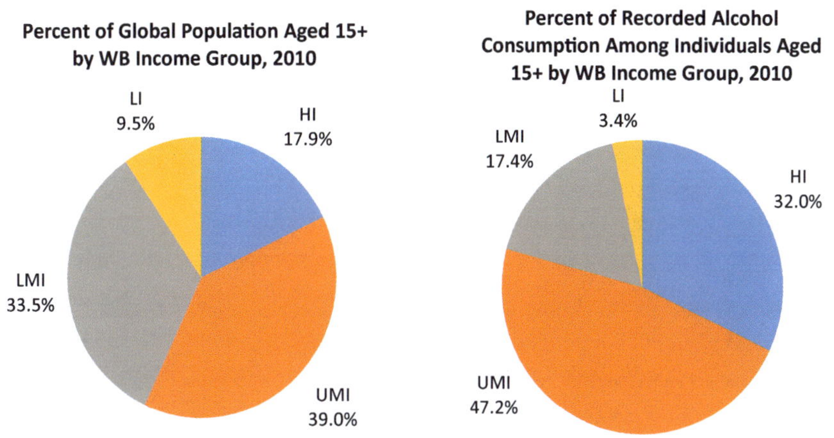

Figure 34. Percent of global population and percent of recorded alcohol consumption by WB Income Group, 2010

Sources: WHO GISAH and UN Department of Economic and Social Affairs, Population Division (2013), World Population Prospects: The 2012 Revision, DVD Edition.

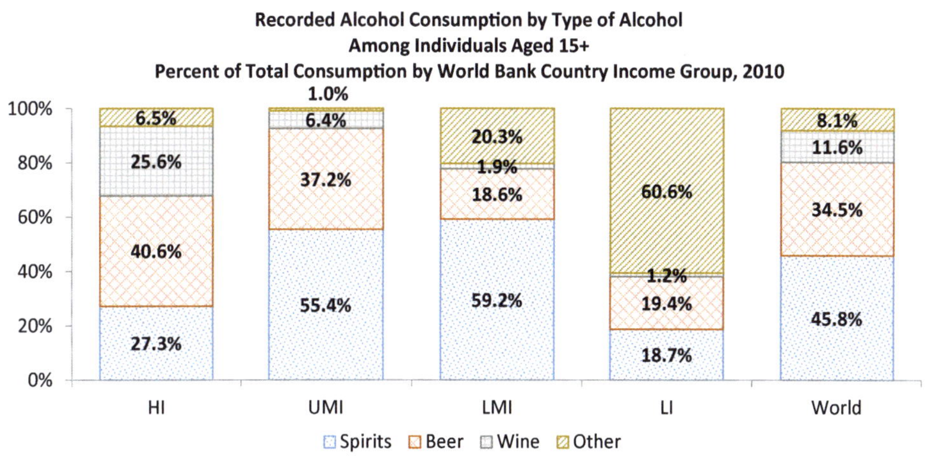

Figure 35. Recorded alcohol consumption by type of alcoholic beverage among individuals aged 15+, percent of total consumption by WB Income Group, 2010

Sources: WHO GISAH and UN Department of Economic and Social Affairs, Population Division (2013), World Population Prospects: The 2012 Revision, DVD Edition.

Figure 35 shows the percent of recorded alcohol consumption by product type in each WB income group in 2010. As was the case in presenting this data for WHO regions (Figure 29), there are wide variations among the income groups in consumption by product types.

Countries in the HI income group consumed 40.6% of its recorded alcohol in the form of beer, while those in the UMI and LMI income groups showed majority

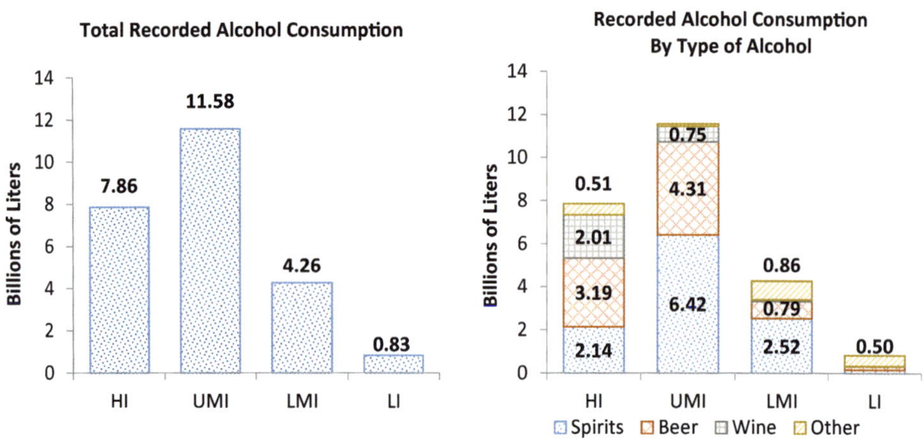

Figure 36. Recorded alcohol consumption by WB income group, among individuals aged 15+, 2010

Sources: WHO GISAH and UN Department of Economic and Social Affairs, Population Division (2013), World Population Prospects: The 2012 Revision, DVD Edition.

preference in spirits (55.4% and 59.2%, respectively, of total recorded alcohol consumption). The LI group consumed 60.6% of its recorded alcohol in the form of other alcohol products. This is partly due to the fact that many of LI countries are in the AFR Region, which accounted for much of the global recorded consumption of other alcohol products in 2010.

Figure 36 shows the total recorded alcohol consumption by WB income group, and the consumption levels by product type. While we can visually see that in both the UMI and LMI regions, spirits consumption in 2010 did indeed account for over 50% of those groups' total recorded alcohol consumption, the UMI group consumed far more spirits in actual volume. In the case of beer consumption, while the HI group consumed 40.6% of its recorded alcohol consumption in the form of beer in 2010, and that percentage for the UMI group was 37.2%, the UMI group actually consumed more liters of beer than the HI group in 2010.

As we did in Figure 31 for the WHO regions, in Figure 37, we show the percent of recorded alcohol consumption in each WB income group, by product type in 2010. The UMI group accounted for 57.1% of global recorded spirits consumption and 50.9% of global recorded beer consumption. The HI group consumed 70.6% of global recorded wine consumption. In the case of other alcohol products, the LMI group accounted for 43.4% of global recorded consumption, while the LI and HI groups registered similar percentages, at 25.3% and 25.8%, respectively.

On a per capita basis, we see from Figure 38 that countries in higher income groups consumed more recorded alcohol than those in lower income groups. This

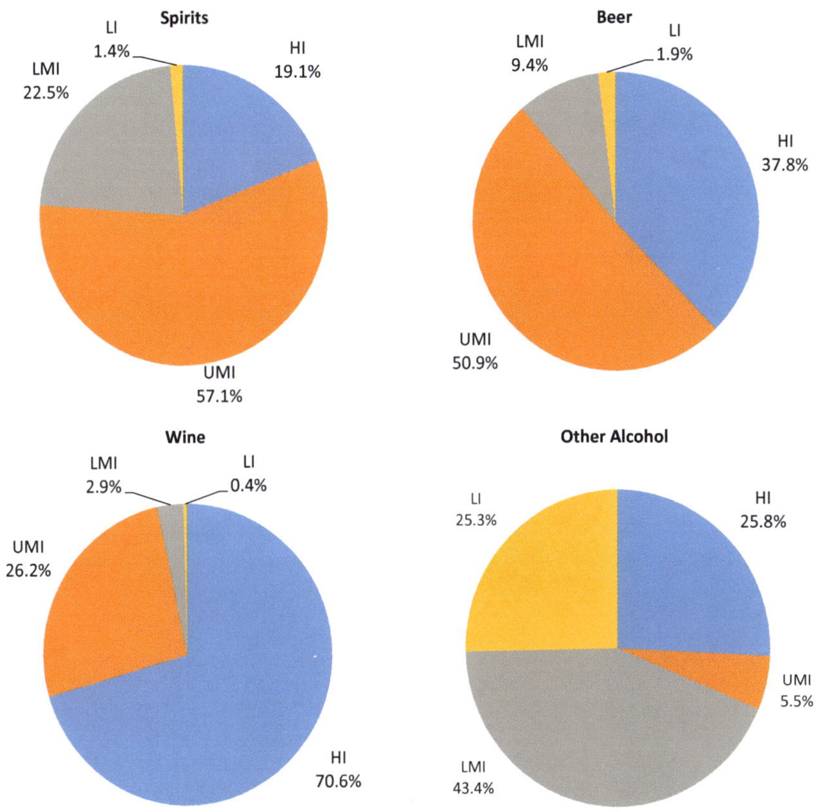

Figure 37. Percent of recorded alcohol consumption by type of alcohol beverage and by WB Income group, among individuals aged 15+, 2010

Sources: WHO GISAH and UN Department of Economic and Social Affairs, Population Division (2013), World Population Prospects: The 2012 Revision, DVD Edition.

data is consistent with what we saw in Figure 11, which showed a similar chart but for total (i.e., recorded plus unrecorded) alcohol consumption in 2010. Figure 38 also shows the break-down of APC recorded consumption by product type. The details of the product type break-down are presented in Figure 39.

Figure 39 shows the APC consumption of recoded alcohol for each product type by WB income group. In 2010, the UMI group consumed the most recorded spirits per capita, at 3.26 liters of pure alcohol. The 2.37 liters registered by the HI group was also above the global average. For beer consumption, the HI group totaled 3.53 liters per capita, more than twice the global average, while the UMI group totaled 2.19 liters per capita, significantly above the global average of 1.68. Wine consumption was dominated by the HI group in 2010, while the LI group registered APC recorded consumption of other alcohol products of 1.05 liters, more than twice the next closest groups (the HI group at 0.57 liters, and the LMI group at 0.51 liters).

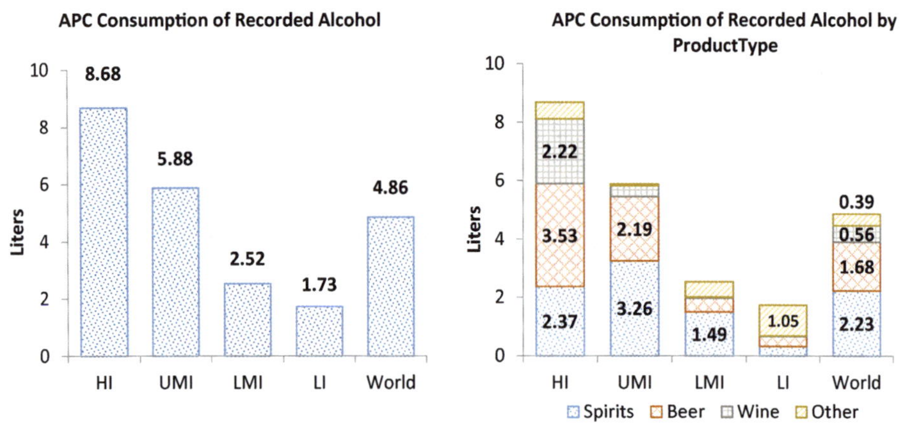

Figure 38. APC consumption of recorded alcohol by WB Income Group, among individuals aged 15+, in liters, 2010

Sources: WHO GISAH and UN Department of Economic and Social Affairs, Population Division (2013), World Population Prospects: The 2012 Revision, DVD Edition.

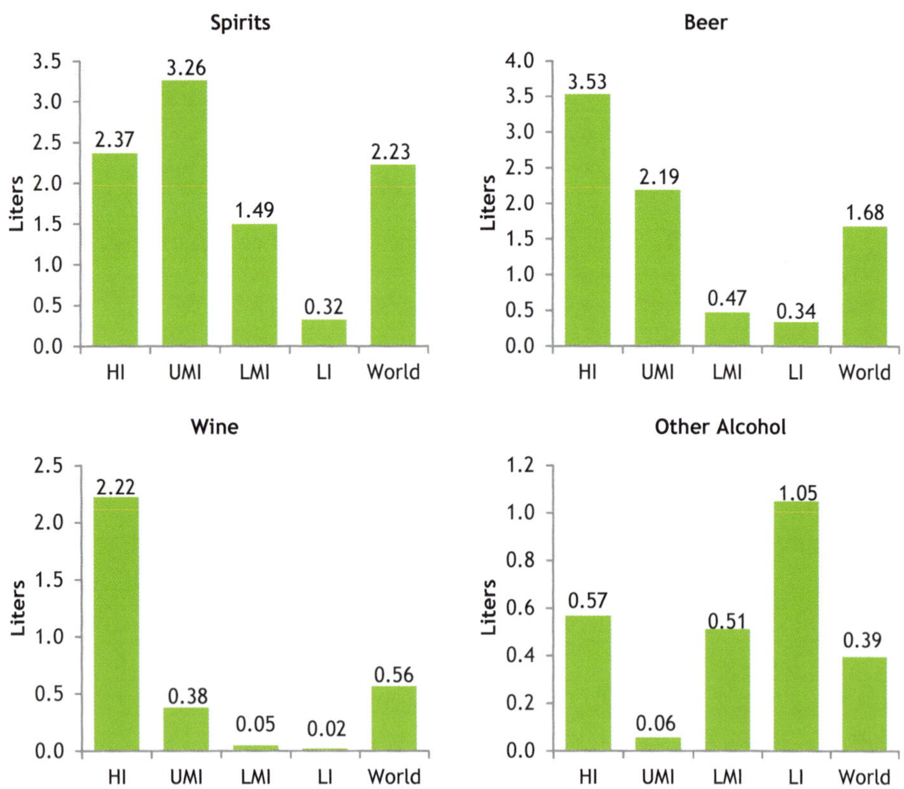

Figure 39. APC consumption of recorded alcohol by type of alcohol beverage and by WB Income Group, among individuals aged 15+, in liters of pure alcohol, 2010

Sources: WHO GISAH and UN Department of Economic and Social Affairs, Population Division (2013), World Population Prospects: The 2012 Revision, DVD Edition.

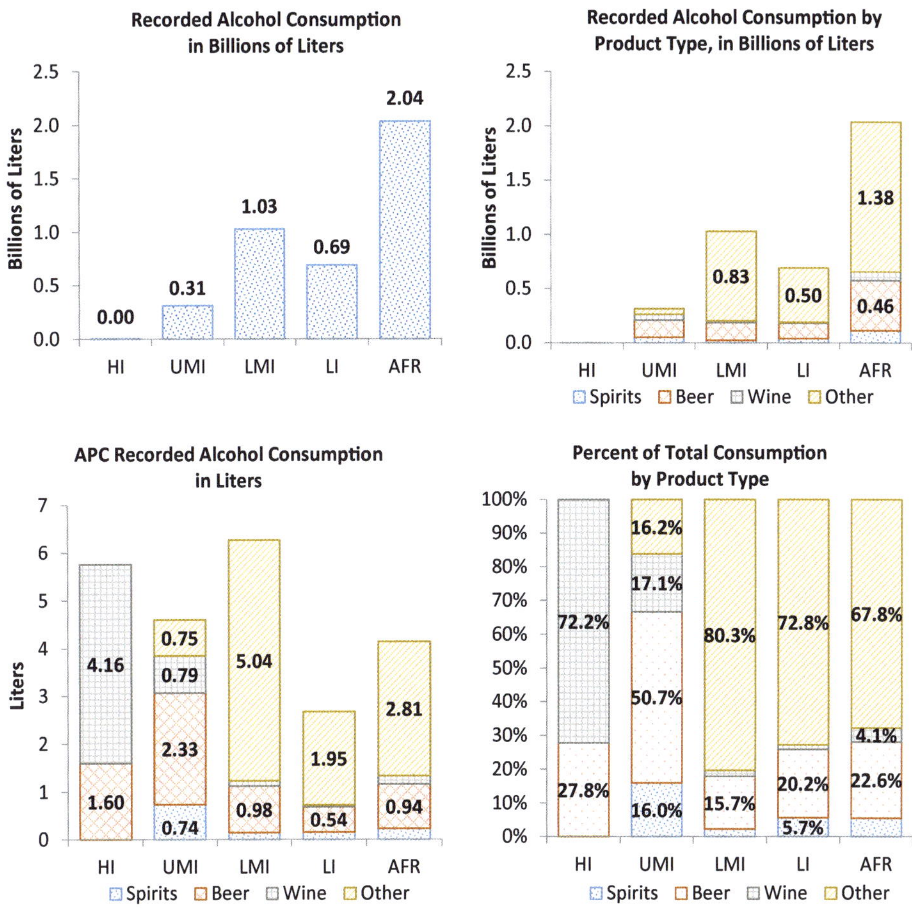

Figure 40. Recorded alcohol consumption by WB Income Group and type of alcohol, among individuals aged 15+, AFR Region, 2010

Sources: WHO GISAH and UN Department of Economic and Social Affairs, Population Division (2013), World Population Prospects: The 2012 Revision, DVD Edition.

The next series of charts, Figures 40–45, shows the break-down of total and APC recorded alcohol consumption by WB income group and by product type in 2010, within each WHO Region.

In the AFR Region, there was little total recorded alcohol consumption in the HI group in 2010. However, among the very few in this region that are in the HI group, 72.2% of recorded alcohol consumption was in the form of wine, and the rest in beer. Beer was the alcoholic beverage of choice among the UMI countries in this region. Other alcoholic beverages were the most popular form of recorded alcohol consumption, especially in the LMI and LI groups. South Africa, a UMI country, with 7.4% of the region's 15+ population, accounted for 41.5% of the region's recorded spirits consumption. For beer and wine, its share of recorded consumption in 2010 was 29.4% and 60.3%, respectively.

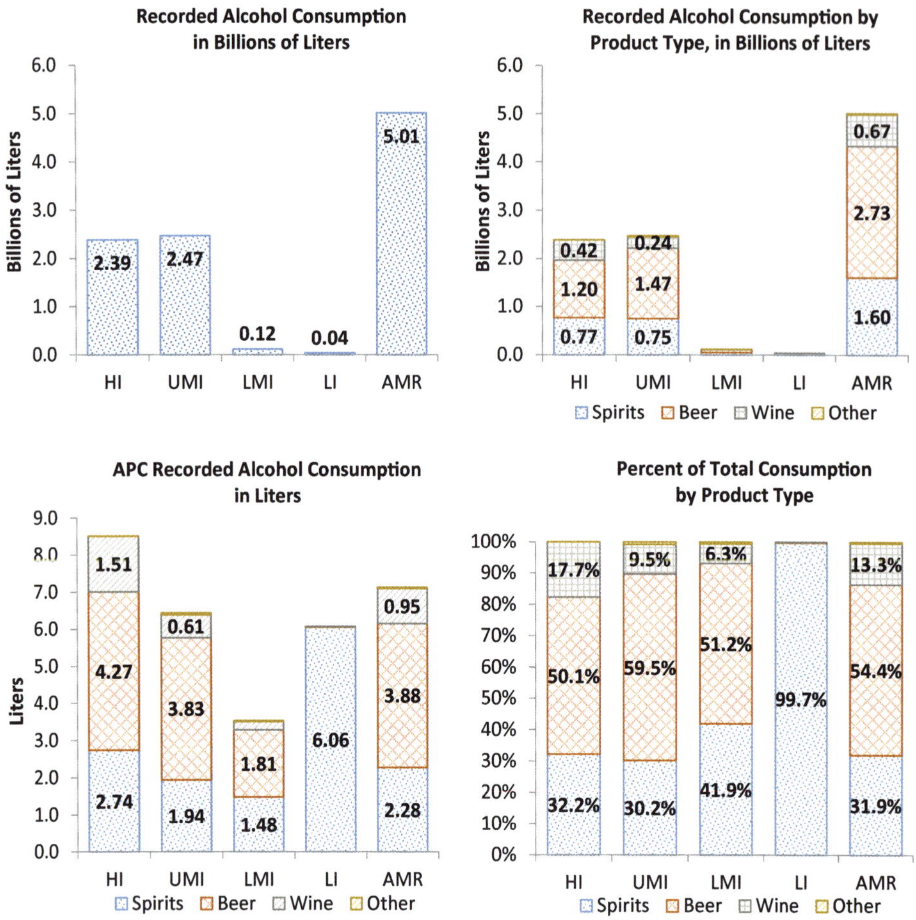

Figure 41. Recorded alcohol consumption by WB Income Group and type of alcohol, among individuals aged 15+, AMR Region, 2010

Sources: WHO GISAH and UN Department of Economic and Social Affairs, Population Division (2013), World Population Prospects: The 2012 Revision, DVD Edition.

In the AMR Region, the vast majority of recorded alcohol consumption in 2010 was in the HI and UMI groups of countries. It should be noted that there are very few countries classified in the LMI and LI groups in this region. Beer was the preferred alcoholic beverage in this region among the HI and UMI countries, in both total and APC recorded consumption. The United States (US), a HI income group country, is the dominant alcohol consumer in this region. With about 35% of the region's 15+ population, the US's share of the region's recorded consumption in 2010 were 44% for spirits, 39% for beer, and 56% for wine. There was no recorded other alcohol consumption in the US in 2010.

In the SEAR region, there was no country classified in the HI group in 2010, therefore there was no recorded alcohol consumption in that group. As Figure 42

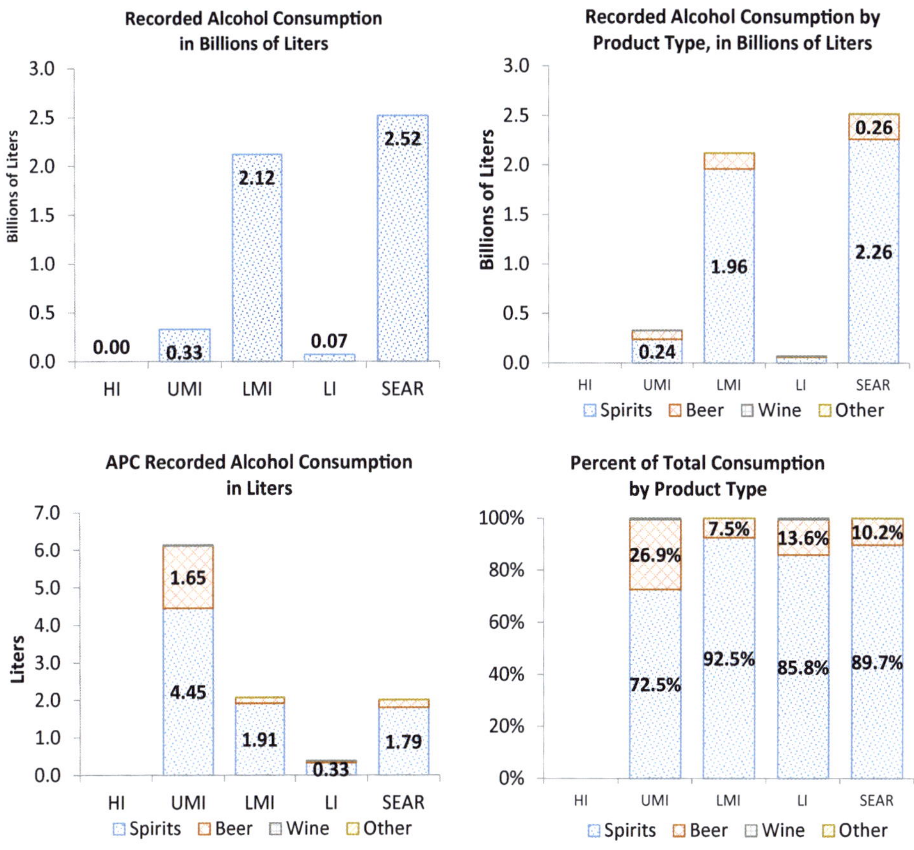

Figure 42. Recorded alcohol consumption by WB Income Group and type of alcohol, among individuals aged 15+, SEAR Region, 2010

Sources: WHO GISAH and UN Department of Economic and Social Affairs, Population Division (2013), World Population Prospects: The 2012 Revision, DVD Edition.

shows, most of recorded alcohol consumption in this region in 2010 was in the form of spirits. Beer did register a significant amount, especially in the UMI group, but was in a very distant second place behind spirits. As noted before, India, a LMI country, is in this region, and is home to almost 67% of the region's 15+ population. India's consumption of recorded spirits accounted for over 85% of the region's consumption in this category in 2010. For beer, India's share of the region's recorded consumption in 2010 was about 56%. Thailand, a UMI country with about 4% of the region's 15+ population, accounted for almost 35% of the region's recorded beer consumption in 2010.

In the EUR region, very few countries were in the LMI and LI groups in 2010. Total recorded alcohol consumption, not surprisingly, occurred mostly in the HI and UMI groups. This was true also for total recorded alcohol consumption by product type. On a per capita basis, however, the UMI group consumed 3.81 liters

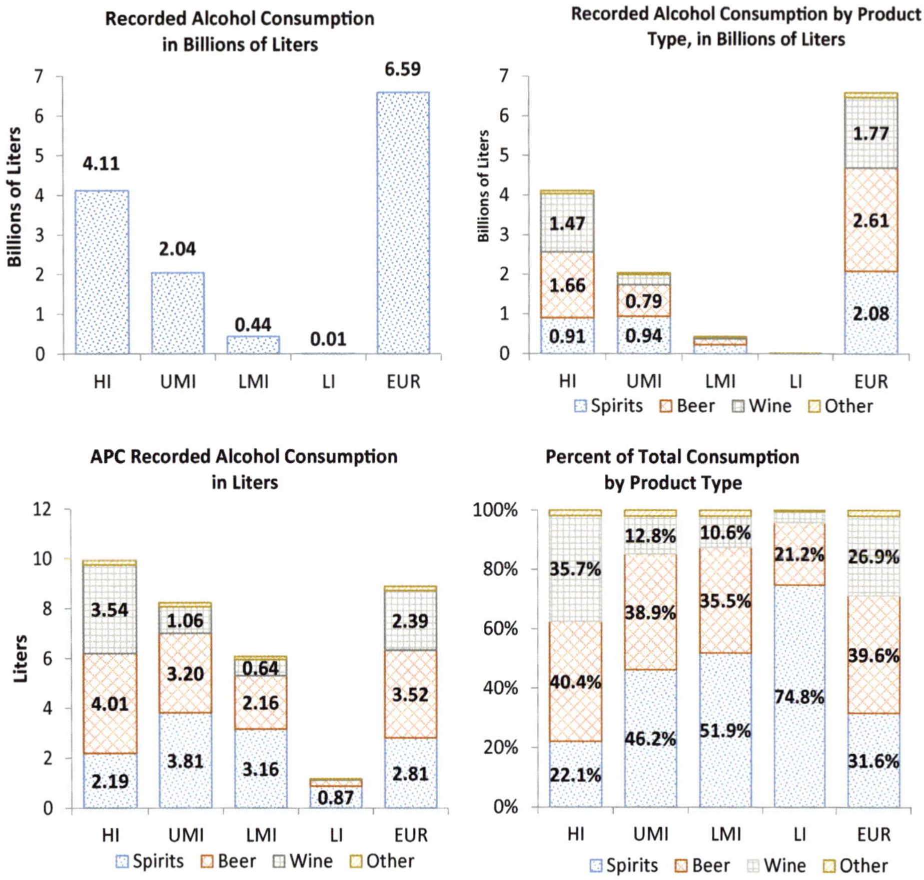

Figure 43. Recorded alcohol consumption by WB Income Group and type of alcohol, among individuals aged 15+, EUR Region, 2010

Sources: WHO GISAH and UN Department of Economic and Social Affairs, Population Division (2013), World Population Prospects: The 2012 Revision, DVD Edition.

of pure alcohol in the form of spirits, compared with the 2.19 liters recorded for the HI group. The HI group registered the highest APC recorded consumption among all income groups in the region for beer and wine consumption. Russia (in the UMI group), with about 16% of the region's 15+ population, accounted for 33% of the region's recorded spirits consumption in 2010. France (HI group), home to 7% of the regions 15+ population, accounted for over 19% of the region's recorded wine consumption in 2010.

The EMR Region consumed the least amount of alcohol among all WHO regions in 2010. While there are LI countries in this region, those countries did not report any recorded alcohol consumption in 2010. Countries in the LMI group in this region consumed the most recorded alcohol in 2010. Those in the HI group,

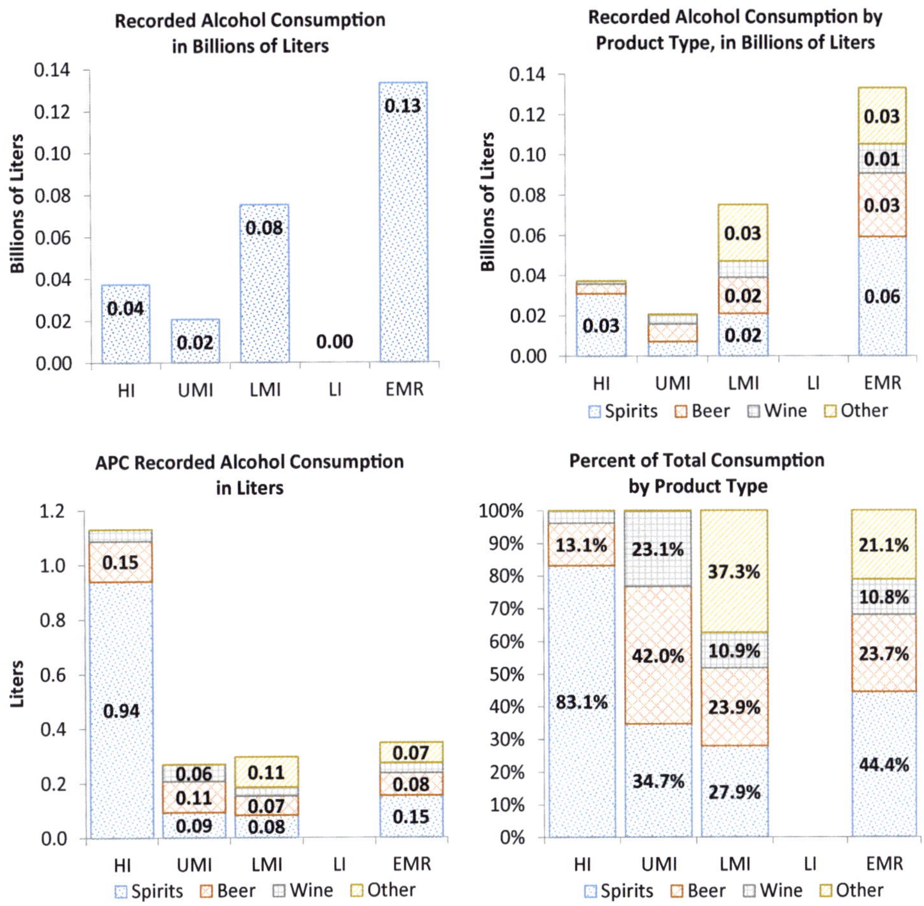

Figure 44. Recorded alcohol consumption by WB Income Group and type of alcohol, among individuals aged 15+, EMR Region, 2010

Sources: WHO GISAH and UN Department of Economic and Social Affairs, Population Division (2013), World Population Prospects: The 2012 Revision, DVD Edition.

however, consumed the most spirits, in terms of both total recorded consumption and APC recorded consumption.

In 2010, the WPR Region consumed the most recorded alcohol among all WHO regions. Figure 45 shows that the vast majority of that consumption took place in the UMI countries in this region, and within this income group, 69.1% of recorded alcohol consumption was in the form of spirits. As note before, China is in this region, in the UMI group. Total recorded alcohol consumption of spirits account for more than 85% of the region's total recorded spirits consumption in 2010. For beer and wine, China's share in the region were 75% and 61%, respectively. China reported no recorded consumption of other alcoholic beverages in 2010. Most of

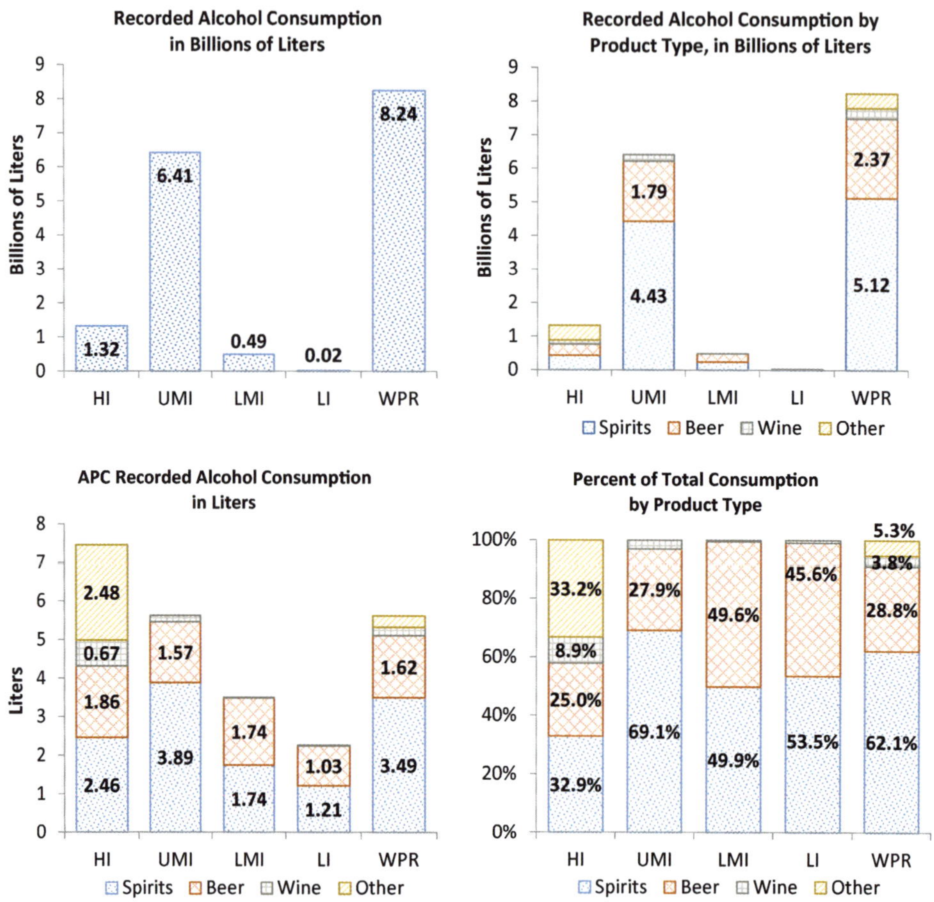

Figure 45. Recorded alcohol consumption by WB Income Group and type of alcohol, among individuals aged 15+, WPR Region, 2010

Sources: WHO GISAH and UN Department of Economic and Social Affairs, Population Division (2013), World Population Prospects: The 2012 Revision, DVD Edition.

the recorded other alcohol consumption in this region in 2010 took place in Australia, Japan and the Republic of Korea, all HI group countries.

Total and per capita consumption of recorded alcohol by product type, 2001–2010

In this final section on recorded alcohol consumption levels and patterns, we will examine the changes in consumption from 2001 to 2010, in terms of both total consumption and APC consumption.

From Figure 46, we see that there has been a steady increase in total recorded alcohol consumption from 2001 to 2010, with a minor but notable decline from

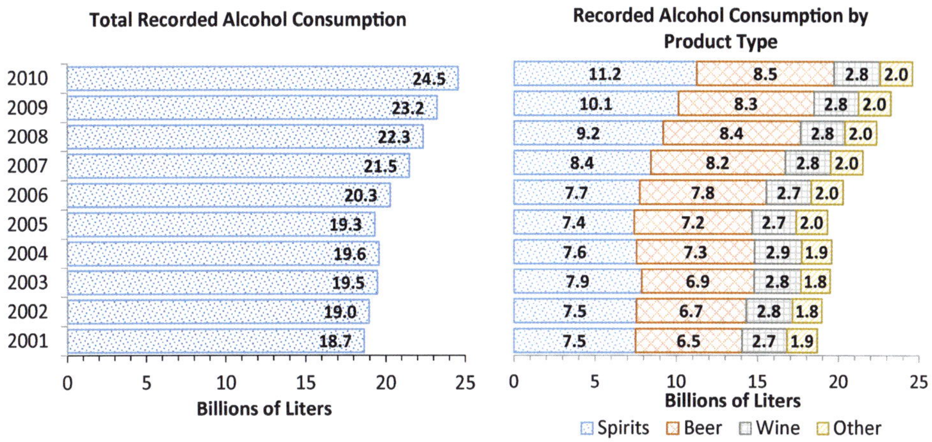

Figure 46. Recorded alcohol consumption, total and by product type, among individuals aged 15+, in billions of liters of pure alcohol, 2001–2010

Sources: WHO GISAH and UN Department of Economic and Social Affairs, Population Division (2013), World Population Prospects: The 2012 Revision, DVD Edition.

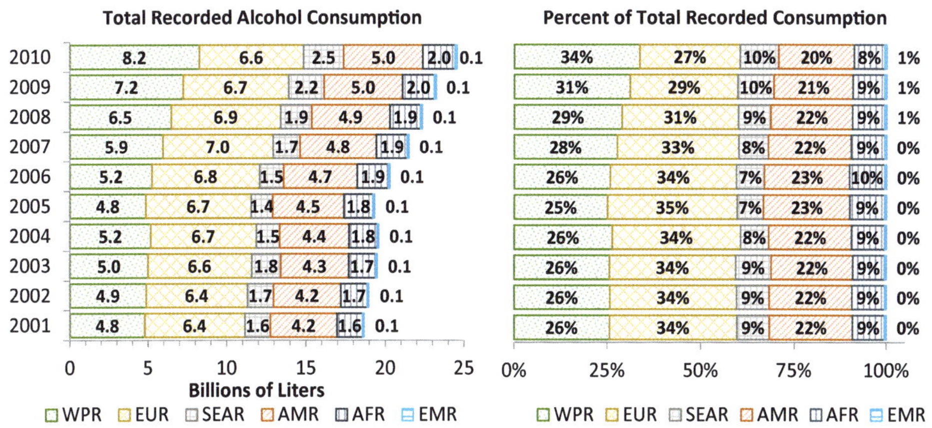

Figure 47. Recorded alcohol consumption by WHO Region, total in billions of liters of pure alcohol and percent of total recorded consumption, among individuals aged 15+, 2001–2010

Sources: WHO GISAH and UN Department of Economic and Social Affairs, Population Division (2013), World Population Prospects: The 2012 Revision, DVD Edition.

2004 to 2005. By product type, both spirits and beer show steady increases in recorded consumption from 2001 to 2010. Wine and other alcoholic beverages, on their parts, appear to be maintaining their total recorded consumption levels, but are not experiencing volume growth.

Figure 47 shows the same 2001–2010 recorded consumption trend by WHO regions. Clearly the WPR Region has experienced increasing total recorded alcohol consumption in terms of billions of liters of pure alcohol. That region's recorded alcohol consumption has also been gaining share of global recorded alcohol consumption — from 26% in 2006 to 34% in 2010, after 6 years of holding steady around 26% from 2001 to 2006. EUR, for its part, has seen its share of global recorded alcohol consumption drop from 34% in 2006 to 27% in 2010. Figure 47 also shows EUR to be the only region with actual decline in total recorded alcohol consumption from 2007 to 2010.

Figure 48 shows the changes in recorded alcohol consumption by WHO region in 2010, for each product type. In cases where a region's recorded consumption did not register a meaningful level, the corresponding data labels

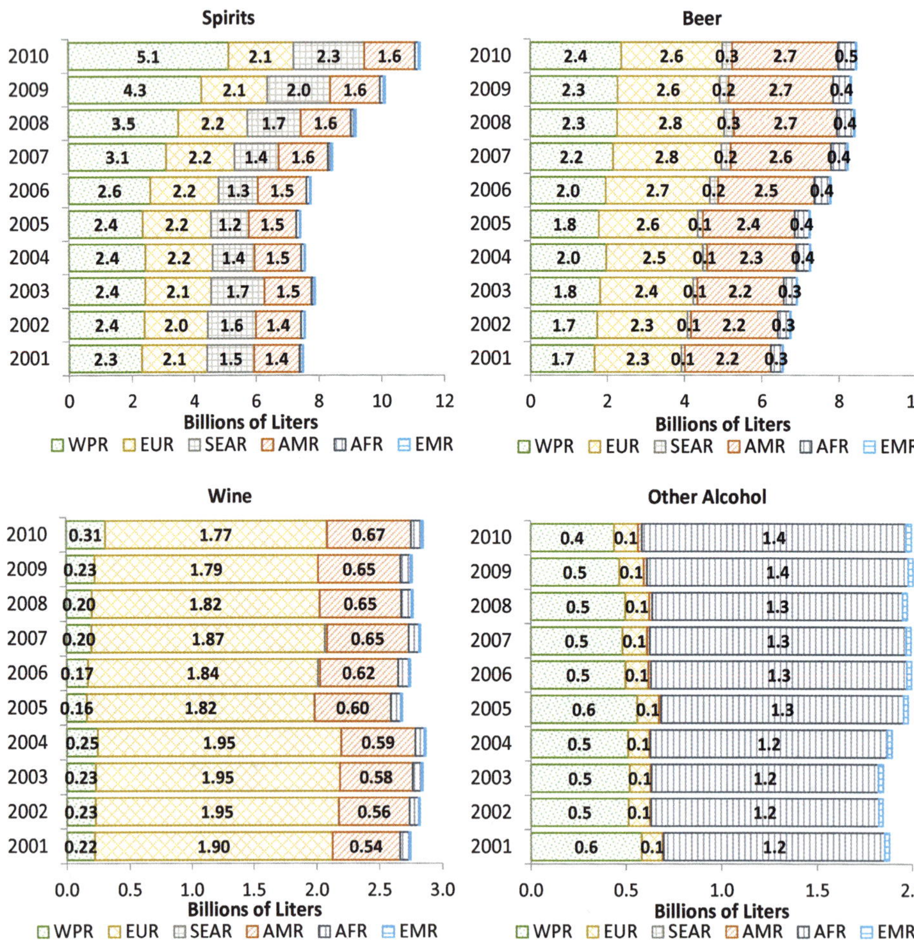

Figure 48. Recorded alcohol consumption by WHO Region for each product type, among individuals aged 15+, in billions of liters of pure alcohol, 2001–2010

have been omitted in the charts. This is true for the EMR region for all product types. From 2001 to 2010, recorded spirits consumption has shown the greatest increase in the WPR region. SEAR's recorded spirits consumption has also shown significant increases from 2007. Recorded beer consumption is also showing steady increases since 2010 in all regions, though Figure 48 suggests that perhaps that increase is coming to a halt in the AMR and EUR regions.

Recorded wine consumption globally does not appear to be growing. There is significant growth in recorded wine consumption in the WPR region from 2005 to 2010, albeit the actual consumption volume is still very low. There is also modest growth in the AMR Region. In the EUR Region, recorded total wine consumption has been on a slow but steady decline from 2001 to 2010.

Figure 49 shows changes in total recorded alcohol from 2001 to 2010 by WB income group. The HI income group has shown steady total recorded alcohol consumption over the period, but has seen its share of global total recorded alcohol consumption decline from 42% in 2001 to 32% in 2010. The most significant gainer in this period is the UMI group of countries — its total recorded alcohol consumption increased from 7.4 billion liters of pure alcohol in 2001 to 11.6 liters in 2010, while its share of global consumption increased from 40% in 2001 to 47% in 2010.

As for changes in recorded alcohol consumption by WB income group in each product type, Figure 50 shows that the UMI group has been leading the way in

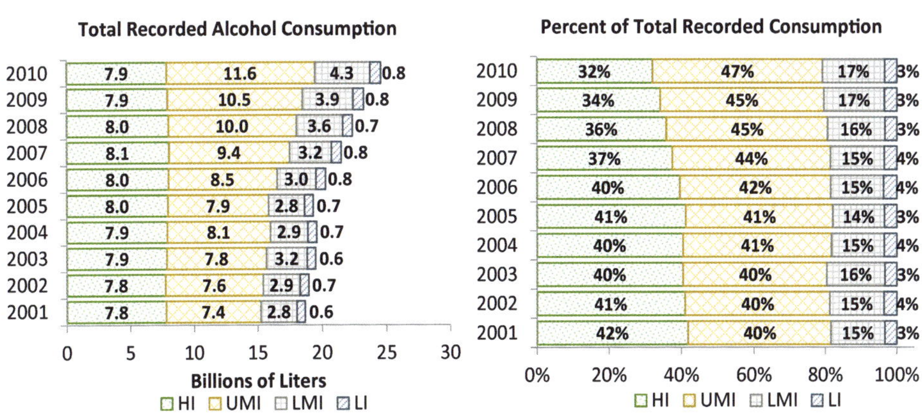

Figure 49. Recorded alcohol consumption by WB Income Group, total in billions of liters of pure alcohol and percent of total recorded consumption, among individuals aged 15+, 2001–2010

Sources: WHO GISAH and UN Department of Economic and Social Affairs, Population Division (2013), World Population Prospects: The 2012 Revision, DVD Edition.

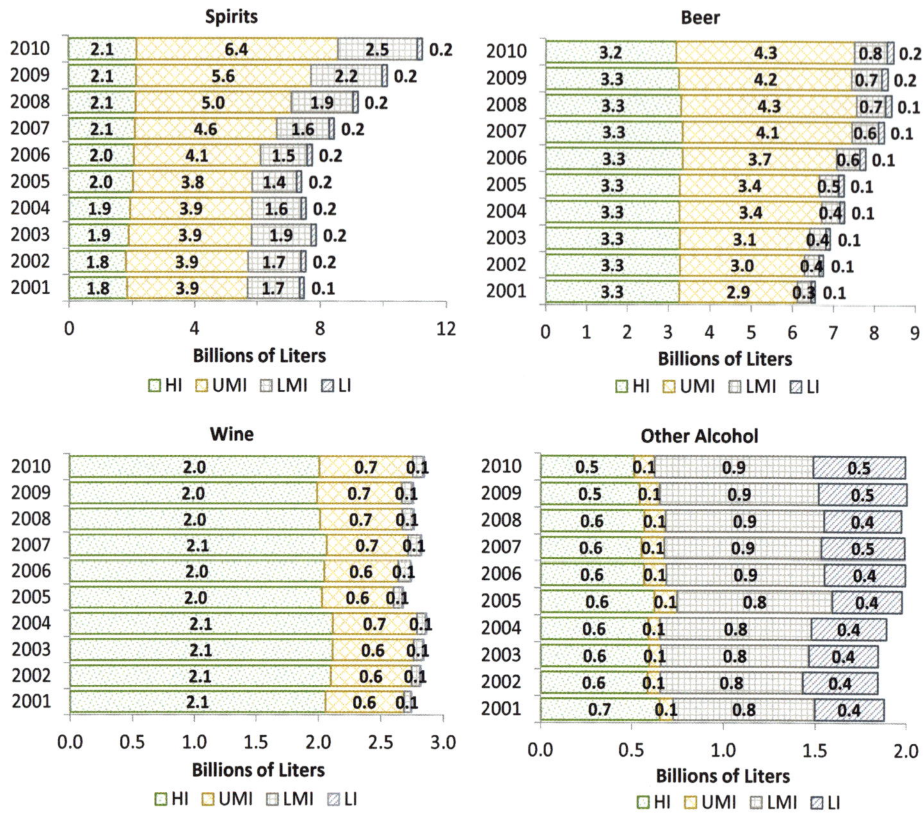

Figure 50. Recorded alcohol consumption by WB Income Group for each product type, among individuals aged 15+, in billions of liters of pure alcohol, 2001–2010

Sources: WHO GISAH and UN Department of Economic and Social Affairs, Population Division (2013), World Population Prospects: The 2012 Revision, DVD Edition.

increased total recorded spirits consumption from 2001 to 2010. The LMI group has also shown significant increases in recorded spirits consumption in that same period. Changes in recorded beer consumption seems to follow the same story line as that of recorded spirits consumption, with the UMI and LMI regions registering increases from 2001 to 2010, while the HI group has been holding steady.

Recorded wine consumption has not changed dramatically between 2001 and 2010. There have been minor decreases in the HI group, and minor increases in the UMI group. In the case of recorded consumption of other alcohol, Figure 50 shows that the HI group has consumed progressively less other alcohol from 2001 to 2010, while there has been modest increases in the LMI and LI regions.

On a per capita basis, Figure 51 shows that APC recorded alcohol consumption has been on a steady rise from 2001 to 2010, again with a notable drop between 2004 and 2005. In terms of APC consumption by product, spirits had the

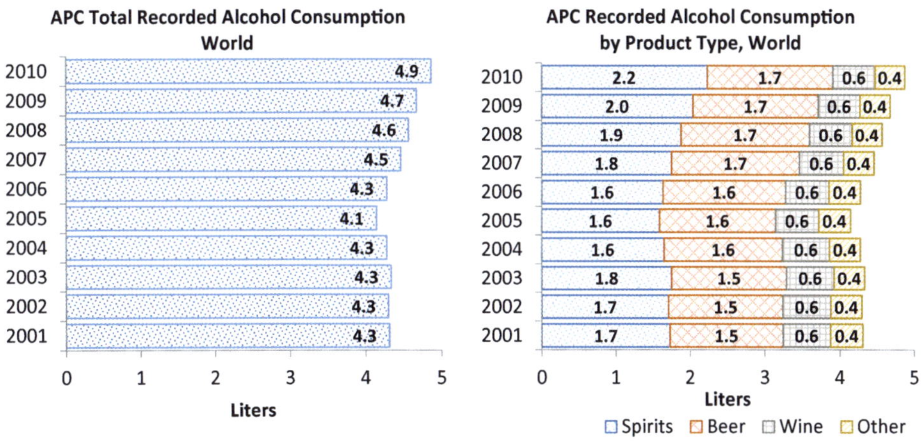

Figure 51. APC recorded alcohol consumption among individuals aged 15+, total and by product type, in liters of pure alcohol, 2001–2010

Sources: WHO GISAH and UN Department of Economic and Social Affairs, Population Division (2013), World Population Prospects: The 2012 Revision, DVD Edition.

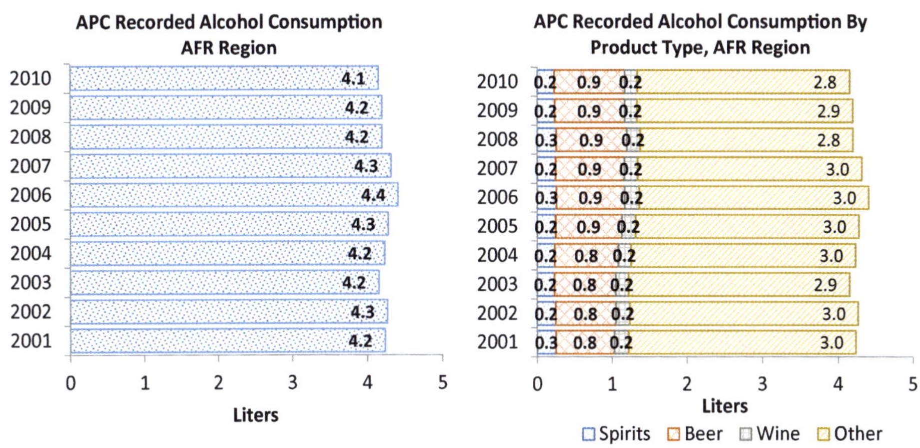

Figure 52. APC recorded alcohol consumption among individuals aged 15+, AFR Region, total and by product type, in liters of pure alcohol, 2001–2010

Sources: WHO GISAH and UN Department of Economic and Social Affairs, Population Division (2013), World Population Prospects: The 2012 Revision, DVD Edition.

greatest increase, from 1.7 liters of pure alcohol in 2001 to 2.2 liters in 2010. Beer also saw meaningful APC recorded consumption increase in the same period, from 1.5 liters in 2001 to 1.7 liters in 2010. APC recorded consumption of wine and other alcohol did not experience meaningful increase from 2001 to 2010.

Figures 52–57 show the changes in APC recorded alcohol consumption in each WHO region, in terms to total APC consumption and APC consumption by

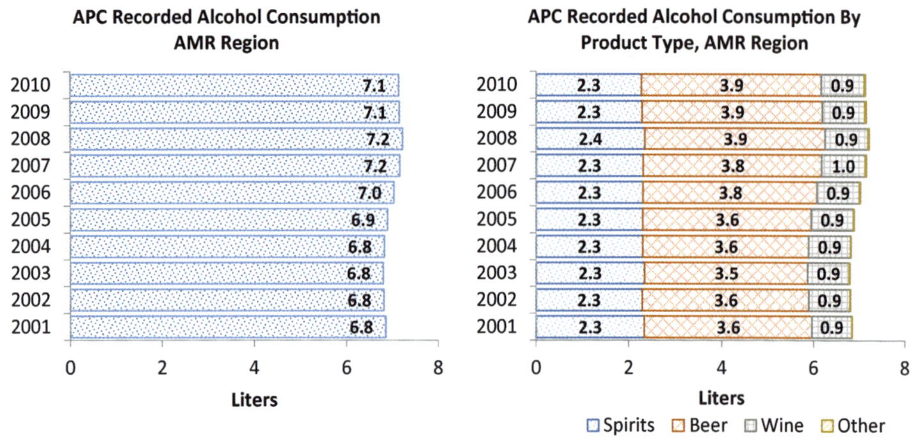

Figure 53. APC recorded alcohol consumption among individuals aged 15+, AMR Region, total and by product type, in liters of pure alcohol, 2001–2010

Sources: WHO GISAH and UN Department of Economic and Social Affairs, Population Division (2013), World Population Prospects: The 2012 Revision, DVD Edition.

product type. In the AFR Region, fluctuations of total APC recorded alcohol consumption between 2001 and 2010 were primarily due to changes in APC recorded other alcohol consumption.

In the AMR Region, APC recorded consumption of beer saw a slow yet steady increase between 2001 and 2010. Wine enjoyed a slight increase from 2006 to 2007, as did spirits between 2007 and 2008. In both those cases the increases were short-lived, but there has been no dramatic decrease in APC recorded consumption of those two products from 2001 to 2010.

The SEAR region has seen dramatic changes in APC recorded alcohol consumption between 2001 and 2010. Total APC recorded consumption declined from 1.5 liters of pure alcohol in 2001 to 1.2 liters in 2005, but has since then been on a steady annual increase, to its 2010 level of 2.0 liters of pure alcohol. Figure 54 shows that for this region, changes in APC recorded alcohol consumption over time have primarily been due to changes in APC recorded spirits consumption. The only other alcohol type of significance in the region is beer, and that has remained a very small fraction of total and APR alcohol consumption in the SEAR.

APC recorded alcohol consumption in the EUR region increased from 9.1 liters of pure alcohol in 2001 to 9.6 liters in 2007, but has since been on a steady decline, to its 2010 level of 8.9 liters. APC recorded consumption of spirits, beer and wine all decreased between 2007 and 2010 in the EUR Region. Only beer showed an increase in APC recorded consumption from 2001 to 2010.

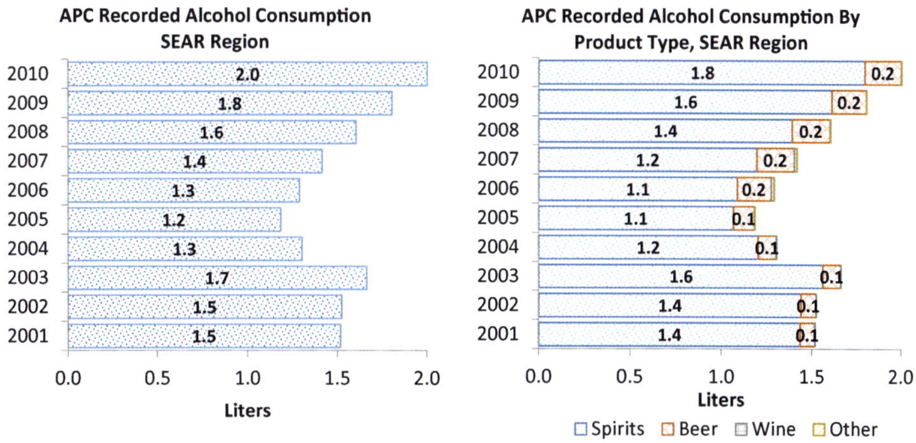

Figure 54. APC recorded alcohol consumption among individuals aged 15+, SEAR Region, total and by product type, in liters of pure alcohol, 2001–2010

Sources: WHO GISAH and UN Department of Economic and Social Affairs, Population Division (2013), World Population Prospects: The 2012 Revision, DVD Edition.

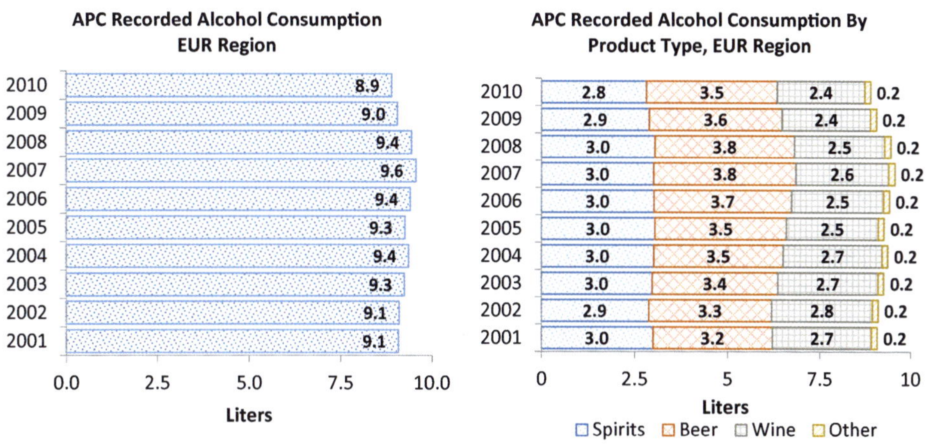

Figure 55. APC recorded alcohol consumption among individuals aged 15+, EUR Region, total and by product type, in liters of pure alcohol, 2001–2010

Sources: WHO GISAH and UN Department of Economic and Social Affairs, Population Division (2013), World Population Prospects: The 2012 Revision, DVD Edition.

The EMR Region, which consistently has very low levels of recorded alcohol consumption, has shown modest increases in APC recorded alcohol consumption between 2001 and 2010. Figure 56 shows that increase in APC recorded spirits consumption is primarily responsible for the increase.

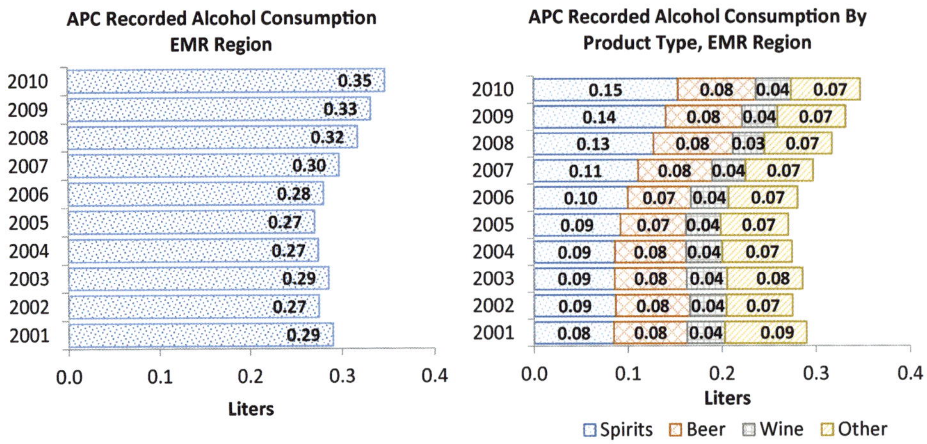

Figure 56. APC recorded alcohol consumption among individuals aged 15+, EMR Region, total and by product type, in liters of pure alcohol, 2001–2010

Sources: WHO GISAH and UN Department of Economic and Social Affairs, Population Division (2013), World Population Prospects: The 2012 Revision, DVD Edition.

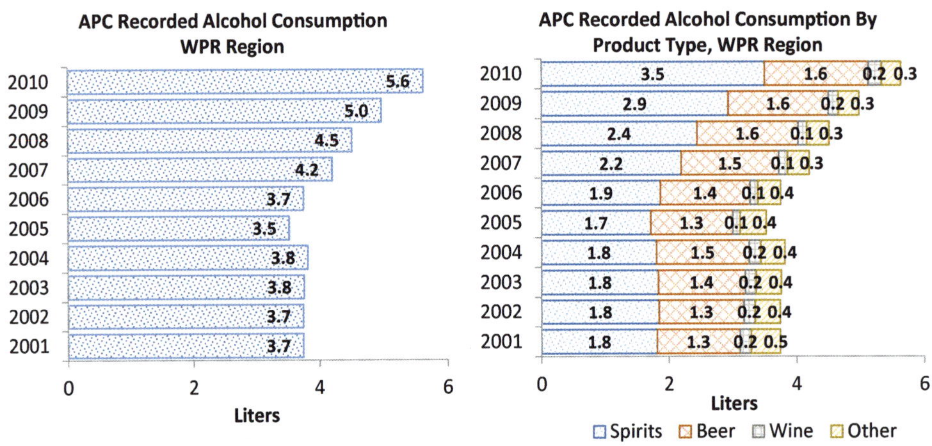

Figure 57. APC recorded alcohol consumption among individuals aged 15+, WPR Region, total and by product type, in liters of pure alcohol, 2001–2010

Sources: WHO GISAH and UN Department of Economic and Social Affairs, Population Division (2013), World Population Prospects: The 2012 Revision, DVD Edition.

Among all the WHO regions, the WPR region has shown the most dramatic increase in APC recorded alcohol consumption between 2001 and 2010. Figure 57 shows that APC recorded alcohol consumption has increased from 3.7 liters of pure alcohol in 2001 to 5.6 liters in 2010. There was a drop in APC recorded alcohol consumption between 2004 and 2005, but it has been on an impressive annual increase ever since. Figure 57 also shows that changes in APC recorded spirits consumption has accounted for most of the overall APC increase in this region. Beer contributed the rest of the increase. APC recorded consumption of other alcohol actually decreased from 0.5 liters in 2001 to 0.3 liters in 2010.

Finally, we examine the changes in APC recorded alcohol consumption between 2001 and 2010, in terms of total APC consumption and APC consumption by product type, for each WB income group.

Countries in the HI income group experienced a decline in APC recorded alcohol consumption, from 9.4 liters of pure alcohol in 2001 to 8.7 liters in 2010 (see Figure 58). Among the product types, APC recorded spirits consumption registered an increase from 2.2 liters in 2001 to 2.4 liters in 2010. All three of the other product types — beer, wine and other alcohol — saw decreases in APC recorded alcohol consumption from 2001 to 2010.

For the UMI group, APC recorded alcohol consumption increased from 4.3 liters of pure alcohol in 2001 to 5.9 liters in 2010. Figure 59 shows that APC recorded spirits consumption contributed 1.1 liters of that total increase from 2001 to 2010, while APC recorded beer consumption contributed 0.5 liters toward the total APC increase.

For the countries in the LMI group, APC recorded alcohol consumption increased from 2 liters of pure alcohol in 2001 to 2.5 liters in 2010, after a drop to

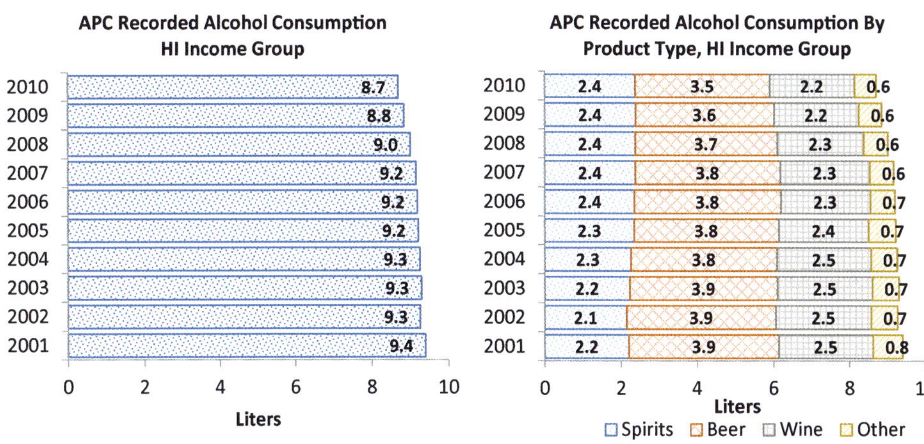

Figure 58. APC recorded alcohol consumption among individuals aged 15+, HI Income Group, total and by product type, in liters of pure alcohol, 2001–2010

Sources: WHO GISAH and UN Department of Economic and Social Affairs, Population Division (2013), World Population Prospects: The 2012 Revision, DVD Edition.

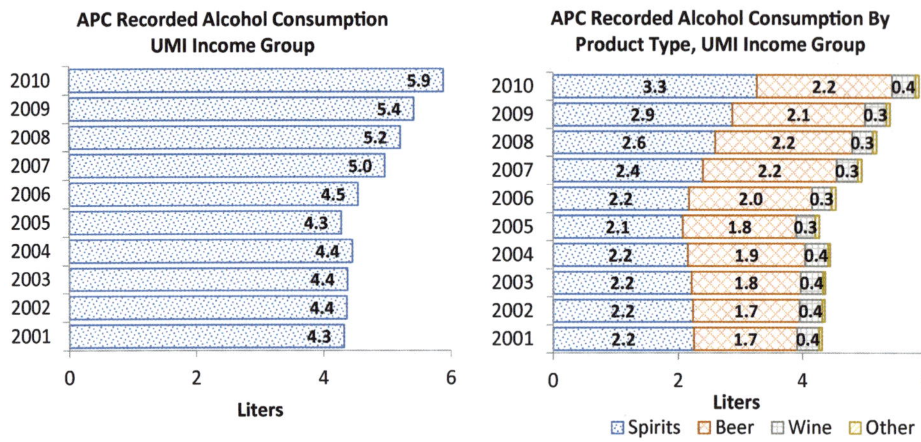

Figure 59. APC recorded alcohol consumption among individuals aged 15+, UMI Income Group, total and by product type, in liters of pure alcohol, 2001–2010

Sources: WHO GISAH and UN Department of Economic and Social Affairs, Population Division (2013), World Population Prospects: The 2012 Revision, DVD Edition.

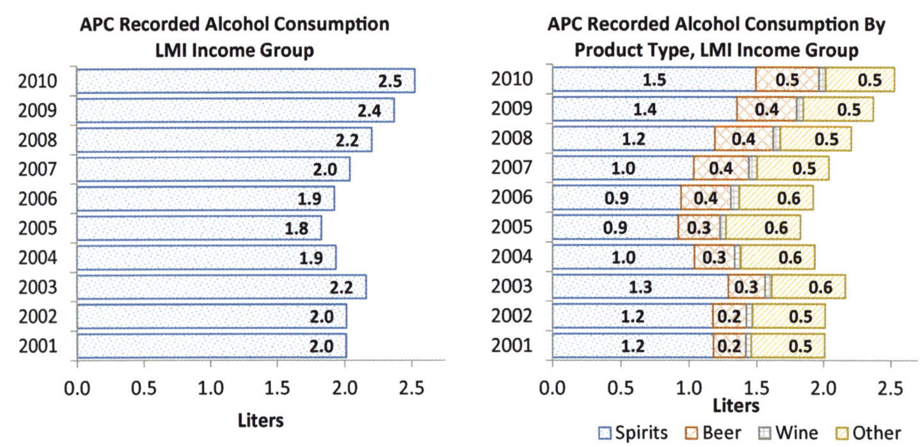

Figure 60. APC recorded alcohol consumption among individuals aged 15+, LMI Income Group, total and by product type, in liters of pure alcohol, 2001–2010

Sources: WHO GISAH and UN Department of Economic and Social Affairs, Population Division (2013), World Population Prospects: The 2012 Revision, DVD Edition.

1.8 liters in 2005. Figure 60 shows that changes in APC recorded consumption of spirits and beer contributed approximately evenly to the total APC increase.

For the LI group, there has been no significant change in total APC recorded alcohol consumption between 2001 and 2010. Fluctuations from year to year have been accounted for primarily by minor changes in APC recorded consumption of spirits and other alcohol.

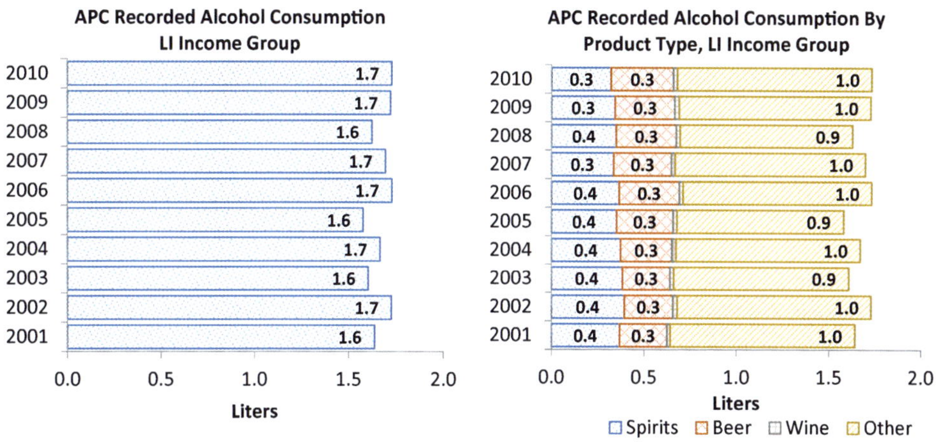

Figure 61. APC recorded alcohol consumption among individuals aged 15+, LI Income Group, total and by product type, in liters of pure alcohol, 2001–2010

Sources: WHO GISAH and UN Department of Economic and Social Affairs, Population Division (2013), World Population Prospects: The 2012 Revision, DVD Edition.

Global Alcohol Production

Data on global alcohol production is hard to come by, with most reports controlled by marketing associations. However, data that is available indicates that Europe (the EU) plays a major role: It is the source of 25% of spirits production and 50% of wine production. Member countries of the EU are involved in 70% of worldwide alcohol exports though around half of these exports are to other countries within the EU; alcohol contributes €9 billion to the EU's balance of payments. Alcohol was responsible for €25 billion of tax revenues in 2001 and contributes 750,000 jobs in production alone.

The industry has become increasingly concentrated, with the top producers accounting for 60% of the global volume of branded beer. When commodity beer is looked at however, small production dominates, accounting for 62% of total production. Global brewers have been investing in Brazil, Russia, China and India, mainly through strategic partnerships. World beer sales were 157.8 billion liters in 2005 (ICAP, 2006).

This pattern of mergers and acquisitions can also be seen in the distilled spirits industry, but again the market continues to have numerous small local producers due to prices and local customs which prefer the local brand. Premium Western-style spirit production is dominated by large players, but they only produce about 20% of the total global spirits market. Diageo — a leading international alcoholic beverages company headquartered in London — produces close to 15% of global Western-style spirits (spirits produced in accordance with international standards) but accounts for less than 5% of total spirits production. Wine production is concentrated in Europe and provides close to 3 million jobs, or 2% of EU civilian employment when both direct and indirect employment are summed together. In the US, the beer industry is responsible for $54 billion in wages and benefits, employing 1.8 million people (ICAP, 2006).

The U.S. alcoholic beverage industry in 2010 contributed $400 billion to the US economy, $90 billion in wages, 3.9 million jobs, and $21 billion in direct state and local revenues, with distilled spirits making up 41% of this direct revenue. Indirect revenue (mainly property and personal taxes) added another $20 billion (Distilled Spirits Council of the United States, 2010).

Health Benefits of Alcohol Consumption

While the public health perspective of alcohol consumption focuses on harmful effects, there is evidence that alcohol consumption can also positively impact health. The physical health benefits of consumption follow a J or U-shaped curve: they are closely linked to the amount of alcohol consumed, and may be linked to the type of alcohol, with red wine perhaps the most beneficial quaff. Mental health benefits from alcohol consumption are difficult to support empirically at this time (Ferreira MP, 2008).

Moderate alcohol consumption has been shown to have positive health benefits, reducing the risk of cardiovascular disease, extending longevity and increasing activity in later life. Both Ferreira and Weems (2008) and Gaziano *et al.* (2000), identify a U-shaped relationship between alcohol consumption and mortality in middle-aged (age 45–65) and older Americans. Gaziano *et al.* surveyed over 260,000 male physicians in the United States who were between 40 and 82 years of age and received responses from just over 112,000. They observed a statistically significant decrease in total mortality of light to moderate drinkers (<2 drinks per day) versus abstainers, adjusted for age and multiple variables. After multivariate adjustment, no significant increases or decreases in risk of lung, colon, prostate, pancreatic or hematologic (lymphoma or leukemia) were apparent in any drinking category. The positive effects were linked to reduction in cardiovascular disease. Additionally, in a study of postmenopausal women, moderate alcohol use (approximately 4–5 drinks per week), was linked to higher serum estradiol levels which in turn are linked to lower risk of cardiovascular disease (Gavaler and Van Thiel, 1992). A study that used nurses for its data found that moderate alcohol consumption decreased the risk of stroke and coronary heart disease but increased the risk of subarachnoid hemorrhage (Stampfer *et al.*, 1988). On the mobility front, a study of close to 8,000 men and women over 65 years old found the risk of losing mobility was lower for those who consumed small-to-moderate amounts of alcohol, compared to subjects who did not consume alcohol (LaCroix *et al.*, 1993).

Other research has focused on the effects of wine, or wine and beer, versus consumption of other spirits and found relatively higher benefits on health. The French paradox is a term from 1992 that refers to the high saturated fat diet of the French yet low incidence of coronary disease (Giuseppe Lippi, 2010). It may be attributable to the consumption of red wine. Isolating the effects of the numerous compounds in red wine from each other and from the societal factors that stratify wine drinkers from others in the population is difficult. However, "scientific research has demonstrated that the molecules present in grapes and in wine alter cellular metabolism and signaling, which is consistent mechanistically with reducing arterial disease" (German and Walzem, 2000). Additionally, red wine has an abundance of phenolic acids and polyphenols which may have health benefits (German and Walzem, 2000).

Other research states conclusively that "alcohol by itself has favorable effects on the level of high-density lipoprotein cholesterol, and inhibition of platelet aggregation. Wine, particularly red wine, has high levels of phenolic compounds that favorably influence multiple biochemical systems, such as increased high-density lipoprotein cholesterol, antioxidant activity, decreased platelet aggregation and endothelial adhesion, suppression of cancer cell growth, and promotion of nitric oxide production" (Alfred and de Lorimier, 2000). However, since reprints of this article are available from the author c/o the de Lorimier Winery, some amount of skepticism should color the weight given to this author's assertions.

More reliable is a meta-analysis of 26 studies, which pooled data on wine and beer consumption and vascular disease. The relative risk of vascular disease was 0.68 for wine drinkers compared to abstainers. Data from 10 studies supported a J curve, with moderate wine consumption reducing vascular disease. Moderate beer drinking also was negatively associated with vascular disease (0.78 risk), but no relationship between specific amounts of beer consumption and risk were discovered (Since some of the studies excluded ex-drinkers while some controlled for selection bias, the authors feel that overall the meta-analysis results are reliable.) (Castelnuovo *et al.*, 2002).

Wine also scores best when serum uric acid levels are added to the equation: A study of close to 15,000 participants found that serum uric acid levels (which can lead to gout), increased as beer and liquor intake increased, but not with wine consumption. In fact, a negative relationship was found between wine consumption and uric acid levels. (Choi, 2004) The studies cited above are US-based; other evidence points to similar benefits globally for the most part. However, cardio protective effects disappear in Russia and are lower in Central East and Eastern Europe than the rest of Europe (Rehm *et al.*, 2012). Looking at beer alone, in Africa, sorghum beer seems to have additional health benefits, providing manganese and potassium (van Heerden and Parry, 2001).

The health benefits mentioned so far relate to decreasing mortality and/or morbidity. A general population study in Finland expands the focus to look at the effects of alcohol consumption on quality of life (Qol), examining associations between alcohol consumption and utility-based health-related quality of life (HRQoL), subjective QoL, self-rated health (SRH), and mental distress. HRQoL was better for moderate drinkers, but the relation mostly disappeared when controls for socio-demographic differences (age, education, income), were added. For women, moderate alcohol consumption was positively correlated with better self-reported health and a higher outcome on one of the health utility measures employed but the results were clinically insignificant (Samuli and Saarni, 2008).

Similar to the theory of the J- or U-shaped curve of the physical health benefits of alcohol consumption is a hypothesis of an inverted J- or U-shaped relationship between consumption and psychological wellbeing.[3] A Russian study did find a J-shape for men and a U-shaped curve for women, but as in the work by Samuli and Saarni cited above, once other variables were added, the shapes flattened considerably. Results for women alone lost significance, while the quadratic relationship remained for the full sample and men (Massin and Kopp, 2014).

That the health results of alcohol consumption may be gender-specific is supported by a paper that looks at life satisfaction and alcohol consumption among college students. The researchers found alcohol use was associated with lower general satisfaction and anticipated future satisfaction among women but a positive, curvilinear relation to social satisfaction (not other measures of life satisfaction), among men (Murphy *et al.*, 2005).

So, while attempts to link mental health and moderate drinking have not produced robust results, the much stronger evidence for physical health benefits in the research cited above have also not been readily accepted. However, research by Klatsky and Friedman put to bed the main arguments against accepting that moderate alcohol consumption has public health benefits. They control for effects of smoking and incorporate research using twins, which refutes the genetic constitution argument that abstainers have constitutions which increase mortality risk. A plausible biological mechanism for better health of light to moderate drinkers is higher high-density lipoprotein cholesterol in drinkers. Light drinkers have a 30–40% lower coronary heart disease mortality risk and a 10% overall lower mortality risk. They conclude that even though heavy drinking causes harm, it is not

[3]The J- or U-shaped curve of physical benefits has drinks per day on the x-axis and risk of adverse health conditions on the y-axis and suggests risk decreases as moderate consumption occurs, but bottoms out at 1–2 drinks per day, then rises. The inverted curve related to mental health has alcohol consumed on the x-axis and mental well-being on the y-axis. In this case, mental health improves with moderate consumption, then plateaus at the top of the inverted u and begins to worsen.

wise to promote general abstinence. This does not mean that all abstainers should be advised to drink: health care practitioners need to look at individuals' personal histories and characteristics (Klatsky, 1995).

Ferreira and Weems contend that US national guidelines for alcohol consumption specific to older adults (e.g., those offered by the National Institute on Alcohol Abuse) may be too restrictive, given the current literature (Ferreira, 2008). This is of importance since: (1) Older adults are the fastest growing segment of the population, and (2) total alcohol intake decreases after retirement. In a study of residents in three US retirement communities, moderate alcohol consumption was associated with improved social interactions and self-reported health status. Similarly, moderate alcohol consumption was positively related to health quality of life in Australian women over 70 years of age. In this same cohort, abstention and infrequent drinking were negatively associated with quality of life and survival (Ferreira, 2008).

Adverse Health and Economic Consequences of Alcohol Consumption and Alcohol Control

The three main pathways from alcohol consumption to harm include: Toxic effects on organs and tissues, intoxication which in turn leads to impairment of physical and mental functioning, and dependence on alcohol such that an individual's control over his consumption is impaired.

The WHO, using 2012 data, attributes 3.3 million deaths a year to alcohol consumption globally and links it to more than 200 diseases/injury conditions. This equates to just under 6% of all deaths. The diseases/conditions include neuropsychiatric, gastrointestinal, and cardiovascular conditions, cancers, fetal alcohol syndrome, and diabetes mellitus. Alcohol use disorders and fetal alcohol syndrome are 100% attributable to alcohol. Evidence now links alcohol causally to infectious diseases such as tuberculosis and pneumonia, though this relationship may require consumption above a certain level. Alcohol consumption can also lead to intentional and unintentional injuries (WHO, 2014).

The percentage of all deaths linked to alcohol is highest in the WHO European Region, which also has the highest alcohol consumption. However, the statistic is driven by Eastern Europe. The lowest proportion of deaths attributed to alcohol occur in the Eastern Mediterranean Region (0.9%), followed by Africa (3.3%). The former is due to abstinence in many Muslim countries, that latter unfortunately due to low overall life expectancy.

Besides being a direct cause of death, alcohol consumption is the attributed cause of 5.1% of the global burden of disease and injury in 2012 (WHO, 2014). The disease perhaps most associated with alcohol is cirrhosis of the liver, but the exact relationship is not well understood. Low to moderate alcohol consumption is not associated with statistically significant increases in liver cirrhosis, but if cirrhosis develops (from alcohol consumption or other causes), even moderate drinking increases the risk of dying (WHO, 2014). Supporting this is the systematic review and meta-analysis covering research from 1980 to 2008 done by Rehm *et al.* which discovered that the impact on mortality of liver cirrhosis was higher than morbidity, that the same average consumption caused a higher risk of cirrhosis for women versus men, and that threshold effects seems to exist (Rehm *et al.*, 2010).

Alcohol consumption is also linked to HIV and other sexually transmitted diseases. This is an indirect relationship and can be confounded by both excessive drinking and unsafe sex representing risky behaviors. Alcohol consumption has been linked to lower adherence to HIV treatment and is even called the "Forgotten Drug in HIV/AIDS" (Fritz *et al.*, 2010).

Similar to STD incidence, there are other negative effects of alcohol consumption that can only be indirectly linked to health — namely, the socioeconomic consequences of heavy drinking. The WHO (2014) describes these socioeconomic consequences as the reactions of others to the drinker's behavior, such as loss of earnings, unemployment, family problems, stigma, and barriers to accessing health care. The report points out that resources spent on alcohol may harm the financial wellbeing of a family or community, and that drunkenness will impair job performance and therefore income. Additionally, surveys conducted around the world show that heavy drinkers may be marginalized by society and not given the same access to health care and other resources.

From a health economics perspective, an individual's health is a stock good that can be increased through investment or decreased through adverse behaviors or external negative factors (Grossman, 2000). Investment in health takes the form of both positive non-monetary health behaviors and monetary investment in the form of purchasing proper nutrients and accessing health care. The direction of the causal relationship between health and economic well-being can go both ways. Good health leads to fewer sick days, greater productivity, and increased school attendance, which results in greater formation of human capital and therefore greater wealth. Causality can also run from wealth to health: Greater wealth provides access to better nutrition, increased knowledge about health, and access to more and better health care. Low wealth and poor health can therefore become intertwined, placing individuals into a cycle of ill-health and low socioeconomic status that can be difficult if not impossible to break free.

One very troubling example of people trapped in cycles of poverty arises from the "dop" system in South Africa — named after the Afrikaans word for alcoholic drink where farm workers were paid partially in alcohol. Though this practice has been outlawed, one-fifth of workers interviewed for a 2000 study reported that the dop system was still being used. Almost 50% of these workers consumed more alcohol than is considered safe and over 9% consumed amounts categorized as dangerous (London, 2000).

Other concerning information about health and alcohol that is emerging relates to consumption patterns. Overall consumption has decreased, but health problems have increased, which may be due to binge drinking. A study in Japan states that, although the available data are not robust enough to conclude why health problems are increasing, the data do point to increased drinking among women while overall consumption is down (Higuchi *et al.*, 2007). Sweden has also seen declines in per capita consumption and risk factors in a study of its youth from 2000 to 2010, but saw a sharp increase in alcohol-related hospitalizations, most likely due to polarized drinking habits (Hallgren *et al.*, 2012).

The results of these specific country findings are supported by Rehm *et al.*, who reported that 1 in 7 deaths for men and 1 in 13 for women (between the ages of 15 and 64), in the EU in 2004 were caused by alcohol. The protective effects of alcohol have been netted out of these numbers. The alcohol-attributed mortality numbers for Eastern Europe and Central-East Europe are the highest within Europe, which the authors partially attribute to lower economic wealth. Liver cirrhosis accounts for over 75% of the alcohol attributable deaths, with the next largest categories intentional injury and mental and neurological diseases. This last category has significantly lower prevalence in Southern European men (Rehm *et al.*, 2012).

Another measure of the public health effects of alcohol is the potential years of life lost (PYLL) due to alcohol. This is an estimate of the additional years a person would have lived had they not died prematurely. In 2004 in the EU, just over 2 million years of life were estimated to be lost due to alcohol. This number is important in that it underlines that these fatalities occur earlier in life than other fatalities, on average. Again, the highest PYLL are in Central-East and Eastern Europe, with the gap between men and women the largest in those regions compared to other parts of Europe (Rehm *et al*, 2012). (For comparison, on average, during 2000–2004 smoking accounted for an estimated 3.1 million years of potential life lost for males and 2 million years of potential life lost for females annually in the United States.) (CDC, 2008).

Costs of alcohol consumption

As mentioned above, the economic costs of alcohol consumption are intertwined with its health costs and include the costs of treating the resultant disease or injury and lost productivity, as well as the effect on the next generation's nutrition and education when caregivers are unable to give care due to alcohol use — all of which cause less investment in health stock. The CDC estimates excessive drinking cost the US$223.5 billion in 2006, which equates to $1.90 per drink. The CDC attributes 75% of this cost to binge drinking. Lost productivity accounts for 72% of the cost, with health care making up another 11%, law enforcement and court costs 9%, and car accidents 6%.

Total costs to society

The WHO has attempted to aggregate the societal costs of drinking, adding up three categories. First is the direct economic costs of alcohol consumption, which include the costs of health care services, damaged property, arrests, and increased crime. Second is indirect costs that arise from lost productivity due to unemployment, absenteeism, reduced productivity, and lost working years. Estimates of these social costs range from 21 billion pounds in the UK and Northern Ireland to €125 billion in the EU, to over $233 billion in the United States. In South Africa, these costs were thought to amount to 10–12% of GDP in 2009 (WHO, 2014). The third category is intangibles and includes pain and suffering and diminished quality of life for the drinker, his family, and possibly others he interacts with. Measuring this third category is very difficult (WHO, 2014).

A Swedish study does an exhaustive job of estimating and compiling the many societal costs of alcohol for the year 2002 in an attempt to establish a prototype for other countries to follow. It concludes that a conservative estimate is 1% of Sweden's GDP. The largest portion of this (approximately 25%) comes from lost productivity due to mortality, with another 5% from health care costs. If all effects on productivity are tallied together, lost productivity represents 50% of the total societal cost of alcohol consumption. (Johansson *et al.*, 2006). This is of particular interest since lost productivity is not commonly the main ill one thinks about in relation to alcohol consumption. The problem with the methodology is that, since many of the costs of alcohol consumption are not tracked per se, the authors must extrapolate extensively from available data and rely heavily on assumptions.

An earlier study in New Zealand underlines the gargantuan task of isolating the full burden that alcohol imposes on society by estimating that the sum of social costs range from $1 to $4 billion in 1991: However, with a range this wide it is hard to give credence to the numbers. Their range for direct costs is a little more narrow, $341 million to $589 million, but still quite broad (Devlin *et al.*, 1997).

Cost/Benefit Analysis of Alcohol Control Policies

For centuries, governments have formulated and attempted to enforce polices to limit alcohol consumption. The policies attempt to dampen demand or limit supply or a combination of the two. Therefore, all discussions of the effectiveness of these policies need to incorporate the central economic principle of the interaction of demand and supply. This section will attempt to outline the effectiveness of these policies, relying on the WHO's 2014 Report for identification of the main categories of policies. We will then attempt to weigh the costs of these policies against their benefits. We will also summarize the formulation of an index to measure the effectiveness of policies on a comprehensive basis.

In order to fulfill its objective to reduce the harmful use of alcohol by 10% by 2025, the WHO has identified the main methods undertaken around the globe at the national and local levels to educate consumers so that they voluntarily use alcohol in a more responsible manner (demand-side interventions), and also efforts to reduce availability and restrict sales of alcohol (supply-side interventions). Examples include: Outright bans, limits on the density of outlets, limits on hours/days/volume of sales, licensing requirements, blood alcohol content (BAC) limits for drivers, legal drinking age restrictions, and crackdowns on illicit production. Most involve controls on supply and we therefore will first discuss supply-side efforts. However, our review of existing studies, as outlined below, will point toward policies moderating demand as being more effective.

Supply-Side Alcohol Policies

According to the *Encyclopedia Britannica*, some form of prohibition — a legal restriction on the sale, manufacturing and/or transport of alcohol — has been made in numerous societies dating back to the Aztecs and ancient China, but only a few Muslim countries have maintained total bans in the present day. Prohibition was tried as recently as the early 20th Century in the US. While widely perceived as a failure, scholarly articles debating its merits and pitfalls have been produced. Blocker, for example, argues that it lowered per capita consumption but that, "Its political failure is attributable more to a changing context than to characteristics of the innovation itself" (Jack and Blocker, 2006). However, since the amendment establishing Prohibition is the only amendment to ever be repealed, and American whiskey sales were up 34% from 2008 to 2013, according to the Distilled Spirits Council of the United States, and up more than 100% for super-premium whiskey (Risen, 2014), it seems pointless to debate the merits of Prohibition here. Instead, we concentrate on more relevant methods of controlling alcohol consumption than attempting to eliminate or even severely constrict supply.

Current restrictions on alcohol sales include blue laws, which ban alcohol sales on Sundays in retail establishments. Available research on the topic is not conclusive as to whether these laws are effective in reducing the negative effects of alcohol consumption (Steefel, 2011; Yoruk, 2014). As sports watching at sports bars on Sundays seems to be growing in popularity, more Sunday bans on store-based alcohol sales do not hold much promise as a preventive method.

A similar method is to restrict the hours of operation of places where alcohol is both sold and consumed, i.e., on premise establishments such as bars and restaurants. A synthesis of studies on the effectiveness of such policies found 10 out of 14 studies supporting that increasing the hours of operation (by 2 or more hours) increases alcohol-related harm. Alcohol-related harm was measured mainly in the form of increased DUI and motor vehicle crashes. These studies were all done in high-income countries other than the United States. Whether or not this evidence supports the converse — that reducing hours will reduce harm, as the researchers suggest (Middleton *et al.*, 2010) — is questionable.

Another method is to limit the number of establishments that sell alcohol. Countries and states have myriad policies for licensing these establishments, and governments keep varying amounts of control over their licensing practices. Some of the regulations limit the geographic density of establishments while factoring in the population of the area. Empirical evidence, mostly from outside the US, does point to density as a contributing factor in the harmful effects of alcohol (Gruenewald, 2011; Stevenson *et al.*, 1999; Stockwell *et al.*, 2009). Most of the harm recorded is related to increased violence in areas with high density of alcohol establishments. The counterfactual — in other words, what would happen to neighboring areas and the prevalence of alcohol's harmful effects when density is reduced — has not been studied, which limits the ability to draw a causal relationship.

Demand-Side Alcohol Policies

A review of past work in this area, (Moskowitz, 1989), found that three government actions that change demand are most effective at reducing alcohol consumption. These are: Increasing alcohol taxes, raising the minimum legal drinking age to 21, and increasing the enforcement of drinking-driving laws. This section will therefore concentrate on these policies.

Before delving into these policies, it is best to lay out the theory of rational addiction, which supports a downward sloping demand curve, even in the case of addictive substances (Becker *et al.*, 1991). This theory is important since common sense would lead one to conclude that price changes would not alter demand for addictive substances: The addiction would drive demand, and efforts to control consumption through price would therefore be futile. If this were true, then raising prices through taxation would curtail alcohol consumption among low- to moderate-drinking consumers, whose drinking habits are possibly providing health benefits, but not decrease consumption among dependent drinkers. Rather, higher prices would instill a higher economic burden on addicted drinkers, making them less likely to invest in their health.

Becker *et al.*'s model of rational addiction makes clear that this does not have to be the case. They explain how addictive behavior involves reinforcement and tolerance. Past drinking reinforces the desire for current consumption and also reduces the utility derived from current consumption, since the consumer has built up a tolerance for the addictive substance. Reinforcement raises the marginal utility of current consumption; tolerance has the opposite effect. A rational, addicted person will therefore drink less now if prices were higher in the past or are expected to be higher in the future, and consumption across time periods are complementary goods. (That is: higher drinking in one period means higher drinking in other periods and vice versa.) Additionally, the rational consumer realizes that the cost of alcohol is not just the price paid, but also the negative effects on current and future health and current and future earnings if the consumption interferes with the productivity of the consumer (Becker *et al.*, 1991).

The rational model of addiction produces this demand function:

$$C_t = f(P_t, C_{t-1}, C_{t+1}, Z_t).$$

Consumption is a function of the current price, consumption in the prior period, consumption in the future period, and other traits relating to tastes (Z_t) (Chaloupka, 1990).

Empirical evidence supports the relationship between price and demand that the rational addiction model predicts: Even for this addictive substance, evidence points to a downward-sloping demand curve. A relatively recent US study exploited the differences in state alcohol sales taxes to test this theory and found that respondents to surveys in states with higher taxes are less likely to drink and less likely to binge, though the average number of drinks for those who do drink are not affected. (The average is not affected since both numerator and denominator decrease: The numerator due to less binge drinking and denominator because some people do not drink at all who otherwise would have in the absence of the higher taxes.) A 10-cent increase in excise tax reduces the odds of drinking by 28% for men (Cook, 2007).

Chaloupka *et al.* explain that excise taxes are the primary means of influencing the price of alcohol. The US Federal Government taxes distilled spirits, wine, and beer by volume. All states tax beer; most tax wine and distilled spirits also. Overall taxes on alcohol, once adjusted for inflation, have declined significantly over the years in the US. While the research examined has varying estimates of price elasticity, there is consensus that beer consumption is the least price elastic, distilled spirits the most elastic. This follows the substitution to lower priced goods: Since beer is the least expensive, there is less substitution available. Most research also finds long-term elasticity to be higher than short-term (Xu and Chaloupka, 2011). A 1998 study by Grossman *et al.* of high school seniors found a short-run price elasticity of alcohol of −0.41 and long-run elasticity of −0.65. The ratio of short-run to long-run elasticity is greater for more addictive goods. This ratio is higher for cigarettes than alcohol, suggesting cigarettes are more addictive (Grossman *et al.*, 1998).

If policymakers wish to minimize the deadweight loss of taxes, then the least price-elastic alcohols should be taxed the most, which, from the evidence cited above, would suggest beer be taxed the most. However, since excise taxes on alcohol beverages have two objectives, raising revenue and reducing the negative impact of alcohol consumption on public health, how the taxes should be applied has been much debated.

Again, we turn to Chaloupka, this time partnering with Saffer, to lay out a framework for the debate on whether excise taxes on alcohol should be equalized or differentiated across beverage type (Saffer and Chaloupka, 1994). Many jurisdictions tax beer and wine less heavily than distilled spirits, due to different public health effects attributed to the different beverages. The US budget deficit reduction act in 1990 raised taxes on beer the most, wine the next highest amount, and distilled spirits the least, almost equalizing the excise tax across the three categories. Saffer and Chaloupka develop a theoretical model to simulate the optimal tax on each of the beverage types. They employ data on consumption and own price elasticities of the three beverage types and estimate cross price elasticities as fractions of own price elasticities. The results of their simulations would dictate that beer be taxed 25% more than spirits, and wine 8% more than spirits. Since their results run counter to prevailing policies, they conclude that equalization, or something close to equalization of excise taxes on beer, wine and distilled spirits may be the optimal tax policy, which has its own perverse logic.

However, in the UK, taxes imposed in 2012 that are based on alcohol content seem to have encouraged the consumption of beer over other spirits and reduced alcohol consumption by 8 billion grams (Rehm *et al.*, 2012). This latter study is important since different alcoholic beverages are substitutes for one another: when the price of a particular type of alcoholic beverage increases, consumers may substitute another alcoholic beverage (generally of lower quality/lower price).

A Swedish study of the interaction of price increases and consumption of various alcoholic products adds valuable findings to the debate. Overall, price increases decrease consumption significantly, but there is substitution from higher priced to lower priced beverages in general. The researchers broke each of wine, beer and spirits into quality categories by price and looked at own and cross-price effects. Higher prices decreased consumption. Higher prices on higher quality beverages increased consumption of lower quality beverages within each type (wine, beer, spirits). Only for beer did higher prices on low quality beers increase consumption of higher quality beers. Price increases on high quality beer and wine increased consumption of low quality spirits. Price increases on beer and spirits decreased sales of high quality wine and increased sales of lower quality wine. Similar results occurred for beer: price increases on wine and spirits decreased sales of high quality beer and increased sales of lower quality beer. If policymakers are imposing taxes to decrease consumption, it might make sense to concentrate on taxing the lowest price goods the most, since there can be no substitution down from the bottom (Gruenwald *et al.*, 2006).

Grunewald *et al.* are clear that they assess quality for their study on price and much of the price differential is due to taste. A caveat to their findings from a health perspective is whether or not lower quality spirits may also have more negative health effects. Clearly, substitution to illegal alcohol products which do not pass FDA controls may have negative health effects; to the extent that taxes push consumers into the arms of home/illicit producers, the positive effects of lower consumption may be muted. Additionally, as explained above, wine does seem to have the most positive health effects, and taxes on wine do lead consumers to substitute beer and spirits, which may be undesirable from a health perspective.

A UK study (Purshouse *et al.*, 2010) supports Grunewald *et al.*'s findings of the effectiveness of taxes in reducing consumption. This research contributes to the policy debate by showing that instituting a minimum price is more effective than price increases: The minimum price has less of an effect on consumption by moderate drinkers and a larger effect on harmful drinkers than a tax that raises prices in general.

Other researchers (Kuo *et al.*, 2003) took advantage of tax reform in Switzerland that occurred in accordance with a WTO agreement. They measured consumption both while tariffs were in effect and after tariffs were lifted. They found that alcohol consumption across all age groups (except those over 60 years of age) responded positively to lower prices, i.e., increased consumption. While this supports Gruenwald *et al.* and Purshouse *et al.* caution should be used in assuming that the response to a price decrease when tariffs are lifted can be used to project consumers' responses to a price increase: Consumers' reaction may be more heterogeneous. The lifting of tariffs most likely changed price differentials between different alcohol beverages and may have caused a temporary increase in consumption as consumers tried imported alcohol.

Stockwell and Crosbie (2001) present a case study of the alcohol market in Australia which highlights the interplay between industry forces and tax policy. Cask wine and alcohol pop drinks have grown in popularity and are seen as contributing to alcohol related harm since these products have high alcohol content relative to price. Tax policies beneficial to wine producers in order to support exports have contributed to the growth of cask wine. On a positive note, tax policies also favor low alcohol beer; consumption of low alcohol beer has also increased and is seen as reducing harm attributed to alcohol.

Since those buying the lowest price alcohol tend to be those with the lowest income, taxes on alcohol do seem to burden those of lower socioeconomic status more, which does reduce equity within society. However, since the studies show that people of lower socioeconomic status have higher price elasticity of demand due to alcohol prices being a larger share of their overall budget (Becker *et al.*, 1991), taxes which impact the more price elastic consumer do have more effect, if the aim is to reduce consumption. If the aim of the tax is to raise revenue, then a tax whose burden falls on those with higher elasticity is not optimal.

The studies referenced above have been conducted in developed, high-income countries, but elasticities may be different in less developed, lower-income economies. Research on the links between economic development and alcohol consumption and alcohol-related harm has found that higher levels of wealth are associated with higher consumption/less abstention. The income elasticity of demand for alcohol seems to support alcohol overall being a normal good, with higher quality alcohol being a luxury good. However, the alcohol-related harm for a given pattern of drinking is generally greater in less developed economies than in more developed economies. This is most likely attributable to worse overall health and health care, more particularly the lack of health care to address alcohol dependence, and less safe roads and vehicles. This relates to health being a stock variable that needs to be invested in if it is to be maintained in prime condition. We therefore need to look at the effectiveness of policies for different socioeconomic groups separately, to the extent that data are available.

Tian and Liu tested the effect of price on alcohol consumption in China and found very little response: price elasticity was close to zero for beer and −0.12 for liquor (Tian and Liu, 2011). However, a meta-analysis of past research on the relation between price and consumption in low- to middle-income countries found elasticity of −0.64 for total consumption of alcohol, −0.50 for consumption of beer, and −0.79 for consumption of other alcoholic beverages. They contrast these elasticities against the price elasticities in high-income countries, which are −0.77 for alcohol overall, −0.46 for beer, and −0.69 for wine (Sornpaisarn *et al.*, 2013).

This work by Sornpaisan *et al.* produced the following weighted elasticities by country in Table 1.

Another 2013 meta-analysis, however, argues that after correcting for publication bias and outliers, the past estimates on both price elasticity and income elasticity of alcohol are not born out. Nelson (2013) finds alcohol price elasticity to be −0.49 and income elasticity to be 0.59. The lower price elasticity means that raising tariffs will be less effective than previously thought.

Table 1. Price elasticity of demand — low-to-middle income countries

Country	Elasticity — Total Alcohol
China	−1.53
Colombia	−0.20
Ecuador	−0.16
Fiji	−1.04
Greece	−0.32
Honduras	−0.86
India	−1.24
Jamaica	−0.88
Korea	−0.86
Malta	−1.21
Mexico	−0.31
Philippines	0.02
Portugal	−0.02
Puerto Rico	−1.38
Russia	−0.65
South Africa	−0.54
Sri Lanka	0.35
Taiwan	−0.13
Thailand	−0.90
Venezuela	−0.91
Zimbabwe	−0.67
Overall	−0.64

Source: Sornpaisarn *et al.* (2013).

Another way to control demand is to make drinking illegal for certain groups. A major restriction on sales is to enact/enforce a minimum legal drinking age (MLDA). While perhaps one of the most controversial policies, the increase of MLDA to age 21 in the United Sates has been shown to save lives in studies too numerous to list. (The controversies are mainly off-topic, relating less to the health effects and more to cultural and ethical questions of measures of adulthood, the ability to serve in the armed forces before reaching the legal drinking age, and learning to drink while under parental/college supervision.) The positive effect of the increase in MLDA is closely linked to driving while intoxicated. In that vein, Chaloupka *et al.* have found stronger drunk driving laws to be effective deterrents to drinking and driving. In particular, they advocate 1-year mandatory license suspensions and harsh minimum mandatory fines. Laws which don't involve court proceedings are more effective (Chaloupka *et al.*,

1993). The problem with revoking driving licenses is that it also severely restricts the ability to have a job in many parts of the US and may sink the offender and the offender's family into poverty.

(As an aside, much of the work on rational addiction and price elasticity predates the higher MLDA. Since this work found elasticity higher for younger consumers, the overall elasticity may currently be lower than these studies conclude.)

Educational policy interventions, including school-based, to change drinking patterns have not shown strong results. Public service campaigns seem to be countered by the alcohol industry with more advertising. Reduction of advertising seems to hold some promise, though if the ban only applies to one type of alcohol advertising, then the effect is muted. Saffer explains that as advertising increases, so does consumption, until it reaches a tapering off point — i.e., there are diminishing marginal returns. A ban in one media outlet causes more advertising in other media forms. For the same advertising expenditure, sales will be lower when advertising is concentrated among fewer outlets due to bans on other outlets. However, the alcohol industry may increase advertising dollars to mitigate the loss in sales. Three studies in Canada showed no effect of advertising bans, although Canadian residents may have still been exposed to advertisements from the US. A longer study of 17 OECD countries saw bans reduce indicators of alcohol abuse (Saffer, 1991). Bans on advertising combined with public service spots on harms are predicted to have strongest results. Also, there seems to be a catch-22 effect with advertising bans. Once the bans decrease alcohol consumption, the bans are often lifted. This relationship was observed in a study of data from 20 countries over 26 years (Saffer and Dave, 2002). Bans have been lifted in Canada, Denmark, New Zealand and Finland. Whether alcohol consumption increased back to pre-ban levels has not been tested (Saffer and Dave, 2002).

Another method to counteract or control harmful alcohol consumption involves health interventions. This method attempts to decrease and/or eliminate demand for alcohol among the segment of the population already identified as having excessive alcohol consumption habits, or being at-risk for excessive consumption.

Some health interventions involve the use of drugs. According to Rehm *et al.*, pharmacotherapy is the most effective intervention. If 40% of alcohol dependents were treated with pharmacotherapy, there would be 11,740 fewer deaths in the first year in the EU (Rehm *et al.*, 2012). In the same report, alcohol attributable societal costs are tallied to equal €155.8 billion per year in Europe.

In the UK, the National Health Service puts hard numbers on health care interventions to mitigate the harmful effects of alcohol, using cost–benefit analyses, and asserts that for every pound spent on treatment, five pounds are saved.

A clinical trial compared the effectiveness of social behavior and network therapy with motivational enhancement therapy and found them equally effective from an economic perspective. That is, both types of treatment saved five times the social costs that would have been incurred without the treatment. The actual cost of the motivational therapy was lower, but follow-up costs were higher than for the social behavior and network therapy, thereby equalizing them from a cost–benefit analysis perspective (UKATT Research Team, 2005).

Anderson *et al.* report the international dollar cost per disability-adjusted life year (DALY) saved by 10 distinct policies and a combination strategy employed within three WHO subregions. The three subregions were identified as places in which alcohol use is a significant public health problem. They are Brazil/Mexico, Russia/Ukraine, and China/Vietnam. Increasing excise taxes by 50% was shown to be the most cost-effective policy in all three regions. That is, the most harm reduction occurred per expense incurred on the policy. For two of the subregions: Brazil/Mexico and Russia/Ukraine, increasing excise taxes by 20% was almost as effective, but for China/Vietnam, the second most effective method was legislation on drinking and driving coupled with enforcement. For Brazil/Mexico and Russia/Ukraine, the most inefficient method was brief intervention for heavy drinkers; for China/Vietnam, tax enforcement was the most expensive per DALY saved (Anderson *et al.*, 2009).

It is clear that one policy will not be the answer, nor will the policies that work best in one region be effective in another region. The development of an Alcohol Policy Index to measure the strength of a country's policies is therefore intriguing. The index developed by Brand *et al.* generates a score based on policies regarding the physical availability of alcohol, drinking context, alcohol prices, alcohol advertising, and operation of motor vehicles. This index was applied to assess alcohol policies in the 30 countries in the OECD. Each score was compared to alcohol consumption, and a strong negative correlation was discovered. Countries can therefore use the index to predict the impact of changes to one or more of their alcohol policies and measure the result on alcohol consumption generated by the model (Brand *et al.*, 2007).

Interactions Between Alcohol and Other Abused Substances

Cigarettes and alcohol have been shown to be complements, so there is hope that campaigns to reduce smoking will also reduce alcohol. However, to date, studies have not shown definitive results on this front; for example, studies have not shown a reduction in US restaurant alcohol sales after many states banned smoking in restaurants.

On the marijuana front, studies have found that the legalization of medical marijuana reduces the number of drinks consumed, especially by 20–29 year olds. (The most prescribed reason is for chronic pain: There's some evidence of prescription mills where obtaining a prescription is a quick and easy process and may not be truly related to a medical need.) Using data from the Beer Institute, researchers have discovered that beer sales fall when Medical Marijuana Legalization (MML) is passed. And while marijuana does impair driving, it seems that drivers who have used marijuana compensate for the ill effects by driving more slowly and avoiding risky maneuvers. MML is credited with reducing fatalities by 19% for 20–29 year olds and by 9% overall (Mark Anderson, 2011).

The use of medical marijuana in the US is relatively new, so the full results are hard to quantify. Marijuana is the most prevalently used illegal drug in the US with 12% of people polled reporting use in the last 12 months. Nine percent of those who use marijuana become addicted. Marijuana does impair driving: Those with high concentrations of marijuana in their blood are 3 to 7 times more likely than those who have not used marijuana to be involved in a vehicular accident. Adults who smoked marijuana regularly in their youth are more likely to suffer from impaired neural connectivity (Volkow *et al.*, 2014).

Policy Implications of Findings

After reviewing global consumption and production, health benefits and harms, and the myriad policies enacted over the centuries, our most salient findings for policymakers are as follows:

(1) **Alcohol is a normal good.** Consumption increases with income both on an individual and macro level. An unintended consequence of improvement in incomes is therefore higher alcohol consumption. The news is not all bad, though, since higher income countries have lower consumption of unrecorded alcohol, and unrecorded alcohol can cause more harm and is harder to control through government policies. Alcohol consumption is increasing most rapidly in the Western Pacific Region and Southeast Asia Region. As auto ownership also increases in these areas but road and auto safety standards do not, the combination can cause increasing loss of productive life years, unless policies are enacted that curtail impaired driving.

(2) **The empirical evidence on policies that aim to reduce harmful alcohol consumption points to a higher minimum drinking age and stiff drunk driving penalties as the most effective deterrents.** On the other hand, for those already abusing alcohol, the three most effective interventions are

pharmacopeia, motivational therapy, and social behavior and network therapy, with the latter two providing optimal cost–benefit tradeoffs. Since views on consumption and consumption patterns differ by ethnicity and socioeconomic status, there will never be a one-policy-fits-all solution. Binge drinking seems to be a growing problem around the world, especially among the young. While education has not been seen to have a large effect on reducing the harm of alcohol, it may be due to the amount of time it takes to change attitudes. Since the young are generally still in school, promoting curricula which explain the harmful effects of heavy drinking seems a prudent course of action.

Conclusion

This chapter begins to quantify the health effects of alcohol consumption globally, although it should be noted that most of the available research is from developed nations. From the perspective of reducing consumption and the harmful health effects associated with excessive use, prohibition is not a viable option since alcohol is a deeply rooted part of the culture in most places around the globe.

As is clear in Section "Global Alcohol Market: An Overview", alcohol consumption has been on the rise around the globe, except in Europe. It is positively correlated with income on a macroeconomic level: Higher income level countries/regions tend to consume more alcohol. A positive trend of increased income is movement away from non-recorded alcohol to recorded alcohol, which tends to be safer to consume due to government controls on the industry's production. However, a negative is the increased consumption of spirits as opposed to beer and wine: as Section "Health Benefits of Alcohol Consumption" explains, beer and wine seem to have more health benefits than spirit consumption.

Additionally, the health benefits from moderate consumption are such that some researchers now feel that abstention is not the best policy recommendation for the entire populace. Policies aimed at reducing demand, such as raising the MLDA, increasing the price via taxation, and tougher drunk driving sanctions seem the most practical and effective options. Greater use of treatments such as brief interventions seem appropriate from a cost–benefit perspective in places where the number of high-risk drinkers is lower. In areas or regions with high levels of hazardous drinking, reliance on taxes and stiffer drunk driving penalties seem the best policies. Two hindrances to policy implementation are the expense imposed on the individual and the social stigma: If alcohol abuse continues to be viewed as something the abuser can control on his own, the right treatments will not be available or at least not widely enough. And while the rational addiction model shows that the abuser has some conscience control over his actions, the fact that alcohol is addictive means that abusers have a physiological response that is very difficult to control. On a positive note, social views on alcohol abuse have been changing in ways that could help prevent or mitigate the harmful effects. For example, driving drunk is no longer as socially acceptable as it once was, with stricter laws being adopted globally. Alcoholism is now classified as a disease by the American Medical Association and the World Health Organization. This classification lifts part of the stigma associated with alcohol abuse and makes more funding available to combat abuse.

Alcohol consumption will continue to be a polarizing topic, but as the topic continues to be studied and the world shares policy results, hopefully the positive effects will be more widely recognized and the negative effects more effectively controlled. Further research on controlling binge drinking should also be a priority, as this could contribute to efforts to decrease the prevalence of this problem among the young.

References

Alfred A, de Lorimier M. 2000. Alcohol, wine, and health. *The American Journal of Surgery,* November, 180(5): 357–361.

Anderson D. Mark, DIR. 2011. Medical Marijuana Laws, Traffic Fatalities, and Alcohol Consumption. *IZA,* November. *Volume Discussion Paper* 6112.

Anderson P, Baumberg B. 2006. *Alcohol in Europe.* London: Institute of Alcohol Studies.

Anderson P, Chisholm D, Fuhr DC. 2009. Effectiveness and cost-effectiveness of policies and programmes to reduce harm caused by alcohol. *Lancet* 2234–2246.

Becker GS, Grossman M, Murphy KM. 1991. Rational Addiction and the Effect of Price on Consumption. *Working Paper No. 68; Center for the Study of the Economy, U of Chicago.*

Brand DA *et al.* 2007. Comparative analysis of alcohol control policies in 30 countries. *Plos Medicine* 4(4): 151.

Castelnuovo AD *et al.* 2002. Meta-analysis of wine and beer consumption in relation to vascular risk. *Circulation* May, 105: 2836–2844.

CDC. 2008. *Smoking-Attributable Mortality, Years of Potential Life Lost, and Productivity Losses — United States. 2000–2004*, November 14, 2008, 57(45): 1226–1228, http://www.cdc.gov/mmwr.

Chaloupka FJ, Saffer H, Grossman M. 1993. Alcohol control policies and motor vehicle fatalaties. *Journal of Legal Studies* January: 161–186.

Chaloupka FJ. 1990. Rational Addictive Behavior and Cigarette Smoking, *Working Paper No. 3268, National Bureau of Economic Research*, http://www.nber.org/papers/w3268.

Chaloupka FJ, Grossman M. 1998. A survey of economic models of addictive behavior. *Journal of Drug Issues* 8(3): 631–643.

Choi, HKaCG. 2004. Beer, liquor, and wine consumption and serum uric acid level: The Third National Health and Nutrition Examination Survey. *Arthritis & Rheumatism* 51: 1023–1029.

Cook PJ. 2007. *Paying the Tab: The Costs and Benefits of Alcohol Control.* Princeton: Princeton University Press.

Devlin NJ, Scuffham PA, Bunt LJ. 1997. The social costs of alcohol abuse in New Zealand. *Addiction* 92(11): 1491–1505.

Distilled Spirits Council of the United States. 2010. *Discus.org.* [Online] Available at: http://www.discus.org/assets/1/7/ContributionFactSheet.pdf [Accessed 15 December 2014].

Ferreira MP, Weems MKS. 2008. Alcohol consumption by aging adults in the United States: health benefits and detriments. *Journal of the American Dietetic Association,* October, 108(10): 68–76.

Fritz K, Morojele N, Kalichman S. 2010. Alcohol: The forgotten drug in HIV/AIDS. *The Lancet,* August, 376(9739): 398–400.

Gavaler JS, Van Thiel D. 1992. The Association between moderate alcoholic beverage consumption and serum estradiol and testosterone levels in normal postmenopausal women: Relationship to the literature. *Alcoholism: Clinical and Experimental Research* 16: 87–92.

Gaziano MJ, *et al.* 2000. Light-to-moderate alcohol consumption and mortality in the physicians' health study enrollment cohort. *Journal of the American College of Cardiology* 35(1): 96–105.

German JB, Walzem RL. 2000. The health benefits of wine. *Annual Review of Nutrition* 20: 561–593.

Giuseppe Lippi MF, EJF, GT. 2010. Moderate red wine consumption and cardiovascular disease risk: Beyond the "French Paradox". *Seminars in Thrombosis and Hemostasis,* 36(1): 59–70.

Grossman M, Chaloupka FJ, Sirtalan I. 1998. An empirical analysis of alcohol addiction: Results from the Monitoring the Future panels. *Economic Inquiry* 36(1): 39–48.

Grossman M. 2000. Chapter 7: The Human Capital Model. In: Culyer AJ, Newhouse JP. (eds.). *Handbook of Health Economics.* Amseterdam: North Holland, 34–408.

Gruenewald Paul J. 2011. Regulating availability: How access to alcohol affects drinking and problems in youth and adults. *Alcohol Research and Health* 34(2): 248–256.

Hallgren M, Leifman H, Andreasson S. 2012. Drinking less but greater harm: Could polarized drinking habits explain the divergence between alcohol consumption and harms among youth? *Alcohol,* 47(5): 581–590.

Hanson DJ. 1995. *Preventing Alcohol Abuse: Alcohol, Culture and Control.* Westport, CT: Praeger.

Hanson DJ. n.d. *potsdam.edu.* [Online] Available at: http://www2.potsdam.edu/alcohol/LegalDrinkingAge.html#.VKNVXnvl-dw.

Higuchi S, Matsushita S, Maesato H, Osaki Y. 2007. Japan: Alcohol Today. *Addiction,* December, 102(7): 1849–1862.

International Center for Alcohol Policies 2006. The Structure of the Beverage Alcohol Industry, *ICAP Reports* 17 March 2006, http://www.icap.org/Publications/ICAPReports.

Jack S, Blocker J. 2006. Did prohibition really work? Alcohol prohibition as a public health innovation. *American Journal of Public Health,* February, 96(2): 233–243.

Johansson P *et al.* 2006. *The Social Costs of Alcohol in Sweden 2002,* Stockholm: SoRad.

Klatsky ALFGD. 1995. Annotation: Alcohol and longevity. *American Journal of Public Health* 85(1): 16–18.

Kuo M, Heeb J-L, Gmel G, Rehm J. 2003. Does price matter? The effect of decreased price on spirits consumption in Switzerland. *Alcoholism: Clinical and Experimental Research* 27(4): 720–725.

LaCroix AZ *et al.* 1993. Maintaining mobility in late life. II. Smoking, alcohol consumption, physical activity, and body mass index. *American Journal of Epidemiolgy* 137(8): 858–869.

London L. 2000. Alcohol consumption amongst South African farm workers: A challenge for post-apartheid health sector transformation. *Drug and Alcohol Dependence* 59(2): 199–206.

Massin S, Kopp P. 2014. Is life satisfaction hump-shaped with alcohol consumption? Evidence from Russian panel data. *Addictive Behaviors* 39: 803–810.

Middleton JC, *et al.* 2010. Effectiveness of policies maintaining or restricting days of alcohol sales on excesive alcohol consumption and realted harms. *American Jouranl of Preventive Medicine* 39(6): 575–589.

Moskowitz JM. 1989. The primary prevention of alcohol problems: A critical review of the research literature. *Journal of Studies on Alcohol* 50(1): 54–88.

Murphy JG, McDevitt-Murphy ME, Barnett NP. 2005. Drink and Be Merry? Gender, life satisfaction, and alcohol consumption among college students. *Psychology of Addicitve Behaviors* 19(2): 184–191.

Nelson JP. 2013. Meta-analysis of alcohol price and income elasticities — with correction for publication bias. *Health Economics Review* 3(17): 1–10.

OECD. 2011. *Health at a Glance 2011: OECD Indicators,* s.l.: OECD Publishing.

Purshouse RC, Meier PS, Brennan A, Taylor KB. 2010. Estimated effect of alcohol pricing policies on health and health economic outcomes in England: An epidemiological model. *The Lancet,* April, 375(9723): 1355–1364.

Rehm J, Gmel G, Sempos CT, Trevisan M. 2003. *Alcohol–Related Morbidity and Mortality.* [Online] Available at: http://pubs.niaaa.nih.gov/publications/arh27-1/39-51.htm.

Rehm J, *et al.* 2010. Alcohol as a risk factor for liver cirrhosis: A systematic review and meta-analysis. *Drug and Alcohol Review* July, 29(4): 437–445.

Rehm J, *et al.* 2009. Alcohol and Global Health 1. *The Lancet* 2009(373): 2223–2233.

Rehm J, Shield K, Rehm M, Gmel G, Frick U. 2012. *Alcohol Consumption, Alcohol Dependence and Attributable Burden of Disease in Europe: Potential Gains from Effective Interventions for Alcohol Dependence.* Toronto: Centre for Addiction and Mental Health.

Risen C. 2014. How Dreams and Money Didn't Mix at a Texas Distillery. *The New York Times*, 28 December, p. BU1.

Room R. 1984. Alcohol Control and Public Health. *Annual Review of Public Health* 5: 293–317.

Saffer H. 1991. Alcohol advertising bans and alcohol abuse: An international perspective. *Journal of Health Economics* 10.

Saffer H, Chaloupka F. 1994. Alcohol tax equalization and social costs. *Eastern Economic Journal* 20(1): 33–43.

Saffer H, Dave D. 2002. Alcohol consumption and alcohol advertising bans. *Applied Economics* 34(11): 1325–1334.

Samuli I, Saarni KJSKJSSPHSKPJL. 2008. Alcohol consumption, abstaining, health utility, and quality of life — a general population survey in Finland. *Alcohol and Alcoholism* 43(3): 376–386.

Sornpaisarn B, *et al.* 2013. Elasticity of alcohol consumption, alcohol-related harms, and drinking initation in low- and middle-income countries: A systemtaic review and meta-analysis. *The International Journal of Alcohol and Drug Research* 2(1): 45–58.

Stampfer M, *et al.* 1988. A prospective study of moderate alcohol consumption and the risk of coronary heart disease and stroke in women. *The New England Journal of Medicine,* 4 August, 319(5): 267–273.

Steefel DP. 2011. Do blue laws save lives? The effect of Sunday alcohol slaes bans on fatal vehicle accidents. *Journal of Policy Analysis and Management,* August, 30(4): 798–820.

Stockwell T, Crosbie D. 2001. Supply and demand for alcohol in Australia: Relationships between industry structures, regulation and the marketplace. *The International Journal of Drug Policy* 12: 139–152.

The Economist. 2001. Uncorking the past. *The Economist*, December.

Tian G, Liu F. 2011. Is the Demand for Alcoholic Beverages in Developing Countries Sensitive to Price? Evidence from China. *International Journal of Environmental Research and Public Health,* June, 8(6): 2124–2131.

UKATT Research Team. 2005. Cost effectiveness of treatment for alcohol problems: Findings of the randomised UK alcohol treatment trial (UKATT). *British Medical Journal* 331–544.

van Heerden IV, Parry CDH. 2001. If You Drink Alcohol, Drink Sensibly. *SAJCN,* September, 14(3): S71–S77.

Volkow ND, Balen RD, Compton WM, Weiss SR. 2014. Adverse health effects of marijuana use. *New England Journal of Medicine,* 5 June, 370: 2219–2227.

WHO. 2014. *Global Status Report on Alcohol and Health.* s.l.: World Health Organization.

Xu X, Chaloupka F. 2011. The effects of prices on alcohol use and its consequences. *Alcohol Research & Health* 34(2): 236–245.

Yoruk B. 2014. Legalization of Sunday alcohol sales and alcohol consumption in the United States. *Addiction* 109: 55–61.

The Health Impacts of Obesity

Franco Sassi, Marion Devaux and Michele Cecchini
OECD, Health Division

An epidemic of obesity has been spreading in countries at all levels of income as a result of new dietary habits and sedentary ways of life, fuelling chronic diseases and premature mortality. The majority of the population, and 1 in 5 children, are today overweight or obese in the OECD area. Rates vary nearly 10-fold across OECD countries alone, but have been growing at similar paces worldwide.

An increased demand for medical care, as well as adverse social and labor market impacts, make obesity a top public health priority and a major cause for concern for governments worldwide. The rationale for government intervention to correct some of the causes of obesity epidemic is still debated, but rests mainly on information failures, social spill-over effects of lifestyle choices, and inconsistent time preferences, as well as on the links between obesity and social disadvantage.

Several population-based prevention policies can be expected to generate substantial health gains and future reductions of health-care expenditures. These include price incentives; health information and communication strategies; measures to regulate the labelling, marketing, and nutritional contents of foods; and measures to increase physical activity, including changes in transportation and living environment.

Keywords: Obesity; Diet; Physical Activity; Market Failure; Inequalities; Prevention; Behavioral Interventions.

Introduction

Before 1980, obesity rates based on the body mass index (BMI) were generally well below 10% worldwide. Since then, rates have doubled or tripled in many countries, and in almost half of OECD countries 50% or more of the population is currently overweight. Mexico's population is one of the most heavily affected worldwide. Between 2000 and 2012, the prevalence of overweight (BMI $\geq$ 25 kg/m^2) increased from 65% to 70%, and the prevalence of obesity from 28% to 33%, before the country enacted one of the most comprehensive strategies to fight obesity (OECD, 2014). In China, where the burden of diet-related illness is rapidly increasing with changes in dietary habits (Baillie, 2008), overweight rates doubled from 13.5% to 26.7% between 1991 and 2006. The rate of obesity tripled over the same period of time (Lu and Goldman, 2010). In Brazil, obesity rates grew 3-fold in men and almost doubled in women between 1975 and 2003 (Monteiro *et al.*, 2007). Smaller increases in overweight were recorded in India (rates for women increased from 10.6 to 12.6 between 1998–1999 and 2005–2006), but increases were much steeper in west urban areas, where rates approached 40% in the early 2000s, almost doubling in less than 10 years (Wang *et al.*, 2009). Overweight and obesity have taken over as the predominant features of malnutrition in South Africa (Puoane *et al.*, 2002), where one-third of women and one-tenth of men are obese with the highest rates among black women and white men. After the political and economic transition, obesity grew also in the Russian Federation, where 1 in 4 women and 1 in 10 men are now obese, and rates are projected to grow fast in the coming years (Cecchini *et al.*, 2010).

The Global Obesity Epidemic and its Public Health Dimensions

Historical trends in height, weight and body mass

Height and weight have been increasing since the 18th century in many of the current OECD countries. Height increases have been closely related with economic growth (Steckel, 1995), although early industrialization brought about periods of slight shrinkage of average height in countries such as Great Britain and the United States (Komlos, 1998). The British were the tallest population in Europe in the 18th century, on an average they were about 5 cm taller and their calorie consumption was 18% larger than that of the French. Americans were even taller, by as much as 6–7 cm over the average height of a Briton, and continued to be the tallest until at least the second half of the 19th century, when their growth in stature slowed down, relative to northern European populations, and the latter took over as the tallest in the 20th century.

Over the same period of time, weight and body mass also increased gradually, until increases in BMI accelerated sharply in many OECD countries starting from the 1980s. Norwegian men aged 50–64 increased their body mass by approximately 1 point in the 18th century, by 3 points in the subsequent century and by a further 3 points between 1870 and 1975 (Fogel, 1994). In the subsequent 25 years alone, average BMI in the same group grew by at least 2 additional points (Strand and Tverdal, 2006; Reas *et al.*, 2007). American men of the same age increased their average BMI by 3.6 points between 1910 and 1985–1988, and by almost the same amount in the following single quarter of a century. Average BMI increased by 1.5 points in England over 15 years, from the early 1990s to the mid-2000s, and by 1 point in France in the same period.

Following the growth in BMI described above, overweight and obesity rates have been increasing consistently over the past three decades at a global level. Obesity has been increasing at a faster pace in countries with historically higher rates, leading to a widening gap among countries over time. Overweight and obese people are a majority today in OECD countries, and 18% of the adult population are obese. The obesity epidemic continues to spread, and no country has seen a reversal of trends since the epidemic began. More than 1 in 3 adults in Mexico, New Zealand and the United States, and more than 1 in 4 in Australia, Canada, Chile, and Hungary are obese. In contrast, rates are just 2 to 4% of adults in Asian countries, when the same BMI thresholds are applied. Rates grew rapidly in Australia, England and the United States since the 1990s, while they grew at a slower pace in other countries, as shown in Figure 1 (OECD, 2014).

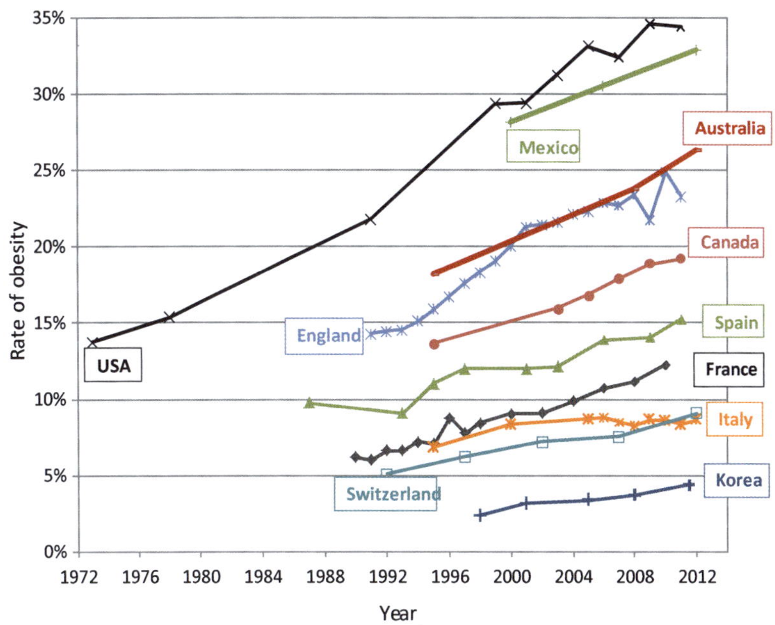

Figure 1. Age-standardized obesity rates

Notes: Age- and gender-adjusted rates of obesity and overweight using the 2005 OECD standard population. Measured height and weight in Australia, England, Korea, Mexico, and USA; self-reported data in other countries. No projection for Australia, Mexico, and Switzerland since they were not produced in 2010.
Source: OECD estimates on national health surveys.

Development of the epidemic: Age, period, and cohort effects

There is substantial evidence of the role of both individual characteristics and environmental influences in the development of overweight and obesity, but less is known about the way these factors have exerted their influences over time, and on the relative contribution they have made to the current obesity epidemic.

An age–period–cohort (APC) analysis based on individual-level health survey data for around 1.8 million individuals aged 15–65 in 6 OECD countries (Canada, England, France, Italy, Korea and the United States) helps to disentangle the relative contributions to the epidemic of different groups of factors (e.g., individual versus environmental). The three time-related factors in the analysis were:

(a) *Age*: Biological and lifestyle changes typically characterize a given age group, for example, physiological capacities, accumulation of social experience or time spent on different activities such as exercise.
(b) *Period of observation*: Period effects reflect events experienced at a given point in time, including cultural, economic, or environmental changes, which affect all individuals simultaneously. Environmental factors also affect every individual in a population at the periods when the surveys were undertaken.
(c) *Birth cohort*: Individuals in a cohort are exposed to similar influences at key stages throughout their lives, for example, nutrition received in the early years of life or the type of education, and share a number of characteristics that vary over time.

The APC analysis confirms the importance of period effects (an actual increase in the prevalence of overweight and obesity in all 6 countries over the periods surveyed) but suggests that the pace of the increase in overweight and obesity may be underestimated in analyses which do not fully account for age and cohort effects.

Factors and dynamics that have characterized recent decades have sharply increased everyone's likelihood of becoming overweight or obese, regardless of their age or birth cohort, reflecting the powerful influences of physical, social and economic environments that favor obesity.

On the other hand, the underlying probability of obesity of successive birth cohorts was generally declining in the earlier part of the 20th century, with signs of an upturn in Canada, France, and the United States (and possibly Korea) from the 1960s. This was not observed for overweight, where cohort trends consistently declined apart from Korea. Declining cohort trends may be explained, for instance, by improvements in education and socioeconomic status (SES) since World War II.

Material living conditions and nutrition are also likely to have been poorer, on an average, for the earliest cohorts. The role of material deprivation, particularly food deprivation, during childhood as a factor that may increase the likelihood of obesity in later life is highlighted in a number of studies, and this effect may be stronger in women than in men (Case and Menendez, 2007).

Negatively sloped and relatively small cohort effects suggest that the large increases in overweight and obesity rates observed since the 1980s are attributed primarily to the factors and dynamics that have characterized the latter time period, which have sharply increased everyone's likelihood of becoming overweight or obese, regardless of their age or birth cohort. These factors and dynamics reflect the powerful influences of obesogenic environments (aspects of physical, social, and economic environments that favor obesity), which have been consolidating over the course of the past 20–30 years, and are behind the increasing period effects resulting from the APC analysis.

Measuring obesity

According to the WHO, overweight and obesity are meant to reflect abnormal or excessive fat accumulation — also called adiposity — that may impair health. The measurement of adiposity is difficult, therefore proxies are normally used based on more easily measurable anthropometric characteristics. The BMI[1], a measure of body weight-for-height, is the most popular proxy for adiposity, dating back to the 19th century.

Until the 1960s, obesity was defined by reference to an "ideal body weight" derived from life insurance actuarial tables. In 1972, obesity researcher Ancel Keys published the results of a study of almost 7,500 men in 5 countries. Keys compared a number of formulas to see which is the best predictor of body fat measured directly, and the equation proposed by Belgian Scientist Adolphe Quetelet proved more accurate than alternatives such as weight divided by height. Keys renamed Quetelet's index "body mass index". Based on BMI data, the WHO concluded in 1997 that obesity had reached epidemic levels worldwide.

The US National Institutes of Health started defining obesity by BMI in the 1980s. In 1998, they defined a BMI of 25–29.9 as "overweight", and 30 and above as "obesity". Based on these standards, a woman who is 1.65 m (5 feet 5 inches) tall is overweight if she weighs 68 kg, and obese if she weighs 82 kg. A man who is 1.75 m (5 feet 9 inches) tall is overweight if he weighs 77 kg, and obese if he weighs 92 kg. There are suggestions that lower thresholds should be used in Asian

[1]The simple formula for the BMI is weight in kilograms divided by square height in meters.

populations (WHO, 2004), as well as in certain ethnic minority groups, because increasing patterns of health risks have been observed in those populations starting from lower BMI levels.

BMI's main advantages are that it is simple and provides easily remembered cut-off points. But many researchers criticize it for not taking into account important factors such as age, sex and muscularity, so that using BMI alone can contribute to the so called "obesity paradox", where certain degrees of excess weight can even appear to offer protection against some conditions in certain population groups (Lewis *et al.*, 2009). Critics argue that waist measurement, for example, or the waist-to-hip ratio, are better indicators of abdominal fat and associated health risks. Keys himself stressed that BMI was useful for epidemiological research, but warned against using it for individual cases.

Despite continued controversy on the use of BMI as a marker of risk (Cawley and Burkhauser, 2006), a very large study of the link between obesity and mortality concluded that BMI is a strong predictor of mortality, and that different proxy measures of adiposity are more likely to be complements than substitutes, as each can provide additional information relative to others (Prospective Studies Collaboration, 2009).

- *Self-report bias in height and weight measures*

A key challenge in the measurement of obesity is self-report bias, which may arise when people provide self-assessed measures of height and weight. This often leads to an underestimation of BMI. Relatively few national health surveys (e.g., the Health Survey for England, the Korean NHANES, and the US NHANES) include measures of height and weight by clinical examination, although an increasing number of countries are moving in this direction. The gap between self-reported and measured data has a significant impact on assessed levels of obesity and overweight, but a lesser impact on measures of social inequality in obesity (Sassi *et al.*, 2009a; Costa-Font *et al.*, 2014). There is no clear evidence that self-report bias may vary among individuals with different levels of education or SES.

Weight is consistently underestimated by women. In men, underestimation tends to increase with weight (Lakdawalla and Philipson, 2002). A French cohort study found an association between self-report bias and education level, showing that higher educational levels tend to reduce overestimation of height in men, while a higher professional status is associated with an increased overestimation of height in women (Niedhammer *et al.*, 2000).

Based on the approach proposed by Cawley (2000), Figure 2 shows the size of self-report bias by gender, ethnicity, and self-reported BMI level. BMI is underestimated by obese people (BMI>30) and particularly by Mexican-American men

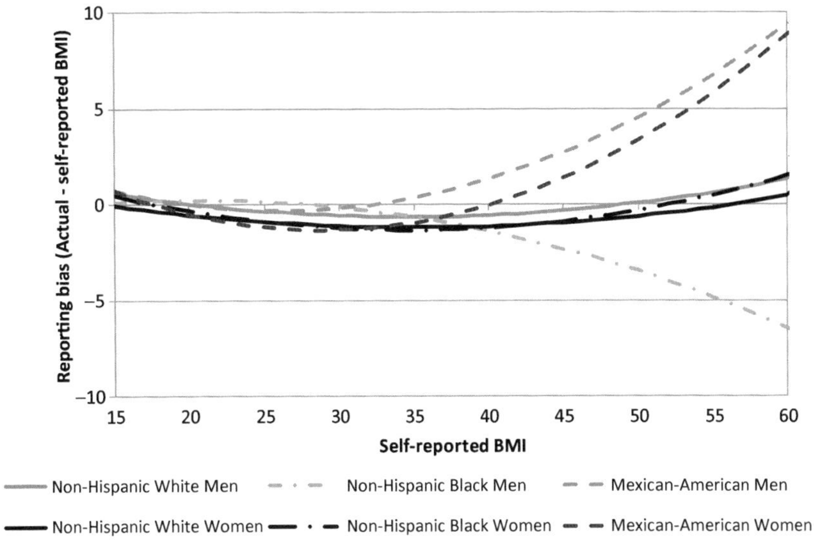

Figure 2. Size of BMI self-report bias by gender and ethnicity
Source: Authors' estimates based on US NHANES data.

and women. On the contrary, non-Hispanic Black men tend to overestimate their BMI. The regression coefficient estimates obtained from this analysis can be used to correct self-reported BMI data from others surveys.

Recent studies have examined changes in self-report bias over time, reaching conclusions that vary by country and period of observation. Hayes *et al.* (2011) found a diminishing self-report bias in BMI in Australia between 1995 and 2008. On the other hand, Irish data show that BMI underestimation increased from 1998 to 2007 (Shiely *et al.*, 2013). Self-report bias in the US was relatively stable from 1976 to 2003/2004, and increased in Canada from 1986 to 2005 (Connor Gorber and Tremblay, 2010), although more recent evidence from Canada suggests that no change occurred between 2005 and 2008 (Shields *et al.*, 2011).

Obesity, disease and longevity

Obesity is a major public health concern because it is a key risk factor for a range of chronic diseases (Malnick and Knobler, 2006; Guh *et al.*, 2009), with diabetes being the most closely linked. The severely obese have a risk of developing type 2 diabetes up to 60 times larger than those at the lower end of the normal weight spectrum. High blood pressure and high cholesterol are also more common as BMI increases. These links make the obese more likely to develop heart disease, particularly coronary artery disease, and stroke, and to die from these diseases.

A large proportion of major cancers such as breast and colorectal cancer is linked to obesity and physical inactivity. Obesity also increases the chances of developing a number of respiratory and gastrointestinal diseases, as well as osteoarthritis, some mental conditions, and many other diseases and complaints, and the list keeps expanding as new epidemiological evidence emerges.

Mortality increases steeply with BMI once individuals cross the 25 kg/m^2 threshold, i.e., the lower limit of the overweight category (Prospective Studies Collaboration, 2009), and especially in those who are severely obese (Kitahara *et al.*, 2014). A BMI between 30 and 35 is associated with a life expectancy loss of 3 to 4 years relative to a person of normal weight. The gap increases to 8 to 10 years for those who are severely obese (BMI 40–45). The link is not as strong beyond the age 70 (Stevens *et al.*, 1998; Corrada *et al.*, 2006). Many cross-sectional studies of older individuals have even found a lower mortality among the overweight and those who are mildly obese than in normal weight individuals, although detailed longitudinal studies have shown that this is mostly an effect of the weight loss associated with chronic diseases (Strandberg *et al.*, 2009).

A growing body of research shows that the impact of obesity on disability is larger than its impact on mortality (Gregg and Guralnik, 2007). In 10 European countries, the odds of disability are nearly twice as large among obese persons as among normal-weight persons, and 3 to 4 times as large in those who are severely obese (Andreyeva *et al.*, 2007). At age 70, an average obese person can expect to live over 40% of their residual life expectancy with diabetes, over 80% with high blood pressure and over 85% with osteoarthritis in the United States, while the corresponding shares for a normal weight person are 17%, 60%, and 68% (Lakdawalla *et al.*, 2005).

The impact of obesity on health care expenditures

A strong association between obesity and chronic diseases suggests that the obese are likely to make a disproportionate use of health care, leading to a substantially larger expenditure relative to normal weight individuals. A wealth of studies has shown this based on data from at least 14 OECD countries and some non-OECD countries, mostly focusing on medical care expenditures. Estimates based on different approaches and methods suggest that obesity is responsible for approximately 1% to 3% of total health expenditure in most countries, with the notable exception of the United States, where several studies estimate that obesity may account for 5% to 10% of health expenditures (Roux and Donaldson, 2004; Konnopka *et al.*, 2011; Tsai *et al.*, 2011). At the individual level, an obese person incurs health care expenditures at least 25% higher than those of a normal weight person, according to a range of studies from a variety of countries (Withrow and Alter, 2010). Additional medical costs caused by obesity in the United States have been quantified as

US$1,270 for men and US$2,530 for women, with annual production losses of US$4,300 to 4,800, on average (Finkelstein *et al.*, 2010). Adding the value of production losses to health care costs, obesity accounts for a fraction of a percentage point of GDP in most countries, and over 1% in the United States.

Popkin *et al.* (2006) have argued that estimates of the costs of obesity often ignore the broader impacts of the patterns of diet and physical activity that lead to obesity. Through a case study of China, they show that accounting for these impacts brings the total cost of overweight and obesity to over 4% of GDP, including estimated production losses in the region of 3.6% of GDP, and projected to rise to over 9% of GDP in 2025 (Popkin *et al.*, 2006). In their analysis, the impacts of dietary and physical activity factors not directly linked with obesity represent 80% of the estimated medical care costs (57% dietary factors, 23% physical activity factors).

However, the question of the economic impact of obesity is not so simple when addressed over the lifetime and at a population level. Because of the time lag between the onset of obesity and related health problems, the rise in obesity over the past two decades will mean higher health care costs in the future. The costs linked to overweight and obesity were estimated to increase by US$48–66 billion per year in the United States and by GBP1.9–2 billion per year in the United Kingdom by 2030 (Wang *et al.*, 2011). Two studies published in 1999, both based on US data, suggest that obesity increases lifetime expenditures (Thompson *et al.*, 1999; Allison *et al.*, 1999). At least one of these studies (Allison *et al.*, 1999) accounts for the disease and health care implications of the longer life expectancy of people who are not obese, reaching the conclusion that after age 80 the expected health care expenditures of a non-obese person outgrow those of an obese person, as the gap in mortality between the two increases with age. A simulation analysis for a cohort of 70-year-olds in the United States found that overweight and obese persons have health care expenditures, respectively, about 7% and 20% higher than those of a normal weight person, during the course of their remaining life spans (Lakdawalla *et al.*, 2005). However, a further study from the Netherlands, found that decreased longevity of the obese makes them likely to incur lower health care expenditures than the non-obese, over a lifetime (van Baal *et al.*, 2008). According to this study, an average obese person, during their entire life span, will incur 13% lower health expenditures than a normal weight person.

The Social Dimensions of Obesity

The social multiplier of obesity

The spread of obesity and overweight within households and social networks is accelerated by a "social multiplier" effect when individual lifestyle choices have an influence on other people's lifestyles.

In England, France, Italy, and Korea, one-sixth to one-fourth of the overall variation in the probability of being obese is determined by differences among households (25% in England, 27% in France, 22% in Italy, and 16% in Korea), rather than among individuals (Sassi *et al.* 2009a). The proportion is up to 50% (similar to what is observed in smoking) for fruit and vegetable consumption and physical activity, and about one-third for fat consumption. Further OECD findings show that when selecting pairs of spouses within households (i.e., *individuals not sharing the same genetic background*), the correlation in BMI levels in each couple was above 12% in all countries except Korea (2%). This correlation was stronger in older-age couples in France, Italy, and Korea, suggesting that the effect is at least in part due to the adoption of common lifestyles and not merely to partner selection.

Genetic factors may also play a part in determining a convergence of BMI levels within households. It has been argued that obesity is the lifestyle-related condition that is most influenced by genetic heritage (Cutler *et al.*, 2003). Studies comparing natural and adopted children with two, one or no obese parents showed that natural children are substantially more likely than adopted ones to resemble their parents in terms of body weight. Silventoinen *et al.* (2010) in a recent review of twin and adoption studies reach the conclusion that both genetic and environmental factors affect BMI variation in childhood, but the effect of common environment disappears in adolescence. However, when selecting only mothers and their children within households (i.e., members who share the same genetic background) in the above health survey data, the correlation in BMI was stronger (or at least equal) than among spouses in all countries, but not so much stronger to suggest that similarities in BMI among household members may be mostly explained by genetic factors. Genetics alone cannot account for the rise in overweight and obesity experienced over the past 20–30 years by all OECD countries. Rather, obesogenic environments appear to have encouraged individuals, especially when culturally and socially vulnerable, to make less healthy lifestyle choices, and those genetically predisposed have tended to become overweight or obese as a result. This interaction between genetic factors and environment appears to be strongly supported by empirical findings.

When accounting for a social multiplier effect, a large proportion of the increase observed in child obesity in recent years can be viewed as a direct effect of increase in adult obesity. Although somewhat alien to economic orthodoxy, the social multiplier effect may be described as an externality, indicating that individual lifestyle choices are likely to have an influence on other people's lifestyles. The impact on other individuals' health may be less direct in this case than, for instance, in the case of passive smoking, but it is no less important. A strong indication emerges that actions targeting individuals outside the social context in which they lead their lives are unlikely to be very effective. A number of countries are increasingly promoting interventions involving peer groups (e.g., school-based, or workplace interventions) or family members (e.g., children and parents). These interventions may better exploit the "social multiplier" effect, turning it into a positive externality which generates favorable influences on health behaviors among members of families and social networks. In addition to providing better chances of interventions being effective in changing behaviors, exploiting the "social multiplier" effect in the way just described may produce faster reductions in overweight and obesity rates than interventions targeting individuals out of their social context.

Obesity, Human Capital and Labor Markets

Education and employment opportunities

An obese person is less likely to have a job than a normal-weight person. The obese have fewer chances of success when they seek employment and they tend to spend longer periods of time unemployed. The probability of regaining employment after a period of unemployment is similarly lower for those with a higher BMI. There is some evidence that the obese are especially disadvantaged in finding employment in occupations involving direct personal contact with customers (Rooth, 2007). The obese are also more likely to be inactive (unemployed and not actively seeking employment) (Cawley and Danziger, 2005; Klarenbach *et al.*, 2006) either because they are in poor health and unable to work, they are discouraged by their lack of success in obtaining employment, or they lack the incentives to pursue a condition (employment) that they may find more distressing and less enjoyable than people of normal weight do, on average. A number of studies provide evidence of a clear link between obesity and employment both in men and in women, and reach the conclusion that the association reflects a causal effect of obesity on labor market outcomes (e.g., Morris, 2007; Tunceli *et al.*, 2006). Other studies have reached different conclusions, finding either a weak link between obesity and employment, type or sector of occupation (Garcia and Quintana-Domeque, 2007), or no link at all (Cawley, 2000; Lindeboom *et al.*, 2010). On the whole, however, the balance of evidence points to a negative influence of obesity on employment, especially, but not exclusively, for women.

Women are more affected than men. Women seem to have a stronger negative association between body weight and employment. In Ireland, for instance, the probability of being employed for obese women (aged over 50) is estimated to be around 8% lower than for normal weight women, while the gap is around 5% in men (Mosca, 2013). Evidence of especially severe outcomes for women is also available from Germany, in terms of both employment and wages (Caliendo and Lee, 2013).

Discrimination against obese people is partly driven by common negative stereotypes about their motivation, self-discipline, and competence. Psychologists and sociologists have tried to ascertain whether the negative influence of obesity on employment is as a result of systematic discrimination by prospective employers. Roehling (1999) reviewed the findings of 17 studies and consistently found discrimination on the basis of weight in all aspects of employment (including selection, placement, compensation, promotion, and discharge).

However, discrimination is a complex phenomenon, which does not always, or not exclusively, reflects prejudicial attitudes. A number of authors have preferred to use the concept of "statistical discrimination" (e.g., Lundborg *et al.*, 2010) to reflect attitudes based on (statistically found) expectations concerning the skills, physical fitness and productivity of obese men and women. Obesity, in this case, becomes a marker of diminished individual potential in the labor market.

Obesity affects employment to different degrees in different racial and ethnic groups. This has been studied mostly in the United States (Cawley, 2000; Cawley and Danziger, 2005) where white women who are severely obese are substantially more likely than average to be out of work (42.2% vs. 31%), while the same condition makes virtually no difference among African-American women. Han *et al.* (2009) found obese white and Hispanic women being less likely to be employed by 1.5% and 4.5% than underweight or normal weight women, whereas obese African-American women did not seem to be affected. Obesity is more common, therefore possibly less stigmatized, among African-American women, and it is not associated with decreased self-esteem in African-American women as much as it is in white women (Averett and Korenman, 1996).

- *Long-term disability and early retirement*

Health problems associated with obesity may lead to temporary or permanent disability. Formal definitions of what is recognized as disability and criteria for awarding state benefits to the disabled vary across countries, but obesity is an increasingly important cause of disability throughout the OECD area. In the United States, the odds of short-term disability episodes are increased by 76% in the obese, and by 26% in those who are overweight but not obese (Arena *et al.*, 2006). The recent growth in obesity rates is a leading cause of increases in disability, accounting for about one-third of increases in 30–45-year-olds (Bhattacharya *et al.*, 2008). In Sweden, a J-shaped relationship was found between BMI and receipt of disability pensions in the working-age population, with the underweight more likely to receive a pension than the overweight (but not obese), but the obese substantially more likely to receive a pension than anyone else, about 2.8 times more likely than a normal-weight person (Månsson *et al.*, 1996). In Finland, BMI is a similarly strong predictor of early work disability, with obese women twice as likely to be in receipt of a work invalidity pension and obese men 1.5 times as likely as their normal-weight counterparts (Rissanen *et al.*, 1990). Obese old people may be forced to withdraw from their job because of their disabilities due to their excessive weight. People with BMI above 35 have higher probability of early retirement or incidence of disability, especially for women (Renna and Thakur, 2010).

- *Wage penalties and productivity gap*

Obese people who are employed often earn less than their colleagues, even when they have equivalent positions and discharge the same tasks. Wage penalties are generally larger in women, although at least one study (Brunello and d'Hombres, 2007) reported larger penalties in men. A study of 450,000 men in Sweden found an exceptionally large 18% wage penalty associated with obesity (Lundborg *et al.*, 2010), although most studies identified pay gaps in the order of 10%.

Obesity affects wages in the private sector but not, or at least not to the same degree, in the public sector, as shown by a study of workers in Denmark (Greve, 2008). There is also evidence from Finland that obese women with higher levels of education and those in higher occupational positions suffer the largest wage disadvantage relative to their normal-weight peers, while the gap is substantially smaller among less educated women and manual workers (Sarlio-Lähteenkorva *et al.*, 2004). Jobs requiring social skills or contact with clients are negatively affected by higher BMI value. For instance, in the United States, White and Hispanic women who are obese suffer larger wage penalties, on average, than African-American women, especially in higher-paid occupation. On the other hand, African-American men, unlike White and Hispanic men, seem to benefit from a higher BMI even in jobs involving social skills and interactions (Johar and Katayama, 2012).

Based on evidence from the United States, racial and ethnic differences mirror those reported above for employment, with obese white women suffering substantial disadvantage in wages, while African-American and Hispanic women are virtually unaffected (Cawley, 2004b; Cawley and Danziger, 2005).

As for the impact of obesity on employment, the role of discrimination in the link between obesity and wages has been the subject of much debate. Discrimination may be associated with lower expected or actual productivity on the job, increased sickness absence and need for medical care, which may be particularly burdensome for employers who are directly responsible for providing health insurance. On the other hand, part of the wage penalty associated with obesity must be caused by the employment disparities. The obese who struggle in the labor market — who may have lower educational qualifications, lower skills and poorer general health — will likely settle for lower paid jobs than their normal-weight counterparts.

The use of different indicators for adiposity (such as BMI, weight, waist circumference, body fat mass and free-fat mass) gives additional insights into the relationship with wages. An inverse U-shaped association between wages and BMI is found among young workers in Germany (Kropfhäußer and Sunder, 2013). In the United States, a one-unit increase in BMI in White women is associated with a 1.1% decrease in wages, and a one-pound increase in body-weight is associated with a 0.18% decrease in wages (Sabia and Rees, 2012). Similarly, a further US study found a one-unit change in BMI to be associated with a 1.83% wage penalty in women, but did not find any association between BMI, or obesity, and wage penalties in men (Han *et al.*, 2011). However, not all findings converge, as for instance workers with higher BMI (or obese workers) do not appear to earn lower wages in Australia (Kortt and Leigh, 2010). Going beyond the BMI measure, a Finnish study shows a negative association between waist circumference and wages (Johansson *et al.*, 2009). Bozoyan and Wolbring (2011) found body fat and fat-free mass to be associated with hourly wages (negative correlation for body fat and positive correlation for fat-free mass), but not BMI and wages.

A further aspect of the impact of obesity on labor markets is differences in productivity between obese and non-obese workers. Differences emerge in connection with absenteeism (sickness absence), but also with productivity and performance at work (presenteeism). The obese are also more likely to claim disability benefits and to become unable to work for extended periods of time, or even permanently.

Evidence from several countries documents differences in absence from work due to sickness among workers with different BMI levels. Overweight or obese workers are more likely than average to be absent from work (Howard and Potter, 2012). Some of the earliest estimates available from the United States suggest that they have twice as many days of sick leave as workers who are not overweight (Burton *et al.*, 1998). The same study also found a progressively increasing likelihood of sick leave with increasing BMI levels. Later, studies provided more detailed measures of this gradient, showing that the increase in days off work due to sickness is larger in women than in men (Finkelstein *et al.*, 2005; Cawley *et al.*, 2007) and that the increase in sick leave starts at higher BMI levels in men (from severe obesity) than in women (Finkelstein *et al.*, 2005). Differences in sick leave between obese and non-obese workers are present in the public, as well as in the private sectors (Bungum *et al.*, 2003). Similar evidence of increased sick leave in obese men and women is available from Belgium (Moens *et al.*, 1999; Moreau *et al.*, 2004), and a statistically significant relationship between obesity and absenteeism was found in female workers in Denmark, Finland, Portugal, and Spain, based on data from the European Community Household Panel survey (Sanz de Galdeano, 2007). In men, obesity leads to increased absenteeism in some types of occupations more than in others. A study based in the United States shows that absenteeism increases with BMI in professional and sales workers, while only morbid obesity is associated with a greater probability of missed work among managers, office workers and equipment operators (Cawley *et al.*, 2007).

A review including studies based on several countries confirmed an existing association between obesity and increased risk and duration of sick leave, which in turn affects workers' productivity (Neovious *et al.*, 2009). Therefore, a lower productivity may generate wage penalties and a reduced likelihood of employment (Dackehag *et al.*, 2011).

Presenteeism is far more difficult to measure than absenteeism or disability. A small number of studies have attempted to quantify reduced productivity for obese workers in the manufacturing sector, mainly through monetary valuations of the impact of self-reported reduced performance on the job due to health reasons. Moderately and severely obese manufacturing workers experience greater difficulties with job-related physical tasks and in completing work demands on time than normal weight workers. Existing estimates suggest that the loss of productivity associated with presenteeism is even larger than that associated with absenteeism, accounting for up to two-thirds of the monetary value of total productivity losses (Ricci and Chee, 2005; Gates *et al.*, 2008). Goetzel *et al.* (2010) found presenteeism to be 10% more likely for overweight employees, and 12% more likely for obese employees, compared with those of normal-weight. In addition, absence from work may not cost employers the full value of the time employees spend off work, to the extent that absence results in unpaid leave or other workers compensate for those who are absent.

Job insecurity is a source of stress that can affect motivation, job satisfaction, efficiency and productivity on the workplace. Being overweight or obese increases perceived job insecurity (measured as the perceived likelihood of losing one's job in the following 2 years). For instance, a statistically significant association between obesity and perceived job insecurity has been observed among German employees (OR 2.55, 95%CI 1.09–5.96) with a direct association in younger obese people (<30 years) and older people (>50 years) (Muenster *et al.*, 2011).

A number of studies have estimated the monetary value of productivity losses associated with obesity. A review of 31 studies (Trogdon *et al.*, 2008) found estimates to be highly heterogeneous across studies, ranging from \$77 to \$1033 per obese person per year depending on the degree of obesity. In the United States, the estimated value of lost productive time by obese workers is \$42.3 billion, exceeding that of normal-weight workers by $11.7 billion (Ricci and Chee, 2005). The incremental per-capita productivity losses due to high BMI (over those of normal-weight workers, including absenteeism and presenteeism) are estimated to range from $470 for overweight men to $4818 for Grade III obese (BMI over 40) men, and from $268 for overweight women to $4299 for Grade III obese women (Finkelstein *et al.* 2010). Based on those estimates, productivity losses due to obesity in the US are projected to reach 1.7–3 million productive person-years by 2030, representing an economic cost as high as $390–580 billion (Wang *et al.*, 2011). In Sweden, the total cost for sick-leave and disability pensions due to absence from work for Swedish obese women is estimated at SEK 10.5 billion per year, which represents an incremental cost of SEK3.6 billion compared with normal-weight women (Narbro *et al.*, 1996).

The changing relationship between affluence and obesity

The social gradient in obesity has changed over time, and the transition has been taking place at different rates in different countries. Early in the 20th century, overweight and obesity were most often associated with wealth and affluence within countries. With rising levels of national income and development, more obesogenic environments, but also greater availability of information on health risks and better opportunities for the well-to-do, obesity has increasingly affected people with less education and lower SES, to the point that the social gradient has been reversed in most high- and middle-income countries (Goryakin and Suhrcke, 2014).

In high-income countries, people with less education and lower SES are more likely to be obese, and the gap is generally larger in women. The social gradient observed in obesity is consistent with gradients in the consumption of less healthy foods and physical inactivity.

Social disparities in overweight and obesity are significant among women, and less pronounced, or absent among men. Estimates of the relative index of inequality in overweight and obesity vary across countries and between genders. Women who are at the bottom of the education ladder are consistently more likely to be overweight or obese than women at the top of the ladder (up to 5 times in Korea), as shown in Figure 3, while smaller or no inequalities are found in men. A virtually identical pattern is observed when assessing overweight and obesity by income or occupation type (Devaux and Sassi, 2013). This gender difference may be explained by several factors. The strength of the association between SES and obesity in women may reflect a stronger reverse causal link (from obesity to SES) in women, at least when SES is measured by income or occupation. The evidence discussed in Section "Obesity, Human Capital and Labor Markets" of higher wage penalties (Garcia Villar and Quintana-Domeque, 2009), and increased likelihood

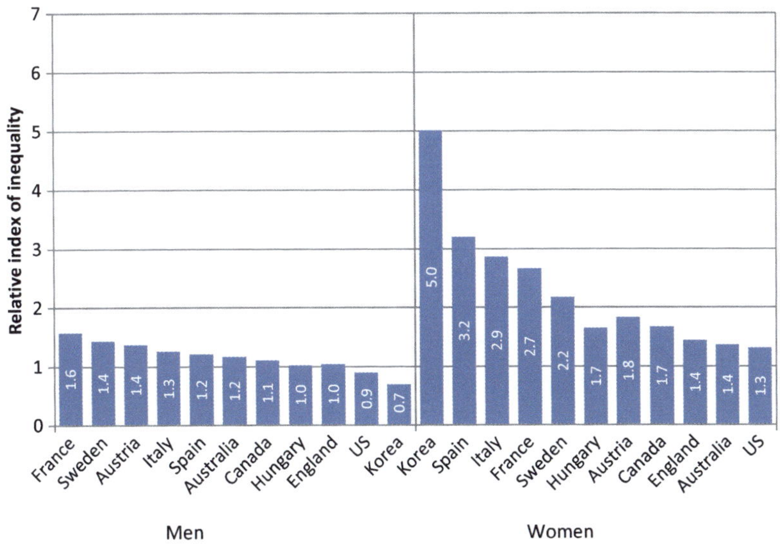

Figure 3. Inequality in overweight by education level

Note: An index value of *n* means that the least educated people in the country are *n* times as likely to be overweight or obese as the most educated. An index value of 1 means that overweight and obesity are equally distributed in people with different levels of education.
Source: OECD estimates based on national survey data.

of unemployment (Morris, 2007; Härkönen *et al.*, 2011) for obese women would seem to support this explanation. Another explanation of the gender gap may come from the different levels of physical activity involved in low-paid jobs held by men and women, with typically male jobs being more physically demanding.

Children in higher SES households are also more prone to be overweight or obese than children in less affluent households (Sassi, 2010). Social disparities in children are a cause of even greater concern, because obesity in early life is linked with obesity and social disadvantage in adult life, along dimensions such as school performance, labor market outcomes, and social inclusion.

In Europe, social disparities in overweight and obesity were found to be associated with national income. A EUR10,000 increase in per-capita GDP corresponded to a 3% increase in overweight and obesity for less educated men, but a 4% decrease for more educated men. No associations with GDP were observed for women (Roskam *et al.*, 2010).

Since 1990, obesity rates have grown more rapidly in low SES groups than in high SES groups in 6 of 8 countries covered in an OECD study (OECD, 2014). However, in the two countries with the highest prevalence of obesity, Mexico and The United States, rates have grown even faster among people with more education, and social gradients have virtually disappeared. A comparative study of Spain and England confirmed a widening of disparities in Spain from 1987 to 2006, while disparities remained virtually stable in England from 1997 to 2007 (Costa-Font *et al.*, 2014). Until 2002, obesity rates increased at a similar pace in all adolescents in the United States, but disparities increased thereafter, as obesity kept rising in lower-SES adolescents and declined slightly in their higher-SES counterparts (Frederick *et al.*, 2014).

People with more education are more likely than those with less education to eat fruit and vegetables daily, based on data from the 2009 European Health Interview Survey (Figure 4).

People with high SES (defined based on income, occupation, education or area of residence) are more likely to engage in moderate to vigorous physical activity than people with lower SES (Dowler, 2001; Gidlow *et al.*, 2006). This may be explained by barriers to physical activity for less affluent social groups, such as living in areas that are less safe (Zubrick *et al.*, 2010) and have fewer green spaces (Crawford *et al.*, 2008; Leslie *et al.*, 2010), or by cost barriers (Cavill *et al.*, 2006). Likely for similar reasons, city dwellers are significantly less likely to meet WHO recommended levels of physical activity compared with people living in rural areas. Social disparities in physical inactivity in 12 EU countries, measured by the relative index of inequality, are shown in Figure 5.

Physical inactivity rates vary with levels of national income (WHO, 2011a; 2011b). In high-income countries rates are over twice as large as in low-income countries. In Europe, a $PPP 10,000 increase in per-capita GDP is associated with a 3% increase in rates of insufficient physical activity, after accounting for sub-regional differences (authors' analysis of EHIS 2009 data).

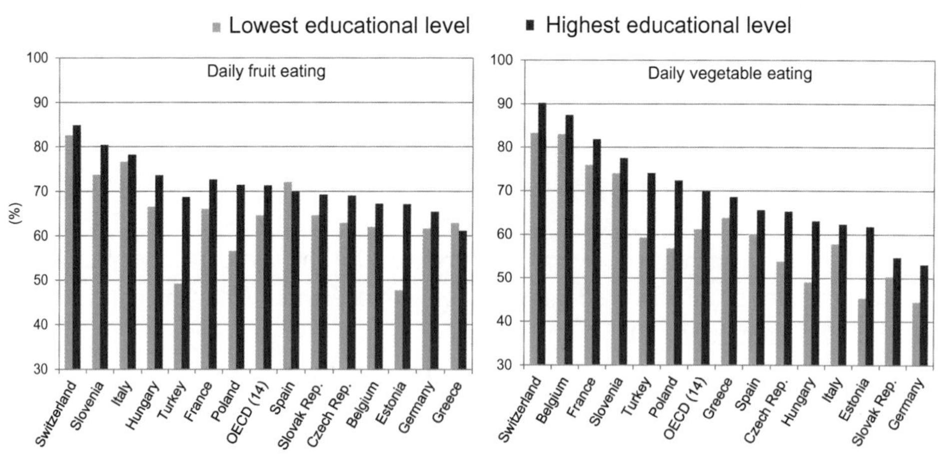

Figure 4. Fruit and vegetable consumption by education level

Source: Authors' analysis of EHIS 2009 data.

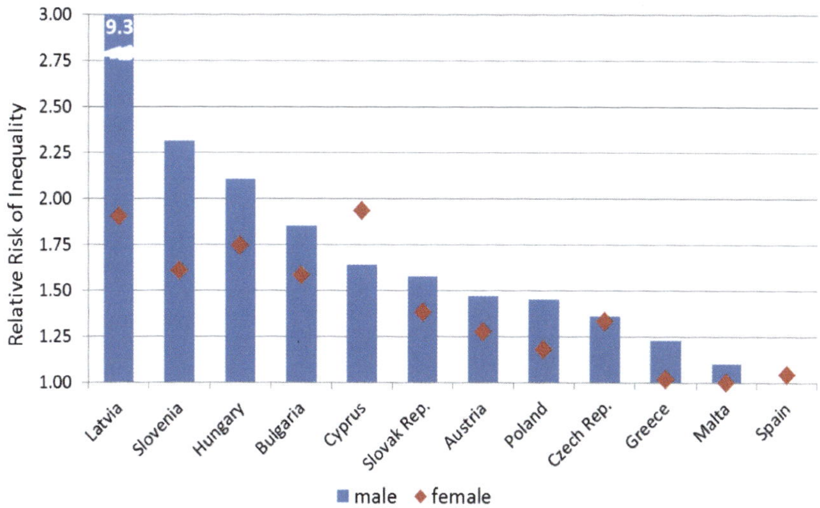

Figure 5. Urban–rural inequalities in insufficient physical activity

Note: An insufficient level of physical activity is defined as less than 150 minutes/week of moderate-intensity aerobic physical activity or equivalent.
Source: Authors' analysis of EHIS 2009 data.

Obesity: Market Failure and Rationality

Who bears the cost of obesity?

Whether obesity causes externalities, and how large these are if they exist, has been a matter of debate. Two possible types of externalities, in particular, have been considered: The fiscal, or insurance, externality, particularly in relation to the demand for collectively funded health care by obese people; and labor market externalities. The evidence presented in Section "The Global Obesity Epidemic and Its Public Health Dimensions" shows that costs increase steeply with BMI. This provides some support to the claim that obesity is associated with insurance externalities (individuals sharing the same risk pool will bear higher costs). However, "a necessary condition for the externality to occur is that the obese incur higher lifetime costs than the non-obese" (Brunello *et al.*, 2008), and there is no conclusive evidence that this is the case, as discussed in Section "The Global Obesity Epidemic and Its Public Health Dimensions." Brunello *et al.* conclude that lifetime costs are higher for the obese, both in the United Stated (8% higher) and in Europe (12% higher), but considering the degree of moral hazard likely associated with those differences, the size of the insurance externality associated with obesity is too small to warrant attention by policy makers. This is in line with empirical evidence produced by Bhattacharya and Sood (2005), who estimated an externality in the order of US$150 per capita, and with Philipson and Posner (2008).

Externalities may also be associated with the labor market outcomes of obesity, discussed extensively in Section "The Social Dimensions of Obesity". In particular, differences in productivity between obese and normal-weight people, often associated with a larger use of disability benefits, represent a potential source of negative externalities. The size of these externalities depends on the characteristics of the relevant labor markets and has not been quantified in detail in existing studies. Further productive inefficiencies may be associated with wages penalties and reduced employment opportunities for obese people, especially women.

The classical tools to address externalities are taxes and subsidies. These may improve the efficiency of market exchanges, but also have distributional impacts. For instance, it may or may not be possible, or desirable, for a government to redistribute the revenues raised from a tax intended to correct negative externalities to those who suffer the consequences of the externalities. Similarly, if a commodity that produces positive externalities is subsidized, it may not be possible to fund the subsidy by charging those who enjoy the positive external effects. From a mere efficiency standpoint, what matters is just that welfare gains exceed any losses, but societies are not indifferent to the distribution of those gains and losses, therefore governments will have to take this into account in assessing the desirability of a policy to address possible externalities.

Information and information failures

Information is critical for markets to operate efficiently. In order to make rational and efficient choices, consumers have to be fully informed about the characteristics and quality of the goods they consume, about the benefits (and harms) they will derive from consumption, and about the opportunity costs they will incur. In the case of diet and physical activity, information on the nature and the size of the associated health risks may be lacking or difficult to use, or it may be concealed or distorted by parties that have a vested interest. Arguably, most people today possess the basic knowledge required for them to broadly discriminate between more and less healthy food options. However, there is evidence that interventions based on the provision of information in various forms, from nutritional labelling to health education campaigns, from health claims in advertising to the dissemination of nutritional guidelines, has at least some impact on individual dietary choices, suggesting that there is still scope for improving consumer information.

The key question for policymakers is whether information failures may warrant some form of corrective action. Brunello *et al.* (2008), as well as Philipson and Posner (2008), do not find that existing evidence of information failures in relation to obesity would justify, *per se*, government action. Cawley (2004a) insists on the "public good" nature of information, which implies that information is underprovided in a market setting justifying governments' involvement in its provision, and suggests that possible failures may be associated with people's ability to process information, rather than with the availability of information.

The direct provision of information by governments (e.g., health education campaigns to improve diets or increase physical activity) or the regulation of information (e.g., limits on advertising, guidelines on food labelling) can be the effective ways of improving consumer information. However, governments are not always equipped for deploying complex communication strategies, and in some cases, their actions may be influenced by the very interests they try to counter. When information failures cannot be fixed, governments may still compensate for the effects of imperfect information by influencing behaviors through appropriate incentives (e.g., fiscal incentives like taxes and subsidies).

Behavioral insights

- *Myopia and inconsistent time preferences*

Understanding the way in which people discount future costs and benefits in making their lifestyle choices is critical to the design of effective policies to counter obesity. A large body of empirical literature about time preferences in relation to a variety of outcomes, including health (e.g., Lipscomb *et al.*, 1996), suggests that there are no good reasons for future health risks associated with lifestyle choices to be discounted at especially high, or especially low, rates. Some characteristics of those choices, such as the relatively small size of the perceived health risks involved, will make people discount future risks more heavily. But other characteristics of the same choices will have the opposite effect. However, empirical evidence from behavioral economics research suggests that health-related behaviors often reflect a wholly different approach to discounting future health risks, in keeping with hyperbolic discounting. Future outcomes are discounted more than exponentially in present judgments, translating into inconsistent preferences over time. This can be framed as a self-control problem, as procrastination is a key feature of hyperbolic discounting. Inconsistency in time preferences is reflected in the discrepancy between the way people think they will discount future outcomes at some later time, and the way they actually discount them when that later time comes. The result is a likely indefinite postponment of the decision to change behavior.

At least some evidence of hyperbolic discounting has been found in relation to obesity: "Time inconsistent preferences regarding weight is a very common problem among teenagers, since the majority of them end up failing to reduce their BMI after having declared to be trying to lose weight" (Brunello *et al.*, 2008). In order to address hyperbolic discounting, governments would need to make judgments on whether people should be pushed to give higher priority to their future self, or long-term preferences, over their present self, or short-term preferences. Alternatively, hyperbolic discounting can be addressed by increasing the availability of "technologies or contracts that facilitate private self-control", such as the fiscal deductibility of private expenditures on devices that may facilitate self-control, like nutrition advice or gym subscriptions (Glaeser, 2006).

- *Habits and addiction*

Certain behaviors involve repeated acts of consumption which are dependent of each other. This may happen because a form of chemical dependence makes it difficult to quit consumption (addiction), or because of psychological mechanisms that encourage the reiteration of consumption (habit). The two often co-exist to varying degrees. The presence of a chemical dependence may strengthen the justification for intervention, but some forms of psychological addiction may also be extremely powerful and potentially damaging.

Once an individual has first engaged in addictive consumption, and borne the initial costs involved, they will tend to continue that consumption and they will need much greater disincentives to be able to quit than those they faced when they started. Lack of self-control and inconsistent time preferences may be seen to produce similar effects. Two psychological mechanisms characterizing habitual behavior represent obstacles to behavior change (Maio *et al.*, 2007). First, is "tunnel vision" and relates to a reduced motivation to seek and use information that may lead to a better understanding of the consequences of the behavior in question, and to a tendency to discount the value of new information that is received, particularly when it highlights risks associated with the habitual behavior. Second, is that people who engage in habitual behavior act on the implicit assumption that if they found the behavior desirable when they first adopted it, it must also be desirable for them to continue to engage in the same behavior.

Habitual behavior can be a source of inefficiency and may lead to sub-optimal outcomes for consumers. Of course, consumers take up habits because they find it convenient to do so. In a short-term perspective, it may be efficient to avoid re-examining the desirability of a certain form of consumption every time consumption is repeated, but in doing so consumers may overlook longer term consequences of that consumption which may well offset any short-term efficiency gains.

The issue of whether specific foods, or ingredients, may have addictive effects is still contentious (for instance, see Avena *et al.* (2008), Benton (2010) on the addictive properties of sugar). While the role of habitual behaviors, combined with strong environmental pressures, in the maintenance of unhealthy eating habits is a potentially important determinant of the obesity epidemic, the existing evidence-base is still too small to support actions specifically aimed at tackling this effect.

Policy Levers to Counter the Obesity Epidemic

Price incentives for healthy eating

The role of food and non-alcoholic beverage taxes in encouraging healthier eating has been debated for over a decade (Jacobson and Brownell, 2000; Marshall, 2000), and many jurisdictions have some form of taxes on specific foods. Denmark introduced a tax on foods containing saturated fats (meat, cheese, butter, edible oils, margarine, spreads, snacks, etc.) in 2011, although it repealed the tax 1 year later. Hungary introduced a tax on selected manufactured foods with high sugar, salt or caffeine content, including carbonated sugary drinks, Finland a tax on confectionery products, combined with a raised excise tax on soft drinks, and France a tax on soft drinks, affecting both drinks with added sugars and drinks with artificial sweeteners. Mexico implemented an 8% tax on high energy density foods, and a tax on sugar-sweetened beverages in 2014.

The evidence-base on the potential effects of taxes on nutrition and health has grown considerably in the past few years. A recent review concluded that taxes have the potential to shift consumer behavior toward healthier dietary patterns, but the effects of taxes depend largely on the details of the policy design (Thow, 2012; Sassi *et al.*, 2013). A review of simulation models concluded that taxes on carbonated drinks and saturated fat and subsidies on fruit and vegetables would be associated with beneficial dietary change (Eyles *et al.*, 2012).

Empirical estimates of the responsiveness of consumers to price changes (price elasticity) in the long-term suggest that taxes would influence food purchases, but to differing degrees depending on the study and nutrient/food in question. However, knock-on effects of taxes on nutrients other than those targeted may offset some of the benefits (Cornelsen *et al.*, 2014). For instance, taxing fats was shown to have a potential for increasing sugar intake (Jensen and Smed, 2007) or salt intake (Mytton *et al.* 2007).

Food subsidies can either be targeted at specific food commodities, or at consumers (all or selected groups). In the former case, the challenge is to ensure that subsidies effectively translate into reduced market prices; in the latter, that consumers spend the extra money to purchase healthy foods. Studies of the effects of population-level food subsidies, reviewed in Thow *et al.* (2010), suggest that subsidies influence consumption in the intended direction, and that taxes are more effective when combined with subsidies. A systematic review of 'prices, demand and body weight outcomes' of a range of fiscal policies found that lower prices of fruit and vegetables were generally associated with lower weight outcomes, especially for children in low-income groups and for those with the highest levels of BMI (Powell *et al.*, 2013).

Incentives at point-of-sale were found to have positive effects on food purchasing patterns in a systematic review (Wall *et al.*, 2006), though the evidence in support of sustained effects is more tenuous. The full range of impacts on consumers is yet to be fully understood and appears to vary with the intervention type.

Existing studies, mostly based on economic models, show that taxes on foods high in salt, sugar and fat, including non-alcoholic beverages, are consistently cost-saving, that is, they cost less to implement than they save in terms of reduced health care expenditures, and they have a favorable health impact at the population level (Smith-Spangler *et al.*, 2010; Sacks *et al.*, 2011). Food taxes are likely to be regressive, although the less well-off also benefit disproportionately from their effects, and need to be designed carefully in order to avoid undesirable substitution effects in food consumption. Both the effectiveness and the distributional impact of taxes appear to be enhanced by coupling them with subsidies targeting healthy foods or disadvantaged consumers (Cecchini *et al.*, 2010; Sassi *et al.*, 2009b; Sassi, 2010). In contrast, modelling analysis in France and Australia suggests that the use of discounts and/or a reduction in VAT or provision of food stamps for fruit and vegetables is not cost-effective (Cobiac *et al.*, 2010a; Dallongeville *et al.*, 2011).

Regulation and industry self-regulation

- *Nutrition labelling and health claims*

Lists of nutrients can be provided on foods, menus, retail shelves, etc. In Europe, the regulations on nutrient labelling changed in 2011. Previously, the provision of a nutrient list was required only when a nutrient claim was made, but nutrient labelling will become mandatory in December 2016 (European Commission, 2011). Other countries, notably the United States, have required mandatory labelling for a much longer time period (Hawkes, 2010). Even though labelling is not yet mandatory in Europe, food companies already supply nutrition lists on the vast majority of their products (Bonsmann *et al.*, 2010).

A significant body of literature on the effects of application of nutrient lists includes five systematic reviews and around 300 papers (Cowburn and Stockley 2005; Grunert and Wills, 2007; Ni Mhurchu and Gorton, 2007; Campos *et al.*, 2011; Mozaffarian *et al.*, 2012). Most evaluations of nutrition labelling are based on experiments assessing different schemes (traffic light, guideline daily amounts, front/back-of-package labels, shelf-labelling system) on a limited set of products and in restricted time and space conditions. Impact on label use and understanding (dietary precursors) are typically measured, rather than dietary intake, with the exception of some more recent studies from the United States. Evidence suggests that food labelling leads to reformulation of food contents — e.g., reduction in salt and fat, increase in fiber (Capacci *et al.*, 2012; Vyth *et al.*, 2012).

There is good evidence that consumers use nutrient lists, but label use is considerably lower among low-SES groups. Food labelling schemes were found to perform better than information campaigns in terms of cost-effectiveness, especially when implemented on a mandatory basis, but the studies available to support this claim are few and vary in the types of schemes assessed and methods applied. Multi-country modelling studies found that mandatory labelling would have a favorable cost-effectiveness ratio in countries at different levels of income (Sassi *et al.*, 2009a; Cecchini *et al.*, 2010). Evidence from Australia on interpretative labels is consistent with these findings. Traffic light labelling was shown to be cost-effective (Sacks *et al.*, 2011) and using a mandatory "tick" symbol to indicate products low in salt, with the expected effect of food companies significantly reducing salt content, was shown to be effective and cost-saving (Cobiac *et al.*, 2010b).

- *Regulation of food advertising to children*

There has been considerable interest in Europe on restricting the commercial promotion of high fat, high sugar, or high salt foods to children. Many countries are developing policies on food marketing to children, although these mainly involve the encouragement of industry self-regulation. At least 22 countries around the world have developed explicit policies on marketing to children, over half of which are in Europe (Hawkes and Lobstein, 2011). Although none are comprehensive, they include specific restrictions and/or require messaging on advertising. The most restrictive approach is found in the United Kingdom, where broadcast advertising of high fat, sugar or salt foods is prohibited to children aged under 16. The food industry has also been active in this area — there are at least 20 pledges by food companies to restrict advertising to children under the age of 12, including the 'EU Pledge', which covers the whole EU Region (Rudd Center for Food Policy and Obesity, 2013).

The development of policies restricting food marketing to children has been based in part on the moderate–strong evidence that food television advertising influences food and beverage preferences, purchase requests, beliefs and dietary intake risk (McGinnis *et al.*, 2006; Cairns *et al.*, 2009). Yet evidence on the actual effectiveness of these policies is still emerging, with no systematic reviews having been conducted on the topic.

Compliance with existing regulations, self-regulations and pledges is generally high (e.g., IFBA, 2009; Landmark Europe, 2010; Accenture, 2012; Tymms, 2012).

Both statutory and self-regulatory restrictions on specific communications channels and marketing techniques have led to decline in advertising according to the criteria adopted in the policy or pledge (e.g., Ofcom, 2010; EU Pledge, 2012; Kim *et al.*, 2013). However, these declines are measured according to the criteria of the policy, rather than declines of total exposure across the marketing mix (e.g., King *et al.*, 2011; Adams *et al.*, 2012; UK Department of Health, 2008; FTC, 2012). All available model-based studies suggest that restrictions can have positive outcomes for dietary intake (e.g., Dhar and Baylis (2011) for fast food) or obesity (Chou *et al.*, 2008; Magnus *et al.*, 2009; Veerman *et al.*, 2009).

Restrictions in the commercial promotion of food, was shown to be cost-effective in a small number of model-based economic studies focusing on restricting food advertising to children. One of these studies compared the cost-effectiveness of restricting commercial promotion through mandatory and self-regulatory approaches in 5 countries (Sassi *et al.*, 2009a; Sassi, 2010; Cecchini *et al.*, 2010). Restrictions were highly cost-effective in the 20 years after implementation, especially in low- and middle-income countries, where they may even be cost-saving in some instances. Even though the statutory regulations were assumed to have a greater health impact, self-regulation (securing half the reduction) was found to be significantly more cost-effective as a result of its significantly lower costs. Also, the extension of existing regulations in Australia to include food advertising during specified children's TV viewing hours was highly cost-effective (Magnus *et al.*, 2009).

- *Food product reformulation*

Potentially, food product reformulation could include any nutrient (or calories), but in practice, action in this area has concentrated on reduction in the level of salt and trans-fats in processed foods, with some attention being paid to portion size. At least 19 European countries have implemented salt reduction strategies (as well as over 10 other countries), all of which include targets for reformulation, usually by voluntary means (Webster *et al.*, 2011). There has been far less action in Europe on trans-fats (Mendis *et al.*, 2011), with the notable exception of Denmark, where the government imposed a maximum level of 2 g/100 g fat on industrially produced trans-fats in 2003. In the Netherlands, there is also a Task Force for the Improvement of the Fatty Acid Composition, which encourages product reformulation on a voluntary basis. Outside of Europe there has been action in trans-fats in Latin America (Monge-Rojas *et al.*, 2011) and North America. In Canada, there are voluntary targets for reduction, and in the United States, there are some local bans on trans-fats. Mandatory labelling of trans-fats has also been reported to have stimulated voluntary reformulation by the food industry (Unnevehr and Jagmanaite, 2008).

Product reformulation policies aimed at reducing the salt content of processed foods were found to be cost-saving or to have a favorable cost-effectiveness ratio in several economic evaluations (Wang and Labarthe, 2011; Barton *et al.*, 2011; Eatwell, 2012). Murray *et al.* (2003) found that reductions in salt from both voluntary and legislative measures would be cost-effective, but legislation more so. In Norway, the effect of industry reformulation combined with an information campaign was modelled; actions would be cost-saving (Selmer *et al.*, 2000). For the United Kingdom, the estimate was made (using actual data) for both voluntary salt reduction by industry and an information campaign. On the basis that the salt reduction initiative saved 44,000 QALYs, it was found to be cost-effective and when savings to the National Health Service are included ($116 million), it was found to be dominant (Eatwell, 2012). In Argentina, reducing salt in bread was found to be cost-saving, and more cost-effective than any of the other interventions analyzed (Rubinstein *et al.*, 2010). A study focused on developing countries found a legislated reduction in salt content of manufactured foods and an accompanying public education campaign would be cost-effective (Willett *et al.*, 2006). The economic evidence on other instances of reformulation (e.g., to reduce trans-fat content) is very limited.

Information, education, and awareness raising

- *Mass media campaigns*

Public awareness campaigns aim to change the consumption of specific foods or nutrients, or to encourage healthy eating more generally. They can be conducted at the national or community level through the mass media, or in specific settings, such as schools, worksites, supermarkets, etc. In Europe, there have been a number of campaigns targeted at specific nutrients, notably salt, fruit, and vegetables (Capacci *et al.*, 2012). Most countries have some form of public awareness campaign for fruits and vegetables, typically based on the 'five portions a day' message (Fulponi, 2009; Capacci *et al.*, 2012).

According to Mozaffarian *et al.* (2012), the weight of evidence suggests that sustained and focused media and educational campaigns, using multiple channels to increase consumption of specific healthy foods (e.g., fruit and vegetables, as well as other 'eat more of' foods, as reviewed below) are likely to be effective at changing knowledge. A systematic review published by the WHO concluded that intensive mass media campaigns using one simple message, and long-term intensive campaigns promoting healthy diets, are moderately effective interventions (Anderson *et al.,* 2009). According to a review of studies based in Europe, most public campaigns were evaluated on the basis of their effects on dietary precursors (knowledge and awareness), rather than on dietary intake, therefore they are not conclusive about the effects of campaigns on behavior and dietary patterns (Capacci *et al.,* 2012).

Several economic analyses of public awareness campaigns are available, some of which assessed campaigns combined with other policy actions, e.g., with interpretive labelling schemes (Sacks *et al.* 2011), or product reformulation (Eatwell, 2012). Most of the evidence from economic studies of information campaigns points to relatively poor cost-effectiveness. Even studies concluding that information campaigns can be cost-effective did so on the basis of the low cost of these actions and confirmed their limited effects at the population level. For example, the effects of a mass media campaign aimed at increasing fruit and vegetable intake, as well as physical activity, were assessed in a multi-country study based on a microsimulation approach (Sassi *et al.*, 2009a; Sassi, 2010). The study found that the campaign would have a favorable cost-effectiveness ratio starting from about 10 years from its initial implementation, but its health effects would be smaller than those of any of the other strategies examined. Worksite information campaigns often accompanied by changes in catering are not effective (Cobiac *et al.*, 2010a; Engbers *et al.*, 2006). In developing country settings, model-based studies found that mass media campaigns for salt, saturated fat and cholesterol reduction had a more favorable cost-effective profile (Ha and Chisholm, 2011; Willett *et al.*, 2006).

- *School-based programs*

Policies aimed at making fruit and vegetables available in schools have been found to have positive, albeit modest, effects on dietary intake. The development of the EU School Fruit Scheme was based on a systematic review of the effects of fruit and vegetable programs in schools (de Sa and Lock, 2008), which concluded that school fruit and vegetable programs are effective in increasing dietary knowledge and intake. Evaluations at the national level suggest that the consumption effect varies between different groups of children — e.g., girls consume more than boys.

A systematic review of 42 school-based interventions in Europe concluded that there is strong evidence of the effect on fruit and vegetable intake for 'multi-component interventions' (i.e., those that combine changes to the food environment with education interventions), with more limited evidence of the effect of interventions that changed provision or provided education alone (Van Cauwenberghe *et al.*, 2010).

Despite the widespread use of measures to promote the availability of fruit and vegetables, and the reasonable large number of evaluations of the effects of these actions, very limited evidence of cost-effectiveness is currently available. Evidence from the Netherlands found these initiatives to be cost-effective, although the finding was sensitive to assumptions regarding the sustainability of dietary changes in the long term (te Velde *et al.*, 2011).

Policies to increase physical activity

A variety of policies and programs have been used to make people more physically active. Mass media campaigns, for instance, have been shown to have a positive, moderate effect on physical activity (Cavill and Bauman, 2004; Kahn *et al.*, 2002; Leavy *et al.*, 2011). Campaigns are generally cost-effective, and can be cost-saving in some settings (Cecchini *et al.*, 2010; Lewis *et al.*, 2010; Sassi *et al.*, 2009a; Vos *et al.*, 2010; WHO, 2011b). School-based programs tend to provide information on the benefits of physical fitness and increased opportunities to undertake physical activity. Some encourage walking and cycling to school (Lee *et al.*, 2008; NICE, 2008). School-based programs can be cost-effective (Lewis *et al.*, 2010; Sassi *et al.*, 2009a); in particular, interventions that combine actions on physical activity and diet seem to be more efficient than interventions on a single domain. Employers can also support active travel by providing adequate facilities (e.g., bike storage, showers), incentives and discounts for fitness clubs, health education programs and individual employee health checks (Bull *et al.*, 2008), with positive effects on physical activity, fitness, body weight and lipids (Proper *et al.*, 2003; Abraham and Graham-Rowe, 2009; Conn *et al.*, 2009; Dugdill *et al.*, 2008). Governments can further incentivise active transport through infrastructure changes and urban planning, such as the extension of bicycle lanes and routes, and traffic-calming measures (e.g., Beale *et al.*, 2007).

Counselling in primary care has positive and moderate effects on reported levels of physical activity (Breckon *et al.*, 2008; Fleming and Godwin, 2008; Williams *et al.*, 2007). In some cases, this can lead to improvements in blood pressure or lipid profile. Primary care interventions are cost-effective, despite the relatively high costs often involved (Garrett *et al.*, 2011; Lewis *et al.*, 2010; Sassi *et al.*, 2009a; WHO, 2011b).

Conclusions

Obesity has risen to epidemic proportions in the OECD area during the past 30 years. Rates are still somewhat lower in major non-OECD countries, but growing at a similarly fast pace as in higher income countries, especially in urban areas.

Height, weight and body mass have been increasing gradually at least since the 18th century, contributing to a steady progress in life expectancy. The rapid acceleration in BMI growth over the past 30 years will likely slow down further progress in longevity.

The obesity epidemic has largely been determined by factors and dynamics that have characterized the last 30 years, which have created obesogenic environments. Improved education and socio-economic conditions have decreased the underlying probability of obesity in successive birth cohorts, but have not been sufficient to offset the effects of environmental changes.

There are important social disparities in overweight and obesity in women and lesser or no disparities in men. Social disparities are also present in children. Disparities in labor market outcomes between obese people and people of normal weight, especially strong in women, likely contribute to the social gradient in overweight and obesity. Obese people are less likely to be a part of the labor force and to be in employment. They are also likely to earn less than people of normal weight, with wage penalties of up to 18%, larger for obese women than men.

Fiscal or insurance externalities deriving from higher health care expenditures for obese people may not be large enough to require specific government intervention. But externalities are also associated with the spread of obesity within families and social networks, revealing a social multiplier effect. Information failures are unlikely to play a major role in the current spread of obesity, but there is a clear role for governments in ensuring an adequate provision of information, especially to vulnerable groups, such children and those in disadvantaged socio-economic circumstances. Inconsistencies in time preferences, leading to poor self-control in health-related consumption, and a biased perception of risk make obesity more likely.

Governments have a wide range of options at their disposal to tackle the rising tide of obesity. They can increase choice by helping to make new healthy options available, or by making existing ones more accessible and affordable. They can use persuasion, education and information to make healthy options more attractive. Regulation and fiscal measures are transparent and contestable interventions, but they hit all consumers indiscriminately, and may be difficult to enact and enforce. Interventions that are less intrusive on individual choices tend to have higher costs of delivery. Interventions that are more intrusive often have higher political and welfare costs.

References

Abraham A, Graham-Rowe E. 2009. Are worksite interventions effective in increasing physical activity? A systematic review and meta-analysis. *Health Psychology Review* 3(1): 108–144.

Accenture. 2012. 2012 Compliance Monitoring Report For the International Food & Beverage Alliance On Global Advertising on Television. Available at https://www.ifballiance.org/sites/default/files/AccentureMonitoringReport2012FINALDecember2012.pdf.

Adams J, Tyrrell R, Adamson AJ, White M. 2012. Effect of restrictions on television food advertising to children on exposure to advertisements for 'less healthy' foods: Repeat cross-sectional study. *Plos One* 7(2): e31578. doi:10.1371/journal.pone.0031578.

Allison DB, Zannolli R, Narayan KM. 1999. The direct health care costs of obesity in the United States. *American Journal of Public Health* 89: 1194–1199.

Anderson J, Parker W, Steyn NP *et al.* 2009. *Interventions on Diet and Physical Activity: What Works*. Geneva: World Health Organization.

Andreyeva T, Michaud PC, van Soest A. 2007. Obesity and health in Europeans aged 50 years and Older. *Public Health* 121(7): 497–509.

Arena VC, *et al.* 2006. The impact of body mass index on short-term disability in the workplace. *Journal of Occupational and Environmental Medicine* 48(11): 1118–1124.

Avena NM, Rada P, Hoebel BG. 2008. Evidence for sugar addiction: Behavioral and neurochemical effects of intermittent, excessive sugar intake. *Neuroscience and Biobehavioral Reviews* 32(1): 20–39.

Averett, S, Korenman S. 1996. The economic reality of the beauty myth. *Journal of Human Resources* 31: 304–330.

Baillie K. 2008. Health implications of transition from a planned to a free-market economy — an overview. *Obesity Reviews* 9(Suppl.)(1): 146–150.

Barton P, Andronis L, Briggs A, McPherson K, Capewell S. 2011. Effectiveness and cost-effectiveness of cardiovascular disease prevention in whole populations: Modelling study. *British Medical Journal* 343: d4044.

Beale S, Bending M, Trueman P. 2007. *An Economic Analysis of Environmental Interventions that Promote Physical Activity*. PDG Report. York: York Health Economic Consortium.

Benton, D. 2010. The plausibility of sugar addiction and its role in obesity and eating disorders. *Clinical Nutrition* 29(3): 288–303.

Bhattacharya J, Choudhry K, Lakdawalla DN. 2008. Chronic disease and trends in severe disability in working age populations. *Medical Care* 46(1): 92–100.

Bhattacharya J, Sood N. 2005. Health Insurance and the Obesity Externality, *NBER Working Paper No. 11529*, National Bureau of Economic Research, Cambridge, MA.

Bonsmann SSG, Celemín LF, Larrañaga A, *et al.* 2010. Penetration of nutrition information on food labels across the EU–27 plus Turkey. *European Journal of Clinical Nutrition* 64(12): 1379–1385.

Bozoyan C, Wolbring T. 2011. Fat, muscles, and wages. *Economics and Human Biology* 9: 356–363.

Breckon JD, Johnston LH, Hutchison A. 2008. Physical activity counselling content and competency: A systematic review. *Journal of Physical Activity and Health* 5(3): 398–417.

Brunello G, d'Hombres B. 2007. Does body weight affect wages: Evidence from Europe. *Economics and Human Biology* 5: 1–19.

Brunello G, Michaud PC, Sanz-de-Galdeano A. 2008. The Rise in Obesity Across the Atlantic: An Economic Perspective. *IZA Discussion Paper* No. 3529, Bonn.

Bull F, Adams E. Hooper P. 2008. Well@Work: Promoting Active and Healthy Workplaces Final Evaluation Report. Loughborough: School of Sport and Exercise Sciences, Loughborough University.

Bungum T, *et al.* 2003. The relationship of body mass index, medical costs, and job absenteeism. *American Journal Health Behavior* 27(4): 456–462.

Burton WN, Chen CY, Schultz AB, Edington DW. 1998. The economic costs associated with body mass index in a workplace. *Journal of Occupational and Environmental Medicine* 40(9): 786–792.

Cairns G, Angus K, Hastings G. 2009. The Extent, Nature and Effects of Food Promotion to Children: A Review of the Evidence to December 2008. Geneva: World Health Organization.

Caliendo M, Lee W-S. 2013. Fat chance! Obesity and the transition from unemployment to employment. *Economics and Human Biology* 11: 121-0133.

Campos S, Doxey J, Hammond D. 2011. Nutrition labels on pre-packaged foods: A systematic review. *Public Health Nutrition* 14(8): 1496–1506.

Capacci S, Mazzocchi M, Shankar B, *et al.* 2012. Policies to promote healthy eating in Europe: A structured review of policies and their effectiveness. *Nutrition Reviews* 70(3): 188–200.

Case A, Menendez A. 2007. Sex Differences in Obesity Rates in Poor Countries: Evidence from South Africa. *NBER Working Paper* No. 13541. Available at: http://www.nber.org/papers/w13541.

Cavill N, Bauman A. 2004. Changing the way people think about health-enhancing physical activity: Do mass media campaigns have a role? *Journal of Sports Sciences* 22(8): 771–90.

Cavill N, Kahlmeier S, Racioppi F. 2006. Physical activity and health in Europe: Evidence for action. Copenhagen: WHO Regional Office for Europe, 2006.

Cawley J. 2000a. Body Weight and Women's Labor Market Outcomes. Cambridge, MA, National Bureau of Economic Research, *Working Paper* No. 7841.

Cawley J. 2000b. An Instrumental Variables Approach to Measuring the Effect of Obesity on Employment Disability. *Health Services Research* 35: 1159–1179.

Cawley J. 2004a. The impact of obesity on wages. *The Journal of Human Resources* 39(2): 451–474.

Cawley J. 2004b. An economic framework for understanding physical activity and eating behaviors. *American Journal of Preventive Medicine* 27(3S): 117–125.

Cawley J, Burkhauser RV. 2006. Beyond BMI: The Value of More Accurate Measures of Fatness and Obesity in Social Science Research. *NBER Working Paper* No. 12291, available on www.nber.org/papers/w12291.

Cawley J, Danziger S. 2005. Morbid obesity and the transition from welfare to work. *Journal of Policy Analysis and Management* 24(4): 727–743.

Cawley J, Rizzo JA and Haas K. 2007. Occupation-specific absenteeism costs associated with obesity and morbid obesity. *Journal of Occupational and Environmental Medicine* 49(12): 1317–1324.

Cecchini M, Sassi F, Lauer JA, Lee YY, Guajardo-Barron V, Chisholm D. 2010. Tackling of unhealthy diets, physical inactivity, and obesity: Health effects and cost-effectiveness. *Lancet* 376(9754):1775–1784.

Chou S-Y, Rashad I, Grossman M. 2008. Fast-food restaurant advertising on television and its influence on childhood obesity. *Journal of Law & Economics* 51(4): 599–618.

Cobiac LJ, Vos T, Veerman JL. 2010a. Cost-effectiveness of interventions to promote fruit and vegetable consumption. *Plos One* 5(11): e14148.

Cobiac LJ, Vos T, Veerman, JL. 2010b. Cost-effectiveness of interventions to reduce dietary salt intake. *Heart* 96(23): 1920–1925.

Conn, VS, Hafdahl, AR, Cooper, PS, Brown, LM, Lusk, SL. 2009. Meta-analysis of workplace physical activity interventions. *American Journal of Preventive Medicine* 37(4): 330–339.

Connor Gorber S, Tremblay MS. 2010. The bias in self-reported obesity from 1976 to 2005: A Canada–US comparison. *Obesity* (Silver Spring) 18(2): 354–361.

Cornelsen L, Green R, Turner R, Dangour AD, Shankar B, Mazzocchi M, Smith RD. 2014. What happens to patterns of food consumption when food prices change? Evidence from a systematic review and meta-analysis of food price elasticities globally. *Health Economics* Sep 18. doi: 10.1002/hec.3107.

Corrada MM, Kawas CH, Mozaffar F, Paganini-Hill A. 2006. Association of body mass index and weight change with all-cause mortality in the elderly. *American Journal of Epidemiology* 163(10): 938–949.

Costa-Font J, Hernández-Quevedo C, Jiménez-Rubio D. 2014. Income inequalities in unhealthy life styles in England and Spain. *Economics & Human Biology* 13: 66–75.

Cowburn G, Stockley L. 2005. Consumer understanding and use of nutrition labelling: A systematic review. *Public Health Nutrition* 8(1): 21–28.

Crawford D, Timperio A, Giles-Corti B, Ball K, Hume C, Roberts R, *et al.* 2008. Do features of public open spaces vary according to neighbourhood socio-economic status? *Health & Place* 14(4): 889–893.

Cutler DM, Glaeser EL, Shapiro JM. 2003. Why have americans become more obese? *Journal of Economic Perspectives* 17(3): 93–118.

Dackehag M, Gerdtham UG, Nordin M. 2011. Productivity or discrimination? An economic analysis of excess-weight penalty in the Swedish labor market. Lund University, Department of Economics, Working Papers 2011:12.

Dallongeville J, Dauchet L, de Mouzon O, Réquillart V, Soler LG. 2011. Increasing fruit and vegetable consumption: A cost-effectiveness analysis of public policies. *European Journal of Public Health* 21(1): 69–73.

de Sa J, Lock K. 2008. Will European agricultural policy for school fruit and vegetables improve public health? A review of school fruit and vegetable programmes. *European Journal of Public Health* 18(6): 558–568.

Devaux M, Sassi F. 2013. Social inequalities in obesity and overweight in eleven OECD countries. *The European Journal of Public Health* 2013; doi: 10.1093/eurpub/ckr058.

Dhar T, Baylis K. 2011. Fast-food consumption and the ban on advertising targeting children: The Quebec experience. *Journal of Marketing Research* 48(5): 799–813.

Dowler E. 2001. Inequalities in diet and physical activity in Europe. *Public Health Nutr*ition 4: 701–709.

Dugdill L, Brettle A, Hulme C, McCluskey S, Long AF. 2008. Workplace physical activity interventions: A systematic review. *International Journal of Workplace Health Management* 1(1): 20–40.

Eatwell. 2012. D2.3: Evaluation of Cost Utility of Policy Interventions. Eatwell Project Report. Reading: Eatwell Project. Available at http://eatwellproject.eu/en/upload/Reports/D2.3_Evaluation_of_cost_utility_of_policy_interventions0%201.pdf.

Engbers L, van Poppel M, Paw M, van Mechelen W. 2006. The effects of a controlled worksite environmental intervention on determinants of dietary behavior and self-reported fruit, vegetable and fat intake. *BMC Public Health* 6: 253.

EU Pledge. 2012. 2012 Monitoring Report. EU Pledge.

European Commission (EC). 2011. Regulation (EU) No 1169/2011 of the European Parliament and of the Council of 25 October 2011 on the provision of food information to consumers. Available at http://eur-lex.europa.eu/LexUriServ/LexUriServ.do?uri=CELEX:32011R1169:EN:NOT.

Eyles H, Ni Mhurchu C, Nghiem N, Blakely T. 2012. Food pricing strategies, population diets, and noncommunicable disease: A systematic review of simulation studies. *PLoS Medicine* 9(12): e1001353. doi: 10.1371/journal.pmed.1001353.

Finkelstein EA, DiBonaventura Md, Burgess SM, Hale BC. 2010. The costs of obesity in the workplace. *Journal of Occupational and Environmental Medicine* 2010 Oct; 52(10): 971–976. doi: 10.1097/JOM.0b013e3181f274d2.

Finkelstein E, Fiebelkorn C, Wang G. 2005. The costs of obesity among full-time employees. *American Journal of Health Promotion* 20(1): 45–51, Sep–Oct.

Fleming P, Godwin M. 2008. Lifestyle interventions in primary care: Systematic review of randomized controlled trials. *Canadian Family Physician Medicine* 54(12): 1706–1713.

Fogel RW. 1994. Economic growth, population theory, and physiology: The bearing of long-term processes on the making of economic policy. *American Economic Review* 84(3): 369–395.

Frederick CB, Snellman K, Putnama R. 2014. Increasing socioeconomic disparities in adolescent obesity. *Proceedings of the National Academy of Sciences USA*. Jan 28; 111(4): 1338–1342.

FTC — Federal Trade Commission. 2012. A Review of Food Marketing to Children and Adolescents: Follow-Up Report. Washington, DC: Federal Trade Commission.

Fulponi L. 2009. Policy Initiatives Concerning Diet, Health and Nutrition. OECD Food, Agriculture and Fisheries Working Papers No. 14. Paris: OECD Publishing.

Garcia J, Quintana-Domeque C. 2007. Obesity, Employment and Wages in Europe. In: Bolin K. Cawley J. (eds.). Advances in Health Economics and Health Services Research. The Economics of Obesity, Vol. 17 Elsevier, Amsterdam, 187–217.

Garcia Villar J, Quintana-Domeque C. 2009. Income and body mass index in Europe. *Economics Human Biology* 7(1): 73–83.

Garrett S, Elley CR, Rose SB, O'Dea D, Lawton BA, Dowell AC. 2011. Are physical activity interventions in primary care and the community cost-effective? A systematic review of the evidence, *British Journal of General Practice* 61(584): e125–e133.

Gates, DM. *et al.* 2008. Obesity and presenteeism: The impact of body mass index on workplace productivity. *Journal of Occupational and Environmental Medicine* 50(1): 39–45.

Gidlow C, Johnston LH, Crone D, Ellis N, James D. 2006. A systematic review of the relationship between socioeconomic position and physical activity. *Health Education Journal* 65: 338–367.

Glaeser E. 2006. Paternalism and Psychology. *University of Chicago Law Review* 73: 133–156.

Goetzel RZ. *et al.* 2010. A multi-worksite analysis of the relationships among body mass index, medical utilization, and worker productivity. *Journal of Occupational & Environmental Medicine* January 2010 52(1S): S52–S58.

Goryakin Y, Suhrcke M. 2014. Economic development, urbanisation, technological change and overweight: What do we learn from 244 demographic and health surveys? *Economics Human Biology* 14: 109–127.

Gregg EW, Guralnik JM. 2007. Is disability obesity's price of longevity? *The Journal of the American Medical Association* 298(17): 2066–2067.

Greve J. 2008. Obesity and labor market outcomes in Denmark. *Economics and Human Biology* 6: 350–362.

Grunert KG, Wills JM. 2007. A review of European research on consumer response to nutrition information on food labels. *Journal of Public Health* 15(5): 385–399.

Guh DP, *et al.* 2009. The incidence of co-morbidities related to obesity and overweight: A systematic review and meta-analysis. *BMC Public Health* 9: 88.

Ha DA, Chisholm D. 2011. Cost-effectiveness analysis of interventions to prevent cardiovascular disease in Vietnam. *Health Policy Plan* 26(3): 210–222.

Han E, Norton EC, Powell LM. 2011. Direct and indirect effects of body weight on adult wages. *Economics and Human Biology* 9: 381–392.

Han E, Norton EC, Stearns SC. 2009. Weight and wages: Fat versus lean paychecks. *Health Economics* 18: 535–548.

Härkönen J, Räsänen P, Näsi M. 2011. Obesity, Unemployment, and Earnings. *Nordic Journal of Working Life Studies* 1(2): 23–38.

Hawkes C. 2010. Government and voluntary policies on nutrition labelling: A global overview. In Albert J. (ed.). *Innovations in Food Labelling*. Woodhead Food Series No. 184. Cambridge: Woodhead Publishing Limited.

Hawkes C, Lobstein T. 2011. Regulating the commercial promotion of food to children: A survey of actions worldwide. *International Journal of Pediatric Obesity* 6(2): 83–94.

Hayes AJ, Philip M Clarke, Tom WC Lung. 2011. Change in bias in self-reported body mass index in Australia between 1995 and 2008 and the evaluation of correction equations. *Population Health Metrics* 9: 53.

Howard JT, Potter LB. 2012. An assessment of the relationships between overweight, obesity, related chronic health conditions and worker absenteeism. *Obesity Research & Clinical Practice* http://dx.doi.org/10.1016/j.orcp.2012.09.002.

IFBA. 2009. Compliance Monitoring of Global Advertising for Television, Print, and Internet for the International Food & Beverage Alliance. Brussels: IBFA. Available at https://www.ifballiance.org/sites/default/files/IFBA%20Compliance%20Monitoring%20Report%2010%20Nov09.pdf.

Jacobson MF, Brownell, KD. 2000. Small taxes on soft drinks and snack foods to promote health. *American Journal of Public Health* 90(6): 854–857.

Jensen JD, Smed S. 2007. Cost-effective design of economic instruments in nutrition policy. *International Journal of Behavioral Nutrition and Physical Activity* 4(10). Available at http://www.ijbnpa.org/content/pdf/1479–5868-4-10.pdf [Accessed September 2014].

Johansson F, *et al.* 2009. Obesity and labour market success in Finland: The difference between having an high BMI and being fat. *Economics Human Biology* 7(1): 36–45.

Johar M, Katayama H. 2012. Quantile regression analysis of body mass and wages. *Health Economics* 21: 597–611.

Kahn EB, Ramsey LT, Brownson RC, *et al.* 2002. The effectiveness of interventions to increase physical activity: A systematic review. *American Journal of Preventive Medicine* 22(4 Suppl.): 73–107.

Kim S, Lee Y, Yoon J, Chung SJ, Lee S. K, Kim H. 2013. Restriction of television food advertising in South Korea: Impact on advertising of food companies. *Health Promotion International* 28(1): 17–25.

Kitahara CM, *et al.* 2014. Association between class III obesity (BMI of 40–59 kg/m^2) and mortality: A pooled analysis of 20 prospective studies. *PLoS Med* 11(7): e1001673.

King L, Hebden L, Grunseit A, Kelly B, Chapman, K, Venugopal, K. 2011. Industry self regulation of television food advertising: Responsible or responsive? *International Journal of Pediatric Obesity* 6(2): 390–398.

Klarenbach S, Padwal R, Chuck A, Jacobs P. 2006. Population-based analysis of obesity and labour force participation. *Obesity* 14: 920–927.

Komlos J. 1998. Shrinking in a growing economy? The mystery of physical stature during the industrial revolution. *Journal of Economic History* 58(3): 779–802.

Konnopka A, Bodemann M, Konig HH. 2011. Health burden and costs of obesity and overweight in Germany. *The European Journal of Health Economics* 12: 345–352.

Kortt M, Leigh A. 2010. Does size matter in Australia? *Economic Record* 86(272): 71–83.

Kropfhäußer F, Sunder M. 2013. A weighty issue revisited: the dynamic effect of body weight on earnings and satisfaction in Germany. Beiträge zur Jahrestagung des Vereins für Socialpolitik 2013: Wettbewerbspolitik und Regulierung in einer globalen Wirtschaftsordnung — Session: SOEP Analysis, No. E11-V2.

Lakdawalla DN, Goldman DP, Shang B. 2005. The health and cost consequences of obesity among the future elderly. *Health Affairs* 24(Suppl. 2): w5r30-41.

Lakdawalla D, Philipson T. 2002. "The Growth of Obesity and Technological Change: A Theoretical and Empirical Examination. *NBER Working Paper* 8946, http://www.nber.org/papers/w8946.

Landmark Europe. 2010. EU Pledge Monitoring Report 2010. Brussels: Landmark Europe. Available at http://www.eu-pledge.eu/.

Leavy JE, Bull FC, Rosenberg M, Bauman A. 2011. Physical activity mass media campaigns and their evaluation: A systematic review of the literature 2003–2010. *Health Education Research* 26(6): 1060–1085.

Lee M, Orenstein M, Richardson M. 2008. Systematic review of active commuting to school and children's physical activity and weight. *Journal of Physical Activity and Health* 5(6): 930–949.

Leslie E, Cerin E, Kremer P. 2010. Perceived neighborhood environment and park use as mediators of the effect of area socio-economic status on walking behaviors. *Journal of Physical Activity & Health* 7(6): 802–810.

Lewis CE, McTigue KM, Burke LE, Poirier P, Eckel RH, Howard BV, Allison DB, Kumanyika S, Pi-Sunyer FX. 2009. Mortality, Health Outcomes, and Body Mass Index in the Overweight Range. *Circulation* 119: 3263–3271, 30 June.

Lewis C, Ubido J, Holford R, Scott-Samuel A. 2010. Prevention Programmes Cost-Effectiveness Review: Physical Activity. Cost Effectiveness Review Series, Number 1. Liverpool: Liverpool Public Health Observatory.

Lindeboom M, Lundborg P, van der Klaauw B. 2010. Assessing the impact of obesity on labor market outcomes. *Economics and Human Biology* 8: 309–319.

Lipscomb J, Weinstein MC, Torrance GW. 1996. "Time Preference", Chapter 7. In Gold MR, Siegel JE, Russell LB and Weinstein MC (eds.). *Cost Effectiveness in Health and Medicine*. Oxford University Press, New York.

Lu Y, Goldman D. 2010. The effects of relative food prices on obesity — evidence from China: 1991–2006. *NBER Working Paper Series*, Vol. w15720.

Lundborg P, Nystedt P, Rooth D. 2010. No Country for Fat Men? Obesity, Earnings, Skills, and Health among 450,000 Swedish Men. *IZA Discussion Paper* No. 4775, available at www.ed.lu.se/papers/iza_lundborg.pdf.

Magnus A, Haby MM, Carter R, Swinburn B. 2009. The cost-effectiveness of removing television advertising of high-fat and/or high-sugar food and beverages to Australian children. *International Journal of Obesity* (Lond), 33(10):1094–1102.

Maio, GR, *et al.* 2007. Tackling Obesities: Future Choices — Lifestyle Change — Evidence Review, Foresight, Department of Innovation Universities and Skills, London.

Malnick SD, Knobler H. 2006. The medical complications of obesity. *QJM* 99(9): 565–579.

Månsson, NO, *et al.* 1996. Body mass index and disability pension in middle-aged men — non-linear relations. *International Journal of Epidemiology* 25(1): 80–85.

Marshall T. 2000. Exploring a fiscal food policy: The case of diet and ischaemic heart disease. *British Medical Journal* 320(7230): 301–305.

McGinnis JM, Gootman JA, Kraak VI. 2006. Food Marketing to Children and Youth: Threat or Opportunity? Washington, DC: National Academies Press.

Mendis S, Puska P, Norrving B. (eds.). 2011. Global Atlas on Cardiovascular Disease Prevention and Control. Geneva: World Health Organization in collaboration with the World Heart Federation and the World Stroke Organization. Available at http://www.world-heart-federation.org/fileadmin/user_upload/documents/Publications/Global_CVD_Atlas.pdf.

Moens G, *et al.* 1999. Body mass index and health among the working population, epidemiological data from Belgium. *European Journal of Public Health* 9(2): 119–123.

Monge-Rojas R, Colón-Ramos U, Jacoby E, Mozaffarian D. 2011. Voluntary reduction of trans-fatty acids in Latin America and the Caribbean: Current situation. *Revista Panamericana de Salud Publica* 29(2): 126–129.

Monteiro CA, Conde WL, Popkin BM. 2007. Income-specific trends in obesity in Brazil: 1975–2003. *American Journal of Public Health* 97: 1808–1812.

Moreau M. *et al.* 2004. Obesity, body fat distribution and incidence of sick leave in the Belgian workforce: The Belstress study. *International Jouranl of Obesity and Related Metabolic Disorders* 28(4): 574–582, April.

Morris S. 2007. The impact of obesity on employment. *Labour Economics* 14: 413–433.

Mosca I. 2013. Body mass index, waist circumference and employment: evidence from older Irish adults. *Economic and Human Biology*, http://dx.doi.org/10.1016/j.ehb.2013.05.002.

Mozaffarian D, Afshin A, Benowitz NL, *et al.* 2012. Population approaches to improve diet, physical activity, and smoking habits: A scientific statement from the American Heart Association. *Circulation* 126(12): 1514–1563.

Muenster E, *et al.* 2011. Association between overweight, obesity and self-perceived job insecurity in German employees. *BMC Public Health* 11: 162.

Murray CJ, Lauer JA, Hutubessy RC, *et al.* 2003. Effectiveness and costs of interventions to lower systolic blood pressure and cholesterol: A global and regional analysis on reduction of cardiovascular-disease risk. *The Lancet* 361(9359): 717–725.

Mytton O, Gray A, Rayner M, Rutter H. 2007. Could targeted food taxes improve health? *Journal of Epidemiology and Community Health* 61(8): 689–694.

Narbro K, Jonsson E, Larsson B, Waaler H, Wedel H, Sjöström L. 1996. Economic consequences of sick-leave and early retirement in obese Swedish women. *International Jouranl of Obesity and Related Metabolic Disorders* 20(10): 895–903.

Neovious K, *et al.* 2009. Obesity status and sick leave: A systematic review. *Obesity Reviews* 10: 17–27.

NICE. 2008. Promoting PA for Children: Review 5 – Active Transport Interventions. NICE Public Health Collaborating Centre – PA. (November 2007, Revised July 2008).

Niedhammer I, Bugel I, Bonenfant S, *et al.* 2000. Validity of self-reported weight and height in the French GAZEL cohort. *International Jouranl of Obesity and Related Metabolic Disorders* 24: 1111–1118.

Ni Mhurchu, C, Gorton, D. 2007. Nutrition labels and claims in New Zealand and Australia: A review of use and understanding. *Australian and New Zealand Journal of Public Health* 31(2): 105–112.

OECD. 2014. OECD Obesity Update 2014. Available online at http://www.oecd.org/els/health-systems/Obesity-Update-2014.pdf.

Ofcom. 2010. HFSS Advertising Restrictions: Final Review. London: Ofcom.

Philipson TJ, Posner RA. 2008. Is the obesity epidemic a public health problem? A review of Zoltan J. Acs and Alan Lyles's obesity, business and public policy. *Journal of Economic Literature* 46(4): 974–982.

Popkin BM, Kim S, Rusev ER, Du S, Zizza C. 2006. Measuring the full economic costs of diet, physical activity and obesity-related chronic diseases. *Obesity Reviews* 7: 271–293.

Powell LM, Chriqui JF, Khan T, Wada R, Chaloupka FJ. 2013. Assessing the potential effectiveness of food and beverage taxes and subsidies for improving public health: A systematic review of prices, demand and body weight outcomes. *Obesity Reviews* 14: 110–128.

Proper KI, Hildebrandt VH, Van der Beek AJ, Twisk JWR, Van Mechelen W. 2003. Effect of individual counseling on physical activity fitness and health: A randomized controlled trial in a workplace setting. *American Journal of Preventive Medicine* 24(3): 218–226.

Puoane T, *et al.* 2002. Obesity in South Africa: the South African demographic and health survey. *Obesity Re*views 10: 1038–1048.

Prospective Studies Collaboration. 2009. Body-mass index and cause-specific mortality in 900 000 adults: Collaborative analyses of 57 prospective studies. *The Lancet* 373(9669): 1083–1096.

Reas DL, Nygård JF, Svensson E, Sørensen T, Sandanger I. 2007. Changes in body mass index by age, gender, and socio-economic status among a Cohort of Norwegian men and women (1990–2001). *BMC Public Health* 7: 269.

Renna F, Thakur N. 2010. Direct and indirect effects of obesity on U.S. labor market outcomes of older working age adults. *Social Science & Medicine* 71: 405–413.

Ricci JA, Chee E. 2005. Lost productive time associated with excess weight in the U.S. workforce. *Journal of Occupational and Environmental Medicine* 47(12): 1227–1234.

Rissanen A, *et al.* 1990. Risk of disability and mortality due to overweight in a finnish population. *British Medical Journal* 301(6756): 835–837.

Roehling MV. 1999. Weight-based discrimination in employment: Psychological and legal aspects. *Personnel Psychology* 52: 969–1017.

Rooth DO. 2007. Evidence of Unequal Treatment in Hiring against Obese Applicants: A Field Experiment. *IZA Discussion Paper* No. 2775, Bonn, available at ftp://repec.iza.org/RePEc/Discussionpaper/dp2775.pdf.

Roskam AJ, Kunst AE, Van Oyen H, Demarest S, Klumbiene J, Regidor E, Helmert U, Jusot F, Dzurova D, Mackenbach JP. 2010. Comparative appraisal of educational inequalities in overweight and obesity among adults in 19 European countries. *International Journal of Epidemiology* 39(2): 392–404.

Roux L, Donaldson C. 2004. "Economics and obesity: costing the problem or evaluating solutions? *Obesity Re*views 12(2): 173–179.

Rubinstein A, Colantonio L, Bardach A. *et al.* 2010. Estimation of the burden of cardiovascular disease attributable to modifiable risk factors and cost-effectiveness analysis of preventative interventions to reduce this burden in Argentina. *BMC Public Health* 10: 627.

Rudd Center for Food Policy and Obesity. 2013. Pledges on food marketing to children worldwide. Online resource available at http://www.yaleruddcenter.org/marketing-pledges/.

Sabia JJ, Rees DI. 2012. Body weight and wages: Evidence from add health. *Economics and Human Biology* 10: 14–19.

Sacks G, Veerman JL, Moodie M, Swinburn B. 2011. 'Traffic-light' nutrition labelling and 'junk-food' tax: A modelled comparison of cost-effectiveness for obesity prevention. *International Journal of Obesity* (*London*) 35(7).

Sanz de Galdeano A. 2007. An Economic Analysis of Obesity in Europe: Health, Medical Care and Absenteeism Costs. *Working Paper* No. 2007-38, FEDEA, Fundacíon de Estudios de Economía Aplicada, Madrid, available at www.fedea.es/pub/Papers/2008/dt2007-38.pdf.

Sarlio-Lähteenkorva S, Silventoinen K, Lahelma E. 2004. Relative Weight and Income at Different Levels of Socioeconomic Status. *American Journal of Public Health* 94(3): 468–472, March.

Sassi F, Belloni A, Capobianco C. 2013. The Role of Fiscal Policies in Health Promotion. *OECD Health Working Papers*, No. 66, OECD Publishing. http://dx.doi.org/10.1787/5k3twr94kvzx-en.

Sassi F, Devaux M, Cecchini M, Rusticelli E. 2009a. The Obesity Epidemic: Analysis of Past and Projected Future Trends in Selected OECD Countries. *OECD Health Working Papers* No. 45, OECD Publishing.

Sassi F, Cecchini M, Lauer J, Chisholm D. 2009b. Improving Lifestyle, Tackling Obesity: The Health And Economic Impact of Prevention Strategies. *OECD Health Working Paper* 48. Paris: OECD Publishing.

Sassi F. 2010. Obesity and the Economics of Prevention: Fit Not Fat. Paris, OECD Publishing and Edward Elgar, 2010.

Selmer RM, Kristiansen IS, Haglerod A. *et al.* 2000. Cost and health consequences of reducing the population intake of salt. *Journal of Epidemiology and Community Health* 54(9): 697–702.

Shields M, Sarah Connor Gorber, Ian Janssen, Mark S Tremblay. 2011. Bias in Self-Reported Estimates of Adult Obesity in Canadian Health Surveys: An Update on Correction Equations for Adults. Statistics Canada, Catalogue no. 82-003-XPE, *Health Reports*, 22(3).

Shiely F, Hayes K, Perry IJ, Kelleher CC. 2013. Height and weight bias: The influence of time. *Plos One* 8(1): e54386. doi:10.1371/journal.pone.0054386.

Silventoinen K, Rokholm B, Kaprio J, Sørensen TI. 2010. The genetic and environmental influences on childhood obesity: A systematic review of twin and adoption studies. *International Journal of Obesity* (*London*) 34(1): 29–40.

Smith-Spangler CM, Juusola JL, Enns EA, Owens DK, Garber AM. 2010. Population strategies to decrease sodium intake and the burden of cardiovascular disease: A cost-effectiveness analysis. *Annals of Internal Medicine* 152(8): 481–487, W170–3.

Steckel RH. 1995. Stature and the Standard of Living. *Journal of Economic Literature* XXXIII(4): 1903–1940.

Stevens J, Cai J, Pamuk ER, Williamson DF, Thun MJ, Wood JL. 1998. The Effect of Age on the association between body mass index and mortality. *New England Journal Medicine* 338: 1–7.

Strand B.H, Tverdal A. 2006. Trends in educational inequalities in cardiovascular risk factors: a longitudinal study among 48000 middle-aged norwegian men and women. *European Journal of Epidemiology* 21(10): 731–739.

Strandberg TE, Strandberg AY, Salomaa VV, Pitkälä KH, Tilvis RS, Sirola J, Miettinen TA. 2009. Explaining the obesity paradox: Cardiovascular risk, weight change, and mortality during long-term follow-up in men. *European Heart Journal* 30(14): 1720–1727.

te Velde SJ, Lennert Veerman J, Tak NI, Bosmans JE, Klepp KI, Brug J. 2011. Modeling the long term health outcomes and cost-effectiveness of two interventions promoting fruit and vegetable intake among schoolchildren. *Economics and Human Biology* 9(1): 14–22.

Thompson D, Edelsberg J, Colditz GA, Bird AP, Oster G. 1999. Lifetime health and economic consequences of obesity. *Archives of Internal Medicine* 159: 2177–2183.

Thow AM. 2012. Fiscal Policy Levers to Improve Diets and Prevent Obesity. AHHA Health Policy Research Institute, Evidence Brief No. 2. Available at http://ahha.asn.au/system/files/docs/publications/20120321_deeble_institute_evidence_brief_fiscal_policy_measures_for_obesity.pdf.

Thow AM, Jan S, Leeder S, Swinburn B. 2010. The effect of fiscal policy on diet, obesity and chronic disease: A systematic review. *Bulletin of the World Health Organization* 88(8): 609–614.

Trogdon, *et al.* 2008. Indirect costs of obesity: a review of the current literature. *Obesity Reviews* 9(5): 489–500.

Tsai AG, Williamson DF, Glick HA. 2011. Direct medical cost of overweight and obesity in the USA: A quantitative systematic review. *Obesity Reviews* 12(1): 50–61.

Tunceli K, Li K, Williams LK. 2006. Long-term Effects of Obesity on Employment and Work Limitations Among U.S. Adults, 1986 to 1999. *Obesity* (Silver Spring) 14(9): 1637–1646.

Tymms S. 2012. Responsible advertising to children: An independent review of the Australian food and beverage industry self-regulatory codes. Available at http://www.afgc.org.au/media-releases1306-industry-surpassing-advertising-to-children-self-regulatory-initiatives.html.

Unnevehr LJ, Jagmanaite E. 2008. Getting rid of trans fats in the US diet: Policies, incentives and progress. *Food Policy* 33(6): 497–503.

UK Department of Health. 2008. Changes in Food and Drink Advertising and Promotion to Children: A Report Outlining the Changes in the Nature and Balance of Food and Drink Advertising and Promotion to Children, from January 2003 to December 2007. London: Department of Health.

van Baal, PHM, Polder JJ, de Wit GA. Hoogenveen RT, Feenstra TL, *et al.* 2008. Lifetime medical costs of obesity: Prevention no cure for increasing health expenditure. *Plos Med* 5(2): e29.

Van Cauwenberghe E, Maes L, Spittaels H. *et al.* 2010. Effectiveness of school-based interventions in Europe to promote healthy nutrition in children and adolescents: Systematic review of published and 'grey' literature. *British Journal of Nutrition* 103(6): 781–797.

Veerman JL, Van Beeck EF, Barendregt JJ, Mackenbach, JP. 2009. By how much would limiting TV food advertising reduce childhood obesity? *European Journal of Public Health* 19(4): 365–369.

Vos T, Carter R, Barendregt J. *et al.* 2010. Assessing Cost-Effectiveness in Prevention (ACE–prevention). Brisbane: University of Queensland.

Vyth EL, Steenhuis IH, Brandt HE, Roodenburg AJ, Brug J, Seidell JC. 2012. Methodological quality of front-of-pack labeling studies: A review plus identification of research challenges. *Nutrition Reviews* 70(12): 709–720.

Wall J, Mhurchu CN, Blakely T, Rodgers A, Wilton J. 2006. Effectiveness of monetary incentives in modifying dietary behavior: A review of randomized, controlled trials. *Nutrition Reviews* 64(12): 518–531.

Wang Y, Chen HJ, Shaikh S, Mathur P. 2009. Is obesity becoming a public health problem in India? Examine the shift from under to overnutrition problems over time. *Obesity Re*views 10: 456–474.

Wang G, Labarthe D. 2011. The cost-effectiveness of interventions designed to reduce sodium intake. *Journal of Hypertension* 29(9): 1693–1699.

Wang YC, McPherson K, Marsh T, Gortmaker SL, Brown M. 2011. Health and economic burden of the projected obesity trends in the USA and the UK. *Lancet* 378(9793): 815–825.

Webster JL, Dunford EK, Hawkes C, Neal BC. 2011. Salt reduction initiatives around the world. *Journal of Hypertension* 29(6): 1043–1050.

WHO Expert Consultation. 2004. Appropriate body-mass index for Asian populations and its implications for policy and intervention strategies. *The Lancet* 363: 157–163.

WHO. 2011a. *Global Status Report* on Noncommunicable Diseases 2010. World Health Organization 2011, Geneva.

WHO. 2011b. Prevention and Control of NCDs: Priorities for Investment. Geneva: World Health Organization.

Willett WC, Koplan JP, Nugent R, Dusenbury C, Puska P, Gaziano TA. 2006. Prevention of chronic disease by means of diet and lifestyle changes, in Jamison DT, Breman JG, Measham AR *et al.* (eds.). Disease Control Priorities in Developing Countries. Washington, DC: World Bank, pp. 833–850.

Williams NH, Hendry M, France B, Lewis R, Wilkinson C. 2007. Effectiveness of exercise-referral schemes to promote physical activity in adults: Systematic review. *The British Journal of General Practice* 57(545): 979–986.

Zubrick SR, Wood L, Villanueve K, Wood G, Giles-Corti B, Christian H. 2010. Nothing to fear but fear itself: parental fear as a determinant of child physical activity and independent mobility, Victorian Health Promotion Foundation (VicHealth), Melbourne.

The Economics of Women's Health in Low- and Middle-Income Countries: A Life Cycle Approach

Marcella Alsan

Department of Medicine, Stanford University. Division of Infectious Disease, Palo Alto Veteran's Administration HealthCare System, National Bureau of Economic Research (NBER-Cambridge), Center for Effective Global Action (CEGA-Berkeley)

Afsan Bhadelia

Department of Global Health and Population, Harvard School of Public Health

Patricia Foo

Department of Economics and School of Medicine, Stanford University

Corinna Haberland

Department of Health Research & Policy, Stanford University School of Medicine

Felicia Knaul

Miami Institute of the Americas and Miller School of Medicine, University of Miami

This chapter highlights evidence that links women's health challenges in LMICs to economics at every stage of life. It advances the notion that discrimination against women persists for sociocultural and economic reasons and is embodied in ill health and disability across the life span.

Beginning in infancy and early childhood, girls face a variety of disadvantages that profoundly affect their health and well-being. These barriers — which include poor access to health care, nutrition and education — continue to affect women, their health, and their economic viability across the life cycle. In adolescence girls face risks associated with gender-based violence and sexually transmitted diseases, while early marriage and early pregnancy contribute to their exit from schooling. Adulthood for women is then marked by a myriad of interrelated issues — including reproductive health concerns, chronic disease, obesity, injury, intimate partner violence (IPV) and mental health problems — which encompass the long-term impact of developmental adversities. Finally, in old age, women's burdens of disease and disability reflect the health inequities faced throughout life and often coincide with a lack of financial security, neglect and abuse. Effectively addressing these challenges requires a comprehensive approach, including efforts to target gender-based inequities, educational campaigns and diagonal health systems strategies.

Keywords: Gender Based Violence; Sexually Transmitted Diseases; Intimate Partner Violence; Sex-Selection; Under-Five Mortality; Health Investments; Child Maltreatment; Child Labor; Street Children; Female Genital Cutting; Female Genital Mutilation; Adolescence; Menstruation; Education; Fertility; Child Marriage; Cervical Cancer; Cash Transfer; Progresa; Nash Cooperative Bargaining.

Introduction

Women in low- and middle-income countries (LMICs) face a wide array of challenges to their emotional and physical health and well-being. Yet, the majority of literature to date on women's health focuses on their reproductive health and, in particular, on curtailing their fertility.

Although reproductive assets are important, we take the view that women's evolving roles in LMICs necessitate a broader assessment of the health challenges that women face across the life cycle, both within and beyond reproduction (Bustreo *et al.*, 2013). We explore women's health over the entire life cycle using an economic lens. In so doing, we advance the notion that reproductive health and fertility cannot be logically separated from the other gender-based inequities — starting with sex-selection and underinvestment in girls' education and nutrition, up through financial insecurity for widows and neglect at the end of life.

This life cycle approach is clearly demarcated in Figure 1, in which we outline in the first column the various life stages and in the first row activities performed. The scheme identifies activities that are appropriate and inappropriate for a given age. For instance, although as a woman ages she should move from care-giving to care-receiving, we frequently observe and provide evidence for the contrary in LMICs.

Throughout the chapter, we highlight evidence that links women's health challenges to economics at every stage of life. We should emphasize that there are broad trends in female labor force participation, political representation and culturally-entrenched gender norms, both inside and outside the field of health care, that are not within the purview of this Handbook chapter. Although we focus on economics, it is important to recognize other approaches, such as a

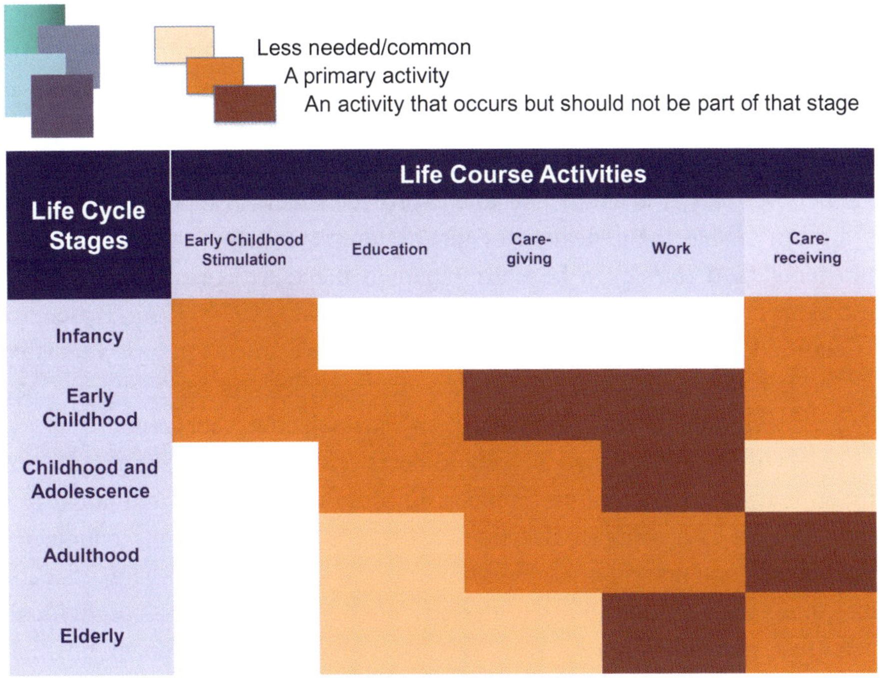

Figure 1. Activities at each stage of the life cycle

rights-based approach to health (UNDHR, 1948; 2014) or the 'women and health' approach.[1] The added value of including the economic lens over the life course is to demonstrate the interactions between women, health, and the labor market over each stage of their life.

The argument we put forward herein is that a significant amount of persistent gender-based health inequities can be understood using basic principles of microeconomic theory. Two models, the unitary model of the household and the Nash cooperative bargaining model, provide key concepts for how economic incentives can give rise to these inequities (Becker, 1974; 1991; Rosenzweig and Schultz, 1982).

In the economic framework, men and women make decisions about their own health inputs or those of their children based on *their perception* of the marginal return to that input, where returns may be measured in terms of the labor market

[1]The 'women and health' perspective is a complementary approach to understanding women's health as more than reproduction. It reflects not only women's health needs but also the role that women play in the health system, whether formally as health care workers or informally as caregivers and primary health decision-makers for their families (Frenk, 2010; Frenk *et al.*, 2012; Langer *et al.*, 2012). It considers women as both targets of interventions to address health needs and as foundational pillars in the social response to these needs.

(e.g., higher wages), the marriage market (e.g., more favorable matches) or the annuities market (e.g., children may serve as a source of income for the aged).

Under the unitary model, the household is described as a single unit with pooled preferences and resources. There is a single decision maker, which may represent the head of household or head of the joint parental unit. If this decision maker believes that girls will not be able to provide financial support to them when they are old or that the education of girl children will not be rewarded by later employment (and may even be detrimental in the marriage market), they will invest more health inputs into boys than girls (Becker, 1974; 1991; Rosenzweig and Schultz, 1982). Thus, the perceived returns to investments in girls versus boys could explain observed gender differences in mortality and schooling in LMICs during early childhood and adolescence, and sex-selective abortions.

Models of Nash-bargained household decisions reflect the notion that women and men may have different preferences. In these models, each individual in the parental couple is a separate decision maker, but collectively, the couple must allocate a common pool of household resources (e.g., food, health care, education, leisure time) with the possibility of dissolution (i.e., divorce). Thus, individual or societal factors that affect a woman's relative threat point (her fallback position if she chooses not to bargain or, in this case, her utility upon dissolving the marriage), determine her relative bargaining power within the union (McElroy and Horney, 1981). For example, if a wife's potential income outside a marriage is higher, a husband is less likely to engage in domestic violence since the wife will be more likely to dissolve the union if he abuses her, given her option to obtain income outside the marriage (Aizer, 2010). These models can also explain differential investments in boys versus girls if wives differ from husbands in their preference for investing in girl children (Blundell *et al.*, 2005). For example, girls may receive less investment if women have a greater preference for investing in girls but have fewer resources to transfer and if men have a greater preference for investing in boys and greater resources to transfer.

This chapter outlines the obstacles girls and women confront every day in LMICs, at every stage of life. We begin by describing the economic forces that impact girls' health in infancy and young childhood and discuss the far-reaching effects such exposures have on their health and well-being as women. Next, we investigate adolescence; this section begins with the onset of menstruation and describes how this biological process affects a young woman's health, educational and economic outcomes in both the short- and long-term. Adulthood is marked by a myriad of interrelated issues in reproduction and beyond reproduction that encompass the long-term impact of developmental adversities. The section on elderly women discusses how their burden of disease reflects health inequities faced throughout life and often collides with their lack of financial security. Finally, the conclusion summarizes the findings and offers policy recommendations that arise from this economic framework.

Women's Health Across the Life Cycle

Infancy and early childhood

Prenatal development, infancy and early childhood are periods of important development and growth for all children. For girls, however, there is the added concern that growth in childhood may affect both their reproductive future and, therefore, the health of their future children, given the significant impact maternal health has on infant outcomes. Active and passive health choices on the part of caregivers and/or external events that impact the health of girls all have the potential to have both immediate and long-term consequences. These, in turn, will impact a girl's length and quality of life, her ability to fully function as a member of her society, and her lifelong health care needs.

- *Under-five mortality*

From a broad, global perspective, girls are no more likely to die under the age of five than boys are, and in some cases, girls may have a certain advantage (Marcoux, 2002; WHO, 2009a; 2009b; 2013a). For example, in some LMICs the under-five mortality rate is lower for girls than for boys, and in the face of equal levels of undernutrition, girls suffer from less stunting and wasting than boys. Similar to boys, the most common cause of mortality in girls under five are infections — such as pneumonia, diarrhea-causing enteric infections, measles, and malaria — which account for about 57% of deaths under age five. Perinatal and neonatal events — such as birth asphyxia and trauma, prematurity, and severe neonatal infections — account for about 30%. Noncommunicable illness and injuries account for 7% and 4%, respectively (WHO, 2009a; 2009b; 2013a). Beyond these more acute conditions, nutritional status greatly affects under-five mortality as well. While nutritional deficiencies by themselves account for a small percentage of deaths, undernutrition and its effects (stunting, severe wasting and intrauterine growth restriction) have been estimated to be the underlying cause of more than 2.1 million child deaths in 2004 (Black *et al.*, 2008; WHO, 2009a; 2009b; 2013a).

- *High-risk areas, sex-selection and economic impact on survival*

There are certain situations and geographic areas, however, in which economic and cultural realities put girls at significantly greater risk for death, disease and malnutrition than their male counterparts. Cultural biases against daughters, especially in the absence of sons, have been shown to have profound impacts on girls' well-being and survival (Arnold *et al.*, 1998; Das Gupta, 2003; Goodkind, 1996; Jha *et al.*, 2011; Sen, 1990; 2003; Zhu *et al.*, 2009).

While in most parts of the world, the ratio of boys to girls at birth is approximately 103–107 boys for every 100 girls born (equivalent to between 1.03 and 1.07:1.00), there are areas in which the ratio is significantly higher. China, for example, had a ratio of 1.17 to 1.00 from 2005 to 2010. Similarly, India's ratio during the same time period was 1.11 to 1.00 (WHO, 2014); Nobel Laureate Economist Amartya Sen highlighted these findings in 1990 (Sen, 1990). Even higher ratios have been found in some regions within these countries where parents view sons as an economic gain for the family whereas daughters might be considered a loss due to her anticipated dowry. There is little doubt that observed skewed sex ratios are the result of a combination of sex-selective abortions and (unreported) female infanticide, with recent data suggesting that the former plays a more important role (Arnold *et al.*, 1998; Das Gupta, 2003; Goodkind, 1996; Jha *et al.*, 2011; Sen, 1990; 2003; Zhu *et al.*, 2009). In addition, birth order and the sex of older siblings seem to have a significant impact on the incidence of prenatal sex selection. Families with one or more girls have been shown to have a significantly higher rate of selective abortion use in subsequent pregnancies. For example, some provinces in China had ratios of over 1.60 to 1.00 for second order births (Jha *et al.*, 2011; Zhu *et al.*, 2009).

At the macroeconomic level, a negative shock to the economy of a developing country has been shown to differentially affect the mortality of infant girls (Baird *et al.*, 2010). Similarly, when male earning potential increased in areas of China while keeping female income constant, survival rates for girls worsened (Qian, 2008). In both India and China, when economic opportunities and women's earnings potential improved, so too did survival rates for girls (Qian, 2008; Rosenzweig and Schultz, 1982).

- *Health investments and their consequences*

Globally, as mentioned above, the rates and severity of illness, undernutrition and their consequences are relatively equal between girls and boys under the age of five (Marcoux, 2002; WHO, 2009a; 2009b), though there are significant differences in some regions, with girls having worse outcomes — especially in Southeast Asia (Arnold *et al.*, 1998; Chakravarty, 2010; Marcoux, 2002; Mishra *et al.*, 2004; Oster, 2009a; 2009b; Pande, 2003). Studies investigating these differences have focused on girls' relatively lower receipt of nutrition and other health inputs within the family. These differences vary in degree based on family composition (e.g., ratio of boys to girls, number of older girl siblings).

Pande looked at data from the National Family Health Survey (NFHS) in India from 1992 to 1993 and found that in rural areas, girls born into a family with older sisters were significantly more likely than boys to suffer from severe stunting, and received few or no immunizations (Pande, 2003). Mishra *et al.* also looked at the NFHS data for 1998–1999 and found that discrimination against girls (especially those later in the birth order) was most visible in families with no living sons. Girls who were later in the birth order in their families (born fourth or later) were also less likely to be breastfed at 24 months and less likely to receive daily milk. Similarly, there was evidence for discrimination against girls in immunization coverage, and for stunting and being underweight when boys were in short supply in the family (Mishra *et al.*, 2004).

Studies investigating Indian immunization initiatives have shown that gender inequities persist in national attempts to increase immunization rates. When immunization centers open in an area, boys are more likely to receive their immunizations before girls. Girls were only able to catch up to boys' rates after the program and its services had been in the region for a longer period of time (Chakravarty, 2010; Oster, 2009a). Lack of immunizations for preventable illness puts infants and young girls at greater risk for severe illness and possible death. When coupled with undernutrition, the risks are even higher and could account for a substantial portion of childhood mortality (Oster, 2009b).

Undernutrition and its consequences are far-reaching. Poor fetal growth or stunting in the first 2 years of life has been shown to reduce adult height, lower educational attainment, and lead to lower adult income. These effects are also intergenerational, with decreased birthweight in the offspring of stunted mothers. Furthermore, short maternal stature, when combined with iron deficiency anemia (often due to a combination of poor nutrition and illness), increases the risk of maternal death during delivery — which also places the infant at greater risk both acutely (e.g., death) and/or long-term (e.g., undernutrition) (Black *et al.*, 2008; Victora *et al.*, 2008).

- *Child labor and street children*

It is estimated that there were some 168 million-child laborers (ages 5 to 17) in the world in 2012. About 85 million of these were undertaking hazardous work (work that directly endangered their health, safety and moral development). In children aged 5 to 11 years reported numbers for laborers were 73 million, with about 18.5 million engaged in hazardous work (International Labour Organization, 2013). These definitions typically exclude household chores, and so they often underestimate children's work, especially that of girls in developing countries, as they tend to perform more household chores than boys (International Labour

Organization, 2013; World Bank, 2005). For those working outside of their family home, there are also gender differences in both the type of work performed and the impact it has on the child's future. For example, girls are more likely than boys to work in domestic service, and, compared to boys, have been found to suffer long-term economic impacts when they drop out of school or split their time between school and work (Knaul *et al.*, 2011). Thus, the primary activities listed in Figure 1 for children and adolescents (such as education) are not occurring, and/or other activities are occurring that should not be part of that life cycle stage (such as work).

Childhood and adolescence are also both threatened by increasing urbanization and political instability in developing countries and the possibility of becoming street children. As described by the WHO manual "Working with Street Children," (WHO, 2000):

> *'Street children are the casualties of economic growth, war, poverty, loss of traditional values, domestic violence, physical and mental abuse. Every street child has a reason for being on the streets. While some children are lured by the promise of excitement and freedom, the majority are pushed onto the street by desperation and a realisation [sic] that they have nowhere else to go ... Street children go through the struggle of providing themselves with basic things such as food, shelter, health and clothing.'*

In the developing world, children as young as eight can be living completely on their own (WHO, 2000). Girls who are on the street might be more likely to be picked up by authorities, recruited to work as domestics or work in the sex industry. Street girls may also simply be less visible, either hiding or disguising themselves as boys (Meinhart, 2013; WHO, 2000).

- *Abuse/sexual abuse*

Child abuse or maltreatment refers to the physical and emotional mistreatment, sexual abuse, exploitation, neglect, and negligent treatment of children. It occurs in many different settings, including the home and the school, and the perpetrators of child maltreatment can be parents, other family members, caregivers, friends, acquaintances, or authority figures (WHO and ISPCAN, 2006). Gender differences in child abuse are striking. While boys are more likely to suffer physical abuse such as beatings, girls are much more likely to be subjected to sexual abuse and exploitation (Colucci and Hassan, 2014; WHO and ISPCAN, 2006). In 2002, the WHO estimated that 150 million girls and 73 million boys under 18 years experienced forced sexual intercourse or other forms of sexual violence involving physical contact (Colucci and Hassan, 2014; UNICEF, 2011; WHO and ISPCAN, 2006).

The health and social consequences of child maltreatment are vast and include major harm to the physical and mental health and development of the victims. Abuse in childhood has been shown to be associated with risk factors and risk-taking behaviors later in life, including violent victimization and the perpetration of violence, depression, smoking, obesity, high-risk sexual behaviors, unintended pregnancy, and alcohol and drug use. These, in turn, can lead to death, disease, and disability due to heart disease, sexually transmitted diseases, cancer and suicide (Pinheiro, 2006; UNICEF, 2011; WHO and ISPCAN, 2006).

Though not unique to the infant/young childhood period in girls' lives, female genital cutting (FGC) or female genital mutilation (FGM) is a form of abuse that has roots in perceived cultural and economic pressures — with FGC/FGM being seen as a "desirable" characteristic in a bride (being more chaste or "clean," more likely to be faithful, etc.) that leads to better and earlier marriages. The procedure, which is predominantly practiced in regions of Africa and the Middle East, can range from partial removal or cutting of the clitoral prepuce to, in its most extreme form, complete removal of all external genitalia and sewing closed the vagina (Chesnokova and Vaithianathan, 2010; WHO, 2011; UNICEF, 2005). The practice has been condemned as a harmful practice and a violation of human rights, with actions at international, regional and national levels, bringing about an apparent decrease in FGC/FGM. Yet in 2008, the World Health Organization estimated that between 100 and 140 million girls and women in the world had undergone such procedures, and 3 million girls were estimated to be at risk of undergoing the procedures every year (WHO, 2006; 2008; 2011a).

Beyond the immediate health impacts and risks — pain, bleeding, infection, shock, and death — FGC/FGM often results in adverse obstetric outcomes. A WHO study from 2001 to 2003 followed over 28,000 women who presented for deliveries in obstetric centers in Africa and found that women with FGC/FGM were at significantly greater risk for caesarean section, postpartum hemorrhage, infant death and low birth weight infants. These risks increased with more extensive FGM (WHO, 2006), and resulted in increased costs for their care (WHO, 2011a).

The health of a woman is inherently linked to the health of the girl she was. Despite some plausible biological advantages in terms of survival and health, girls also face social, cultural and gender-based disadvantages that place their health at risk as children and continue into adolescence and adulthood (WHO, 2009a). As described next, these barriers — which include poor access to health care — continue to affect women, their health, and their economic viability across the life cycle.

Adolescence

Adolescence is a period of marked physiological changes for young women. These changes are often accompanied by transitions in their expected role in society. The most notable physiological change that marks the passage of girls into adolescence is menarche, or the first menstrual cycle. Menstruation takes on different meanings across cultures, but almost universally carries significant cultural weight. Many cultures associate menstruation with uncleanliness, shame or incapacity (Buckley and Gottlieb, 1988; Stubbs, 2008; Szarewski *et al.*, 2012). In LMICs, girls report a fear that they will become the subject of teasing or humiliation if others become aware that they are menstruating (Mason *et al.*, 2013). Some cultures interpret menarche as a signal of physical readiness for sexual activity and early marriage (Grant *et al.*, 2013). Studies have shown that, at home, some girls hide evidence of menarche for fear of being punished for early sexual activity (McMahon *et al.*, 2011; Sommer and Ackatia-Armah, 2012). This period of rapid biologic, social and economic change is influential for women well into adulthood. Adolescents also play a large role in the economic future of LMICs due to their sizable population; in 2010, they were estimated to constitute over a quarter of the population in LMICs on average (Sawyer *et al.*, 2012).

- *Menstruation and education*

After menarche, young women in LMICs often stop attending school at the critical transition from primary to secondary education and begin to carve out economic paths that diverge from those of men in their communities. Although education should be a primary activity during adolescence (see Figure 1), they may begin to divert their time toward caregiving or work instead (Alsan, 2015).

There are multiple barriers that adolescent girls face in pursuing education. In addition to the social stigma of menstruation, adolescent girls in many LMICs cannot obtain adequate sanitary products or do not have access to adequate water or public sanitation facilities to maintain good menstrual hygiene (Maimaiti and Siebert, 2009; Mason *et al.*, 2013). Furthermore, at school, teachers are often male, making it difficult for girls to ask for support and mentoring around menarche in the school environment (McMahon *et al.*, 2011).

Given these potential barriers, it is not surprising that menarche and menstruation are associated with decreased rates of schooling for girls. However, estimating the true causal effect of menstruation on girls' educational attainment is difficult, since several factors that enter into the decision to pursue education (e.g., early marriage and pregnancy) also occur around the age of menarche. Although the World Bank has estimated that girls may miss a many as 10 to 20% of her school days due to menstruation (World Bank, 2005), more recent studies that have attempted to determine rates of absenteeism due to menstruation have found mixed results on whether there is a causal link between menstruation and girls' educational attainment.

These recent studies focus on isolating the effects of specific factors (e.g., factors in the environment, costs of menstrual supplies, puberty education) on absenteeism and their impact on girls' education. Grant *et al.* (2013) found that, in Malawi, menstruation accounted only for a small proportion of all female absenteeism and did not create a gender gap in absenteeism. Similarly, a randomized controlled trial in Nepal found that schoolgirls who received and were instructed on the use of menstrual cups (reusable, silicone devices inserted during menstruation) were not more likely to attend school during their periods, and that the overall rates of absenteeism due to menses were small, roughly 0.6 school days per year. The Nepal study also found no significant effects on test scores, self-reported measures of self-esteem or gynecological health (Oster and Thornton, 2011). In contrast, a pilot randomized controlled trial in Ghana found that, after 5 months of puberty education, schoolgirls between the ages of 12 and 18 had a statistically significant 9% increase in their school attendance compared to the control group. Similar to the findings from the Nepal study, receipt of free sanitary pads in addition to puberty education did not affect school attendance compared to puberty education alone (Montgomery *et al.*, 2012).

The data on the impact of school facilities (i.e., the ability of girls to privately deal with menses-related issues) are also mixed. Grant *et al.* (2013) found no evidence for school-level variance in menstruation-related absenteeism, suggesting that absenteeism due to menstruation was not sensitive to school environments. Rather, co-residence with a grandmother and spending time on schoolwork at home were associated with lower odds of absence during the last menstrual period. However, one study from India found that among adolescent girls (grades 6–8), construction of sex-specific latrines in schools increased girls' enrollment by 10%, while construction of unisex latrines increased girls' enrollment by only 2% (Adukia, 2014). The increase in school enrollment for adolescent boys was similar across unisex or sex-specific latrines.

The mixed results from the provision of menstrual supplies combined with the results on the effect of menstrual education and school environment are consistent with the hypothesis that girls' overall, everyday concerns about health, puberty, and privacy, as well as support at home, are more important than specific sanitary supplies in determining school attendance. As highlighted in a recent systematic review (Sumpter and Torondel, 2013), further high-quality rigorous studies in this area are needed to better understand how combinations of the above interventions might positively impact young women's education and economic potential.

- *Fertility, sexual behavior, and marriage*

The onset of menstruation is a marker of a young woman's reproductive potential. This sets the stage for some of the largest health challenges facing adolescent girls in LMICs — sexually transmitted infections (STIs), early fertility, and child marriage. LMICs have the highest rates of treatable STIs (e.g., syphilis, gonorrhea, chlamydia) and HIV across the globe, with a higher incidence of HIV among young females in regions where HIV is endemic (Patton and Sawyer, 2013). Worldwide, rates of early pregnancy are highest in LMICs (Lloyd *et al.*, 2014). As a consequence, complications of pregnancy and childbirth are the leading cause of death in women aged 15–19 (Patton *et al.*, 2009). Child marriage (defined as marriage before the age of 18) continues to occur at rates as high as 45% for girls in some regions, despite an estimated worldwide 11 percentage point decline over the past 30 years (Nguyen and Wodon, 2012).

These factors have significant effects on women's long-term health and economic outcomes in LMICs. For example, cervical cancer, a disease of adulthood, is caused by STI. Cervical cancer causes more than 270,000 deaths annually worldwide, of which more than 85% occur in low-income countries (Forman *et al.*, 2012; WHO, 2013b). Adolescence is the period in which both prevention against the causative organism, the human papillomavirus (HPV), is most effective. However, vaccination programs are infrequent in LMICs. In 2012, of the 51 countries implementing national HPV vaccination programs, only 6 were LMICs (Cervical Cancer Action, 2012).

Both early marriage and early pregnancy contribute to girls' exit from schooling in adolescence (UNESCO, 2012). Estimating the casual effect of marriage or pregnancy on schooling decisions is difficult due to the fact that education and marriage are decisions that are often made jointly (Duflo, 2012; Jensen, 2012). For example, girls less interested in pursuing education (due to ability, family pressure, etc.) may marry earlier and yet might have dropped out of school even in the absence of marriage. On the other hand, girls who expect a higher return to education (e.g., higher wages) may decide to delay marriage and stay in school. Both of these examples would lead to a negative correlation between marriage or pregnancy and education, but both would be due to an unobserved factor, expected return to education. The best evidence to date of the effect of early marriage on schooling comes from a study by Field and Ambrus (2008) in Bangladesh that uses an instrumental variable strategy. The authors use variation in the timing of menarche to instrument for the age at first marriage. Their empirical strategy is based on the custom that girls in Bangladesh are typically not allowed to marry before reaching puberty. They find that each additional year of delay in the age of marriage increases schooling by 0.22 years and increases the likelihood of literacy of 5.6 percentage points.

• *Effect of increasing education*

As noted previously in discussing the impact of early marriage and pregnancy on education, the relationship between these variables is bidirectional — that is, evidence shows that staying in school protects adolescent girls against early marriage, teen pregnancy and other reproductive and sexual harms including HIV infection (Alsan and Cutler, 2013; Dupas, 2011; Ozier, 2011). Education is also predicted to improve girls' future labor market outcomes, although no study to date has directly documented education's effect on these longitudinal outcomes among women in LMICs.

Several randomized controlled trials have looked at the effect of increasing girls' schooling on the rates of fertility or STIs (Baird *et al.*, 2011; 2012; Duflo, 2012; Hallfors *et al.*, 2011). These studies typically use some intervention to target increased school enrollment or attendance as their primary outcome, and additionally look at the intervention's effect on fertility, early marriage, sexual activity and STI rates.

Several trials use financial incentives, known as cash transfers, to increase girls' educational attainment (for more on incentives and cash transfers, see also Volume 2, Chapter 10 of this Handbook, *Incentivizing Health Care Utilization and Health Outcomes*) (Baird *et al.*, 2011; 2012; Schultz, 2004). Collectively, these studies have shown that cash transfers increase schooling on both the intensive (attendance) and extensive (enrollment) margins as well as reduce rates of early marriage, early pregnancy, sexual activity and STIs.

Among the most influential cash transfer programs was Mexico's PROGRESA program, which showed that a conditional cash transfer (CCT), which paid 50–75% of a household's private economic cost of schooling (conditional on enrollment) increased girls' secondary school enrollment by 14% (Schultz, 2004). Although this early study did not look at the intervention's effect on girls' fertility, early marriage, sexual activity or STI rates, its success led to widespread adoption of cash transfer programs across LMICs and subsequent evaluations of the impact on girls' reproductive health. In a randomized controlled trial in Malawi, Baird *et al.* (2011; 2012) studied the effect of both unconditional and conditional cash transfers. They found that both types of transfers reduced school drop-outs and rates of STIs (specifically, HIV and herpes simplex virus-2). CCTs were more than twice as efficacious at reducing school drop-out rates, but only unconditional cash transfers were efficacious at reducing teen pregnancy and early marriage rates (Baird *et al.*, 2011; 2012).

Other interventions have included provision of in-kind transfers. Hallfors *et al.* (2011) performed a randomized controlled trial of a comprehensive "school support" program for orphan girls in Zimbabwe that provided uniforms and school supplies and paid school fees. Among their sample of 329 girls, they found the intervention reduced school dropout by 82% and marriage by 63% after 2 years. Duflo *et al.* (2012) evaluated a large randomized controlled trial in Kenya in which school subsidies in the form of school uniforms were provided in the last 3 years of primary school. They found that this intervention reduced the teen pregnancy rate by 3 percentage points (from 16% to 13%) within the first 3 years, and that a significant effect on fertility persisted 7 years after the program. However, they found no effect of the education subsidy on STI rates.

- *Gender-based violence*

Adolescence is often the age at which girls become targets for gender-based violence. Measuring the incidence and prevalence of gender-based violence — of which physical IPV and sexual violence are the two most common types — presents several methodological challenges (Bott *et al.*, 2005). Surveys vary in the types of questions asked, and most surveys are only effective at measuring discrete incidences of violence rather than overall patterns of controlling behavior. Furthermore, all surveys are likely to suffer from underreporting due to shame or fear of reprisals (Ellsberg *et al.*, 2001).

Based on what evidence exists, adolescent girls report feeling powerless to resist unwanted and coerced sex in LMICs. Sexual coercion is defined as "an individual woman's lack of choice to pursue other options [to avoid sexual interactions] without severe social and physical consequence" (Heise *et al.*, 1995). Acts of sexual coercion range from verbal harassment to unwanted touch to rape. In some areas, more than one-third of girls report that their first sexual encounter was coerced (WHO, 2012). Sexual coercion may result from forced sex, pressure through money or gifts, verbal aggression or physical threats (Moore *et al.*, 2007; Wood *et al.*, 1998). Girls' sense of being powerless may be reinforced by political and cultural norms. Studies in sub-Saharan Africa have concluded that gender roles in parts of the region sexually disenfranchise girls, making them more vulnerable to sexual assault (Blanc, 2001; Kalichman *et al.*, 2005). For example, some adolescent boys believe that a girl's "no" is a "yes," shrouded by cultural expectations (Varga, 2003). Furthermore, rape is often associated with bringing shame and stigma on oneself and one's family members. These associations are reinforced by legal systems that may define sexual violence to be a private rather than criminal office, fail to pursue perpetrators of coerced sex, or prosecute the victims of sexual violence for adultery or abortion (Bott *et al.*, 2005; Chandra-Mouli *et al.*, 2013).

Sexual coercion in adolescence has immediate and downstream effects on a woman's lifelong health. It is linked to higher rates of suicide, HIV and other sexually transmitted infections, unintended pregnancy, high-risk behavior including multiple partnerships and unprotected sex and future gender-based violence (Gomez, 2011; Heise *et al.*, 1999; Kalichman and Simbayi, 2004; Koenig *et al.*, 2004; Peltzer and Pengpid, 2012; WHO, 2013b). The threat of sexual harassment and abuse can negatively affect girls' downstream health and economic prospects. Several studies in South Asia and sub-Saharan Africa have shown that parents' fears for their daughters' physical and sexual safety is a major reason for withholding girls from school (Mensch and Lloyd, 1998).

Interventions to prevent sexual abuse and coercion are, on the whole, drastically and disproportionately low in LMICs relative to the burden of violence faced by adolescent girls (Jejeebhoy and Boot, 2005). Few interventions have been tried, and even fewer have been documented, providing limited evidence for efficacious interventions. Some countries have begun to reform their law enforcement systems, with public acknowledgement of the legal system's inadequate response to sexual coercion. At the local level, some authorities have tried providing school-based counseling and referral services and found that female students are eager to use these services (Guedes *et al.*, 2002; Mgalla *et al.*, 1998). Other school-based interventions have targeted teachers, trying to change teachers' attitudes toward gender-based violence and providing tools to address gender-based violence in the school setting (Jejeebhoy and Boot, 2005). Similar interventions to change attitudes and increase knowledge have been implemented in the health care setting (Colombini *et al.*, 2008). In addition, there have been anecdotal reports that provision of sex-specific sanitation may improve women's safety from sexual violence (Bott *et al.*, 2005). However, these few interventions may have limited efficacy, stymied by widespread cultural beliefs that are difficult to change.

Adulthood

As women reach adulthood, the focus on their reproductive capacity is increased and their social value becomes further dependent on bearing offspring. In many parts of the developing world, women's social value is related particularly to bearing male offspring (Cohen, 2000; Sen, 2002; Das Gupta, 2003). The pressure on women to utilize their reproductive capacity often stems from pressure within households — mainly husbands and mother-in-laws — and is reinforced by societal norms (Bloom *et al.*, 2001; Das Gupta, 1995). Having (grand)children becomes a rite of passage into womanhood. Partially in response to its prominent societal role, as well as to promote family planning as a method to curb population growth, maternal and reproductive health has traditionally dominated the global health agenda for women, especially once women reach childbearing age. The narrow focus on contraception, in particular, risks not fully incorporating women's other health needs in adulthood.

The United Nations International Conference on Population and Development in Cairo in 1994, recognizing the interconnectedness of population and development, sought to make women's reproductive health and rights a cornerstone for action and to shift the focus from demographic targets to human development with a broader women's health agenda (UNFPA, 1994). This was a milestone event that recognized the need for a life cycle approach as well as the importance of including a focus on diseases such as cancer. Twenty years later, progress on many of the key actions outlined at the conference have yet to be achieved. Furthermore, new health issues, particularly noncommunicable diseases (NCD), are emerging as life expectancies increase in LMICs by 3.9% annually between 2010 and 2015 (UN, 2013).

Between 1990 and 2010, overall deaths from communicable, maternal, neonatal and nutritional related illnesses declined from 34.1% to 24.9%, while noncommunicable causes increased from 57.1% to 65.5% (Lozano *et al.*, 2012). Many LMICs face a double burden of disease, with NCDs growing alongside ongoing concerns of tackling communicable diseases.

- *Reproductive health*

The availability or lack of reproductive care, such as emergency contraception (EC), abortion, care during childbirth and postpartum care, plays an important role in women's reproductive health in LMICs.

EC can significantly minimize unwanted pregnancies by providing women a safeguard after unprotected intercourse or when other forms of contraception have failed. The lack of availability of EC can have an impact on a women's life if an unwanted pregnancy occurs. Efforts to improve access to and increase awareness of EC have been ongoing and slowly increasing in LMIC. In Mexico City, a study evaluating a 3-year program training health professionals and conducting a public education campaign observed that support for EC increased by 10% and client awareness increased by 19%. In many LMICs, however, health providers have limited knowledge of the existence of EC, the forms of EC available and how to correctly prescribe it (Adekunle *et al.*, 2000; Steiner *et al.*, 2000). For instance, a study from Ghana showed that only one-third of health providers had even heard of EC (Steiner *et al.*, 2000). Many countries only provide EC by prescription and this, along with the cost (Van Rossem and Meekers, 2000), can serve as added barriers to EC (Conard and Gold, 2004).

In relation to birth control, a study in Zambia noted that there are inefficiencies in household bargaining (Ashraf *et al.*, 2012). The authors estimated that women offered contraception in the presence of their husband were 19% less likely to accept it than if their husband was not present. The authors interpret this result as evidence that women have different preferences for birth control than men. Extensive evidence suggests that contraception can serve as a highly effective strategy to reduce maternal mortality (Ahmed *et al.*, 2012). Further, increased education is linked to women having further autonomy over their fertility, which in turn leads to improved women's health outcomes (Behrman *et al.*, 2006; Das Gupta, 2013).

When unintended pregnancies do occur, options for safe abortion are also lacking. Among LMICs, there are approximately 29 abortions per 1,000 women aged 15–44 and an estimated 56% are unsafe, as compared to high-income countries, with 17 abortions per 1,000 women with less than 0.5% being unsafe. Removing data on China from the LMIC pool results in 29 abortions per 1,000 women, with 75% of abortions in LMICs being unsafe (Sedgh *et al.*, 2012). The overall incidence across developing regions indicates that every woman will likely have 1 abortion by the age of 44 (Shah and Åhman, 2012), demonstrating an urgent need for comprehensive reproductive services (Sedgh *et al.*, 2012).

Approximately 500,000 women — mostly in developing countries — die annually during pregnancy, at childbirth, or soon thereafter (WHO, 2005). The most common method of reducing maternal deaths is through antenatal care, skilled delivery, and delivery at a medical facility (de Bernis *et al.*, 2003; Gertler *et al.*, 1993; McCaw-Binns *et al.*, 2007). However, significant progress is needed with respect to skilled delivery to meet the Millennium Development Goal (MDG) of reducing the maternal mortality ratio by 75% by 2015 (number of maternal deaths per 100,000 live births within 42 days of delivery) (Kassebaum *et al.*, 2014).

From an economic perspective, the loss of life from maternal mortality has immediate and direct costs, ranging from funeral expenses to hospitalization and emergency service charges. A study from rural China calculated these costs to amount to 37% of annual household income, four times that of what is defined as a catastrophic expense (Ye *et al.*, 2012). The long-term economic costs have been more difficult to calculate. Substantive progress has indeed been made in reducing maternal mortality over the past 20 years (Forouzanfar *et al.*, 2011; Hogan *et al.*, 2010).

- *Beyond reproduction*

As the post-2015 development agenda is drafted, broadening the definition of maternal health would give recognition to the need for a woman to be able live her life to the fullest (Colucci and Hassan, 2014; Knaul, 2013; WHO and ISPCAN, 2006). This would entail better linkage to reproductive and beyond-reproduction health care, which are intrinsically connected. For example, as mentioned previously, the majority of cervical cancer cases are related to HPV, which is acquired through sexual activity and hence relevant for reproductive health. The risk of developing breast cancer is related to age at first pregnancy, parity (number of times that a woman has given birth to a fetus with a gestational age of 24 weeks of more) and breastfeeding (Collaborative Group on Hormonal Factors in Breast Cancer, 2002). Moreover, women with gestational diabetes are at higher risk of Type 2 diabetes (Bellamy *et al.*, 2009). These associations clearly link NCD and chronic disease to reproduction.

An estimated 65% of deaths among women are caused by chronic disease, specifically NCD (WHO, 2008), and the majority of these are in LMICs (WHO, 2011b). Cardiovascular disease (CVD) is the cause of 12.8% and 10.7% of global deaths among men and women, respectively. Approximately, 4.2% of global female deaths are due to breast and cervical cancers, serving as one of seven leading causes of death among women. Overall, evidence suggests that with every 10% increase in NCD, there is a resulting 0.5% decrease in annual economic growth (WHO, 2011b). A 2% annual global reduction in chronic diseases over the next 10 years in the 23 countries which bear 80% of the global NCD burden will avoid 24 million deaths and save approximately US$8 billion.

The four major chronic diseases — CVD, cancer, diabetes and respiratory diseases — pose a challenge for both men and women in LMICs. Where death registry data were available in 2005, age-standardized death rates for men were 54% higher and for women were 86% higher than counterparts in high-income countries. Although women tend to live longer than men, in developing countries, this advantage is outweighed by gender-based discrimination, both in terms of health care utilization and quality of care, reducing not only women's life expectancy but also resulting in unhealthier lives during the years that they do survive (WHO, 2009a).

- *Chronic disease: the case of cancer*

While various chronic diseases afflict women during adulthood, we explore the case of cancer here as an example of the complexities of long-term care.

Recent literature has highlighted the differentials in cancer morbidity and mortality between the rich and poor within and across countries. For instance, mortality figures from breast cancer in LMICs are almost double that in high-income countries. Cervical cancer mortality is similarly concentrated in poorer nations — 230,000 annual deaths in LMICs as compared to 35,000 annual deaths in high income countries (IARC, 2012). This has been termed the "cancer divide" (Knaul *et al.*, 2012). The cancer divide is characterized by the greater concentration of risk factors, stigma and discrimination related to cancer, and higher incidence of and fatality from preventable cancers in LMICs. Additionally, access to opioids for pain control is often limited in poorer countries, leaving millions to suffer (Knaul *et al.*, 2012).

Breast and cervical cancer, both associated with reproductive health, illustrate the cancer transition. The cancer transition reflects the societal and economic advances in many parts of the world that have led to a decline in infection-related cancers and a rise in cancers associated with reproductive, dietary, and hormonal causes (Bray *et al.*, 2012). State-specific data from Mexico illustrate the women's cancer transition. In poorer states, cervical cancer is the main cause of cancer-related deaths among women, whereas breast cancer is the primary cause of cancer mortality among women in richer states (Knaul *et al.*, 2014).

The rise of breast and cervical cancer has notably been among younger women (Villarreal-Garza *et al.*, 2013), with LMICs having double the incidence in women under 50 years than high-income countries (Knaul *et al.*, 2011; 2012). A comparative analysis of breast cancer cases in Brazil, Colombia, Costa Rica and Ecuador found 20–41% of cases to be among women between 20 and 44 years of age, while only 12% of cases were within this age group in the United States and Canada (López-Carrillo *et al.*, 2014b). This is especially relevant for the design and implementation of women's health programs. Changing risk factors in LMICs, such as the trend toward later age of first pregnancy and lower parity, and changing dietary habits will also have implications for programming (Porter, 2008).

Due to gender bias, women face various barriers to accessing care, including cost, long distances to point of care, limited mobility, and lack of female health workers (Farmer *et al.*, 2010; Knaul *et al.*, 2012; 2008). These must be addressed for improved cancer outcomes.

- *Obesity and smoking*

The obesity epidemic is reaching every corner of the globe and, similar to other chronic conditions, it is no longer associated with affluence. Between 2005 and 2025, it is projected that female smoking will double (Amos *et al.*, 2011). Limited research has been conducted to understand the factors impacting why girls and women decide to smoke (Amos *et al.*, 2011). The Framework Convention on Tobacco Control provides guiding measures to reduce initiation, decrease consumption and aid in cessation of tobacco use (Mackay, 2012). These must be adopted along with broader strategies to address chronic diseases (Valdes *et al.*, 2005) (See also Volume 2, Chapter 6 of this Handbook on *Smoking*).

Global estimates show that women have a higher likelihood of being obese than men (WHO, 2011b). In Brazil, projections estimate that by 2015, 12.4% of men and 24.5% of women will be obese (Abegunde *et al.*, 2007). The association between obesity, Type 2 diabetes and high blood pressure imply that differences across gender in prevalence will have far-reaching implications for women's health. Moreover, obesity in early adulthood raises the risk of menstrual problems as well as hypertension during pregnancy and subfertility.

- *Injuries*

Between 15 and 44 years of age, burns have been listed as the seventh leading cause of death and disability among women (Ribeiro *et al.*, 2008). In India, where acid attacks are a devastating reality, one study found that 106,000 out of 163,000 reported burn-related deaths in the country are women (Sanghavi *et al.*, 2009). Stove injuries are another common cause of burns (Peck *et al.*, 2008).

Injuries can lead to physical disability as well prolonged psychological and economic effects on victims and their families (Gosselin, 2009). Injuries often require catastrophic health expenditure (Gosselin, 2009). The cost of burn care — resuscitation, dressings, surgery, adequate nutrition and physical therapy — was estimated in one Indian study to be approximately US$123 per patient (Ahuja and Goswami, 2013). In a country such as India, where millions live on less than US$1 per day, such an expense may be well beyond reach.

- *Mental health*

Globally, WHO estimates from 2005 indicate that majority of 1.2 million annual deaths from neuropsychiatric disorders were related to dementia, Parkinson's disease, and epilepsy, while a much smaller proportion were attributable to mental disorders such as depression, schizophrenia, and post-traumatic stress disorder (Mathers and Loncar, 2006). Data on the prevalence mental illness in developing countries are lacking (Fisher *et al.*, 2009; Lund *et al.*, 2010) — yet existing numbers provide a grim view (Villegas *et al.*, 2011). Some country-specific data, such as that from Pakistan, provide evidence that women are two to three times more likely to suffer mental disorders than men (Mirza and Jenkins, 2004).

Maternal mental health is a common issue among women worldwide with depression accounting for the highest proportion of mental and neurological disorders (Prince *et al.*, 2007; Vos *et al.*, 2012). A global systematic review of women in developing and developed countries found a postpartum depression (PPD) prevalence of 31.3% and 21.5%, respectively (Villegas *et al.*, 2011). In Zimbabwe, among a group of HIV-positive and HIV-negative mothers, 33% overall fell under the clinical criteria for postnatal depression (Chibanda *et al.*, 2013).

Mental health interventions, where undertaken, have resulted in improved economic outcomes (Lund *et al.*, 2011). Group problem-solving therapy was found to be an effective, culturally accepted and programmatically feasible alternative to drug therapy for PPD in Zimbabwe (Chibanda *et al.*, 2013). Women in the Zimbabwe study were screened using the Edinburgh Postnatal Depression Scale (EPDS) and randomized between two intervention groups — group psychotherapy ($n = 30$) and pharmacotherapy ($n = 28$). Results of the study demonstrated a significant EPDS score change from pre- to post-intervention between the groups. EPDS scores changes from 17.3 (±3.7) to 8.22 (±3.6) in the problem-solving group versus 17.9 (±3.9) to 10.7 (±2.7) in the pharmacotherapy group (Chibanda *et al.*, 2013). Studies from India and Lebanon found rates of PPD in their cohorts to be 23% and 21%, respectively (Chaaya *et al.*, 2002; Patel *et al.*, 2002). In the Indian study, poverty and poor marital relationship served as risk factors for PPD while PPD was itself a risk factor for chronic depression. Further, gender of infant was noted as a determinant of PPD. Social determinants, such as gender subjugation within and outside the home, have a greater influence on depression in LMICs (Mendenhall and Weaver, 2014). Mental illness can also impact self-care and childcare and hence has repercussions for many other health outcomes (Mendenhall and Weaver, 2014) (See also Volume 2, Chapter 1 of this Handbook on *Mental Health*).

- *Violence against women*

The majority of cases of violence against women are committed by domestic partners and are more commonly referred to in the literature as IPV, which includes rape, physical assault and stalking (Duvvury *et al.*, 2013; Garcia-Moreno *et al.*, 2006). A WHO multi-country study of 10 countries and 15 sites, interviewing 24,097 women age 15–49 years of age, found the prevalence of IPV in 6 sites to be between 50% and 75% (Garcia-Moreno *et al.*, 2006). IPV also has dramatic effects on mental health (Astbury and Walji, 2014; Bonomi *et al.*, 2006).

Trauma resulting from IPV can lead to work absenteeism, productivity losses and a reduction in household income (Duvvury *et al.*, 2013). The impact on productivity due to lost earnings of women who have experienced IPV is estimated at 1.2%, 2%, and 0.94% of GDP in Chile, Nicaragua, and Vietnam, respectively (Duvvury *et al.*, 2013; Morrison and Orlando, 1999).

There are several correlates of IPV. Education has sometimes been found to be associated with lower IPV (Jewkes, 2002). In India, women without a formal education had a 5.1 times higher chance of IPV compared to college-educated women (Ackerson *et al.*, 2008). Wives of men without formal education had a 1.84 times higher chance of IPV than wives of college-educated men (Ackerson *et al.*, 2008). Krishnan (2005) found gender, caste, and class inequalities to be intrinsically linked with IPV. Evidence from Bolivia supports the causal role of alcohol addiction on violence against women (Jaen-Varas *et al.*, 2014). Women in South India whose dowries have been unsatisfactory to their in-laws and 'love marriages' (those in which marriage is by own choice) similarly pose greater risk of IPV (Rocca *et al.*, 2009). Economic disempowerment, limited education, entrenched patriarchal norms and acceptance of domestic violence were found to be contributing factors in Pakistan (Karmaliani *et al.*, 2012). However, education and employment are not necessarily protective as seen by Rocca *et al.* (2009), who documented that participation in vocational training and employment were associated with a higher risk of IPV for women in South India.

Violence against women can also have spillover effects on children. A Nicaraguan study found that 63.1% of children of female IPV victims had to repeat a school year and these same children dropped out of school four years sooner than their counterparts (Morrison and Orlando, 1999).

Training of health workers on IPV case finding, marital counseling, alcohol consumption support, and community-based awareness campaigns is necessary to counter IPV (Krishnan, 2005). Men must play a central role in and be agents of change within their homes and their communities (Colucci and Hassan, 2014).

Aging

As emphasized in the UN Report, *Between Gender and Ageing: The Status of the World's Older Women*, "the diseases of old age often begin much earlier in life" (UN WomenWatch, 2012). The gender inequity in a society impacts the relative risks men and women face earlier on as well as the resources they have to mitigate risk and cope with acute and chronic health problems in later years. Poor nutrition, poverty, violence, tobacco use, lack of access to education and dangerous work conditions combine to influence health in later years. Given the shift in global demographics, the ill health of the elderly is a public health issue every country will need to address. According to the UN, a combination of falling fertility rates and decreasing mortality rates predicts that the 60+ world population will reach 20% by 2050. This corresponds to nearly 1.5 billion elderly individuals in the developing world (UN WomenWatch, 2012). Furthermore, since women tend to live longer than men, they represent a higher proportion of older adults: 54% of people 60 years of age and older are women, a proportion that rises to almost 60% at age 75 and older, and to 70% at age 90 and older. Although all countries will have to confront the medical concerns of their aging population, the unique challenges facing elderly women living in developing countries is a topic that is relatively underexplored.

- *NCD and disability*

In older age, the NCDs that began to arise in adulthood shift to become the predominant cause of morbidity and mortality. Although often thought of as a "male" disease, CVD is the leading cause of death for older women worldwide. In fact, CVD kills more women than men each year (UN WomenWatch, 2012). According to the report, *A Race Against Time, The Challenge of Cardiovascular Disease in the World*, CVD in South Africa caused the highest portion of years of life lost due to NCD for poor women — 45.5% — compared to 35% for poor men (p. 34). The WHO estimates that nearly half a million women aged 50+ in low-income countries and about 2.1 million in LMIC die from CVD annually (WHO, 2009b).

Sex-related differences in the epidemiology and outcomes of CVD are just now being elucidated. There are several reasons why CVD is a leading cause of death for older women. First, lower awareness of the risk factors for women — on the part of patients and providers — can delay appropriate and timely therapy. Second, presentation of the disease may vary between the sexes, complicating diagnosis. Third, comorbid conditions such as diabetes and atrial fibrillation are associated with higher mortality among women, yet the same primary and secondary prevention strategies are recommended for women and men (Finks, 2010; Pilote *et al.*, 2007). Changing lifestyles are also bolstering women's risk of heart disease in the developing world. A survey of cardiologists in India (Visualizing the Extent of Heart Disease in Indian Women, VEDNA Study, 2013) revealed a 16 to 20% rise in CVD among women in the previous 5 years. The survey implicated stress from the workplace as well as physical inactivity, diabetes and obesity as the primary drivers of the trend.

Disability is also more common in old age and poses a threat to the financial security of older women. Disability can be broadly defined as "limitation in functioning resulting from interactions between the individual's health condition (e.g., diseases, injuries, disorders) and environmental factors" (WHO, 2002). World Health survey data from 57 countries showed that the prevalence of disability among women compared with men aged 50+ years was 40.1% versus 23.8% (Hosseinpoor *et al.*, 2012). The prevalence of disability was compounded by socio-economic status with a rate of 49.3% among women in the lowest quintile of wealth and only 29.5% in the highest quintile. Similar stark differentials were noted for those with no education (47.2%) versus those with college or above (32.5%). Using a Blinder–Oaxaca decomposition, the authors reported that 45% of the sex inequality in disability could be attributed to differences in the distribution of socio-demographic factors between genders, whereas 55% of the inequality resulted from differences in the effects of these socio-demographic factors on the outcomes. One of the potential limitations of studies on disability in women is that it is often self-reported. However, more objective measures of physical disability, such as assessments of activities of daily living (ADLs) or observed physical performance have generally validated the self-reported data (Merrill *et al.*, 1997). Thus, the higher prevalence of disability among women might partially be due to reporting bias, but it also seems to be due to a higher incidence and/or slower recovery of elderly women to health insults.

One study using survey data from India found the gender gap in functional disability reversed sign (but was not significant) after adding controls for economic independence and concluded that "financially empowered older women have better functional health status than men" and "the poor health and lower healthcare utilization noted among older women, compared with men in India, can be largely explained by gender differentials in socioeconomic status and consequent financial empowerment" (Roy and Chaudhuri, 2008, p. 1951).

- *Financial (in)dependence in older age*

Elderly women often co-reside with other family members in LMICs. As shown in Figure 1, at a time when women should be receiving care, they are often still providing it to grandchildren and working. To the extent that pensions are available, evidence suggests that they are often used by other family members and/or for the benefit of grandchildren (Duflo, 2000). In developing countries, pensions are a nontrivial part of government spending and the generosity of the program is often debated (Lloyd-Sherlock, 2000). Data do not support the idea that the pensions that do exist are sufficient or reach the elderly poor who need them most. Their impact on the elderly recipient is often muted by their meager allowance and sharing of the resource within the family unit (International Labour Organization, 2011).

Reforms to pensions have been proposed and often involve the transformation of entitlements to contributory plans. However, elderly women, who are less likely to have had independent, formal employment in LMICs and yet often live longer, would be especially vulnerable to such reforms if special allowances were not made to account for their informal and home-based work.

Inheritance rights may also have a large effect on the financial well-being of elderly women. Whether or not widows can inherit their husbands' assets affects their economic independence. In the absence of such rights, women may be forced to remarry or live with relatives out of desperation and therefore become vulnerable to physical, verbal, psychological/emotional, sexual and financial abuse (WHO, 2008). The WHO estimates that, throughout the world, 1 in 6 to 1 in 15 elderly individuals suffer abuse or neglect. The numbers are difficult to assess given the isolation of elderly individuals, lack of uniform reporting laws as well as the lack of attention and awareness to the issue among health professionals and the general public. Risk factors for elder abuse include dementia and a shared living situation. The WHO notes that, "While older men have the same risk of abuse as women, in some cultures where women have inferior social status, elderly women are at higher risk of neglect through abandonment when they are widowed and their property is seized" (WHO, 2011c).

Screening is a key to detect elder abuse, but to prevent abuse, institutional changes — such as assuring adequate financial independence for men and women as they age — will be key to preventing the vulnerability that permits such abuse to occur.

Conclusion

This chapter has sought to use the lens of economics to view the health of women throughout the life cycle. We have advanced the notion that discrimination against women persists for historical, sociocultural and economic reasons and these forces are embodied in ill health and disability.

Once such a complex view of women's health is edified, policy recommendations cannot be targeted to only one domain (such as reproduction) or one point in the life cycle. The chapter has mentioned several strategies that could influence the more egregious gender-based inequities, such as improving the health of girls in early life, enabling safe childbirth, ending child marriage, prohibiting domestic violence, and ensuring women's legal rights to property and divorce. Gender-based affirmative action policies in education, labor and political leadership also have shown to change aspirations for young girls and their parents. Encouraging girls to remain in school for secondary education may be a particularly important policy lever for delaying first marriage and sexual debut. Diagonal health systems strategies (Frenk, 2006; Sepúlveda *et al.*, 2006) that connect points in the life cycle and cut across health issues will benefit men and women alike as would broader public health interventions. These strategies might target life cycle issues such as gender-based violence, mental health or opportunities to increase women's financial independence and status. Further, they may harness joint platforms such as integrating screening for women's cancers into maternal and child health or into sexual and reproductive health programming.

There are other gender-based norms that will be more difficult to change, such as parental pressures, societal expectations and cultural norms that breed self-doubt and transmit the idea of female inferiority across generations. However, as the labor market changes and the demand for skill rises, the returns on girls' education will also rise, and cultural expectations should respond. Despite the current challenges, gender equity is a goal to be pursued in health as well as in other spheres. Strengthening the health and well-being of women is essential to achieving the objective of equitable human development.

References

Abegunde D, Mathers C, Adam T, Ortegon M, Strong K. 2007. The burden and costs of chronic diseases in low-income and middle-income countries. *Lancet* 370: 1929–1938.

Ackerson LK, Kawachi I, Barbeau EM, Subramanian SV. 2008. Effects of individual and proximate educational context on intimate partner violence: A population-based study of women in India. *American Journal of Public Health* 98: 507–514.

Adekunle A, Arowojolu A, Adedimeji A, Okunlola M. 2000. Emergency contraception: Survey of knowledge, attitudes and practice of health care professionals in Ibadan, Nigeria. *Journal of Obstetrics & Gynaecology* 20: 284–289.

Adukia, A. 2014. Sanitation and Education. URL: http://scholar.harvard.edu/files/adukia/files/adukia_sanitation_and_education.pdf (accessed 9-25-2014).

Ahmed S, Li Q, Liu L, Tsui AO. 2012. Maternal deaths averted by contraceptive use: An analysis of 172 countries. *The Lancet* 380: 111–125. doi:10.1016/S0140-6736(12)60478-4.

Ahuja RB, Goswami P. 2013. Cost of providing inpatient burn care in a tertiary, teaching, hospital of North India. *Burns Journal of International Society of Burn Injuries* 39: 558–564.

Aizer A. 2010. The gender wage gap and domestic violence. *American Economic Review* 100: 1847–1859.

Alsan MM, Cutler DM. 2013. Girls' education and HIV risk: Evidence from Uganda. *Journal of Health Economics* 32: 863–872.

Alsan MM. 2015. The Gendered Impact of Mass Vaccination. *Working Paper.*

Amos A, Greaves L, Nichter M, Bloch M. 2012. Women and tobacco: a call for including gender in tobacco control research, policy and practice. *Tobacco Control* 21: 236–243.

Arnold F, Choe MK, Roy TK. 1998. Son preference, the family-building process and child mortality in India. *Population Studies* 52: 301–315.

Ashraf N, Field E, Lee J. 2012. Household Bargaining and Excess Fertility: An Experimental Study in Zambia.

Astbury J, Walji F. 2014. The prevalence and psychological costs of household violence by family members against women with disabilities in Cambodia. *Journal of Interpersonal Violence* 29(17): 3127–3149.

Baird S, Friedman J, Schady N. 2010. Aggregate income shocks and infant mortality in the developing world. *Review Economics Statistics* 93: 847–856.

Baird S, Garfein RS, McIntosh CT, Özler B. 2012. Effect of a cash transfer programme for schooling on prevalence of HIV and herpes simplex type 2 in Malawi: A custer randomised trial. *The Lancet* 379: 1320–1329.

Baird, S, McIntosh C, Ozler B. 2011. Cash or condition? Evidence from a cash transfer experiment. *Quarterly Journal of Economics* 126: 1709–1753.

Becker GS. 1974. A theory of social interactions. *Journal of Political Economy* 82: 1063–1093.

Becker GS. 1991. *A Treatise on the Family.* Harvard University Press.

Behrman JR, Murphy A, Ramakrishnan U, Yount K, Quisumbing A. 2006. What Is the Real Impact of Schooling on Age of First Union and Age of First Parenting? New Evidence from Guatemala (No. WPS4023). The World Bank.

Bellamy L, Casas J, Hingorani A, Williams D. 2009. Type 2 diabetes mellitus after gestational diabetes: A systematic review and meta-analysis. *The Lancet* 373: 1773–1779.

Black RE, Allen LH, Bhutta ZA, Caulfield LE, de Onis M, Ezzati M, Mathers C, Rivera J. 2008. Maternal and child undernutrition: Global and regional exposures and health consequences. *The Lancet* 371: 243–260.

Blanc A. 2001. The effect of power in sexual relationships on sexual and reproductive health: An examination of the evidence. *Studies in Family Planning* 32: 189–213.

Bloom SS, Wypij D, Das Gupta M. 2001. Dimensions of women's autonomy and the influence on maternal health care utilization in a North Indian City. *Demography* 38: 67–78.

Blundell R, Chiappori P, Meghir C. 2005. Collective labor supply with children. *Journal of Political Economy* 113: 1277–1306.

Bonomi AE, Thompson RS, Anderson M, Reid RJ, Carrell D, Dimer JA, Rivara FP. 2006. Intimate partner violence and women's physical, mental, and social functioning. *American Journal of Preventing Medicine* 30: 458–466.

Bott S, Morrison A, Ellsberg M. 2005. Preventing and Responding to Gender-based Violence in Middle and Low-income Countries: A Global Review and Analysis (*World Bank Policy Research Working Paper* No. 3618).

Bray F, Jemal A, Grey N, Ferlay J, Forman D. 2012. Global cancer transitions according to the human development Index (2008–2030): A population-based study. *Lancet Oncology* 13: 790–801.

Buckley T, Gottlieb A. 1988. *Blood Magic: The Anthropology of Menstruation*. University of California Press, Berkeley.

Bustreo F, Chestnov O, Knaul FM, Araujo de Carvalho I, Merialdi M, Temmerman M, Beard JR. 2013. At the Crossroads: Transforming health systems to address women's health across the life course. *Bulletin of the World Health Organization* 91: 622–622.

Cervical Cancer Action. 2012. Progress in Cervical Cancer Prevention: The CCA Report Card. Cervical Cancer Action.

Chaaya M, Campbell OMR, Kak FE, Shaar D, Harb H, Kaddour A. 2002. Postpartum depression: Prevalence and determinants in lebanon. *Archives of Women's Mental Health* 5: 65–72.

Chakravarty A. 2010. Supply shocks and gender bias in child health investments: Evidence from the ICDS programme in India. *The B.E. Journal of Economic Analysis & Policy.* 10: Article 88.

Chandra-Mouli V, Camacho AV, Michaud PA. 2013. WHO guidelines on preventing early pregnancy and poor reproductive outcomes among adolescents in developing countries. *Journal of Adolescent Health* 52: 517–522.

Chesnokova T, Vaithianathan R. 2010. The economics of female genital cutting. *BE Journal of Economic Analysis & Policy* 10.

Chibanda D, Shetty AK, Tshimanga M, Woelk G, Stranix-Chibanda L, Rusakaniko S. 2013. Group problem-solving therapy for postnatal depression among HIV-positive and HIV-negative mothers in Zimbabwe. *AIDS Care* 13: 335–341.

Cohen A. 2000. Excess female mortality in India: The case of Himachal Pradesh. *American Journal of Public Health* 90: 1369–1371.

Collaborative Group on Hormonal Factors in Breast Cancer. 2002. Breast cancer and breastfeeding: collaborative reanalysis of individual data from 47 epidemiological studies in 30 countries, including 50302 women with breast cancer and 96973 women without the disease. *Lancet* 360(9328): 187–195.

Colombini M, Mayhew S, Watts C. 2008. Health-sector responses to intimate partner violence in low- and middle-income settings: A review of current models, challenges and Opportunities. *Bulletin of the World Health Organization* URL: http://www.who.int/bulletin/volumes/86/8/07-045906/en/.

Colucci E, Hassan G. 2014. Prevention of domestic violence against women and children in low-income and middle-income countries. *Current Opinion in Psychiatry* 27: 350–357.

Conard LAE, Gold MA. 2004. Emergency contraceptive pills: A review of the recent literature. *Current Opinion in Obstetrics and Gynecology* 16: 389–395.

Das Gupta M. 1995. Life course perspectives on women's autonomy and health outcomes. *American Anthropologist* 97: 481–91.

Das Gupta M. 2003. Why is son preference so persistent in East and South Asia? A cross-country study of China, India and the Republic of Korea. *Journal of Devlopment Studies* 40: 153–187.

Das Gupta M. 2013. Women's Empowerment and Fertility: Policy Lessons.

De Bernis L, Sherratt DR, AbouZahr C, Van Lerberghe W. 2003. Skilled attendants for pregnancy, childbirth and postnatal care. *British Medical Bulletin* 39–57.

Duflo E. 2000. Grandmothers and Granddaughters: Old Age Pension and Intra-household Allocation in South Africa (*Working Paper* No. 8061). National Bureau of Economic Research.

Duflo E. 2012. Women's empowerment and economic development. *Journal of Economic Literature* 50(4): 1051–1079.

Duflo E, Dupas P, Kremer M. 2012. Education, HIV, and Early Fertility: Experimental Evidence from Kenya.

Dupas P. 2011. Do teenagers respond to HIV risk information? Evidence from a field Experiment in Kenya. *American Economic Journal Applied Economics* 3: 1–34.

Duvvury N, Callan A, Carney P, Raghavendra S. 2013. Intimate Partner Violence: Economic Costs and Implications for Growth and Development (No. 3), Women's Voice, Agency, & Participation Research Series 2013. The World Bank.

Ellsberg M, Heise L, Pena R, Agurto S, Winkvist A. 2001. Researching domestic violence against women: Methodological and ethical considerations. *Studies in Family Planning* 32: 1–16.

Farmer P, Frenk J, Knaul F, Shulman L, Alleyne G, Armstrong L, Atun R, Blayney D, Chen, L, Feachem R, Gospodarowicz M, Gralow J, Gupta S, Langer A, Lob-Levyt J, Neal, C, Mbewu A, Mired D, Piot P, Reddy K, Sachs J, Sarhan M, Seffrin J. 2010. Expansion of cancer care and control in countries of low and middle income: A call to action. *The Lancet* 376: 1186–1193.

Field E, Ambrus A. 2008. Early marriage, age of menarche, and female schooling attainment in Bangladesh. *Journal of Political Economy* 116: 881–930.

Finks S. 2010. Cardiovascular Disease in Women. PSAP-VII – Cardiology, American College of Clinical Pharmacy. URL: http://www.accp.com/docs/bookstore/psap/p7b01sample03.pdf (accessed 9-24-2014).

Fisher J, de Mello MC, Izutsu T. 2009. Mental Health Aspects of Pregnancy, Childbirth and the Postpartum Period (Chapter 9). In: Chandra PS, Herrman H, Fisher J, Kastrup M, Niaz U, Rondón MB, Okasha A. (eds.). Contemporary Topics in Women's Mental Health: Global Perspectives in a Changing Society. John Wiley & Sons, Ltd., pp. 197–225.

Forman D, de Martel C, Lacey C, Soerjomataram I, Lortet-Tieulent J, Bruni L, Vignat J, Ferlay J, Bray F, Plummer M, Franceschi S. 2012. Global burden of human papillomavirus and related diseases. *Vaccine, Comprehensive Control of HPV Infections and Related Diseases* 30(Suppl. 5): F12–F23.

Forouzanfar MH, Foreman KJ, Delossantos AM, Lozano R, Lopez AD, Murray CJL, Naghavi M. 2011. Breast and cervical cancer in 187 countries between 1980 and 2010: A systematic analysis. *The Lancet* 378: 1461–1484.

Franco-Marina F, López-Carrillo L, Keating N, Arreola-Ornelas H, Knaul F. 2015. Breast cancer age at diagnosis patterns in four Latin American Populations: a comparison with North American countries. Submitted to Cancer Epidemiology.

Frenk J. 2006. Bridging the divide: Global lessons from evidence-based health policy in Mexico. *The Lancet* 368: 954–961.

Frenk J. 2010. A Women and Health Agenda: It's Time. Harvard School of Public Health. URL: http://www.hsph.harvard.edu/news/magazine/spr10womenhealth/ (accessed 9-10-2014).

Frenk J, Gómez-Dantés O, Langer A. 2012. A comprehensive approach to women's health: Lessons from the Mexican health reform. *BMC Womens Health* 12: 42.

Garcia-Moreno C, Jansen HAFM, Ellsberg M, Heise L, Watts CH. 2006. Prevalence of intimate partner violence: Findings from the WHO multi-country study on women's health and domestic violence. *Lancet* 368: 1260–1269.

Gertler P, Rahman O, Feifer C, Ashley D. 1993. Determinants of pregnancy outcomes and targeting of maternal health services in Jamaica. *Social Science & Medicine* 37: 199–211.

Gomez A. 2011. Sexual violence as a predictor of unintended pregnancy, contraceptive use, and unmet need among female youth in Colombia. *Journal of Women's Health* 20: 1349–1356.

Goodkind D. 1996. On substituting sex preference strategies in East Asia: Does Prenatal sex selection reduce postnatal discrimination? *Population Development Review* 22: 111–125.

Gosselin RA. 2009. The increasing burden of injuries in developing countries: Direct and indirect consequences. *Techniques in Orthopaedics* 24: 230–232.

Grant M, Lloyd C, Mensch B. 2013. Menstruation and school absenteeism: Evidence from rural Malawi. *Comparative Education Review* 57: 260–84.

Guedes A, Bott S, Guezmes A, Helzner JF. 2002. Gender-based violence, human rights, and the health sector: Lessons from Latin America. *Health and Human Rights: An International Journal* 6: 177.

Hallfors D, Cho H, Rusakaniko S, Iritani B, Mapfumo J, Halpern C. 2011. Supporting adolescent orphan girls to stay in school as HIV risk prevention: Evidence from a randomized controlled trial in Zimbabwe. *American Journal of Public Health* 101: 1082–1088.

Heise L, Ellsberg M, Gottemoeller M. 1999. Ending Violence Against Women (No. 11), Population Reports. Johns Hopkins University School of Public Health, Baltimore.

Heise L, Moore K, Toubia N. 1995. Sexual coercion and reproductive health: A focus on research. *Population Council* URL: http://www.popcouncil.org/uploads/pdfs/scoer.pdf (accessed 1-28-15).

Hogan MC, Foreman KJ, Naghavi M, Ahn SY, Wang M, Makela SM, Lopez AD, Lozano, R, Murray CJ. 2010. Maternal mortality for 181 countries, 1980–2008: A systematic analysis of progress towards Millennium Development Goal 5. *The Lancet* 375: 1609–1623.

Hosseinpoor A, Williams J, Jann B, Kowal P, Officer A, Posarac A, Chatterji S. 2012. Social determinants of sex differences in disability among older adults: A multi-country decomposition analysis using the World Health Survey. *International Journal for Equity in Health* 11: 52.

IARC. 2012. GLOBOCAN 2012: Estimated Cancer Incidence, Mortality and Prevalence Worldwide in 2012 (WHO) (Fact sheet). International Agency for Research on Cancer (IARC).

International Labour Organization. 2011. Social security and ageing populations in developing countries. World Work 71: 25–27.

International Labour Organization. 2013. Marking Progress Against Child Labour (Report).

Jaen-Varas D, Ribeiro WS, Whitfield J, de Jesus Mari J. 2014. Mental health and Psychiatric Care in Bolivia: What Do We Know? *International Journal of Mental Health Systems* 8: 18.

Jejeebhoy S, Boot S. 2005. Non-consensual sexual experiences of young people in developing countries: An overview. In: Jejeebhoy S, Shah I, Thapa S. (eds.). Sex Without Consent: Young People in Developing Countries. Zed Books, London and New York, p. 384.

Jensen R. 2012. Do labor market opportunities affect young women's work and family decisions? Experimental evidence from India. *Quarterly Journal of Economics* 127: 753–792.

Jewkes R. 2002. Intimate partner violence: Causes and prevention. *The Lancet* 359: 1423–1429.

Jha P, Kesler MA, Kumar R, Ram F, Ram U, Aleksandrowicz L, Bassani DG, Chandra S, Banthia JK. 2011. Trends in selective abortions of girls in India: Analysis of nationally representative birth histories from 1990 to 2005 and census data from 1991 to 2011. *The Lancet* 377: 1921–1928.

Kalichman S, Simbayi L. 2004. Sexual assault history and risks for sexually transmitted infections among women in an African Township in Cape Town, South Africa. *AIDS Care* 16: 681–689.

Kalichman S, Simbayi L, Kaufman M, Cain D, Cherry C, Jooste S, Mathiti V. 2005. Gender attitudes, sexual violence, and HIV/AIDS risks among men and women in Cape Town, South Africa. *Journal of Sex Research* 42: 299–305.

Karmaliani R, Pasha A, Hirani S, Somani R, Hirani S, Asad N, Cassum L, McFarlane J. 2012. Violence against women in Pakistan: Contributing factors and new interventions. *Issues in Mental Health Nursing* 33: 820–826.

Kassebaum N, *et al.* 2014. Global, Regional, and national levels and causes of maternal mortality during 1990–2013: A systematic analysis for the global burden of disease study 2013. *The Lancet* 384: 980–1004.

Knaul F. 2013. What Is Maternal Health? Huffington Post Blog. URL: http://www.huffingtonpost.com/felicia-m-knaul/what-is-maternal-health_b_2830972.html (accessed 11-14-14).

Knaul FM, Bhadelia A, Arreola-Ornelas H, Dos Santos Silva I, Rodin D, Atun R, Langer A, Frenk J. 2014. Women's Reproductive Health in Transition: The Overlapping Challenge of Breast and Cervical Cancer. Cancer Control 2014.

Global Health Dynamics and International Network for Cancer Treatment and Research, Suffolk, UK and Brussels.
Knaul F, Bhadelia A, Gralow J, Arreola-Ornelas H, Langer A, Frenk J. 2012. Meeting the emerging challenge of breast and cervical cancer in low- and middle-income countries. *International Journal of Gynaecology and Obstetrics: The Offical Organ of the International Federation of Gynaecology and Obetetrics* 119(Suppl. 1): S85–88.
Knaul, Felicia M, Frenk J, Shulman L. 2011. The Global Task Force on Expanded Access to Cancer Care and Control in Developing Countries. Closing the Cancer Divide: A Blueprint to Expand Access in Low and Middle Income Countries. Harvard Global Equity Initiative, Boston, MA, November 2011. URL: http://gtfccc.harvard.edu/fs/docs/icb.topic1063570.files/ccd_report_111027.pdf (accessed 11-17-14).
Knaul F, Nigenda G, Lozano R, Arreola-Ornelas H, Langer A, Frenk J. 2008. Breast cancer in Mexico: A pressing priority. *Reproductive Health Matters* 16: 113–123.
Koenig M, Zablotska I, Lutalo T, Nalugoda F, Wagman J, Gray R. 2004. Coerced first intercourse and reproductive health among adolescent women in Rakai, Uganda. *International Family Planning Perspectives* 30: 156–163. doi:10.1363/ifpp.30.156.04.
Krishnan S. 2005. Do structural inequalities contribute to marital violence? Ethnographic evidence from rural South India. *Violence Women* 11: 759–775.
Langer A, Frenk J, Horton R. 2012. Women and health initiative: Integrating needs and response. *The Lancet* 380: 631–632. doi:10.1016/S0140-6736(11)60742-3.
Lloyd C, Aramburu CE, Astone NM, Basu K, Behrman JR, Gage AJ, Jejeebhoy S, Jessor, R, Kuate-Defo B, Lam DA, Magnani RJ, Mensch BS, Singh S, Stromquist NP. 2014. Growing Up Global: The Changing Transitions to Adulthood in Developing Countries. The National Academies Press, Washington, DC.
Lloyd-Sherlock P. 2000. Old age and poverty in developing countries: New policy challenges. *World Development* 28: 2157–2168.
Lozano R, *et al.* 2012. Global and regional mortality from 235 causes of death for 20 age groups in 1990 and 2010: A systematic analysis for the global burden of disease study 2010. *The Lancet* 380: 2095–2128.
Lund C, Breen A, Flisher AJ, Kakuma R, Corrigall J, Joska JA, Swartz L, Patel V. 2010. Poverty and common mental disorders in low and middle income countries: A Systematic Review. *Social Science & Medicine* 1982(71): 517–528.
Lund C, De Silva M, Plagerson S, Cooper S, Chisholm D, Das J, Knapp M, Patel V, 2011. Poverty and mental disorders: Breaking the cycle in low-income and middle-income countries. *The Lancet* 378: 1502–1514.
Mackay J. 2012. The global epidemiology of tobacco and related chronic diseases. *Public Health* 126: 199–201.
Maimaiti Y, Siebert S. 2009. The Gender Education Gap in China: The Power of Water (SSRN Scholarly Paper No. ID 1391760). Social Science Research Network, Rochester, NY.
Marcoux A. 2002. Sex differentials in undernutrition: A look at survey evidence. *Population Development Review* 28: 275–284.
Mason L, Nyothach E, Alexander K, Odhiambo FO, Eleveld A, Vulule J, Rheingans R, Laserson KF, Mohammed A, Phillips-Howard PA. 2013. We keep it secret so no

one should know — A qualitative study to explore young schoolgirls attitudes and experiences with menstruation in rural Western Kenya. *PLoS One* 8: e79132.

Mathers CD, Loncar D. 2006. Projections of global mortality and burden of disease from 2002 to 2030. *PLoS Medicine* 3: e442. doi:10.1371/journal.pmed.0030442.

McCaw-Binns A, Alexander SF, Lindo JLM, Escoffery C, Spence K, Lewis-Bell K, Lewis, G. 2007. Epidemiologic transition in maternal mortality and morbidity: New challenges for Jamaica. *International Journal of Gynaecology and Obstetrics: The Offical Organ of the International Federation of Gynaecology and Obetetrics* 96: 226–232. doi:10.1016/j.ijgo.2006.12.002.

McElroy M, Horney M. 1981. Nash-bargained household decisions: Toward a generalization of the theory of consumer demand. *International Economic Review* 22: 333–349.

McMahon SA, Winch PJ, Caruso BA, Obure AF, Ogutu EA, Ochari IA, Rheingans RD. 2011. "The girl with her period is the one to hang her head" Reflections on menstrual management among schoolgirls in Rural Kenya. *BMC International Health and Human Rights* 11: 7.

Meinhart M. 2013. Sexual Exploitation and Abuse Among Girl Street Children in Developing Countries. Columbia University Partnership for International Development.

Mendenhall E, Weaver LJ. 2014. Reorienting women's health in low- and middle-income countries: The case of depression and Type 2 diabetes. *Global Health Action* 7.

Mensch B, Lloyd C. 1998. Gender differences in the schooling experiences of adolescents in low-income countries: The case of Kenya. *Studies in Family Planning* 29: 167–184.

Merrill SS, Seeman TE, Kasl SV, Berkman LF. 1997. Gender Differences in the comparison of self-reported disability and performance measures *Journals of Gerontology A Biological Sciences & Medical Sciences* 52A: M19–M26.

Mgalla Z, Schapink D, Boerma J. 1998. Protecting school girls against sexual exploitation: A guardian programme in Mwanza, Tanzania. *Reproductive Health Matters* 6: 19–30.

Mirza I, Jenkins R. 2004. Risk factors, prevalence, and treatment of anxiety and depressive disorders in Pakistan: Systematic review. *British Medical Journal* 328: 794. doi:10.1136/bmj.328.7443.794.

Mishra V, Roy TK, Retherford RD. 2004. Sex differentials in childhood feeding, health care, and nutritional status in India. *Population and Development Review* 30: 269–295.

Montgomery P, Ryus CR, Dolan CS, Dopson S, Scott LM. 2012. Sanitary pad interventions for girls' education in Ghana: A pilot study. *PLoS One* 7: e48274.

Moore A, Awusabo-Asare K, Madise N, John-Langba J, Kumi-Kyereme A. 2007. Coerced first sex among adolescent girls in Sub-Saharan Africa: Prevalence and context. *African Journal of Reproductive Health* 11: 62–82.

Morrison AR, Orlando MB. 1999. Social and Economic Costs of Domestic Violence: Chile and Nicaragua (Chapter 3). In: Too Close to Home: Domestic Violence in the Americas. Inter-American Development Bank; Distributed by The Johns Hopkins University Press, p. 206.

Nguyen MC, Wodon Q. 2012. Global Trends in Child Marriage. The World Bank. URL: http://www.ungei.org/files/Child_Marriage_Trends3.pdf (accessed 9-9-14).

Oster E. 2009a. Does increased access increase equality? Gender and child health investments in India. *Journal of Development Economics* 89: 62–76.

Oster E. 2009b. Proximate sources of population sex imbalance in India. *Demography* 46: 325–339.

Oster E, Thornton R. 2011. Menstruation, sanitary products, and school attendance: Evidence from a randomized evaluation. *American Economic Journal Applied Economics* 3: 91–100.

Ozier O. 2011. The Impact of Secondary Schooling in Kenya: A Regression Discontinuity Analysis. The World Bank. URL: http://www-wds.worldbank.org/external/default/WDSContentServer/WDSP/IB/2015/08/06/090224b0830565b7/1_0/Rendered/PDF/The0impact0of00scontinuity0analysis.pdf (accessed 9-16-14).

Pande RP. 2003. Selective gender differences in childhood nutrition and immunization in Rural India: The role of siblings. *Demography* 40: 395–418.

Patel V, Rodrigues M, DeSouza N. 2002. Gender, poverty, and postnatal depression: A study of mothers in Goa, India. *American Journal of Psychiatry* 159: 43–47.

Patton GC, Coffey C, Sawyer SM, Viner RM, Haller DM, Bose K, Vos T, Ferguson J, Mathers CD. 2009. Global patterns of mortality in young people: A systematic analysis of population health data. *The Lancet* 374: 881–892.

Patton GC, Sawyer SM. 2013. Adolescent Health Globally: Issues and Challenges. Nestle Nutrition Institute.

Peck MD, Kruger GE, van der Merwe AE, Godakumbura W, Ahuja RB. 2008. Burns and fires from non-electric domestic appliances in low and middle income countries Part I. The scope of the problem. *Burns Journal of the International Society of Burn Injuries* 34: 303–311.

Peltzer K, Pengpid S. 2012. Suicidal ideation and associated factors among school-going adolescents in Thailand. *International Journal of Environmental Research and Public Health* 9: 462–473.

Pilote L, Dasgupta K, Guru V, Humphries KH, McGrath J, Norris C, Rabi D, Tremblay J, Alamian A, Barnett T, Cox J, Ghali WA, Grace S, Hamet P, Ho T, Kirkland S, Lambert, M, Libersan D, O'Loughlin J, Paradis G, Petrovich M, Tagalakis V. 2007. A comprehensive view of sex-specific issues related to cardiovascular disease. *Canadian Medical Association Journal* 176: S1–44.

Pinheiro P. 2006. World Report on Violence Against Children, Secretary-General's Study on Violence Against Children. United Nations, New York.

Porter P. 2008. "Westernizing" women's risks? Breast cancer in lower-income countries. *New England Journal of Medicine* 358: 213–216.

Prince M, Patel V, Saxena S, Maj M, Maselko J, Phillips MR, Rahman A. 2007. No health without mental health. *Lancet* 370: 859–877. doi:10.1016/S0140-6736(07)61238-0.

Qian N. 2008. Missing women and the price of tea in china: The effect of sex-specific earnings on sex imbalance. *Quarterly Journal of Economics* 123: 1251–1285.

Ribeiro PS, Jacobsen KH, Mathers CD, Garcia-Moreno C. 2008. Priorities for women's health from the global burden of disease study. *International Journal of Gynaecology and Obstetrics: The Offical Organ of the International Federation of Gynaecology and Obetetrics* 102: 82–90.

Rocca CH, Rathod S, Falle T, Pande RP, Krishnan S. 2009. Challenging assumptions about women's empowerment: Social and economic resources and domestic violence among young married women in urban South India. *International Journal of Epidemiology* 38: 577–585.

Rosenzweig MR, Schultz TP. 1982. Market opportunities, genetic endowments, and intra-family resource distribution: Child survival in rural India. *American Economic Review* 72: 803–815.

Roy K, Chaudhuri A. 2008. Influence of socioeconomic status, wealth and financial empowerment on gender differences in health and healthcare utilization in later life: Evidence from India. *Social Science & Medicine* 66: 1951–1962.

Sanghavi P, Bhalla K, Das V. 2009. Fire-related deaths in India in 2001: A retrospective analysis of data. *The Lancet* 373: 1282–1288.

Sawyer SM, Afifi RA, Bearinger LH, Blakemore SJ, Dick B, Ezeh AC, Patton GC. 2012. Adolescence: A foundation for future health. *Lancet* 379: 1630–1640. doi:10.1016/S0140-6736(12)60072-5.

Schultz TP. 2004. School subsidies for the poor: Evaluating the Mexican Progresa Poverty Program. *Journal of Development Economics, New Research on Education in Developing Economies* 74: 199–250.

Sedgh G, Singh S, Shah IH, Åhman E, Henshaw SK, Bankole A. 2012. Induced Abortion: Estimated rates and trends worldwide from 1995 to 2008. *The Lancet* 379: 625–32.

Sen A. 1990. More Than 100 Million Women Are Missing. N. Y. Rev. Books.

Sen A. 2003. Missing women — revisited. *British Medical Journal* 327: 1297–1298.

Sepúlveda J, Bustreo F, Tapia R, Rivera J, Lozano R, Oláiz G, Partida V. García-García L, Valdespino J. 2006. Improvement of child survival in Mexico: The diagonal approach. *Lancet* 368: 2017–2027.

Shah IH, Åhman E. 2012. Unsafe abortion differentials in 2008 by age and developing country region: High burden among young women. *Reproductive Health Matters* 20: 169–173.

Sommer M, Ackatia-Armah NM. 2012. The gendered nature of schooling in Ghana: Hurdles to girls menstrual management in school. *JENdA: A Journal of Culture and African Women Studies*.

Steiner MJ, Raymond E, Attafuah JD, Hays M. 2000. Provider knowledge about emergency contraception in Ghana. *Journal of Biosocial Science* 32: 99–106.

Stubbs ML. 2008. Cultural perceptions and practices around menarche and adolescent menstruation in the United States. *Annals of the New York Academy of Sciences* 1135: 58–66.

Sumpter C, Torondel B. 2013. A systematic review of the health and social effects of menstrual hygiene management. *PLoS One* 8: e62004.

Szarewski A, von Stenglin A, Rybowski S. 2012. Women's attitudes towards monthly bleeding: Results of a global population-based survey. *European Journal of Contraception and Reproductive Health Care Official Journal of the European Socirty of Contraception and Reproductive Health* 17: 270–283.

The World Bank. 2005. Gender Roles and Impact. The World Bank. URL: http://www.wsp.org/Hygiene-Sanitation-Water-Toolkit/BasicPrinciples/GenderRoles.html (accessed 8-6-14).

UN. 1948. The Universal Declaration of Human Rights. UN. URL http://www.un.org/en/documents/udhr/ (accessed 11.18.14).

UN. 2013. World Population Prospects: The 2012 Revision.

UNESCO. 2012. From Access to Equality: Empowering Girls and Women through Literacy and Secondary Education., 2nd ed. UNESCO, Paris, France.

UNFPA. 1994. Master Plans for Development, Summary of the International Conference on Population and Development (ICPD) Programme of Action, Cairo, Egypt. UNFPA. http://www.unfpa.org/public/cache/offonce/home/sitemap/icpd/International-Conference-on-Population-and-Development/ICPD-Summary;jsessionid=ABA2A2D20965E6720644B21923A088E4.jahia01 (accessed 9.5.14).

UNICEF – Innocenti Research Center. 2005. Changing a Harmful Social Convention: Female Genital Mutilation / Cutting. *Innocenti Digest*. URL: http://www.unicef-irc.org/publications/pdf/fgm_eng.pdf (accessed 1-28-15).

UNICEF. 2011. Sexual Violence Against Children. UNICEF. URL: http://www.unicef.org/protection/57929_58006.html (accessed 11.5.14).

UN WomenWatch. 2012. Between Gender and Ageing The Status of the World's Older Women and Progress Since the Madrid International Plan of Action on Ageing. http://www.un.org/womenwatch/osagi/ianwge2012/Between-Gender-Ageing-Report-Executive-Summary-2012.pdf.

Valdes A, Andrew T, Gardner J, Kimura M, Oelsner E, Cherkas L, Aviv A, Spector T, 2005. Obesity, cigarette smoking, and telomere length in women. *The Lancet* 366: 662–664.

Van Rossem R, Meekers D. 2000. An evaluation of the effectiveness of targeted social marketing to promote adolescent and young adult reproductive health in Cameroon. *AIDS Education and Prevention: Official Publication of the International Society of AIDS Education* 12: 383–404.

Varga C. 2003. How gender roles influence sexual and reproductive health among South African adolescents. *Studies in Family Planning* 34: 160–172.

Biocon – Queen of Heart. 2013. VEDNA Study. URL: http://www.slideshare.net/queenof-heartexpress/heart-disease-in-women (accessed 9-23-14).

Victora CG, Adair L, Fall C, Hallal PC, Martorell R, Richter L, Sachdev HS. 2008. Maternal and child undernutrition: Consequences for adult health and human capital. *The Lancet* 371: 340–357.

Villarreal-Garza C, Aguila C, Magallanes-Hoyos MC, Mohar A, Bargalló E, Meneses A, Cazap E, Gomez H, López-Carrillo L, Chávarri-Guerra Y, Murillo R, Barrios C. 2013. Breast cancer in young women in Latin America: An unmet, growing burden. *The Oncologist* 18: 1298–1306.

Villegas L, McKay K, Dennis CL, Ross LE. 2011. Postpartum depression among rural women from developed and developing countries: A systematic review. *Journal of Rural Health:Official Journal of the American Rural Health Association and the National Rural Health Care Association* 27: 278–288.

Vos T, *et al.* 2012. Years lived with disability (YLDs) for 1160 sequelae of 289 diseases and injuries 1990-2010: A systematic analysis for the Global Burden of Disease Study 2010. *Lancet* 380: 2163–2196. doi:10.1016/S0140-6736(12)61729-2.

WHO. 2000. Special Project on Street Children. WHO. URL http://www.who.int/substance_abuse/activities/street_children/en/ (accessed 8.25.14).

WHO. 2002. Towards a Common Language for Functioning, Disability and Health.

WHO. 2005. The World Health Report 2005 — Make Every Mother and Child Count. WHO. URL http://www.who.int/whr/2005/en/ (accessed 9.8.14).

WHO. 2006. Female genital mutilation and obstetric outcome: WHO collaborative prospective study in six African countries. *The Lancet* 367: 1835–1841.

WHO. 2008. Eliminating female genital mutilation: An interagency statement — OHCHR, UNAIDS, UNDP, UNECA, UNESCO, UNFPA, UNHCR, UNICEF, UNIFEM, WHO. WHO. URL: http://www.who.int/reproductivehealth/publications/fgm/9789241596442/en/ (accessed 1.28.15).

WHO. 2009a. Women and Health: Today's Evidence Tomorrow's Agenda. World Health Organization.

WHO. 2009b. Global Health Risks — Mortality and Burden of Disease Attributable to Selected Major Risks. World Health Organization, Geneva.

WHO. 2011a. An Update on WHO's Work on Female Genital Mutilation (FGM). World Health Organization.

WHO. 2011b. Global Status Report on Noncommunicable Diseases 2010. WHO. URL: http://www.who.int/nmh/publications/ncd_report2010/en/ (accessed 3.11.15).

WHO. 2011c. Elder Maltreatment Fact Sheet N°357. WHO Media Cent. URL: http://www.who.int/mediacentre/factsheets/fs357/en/.

WHO. 2012. World Health Statistics 2012. WHO. URL: http://www.who.int/gho/publications/world_health_statistics/2012/en/ (accessed 9.8.14).

WHO. 2013a. Women's Health Fact Sheet N°334. WHO Media Cent. URL: http://www.who.int/mediacentre/factsheets/fs334/en/ (accessed 7.15.14).

WHO. 2013b. Human Papillomavirus (HPV) and Cervical Cancer Fact Sheet N°380. WHO. URL http://www.who.int/mediacentre/factsheets/fs380/en/ (accessed 11.13.14).

WHO. 2014. Countr Profiles on Maternal and Perinatal Health. WHO. URL: http://www.who.int/maternal_child_adolescent/epidemiology/profiles/maternal/en/ (accessed 7.16.14).

WHO. ISPCAN. 2006. Preventing Child Maltreatment: A Guide to Taking Action and Generating Evidence. World Health Organization and International Society for Prevention of Child Abuse and Neglect, Geneva, Switzerland.

Wood K, Maforah F, Jewkes R. 1998. "He forced me to love him": Putting violence on adolescent sexual health agendas. *Social Science & Medicine* 1982(47): 233–242.

Ye F, Wang H, Huntington D, Zhou H, Li Y, You F, Li J, Cui W, Yao M, Wang Y. 2012. The immediate economic impact of maternal deaths on rural Chinese households. *PLoS One* 7: e38467.

Zhu WX, Lu LI, Hesketh T. 2009. China's excess males, sex selective abortion, and one child policy: Analysis of data from 2005 National Intercensus Survey. *British Medical Journal* 338: b1211.

The Role of Policy Making for Investing in Women's and Children's Health*

Flavia Bustreo
Assistant Director-General
Family, Women's and Children's Health, World Health Organization

Jennifer Franz-Vasdeki
Consultant, Partnership for Maternal Newborn and Child Health

Shyama Kuruvilla
Senior Strategic Adviser
Family, Women's and Children's Health, World Health Organization

Blerta Maliqi
Senior Technical Officer
Department of Maternal, Newborn, Child and Adolescent Health, World Health Organization

Rachael Hinton
Technical Officer
Partnership for Maternal Newborn and Child Health

As we move into the post-2015 era, continued momentum is needed to ensure that progress made in women's and children's health under the Millennium Development Goals (MDGs) is continued and accelerated over the next 20 years. To this end, this chapter focuses on the enabling polices necessary to optimize investments in women's and children's health. Key investments that are needed are to support health systems, engagement with communities and further innovation

* The Policy Compendium and Global Investment Framework to which this paper refers are the result of collaborative work among key partners and constituencies working on policies and programs which affect the health of women, newborns, children and adolescents. These partners and experts in maternal, newborn and child health are gratefully acknowledged. We would also like to thank the WHO interns for their contribution to the drafting of this chapter.

and technology to improve access to effective interventions and services. We use the findings brought together by the *Global Investment Framework* and the *Policy Guide for Implementing Essential Interventions for Reproductive, Maternal, Newborn and Child Health.* These two resources offer a complementary approach to identifying the investments and policy environment required to maximize health and wellbeing — both as a right in and of itself and also for the many social, economic and environmental benefits for countries. To demonstrate this, we evidence a range of examples primarily from low- and middle-income countries that have developed policies, strategies and applied guiding principles. As a result, their success is due not only to actions and policies directly developed and implemented by the health sector, but also by health-enhancing sectors, such as education, water and sanitation and nutrition.

Keywords: Health Policy; Public Policy; Reproductive Health; Healthcare Financing; Health Planning Support; Maternal Health; Child Health; Universal Health Coverage.

Introduction

More than 20 years ago, the World Development Report highlighted the importance of investing in health (World Bank, 1993). The report brought significant public attention to the issue and the accompanying policies required to improve economic development. Two decades later, the Commission on Investing in Health (CIH) demonstrated that investing in health is even more beneficial to society than even previously estimated (Jamison *et al.*, 2013). These benefits include greater GDP growth through improved productivity and substantial reductions in preventable deaths. In fact, returns on investing in health have accounted for as much as 11% of economic growth in low- and middle-income countries in recent years (Jamison *et al.*, 2003; Stenberg *et al.*, 2014). This is possible because healthier people are better able to acquire education and skills, participate in the labor force and are more productive, both economically and socially. Healthy families are less exposed to financial risk from medical bills and lost income from illness. This translates into more money available for savings and increased economic activity (Frenk and de Ferranti, 2012).

In response to the CIH's findings, the Global Investment Framework (GIF) for Women's and Children's Health was developed to further investigate the particular economic and social benefits of investing in women's and children's health (Stenberg *et al.*, 2014; UNSG, 2010). The GIF found that an additional US$5 per person per year to 2035 could lead to nearly US$9 in economic and social benefits as a result of lower morbidity and mortality among women and children (Stenberg *et al.*, 2014). It could also mean avoiding the preventable deaths of 147 million children, 32 million stillbirths, and 5 million women between 2013 and 2035. This is possible in part because economic growth enables further resource mobilization

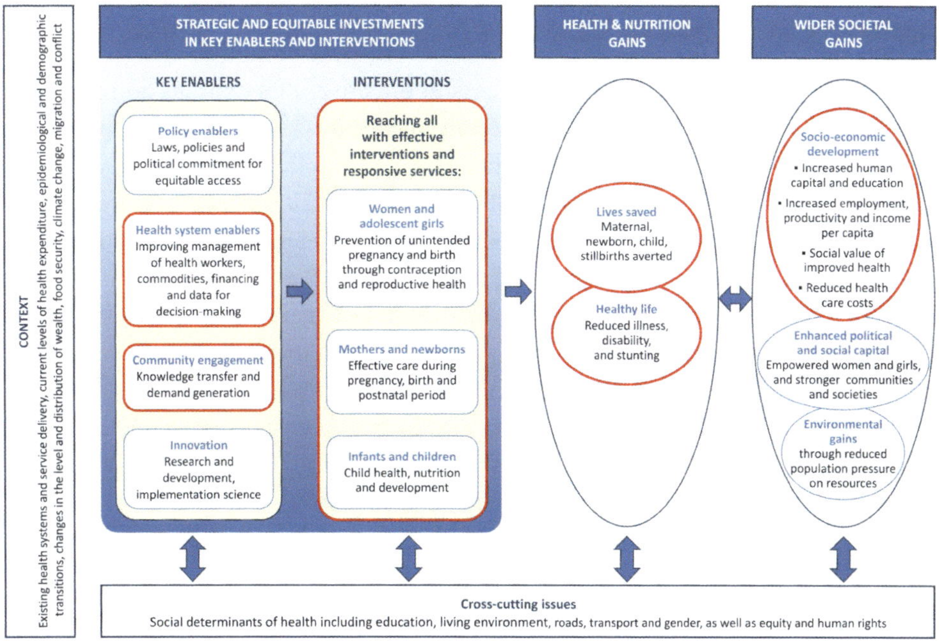

Figure 1. Global investment framework conceptual framework

Source: Stenberg *et al.* (2014).

for health. When combined with further development and delivery of new health technologies, it is possible to reduce infectious, child and maternal mortality rates to universally low levels. Even more promising, all of this could be achieved within a generation (Jamison *et al.*, 2013).

As we move into the post-2015 era, continued momentum is needed to ensure that key progress made in women's and children's health under the Millennium Development Goals (MDGs) is carried forward and accelerated over the next 20 years. We also need to continue learning from evidence that has been gained over the previous two decades. Key to the MDGs is having the right policy environment in which to make the best investments for individuals' health and wellbeing. This is also essential for ensuring the maximum social, economic and environmental benefits — particularly in light of the Sustainable Development Goals (SDGs) and the updated Global Strategy for Women's and Children's and Adolescents' health (United Nations Foundations, 2015).

To this end, this chapter focuses on the enabling polices necessary to maximize investments in women's and children's health. An enabling policy environment supports the strengthening of health systems, engagement with communities and encourages innovation and technology as well as interaction with other sectors that determine social and economic development of countries (Figure 1). Key to an enabling policy environment for women's and children's health along the continuum of care are the appropriate laws and political commitments required to ensure all women and children have access to effective interventions and services. We evidence a range of examples primarily from low- and middle-income countries that have developed policies, strategies and applied guiding principles to improve women's and children's health over the last 20 years. In particular, we focus on policy stories from Bangladesh, Cambodia, China, Egypt, Ethiopia, Lao PDR, Nepal, Peru, Rwanda and Vietnam. These 10 countries are part of the *Success Factors* series that highlights *how* these countries have adopted a multisectoral approach to improve maternal and child mortality (Kuruvilla *et al.*, 2014). As a result, their success is due not only to actions and policies directly developed and implemented by the health sector, but also by health-enhancing sectors including education, water and sanitation and nutrition. Economic development and good governance also underpinned progress in these countries.

As a framework for how the right policy environment enables investments and the resulting health and socioeconomic benefits, we use the findings brought together by the GIF and the Policy guide for Implementing Essential Interventions for Reproductive, Maternal, Newborn and Child Health. These two resources complement one another in identifying the investments and policy environment required to maximize health and wellbeing — both as a right in and of itself and also for the many social, economic and environmental benefits for countries.

The global investment framework for women's and children's health

Globally, there is widespread understanding of the most effective interventions to improve women's and children's health. Less well understood is *how* to achieve better health outcomes. The conceptual Global Investment Framework (GIF) makes the links between implementation of the Reproductive, Maternal, Newborn and Child Health (RMNCH) evidence-based interventions *and* the achievement of health and wider societal gains. This implementation is informed by four 'key enablers' that make it possible to identify and scale the relevant RMNCH essential interventions based on local context and in a way that is politically, financially, technically and socially sustainable (Stenberg *et al.*, 2014).

The GIF was developed in response to a recommendation by the UN Independent Expert Review Group (iERG) on information and accountability for women's and children's health, World Health Organization (WHO), the Partnership for Maternal, Newborn & Child Health (PMNCH), and *The Lancet* Commission on Investing in Health. The analysis reviews key interventions related to RMNCH. It also highlights how investing in the health sector, combined with other investments in physical infrastructure, including roads, can work to improve RMNCH.

Within this context, the analysis estimated the potential health, social and economic benefits of investing in health systems between 2013 and 2035. The study focused on the delivery of six packages of evidence-based essential RMNCH interventions: Family planning, maternal and newborn health, malaria, HIV, immunization and child health (PMNCH, 2011a; Stenberg *et al.*, 2014). The focus of the study was the 74 low- and middle-income countries that account for more than 95% of maternal and child deaths.

Three different investment scenarios were modeled: low, medium and high. The 'low' scenario maintains coverage levels as they are currently. The other two scenarios estimate benefits of accelerating levels of investment: 'medium' assumes increased levels of coverage based on historical country trends; the 'high' applies the best performance trends seen in coverage from 1990 to 2010 (Stenberg *et al.*, 2014). While costs vary across regions and countries depending on different levels of existing infrastructure and local costs, the GIF analysis demonstrates that modest investments have the potential to bring about substantial health benefits — particularly for newborns and children.

The GIF offers valuable findings on how investing in the health sector, combined with other investments in physical infrastructure, including roads, can work to improve RMNCH (Stenberg *et al.*, 2014). While costs vary across regions and countries depending on different levels of existing infrastructure and local costs, the GIF analysis demonstrates that modest investments have the potential to bring about substantial health benefits — particularly for newborns and children.

Investments are essential to achieving better health outcomes for women and children. However, money alone is not the solution. The GIF emphasizes that the right policies supporting evidence-based, high-impact interventions, both health and non-health related, are essential for sustainable improvements in women's and children's health. The GIF reaffirms that an increase in appropriate and adequate financing is essential not only to ensure that women and children achieve the most basic right to life, but also to live healthy and happy lives through improved access to essential packages of interventions. For example, around one-half of all maternal and child deaths prevented can be attributed to better access to contraceptives and thus fewer unintended pregnancies. The majority of these averted deaths would be in Sub-Saharan Africa and South Asia (Stenberg *et al.*, 2014).

Policy guide for implementing essential interventions for reproductive, maternal, newborn and child health: A multisectoral policy compendium for RMNCH

The Policy Compendium is a companion document to the Essential Interventions, Commodities and Guidelines for RMNCH (PMNCH, 2011b). It highlights key health-systems-related policies known to support the delivery of proven interventions for women and children's health. It focuses on policies related to the economic, social, technological and environmental factors that influence health outcomes and service delivery. The Policy Compendium is designed for policymakers and managers in charge of developing, implementing and evaluating RMNCH strategies, plans and programmes — from both health and non health sectors (including finance, agriculture, education, transportation, energy, etc.) (WHO, 2014). The Policy Compendium combines evidence and consensus-based policy recommendations and guidance to support the implementation of essential RMNCH interventions in the areas of health systems, RMNCH policies, international agreements, multisectoral policies that influence RMNCH service delivery and outcomes, including water and sanitation, food security, education and infrastructure.

Health-Related Policies that Enable RMNCH Investments for Better Results

The GIF and Policy Compendium offer important findings for policymakers on the importance of health interventions in reducing mortality and morbidity among women and children. Investments are essential to achieving better health outcomes for women and children. However, money alone is not the solution. The right policies, both health and non-health related, are essential for sustainable improvements in women's and children's health.

Outlined below are the different types of health-related policies required for supporting the delivery of RMNCH interventions. In order to improve the health of women and children, the following health policy areas are required: Constitutional and legal entitlements that support RMNCH programming; Universal health coverage; Strategies, plans and mechanisms to guide RMNCH programme implementation; Community mobilization and engagement; Accountability for results and high-impact health interventions (Table 1) (WHO, 2014).

Constitutional and Legal Entitlements that Support RMNCH

A strong legal and policy environment that promotes the enjoyment of the right to health by all women, children and adolescents is required to effectively implement the RMNCH interventions. The WHO Constitution declares health a fundamental human right (WHO, 1946).

Many countries have defined health and access to health as a legal entitlement for its citizens, specifying the enjoyment of the highest attainable standard of health as one of the fundamental rights of every human being without distinction in national constitutions and national legal frameworks (Bustreo and Hunt, 2014).

Table 1. Health related policies for supporting the delivery of RMNCH interventions

Policy topic areas	Policy on
Constitutional and legal entitlements that support RMNCH	• Right to the highest attainable standard of health • Universal access to health care and services
Universal health coverage	• Adequate and sustainable RMNCH resource allocation and expenditure • Elimination of financial barriers • RMNCH resource reporting and tracking
Strategies, plans and mechanisms to guide implementation of RMNCH interventions and programs	• RMNCH strategies, plans and mechanisms • Evidence-based, equitable and quality RMNCH services • Health workforce • Essential health infrastructure and commodities
Community mobilization and engagement	• Community participation • Community mobilization and health education
Accountability for results	• Civil registration and vital statistics • Birth registration, death notification and maternal death reviews • Well-functioning health information systems, definition of key RMNCH indicators and targets • Multi-stakeholder data review
High-impact health interventions	• Quality care at birth • Immunization • Family planning

Source: World Health Organization, Geneva (2014).

This implies women and children have a legal entitlement to health, including access, and to achieve their highest health potential. In addition, a number of legal instruments specific to the health of women children have been negotiated, agreed upon and adopted by countries. Some of the most relevant legal instruments are the Universal Declaration of Human Rights (UN, 1948). The Convention on the Rights of the Child (Conventions on the Right of the Child, 1989) and the Convention on the Elimination of All Forms of Discrimination Against Women (CEDAW) among others (CEDAW, 1979).

To ensure an enabling policy environment for women's and children's health, national legal and policy frameworks must also specify guaranteed legislated access to the comprehensive package of essential interventions as highlighted by the GIF, as well as more costly specialized interventions (WHO, 2014). Brazil, for example, explicitly addresses 'health … and the protection of motherhood' in its Constitution (Ferraz, 2009). Nepal has similarly recognized every citizen's right to basic, free health services, economic, social and cultural rights — including the right to health (Bustreo and Hunt, 2014; Ministry of Health Ethopia *et al.*, 2014). Malawi, similarly a low-income country, has made tremendous progress in improving maternal and child health outcomes. Malawi's adoption of a democratic Constitution, which has a special provision for women and children, has been key to the promotion and protection of women's and children's health (Bustreo and Hunt, 2014).

Universal Health Coverage

Availability and access of health care by women and children underpins the goal of Universal Health Coverage (UHC) (WHO, 2014). UHC is meant to ensure that all people, including women and children, obtain the health services they need without experiencing financial hardship to pay for them. Access to health services enables women and children to be active contributors to their family. Protection from financial risks also prevents them from being pushed into poverty when they require essential services. UHC is thus a critical element of any effort to reduce social inequities and the hallmark of a government's commitment to improve the wellbeing of all citizens (WHO, 1946; 1978).

The policy framework should ensure that financing for RMNCH is sustainable and accounted for; this requires the identification of funding sources and provision for guidelines on mobilizing public and private resources for RMNCH. Policies also need to have mechanisms in place to demonstrate value for money and specify accountability (PMNCH, 2012; 2012a; 2012b; 2013; WHO, 2011a; 2010b). The policy framework and related instruments need to allow for specification and monitoring of per capita total expenditure and general government expenditure on RMNCH. Ideally this should be disaggregated by income level, age, place of residence, ethnic origin, etc., to identify any inequities and barriers to access (United Nations Foundation, 2015; WHO, 2001; 2010b, 2011; Organization of African Unity, 2001). RMNCH resources should also be reported and tracked to ensure support of RMNCH interventions. This includes policy provisions for RMNCH resource allocation and expenditure to be reported in a separate budget line. Ideally, National health Accounts must be able to track financial resources allocated to RMNCH. Particularly in instances where donors play an important role in financing health care, policies on resource reporting must set out requirements to formally establish how governments and partners will report commitments and disbursements — and, in particular, flows for RMNCH (IHP+, 2012; UN, 2011; World Bank *et al.*, 2003; WHO, 2008; 2011a; 2012). Only in this way policymakers and the public will be able to demonstrate that health needs of women and children's are met with resources.

The effectiveness of laws and how well a country manages difficulties within the health sector and beyond can lead to dramatic differences in health outcomes

Box 1. The impact of universal health coverage: Evidence from South and East Asia

Although not one of the 74 high burden countries, Thailand has had universal health coverage in place since 2002 and has achieved a health delivery model that reaches even the most remote areas. Interventions essential to child survival and maternal health, including free antenatal care, skilled birth attendance, family planning, and immunization reached universal coverage by the 1990's and all health MDGs were achieved by the early 1990's (Patcharanarumol *et al.*, 2011). Thailand's significant strides in the health sector have both benefitted from and arguably contributed to economic growth and poverty reduction in the country.

While classified as high burden countries for maternal and child mortality, in recent years Bangladesh and Vietnam have demonstrated strong leadership in the area of affordable health coverage for women and children. In Bangladesh, this has been achieved in part through a voucher scheme designed to improve access and utilization of maternal health services through the reduction of financial barriers and provision of incentives (Ahmed and Khan, 2011). The scheme has resulted in higher rates of skilled birth attendance, institutional deliveries and postnatal care visits, particularly among the poor (Hatt *et al.*, 2010). A program in Vietnam was created to increase access to health services for poor and marginalized sections of the population. Children under the age of six are target beneficiaries of the program and are issued a free card for accessing services. The program has been successful in increasing the utilization of services while reducing the risk of catastrophic out-of-pocket spending for an estimated 15 million people in the country (Ministry of Health Vietnam *et al.*, 2014).

between countries with similar per head income levels. The provision of universal health coverage provides particularly revealing evidence of what a country can achieve, despite income level (See Box 1) (Frenk and de Ferranti, 2012).

Policies for Effective Interventions, Equitable Coverage and Strong Health Workforce and Systems

Health strategies and plans are evidenced-based and address equity and quality

In order to make any progress in improving the health of women and children, the policies adopted by the health sector must be evidence-based, and ensure that essential RMNCH interventions are made available, accessible, acceptable and of quality. RMNCH interventions, indicators and targets need to be specified in the national health strategy and plan and also reflected in the overall national development plan and budget (AU, 2006; 2007; Organization of African Unity, 2001; Reports and Articles, 2014; UNSG, 2010; WHO, 2008; Wismar *et al.*, 2008). Policies also need to specify the involvement and approval process by key stakeholders and set out guidance for public–private partnerships (ECOSOC, 2007; IHP+, 2011; PMNCH, 2012c; WHO, 2011a). Cambodia has put in place policies and programs in part based on the development of technical standards and mechanisms for improving coordination of RMNCH interventions. Systems policies and program inputs have focused on better health care financing, the health workforce and using data for tracking progress. These efforts have improved access to essential RMNCH services and reduced inequity (Ministry of Health Cambodia *et al.*, 2014).

Policies that regulate planning processes in the health sector must allow for the development of plans that meet priority health needs for women and children. This can be done through people-centered, integrated approaches and by informing and encouraging women and children to stay healthy and prevent illness. Plans should address issues of availability, access and affordability of care and services, including access to evidence-based interventions and essential medicines and technologies to diagnose and treat medical problems. In Egypt, the government focused on reducing the risk factors causing maternal and neonatal deaths in the poorest areas of the country (Ministry of Health Egypt *et al.*, 2014). This was achieved through interventions that integrated policy, technical management and community-based factors. These efforts contributed to better access to essential obstetric and neonatal care for over 2.6 million women of reproductive age and 660,000 children under 5.

The ability to access services is oftentimes greatly influenced by socioeconomic status. A large part of the unfinished business in RMNCH is addressing pervasive inequity and ensuring that all women and children receive the services they need, regardless of differences in wealth, gender, ethnic group or geography. Among the 74 countries that globally count for 95% or maternal and child deaths, the coverage score of RMNCH essential interventions among the richest — generally above 60%, and often above 80% — far exceeds coverage among the poor. If such high coverage can be achieved among the wealthy, it should be possible to do the same across the whole population (Reports and Articles, 2014). Health Policies aiming to improve the health of women and children must assure that their needs are addressed despite their socioeconomic status. These policies should make provisions for equitable access to evidence based interventions and appropriate care, and make it possible for them to participate in decisions affecting their care. To do so, policies need to be in place to address the access barriers for women and children.

An enabling policy environment must make provisions to ensure well-known evidence-based interventions are part of any service delivery package or platform for women and children. This is also the case for high-impact interventions, including immunization, quality care at birth and family planning. Globally agreed evidence-based guidelines, standards and protocols must inform national policies and standards on quality of RMNCH care; these must also be periodically updated and integrated into training materials (Fervers *et al.*, 2006; Moran *et al.*, 2012; WHO, 2011b). Policies must ensure that all RMNCH interventions are delivered with quality and reach all women and children in need. Policies that regulate service delivery must allow for local adaptation of RMNCH interventions. In order to respect cultural preferences, the Ministry of Health in Peru approved regulation to allow women to exert the right to choose their preferred delivery position. This enabled health care facilities to accommodate vertical childbirth. The strategy has contributed to an increase in institutional delivery rates in rural areas (Ministry of Health Peru *et al.*, 2014).

Policies must include mechanisms to allow for quality assessment, improvement and assurance. In Cambodia, the government implemented multiple approaches to sector-wide management and has subsequently improved coordination for financing of health services. This approach has improved the development of guidelines, planning and tracking progress in specific RMNCH areas and has helped ensure that development partners align with government priorities and plans. It has also contributed to increased resource allocation and action in RMNCH (Ministry of Health Cambodia *et al.*, 2014).

In Bangladesh, health sector development strategies have shifted the focus of health and population programmes towards a sector-wide approach and the decentralisation of delivery of essential service packages (Ministry of Health Bangladesh *et al.*, 2014). As a result, remarkable improvements were achieved primarily through better vaccine coverage, improved access to family planning, policies focused on newborn health interventions, emergency obstetrical care, making prenatal care and births more affordable, and the expansion of the IT sector (Ministry of Health Bangladesh *et al.*, 2014). Rapid progress was possible due in large part to different actors across society collaborating for the improvement of women's and children's health.

Workforce policies that enhance RMNCH outcomes

A competent health workforce is one of the most critical determinants of the survival of women and children. Many countries suffer from an insufficient workforce either because it is too small or because workers are not in the right place at the right time. Therefore, it is very important that workforce policies that regulate the numbers, deployment and retention of the workforce at all levels of the health-care system (i.e., referral, first level and community, in all geographic areas) take into consideration RMNCH needs. Implementation plans must also be costed and linked to the national health workforce strategic plan. Policies must set out standards for retaining and motivating the health workforce, including public and private health workers, in a way that responds to RMNCH goals and targets (GHWA, 2008; 2011; WHO, 2006; 2010c; 2011c; 2012a).

Workforce policies in relation to RMNCH must respond to the contexts they serve. This requires that the regulatory policy framework specifies what each cadre of the health workforce is authorized to provide. In many countries where scaling up of provision of RMNCH services by health professionals across all levels and geographies is not yet possible, innovative strategies around health workforce must be explored. Rwanda has developed an innovative approach to reduce RMNCH workforce shortages in the country. Over 45,000 Community Health Workers (CHWs) provide essential health services at the village level. CHWs are in charge of integrated case management of childhood illness and family planning. Female community health works are in charge of maternal and new-born care. Health facility staff and CHWs receive financial incentives in addition to their monthly salary. These incentives enhance staff commitment and quality standards, and are based on health service delivery (Ministry of Health Rwanda *et al.*, 2014). Similarly, in Ethiopia, salaried health extension workers implement a community-based care program. These workers are mostly female and selected by their communities (Ministry of Health Ethopia *et al.*, 2014a).

Box 2 provides an example of how Rwanda has developed a triple planning approach to address immediate needs with community health workers, investing in the long-term vision of a professional health workforce and building capacity to adapt to change and emergencies (Ministry of Health Rwanda *et al.*, 2014).

Box 2.

The government of Rwanda has increased its efforts to address the challenge of the human resource shortage through various reforms and initiatives. After the genocide, in 1994, Rwanda deployed community health workers (CHWs) and volunteers for urgent health needs. Rwanda's 45,000 CHWs provide essential health services at the village level. At the same time, Rwanda promoted investments in a long-term vision to build its professional health workforce and health facilities with medical colleges, referral hospitals and international academic and professional collaborations (HRH, 2014; Ministry of Health Rwanda *et al.*, 2014; Van Rooyen *et al.*, 1997).

Box 3. Improving the quality of health care in China and Lao

In the 1990's, the 'contract responsibility system' and 'target responsibility agreements' were introduced in China to improve the quality of health care at all levels, as well as to monitor supply-side performance. The contract responsibility system primarily focuses on the Expanded Programme of Immunization and Prenatal Care. The target agreements were signed between the country health bureau, the township health centre, and the country MCH hospital to monitor their performance on delivery and services (Ministry of Health China *et al.*, 2014).

In Lao, an essential medicine list for all RMNCH activities has been defined and overseen by a Food and Drug Administration. A Medical Product Supply Centre is responsible for logistics managements. Monthly reports on stock availability are reported to the Centre for tracking. This has helped establish a unified centralized system that has improved the availability and quality of drugs in the country at all levels (Ministry of Health Lao PDR *et al.*, 2014).

Policy to regulate infrastructure and commodities for RMNCH

There is essential infrastructure required for effective, timely and equitable delivery of RMNCH services and commodities — both within and outside the health sector. A large population of pregnant women may have access to childbirth services, however, if health workers lack essential medicines and commodities necessary to deliver the RMNCH interventions, the positive impact from having and accessing these services remains uncertain. Likewise, there is no quality service if essential health infrastructure, facilities and appropriate commodities are not in place. Without quality, the chances of reducing maternal and child health mortality are very low. Therefore, policies must make provisions for services to be and remain of quality and supported by adequate resources (see Box 3).

Community Mobilization and Engagement

Women and children are critical members of the community and key drivers of social, economic and environmental development. Over 500 million women have joined the workforce over the previous three decades as a result of better female education, improved access to contraception and improved gender equity (World Bank, 2012). For example, increased use of family planning leads to fewer births and deaths, and reduces population pressure with a range of environmental benefits. In high fertility countries, rates of return from better access to contraception are estimated to exceed 8% of GDP by 2035 (Frenk and de Ferranti, 2012). In fact, declining fertility rates and increasing child survival explain 30% to 50% of South-Eastern Asia's dramatic economic growth between 1965 and 1990 (Bloom and Williamson, 1997). Improved nutrition of women and children reduces stunting and low birthweight — this leads to healthier adults with the potential for long-term economic productivity with intergenerational benefits. Today's healthy children are tomorrow's workforce; they will grow up to be more productive citizens with a higher lifetime earning potential than those who are not (Presern, 2013).

Nonetheless, social norms oftentimes may make it more difficult for women and children to participate in decisions that affect their health and the health of their families, as well as access and use services when and where needed. Ensuring community awareness and participation, including that of women and children, is therefore a starting point for many countries to improve health. An enabling policy for women's and children's health is one that allows for them to participate, be informed and make decisions about what kind of care they need and how they access it. Information sharing, education and peer support are necessary to unblock social and cultural bottlenecks to health provision for women and children. Health sector policies, and more specifically RMNCH-related policies, must clearly provide opportunities for communities to participate in tailoring health sector's response to their health needs. Improving utilization and eliminating delays in care requires communities to be empowered and engaged in RMNCH. Mechanisms must be set out by policies to allow community involvement and broad stakeholder consultation on RMNCH-strategies, implementation and evaluation at different levels of the health system (Marston *et al.*, 2013; McCoy *et al.*, 2012). In designing these policies, communities should help to define and prioritize local RMNCH priorities and be fully aware of the short- and long-term consequence of women and children's health. When communities feel ownership of interventions and outcomes, access to RMNCH improves. Oftentimes equity issues are masked at the national level. Community engagement can help to promote better outcomes across the country. It can also illuminate potential grassroots sources of funding and resource mobilization (AU, 2013). Community health workers in Rwanda are essential in the increased registration of births and maternal and child deaths in the country. Likewise, community committees monitor and report on health service provision (Ministry of Health Rwanda *et al.*, 2014). In Bangladesh, a remarkable decline in fertility has been due in part to campaigns to increase demand for family planning services. Female frontline community health workers have been central to this effort by brining a range of contraceptive options and information to the doorsteps of village households (Ministry of Health Bangladesh *et al.*, 2014).

Policies on community mobilization and health education must set out key messages, channels, activities and audiences based on priority areas of the RMNCH strategies. Furthermore, policy guidance and provisions must be made to ensure financial, staffing, administration and infrastructure resources to support community mobilization and engagement (see Boxes 4 and 5) (Lassi *et al.*, 2010; Lee *et al.*, 2009; Ottawa, 1986; Prost *et al.*, 2013; Storey *et al.*, 2011; WHO, 2010d; 2012a).

Box 4. Advocating for better health through the media

A mass-media campaign in Cambodia was developed by the MoH and the National Centre for Health Promotion, focusing on the themes of diarrhoea, acute respiratory illness, immunization and child nutrition. It included the promotion of early initiation and exclusive breastfeeding (Ottawa, 1986; UN, 1948; WHO, 2008a; 2010d) and pre- and postnatal care. Communication methods included: TV spots with messages on exclusive breastfeeding emphasizing that "not even water" should be given to young infants; radio spots using a "breastfeeding song"; and a 24-episode TV soap opera, which included breastfeeding messages. As a result of these efforts, the proportion of respondents who believed children should receive food or liquids other than breast milk decreased from 60% to 18% and knowledge of immediate breastfeeding increased from 38% to 67%. Health system support to train health staff in nutrition and breastfeeding topics also began in earnest in the early 2000s with efforts to scale up training to all health staff over the next decade (Ministry of Health Cambodia *et al.*, 2014).

Box 5. Community-based solutions to efficient service delivery

In Nepal, there has also been an important emphasis on community-based approaches to deliver maternal and child health services, and to address human resource shortages and the challenges of remote areas (Ministry of Health Nepal *et al.*, 2014). Targeted free health care services and programs to improve community engagement and empowerment have also been used to reach poor, marginalized, socially excluded and underserved populations. For example, the use of nearly 50,000 female community health volunteers to provide community-based care in Nepal has further relieved the burden. This includes the community-based integrated management of childhood illness program (Ministry of Health Nepal *et al.*, 2014).

Accountability for Results

Oversight and accountability are key to improving women's and children's health. Accountability allows transparency on the timeliness of how resources are spent and where and whether desired results are achieved (United Nations Foundations, 2015). Countries must be able to develop and implement policies that allow for this accountability to happen (UN, 2011). Enacting accountability implies working in three policy areas: monitoring, review, and remedy (or action). First, any health related policy must provide for the monitoring of the results that it aims to achieve. In this way it can be established what is happening, where and to whom. The MDGs monitoring provided countries with an entry point to streamline the information and metrics used for women's and children's health. However, this is not enough. Health policies, especially those related to monitoring and regulating health of women and children must make provisions that allow for the information to be analyzed and reviewed. In this way it is possible to learn if plans have been implemented as designed and what was achieved. Finally, policies need to provide for enacting accountability and remedy (or action); this allows for putting things right when and where necessary.

A starting point in the accountability for women and children's health is civil registration and vital statistics. Changes and improvements in the health of women and children will not be measured if all births, deaths and their underlining causes are not accounted for. It is a human right for anyone to be registered at birth and have a birth certificate. However, in many countries children arrive at their 18th birthday without ever being registered or acknowledged and, as a result, are denied access to health, education and society. An enabling policy environment will ensure that by law all births are registered within 24 hours of delivery or as soon as possible thereafter (up to 1 month), including notification of stillbirths (Child, 2011).

Another crucial part of vital information is death registration and notification. The policy must indicate that all maternal, newborn and child deaths should be registered within 24 hours of death with the cause of death recorded using most updated ICD codes (Health Metrics Network and WHO, 2008). Interrelated to death notification are policies that require the review of maternal and child deaths. These policies exist in many countries, however, in many parts of the world where the number of deaths is unaccounted for they need to be further strengthened and implemented at scale. The reason behind this is that policies on review of cause of death for mothers and children and reasons that brought about tragedies, have the potential to save the lives of many more by identifying the gaps in accessing and using the services in addition to gaps in their quality and response. Death reviews require an analysis of the circumstances of each maternal and child death, identification of avoidable factors, and actions to improve

Box 6. Ensuring accountability for health in Nepal

In Nepal, a country without a functioning vital registration system, data from censuses, studies and surveys are used to monitor mortality rates and inform program design. A national health management information system tracks service use, enables monitoring of results and shaping of priorities and plans. Disaggregated data are used to assess progress against targets. Areas of poor performance are flagged during annual reviews so that action can be taken. Maternal death reviews have also been used to understand the causes of institutional deaths in selected referral hospitals and there are efforts to link findings to government policy decisions (Ministry of Health Nepal *et al.*, 2014).

care at all levels of the health system — from home to hospital. Nepal provides a good look at how collecting accurate and reliable health information demands long-term political commitment and investment (Box 6). (PMNCH, 2013a; WHO *et al.*, 2004; 2010). Likewise, Egypt provides an excellent example of how results from a mortality survey helped to launch a national campaign to improve maternal health (See Box 7).

Box 7. Using evidence to promote maternal health in Egypt

As political momentum for maternal and child health in Egypt was building in the early 1990's, the results from the Maternal Mortality Survey (MMS) 1993 provided an important platform and momentum from which comprehensive programs were launched to address not only maternal but also child health. Results from the MMS highlighted the majority of maternal deaths in the country were avoidable. In response, an essential package of maternal and child health services and standards were developed for antenatal and postnatal care, delivery, obstetric care, neonatal care, and preventive services for child health. Results from the MMS also ushered in a wide range of activities to raise standards through improved training and supervision, and by upgrading facilities and equipment. An enabling policy environment had been created under which investments in social and economic development were being made. The MMS also enabled the Government of Egypt to tackle health-system wide problems including making linkages between antenatal, delivery and postpartum care, strengthening referral systems, ensuring improved oversight and regulation of the private sector, reducing deficiencies in hospital management and systems, and better training (Ministry of Health Egypt *et al.*, 2014).

Multisectoral Policies and Women's and Children's Health

The GIF clearly recognizes the interdependency between health results for women and children and the broader determinants of social and economic development. While the policies and policy making related to these broader determinants may well be beyond the immediate scope and practice of implementation of RMNCH programs, it is of a paramount importance to recognize them and pay special attention. This section highlights some of the key determinants and sectors influencing women's and children's health and the policies required to address them. We focus on the broad area of inclusive economic development and governance, as well as specific sectors and policies that directly influence and impact health for women and children.

Although the health sector may be primarily responsible for delivering health care, experience demonstrates that long-term health improvements require actions from all parts of society. The most successful countries are those that have had strong political vision and guiding principles, who have implemented evidence-based policies and strategies for decision-making and accountability, and have financed investments within and beyond the health sector. (Kuruvilla *et al.*, 2014). In fact, as much as 50% of the reduction in maternal and child mortality in low- and middle-income countries since 1990 occurred from health-influencing sectors such as education, WASH, gender (including women's political and economic participation, infrastructure (including roads, electricity and technologies) (Ministry of Health Rwanda *et al.*, 2014).

While economic growth underpins multisectoral progress, it is not sufficient (Bishai *et al.*, 2014). In particular, economic development must be inclusive if it is to reduce poverty, hunger, improve environmental sustainability and promote peace and security. Over the last two decades, it has not necessarily been countries with the highest Gross National Product (GNP) that have improved their RMNCH, but rather countries that have demonstrated strong policies within and outside the health sector to promote equitable growth and health outcomes (Frenk and de Ferrante, 2012). Cambodia offers a good example of how policies outside the health sector focused on disadvantaged populations have supported sustainable development in the country (Box 8).

Good Governance

Good governance and, in particular, control of corruption is associated with better health comes and especially in the area of women's and children's health (Kuruvilla *et al.*, 2014). Good governance enables effective policy making and helps to ensure the quality of public services and policy formulation, as well as

Box 8. Investing in the poor in Cambodia

In Cambodia, policies to reduce poverty and support pro-poor development reinforced improvements in people's existing work, i.e., principally cultivation of land and labor. Poverty reduction was driven by policies that removed price controls and taxes on rice production — the country's staple crop. Policies to improve rural infrastructure, including roads, communication and rural irrigation also lead to better productivity. Improvements in industrial production were driven by business-friendly industrial policies, which promoted investments in industry. (Ministry of Health Cambodia *et al.*, 2014). Maternal and child mortality have declined in the country due in part to reduced poverty and improved infrastructure.

implementation and evaluation (Transparency Accountability Initiative, 2011). Political vision and social commitment at all levels in society are important for improving women's, children's and adolescents' health. In particular, political direction and leadership needs to reach a critical mass to effect national change. Guiding principles such as human rights and aid effectiveness help shape government strategies, align stakeholder action and orient progress towards agreed results. Ensuring value for money is also a key feature of enabling governance. Countries such as Bangladesh, Ethiopia, Kyrgyzstan, India and Thailand that have shown greatest improvements in women's and children's health over the past 20 years are also those countries that improved health outcomes despite relatively low levels of investment (Kuruvilla *et al.*, 2014; Patcharanarumol *et al.*, 2011).

Rwanda has prioritized good governance and made it a pillar of its policy-making towards equitable social and economic development. There is a government-wide emphasis on cross-sector collaboration, decentralization, the sector-wide approach (SWAP) framework, and better accountability between the local and national level. Rwanda's performance-based environment and zero tolerance policy on corruption have further strengthened accountability among actors and institutions. The Government of Rwanda has also instituted a national gender policy, structures to empower women and to prevent gender-based violence. Female representation within the parliament is high, with women currently holding a majority of seats (64% in the lower house and 40% in the Senate) (Ministry of Health Rwanda *et al.*, 2014).

Although it can be difficult to establish causal links between policy and program inputs and health impact, studies have shown that among countries that have made rapid progress, 50% was accredited to investments outside of the health sector. These sectors are often referred to as 'health-enhancing sectors' (Kuruvilla *et al.*, 2014). Efforts to reduce preventable maternal and child deaths require country-level planning that adopts a multisectoral approach across these different sectors. It is the broader socio-economic and cultural context that defines the behavior towards and access to health by communities, families and, by women and children. This means health sector policies alone are not sufficient to improve the health of women and children. Countries that are making accelerated progress towards improving health related MDGs, are also making progress on most of the other MDGs, including to decrease poverty and hunger, improve education, gender quality and environmental sustainability (Kuruvilla *et al.*, 2014).

Despite these findings, quantifying the specific impact of 'health-enhancing sectors' remains a challenge. However, among all the multisectoral policies, the GIF specifically recognizes and quantifies women's and children's health gains that can be made by working in three areas: nutrition, education and water and sanitation (Figure 1).

Nutrition

Adequate nutrition remains a very important determinant of health for women and children. Malnutrition in all forms is a major contributor to disease and early deaths for women and children. Undernutrition can lead to health problems across generations, particularly among the most vulnerable populations (PMNCH, 2014). Roughly half of all deaths among children under the age of are due to undernutrition. In 42 of the 62 *Countdown* countries where data are available, more than 30% of children are stunted (Reports and Articles, 2014). Likewise, poor nutrition harms women's health and increases the risk of stillbirths and low birth weight babies (Reports and Articles, 2014). Regulations and strategies should protect the right of all to have access to sufficient, safe, affordable, and nutritious food. Policymakers should make sure these policies provide a package of nutrition-specific and culturally sensitive, cost-effective, evidence-based interventions, such as the promotion of exclusive breastfeeding, access to supplements and fortification, and therapeutic feeding for severe undernutrition. Furthermore, nutrition literacy should be promoted from school age, and communities need to have adequate information about how to prepare adequately nutrient-dense food, particularly for children (PMNCH, 2014).

Particularly in poor, rural areas proper nutrition provision can be a major challenge to improving health outcomes. In Lao, government policies to promote better food security and nutrition in highland areas support farmer organizations and are working to increase commercialization of the agricultural sector and provide better support for the production of cash crops (Ministry of Health Lao

PDR *et al.*, 2014). In Ethiopia, the National Nutrition Programme uses multisector partnerships to tackle undernutrition through social protection, food security, community nutrition programs, micronutrient supplementation, treatment of severe acute malnutrition and a package of free health services. The country is now on track to achieve MDG 1C to reduce hunger (Ministry of Health Lao PDR *et al.*, 2014).

Education

Schooling and education are critical determinants that define health of a population in general and that of women and children in particular. It is through school and in school where the young generation gets its information about health and healthy life. Girls' education and the length of their schooling are closely related to increased child survival, lower fertility rates, higher levels of employment for women and income generation. Therefore, any policy that encourages universal education for girls and boys, and which provides mechanisms to assure that girls can attend school as long as possible throughout their teenage years, will have only a positive impact in the health of women and children. Although largely ignored by the broader public health discourse, early childhood education is another key aspect of education. The higher the quality of education, the better are the health and economic outcomes. Policies must ensure that health education is part of the broader education agenda, which is regulated and monitored. For this to happen, policies must set out regulations and strategies to protect the right of all children to education, including ensuring every child has access to and completes pre-primary and primary education and access to lower secondary education. Availability and access to education services should be improved through infrastructure, human resources, adequate financing, and addressing social, cultural and other barriers to attendance. Also, skills gaps, such as gender and urban/rural gaps in the use of new technologies have to be tackled through policies (UN, 1948; Conventions on the Rights of the Child, 1989; UNESCO, 1990; WHO, 2011d; World Education Forum, 2000).

Ethiopia has seen unprecedented expansion of its education system. Better access to education has worked to reduce the gender gap, especially among the poorest and almost full gender parity has been achieved in schools. Many factors have contributed to better access to education in Ethiopia, including sustained government commitment. Ethiopia has also endorsed pro-poor education policies such as abolition of school fees for primary and lower secondary schools; alternative basic education for out-of-school children in remote areas; adult literacy programs; and school feeding programs (Ministry of Health Ethiopia *et al.*, 2014).

Water and Sanitation

Access to clean water and sanitation facilities translates into direct health and economic benefits. Women and children usually bare the burden of water collection and are at greatest risk to personal safety and health in the absence of appropriate sanitation facilities. Worldwide, 780 million individuals lack access to improved (drinking-water) and 2.5 billion lack improved sanitation. Diarrhoea due to infection is widespread throughout developing countries. Diarrhoeal disease is the second leading cause of death in children under 5 years old. Each year diarrhea kills around 7,60,000 children under 5 years of age while globally, there are nearly 1.7 billion cases of diarrhoeal disease every year (WHO, 2015). A causal relationship has been established between access to water supply and higher-income levels. This means that better access to water and basic sanitation services can actually drive economic growth. In the poorest countries where there is improved access to clean water and sanitation services, annual average growth has been found to be 3.6% higher than in similarly poor countries without improved access (WHO, 2004). These include economic gains generated due to less time being ill, fewer health sector and patient costs due to less treatment of diarrhoeal diseases, and the value of prevented deaths (Hutton, 2004). The economic benefits of making these improvements nearly always outweighs the costs, and in same cases, by orders of magnitude (Hutton, 2004).

Vietnam demonstrates the benefits of upgrading infrastructure for drinking water and sanitation to serve all levels of society. As part of its multisector effort to improve nutrition, the country has focused on better sanitation and improved supplies of safe drinking water. Improved access has also been equitable and the gap between rural and urban populations with access to improved water sources has grown smaller. By 2010, 93% of the rural population had access to an improved drinking-water source, compared to 99% of the urban population (Ministry of Health Vietnam *et al.*, 2014).

Discussion/Conclusions

An enabling policy environment is required to make the best investments both within and outside the health sector. Together with good governance, it is an essential starting point for reaching women and children in all socio-economic and geographic strata of society. Also required are investments for women's and children's health to be made with human rights as a key-driver, in addition to social and economic benefits. Unfortunately, of the countries with the highest burden of maternal and child deaths, some key policies related to maternal and child health are not widely in place (Conventions on the Rights of the child, 1989). This gives us an idea of country progress in adopting key policy measures required to improve maternal and child health outcomes — and there is much more work to be done. We have discussed here the importance of addressing reproductive, maternal and child health to improve the lives and health of women and children around the world. Many women and children in the lowest income countries now bare a triple burden of ill health related to pregnancy and childbirth, to communicable diseases, and to the rise in non-communicable diseases.

Health policies are at the core of informing and shaping health improvements. Multisector policies are similarly at the heart of accelerating positive health outcomes, particularly for women and children. It is the shared goals and investments, both within and outside the health sector, which can produce sustainable health outcomes. Trying to implement only health interventions without social mobilization or promoting economic development without addressing social and health dimensions will never yield full health benefits. Best results are achieved when all sectors are working in synergy. This goes back to the shared vision of equitable and sustainable development in the post-2015 era. This requires social, economic and environmental action and investing in the right strategies, in the right context, and at the right level as a pre-condition of achieving the post-2015 vision.

The Global Investment Framework for Women's and Children's Health, together with the Policy Guide for Implementing Essential Interventions for Reproductive, Maternal, Newborn and Child Health, can assist countries in identifying investments that drive forward the impact of national health and development plans. Together they show us that it is possible to understand, estimate and ultimately improve the health of women and children. In this way, it becomes possible to improve economic development and the health of entire generations. Investments in health are not only highly affordable but generate a multitude of health and economic benefits — this makes them of excellent value. Making greater investments in children's health leads to better educated and more productive adults. This leads to better demographic outcomes as healthier children will be more productive over the course of their lifetime. Investing in health can help break the poverty-cycle and thus is a key mechanism for reducing the intergenerational transmission of poverty (Belli *et al.*, 2005). Policies and policymakers that communicate the importance of investing in health and monitor such investments will help countries become more accountable for the health and well-being of their citizens. A high level of communication also promotes the essential cross-sector collaboration that is necessary to produce full health benefits. Strong policies and leadership can also help to overcome the many institutional barriers that often exist with multisector collaboration (Kuruvilla *et al.*, 2014).

Despite global campaigns to raise awareness and funding for the health of women and children, investments are insufficient. The GIF helps us further demonstrate not only the many benefits of investing in RMNCH, but also the continued social and economic losses of not investing enough, or adequately. Women and children will continue to die in unacceptably high numbers of preventable illnesses, medical costs continue to rise and productivity remains low. Making the case for investing in women's and children's health, therefore, is also making a case for strengthening social and economic development.

Tremendous progress has been made in reducing preventable deaths among women and children over the past 20 years. Globally, maternal and child mortality have been reduced by nearly 50% (United Nations Foundations, 2015). This demonstrates that change is possible. Nonetheless, the MDGs 4 and 5 will not be met by all countries by 2015. More investment is needed to ensure the success that has been made over the past 20 years can continue. There are many encouraging examples of countries that have been successful in reducing maternal and child deaths under challenging circumstances, while improving overall health and wellbeing of women and children. Many of the countries highlighted in this chapter improved health outcomes for women and children despite low health expenditures and GDP per capita. Oftentimes these gains have been made in the face of political and socioeconomic challenges. What these countries help demonstrate is that making gains in health is not about how much money is invested but *how* the money is invested. The GIF shows how investments in a range of essential packages with high impact are key to reducing mortality. Good governance, political will and a sensible allocation of resources are crucial requirements for the Sustainable Development Goals being developed for the post-2015 agenda. With the right leadership, desire, policies and action, substantial improvements in women's and children's health can and will be made over the next 20 years.

References

Ahmed S, Khan MM. 2011. Is demand-side financing equity enhancing? Lessons from a maternal health voucher scheme in Bangladesh. *Social Science & Medicine* 72: 1704–1710.

AU. 2006. Maputo Plan of Action: Universal Access to Comprehensive Sexual and Reproductive Health Services in Africa.

AU. 2007. CARMMA. African Health Strategy. (African Union, Johannesburg).

AU. 2013. Policy Brief: Community Engagement and Reproductive, Maternal, Newborn and Child Health. AU, Johannesburg.

Belli PC, Bustreo F, Preker A. 2005. Investing in children's health: What are the economic benefits? *Bulletin of the World Health Organization* 83: 777–784, doi:/S0042-96862005001000015.

Bishai D, Cohen R, Alfonso YN, Adam T, Kuruvilla S, Schweitzer J. 2014. Factors contributing to child mortality reductions in 142 low- and middle- income countries between 1990 and 2010. Paper presented at the *Population Association of America, Annual Meeting, Boston*. Available at http://www.thelancet.com/pdfs/journals/lancet/PIIS0140-6736(14)60075-1.pdf.

Bloom DE, Williamson JG. 1997. Demographic transitions and economic miracles in emerging Asia. National Bureau of Economic Research, *NBER Working Paper No.* 6268.

Bustreo F, Hunt P. 2014. Women's and Children's Health: Evidence of Impact of Human Rights. (World Health Organization, Geneva, 2014).

CEDAW. 1979. Convention on the Elimination of all forms of Discrimination against Women (CEDAW).

Child EWE. 2011. Commission on Information and Accountability for Women's and Children's Health.

Convention on the Rights of the Child. (1989). Available at https://treaties.un.org/pages/viewdetails.aspx?src=treaty&mtdsg_no=iv-11&chapter=4&lang=en.

ECOSOC. 2007. United Nations Public–Private Alliance for Rural Development: Resolution 2007/36. (ed World Bank) (Washington DC, 2014).

European Observatory on Health Systems and Policies. Health Targets in Europe: Learning from Experience. (World Health Organization, Geneva, 2008).

Every Woman Every Child. Global Strategy 2.0. (United Nations Foundation, Washington DC, 2015).

Ferraz OL. 2009. The right to health in the courts of Brazil: Worsening health inequities? *Health and Human Rights* 11: 33–45.

Fervers B, *et al.* 2006. Adaptation of clinical guidelines: Literature review and proposition for a framework and procedure. *International Journal for Quality in Health Care: Journal of the International Society for Quality in Health Care/ISQua* 18: 167–176, doi:10.1093/intqhc/mzi108.

Frenk J, de Ferranti D. 2012. Universal health coverage: Good health, good economics. *Lancet* 380: 862–864. doi:10.1016/S0140-6736(12)61341-5.

Fulfilling the Health Agenda for Women and Children. *The 2014 Report, Countdown to 2015.* Available at http://www.countdown2015mnch.org/documents/2014Report/Countdown_to_2015-Fulfilling%20the%20Health_Agenda_for_Women_and_Children-The_2014_Report-Conference_Draft.pdf.

GHWA. 2008. The Kampala Declaration and Agenda for Global Action. (WHO/GHWA, Geneva, 2008).

GHWA. 2011. Workforce Country Coordination and Facilitation. (WHO, Geneva, 2011).

Hatt L, *et al.* 2010. Economic Evaluation of Demand-Side Financing (DSF) for Maternal Health in Bangladesh. Bethesda MD: Review, Analysis and Assessment of Issues Related to Health Care Financing and Health Economics in Bangladesh, Abt Associates Inc.

Health Metrics Network and WHO. 2008. Framework and Standards for Country Health Information Systems. Second Edition. WHO, Geneva, 2008.

HRH. 2014. *Human Resources for Health Program Rwanda: Program Overview*, <http://www.hrhconsortium.moh.gov.rw/about-hrh/program-overview/>.

Hutton GHL. 2004. Evaluation of the Costs and Benefits of Water and Sanitation Improvements at the Global Level. WHO, Geneva.

IHP+. 2011. Joint Assessment of National Health Strategies and Plans. Version 2.

IHP+. Developing a Country Compact: What Does It Take and What are the Gains. (International Health Partnership, London, 2012).

Jamison DT, *et al.* 2013. Global health. 2035: A world converging within a generation. *Lancet* 382: 1898–1955. doi:10.1016/S0140-6736(13)62105-4.

Kuruvilla S, *et al.* 2014. Success factors for reducing maternal and child mortality. *Bulletin of the World Health Organization* 92: 533–544B. doi:10.2471/BLT.14.138131.

Lassi ZS, Haider BA, Bhutta ZA. 2010. Community-based intervention packages for reducing maternal and neonatal morbidity and mortality and improving neonatal outcomes. *The Cochrane Database of Systematic Reviews*, CD007754. doi:10.1002/14651858.CD007754.pub2.

Lee AC, *et al.* 2009. Linking families and facilities for care at birth: What works to avert intrapartum-related deaths? *International Journal of Gynaecology and Obstetrics: The Official Organ of the International Federation of Gynaecology and Obstetrics* 107 (Suppl. 1), S65–S85, S86–S68. doi:10.1016/j.ijgo.2009.07.012.

Marston C, RA, McGowan CR, Portela A. 2013. Effects of community participation on improving uptake of skilled care for maternal and newborn health: A systematic review. *Community Participation Systematic Review* 8: 1–9.

McCoy DC, Hall JA, Ridge M. 2012. A systematic review of the literature for evidence on health facility committees in low- and middle-income countries. *Health Policy and Planning* 27: 449–466, doi:10.1093/heapol/czr077.

Ministry of Health Bangladesh, P, WHO, World Bank, AHPSR and Participants in the Bangladesh Multistakeholder Policy Review. 2014. Success Factors for Women's and Children's Health: Bangladesh. (PMNCH, Geneva, 2014).

Ministry of Health Cambodia, P, WHO, World Bank, AHPSR and Participants in the Cambodia Multistakeholder Policy Review. 2014. Success Factors for Women's and Children's Health: Cambodia. (PMNCH, Geneva, 2014).

Ministry of Health China P, WHO, World Bank, AHPSR and Participants in the China Multistakeholder Policy Review. 2014. Success Factors for Women's and Children's Health: China. (PMNCH, Geneva, 2014).

Ministry of Health Egypt P, WHO, World Bank, and AHPSR and Participants in the Egypt Multistakeholder Policy Review. 2014. Success Factors for Women's and Children's Health: Egypt. (PMNCH, Geneva, 2014).

Ministry of Health Ethiopia, P, WHO, World Bank, AHPSR and Participants in the Ethiopia Multistakeholder Policy Review. 2014. Success Factors for Women's and Children's Health: Ethiopia. (PMNCH, Geneva, 2014).

Ministry of Health Lao PDR, P, WHO, World Bank, AHPSR and Participants in the Lao PDR Multistakeholder Policy Review. 2014. Success Factors for Women's and Children's Health: Lao PDR. (PMNCH, Geneva, 2014).

Ministry of Health Nepal, P, WHO, World Bank, AHPSR and Participants in the Nepal Multistakeholder Policy Review. 2014. Success Factors for Women's and Children's Health: Nepal. PMNCH, Geneva, 2014.

Ministry of Health Peru P, WHO, World Bank, AHPSR and Participants in the Peru Multistakeholder Policy Review. 2014. Success Factors for Women's and Children's Health: Peru. (PMNCH, Geneva, 2014).

Ministry of Health Rwanda, P, WHO, World Bank, AHPSR and Participants in the Rwanda Multistakeholder Policy Review. 2014. Success Factors for Women's and Children's Health: Rwanda (PMNCH, Geneva, 2014).

Ministry of Health Vietnam & PMNCH, W., World Bank, AHPSR and Participants in the Viet Nam Multistakeholder Policy Review. 2014. Success Factors for Women's and Children's Health: Viet Nam (PMNCH, Geneva, 2014).

Moran AC, *et al.* 2012. Benchmarks to measure readiness to integrate and scale up newborn survival interventions. *Health Policy and Planning* 27(Suppl 3), iii29–39. doi:10.1093/heapol/czs046.

Organization of African Unity. 2001. Abuja declaration on HIV/AIDS, Tuberculosis, and other infectious diseases.

Ottawa. 1986. The Ottawa Charter for Health Promotion. First International Conference on Health Promotion.

Patcharanarumol W, Tangcharoensathien V, Limwattananon S, Panichkriangkrai W, Pachanee K, Poungkantha W, *et al.* 2011. In McKee M, Balabanova D, Mills A. (eds.). *'Good Health at Low Cost': 25 Years On: What Makes a Successful Health System?* (The London School of Hygiene & Tropical Medicine, 2011).

PMNCH I. 2012c. Private Enterprise for Public Health. Every Women Every Child. (Geneva, 2012).

PMNCH. 2011a. A Global Review of the Key Interventions Related to Reproductive, Maternal, Newborn and Child Health (RMNCH). (The Partnership for Maternal, Newborn & Child Health, Geneva, 2011a).

PMNCH. 2011b. Essential Interventions, Commodities and Guidelines for RMNCH. A Global Review of the Key Interventions Related to Reproductive, Maternal, Newborn and Child Health (RMNCH). (The Partnership for Reproductive, Maternal, Newborn & Child Health, Geneva, 2011b).

PMNCH. 2012. Promising Mechanisms to Strengthen Domestic Financing for Women's and Children's Health. (Partnership for Maternal, Newborn and Child Health, Geneva, 2012).

PMNCH. 2012a. Knowledge Summary 21: Strengthen National Financing. (Partnership for Maternal, Newborn and Child Health, Geneva, 2012).

PMNCH. 2012b. Knowledge Summary: Nutrition. PMNCH, Geneva.

PMNCH. 2012b. Financing Access to RMNCH Interventions for Universal Health Coverage SB17. (Partnership for Maternal, Newborn and Child Health, Geneva, 2012).

PMNCH. 2013a. Knowledge Summary 27: Death Reviews: Maternal, Perinatal and Child PMNCH, Geneva, 2013.

PMNCH. Knowledge Summary 24: Economic Case for Investment in RMNCH. (Partnership for Maternal, Newborn and Child Health, Geneva, 2013).

Presern C. 2013. Placing populations' health at the heart of the post-2015 agenda. *Bulletin of the World Health Organization* 91: 467–467A. doi:10.2471/BLT.13.125146.

Prost A, *et al.* 2013. Women's groups practising participatory learning and action to improve maternal and newborn health in low-resource settings: A systematic review and meta-analysis. *Lancet* 381: 1736–1746. doi:10.1016/S0140-6736(13)60685-6.

Stenberg K, *et al.* 2014. Advancing social and economic development by investing in women's and children's health: A new global investment framework. *Lancet* 383: 1333–1354. doi:10.1016/S0140-6736(13)62231-X.

Storey D, *et al.* 2011. Social and Behaviour Change Interventions Landscaping Study: A Global Review. Department of Health, Behavior & Society, Johns Hopkins Bloomberg School of Public Health, Baltimore.

Transparency Accountability Initiative. 2011. Opening Government. A Guide to Best Practice in Transparency, Accountability and Civic Engagement Across the Public Sector. London.

UN. 1948. Universal Declaration of Human Rights. Article 25, Para 1. (UN, New York, 1948).

UN. Commission on Information and Accountability for Women's and Children's Health. Keeping Promises, Measuring Results. (United Nations, New York, 2011).

UNESCO. 1990. World Declaration on Education for All.

UNSG. Global Strategy for Women's and Children's Health. (United Nations Secretary General, Geneva, 2010).

VanRooyen MJ, *et al.* 1997. Health Care in post-war Rwanda: Re-establishing a national hospital using a mentor approach. *The Journal of Health Administration Education* 15: 101–111.

WHO H. 2008. Assessing the National Health Information System: An Assessment tool (Version 4). Geneva. (World Health Organization, Geneva, 2008).

WHO S. o. P. H., University of Queensland. 2010. Improving the Quality and Use of Birth, Death and Cause of Death Information: Guidance for a Standards Based Review of Country Practices. WHO, Geneva, 2010.

WHO. 1978. Declaration of Alma-Ata: International Conference on Primary Health Care, Alma-Ata, USSR, 6–12 September 1978. (World Health Organization, 1978).

WHO. 2004. Beyond the Numbers: Reviewing Maternal Deaths and Complications to Make Pregnancy Safer. WHO, Geneva, 2004.

WHO. 2004. Making Water a Part of Economic Development: The Economic Benefits of Improved Water Management and Services. WHO/SIWI.

WHO. 2008a. Closing the Gap in a Generation: Health Equity Through Action on the Social Determinants of Health. Final Report of the CSDH. Commission on Social Determinants of Health. WHO, Geneva, 2008.

WHO. 2009. Guide to Producing Reproductive Health Subaccounts within the National Health Accounts. (World Health Organization, Geneva, 2009). Available at http://apps.who.int/nha/developments/Guide_to_RH_subaccounts.pdf?ua=1.

WHO. 2010b. World Health Report: Health systems financing: The path to universal coverage. (World Health Organization, Geneva, 2010b).

WHO. 2010c. The WHO Global Code of Practice on the International Recruitment of Health Personnel. (WHO, Genvea, 2010).

WHO. 2010d. Working with Individuals, Families and Communities to Improve Maternal and Newborn Health. WHO, Geneva, 2010.

WHO. 2011a. The Abuja Declaration: Ten Years On. (World Health Organization, Geneva, 2011).
WHO. 2011b. Adapting WHO Normative HIV Guidelines for National Programs. Essential Principles and Processes. (WHO, Geneva, 2011).
WHO. 2011c. WHA Resolution EB128.R9: Health Workforce Strengthening. (WHO, Geneva, 2011).
WHO. 2011d. Education: Shared Interests in Well-Being and Development. WHO, Geneva.
WHO. 2012. Guide to producing Child Health Subaccounts within the National Health Accounts. (World Health Organization, Geneva, 2012).
WHO. 2012a. Optimizing Health Worker Roles for Maternal and Newborn Health. (WHO, Geneva, 2012).
WHO. 2015. *Water Sanitation Health: Burden of Disease and Cost-Effectiveness Estimates*.
WHO. A Policy Guide for Implementing Essential Interventions for Reproductive, Maternal, Newborn and Child Health (RMNCH): A Multisectoral Policy Compendium for RMNCH. (World Health Organization, Geneva, 2014).
WHO. Constitution of the World Health Organization. (World Health Organization, Geneva, 1946).
WHO. Macroeconomics and Health: Investing in Health for Economic Development. (World Health Organization, Geneva, 2001).
WHO. 2006. World Health Report 2006: Working Together for Health. (WHO, Geneva, 2006).
Wismar MMM, Ernst K, Sricastava D, Busse R. 2008. Health Targets in Europe Learning from Experience. (WHO, Geneva, 2008).
World Bank, WHO and USAID. 2003. Guide to producing National Health Accounts — with Special Application for Low-Income and Middle-Income Countries. (World Health Organization, Geneva, 2003).
World Bank. 1993. World Development Report: Investing in Health, Volume 1. (World Bank, Washington DC, 1993).
World Education Forum. 2000. The Dakar Framework for Action. Education for all. Meeting our Collective Commitments. UNESCO, France.
World Bank. 2012. World Bank Development Report 2012: Gender Equality and Development. (World Bank, Washington DC, 2012).

Behavioral Economics: Health Applications in the US

Douglas E. Hough

Johns Hopkins University, Bloomberg School of Public Health

Behavioral economics provides a theoretical framework that can explain and predict the behavior of patients, physicians, and policymakers in health care in the US, better than standard, neoclassical economics. In this chapter, we explore the contribution that behavioral economics is beginning to make in health care. First, we discuss a set of robust concepts in the field, the most prominent of which are: loss aversion, the endowment effect, framing, the power of the default, hyperbolic discounting, and System 1 vs. System 2 thinking. Next, we discuss the kinds of interventions and policy levers that have been employed to improve decision-making and actions in health care. Then, we focus on specific situations in which the tenets and tools of behavioral economics have been applied to a number of critical health care issues in the US: Smoking cessation, weight loss, overeating, and substance abuse. In addition, we consider potential applications of behavioral economics in policymaking, patient behavior, and physician behavior. Finally, we consider the challenges that face behavioral economics.

Keywords: Loss Aversion; Endowment Effect; Framing; Hyperbolic Discounting.

Health economists have struggled for decades with explaining and predicting the behavior of patients and physicians in the US health care system. They do not behave the way that utility maximizers and profit maximizers are supposed to act. As a result, very accomplished and creative economists have had to formulate intricate theories to explain the behavior of seemingly irrational economic actors in health care. The problem may lay not with the skills of these economists, but rather, the theoretical frameworks that they are using. Mainstream, neoclassical economics may not be sufficiently inclusive to accommodate how patients, physicians, and even health policymakers make decisions and take actions. Instead, the emerging discipline of behavioral economics may be better positioned to explain and predict how those in the health care sector will behave.

This chapter will examine behavioral economics and describe how the tenets of this field have been applied to health care issues in the US. We will begin by briefly discussing the deficiencies of neoclassical economics in health care. We will then describe concepts in behavioral economics that have been tested repeatedly and have been found to be robust. Then, we will explore how behavioral economics has been applied generally in the US. Next, we will describe current applications of behavioral economics in health care in the US and consider how the discipline could be used in other ways in the future to describe and predict behavior in health care. Finally, we will describe the criticisms of behavioral economics, and confront the challenges that this field will have in demonstrating its value in the economics of health care.

Why Neoclassical Economics Often Fails to Explain Behavior in Health Care

One difficulty that neoclassical economics has in explaining behavior in health care is that its fundamental assumptions do not align with how people act in this arena. The most problematic assumptions are:

- All participants in economic transactions are rational, that is, they always act to advance their self-interest.
- All participants know their preferences.
- All participants have full information about the goods and services that they are selling or buying.
- Decisions are path-independent, that is, the decisions that producers and consumers make do not depend on the process they use to make the decisions.
- If market participants do make mistakes, they make random mistakes.

Unfortunately, these assumptions often do not hold in health care. People actively trying to lose weight will go on a Krispy Kreme doughnut binge. Physicians will not offer services that do not maximize their profits. Patients — even with extensive informed consent procedures — may not know which forms of cancer treatment they prefer. Patients often will not know — again, even with informed consent, informational brochures, and the Internet — the potential benefits and risks of surgery for lower back pain. A physician knows very well that her patients will make different decisions if she frames the potential outcomes and alternative treatments in different ways. And, as behavioral economics has demonstrated, when people make mistakes, they often make systematic mistakes.

As Milton Friedman and Leonard Savage argued over 60 years ago (Friedman and Savage, 1948), the quality of a theory should be based on the accuracy of its explanations and predictions, not on the realism of its assumptions. Unfortunately, the uneven performance of neoclassical economics in explaining and predicting behavior in health care makes it vulnerable to competition with alternative theories of behavior.

Behavioral economics claims to overcome many of the deficiencies inherent in neoclassical economics, primarily by incorporating the findings of research in behavioral psychology. As several behavioral economists have argued, economics and psychology used to be more tightly connected (Ashraf *et al.*, 2005). With the marginalist revolution, psychology was pushed aside in favor of mathematical rigor. Behavioral economics reintroduces psychology into the analysis, as reflected in its fundamental assumptions:

- All participants in economic transactions are not always rational. They may not be irrational, but sometimes rationality does not play a large part in decision-making.
- Participants often do not know their preferences, but learn them through experience and trial-and-error.
- Participants often have incomplete information about the goods and services that they are selling or buying, and often fill that gap with heuristics.[1]
- Decisions are path-dependent; producers and consumers make different decisions based on how the alternatives are framed.
- When people make mistakes (that is, when they do not act in their best interest), they often make systematic mistakes (which can be predicted).

These assumptions are more consonant with the behavior of patients and physicians described above. In addition, as we shall see, the assumptions and tenets of behavioral economics better explain arguments made in the fierce debate in the United States over the Affordable Care Act.[2] These include the tirade by a South Carolina constituent in a town hall meeting, "Keep your government hands off my Medicare," (even though Medicare has always been a government program) and President Barack Obama's promise that, "If you like your health plan, you can

[1] Heuristics are strategies for decision making that use a relatively small number of simple and readily accessible rules rather than engaging the full gamut of possibilities. Heuristics can be as simple as "rules of thumb" (such as "You should follow another car no closer than the distance you will drive in two seconds") or as complex as multilevel decision trees.

[2] The Patient Protection and Affordable Care Act of 2010, often called the "Affordable Care Act" or "Obamacare," is the US Health Reform Law that was enacted after much acrimonious debate. The law continues to be divisive, with ongoing court challenges and threats of repeal. Key features of the law can be found at: www.hhs.gov/healthcare/facts/timeline/timeline-text.html.

keep it" (since many people were concerned that they would be forced to change health plans).

Robust Concepts in Behavioral Economics

Behavioral economics as a field is a little more than thirty years old, with the "birth" often attributed to the path-breaking article, "Prospect Theory: An Analysis of Decision Under Risk," by Daniel Kahneman and Amos Tversky, published in *Econometrica* in 1979 (Kahneman and Tversky, 1979). Over that time, a number of hypotheses have been proposed and tested. Some have held up; others were refuted by later research. In some sense, behavioral economics is still in search of a unified theory and a set of universal constructs. Nevertheless, there are a handful of fundamental tenets that have been sufficiently tested and validated that they can be applied with confidence. The ones of most interest here include:

- Loss aversion.
- Endowment effect.
- Framing.
- The power of the default.
- Hyperbolic discounting.
- System 1 vs. System 2 thinking.

Following is a brief description of each tenet.

Loss aversion. Behavioral economics begins with the observation that people hate losses; in fact, evidence suggests that they hate losses almost twice as much as they like gains. This behavior, which Kahneman and Tversky (1979) termed "loss aversion," contradicts the contention of neoclassical economics that people maximize the expected utility of gains and losses. The exact form of this behavior is shown in Figure 1. The first thing to notice is that behavioral economics does not assume that consumers have a full-formed utility function (as neoclassical economics contends). Rather, consumers make a decision based on their current position, or reference point. As a result, consumers making decisions are evaluating changes in their situation — gains or losses. Based on observations of consumers' behavior, Kahneman and Tversky argue that people tend to be risk-averse in gains (hence, their tendency to sell winning stocks too early), but risk-loving in losses (hence, the tendency of gamblers to "go for broke" when they are losing). In addition, the figure shows that consumers receive much lower value from a gain of x than the value they would give up by the loss of x, hence, loss aversion. A vivid illustration of this phenomenon is from tennis Great Andre Agassi, who in his

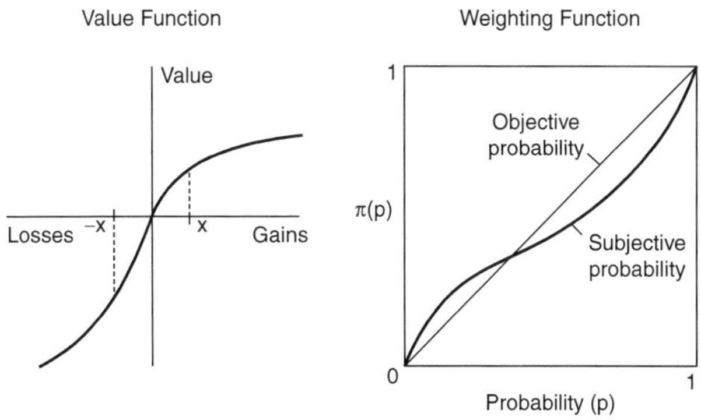

Figure 1: The simple analytics of behavioral economics

Source: Kahneman D, Tversky A. (1979). Prospect theory: An analysis of decision under risk. *Econometrica* 47(2): 263–292. Used by permission.

autobiography wrote, "Now that I've won a slam, I know something that very few people are permitted to know. A win doesn't feel as good as a loss feels bad, and the good feeling doesn't last as long as the bad. Not even close" (Agassi, 2009).

The figure on the right-hand side shows another aspect of loss aversion: People are not calculating machines when they evaluate risks; they make their own interpretations of probabilities. In particular, they tend to overweight small probabilities and underweight large probabilities. For example, a number of studies (e.g., Kunreuther *et al.*, 2001) have shown that people do not meaningfully distinguish among a one in 10,000 chance, a one in 100,000 chance, and a one in a million chance, despite the 10-fold difference in each of these probabilities. If that mistake is pervasive, then the expected utility theory of neoclassical economics breaks down.

The endowment effect. One illustration of loss aversion is a concept known as the "endowment effect." People tend to value something — a thing, a product, an idea — more highly once they have it. Behavioral economists have found the endowment effect in a wide variety of situations. The experiment that demonstrated this effect first in economics was conducted by Jack Knetsch with three classes of students (Knetsch, 1989). In the first class, students were given a coffee mug, and told that it was in compensation for their completing a short questionnaire. When they handed in the questionnaire, they were given the option to trade their mug for a bar of Swiss chocolate (which had about the same retail value as the coffee mug). In the second class, students were given the bar of Swiss chocolate and then asked to complete the same short questionnaire. When they were finished, they were given the option to trade their chocolate bar for a coffee mug. Finally, students in the third class were given a choice between the mug and the chocolate bar before they completed the questionnaire (and were not allowed to trade it after handing in the completed questionnaire). Neoclassical economists would predict that roughly the same percentage of students in each class would select the coffee mug, because the students would know their preferences between chocolate bars and coffee mugs before walking into class. That did not happen, however. Although 56% of those in the third class chose a coffee mug, 89% of those in the first class chose to keep their coffee mug, and only 10% of those in the second class chose to trade their chocolate bar for the mug.

Why the difference? Knetsch concluded that possession of the coffee mug or the chocolate bar changed the students' perception of the value of the product, even for the few minutes that they were completing the questionnaire. Perhaps, they felt that they "earned" what they were given, or that having to make a decision between the two was too taxing. Or, perhaps they felt that surrendering what they had just been given represented a loss, one that was greater than the expected gain from acquiring the other object. That is, they felt loss aversion.

Framing. For millennia, politicians and marketers have understood that they can influence people's decisions by the way that issues are framed, perhaps more than the content of their message. Tverksy and Kahneman argued that "framing is controlled by the manner in which the choice problem is presented as well as by norms, habits, and expectancies of the decision maker" (Tversky and Kahneman, 1986). As noted above, neoclassical economists contend that rational individuals will see through the framing and focus on the content of the message. This assumption, however, has been refuted in a number of research studies.

Barbara McNeil and her colleagues conducted a classical study on framing in health care more than 30 years ago (McNeil *et al.*, 1982). They engaged three distinct groups — 238 men with chronic medical problems, 424 radiologists, and 491 MBA students from Stanford Business School. The participants were told to imagine that they were informed that they had lung cancer, which was treatable by either surgery or radiation therapy. Half of each group was given the following statistics: "Of 100 people having surgery, 90 live through the post-operative period, 68 are alive at the end of the 1st year and 34 are alive at the end of 5 years. Of 100 people having radiation therapy all live through the therapy period, 77 are alive at the end of the 1st year and 22 are alive at the end of 5 years." The other half was told the following: "Of 100 people having surgery 10 die during surgery or the post-operative period, 32 die by the end of the 1st year and 66 die by the end of 5 years. Of 100 people having radiation therapy none die during the therapy period, 23 die by the end of the 1st year and 78 die by the end of 5 years." A careful reader will note that the content of each presentation is identical, except that the first was done in a survival frame and the second in a mortality frame. Despite the expectations of neoclassical economics that individuals ought to be able to make the same decision regardless of the presentation frame, 18% preferred radiation therapy in the survival frame and 44% preferred that treatment in the mortality frame. Perhaps as surprising, there were no statistically significant differences in results among the participants — physicians, patients, and students — despite their diversity in age, income, education, and experience with illness. All were affected by framing.

Power of the default. In many situations, a decision needs to be made about an initial position: We drive on the left or the right; automatic transmissions are either standard or optional; sales tax is either added at the end (as it is in the US) or incorporated into the price of the product (as in the UK). Sometimes, the initial — or default — position is easy to change, as in the case of standard versus optional features on a car; sometimes, it is more difficult, such as which side of the road to drive on. What behavioral economists have discovered is that where you start makes a remarkably big difference, even if people would be expected to have distinct preferences and if it is easy for them to change from the default.

A famous study illustrates this point. Eric Johnson and Daniel Goldstein examined the rate at which adults in European countries register to be potential organ donors (Johnson and Goldstein, 2003). In four of the countries — Denmark, the Netherlands, the United Kingdom and Germany — between 4% and 27% of adults were registered organ donors. In the other seven countries — Austria, Belgium, France, Hungary, Poland, Portugal and Sweden — the organ donation rate was between 86% and 99%. Although there are some cultural and historical differences among these countries, there is seemingly nothing that could explain these extraordinary differences. Johnson and Goldstein discovered that the two sets of countries used different defaults. In the first four countries, adults who wanted to be organ donors must sign up; that is, they had to "opt-in" or give their explicit consent to be an organ donor. In the other countries, adults were automatically enrolled as organ donors (or what is known as "presumed consent"), but could "opt-out" of the program if they wished. Neoclassical economists would argue that such differences would persist only if transactions costs — in time or money — were high, or if people were not told about their organ donor status. It turns out that none of these explanations addresses the seemingly anomalous behavior. It is fairly easy to change from the default position in any these countries.

How, then, to explain this dramatic difference in behavior? Johnson and Goldstein (and others who have examined this issue) offer several explanations. First, the default can act as an implicit recommendation or endorsement by the government or society. ("Everyone else is registered as an organ donor. I haven't thought about it much, but I guess that is what everyone does here.") A second factor may just be inertia. People in Hungary and Poland may want to opt out, but never quite get around to doing so. Third, the default could be an example of the endowment effect; the default position becomes the endowment, and people will change from the default only if the alternative is demonstrably better. Finally, Richard Thaler and Cass Sunstein, in their book *Nudge*, argue that defaults are a way by which the ambiguous preferences of people can be given a push — a "nudge" — to what presumably they would have chosen themselves had they thought about it (Thaler and Sunstein, 2008).

Hyperbolic discounting. People prefer the present to the future; that is, they discount the future relative to the present. That is one significant reason why people demand a premium (i.e., an interest rate) to forego money today for money in the future. Economists have typically assumed that people have an exponential discount rate. Such a discount rate has several attractive properties: It is constant over time, and value declines proportionally over time. The second property of proportional declines in value means that if an individual prefers \$100 today to \$200 two years from now, he would also prefer \$100 eight years from now to \$200 ten years from now. As it turns out, this behavior often does not happen, and, as has been demonstrated, (Ainslie and Haslam, 1992) an individual is more likely to prefer the \$200 in 10 years from now to the \$100 in 8 years. In this case, his preferences are "time inconsistent" and he follows what is called a "hyperbolic discount" function. People who exhibit hyperbolic discounting have a high discount rate in the shortterm and a much lower discount rate in the long-term. One consequence of hyperbolic discounting is that people will make decisions (often implicitly) about their future that they will regret once that future becomes the present. Witness our inability to lose enough weight before our high school reunion. Or, more profoundly, the regret that people often have when they are close to retirement and find that they have failed to save enough in their younger years to support their planned lifestyle.

System 1 vs. System 2 thinking. Another difference between behavioral and neoclassical economics involves assumptions about the process by which people make decisions. Daniel Kahneman posits two distinct approaches to decision-making: System 1 and System 2. System 1 thinking is fast, effortless, and automatic, and often is used when the decision-maker is skilled and experienced in the task at hand. In fact, she might be so skilled and experienced that she cannot explain how she made the decision. System 2 thinking, on the other hand, is relatively slow, effortful, controlled, and deductive. The decision-maker can explain — sometimes in great detail — how he made the decision (Kahneman, 2011). Neoclassical economics implicitly assumes that people always use System 2, as it reflects a deliberate, calculating mode of thinking. Behavioral economics allows for both systems of thought. As Kahneman and others have demonstrated, System 1 — although very fast and energy-conserving — can promote biases and create decision errors. System 1 thinking relies on heuristics and rules of thumb. Although many heuristics are based in reality, they do not work all the time; indiscriminant use of heuristics will blind decision-makers to nuances that need to be recognized. Otherwise, people will make assumptions and take actions that will not be in their best interest.

General Applications of Behavioral Economics

In neoclassical economics, prices and costs are the primary drivers of behavior. As a result, the economist's toolbox for influencing behavior contains essentially those two items. However, as we have already seen, people — and even organizations — can be driven by factors that are outside of this calculus. Because it acknowledges and incorporates factors beyond price and cost, behavioral economics gives decision-makers — at the government and organizational levels — additional levers to influence behavior. In this section, we will discuss these levers and how they have been studied and applied in the US a word of caution, however. Behavioral economics has become very popular of late, and there is a danger that researchers and policymakers will think that it can solve all social problems. One must recognize that behavioral economics is still a young field, and much work needs to be done to calibrate its findings. In addition, it is important to appreciate that human beings sometimes work in mysterious ways, and their behavior cannot always be predicted and influenced. (We should remember Nobel laureate physicist Murray Gell-Mann's statement, "Think how hard physics would be if particles could think.")

There is a spectrum of approaches that can be taken to influence behavior. Yashar Saghai has developed a particularly useful taxonomy in this regard (Saghai, 2013). The first approach is information or education, which supposes that individuals intend to "do the right thing" but lack sufficient information to do so, in terms of either motivation or process. The second is persuasion: In addition to information, the individual needs to be convinced to do the right thing. The third — which has been widely adopted in manufacturing, air travel, and, more recently, health care — is guidelines or checklists. Guidelines can represent either the consensus or "best practice" methods used by experienced practitioners. Checklists require practitioners to engage System 2 thinking on tasks that they routinely perform and, thus, would usually use System 1 thinking for. The concept is that the checklist will ensure that the practitioner (e.g., airline pilot) addresses all salient and material issues involved in a procedure (e.g., pre-flight safety checks) for which errors may have disastrous results.

A fourth approach to influencing behavior, penalties and rewards, is the favorite approach of most neoclassical economists. People can be rewarded for good performance, or penalized for poor performance. Penalties and rewards can be denominated in money, near-money (e.g., gift cards), tangible goods or services, or time. By manipulating the size of the penalty or reward, policymakers can change an individual's calculations of marginal benefits and marginal costs and, thus, their decisions.

Behavioral economics provides several additional policy levers. The first is commitment devices. These are voluntary programs in which people in their rational, calculating state use their System 2 thinking to prepare for situations in which they know that they will be less likely to behave rationally. For example, in the first half of the last century, people would participate in what was known as "Christmas Clubs." They would deposit money on a regular basis in a low- (or no-) interest-bearing savings account, from which they would not be able to withdraw until it was time to buy Christmas presents. The programs gave participants the discipline they needed to save.

The second policy lever from behavioral economics is defaults. As discussed earlier, defaults are based on the premise that, in many cases, some starting point must be established. Given the power of many defaults, Thaler and Sunstein assert that policymakers have an important role in creating what they call "choice architecture" (Thaler and Sunstein, 2008). Choice architecture involves: The form of the default, the criteria for establishing the default, the degree of transparency of the default (so that the individuals can recognize that a default choice has been made for them), and the ease with which individuals can opt out of the default. As may be obvious, the wrong choice architecture can transform a friendly nudge into a coercive shove.

A variation on defaults is the forced choice. Instead of an opt-in or opt-out structure, the individual could be forced to make a choice, and thus reveal his true preference. For example, the Department of Motor Vehicles could require a motorist to choose whether or not to be an organ donor before receiving his driver's license. This approach has the advantage of eliciting an individual's preferences directly rather than inferring or interfering with those preferences.[3]

Beyond these levers from behavioral economics, Saghai offers two others. The first is a mandate, which removes choice but often leaves a loophole (if enforcement

[3]Two downsides of this approach are that an individual may not be ready to make such a choice at that moment, or she may make a hasty choice just to accomplish her original goal (i.e., obtain a driver's license).

is lax). In some sense, a mandate is a default without the opportunity to change the default. A mandate is useful if the consequences of voluntary action are not sufficient. For example, parents might be mandated to have their children vaccinated, to ensure that communicable diseases are not spread throughout a community. The other lever is coercion or compulsion. This approach — although extreme — could be appropriate (even in a democratic society) if the consequences of noncompliance threatened the society. An example would be a quarantine for those infected with an extremely infectious disease.

Organizations are beginning to apply insights from behavioral economics to improve their performance, and that of their employees and customers. (In fact, for centuries marketers have exploited what is now known as behavioral economics to entice potential customers.) Examples include:

- Employers are switching from opt-in to opt-out systems in their defined contribution retirement plans, to encourage employee participation in the plans.[4] Madrian and Shea (2001) found that one large employer experienced a 3-fold increase in plan take-up among new employees when it changed its default to opt-out.
- Health clubs find that members prefer monthly, all-inclusive rates to per-use fees, even if per-use fees are less costly (DellaVigna and Malmendier, 2006).
- An experiment in Chicago Heights, Illinois, found that student achievement scores increased significantly when teachers were given a $4,000 bonus at the beginning of the year (which they had to return if the students had not improved their performance) (Fryer *et al.*, 2012).
- A contemporary version of the Christmas Club is stickK.com, a website launched in 2008, in which people interested in achieving a goal create a commitment contract, specifying their goals, the stakes for not achieving the goals (money, reputation), the recipient of the stakes, a designated referee, and a support group. The website claims to have facilitated over 270,000 commitments, and have tens of millions of dollars of commitment contracts active at any one time. Actual commitment contracts at stickK.com have included: "exercise for one hour every day," "read a book a month," "publish a book within one year," "lose 36 pounds in 24 weeks," "quit smoking for 28 days," "arrive to church on time," and "stay off reddit." To increase the

[4]In defined contribution retirement plans in the US, employers contribute a pre-determined amount (either in absolute dollar amount or in a percentage of employee income) to a retirement fund for an employee. The employee is responsible for managing the account in terms of investment mix and ultimate payout. In more traditional, defined benefit retirement plans (also called pension plans), it is the employer that sets the level of benefits that an employer will receive in retirement (often based on the employee's tenure with the employer and income history).

power of the commitment, some participants will designate a cause that they hate as the recipient of the stakes should they not keep their commitment.

- The growth in popularity of automatic bill payment plans stems (at least in part) from the finding in behavioral economics that lack of salience or visibility of the amount due improves the ability of sellers to pass on price increases. What a consumer gains in convenience by not having to physically pay a bill is at least partially offset by the potential for the seller to increase prices or introduce fees without the consumer noticing. For example, Finkelstein (2009) found that highway tolls increased faster in states that had EZ-Pass systems that enabled drivers to avoid stopping at a toll booth and having to pay a toll in cash.
- The changing role of deductibles and rebates in insurance can be explained through loss aversion, where deductibles are typically seen as losses and rebates as gains. Both research (Johnson *et al.*, 1993) and changing marketing practices in auto insurance (e.g., Allstate's semi-annual "bonus checks" to safe drivers) have revealed that consumers much prefer rebates to deductibles, even when the dollar values are identical. That is, consumers frame deductibles as losses, because they have to pay part of an insurance claim themselves. On the other hand, a rebate is perceived as a gift.[5]
- The federal income tax withholding system may be an example of a (mandated) commitment device, but it also demonstrates the power of rebates over discounts. Of the 145 million federal income tax returns filed in 2012, 120 million (83%) received refunds, in effect, an interest-free loan to the government (Internal Revenue Service, 2014).

Current Applications of Behavioral Economics in Health Care

As I have examined in another work (Hough, 2013), behavioral economics is just beginning to be applied in health care. There are three contexts in which the discipline is being applied. The initial context relates to consumer — or patient — behavior. The second is in understanding and influencing physician behavior, and the third is in the application of behavioral economics in health policy. The most extensive application of behavioral economics in health care has been in trying to influence patient behavior — losing weight, stopping smoking, curbing drug abuse, maintaining HbA1c levels for diabetics, and improving medication adherence. In this section, we will consider a number of these studies, more as illustration of the work that is being done than an encyclopedic review of the research and policy literature. We will cover four areas: Smoking, obesity, overeating, and substance abuse.

[5]The same behavior can be seen with federal income tax returns. Of the 146 million individual income tax returns filed in the US in 2012, 112 million (76%) received a refund, averaging $2,800 per filer. http://www.irs.gov/uac/SOI-Tax-Stats-Tax-Stats-at-a-Glance.

Smoking cessation. Kevin Volpp, a physician, health economist and Director of the Center for Health Incentives and Behavioral Economics at the University of Pennsylvania, has been the most prolific researcher in the application of behavioral economics to health care. Two of his studies will be described here. The first study examined the impact of financial incentives on smoking cessation (Volpp *et al.*, 2009). Volpp and his team recruited 878 employees at General Electric who were smokers and interested in quitting. Half were randomly assigned to receive only information about community-based smoking-cessation programs, and the other half were given a series of financial incentives. The financial incentives were: $100 for completing the community-based program, $250 for smoking cessation for 6 months after the program, and another $400 for an additional 6 months of smoking cessation. The results were that the incentivized group had almost three times the quit rate as the control group. However, the quit rate was still rather small: 14.7% vs. 5.0% for the first round of cessation, and 9.4% vs. 3.6% for the second round. In a sense, this experiment was very much within the realm of neoclassical economics, with participants expected to make decisions based on marginal benefits and marginal costs. However, behavioral economics has demonstrated that human decision-making is much more complex than anticipated in standard economic models, and as Volpp and his team noted in their study, interventions more sophisticated than price need to be applied.

Several researchers have found that financial incentives for smoking cessation are especially effective when directed at pregnant women. Stephen Higgins and his colleagues at the University of Vermont and Rebecca Donatelle and her colleagues at Oregon State University have been most active in this regard. Higgins *et al.* (2012) reported on the results of six randomized controlled trials on the application of financial incentives among economically disadvantaged pregnant smokers. Quit rates during the *antepartum* period ranged from 19% to 41% for those given a financial incentive and from 0% to 12% for those not given a financial incentive.[6] The researchers found that the incentives were more effective:

- The more frequent the incentives were distributed.
- The higher the incentives (in particular, $50 was much more effective than $25).
- The more that graduated incentives were given (to reward persistent smoking cessation).

[6] In all six studies, the participants were given usual care regarding smoking cessation by their obstetric provider. Three studies also provided pregnancy-specific smoking cessation pamphlets, one study provided a pregnancy-specific smoking cessation self-help kit to all participants, and one study provided "best-practice 5As" (ask, advise, assess, assist, arrange).

These results support several of the behavioral economics concepts discussed earlier in this chapter. Smoking cessation faces the challenge of hyperbolic discounting. The pleasure of a cigarette often outweighs the long-term benefits of cessation. Frequent incentives helps to counter that problem, as does the prospect of increasing incentives with persistence, and as does the prospect of improving the health of the soon-to-be-born child.[7] In addition, the graduated incentive plays on loss aversion, as the participant knows that she will have to go back to the base incentive if she smokes a cigarette.

Stacey Sigmon and Mollie Patrick recently published a narrative review of hundreds of studies conducted on smoking cessation experiments (Sigmon and Patrick, 2012). Overall, they found that financial incentives were more effective than other cessation methods (such as education, peer groups, and nicotine patches). Financial incentives were effective for special populations — substance abusers, adolescents, patients with chronic obstructive pulmonary disease (COPD). They confirmed the findings described above for pregnant women: Larger magnitude incentives, more frequent incentives, and escalating incentives were the most effective. They note that financial incentive programs face a number of challenges. The first is the maintenance of smoking abstinence after the intervention ends; the evidence is mixed on the long-term effectiveness of all intervention programs (even incentive-driven ones). The authors suggest that a less intensive, long-term incentive program might be effective after the initial intervention. This challenge leads to the second: The cost of financial incentive programs, especially if they are scaled up to large populations. Although the programs often can be shown to be cost-effective, the magnitude of program outlays may be daunting for employer-based and public programs (such as Medicaid).

Weight loss. Kevin Volpp and his colleagues conducted an interesting experiment involving weight loss (Volpp *et al.*, 2008). They randomly assigned 57 healthy individuals with a body mass index between 30 and 40 into three groups, each with a goal to lose 16 pounds in 16 weeks. The first group was the control, with the participants enrolled in a weight-monitoring program with monthly weigh-ins. Those in the second group were enrolled in the same weight-loss program, but with a daily lottery if the participant met his or her weight loss goal (which tests the participants' sense of loss aversion). The third group was given a "deposit contract," a kind of commitment device, in which the participants had to contribute some of their own money (between $0.01 and

[7]The fact that the pregnancy is a short-term (rather than lifelong) event also helps to attenuate hyperbolic discounting.

$3.00 per day) which was matched by the program but was at risk if a participant failed to meet the stated weight loss goal. The study found that those in the incentive groups lost more weight after 16 weeks than did those in the control group (14.0 pounds for the deposit contract group and 13.1 pounds for the lottery group, vs. 3.9 pounds for the control group). Unfortunately, three months after the end of the program, participants in the incentive groups gained back some of their weight, although the mean total weight loss was still greater than in the control group.

Jeffrey Kullgren and his colleagues (which included Kevin Volpp) conducted a clever variation on financial incentives for weight loss (Kullgren *et al.*, 2013). They recruited 105 employees of Children's Hospital of Philadelphia who had a BMI between 30 and 40, and who were willing to try to lose 24 pounds over 24 weeks. The volunteers were divided into three groups: A control group, who were given a link to a national weight-control network; a group in which participants would receive $100 at baseline and in 4-week intervals if they met their weight loss goals; and a group that was subdivided into groups of 5 unidentified participants who were to share in a pool of money. At each 4-week interval, each group would divide its pool of $500 among those in the group that met their weight-loss goals; clearly, a participant would benefit in this group if he achieved his weight-loss goal and the others in his group did not.

After 24 weeks, those in the control group had lost an average of 1.1 pounds, compared to 3.7 pounds for the individual-incentive group and 10.6 pounds for the group-incentive group. The differential persisted 12 weeks after the incentives stopped, with the control group gaining back an average of 0.2 pounds, the individual-incentive group gaining back 1.9 pounds (that is, about half of the incented weight loss) and the group-incentive group gaining back 3.1 pounds (30% of the original weight loss). The difference in weight loss between the group-incentive and control groups (at both 24 and 36 weeks) was statistically significant, but not that between the individual-incentive and control groups. The researchers speculate that the potential to earn higher stakes in the group setting engaged the participants, and exploited their optimism bias.[8] Note, however, that the average weight loss of all groups was dramatically less than the goal of 24 pounds. (In fact, only 5 of the 105 participants lost 24 or more pounds.) Also note that the weight loss was much less than in the previous study, which Kullgren *et al.* attribute to the monthly (rather than daily) rewards for weight loss. Thus, as has been mentioned throughout this chapter, financial incentives and the tenets of behavioral econom-

---

[8]Those in the group-incentive group earned an average of $514.70, compared to only $128.60 in the individual-incentive group.

ics may make an impact on human behavior, but are likely not sufficient to accomplish most goals.

The interest in weight loss has gone far beyond research projects. Many employers are offering employee wellness programs, including weight loss. John Cawley and Joshua Price analyzed the effectiveness of financial incentive programs administered by a company that runs wellness programs for employers (Cawley and Price, 2013). They had access to incentivized weight loss programs for 2,635 employees over 24 worksites. Fortunately for the researchers, the wellness company used incentive programs that had payment systems and commitment devices. Four such programs were examined:

- "Continuous Payment," in which participants received quarterly payments based on the percentage of baseline weight lost.
- "Deposit Contract with Lump Sum Repayment," in which each participant had to pay $9.95 per month (which was refunded if the participant lost 5% of baseline weight by the end of 1 year, plus a $100 payout if the participant lost at least 10% of baseline weight).
- "Deposit Contract with Continuous Repayment," in which each participant had to pay $9.95 per month, but is rewarded quarterly on a sliding scale based on the percent of baseline weight lost (from 1% to 20%).
- "Control," in which participants are given a flat $20 at the end of the year (that is, with no incremental incentives for weight loss).

Cawley and Price note that the incentive design suffers from numerous experimental flaws (e.g., lack of randomization, lack of controls for attrition), but the situations provide a real-world, full-scale element that smaller, carefully-designed research studies do not.

Their findings should give pause to those eager to employ incentives and behavioral economics to wellness programs. First, 43% of the participants dropped out of the programs at the end of the first quarter, and 68% quit by the end of the year; these rates were unaffected by the presence of either incentives or commitment devices. Second, at year end, weight loss in the Continuous Payment group was not significantly different from the Control group. Third, weight loss in the Deposit Contract groups at the end of the year was significantly higher than that of either the Continuous Payment or Control groups. Fourth, most of the weight loss occurred in the first two quarters of the programs. Fifth, given the high attrition rates, the net reward paid to participants in the Deposit Contract with Lump Sum Repayment program was negative: on average participants paid (rather than earned) $19.42 for every pound that they lost. Cawley and Price conclude that real-world weight loss programs need to be much better designed and executed — to avoid wholesale attrition, confusing deposit and payout schemes, and attenuation of incentive effectiveness — in order for the tenets of behavioral economics to be applied correctly. In effect, much more calibration needs to be done before the use of creative financial incentives can be deployed on a large scale.

Overeating. It is widely known that two-thirds of Americans are overweight, and one-third are obese (Weight-Control Information Network, 2012). Marketing researchers and behavioral economists have established that, not only is it difficult to lose weight, it is remarkably easy to overeat. Brian Wansink, Professor of Marketing and Director of the Food and Brand Lab at Cornell University, has devoted his career to demonstrating how Americans succumb to what he calls "mindless eating" (Wansink, 2006). His research has shown that:

- People will eat more popcorn — even five-day old popcorn — if it is placed in front of them.
- People will eat more soup from a bowl that refills itself.
- Children will eat more healthy foods if the foods are conveniently located in the school cafeteria (and the unhealthy foods are hard to get to).
- Consumption at buffets is highly correlated with the size of plates, the visibility of the buffet, the distance from the tables and the buffet, and even the orientation of the tables.

In some sense, these findings are obvious. What Wansink and his colleagues have found is that diners are unaware — and even dismissive — of the power of these forces. From a behavioral economics perspective, Wansink's findings illustrate the impact of framing, hyperbolic discounting, and System 1 vs. System 2 thinking on how people eat.

The strength of these forces presents both a problem and an opportunity. The problem is that the source of eating behavior is deep-seated and challenging to modify. The opportunity is that the unhealthy behaviors might be dislodged by using — rather than trying to overcome — these same forces. Thaler and Sunstein (2008) call this process the development of "choice architecture." Eric Johnson and his colleagues (including Brian Wansink) have created a taxonomy of choice architecture tools that are helpful in this regard (Johnson *et al.*, 2012). The tools include:

- Managing the number and kinds of options to steer people toward healthy choices (such as providing six rather than 24 kinds of yogurt in a grocery store, or placing bananas rather than sugary applesauce near the desserts in a buffet).

- Providing decision aids and recommendations (such as calorie counts for healthy and unhealthy foods in a restaurant).
- Creating defaults (such as visible displays of healthy foods and obstructed views of desserts and fatty foods).
- Partitioning options (such as designating part of a grocery cart for fruits and vegetables, or segregating healthy food options and combining unhealthy foods on a menu).
- Manipulating attributes (such as making healthy foods more attractive [e.g., through celebrity endorsements] and making unhealthy foods less desirable [e.g., by showing how long someone would have to exercise to burn off the calories]).

Although these tools can appear at first glance to be trivial, Wansink and others have demonstrated that these nudges can significantly influence eating behavior. For example, a middle school cafeteria in Corning, New York increased salad sales by 21% by rotating the salad bar by 90 degrees and moving it to the middle of the lunch room. Another school cafeteria requires students to pay cash for all desserts and soft drinks (which creates a negative attribute for the junk food and increases the salience of the purchase compared to using a debit or credit card) (Just and Wansink, 2009). Sara Bleich and her colleagues at Johns Hopkins University tested how adolescents in Baltimore reacted to different information regarding sugar-sweetened beverages: Number of calories and teaspoons of sugar, and minutes of running required and miles of walking required to burn off the calories in those beverages. They found that the number of miles walked had the biggest impact, with a 12% reduction in consumption. They also found that adolescents bought smaller serving sizes (Bleich *et al.*, 2014).

Substance abuse. The abuse of legal and illegal drugs would appear to be a rich subject for exploration by behavioral economists (although Nobel Laureate Gary Becker and Kevin Murphy (1988) have led a neoclassical approach to analyzing addiction). George Loewenstein in particular (Loewenstein, 1988; 1996; 2005) has formulated a variation of hyperbolic discounting, called the "hot-cold empathy gap." Individuals (such as drug users) make different decisions when they are in a "cold" state (that is, when they are driven by rational, calculating thought) than when they are in a "hot" state (when they are driven by emotions). As importantly, Loewenstein hypothesizes, people do not recognize that they will make different decisions when they are in the other state; as a result, their decisions and actions will be inconsistent.

In a recent extensive review, Bickel *et al.* (2014) interpret what psychologists call "reinforcer pathology" from the lens of behavioral economics. They cite study after study that demonstrates the connections: "Steep delay and probability discounting (what behavioral economics calls hyperbolic discounting and loss aversion) may reflect a maladaptive decision-making bias, and individuals who devalue delayed or uncertain outcomes may prefer drug use relative to many alternative behaviors." (p. 649). Examples include:

- Higher demand for alcohol among heavy drinkers is associated with greater hyperbolic discounting.
- Hyperbolic discounting is prevalent in those addicted to alcohol, cocaine, tobacco, opioids, and methamphetamines.
- Those who exhibit hyperbolic discounting prior to drug use have a higher probability of becoming addicted (which suggests a complex causal relationship between rates of time preference and drug use).
- The highest rates of substance abuse occur when there are the fewest substance-free reinforcers, that is, when there are fewer alternatives to the abusive activity (think "mindless eating").

As we have discussed throughout this section, Bickel *et al.* identify the policy levers from behavioral economics that have been shown in experimental and field studies to influence the behavior of substance abusers: Incentives to quit (or what psychologists call "contingency management"); reduction in availability or increase in price of the abused substance (what psychologists call "community reinforcement approach"); increased awareness (or "salience") by the abusers of the costs to themselves and others of their substance abuse (what psychologists call "brief motivational intervention"); and even procedures to modify an individual's discount rate (such as through deposit contracts).

What the review by Bickel *et al.* illustrates is — once again — the twin promise and challenge of behavioral economics. The discipline provides a new and complementary lens for understanding human behavior, one that combines the perspective of both standard economics and behavioral psychology. In addition, it offers some policy levers to influence behavior; to date these tools have shown potential, but the evidence is not overwhelming to support their wholesale application.

Potential Applications of Behavioral Economics in Health Care

Behavioral economics is still a young field, but as George Loewenstein has said, it is "actually quite impressive how far it has come in such a short period of time" (Hough, 2013). The same could be said for the application of behavioral economics to health care. As noted in the previous section, a lot of work has been done in exploring the usefulness of behavioral economics in explaining the seemingly irrational behavior of those who smoke, overeat, or abuse drugs. Nevertheless, these studies need to be replicated, both to ensure that the results are robust and to calibrate the dosage of interventions.

In addition, there are a number of patient behaviors that still need to be addressed. The most pressing is medication adherence. Only three-fourth of patients fill new prescriptions, and only three-fourth of those take the pills as prescribed (DiMatteo, 2004; Fischer *et al.*, 2010). Both neoclassical economics (price, transactions costs) and behavioral economics (lack of salience in treating asymptomatic disease, or declining affect in treating chronic disease) have plausible explanations for this behavior. Laboratory and field experiments need to be undertaken (perhaps in an adversarial collaboration) to test which explanations are more accurate, and — once that occurs — determine the most effective mechanisms for improving medication adherence.

With the implementation of the Affordable Care Act, it is important to understand what causes people to enroll in which health insurance plans: Do they look at the total cost of health care (including deductibles and copays), or do they fixate on the monthly premium (as behavioral economics would suggest)? Do they like lots of plan choices, or do they struggle when faced with many choices (as the work of Sheena Iyengar (2010) and others indicate)? Will many people switch plans, or will they stay with the one they have had (as predicted by the endowment effect) even if few others are switching to their plan?

In addition, it would be interesting to explore the impact of opt-out systems in the US. Would many people object or balk if they were automatically enrolled as organ donors (given sufficient information and easy opt-out mechanisms)? Liberal states such as Maryland, Massachusetts and New York could act as test cases. Also, the provisions of the Affordable Care Act could be amended to change mandated health insurance to a default in which uninsured individuals or households would be automatically enrolled in a plan, which could be easily changed. Again, state experiments would be helpful in this regard.

Finally, regarding patient and consumer behavior, it would be instructive to examine why action bias occurs. That is, why do patients insist on getting a prescription, lab test, or other procedure — even when such actions would do little or nothing to diagnose or treat their problem? The ABIM Foundation, through its Choosing Wisely campaign, has compiled a list of tests and procedures that physician specialty associations have determined have little or no diagnostic or therapeutic value (such as CT scans or electromyography for low-back pain) (ABIM Foundation, 2014). Patients still request some of these, and behavioral economics has some potential explanations that would be worthy of testing.

The issue of low- or no-value tests and procedures also raises questions about physician behavior that is relevant to behavioral economics. As noted earlier, physicians engage System 1 thinking in order to provide care to their daily schedule of patients. This approach works remarkably well. However, there are times — such as when they write unnecessary prescriptions or order unnecessary tests out of habit — when System 1 fails. Exploring the explicit and implicit reasons why physicians do so could then inform interventions to improve physician decision-making.

Likewise, physicians understand the power of framing when they present the benefits and risks of treatment options to their patients. They must present one before the other, and they know that which comes first will drive patient decisions. As a result, a potentially fruitful line of research would examine the optimal "choice architecture" of treatment presentations. (Of course, a first step would involve defining "optimal" and from whose perspective.) This research would modify: the relative timing of benefit and risk presentations; the relative number of benefits and risks presented; the person making the presentation (e.g., the physician herself, another provider in the practice, an outside expert); and the format of the presentations (e.g., live, video, paper).

The initiatives described in this section are a sample of behaviors in health care that can be research projects and/or policy interventions employing the concepts and tools of behavioral economics. They represent the intersection of the more robust tenets of the discipline with issues that have vexed the US health care system. Of course, there are a myriad of other health care issues that might be responsive to behavioral economics, but the field needs to establish its validity in core areas before branching out.

Challenges Facing the Application of Behavioral Economics in Health Care

As noted earlier, there is considerable excitement among behavioral economists in general, and an interest in applying the tools of the discipline to many situations — including health care. Although the field would benefit from attention, there are a number of challenges that need to be overcome before it should be applied on a widespread basis. The first, and most important, is that the discipline needs a complete, comprehensive theory of consumer/patient behavior. At this point, there are a number of interconnected elements of a theory, but the field lacks a single, unifying theory with a recognized nomenclature. Second, which is not as critical in health care, is any kind of theory of supply. Perhaps, producers act enough like profit-maximizers (or satisficers) that an alternative to the neoclassical model is unnecessary, but work needs to be done to make that determination. Third, the application of behavioral economics to date has revealed that the financial interventions that have been employed may have a short-term impact, but the impact is greatly attenuated over time. If this is an endemic result, then more caution needs to be exercised in applying such interventions in circumstances that require long-term behavioral change.

The fourth challenge for behavioral economics is actually a danger. Edward Deci has long argued that interventions that are based on extrinsic motivation (such as financial incentives) run the risk of crowding out intrinsic motivation (Deci, 1971; Deci and Ryan, 1985; Deci *et al.*, 1999). If true, then short-term interventions will fail to propel participants to sustained behavior change once the interventions are discontinued. The result will be disappointment on the part of the researchers and disillusionment on the part of funders and policymakers.

The final challenge for behavioral economics (or neoclassical economics, for that matter) is the potential that economic norms, once applied, can replace social norms. As a result, what people do because of their obligation to society or feelings of solidarity within a community is replaced by the pursuit of economic gains. Uri Gneezy and Aldo Rustichini have discovered this phenomenon in both laboratory and naturally occurring experiments (Gneezy and Rustichini, 2000a; 2000b). Dan Ariely has argued that once a community shifts from social to economic norms, it is practically impossible to reverse course. Therefore, policymakers need to be cautious in introducing economic incentives into situations that have traditionally been handled through other means; the consequences may be profound.

Conclusion

Behavioral economics is a relatively new branch of economic thought, one that has reintroduced principles of psychology to the field. As a result, economic theory gives a more complete and accurate portrayal of human decision-making. By no longer assuming that individuals are rational all the time, behavioral economics expands the reach of economics. This extension benefits the analysis of the US health care sector, for which standard, neoclassical economics has been inadequate in explaining the behavior of patients, physicians, and policymakers. Behavioral economics has introduced such concepts as loss aversion, the endowment effect, framing, the power of the default, hyperbolic discounting, and System 1 vs. System 2 thinking. As we have seen in this chapter, these concepts enlighten our understanding of why people make seemingly irrational decisions such as becoming addicts, or failing to lose weight or quit smoking despite their best intentions. They help us to clarify why patients demand a prescription for a drug when they come to a physician's office, yet will not adhere to the medication regimen. They show why physicians will sometimes not perform in their patients' — or their own — best interests. From a global perspective, these concepts and their potential applications are also increasingly being recognized as critical levers for health and development policy, as described by the World Bank Group in its *World Development Report 2015: Mind, Society, and Behavior.*

The field of behavioral economics is less than three decades old, and has been applied to health care for just a decade. Nevertheless, the field offers great promise in understanding the behavior of decision-makers. Yet, much still needs to be done — to unify the theory and to validate the hypotheses through multiple empirical tests. We all must be cautious about applying these new and barely tested theories to any and all situations. But, with patience, we might be able to learn more about human behavior in general and the health care sector in particular.

References

ABIM Foundation. 2014. Choosing wisely. Retrieved from http://www.choosingwisely.org/.

Agassi A. 2009. *Open: An Autobiography*. New York: Alfred A. Knopf.

Ainslie G, Haslam N. 1992. Hyperbolic Discounting. In Loewenstein G, Elster J (eds.). *Choice Over Time* (pp. 57–92). New York, NY: Russell Sage Foundation.

Ashraf N, Camerer CF, Loewenstein G. 2005. Adam Smith, behavioral economist. *Journal of Economic Perspectives* 19(3): 131–145.

Becker GS, Murphy KM. 1988. A theory of rational addiction. *Journal of Political Economy* 96(4): 675–700.

Bickel WK, Johnson MW, Koffarnus MN, MacKillop J, Murphy JG. 2014. The behavioral economics of substance use disorders: Reinforcement pathologies and their repair. *Annual Review of Clinical Psychology* 10(1): 641–677.

Bleich SN, Barry CL, Gary-Webb TL, Herring BJ. 2014. Reducing sugar-sweetened beverage consumption by providing caloric information: How black adolescents alter their purchases and whether the effects persist. *American Journal of Public Health* 104(12): 2417–2424.

Cawley J, Price JA. 2013. A case study of a workplace wellness program that offers financial incentives for weight loss. *Journal of Health Economics* 32(5): 794–803.

Deci EL. 1971. Effects of externally mediated rewards on intrinsic motivation. *Journal of Personality and Social Psychology* 18(1): 105–115. doi:10.1037/h0030644.

Deci EL, Koestner R, Ryan RM. 1999. A meta-analytic review of experiments examining the effects of extrinsic rewards on intrinsic motivation. *Psychological Bulletin* 125(6): 627–668.

Deci EL, Ryan RM. 1985. *Intrinsic Motivation and Self-Determination in Human Behavior*. New York: Plenum.

DellaVigna S, Malmendier U. 2006. Paying not to go to the gym. *American Economic Review* 96(3): 694–719.

DiMatteo MR. 2004. Variations in patients' adherence to medical recommendations: A quantitative review of 50 years of research. *Medical Care* 42(3): 200–209.

Finkelstein A. 2009. E-ZTax: Tax salience and tax rates. *Quarterly Journal of Economics* 124(3): 969–1010.

Fischer MA, Stedman MR, Lii J, Vogeli C, Shrank WH, Brookhart MA, Weissman JS. 2010. Primary medication non-adherence: Analysis of 195,930 electronic prescriptions. *JGIM: Journal of General Internal Medicine* 25(4): 284–290.

Friedman M, Savage LJ. 1948. The utility analysis of choices involving risk. *Journal of Political Economy* 56(4): 279–304.

Fryer RG, Levitt SD, List J, Sadof S. 2012. *Enhancing the Efficacy of Teacher Incentives through Loss Aversion: A Field Experiment.* (*Working Paper* 18237). Cambridge, MA: National Bureau of Economic Research.

Gneezy U, Rustichini A. 2000a. A fine is a price. *The Journal of Legal Studies* 29(1): 1–17.

Gneezy U, Rustichini A. 2000b. Pay enough or don't pay at all. *Quarterly Journal of Economics* 115(3): 791–810.

Higgins ST, Washio Y, Heil SH, Solomon LJ, Gaalema DE, Higgins TM, Bernstein IM. 2012. Financial incentives for smoking cessation among pregnant and newly postpartum women. *Preventive Medicine* 55(Suppl): S33–S40.

Hough D. 2013. *Irrationality in Health Care: What Behavioral Economics Reveals about What We Do and Why*. Stanford, CA: Stanford University Press.

Internal Revenue Service. 2014. Retrieved from www.irs.gov.

Iyengar S. 2010. *The Art of Choosing*. New York: Twelve.

Johnson EJ, Goldstein D. 2003. Do defaults save lives? *Science* 302(5649): 1338–1339.

Johnson EJ, Hershey J, Meszaros J, Kunreuther H. 1993. Framing, probability distortions, and insurance decisions. *Journal of Risk and Uncertainty* 7(1): 35–51.

Johnson EJ, Shu SB, Dellaert BG, Fox C, Goldstein DG, Häubl G, Larrick RP, Payne JW, Peters E, Schkade D, Wansink B, Weber EU. Beyond nudges: Tools of a choice architecture. *Marketing Letters* 23(2): 487–504.

Just DR, Wansink B. 2009. Smarter lunchrooms: Using behavioral economics to improve meal selection. *Choices* 24(3).

Kahneman D. 2011. *Thinking, Fast and Slow* (1st ed.). New York: Farrar, Straus and Giroux.

Kahneman D, Tversky A. 1979. Prospect theory: An analysis of decision under risk. *Econometrica* 47(2): 263–292.

Knetsch JL. 1989. The endowment effect and evidence of nonreversible indifference curves. *American Economic Review* 79(5): 1277–1284.

Kullgren, JT, Troxel AB, Loewenstein G, Asch DA, Norton LA, Wesby L, Tao Y, Zhu J, Volpp KG. 2013. Individual- versus group-based financial incentives for weight loss: A randomized, controlled trial. *Annals of Internal Medicine* 158(7): 505–514.

Kunreuther H, Novemsky N, Kahneman D. 2001. Making low probabilities useful. *Journal of Risk and Uncertainty* 23(2): 103–120.

Loewenstein G. 1996. Out of control: Visceral influences on behavior. *Organizational Behavior and Human Decision Processes* 65(3): 272–292.

Loewenstein G. 2005. Hot–cold empathy gaps and medical decision making. *Health Psychology* 24(4): S49–S56.

Loewenstein GF. 1988. Frames of mind in intertemporal choice. *Management Science* 34(2): 200–214.

Madrian BC, Shea DF. 2001. The power of suggestion: Inertia in 401(k) participation and savings behavior. *Quarterly Journal of Economics* 116(4): 1149–1187.

McNeil B, Pauker S, Sox H, Tversky A. 1982. On the elicitation of preferences for alternative therapies. *The New England Journal of Medicine* 306(21): 1259–1262.

Saghai Y. 2013. Salvaging the concept of nudge. *Journal of Medical Ethics* 39(8): 487–493.

Sigmon SC, Patrick ME. 2012. The use of financial incentives in promoting smoking cessation. *Preventive Medicine* 55(Suppl): S24–S32.

Thaler RH, Sunstein CR. 2008. *Nudge: Improving Decisions About Health, Wealth, and Happiness*. New Haven: Yale University Press.

Tversky A, Kahneman D. 1986. Rational choice and the framing of decisions. *Journal of Business* 59(4): S251–S278.

Volpp KG, John LK, Troxel AB, Norton L, Fassbender J, Loewenstein G. 2008. Financial incentive-based approaches for weight loss: A randomized trial. *JAMA: The Journal of the American Medical Association* 300(22): 2631–2637.

Volpp KG, Troxel AB, Pauly MV, Glick HA, Puig A, Asch DA, Galvin R, Zhu J, Wan F, DeGuzman J, Corbett E, Weiner J, Audrain-McGovern J. 2009. A randomized, controlled trial of financial incentives for smoking cessation. *The New England Journal of Medicine* 360(7): 699–709.

Wansink B. 2006. *Mindless Eating: Why We Eat More than We Think.* New York: Bantam Books.

Weight-Control Information Network. 2012. *Overweight and Obesity Statistics* (No. NIH Publication No. 04-4158). Bethesda, MD: National Institute of Diabetes and Digestive and Kidney Diseases.

World Bank Group. 2015. *World Development Report 2015: Mind, Society, and Behavior.* Washington, DC: World Bank. Retrieved from: https://openknowledge.worldbank.org/handle/10986/20597.

Behavioral Economics: Health Applications in the UK

Adam Oliver*

Department of Social Policy, London School of Economics and Political Science

Over the past five years, the use of behavioral economics as an input into policy design generally, and health policy specifically, has been topical in the UK. This chapter details the genesis of this interest, and emphasizes that, according to UK Government rhetoric, the use of behavioral economics to influence the behavior of citizens — that is to say, nudge policy — has been the favored approach. The chapter then summarizes the health policy interventions that have been proposed by the Government's Behavioral Insights Team, and finds that the reasoning given for introducing these interventions often do not match the original conceptual requirements of the nudge approach, namely that an intervention ought to be anti-regulatory, be informed by behavioral economics and be focused on addressing negative internalities. In the area of behavioral economic policy, the Government's rhetoric therefore appears to be somewhat at odds with practice. The chapter finishes with a discussion of an alternative use of behavioral economics in policy, that of using the findings of the subdiscipline not to influence demand side behavior, but to regulate against pernicious activities on the supply side.

Keywords: Budge; Libertarian Paternalism; Nudge.

Introduction

Behavioral economics is really nothing more than the study of how people make decisions. Insofar that humans have always presumably been interested in this question, although perhaps not labeled as such, the discipline has been around since time immemorial. More recently and formally, it preoccupied at least some of those who laid the foundations of economics. Adam Smith's *Theory of Moral Sentiments*, for instance, is in part a book — or, rather, a master class — on

*Houghton Street, London WC2A 2AE, UK. Tel: +44 (0) 20-7955-6471; E-mail: a.j.oliver@lse.ac.uk.

intuitive behavioral economics (Smith, 1759). These days, behavioral economics is generally thought of as a systematic critique of the (albeit originally normative) assumption that people are self-interested, fully rational, utility-maximizing agents that came to dominate economics over the past century, although perhaps the most famous economist of the 20th century fully recognized that people are not as rational as many subsequent economists supposed, when he wrote that "the full consequences [of our decisions] ... can only be taken as the result of animal spirits — a spontaneous urge to action rather than inaction, and not as the outcome of a weighted average of quantitative benefits multiplied by quantitative probabilities" (Keynes, 1936).

The contribution of modern behavioral economists has to date principally been to go beyond intuition by observing, in controlled settings, the systematic tendencies by which people violate the assumptions of the mainstream neoclassical model of economics, and in some circumstances to estimate numerical parameters of specific behavioral economic phenomena, such as loss aversion. The French economist and Nobel laureate, Maurice Allais, was arguably the first person to contribute towards this effort in his famous critique of the independence axiom of expected utility theory, the theory that, when presented with risky options, decision-makers will choose the option from which they expect to derive the highest utility. Specifically, Allais (1953) argued that when presented with two or more options, people will, in particular circumstances, often systematically fail to perceive any outcome that is common among the options as irrelevant to their decision. This effect he attributed to the high weight people tend to attach to certainty, which may in itself be driven by a strong aversion to potential losses. The so-called Allais paradox predictably faced strong resistance from *l'Ecole Américaine*, leading him later to state pointedly that for "nearly 40 years the supporters of the neo-Bernoullian formulation (i.e., expected utility theory) have exerted a dogmatic and intolerant, powerful and tyrannical domination over the academic world; only in very recent years has a growing reaction began to appear. This is not the first example of the opposition of the 'establishments' of any kind to scientific progress, nor will it be the last" (Allais, 1990). Nonetheless, in subsequent decades, and particularly since the 1970s, behavioral economics has been dominated by Americans, and American-based Israelis.

Of all the many scientific contributions made by behavioral economists over the past 40 years, the most significant is probably prospect theory, developed by psychologists Daniel Kahneman and Amos Tversky, for which the former collected the 2002 Memorial Prize in Economics Sciences and which the latter would have surely shared but for his premature death. Prospect theory, unlike standard models of rational choice, was proposed as a purely descriptive theory. In prospect theory, Kahneman and Tversky (1979) and Tversky and Kahneman (1992) proposed two major modifications to expected utility theory: First, the carriers of value are gains and losses around a reference point rather than final assets, and losses are, through empirical observation, weighted substantially more than — at least twice as much as — gains of the same magnitude; second, people transform probabilities in an inverse S-shaped pattern, such that they overweight small probabilities, underweight large probabilities, and perceive subjective probability to equal objective probability at approximately 0.4. Kahneman and Tversky claimed that prospect theory could account for the major violations of expected utility theory, including the Allais paradox, and they asserted that the most distinctive implication of their theory is a predicted 4-fold pattern of risk attitudes, such that people will be risk averse when faced with small probabilities of losses and large probabilities of gains, and risk seeking when faced with large probabilities of losses and small probabilities of gains. Thus, prospect theory possibly at least partially explains why people demonstrate inconsistent risk attitudes by purchasing insurance (risk aversion in the face of a small probability of losses) *and* lottery tickets (risk seeking in the face of a small probability of gains), an inconsistency that has challenged generations of economists.

Kahneman and Tversky served as figureheads for the cadre of behavioral economists who emerged with and after them, and there is now a large body of behavioral economic research, much of which is broadly, if sometimes reluctantly, accepted by the mainstream economics community. It is only in relatively recent years, however, that behavioral economic observations have been applied substantively to practical policy concerns. These policy efforts have been underpinned by philosophical frameworks — principally soft forms of paternalism (or approaches against anti-paternalism that purportedly do not advocate paternalism) — developed by some of the world's leading behavioral economists, and include asymmetric paternalism, formulated by Camerer *et al.* (2003), and libertarian paternalism, developed by Thaler and Sunstein (2003; 2008). Asymmetric paternalism incentivizes irrational decision-makers to instead make rational choices, without harming rational decision-makers. It is asymmetric in the sense that those who already make rational choices are minimally affected while those who make irrational choices have the opportunity to reap larger benefits. Similarly, libertarian paternalism aims to steer people toward welfare-promoting choices (for example, by reframing the choices or changing the default option) while maintaining individuals' freedom of choice. These two approaches are very similar to each other: Both focus upon influencing behavior on the demand-side (i.e., the consumer or the citizen), but asymmetric paternalism is more open than libertarian paternalism to regulatory intervention. Both theories are also minor modifications of welfare economics, in that they retain wellbeing as the normative criterion but detach the achievement of wellbeing from individual choice.[1] Libertarian paternalism has been much more influential in policy circles, partly perhaps because the policies aligned to it have been assigned a catchy buzzword — *nudges* — and possibly partly because the approach was outlined in Thaler and Sunstein's popular science book "Nudge" with a dust jacket that depicted an elephant nudging a smaller elephant, and has thus, for better or for worse, transcended the narrower confines of the academic discourse.

To the uninitiated, libertarian paternalism may sound like an oxymoron, but Thaler and Sunstein use the term libertarian to modify the word paternalism in order to signify that their approach is liberty-preserving. There should be no burden on those who choose their pre-existing behaviors rationally and thus wish to continue with those behaviors. Therefore, the approach does not allow regulation or bans, which is another possible reason why it may be a more attractive philosophy than asymmetric paternalism to many contemporary policymakers. The approach is only paternalistic in the sense of wanting to motivate behavior change among those who, on reflection, would have liked to have made different choices for themselves. That is, a nudge is meant to bring the instantaneous decisions of those who, on reflection, think that their non-reflective actions are irrational into better alignment with their deliberative preferences (and thus relies on the heavy assumption that deliberative preference is necessarily rational). Thus, the focus is on reducing negative internalities — the longer-term harms that a person himself or herself experiences due to their own ill-considered automatic decisions. Libertarian paternalism rules out using significant financial incentives or overt persuasion to change behavior; the essence of the approach is that behavioral economic insights — such as loss aversion, probability weighting and present bias (the observation that people place a heavy emphasis on the immediate moment) — can and should inform the design of what Thaler and Sunstein call the choice architecture, or in other words, the context or the environment, so that more people make automatic decisions that, on reflection, they would like to make and yet, due to bounds on their economically-defined rationality and human error, ordinarily fail to do so. By appealing to the cognitive affects and processes that people employ when making automatic decisions, we might expect that behavioral economic informed interventions will have more effect than interventions that are otherwise informed.

The concept of libertarian paternalism and its application in the form of nudges has attracted the attention of governments in a number of countries, but none more so than that of the United Kingdom (UK), where a right of center

[1] Sugden (2013) advocates an opposing approach by proposing that opportunity to choose should be the normative criterion, without claiming that increases in opportunity necessarily improve wellbeing.

Coalition Government lauded the apparent promise of the approach to offer non-regulatory inexpensive demand-side solutions to some of the most profound problems in contemporary societies. "This new approach," according to a 2010 Government Report, "represents an important part of the Coalition Government's commitment to reducing regulatory burdens on business and society, and achieving its policy goals as cheaply and effectively as possible" (Behavioural Insights Team, 2010). Nudge policy, taken at face value, offers an alternative to regulating the sometimes pernicious activities of the supply-side. Soon after being appointed Prime Minister in 2010, David Cameron established the Behavioral Insights Team (BIT), colloquially known as the Nudge Unit, with Thaler serving as an advisor. The BIT (https://www.gov.uk/government/organisations/behavioural-insights-team) has only a handful of staff and has arguably experienced diminishing influence over time — which may cause some to worry, and others to hope, that the approach is a fad. Yet it remains, from a central government policy perspective (despite the unit being in part turned into a private consultancy in 2013), a global leader in developing and piloting behavioral economic-informed policy interventions.

Two months prior to the Coalition Government's election to office, a number of those who would go on to work for the BIT in various capacities published the intellectual foundation for the approach that was subsequently adopted. This document is known as the *Mindspace Report* (Cabinet Office and Institute for Government, 2010). Given its importance to the foundation of the BIT, it is worth critically considering the document in some detail.

The Mindspace Report

'Mindspace' is a somewhat convenient mnemonic, comprised of the following characteristics that are, according to the authors of the report, of relevance when considering behavior change interventions:

Messenger: We are heavily influenced by who communicates information.
Incentives: Our responses to incentives are shaped by predictable mental shortcuts.
Norms: We are strongly influenced by what others do.
Defaults: We go with the flow of pre-set options.
Salience: Our attention is drawn to what is novel and seems relevant to us.
Priming: Our acts are often influenced by sub-conscious cues.
Affect: Our emotional associations can powerfully shape our actions.
Commitments: We seek to be consistent with our public promises, and reciprocate acts.
Ego: We act in ways that make us feel better about ourselves.

The mnemonic, as intended, is quite easy to memorize, but grouping behavioral drivers in this way may risk some confusion. For instance, some of the factors appear highly interconnected — Messenger and Norms, for example, both seem to be driven in part by trust, and Norms, Defaults, Salience and Priming are associated with giving people clear reference points or anchors. Affect and Priming are not always readily distinguishable, and Commitments and Priming may gain their effect from, and be used to tackle, the mental shortcuts, such as loss aversion and present bias, which the authors of *Mindspace* group under Incentives. Close inspection of the mnemonic therefore creates a somewhat hazy impression, offering little specific clarity on where each characteristic can be used and to what effect, although, admittedly, the list does give a broad indication of the types of influences that may be of import.

The *Mindspace* approach is presumably meant to be a form of soft paternalism and, particularly when it was adopted by the BIT with Thaler serving as an advisor, libertarian paternalism. Indeed, the authors state that "We are interested in the soft touch of policy rather than its heavy hand: going with the grain of human nature, rather than rubbing us up the wrong way." Yet, confusions arise here too. Thaler and Sunstein's approach focused upon addressing negative internalities — that is, altering personal lifestyle behaviors so as to improve the lives of those engaged in these behaviors, as judged by these people themselves (i.e., paternalism). The authors of *Mindspace*, however, propose using the approach to address negative internalities *and* externalities, and thus the remit of nudging became very quickly confused in UK (and global) academic and policy circles. This confusion perhaps arose partly due to reasons of political expediency, in that attempts by public policymakers to curtail private behaviors that are harmful to others are likely to gain broader general public support than attempts to alter personal lifestyle behaviors that present no external harms, particularly if those whose support is being solicited feel at risk of being nudged. As acknowledged by the authors of *Mindspace*, public permission for the nudge approach matters. Unfortunately, public permission, unless garnered for the policy at only a very general level, may undermine the effectiveness of interventions that rely on a covert influence on automatic choice behaviors. The question then is whether public permission at a very general level of policy, rather than at the level of each individual intervention, is sufficient to legitimize the approach.

The LSE Philosopher, Luc Bovens, has argued that ethical acceptability does not require governments to explain that an intervention has been implemented, particularly if full transparency limits the effectiveness of the intervention, so long as those being nudged have the ability to discern its implementation (House of Lords, 2011). Boven's view, however, can be quite readily challenged, in that behavioral economic policy potentially covers a large range of qualitatively different interventions, from the profound and, for many, unacceptably intrusive (e.g., defaulting people into actions, such as organ donation, that they would rather not do but are not fully cognizant that they are now enrolled into), to the seemingly innocuous (e.g., moving food items around on canteen shelves). People might not fully appreciate the extent to which libertarian paternalism could plausibly offer governments the legitimacy to manipulate behavior covertly. In democracies, where public policymakers ought to be at least held up to standards of transparency, requiring public permission at only the general policy level would allow governments much scope to overstep what many would feel to be the limits of their authority. The *Mindspace* authors acknowledge that whenever the effectiveness of public policy interventions depends on triggering the automatic system, governments will leave themselves open to charges of manipulation, and they intimate that there needs to be a public discussion on the proper role of the state. They also maintain that the extent to which the *Mindspace* approach preserves substantive freedoms is likely to come down to political judgment. That may well be the case, but the political decision to implement covert policy interventions ought to be informed by public opinion and not solely by the judgment of the few who hold power, and the public debate on this issue has yet to be had.

The *Mindspace* authors also highlight a further problem that is endemic to the nudge approach, which is that very few behavioral interventions of this sort have been assessed for their sustained effect. Some interventions, such as changing default positions from having to opt-in to a particular activity to being required to opt-out, rely on sustained inertia rather than sustained action for their effectiveness, and since human beings are quite good at being inert, their longer-term effectiveness is likely to be secure. However, the majority of purported nudges, many of which will be detailed later in relation to smoking cessation and exercise, for example, require sustained action rather than inaction. It is unfortunate that many contemporary advocates for behavioral change interventions have not adopted the *Mindspace* authors' cautionary stance on sustainability, and have been sometimes guilty of overselling policies based on flimsy evidence of effect (there are also more than a few policymakers who tend to overbuy the promise that these interventions offer). This overselling is arguably understandable because behaviouralists of various stripes have been, and are, fighting hard to get their ideas accepted in policy circles and have thus, over recent years, sensed and seized their opportunity. However, some have become so enamored with their general approach that they have placed insufficient emphasis on self-criticism. One of the decision-making heuristics that psychologists and behavioral economists have laid claim to over the last 40 years is called confirmation bias: That is, the finding that people search for and anchor on evidence that supports their own theories, overlooking evidence that places their ideas in a less favorable light. Knowledge of this phenomena was of course well known before behavioral economists laid claim to it; Karl Popper (1957), for instance, in *The Poverty of Historicism* wrote that "if we are uncritical we shall always find what we want: We shall look for, and find, confirmations, and we shall look away from, and not see, whatever might be dangerous to our pet theories. In this way it is only too easy to obtain what appears to be overwhelming evidence in favor of a theory which, if approached critically, would have been refuted." Nonetheless, it is somewhat ironic that confirmation bias contaminates the contemporary discourse on behavioral interventions, not least because a self-critical exposition of the general approach may well be more convincing to those who might otherwise resist.

In terms of possible policy applications, it may therefore be prudent to stick with the behavioral economic findings for which there is a substantial evidence base. The *Mindspace* Report lists these as predictable mental shortcuts under 'Incentives,' and they include loss aversion around a reference point, present bias, and the overweighting of small probabilities. This limited number of substantive behavioral economic tools would at least help analysts to retain a degree of intellectual clarity, and lend reasonable theoretical and methodological justification to what they are trying to do. An assessment of whether interventions that are popularly being advocated as nudges comply with the original requirements of libertarian paternalism laid out by Thaler and Sunstein would also dispel some of the confusion that has infected the whole approach. It is, furthermore, surely important to try to hold governments accountable for their rhetoric, and it is to this we now turn.

A Three-Dimensional Space

As aforementioned, libertarian paternalism and nudge policy appear to be based on a number of premises — for example, the non-use of significant financial incentives and an absence of persuasion, with a preference instead for redesigning choice environments in light of extant human cognitive processes such that people are more likely to make automatic decisions that better align with their deliberative preferences. Three core features of libertarian paternalism, each represented on an axis in Figure 1, are that it addresses internalities rather than externalities, that it preserves liberty and is therefore anti-regulatory, and that its applications are informed by behavioral economics rather than the standard model of rational choice.

A classic nudge would be placed at the origin in Figure 1, which indicates that the intervention would preserve liberty, be informed by behavioral economics, and be focused on addressing negative internalities. An example of such an intervention might be to place apples rather than chocolate bars at supermarket checkout

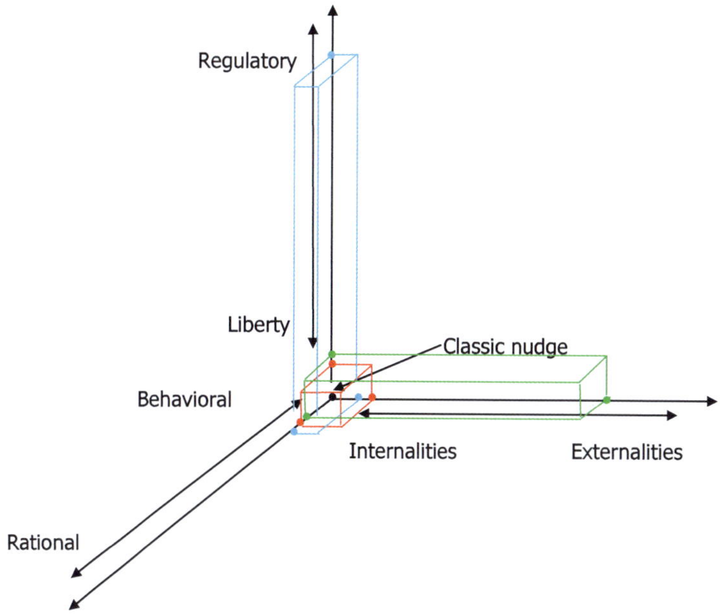

Figure 1. The libertarian paternalism space

counters — in such circumstances, a shopper is not required to buy the apples but might, on reflection, prefer to buy an apple rather than a chocolate bar, and is more likely to now buy an apple because the presence of the apple near to the checkout has invaded his immediate and automatic decision making mental apparatus. Movements up the vertical axis in Figure 1 indicate that an intervention adopts a more regulatory stance, movements along the horizontal axis indicate the extent to which the intervention is focused upon addressing externalities rather than internalities, and movements along the axis that is diagonally depicted show the degree to which the intervention is informed by rational choice theory. Nudge policies should therefore cluster around the origin. Hypothetical policies that are not aligned with the nudge approach are indicated by the tall and long boxes in Figure 1, the tall box because it is highly regulatory (such as compulsory seat-belts), and the long box because it focuses on addressing negative externalities (such as motivating reduced hospital waiting times).

The three-dimensional space depicted in Figure 1 can thus be used to give a visual representation of the extent to which actual interventions that are purported to be motivated by the nudge approach align with the requirements of libertarian paternalism. Soon after it was established, the BIT released a discussion paper on behavioral interventions intended to improve personal health-related choices (Behavioural Insights Team, 2010). It is noteworthy, and laudable, that the BIT has adopted a scientific approach with the interventions that it has proposed for consideration, and has at this stage called for piloting, rather than a national roll-out, of these policies. As such, little will be said about the effectiveness of these interventions here, for the good reason that their effectiveness, particularly their sustained effectiveness, is generally not yet known. Figures 2 and 3 depict

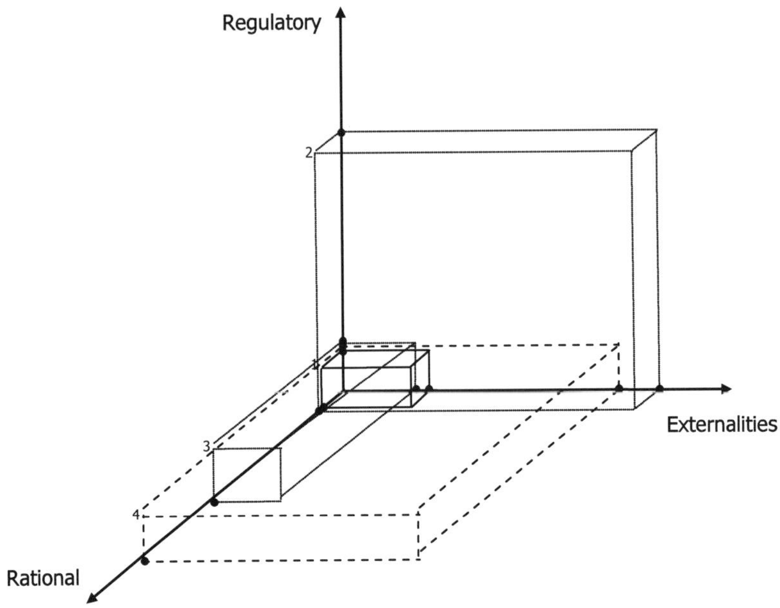

Figure 2. The BIT health proposals

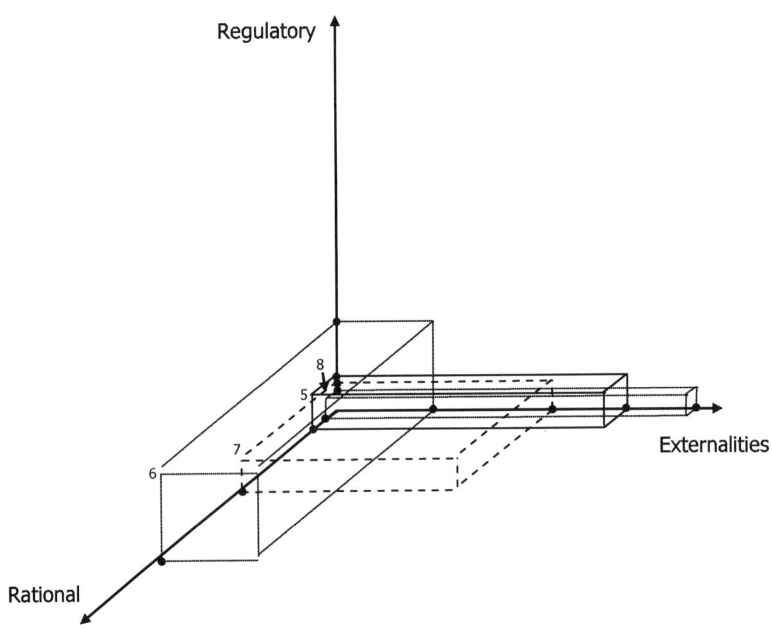

Figure 3. The BIT health proposals continued

these interventions in the three dimensional space. The top left corner of each box within the spaces is assigned a number that aligns with the numbered interventions listed in Table 1. The distances from the origin on each dimension of course rely on judgment, but a balanced judgment nevertheless offers an indication of the extent to which the nudge approach that was embraced so enthusiastically in Prime Minister David Cameron's rhetoric has actually informed the interventions proposed by the BIT unit that was formed partly on the basis of that rhetoric.

To reiterate, the depictions of the various interventions in Figures 2 and 3 are necessarily approximations based on judgment, but they do offer a diagrammatic visualization of the extent to which the BIT proposals satisfy the original theoretical requirements of libertarian paternalism. It is, one hopes, reasonably clear that while the BIT's proposed health-related interventions do not, for the most part, rely on regulation, their use of behavioral economics is sometimes not obvious and they often appear to focus upon addressing externalities rather than internalities. The tendency towards a focus on negative externalities is consistent with the *Mindspace Report*, but the drift away from the original nudge requirements breeds confusion; as noted earlier, however, it is perhaps understandable, due to the reluctance shown by many contemporary politicians to avoid accusations of nannying, that they do not wish to create the perception that they are interfering in personal lifestyle choices, unless, of course, those choices impose real or imagined harms on others.

Although this particular chapter focuses on health-related policy interventions, the three-dimensional space can also be used to map purported nudges in other sectors to ascertain to some degree the extent to which these are actual nudges, strictly defined. For example, Figure 4 depicts some selected interventions outlined in the BIT (2011) report on personal energy use. These interventions, which are targeted at improving environmental consciousness and reducing carbon emissions, are principally focused on externalities, although some consideration of internalities does come into play since individuals can save themselves money by acting upon at least some of the proposed initiatives (moreover, an increasing number of people are probably internally motivated to reduce their negative externalities in this context). Intervention (1) in Figure 4 is the proposal to introduce upfront incentives for environmentally beneficial behavior, which may appeal to notions of present bias by offsetting the immediate costs associated with being more energy conscious. For example, the BIT propose a one-month holiday from council tax payments (the tax that residents pay to their local government authorities for the provision of services, which varies across geographical areas but is typically in the region of £1,000 per month) for those who agree to insulate their lofts, a subsidy that may be somewhat galling to those who have already undertaken this task. Similarly, the government introduced a policy of providing financial support to those choosing to install renewable heating technologies in place of

Table 1. BIT health proposals

1. **Smoking Cessation:** The BIT proposed commitment devices, otherwise known as default contracts, to incentivize smoking cessation. These interventions require smokers to voluntarily pre-commit small amounts of their own money to a smoking cessation programme, which is returned to them if they remain abstinent. Admittedly, getting people to pre-commit even small amounts of money may be particularly difficult among those groups where smoking is most prevalent (such as the poor), but the intended behavioral motivation is that people will not want to lose even small amounts of money, and thus, via loss aversion, will be keen to meet the programme's objectives, a device that has received much attention in other contexts (e.g., see www.stickK.com). The intervention is therefore behaviorally motivated, is non-compulsory, and, assuming quite reasonably that those who enroll in these types of programmes wish to change their behaviors, is focused on addressing negative internalities (although a concern with saving money for the National Health Service (NHS) by reducing smoking rates lends an element of externality consideration to this intervention). Agreeing to a commitment device appears to require more conscious deliberation than a simple alteration of the choice architecture entails, but in terms of the three-dimensional space, it conforms reasonably closely to the characteristics of a nudge.
2. **Organ Donation:** In order to increase the number of people on the organ donor register, the BIT proposed piloting a move from an opt-in system to one of prompted choice, where, for instance, people have to state whether or not they wish to be a donor at the time of purchasing or renewing their driving license. This change in the default position, a form of reference point, has had some success in increasing the number of people on the register in other contexts, and is behaviorally motivated. An important aside, however, is that requiring next of kin consent for the use of organs at the time of death reduces the effectiveness of prompted choice to increase the number of available organs. At face value, prompted choice preserves autonomy in that people are free to refrain from being on the register if they so wish, although many might feel they are being somewhat coerced by the use of such a mechanism and a national roll-out of the intervention would presumably require regulation. The policy appears to be driven by externality considerations (others may benefit if one registers), although considerations of reciprocity may play a role (if more people register, we all may benefit). The BIT is testing, with some success, whether emphasizing reciprocity is more likely to encourage people to register (Behavioural Insights Team, 2013). This intervention, nonetheless, in Figure 2 is likely to be further along the regulatory and externality axes than a classic nudge.
3. **Teenage Pregnancy:** The BIT suggested that teenagers mentor toddlers in an attempt to reduce the rate of teenage pregnancy. Presumably, the targeted teenagers would be able to opt out of the programme if they so wish (and thus, as with commitment devices, enrollment appears to rely on conscious choice). If so, autonomy is preserved. Moreover, the intervention, although driven to some extent by externality concerns, addresses negative internalities under the arguable assumption that the young women in question, on reflection, genuinely would rather not have a child during their teenage years. However, the intervention seems only tenuously linked to behavioral economics, with a possible association with Akerlof and Kranton's (2010) work on identity economics, where a closer identification with a particular situation might be expected to lead to a change in individual behavior (i.e., greater identification with all that is required of a mother may motivate some teenagers to more carefully avoid pregnancy). That said, this particular intervention may equally be informed by rational choice

(*Continued*)

Table 1. (*Continued*)

theory, where more knowledge and information might lead to different decisions, and is therefore further along the rational axis in Figure 2 than a classic nudge.

4. **Alcohol Consumption:** Due to some evidence that students think their peers drink more alcohol than they actually do, and that this in turn increases average drinking levels in this population, the BIT propose to communicate accurate drinking levels to university students. Although the inaccurate perceptions of alcohol consumption imply a misaligned reference point and the intervention perhaps involves correcting this, the provision of better information also appears to appeal to rational decision making. Moreover, although there is some concern with negative internalities, the thrust of the approach focuses on addressing externalities, in particular costs to the NHS. The intervention does not require regulation and leaves students at liberty to drink what they wish, but one may then question whether the intervention would address substantially the problem (if excessive drinking by students is indeed a problem) to which it is targeted. This intervention is more rational and addresses more externalities than a classic nudge.
5. **Healthy Eating:** Manipulation of the reference point by putting markings on supermarket trolleys to define areas where fruit and vegetables are placed is proposed as a means of encouraging increased purchasing of these products (whether increased purchasing necessarily leads to increased consumption is a moot point), but the BIT's motivation for encouraging healthier eating habits is again that of an externality concern — i.e., how much obesity costs the NHS — and is therefore quite far along the externality axis in Figure 3. Consumers would remain free in relation to their fruit and vegetable purchasing patterns, and the BIT is not proposing that supermarkets be required to use the visual prompts. The supermarkets are unlikely to use the prompts if they think they are harming profits, but may comply with what they might consider to be a rather trivial intervention as a means of warding off stronger government regulation.
6. **Children's Health:** The use of small incentives to effect behavior change in children is proposed for more than one intervention by the BIT. For instance, they announced a partnership with *LazyTown*, an initiative that has been operating nationally in Iceland since 1996, in which young children sign contracts with their parents that rewards them for eating healthily, going to bed early and being active. A further initiative allows diabetic children to claim points, exchangeable for computer games, for consenting to blood sugar measurements. Some might question whether good behavior among children ought to be motivated with what may be construed as bribes, although others may contend that manipulating the actions of those who lack full agency (e.g., children) is more justifiable than doing similarly with most adults, which strengthens the argument for attempting to address negative internalities in this case. It may also be contended justifiably that incentives such as these are tools of rational economic theory (hence its placement along the rational axis in Figure 3), although if the incentives are very small with their objective primarily being that of engaging children in the immediate moment, then, arguably, they feed on notions of present bias and are thus informed by behavioral economics. Moreover, depending on the strictness of the parents, these methods may preserve liberty, and do not have to involve overly overt methods of persuasion, although, like some of the other interventions discussed above, they probably require more conscious deliberation than that entailed by a simple alteration of the choice architecture.
7. **Promoting Activity:** Warming to the theme of incentives, the BIT propose consideration of piano stairs — that is, embedding sensors in stairs so that people can make sounds with their feet — so as to encourage people to be more active. Piano stairs fall under the rubric of fun

(*Continued*)

Table 1. (*Continued*)

theory, or the making of unpleasant but healthy tasks more enjoyable in the immediate moment, and may therefore be associated with present bias to a slightly stronger degree than with Intervention 6. Such interventions do not force people to do anything, and pre-existing behaviors can be pursued if they are (and even if they are not) rational. BIT's emphasis in relation to this intervention again seems to be on saving money for the NHS, and is thus focused on externalities, although an internality argument can also be made. In Figure 3, this intervention is likely to be more rational and to be more externality-drive than a classic nudge.

8. **Food Hygiene**: The BIT expresses enthusiasm for the UK's National Food Hygiene Rating Scheme, where food outlets post voluntarily on their entrances their food hygiene rating in the form of a standardized sticker, from five points for very good, to zero points for 'urgent improvement necessary', a scheme that has also been used with some success in other countries (e.g., see Thaler and Sunstein, 2008). Although voluntary, one might expect the intervention to be more effective if it were compulsory and thus involved the regulation of the supply-side. Nonetheless, it is seemingly informed by behavioral economics in that food outlets may take a middling score (say, three to four points) as their reference point of acceptability, and might thus be particularly motivated to avoid the psychological loss associated with scores worse than that. It is perhaps important to note that substantial improvements in performance have been observed following the use of similar instruments of public reporting in environments where consumer choice is absent, including the hospital sector in some health care systems, and therefore such improvements are not merely rational, demand-led responses towards yet another intervention that appears to be focused on addressing negative externalities. In Figure 3, this intervention is placed far along the horizontal externalities axis.

those that use fossil fuels. As with the health-related incentives, these interventions do not seem to be targeting non-deliberative decision making, a key feature of libertarian paternalism, and some may contend that they introduce an element of coercion. The BIT also highlight the potential usefulness of smart electricity meters (represented by (2) in Figure 4), which offer a reading of the average energy consumption of similar households in addition to one's own electricity use. This additional information can of course be ignored and therefore may not impinge substantially upon autonomy, but it could reasonably be contended that the smart meters are merely providing additional information and are hence forms of persuasion rather than nudges. However, it could equally be argued that the average consumption level of similar households is behavioral economic informed in the sense that this may provide a reference point, against which the consumer might perceive higher energy consumption as a loss, motivating them to use less electricity. Further, in an effort to encourage its departments to conserve energy, the government is experimenting with changing default settings in heating and cooling systems (intervention (3)). Changing the default requires regulation of sorts, but if the employees within these departments have the capacity to override the default settings and face no internal or external sanction should they wish to

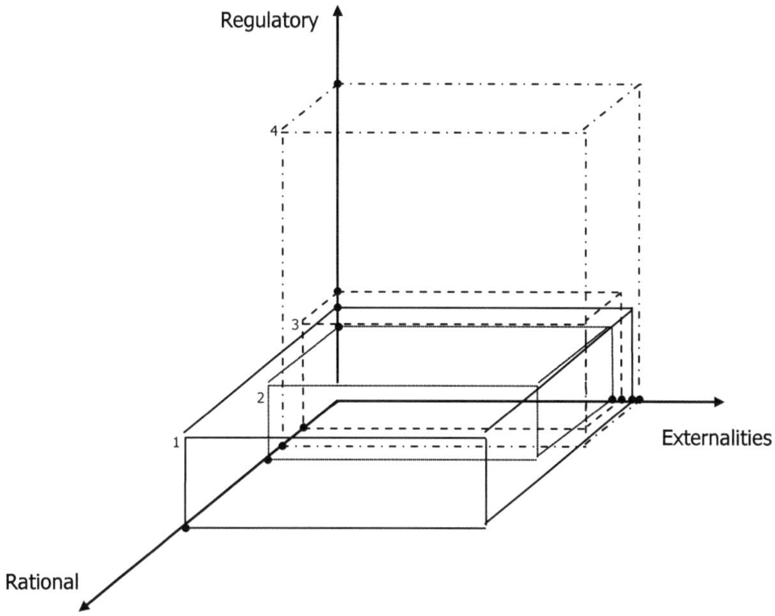

Figure 4. Selected BIT energy saving proposals

do so, then their autonomy is for the most part retained, and, as already noted, default manipulation is behaviorally motivated. Finally for here, the government is publishing league tables that show the extent to which each department is demonstrating progress towards a pan-government energy saving target (intervention (4)). The autonomy of each department appears compromised by this initiative in that their performance is involuntary recorded for all to see, but the intervention is behaviorally informed if, as seems reasonable, each department perceives average (or higher) performance as the reference point, and any performance lower than this as, in some sense, a loss.

By and large, the self-proclaimed nudgers are often not, strictly speaking, nudging. This matters because it draws a mist over the intellectual clarity of applied nudge policy and policymakers are seemingly not acting consistently with their rhetoric. This being said, a reasonable argument can be made that behavioral economic policy might in any case be more appropriate and profound if its parameters were quite different to the constraints laid out by nudge.

An Alternative to Nudging

Libertarian paternalism postulates much that is contentious, perhaps the most important point of which is the question of whether we should make it legitimate for governments to introduce (or extend their range of) policies that provoke unconscious behavior change that presumably must rely on covert policy design (with interventions not necessarily hidden, but unnoticed), particularly policies that are meant to be limited to addressing internalities. Libertarian paternalists would argue that they wish only to nudge people towards their own deliberative preferences — what people themselves, on reflection, say that they want. However, some contend that there is no guarantee that deliberative preferences exist (Sugden, 2009), and even if they do, it may be the case that people would not want their behaviors manipulated covertly towards any objective; in short, that the ends do not justify the means. It thus seems reasonable to contest that libertarian paternalism may be at odds with open deliberative democracy. The very idea of paternalistic intervention by government is inconsistent with many people's perception of what it means to be a free society, although some explicit policies that interfere in personal choice to limit the extent to which people might otherwise harm themselves — e.g., mandatory seatbelt and motorcycle helmet legislation — appear to attract broad public support. As reflected by the predominant motivation for most of the BIT's proposals, it is likely that people feel more comfortable with government action that limits the extent to which people harm others; in essence, the application of Mill's (1869) harm principle. Which begs the question, if people are imposing negative externalities on others, why should we feel beholden to protect their liberty?

Although the authors of the *Mindspace Report* argue that their preferred form of behavioral economic policy ought to be used alongside other policy tools, such as regulation, they do not discuss the possibility of using behavioral economics as an intellectual justification of where and how to regulate. It is my contention that the use of behavioral economics to inform, following a period of open public discussion, the explicit regulation against harms imposed by the supply side might offer a more profound use of this subdiscipline than that of attempting to manipulate the demand side, an approach that I have elsewhere labeled 'budge' (Oliver, 2013). A key distinction between the nudge and budge approaches is that nudges counter the profit-maximizing, behavioral economic-informed manipulation of consumers and citizens by private organizations with similar welfare-maximizing interventions introduced by the public sector, whereas budges openly regulate against these private sector activities.

In common with nudges, the fundamental requirements of budge policy can also be depicted on a three dimensional diagram. In Figure 5, the behavioral-to-rational axis is identical to that in Figure 1. Budges rely on knowledge of behavioral economics to detect when the private sector is essentially using profit-maximizing nudges that exploit the individual consumer. For example, confectionary companies, due to their implicit knowledge of the power of present bias and salience on individual choice behavior, have traditionally paid supermarkets substantial

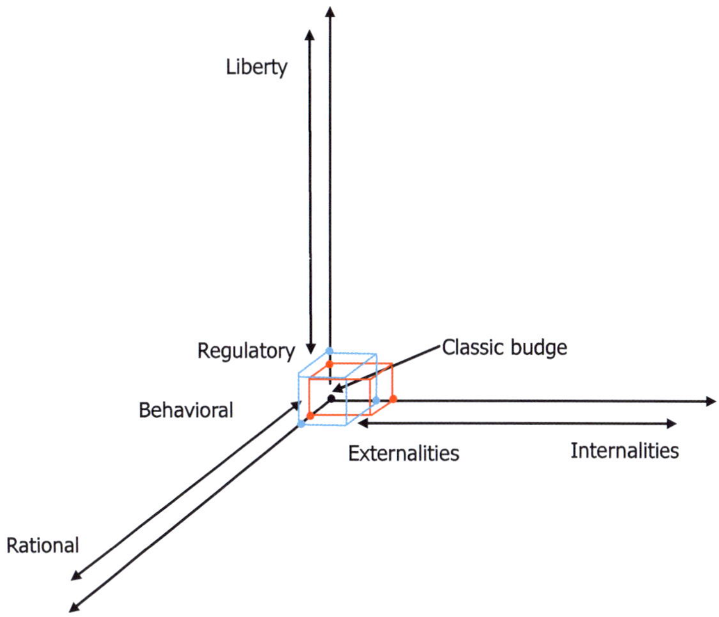

Figure 5. The budge space

amounts of money to display their products next to cashier counters. If policymakers recognized that these behavioral economic characteristics were being exploited so as to encourage people to buy more of these products than is good for them (i.e., that the confectioners are essentially imposing harms on the consumer), they would have an intellectual justification for at least having an open discussion as to whether this activity ought to be regulated against. In this case, the design of the regulation would not be informed by behavioral economics in the way that the design of nudges are meant to be informed as such, but knowledge of the behavioral economic findings is required in order to detect when private sector interests are using them for their own, sometimes objectionable, ends. In other instances, the design of the regulation itself can also be informed by behavioral economics so as to attempt to strengthen its effect (and one such example will be discussed below), but this is not a requirement for budge policy. The liberty-to-regulatory and internalities-to-externalities axes of Figure 1 are inverted in Figure 5, to depict that a budge is meant to regulate openly against external harms. A classic budge, such as (perhaps) banning supermarkets from placing chocolate bars at cashier checkouts or prohibiting cereal manufacturers from advertising or even producing high-chocolate-content breakfast products for children, would thus be placed close to the origin.

Nudges leave the supply-side alone and manipulate the demand-side; budge policies leave the demand-side alone and regulate the supply-side. As aforementioned, one of the reasons for the current popularity of the nudge approach in UK policy is because it aligns with the antiregulatory positioning of the government. This is indicated in the BIT (2010) report on health, which specifies that the Public Health Responsibility Deal is an example of the government working with other organizations to ensure that we all live up to our responsibilities in supporting healthier lifestyles. The Public Health Responsibility Deal between the government and the food and drinks industries entailed the latter agreeing voluntarily to make efforts to encourage healthier consumption patterns so as to avoid heavier forms of regulation. Unfortunately, the effectiveness of the Deal has proved inauspicious (House of Lords, 2011), principally because profit-making businesses are driven, quite rationally, by profit maximization, and they know how to present an image of compliance with the Deal that will not fundamentally undermine their overriding priority.

For example, consider the policy of labeling food products with traffic light symbols, such as red, amber and green signs to indicate high, intermediate and low energy dense foods, respectively. From behavioral economics, we might hypothesize that people will select amber signs as their reference point, and thus be particularly motivated to avoid those foods with red symbols, judging them to be, in some respect, losses. Indeed, traffic light labeling of this sort has been shown to work (House of Lords, 2011), provided that the labeling is not too complex (such labeling may also have negative consequences, such as a processed cheese being labeled as healthier than a naturally produced cheese, but we shall leave those concerns aside here). Those industries that produce foods that would be given a red symbol, such as cheese and chocolate manufacturers, naturally resist such labeling, and indeed implicitly use the human tendency towards present bias when marketing their products, highlighting the immediate pleasures that these goods offer and overlooking their potential longer term harms. If an open public discussion reached the conclusion that these harms are substantive, the government would have a strong intellectual justification for mandating food manufacturers and supermarkets to place simple traffic light symbols on all of the products that they sell. This would then be a budge policy where both the reason for regulating and the design of the regulation are informed by behavioral economics, and is represented by the box positioned marginally closest to the origin. In order to avoid a budge of this kind, many supermarkets voluntarily place traffic light symbols on their products, ostensibly in compliance with the Responsibility Deal. However, the labels that they apply tend to be too complex to have a discernable effect on consumer choice (particularly perhaps among those groups for whom healthier eating habits are likely to be most beneficial), and thus do not pose a threat to profits. We can speculate reasonably that supermarkets are aware that too much complexity negates the effectiveness of this particular intervention.

Like nudges, budges can of course be applied beyond health-related considerations, and extend to all sectors of public policy. For example, payday loan companies heavily market their services, often towards relatively poor people, at invariably barely revealed interest rates measuring many thousands of percent in the UK. These companies appeal to present bias — the heavy emphasis on the short term pleasure of spending and the underweighting of the longer term pain of repayment — and in the process, harm many people. An open discussion of these activities, motivations and consequences might reveal widely held support for a more heavily regulated pay day loan market which, if not extending to an outright ban on the provision of these services, might at least lead to the imposition of more reasonable maximum interest rate charges. Such regulation, motivated by the knowledge that payday loan companies implicitly use behavioral economic phenomenon to exploit and impose harms on others, would be a budge, and is represented by the other box in Figure 5.

Conclusion

Behavioral economics has captured the imagination of many of those working in UK policy over the past several years, demonstrated principally by the popularity of the nudge approach. This particular branch of behavioral economic-informed policy retains individual utility maximization as the normative goal, but unlike the standard theory of rational choice, assumes that people make errors in that their automatic decisions often conflict with their deliberative preferences. These errors, it is postulated by libertarian paternalists, can often be rectified if the environment — the choice architecture — is redesigned according to the findings of behavioral economics. Since the basic assumption is that such a redesign will cause people to make better choices for themselves as judged by themselves, and that they will make these choices automatically and unconsciously, the approach, via covert policy intervention, addresses negative internalities.

In democracies, it can be contested quite reasonably that it is somewhat objectionable to give governments authority to manipulate covertly individual behaviors appertaining to personal lifestyles that have no bearing on others. This contention, and the possibility that many purported nudges, such as placing internal markings on supermarket trolleys and the introduction of piano stairs, are merely scratching at the surface of deep societal problems, might lead one to conclude that overt regulation of those who persuade boundedly rational individuals to consume more of some products than is good for them is a more appropriate and profound course for policy action. Behavioral economic findings, including present bias, reference points and loss aversion, can sometimes be used as an intellectual justification for where and how to regulate, which forms the policy approach known as budge.

Whichever approach one prefers, there ought to be clarity and consistency in and between what one is proposing and what one is doing. Many purported nudge interventions in UK policy do not seem to comply with the original tenets of libertarian paternalism; in particular, they often seem to be motivated by externality concerns, and they sometimes appear to be informed by rational choice theory. Whether or not one agrees with the approach adopted by governments, we ought to hold them accountable for their rhetoric. Part of the confusion in the area is consequent on the current fashion for nudge policy, such that a whole spectrum of policies, some of which are informed by very weak evidence bases, and others of which are divorced from the original requirements of libertarian paternalism, are being labeled under this generic term. The rise of behavioral economics in policy discussions over the past few years has been very good for those of us who were involved in the area even before it became popular. For this, much credit has to go to the libertarian paternalists, in particular Thaler and Sunstein. But nudge is being oversold by many researchers, and overbought by some in policy, such that the intellectual clarity of the approach has been lost. This is a mistake, because it risks trivializing the substantive practical, albeit still largely potential, contribution that behavioral economics can make to policy design and implementation.

References

Akerlof GA, Kranton RE. 2010. *Identity Economics: How Our Identities Shape Our Work, Wages, and Well-Being*. Princeton: Princeton University Press.

Allais M. 1953. Le Comportement de l'Homme Rationnel Devant le Risque: Critique des Postulats et Axiomes de l'Ecole Américaine. *Econometrica* 21: 503–546.

Allais M. 1990. Allais Paradox. In Eatwell J, Milgate M, Newman P (eds.). *The New Palgrave. Utility and Probability*. New York: Macmillan Press.

Behavioural Insights Team. 2010. *Applying Behavioural Insight to Health*. London: Cabinet Office.

Behavioural Insights Team. 2011. *Behaviour Change and Energy Use*. London: Cabinet Office.

Behavioural Insights Team. 2013. *Applying Behavioural Insight to Organ Donation: Preliminary Results from a Randomised Controlled Trial*. London: Cabinet Office.

Cabinet Office and Institute for Government. 2010. *MINDSPACE: Influencing Behaviour through Public Policy. London*: Cabinet Office and Institute for Government.

Camerer C, Issacharoff S, Loewenstein G, O'Donoghue T, Rabin M. 2003. Regulation for conservatives: Behavioral economics and the case for 'Asymmetric Paternalism'. *University of Pennsylvania Law Review* 1151: 1211–1254.

House of Lords. 2011. *Behaviour Change*. London: The Stationery Office.

Kahneman D, Tversky A. 1979. Prospect theory: An analysis of decision under risk. *Econometrica* 47(2): 263–292.

Keynes JM. 1936. *The General Theory of Employment, Interest and Money*. London: Macmillan.

Mill JS. 1869. *On Liberty*. London: Penguin Classics (1982).

Oliver A. 2013. From nudging to budging: Using behavioural economics to inform public sector policy. *Journal of Social Policy* 42: 685–700.

Popper K. 1957. *The Poverty of Historicism*. New York: Routledge Classics (2002).

Smith A. 1759. *The Theory of Moral Sentiments*. London: Penguin Classics (2010).

Sugden R. 2009. On Nudging. A review of nudge: Improving decisions about health, wealth and happiness by Richard H. Thaler and Cass R. Sunstein. *International Journal of the Economics of Business* 16: 365–373.

Sugden R. 2013. A Response to Sah, Cain and Loewenstein. In Oliver A. (ed.). *Behavioural Public Policy*. Cambridge University Press: Cambridge.

Thaler RH and Sunstein CR. 2003. Libertarian paternalism. *The American Economic Review* 93: 175–179.

Thaler RH, Sunstein CR. 2008. *Nudge: Improving Decisions About Health, Wealth and Happiness*. New Haven: Yale University Press.

Tversky A, Kahneman D. 1992. Advances in prospect theory: Cumulative representation of uncertainty. *Journal of Rick and Uncertainty* 5(4): 297–323.

Index

A
Abortion, 400, 402, 410, 412–413
Absenteeism, 6, 8, 11, 13, 28, 219, 338, 368–370, 407, 417
Acute Malnutrition, 453
Addiction, 22, 226, 233, 340–341, 346, 349, 376, 417, 480
Addictive Behavior, 226, 341
Addictive Consumption, 376
Adiposity, 359–360, 368
Adolescence, 2, 4, 6–7, 11, 13, 87, 364, 397–410
Adult Dental Care Use, 107
Adult Literacy Programs, 453
Adulthood, 1–7, 13, 16, 83, 113, 345, 398–418
Affordability Concept, 262–263
Affordability in South Africa, 265
Affordability Measurements, 263
Affordability of Dental Care, 105, 107–108, 113
Affordability of Tobacco Products, 192, 205
Affordable Care Act, 22, 97, 465, 482
African Region (*see also* AFR)
    cigarette excise tax rates, 242
    countries' status, 242
    retail prices, 242
Age–Period–Cohort (*see also* APC) Analysis, 358
Age-Standardized Obesity Rates, 357
Aggregate Level Studies, 232–233
Aging, 4–5, 43–52, 63–65, 70–76, 89, 107, 113, 418
Alcohol Abuse, 287, 335, 346, 349–350
Alcohol Consumption
    by WHO region, 289–291, 296–300, 305, 307, 321–322
    data, 287–288, 305
    per capita (*see also* APC), 288, 291–292, 295–296, 298–301, 304–305, 309–320, 324–331
    economic costs, 337
    moderate consumption, 287, 332–336
    negative effects, 285, 336, 339
    recorded alcohol consumption, 289, 298, 303, 305–329
    total alcohol consumption, 289–306
    unrecorded alcohol consumption, 289–291, 294, 296, 298, 302, 305, 313
Alcohol Control Policies, 338
Alcohol Market in Australia, 343
Alcohol Policy Index, 347
Alcohol-attributed Mortality, 337
Alcoholic Beverages, 285, 288, 305–306, 315, 319, 321, 342, 344, 378
Alcoholism, 350
Alternative Dental Care Systems, 108

American Medical Association, 350
American Region (*see also* AMR), 291, 298, 302–303, 308, 316, 323, 326
  cigarette excise tax rates, 243
  countries' status, 243
  retail prices, 243
Antenatal Care, 413, 441
Antepartum Period, 475
Asset-Based Community Development Institute (*see also* ABCD), 170, 176
Asymmetric Paternalism, 491–492
Austria's Compulsory Health Insurance, 101
Average Number of Dentist and Physician Visits, 104
Average Price, 240–246, 266

B

Banning Promotion, 224
Banning Sponsorship Policies, 224
Banning Tobacco Advertising, 224
Bans, 155, 162, 220, 223–225, 251, 339, 346, 381, 492
Beer Consumption, 308, 312–313, 317, 323–324, 329, 333, 341, 344
Beer Industry, 332
Beer Institute, 348
Behavioral Economic Policy, 489, 494, 504
Behavioral Economists, 465, 469, 479–480, 483, 490–491, 495–496
Behavioral Insights Team (*see also* BIT), 489, 493–506
Behavioral Interventions, 355, 495–497
Behaviors, 8, 12, 17, 155, 157, 159, 336, 365, 376–377, 405, 479, 481–483, 492, 494, 500–507
Bidis (*see also* Biris), 193–194, 197, 200, 234, 238,
Binge Drinking, 285–287, 338, 341, 349–350
Birth Control, 412
Blue Laws, 339
Body Mass Index (*see also* BMI)
  BMI self-report bias, 361
  BMI thresholds, 357
Body Weight and Employment, 365
Brazil/Mexico, 347
Brazilian Oral Health Policy, 100
Breakdown of Illicit Trade in Tobacco, 252
Breast Cancer, 125, 127, 137–145, 414–415
Breastfeeding, 414, 447, 452
British American Tobacco (*see also* BAT), 207
Budge, 489, 504–507

C

Caesarean Section, 405
California's Tobacco Control Program, 249
Campaigns, 17, 62, 170, 172, 179, 221, 224, 251, 346–347, 374–375, 379, 381–383, 398
Canadian Health Care System, 99
Cancer Divide, 414
Cardiovascular Disease, 8, 19, 332, 414, 418
Caries-Active Group, 88
Cash Transfer, 18, 398, 409
Cervical Cancer, 398, 408, 413–415
Changing Market Share of Cigarette Price Band, 228
Charcoal Filter Cigarette Sales 2007–2012, 213
Cheap White Cigarettes, 253
Child Health, 179, 421, 433–436, 440, 445–449, 453, 455
Child Labor, 398, 403
Child Maltreatment, 398, 404–405
Child Marriage, 398, 408, 421
China/Vietnam, 347
Choice Architecture, 472, 479, 483, 492, 500–501, 507
Christmas Clubs, 472

Chronic Disease, 45, 49, 83–84, 109–110, 398, 414, 482
Chronic Medical Problems, 468
Chronic Obstructive Pulmonary Disease (*see also* COPD), 219, 476
Cigarette Consumption, 194, 199, 227, 236, 250, 252, 256, 261, 265, 268
Cigarette Export Volume, 255
Cigarette Industry's Pricing Behavior, 259
Cigarette Pack Health Warnings, 222
Cigarette Prevalence, 202
Cigarette Production, 208, 261
Cigarette Sales, 195–196, 212–213, 258
Cigarette Taxation, 263
Cigarette Trade Balance, 272
City Dwellers, 372
Classical Models of Demand, 225
Clinical Trial, 347
Coalition Government, 493
Cognitive Affects and Processes, 492
Combusted Products, 193
Commission on Investing in Health (*see also* CIH), 434, 436
Commitment Mechanism, 248
Commitments and Disbursements, 440
Commonwealth Fund, 105–106
Community Dental Health Coordinator, 112
Community Health Workers (*see also* CHWs), 444
Community Mobilization, 176, 438–439, 445, 447
Community Periodontal Index, 86
Compensatory Behavior of Smokers, 232
Complementary Health Insurance (*see also* CHI), 99
Conditional Cash Transfer (*see also* CCT), 409
Confectioners, 505
Consumer Preferences, 227
Consumption of Cigarettes, 192, 261
Consumption Pattern, 247
Contingency Management, 481
Contract Responsibility System, 445
Convention on the Elimination of All Forms of Discrimination against Women, 439
Copayments, 98, 102–103
Corlett–Hague Rule, 236
Corrective Tax, 235
Correlation between
  illicit trade, cigarette price and excise tax, 258
  cigarette taxes and the market share of illicit trade, 259
  corruption and illicit trade, 260
  cigarette consumption and excise tax revenues, 261
  income level and level of alcohol consumption, 295
Corruption, 161, 163, 258–260, 450–451
Cost of the Tax Burden, 229
Cost–Benefit Analysis, 24, 66, 127, 347
Costs of Obesity, 363
Premium Brand Cigarettes, 228
CT Scans, 482
Customs Seizures, 254

D

Decrease in Global Demand for Cigarettes, 212
Delivering, 43, 45, 53, 63, 78, 113–114, 450
Demand and Supply, 45, 339
Demand-Side Alcohol Policies, 340
Demographic Variables, 164
Denmark's NHS, 102
Dental Assistant Roles, 111
Dental Care
  delivery systems, 108
  financing, 83, 85, 107–108, 113
  system challenges, 108, 113
  systems around the world, 85, 92, 108, 113
  systems in OECD countries, 93

Dental Caries, 84, 86–87, 109
Dental Disease, 84–86, 92, 109
Dental Epidemiology, 87
Dental Insurance Coverage, 97, 100–101, 103–104, 108, 112–113
Dental Personnel per 10,000 Population, 96
Dental School Capacity, 110
Dental Spending, 92–98, 101, 105
Dental Workforce, 110–111
Department of Motor Vehicles, 472
Deposit Contract, 476–478
Developing Countries, 83, 85, 87, 95, 108–110, 113, 151–156, 179–180, 194, 196, 203–209, 215, 220, 231, 260, 262, 264, 268, 270
Diabetes, 8–11, 19, 83–84, 110, 335, 361–362, 414–415, 419
Diagonal Health Systems Strategies, 398, 421
Diarrhoeal Disease, 454
Diet, 109, 247, 333, 355–356, 363, 374, 383
Dietary and Physical Activity Factors, 363
Diet-related Illness, 356
Direct Costs, 25, 217, 220, 285, 338, 413
Direct Costs of Smoking, 220
Disability
    benefits, 368, 374
    pensions, 366, 370
    adjusted life years (*see also* dalys), 5, 88–90
    dalys per capita, 89–91
Discrimination, 2, 17, 30–31, 366–367, 397, 403, 414, 421, 439
Disillusionment, 484
Decayed, Missing and Filled Teeth (*see also* DMFT) Index
Dental caries trends, 87
DMFT index for children, 92
Domestication of Cereal Crops, 286
Dop System, 336–337
Drunk Driving Penalties, 348–349
DT, 112

E

Early Marriage, 397, 406, 408–409
Early Pregnancy, 397, 408–409
Eastern Mediterranean Region (*see also* EMR), 195–202, 241, 243–244, 288–309, 318–328, 335
Econometric Methods, 233
Econometric Studies, 227
Economic Assessment, 131
Economic Cost of Smoking, 218–219
Economic Disempowerment, 417
Economic Evaluation, 1, 3, 23–29, 71, 75, 123–129, 140, 145–146
Economic Evidence, 16, 27, 126–128, 133, 247, 381
Economic Impact, 28, 124–125, 130, 136, 218, 363, 401
Economic Model, 142, 144
Economic Value, 127, 130–132, 141, 144, 146, 149
Education, 2–18, 30–31, 61–69, 83, 110–112, 130, 153–177, 205, 219, 247, 271, 334, 349, 358, 360–375, 381–387, 397–421, 434, 436, 438–450, 452–476
Socioeconomic Status (*see also* SES), 205, 235, 358–372, 379
Effect of Price on Tobacco Demand, 229
Effect of Tobacco Excise Taxes, 249
Effective Interventions, 25, 348, 382, 434, 436, 441
Effects of Poor Mental Health, 2
Effects of Wine, or Wine and Beer, 333
Elderly Women, 400, 418–420
Electromyography, 482
Electronic Cargo Tracking System, 261
Emergency Contraception, 412
Empirical Observation, 491
Employment, 2, 4, 7–30, 56, 66–71, 77, 100, 111–112, 267–269, 332, 365–374, 400, 418, 420, 453
Endowment Effect, 463, 466–470, 482, 484
Epidemiological Studies, 214, 217
Equitable Human Development, 421

European Union (*see also* EU)
EU pledge, 379–380
EU School Fruit Scheme, 382
Excise tax revenues of cigarettes in EU, 261
Fine cut tobacco in the European Union, 239
European Region (*see also* EUR)
EUR cigarette excise tax rates, 245
EUR region, 289, 291, 297, 300–302, 309, 317–323, 327
EUR retail prices, 245
Eurmonitor data, 262
Evolution of smokers, 203
Excise Tax in PPP$, 240
Expanded Programme of Immunization and Prenatal Care, 445
Expenditure, 3, 9, 18–22, 45, 49–70, 77, 94–100, 136, 164, 205–206, 218, 245, 346, 362, 416, 439, 446
Export Value of Unmanufactured Tobacco, 209
External and Internal Costs, 235
Externalities, 155, 235, 240, 373–374, 384, 497–505

F

Family Planning, 411, 437, 439–446
Female Genital Cutting, 398, 405
Female Genital Mutilation, 398, 405
Female Prevalence of Smoking, 214
Female Smokers, 205, 213, 235
Fertility, 47, 90, 398, 408–418, 446, 453
Financial Barriers to Dental Care
Financial Incentives, 170–173, 179, 409, 444, 475–479, 492, 496
Financial Security, 398, 400, 419
Financing, 1, 3, 18–23, 43, 45, 54–66, 76, 87, 107, 113, 137, 440, 443
Finland's BMI, 367
Finland's Health Care, 102
Fiscal Incentives, 375
Fiscal Policies, 378
Food Advertising, 379–380
Food Deprivation, 359
Food Hygiene, 502
Food Labelling Schemes, 379
Food Product Reformulation, 380
Food Subsidies, 377
Food Taxes, 378
Framing, 141, 463, 466–469, 479, 484, 491
French Health Care System, 99
Fruit and Vegetable Consumption, 364, 372

G

GBD 2010 Study
291 conditions, 85
Gender Gap, 371, 407, 419, 453
Gender-Based Inequities Educational Campaigns, 398
Gender-Based Violence, 397, 410–411, 451
Generalized Trust, 151–164
Genetic Factors, 364
Genetics, 124, 144
Genomic-Based Medicine, 123, 125
Germany's Health Care, 102
Girls' Education and Nutrition, 398
Global Adult Tobacco Surveys (*see also* GATS), 197, 200–211, 234
Global Alcohol Production, 331
Global Cigarette Consumption, 194, 252
Global Cigarette Market, 207, 212, 216, 250
Global Export of Cigarettes and Trade Discrepancy, 254
Global Import of Cigarettes and Trade Discrepancy, 254
Global Investment Framework (*see also* GIF), 433–438, 450–456
Global Tobacco Epidemic, 199–202, 205, 214, 221, 238, 241–246
Global Tobacco Export Value, 209
Global Tobacco Exports, 209

Global Tobacco Leaf Production, 208
Global Trade Discrepancy of Cigarettes, 255
Globalization of the Tobacco Market, 206
Greece's Health Care, 102
Gross Domestic Product (*see also* GDP), 11, 19, 44, 52–53, 93–95, 219–228, 263, 285–286, 338, 363, 371, 417, 446
Gross National Product (*see also* GNP), 450
Gum Disease, 84–85
GYTS Data, 204

H

Habit, 109, 205, 233, 376, 483
Habitual Behavior, 376
Harmful Consequences of Tobacco, 248
HbA1c Levels for Diabetics, 474
Health Care
  and/or psychological support, 154
  costs, 8–11, 17, 25, 113, 126, 204, 338, 363, 385
  financing, 19, 23, 113, 442
  services, 19, 71, 75, 99–101, 109, 113, 126, 133, 156, 159, 447
Health Checks, 383
Health Financing, 3, 23, 34
Health Investments, 398, 402
Health Planning Support, 434
Health Policies, 3, 23, 119, 442, 448, 455
Health Policymakers, 463
Health Risks, 205, 360, 374–375
Health Spending, Dental Spending, and GDP, 95
Health-Enhancing Sectors, 434, 436, 451–452
Healthy Eating, 377, 381, 501
Healthy Foods, 370, 377–381, 479–480
Healthy Gums, 83–84
Heating and Cooling Systems, 502
Heavy Drinking, 287, 334, 336, 349
HI Countries, 208–209, 294, 304
HI Group, 296, 301, 304–305, 312–318, 320, 324
HI Income Group, 296, 310–311, 316, 323, 329
High Blood Pressure, 361–362, 415
High Cholesterol, 361
Higher Drinking, 341
Higher Minimum Drinking Age, 348
Highest Changes in RYO Sales, 198
High-Income Countries (*see also* HICs), 5–10, 18–20, 23, 27, 113, 152, 167, 169, 194, 204, 218, 227, 233–235, 250, 252, 266, 270, 302, 340, 372, 413–415
Historical Trends in Height, Weight and Body Mass, 356
HIV/AIDS
  forgotten drug in HIV/AIDS, 336
  HIV-positive and HIV-negative mothers, 416
Hot-Cold Empathy Gap, 480
Household Characteristics, 162–165
Human Capital, 13, 154–159, 336, 365, 370
Human Papillomavirus (*see also* HPV), 408
Hyperbolic Discounting, 227, 375–376, 463, 466, 470, 476, 479–481
Hypothetical Policies, 53, 497

I

Ideal Body Weight, 359
Illicit Cigarette Market, 253, 255, 259
Illicit Cigarette Trade Volume and Customs Seizures, 254
Illicit Cross-Border Shopping, 256
Illicit Trade in Tobacco, 252–253, 262
Illicit Trade Market and Corruption, 260
Immunization, 403, 437, 439, 441–447
Impact of Increasing Cigarette Excise Tax, 250
Impact of Obesity, 362–363, 367–368
Impact of Price on Tobacco Demand, 232
Impact of Smoking on Health Spending, 218
Impact of Tobacco Taxes on the Poor, 245
Imperial Tobacco (*see also* IT), 207

Import Duties, 209, 236–237
Incentives, 30, 58, 64, 67–77, 170–177, 252, 355, 365, 375–378, 383, 399, 409, 441, 444, 475–484, 496–502
Independent Expert Review Group (*see also* iERG), 436
Indian Immunization Initiatives, 403
Indirect Costs, 10, 12, 19, 25–26, 217–219, 285–286, 338
Individual Beliefs, 163
Individual Beliefs and Values, 153, 163
Individual Compliance, 155
Inequalities, 2, 9, 16–18, 97, 99, 107, 355, 370, 373, 417
Inequality in Overweight by Education Level, 371
Infant Death, 405
Inflation-Adjusted Price of Cigarettes, 224
Inflationary Impact of Tobacco Tax Increase, 270
Informal Labor, 268
Information Failures, 355, 374–375, 384
Insurance Externality, 373
Internalities, 235, 489, 492, 494, 496–507
Intimate Partner Violence, 398, 421
Italy's Health Care, 103

J

J or U-Shaped Curve, 332, 334
Japan Tobacco International (*see also* JTI), 207
Job Insecurity, 13, 16, 369
J-Shaped Relationship, 366

K

Kretek, 193–197, 200, 202
Krispy Kreme Doughnut Binge, 464

L

Labor Market, 66, 110, 171, 355, 365–374, 399, 409
Lack of Controls for Attrition, 478
Lack of Randomization, 478
Large Cigarette Consuming Countries, 197
Level of Smuggling, 261
LI Group, 296, 300, 303, 312–316, 330
Libertarian Paternalism, 489–496, 501–505, 509
Life Expectancy, 8, 45, 49, 52, 76, 88, 91, 216, 362–363, 384, 414
Lifestyle Choices, 355, 363–364, 375, 499
Lifestyles, 71, 363–364, 419, 506–507
Lifetime Expenditures, 363
Limited Dependent Variable Techniques, 234
Littered Cigarette Packs, 257
LMI Countries, 303, 317
Longevity, 49, 89, 91, 332, 361, 363, 384
Long-Term Care (*see also* LTC), 43–58, 60–64, 68, 70–76
Long-Term Elasticity, 341
Loss Aversion, 463, 466–468, 474, 484, 490–500, 507
Low- and Middle-Income Countries (*see also* LMICs), 5, 155, 191–201, 205, 208, 215, 218, 234, 271, 398, 427, 434–437
Low Birth Weight Infants, 405
Low Tar Cigarettes, 212–214
Low-Income Countries (*see also* LICs), 20–23, 31, 89, 152, 165–169, 179, 227, 240, 247, 250–252, 266, 271, 372, 408, 419
Lung Cancers, 88, 214

M

Malaria, 401, 437
Manufacture and Consumption of Cigarettes, 192
Manufactured Cigarettes, 193, 200
Marijuana, 348
Market Failure, 355, 373
Market Share of Combusted Tobacco Products, 194
Marshallian Law of Demand, 228
Material Living Conditions, 359
Maternal and Child Mortality, 436, 441, 450–451, 456, 458

Maternal and Newborn Health, 437
Maternal Health, 401, 441, 449
Maternal Mortality Survey (*see also* MMS), 449
Mean-Age-of-Death Measure, 90
Mechanisms of Informal Assistance, 154
Medicaid, 74–75, 97, 104, 107, 476
Medical Marijuana Legalization (*see also* MML), 348
Medicare, 97, 100, 465
Menstruation, 398, 400, 406–408
Mental Health Area, 3, 30
Mental Health Disorders, 3
Mental Health Field, 1–3, 10, 25
Mental Health Interventions, 1, 3, 31, 416
Mental Health Issues, 1–2, 10, 30
Mental Health Needs, 1, 9, 18, 22, 29–31
Mental Health Problems, 1–31, 169, 398
Mental Illness, 1–31, 416–417
Microfinance, 171, 173, 176, 179
Micro-level Studies, 233
Millennium Development Goals (*see also* MDGs), 433, 435, 441, 448, 452, 456
Mindspace, 493–499, 504
Minimum Legal Drinking Age (*see also* MLDA), 340, 345–346, 349
Mortality, 1–8, 88–90, 109, 160, 204, 215–219, 249–251, 334–338, 360–364, 400–412, 434–441, 450–458
Mortality Frame, 468–469
Motivational Therapy, 347–349
MPOWER, 220–221, 225
Multi-Component Interventions, 382
Multinational Tobacco Companies (*see also* MTCs), 207

N

Narodowy Fundusz Zdrowia (*see also* NFZ), 103
Nash Cooperative Bargaining Model, 399
National Board of Revenue (*see also* NBR), 267
National Family Health Survey (*see also* NFHS), 403
National Health Insurance, 100, 113, 249
National Health Service (*see also* NHS), 26, 97, 132, 219, 346, 381
National Institute on Alcohol Abuse and Alcoholism (*see also* NIAAA), 287
Negative Impact of Excise Tax Increase, 244
Negative Influence of Obesity, 365–366
Neo-Bernoullian Formulation, 490
Non-Combusted Products, 193
Non-Communicable Disease (*see also* NCDs), 11, 19, 88–91, 113, 192, 215, 251, 412, 414, 418–419
Non-price Factors, 259
Non-price Interventions, 224
Nudge, 470, 472, 480, 489, 492–508
Nutrition, 84, 336–337, 359, 377, 402, 418, 434, 436, 446–447, 452–454
Nutrition Labelling, 378

O

Obese Person, 362–363, 365, 369
Obese Workers, 368–369
Obesity and Chronic Diseases, 362
Obesity Epidemic, 355–358, 377, 384
Obesity Paradox, 360
Obesity Rates, 355–359, 365–366, 371–372
Obesogenic Environments, 359, 364, 370, 384
OECD Countries, 11, 44–48, 50–55, 60–65, 90–94, 101, 104–106, 233, 286, 355–358, 383
OECD Health Data 2013, 92
Optimal Tax Theory, 236
Oral Conditions, 83, 85–90, 109
Oral Health, 83–87, 92–114
Oral Health Regimen, 85
Ordinary Least Squares (*see also* OLS) Technique, 159, 161, 234
Ordre National des Chirugiens-Dentistes, 99

Organ Donation, 153, 163, 469, 495, 500
Osteoarthritis, 362
Out-of-Pocket Spending, 94, 106, 441
Overeating, 463, 474, 479
Overweight, 2, 355–371, 384, 467, 479, 491
Ownership Status of Producers, 206–207

P

Pan-Government Energy Saving Target, 503
Partner Violence, 398
Partnership for Maternal, Newborn and Child Health (*see also* PMNCH), 436
Patient Protection and Affordable Care Act of 2010, 22, 465
Payday Loan Companies, 507
People's Awareness on Tobacco Use, 211
Per-Capita GDP, 371–372
Percent of Global Population, 289, 293, 296, 301, 305, 311
Percentage Change in Smokeless Tobacco Sales, 198
Percentage Change of Total Cigarette sales, 196
Personalized Medicine, 123–129, 132, 140–142
Philip Morris International (*see also* PMI), 207
Physical Activity, 159, 355, 363, 371–373, 382–384
Physical Inactivity, 419, 362, 370, 372
Physically Active, 383
Piano Stairs, 501, 507
Pipe Tobacco Consumption, 197
Pipe Tobacco Sales, 198
Policy Compendium, 433, 437–438
Polish Health Care System, 103
Population Growth, 5, 89, 300, 411
Population Size, 88–89, 289, 298
Population-Weighted Average, 287, 291
Postnatal Care Visits, 441
Postnatal Depression, 416
Postpartum Hemorrhage, 405
Potential Years of Life Lost (*see also* PYLL), 337
Poverty-Cycle, 455
Power of the Default, 463, 466, 469, 484
Premature Mortality, 2, 5, 8, 88, 204, 355
Presenteeism, 6, 13, 28, 368–370
Prevalence of
  cigarette smoking by income group, 199
  cigarettes and RYO among current smokers, 201
  health conditions, 86
  tobacco use and smoking cigarettes, 202
  youth consuming tobacco, 204
Prevention, 3, 27–31, 45, 49, 53, 70–88, 102–112, 126, 131, 149, 176, 220, 251, 355
Price Elasticity, 228, 231–238, 247, 344–346
Price Incentives, 355, 377
Prices in South Africa, 265
Pricing Policies and Control of Tobacco in Europe (*see also* PPACTE), 257
Primary Care
  interventions, 383
  providers, 111
Priority Action Areas, 109
Producers, 206–210, 228–232, 240, 253, 331, 343, 465, 483
Production Function Framework, 107
Productivity, 12–18, 25, 28–29, 52, 64–77, 204, 218–219, 247, 286, 336–341, 366–370, 446, 451, 456
Productivity Losses, 7, 11, 14, 19, 369–370, 417
Profit Maximizers, 463, 483
PROGRESA, 398, 409
Progress in Select Tobacco Control Measures, 221
Prohibition, 339, 349
Prospect Theory, 466–467, 490–491
Protocol to Eliminate Illicit Trade in Tobacco Products, 262

Public Dental Service (*see also* PDS), 99, 102–103
Public Good, 155, 375
Public Health Responsibility Deal, 506
Purchasing Power Parity (*see also* PPP), 92–93
Purchasing Power Parity Dollars (*see also* PPP$), 240–246, 372
Pure Alcohol, 288–331

Q

Quality Assessment, 443
Quality of Life, 4–13, 23–30, 68–80, 139, 248, 286334–338, 401

R

Racial and Ethnic Diffcrcnccs, 367
Radiation Therapy, 468–469
Radiologists, 468
Rational Addiction Framework, 226
Rational Addiction Model, 226, 341, 349
Rational Choice Theory, 497, 508
Reductions in Salt, 381
Regulating, 43, 45, 54, 67–70, 78, 100, 448
Reinforcer Pathology, 480
Relative Income Price (*see also* RIP)
  average annual percentage change, 264, 273
  decomposition of annual percentage change, 273
  of cigarettes, 266, 272
Reproductive Health, 398, 409, 411–412, 414–415, 421, 434
Reproductive, Maternal, Newborn and Child Health (*see also* RMNCH)
  Policy guide for implementing essential interventions, 434, 436–437, 455
  interventions, 437–445
  policies, 438, 440
  programming, 438
  service delivery and outcomes, 438
Risk Averse, 466, 491
Risk Factors for Oral Diseases, 110
Roll your own (*see also* RYO), 193–201, 238–239
Russia/Ukraine, 347

S

School Support Program, 409
School-Based Programs, 382–383
Screening, 14, 98, 124, 141, 420–421
South-East Asia Region (*see also* SEAR)
  cigarette excise tax rates, 246
  region, 289–290, 309, 316–317, 326–327
  retail prices, 246
Second National Health and Nutrition Examination Survey, 226
Second-IIand Smokc, 215, 221, 235
Sector-Wide Approach (*see also* SWAP) Framework, 443, 451
Self-Rated Health (*see also* SRH), 158, 334
Self-Report Bias, 360–361
Self-Reported BMI Level, 360
Sex-Selection, 398, 401
Sex-Selective Abortions, 400, 402
Sexual and Reproductive Health Programming, 421
Sexual Coercion, 410–411
Sexually Transmitted Diseases, 336, 397–398, 405
Sexually Transmitted Infections (*see also* STIs), 408, 410
Share of Excise and Total Tax, 241
Share of Low and Ultra-Low Tar Cigarette Market, 214
Short Maternal Stature, 403
Short-Run Price Elasticity, 233, 342
Sick Fund Membership, 102
Sick Leave, 368–370
SimSmoke Model, 224
Sistema Único de Saúde (*see also* SUS), 100
Skilled Birth Attendance, 441
Smart Electricity Meters, 502

Smokeless Tobacco, 193, 197–202, 215, 234
Smoking
  attributable death rate, 218
  attributable deaths, 215–216, 224, 251
  attributable diseases, 216–219, 224
  attributable mortality, 219, 249
  and socioeconomic status, 205
  bans, 155, 162
  cessation, 234, 463, 475–476, 495, 500
Smuggled Cigarettes, 253, 257–258
Social Capital, 18, 151–180
Social Determinants, 151, 417
Social Disparities, 370–372, 384
Social Mobilization, 455
Social Multiplier Effect, 363–365, 384
Societal Costs of Drinking, 338
Socio-Demographic Factors, 419
Socioeconomic Consequences, 336
Socioeconomic Status (*see also* SES), 205, 235, 358–372, 379
Sorghum Beer, 333
Spain's Health Care, 103
Spirits Consumption, 307–312, 315–319, 323–329
State Tobacco Monopoly Administration (*see also* STMA), 229, 472–473
Statistical Discrimination, 366
Statutory Health Insurance (*see also* SHI), 99, 102
Street Children, 398, 403–404
Stress, 2–10, 14, 30, 66, 155, 169, 236, 334, 360, 365, 369, 419
Sub-Saharan Africa, 90–91, 156, 410–411, 437
Substance Abuse, 3, 7, 15, 22, 287, 463, 474, 480–481
Supermarket Trolleys, 501, 507
Supply-Side Alcohol Policies, 339
Survival Frame, 468–469
Sustainable Development Goals (*see also* SDGs), 435, 456
Sustained Effectiveness, 498
Swedish Health Care System, 98

T
Target Responsibility Agreements, 445
Task Force for Improving Fatty Acid Composition, 380
Task-Shifting, 110
Tax and Price, 229, 231–235, 257
Tax and Smoking, 234–235
Tax and Youth Smoking, 234
Tax Increase, 229, 231, 241, 245, 261, 269
Tax Policies, 343
Tax Reform, 343
Taxes and Subsidies, 374–375
Taxes on Nutrients, 377
Tax-induced smuggling, 260
Teenage Pregnancy, 500
Teledentistry, 110
The Netherlands, 56, 65, 74, 106, 124, 128, 136–140, 158, 178, 197, 209, 363, 383, 469
Three Time-Related Factors, 358
Three-Dimensional Space, 497, 499–500
Tobacco
  attributable diseases, 219
  related employment, 267
  trade balance in value, 210
  trade balance in volume, 210
  consumers, 235
  consumption, 193, 197, 228, 231–237, 247, 249, 263, 267
  control measures, 192, 211–212, 221, 224, 231, 251, 261
  control policies, 207, 212, 230, 268
  epidemic, 192, 199–202, 205, 214, 218–228, 231, 240–248, 266, 271
  excise taxes, 228, 231, 237, 249
  smoking by income group, 206
  smoking by income quintile, 206
  tax administration, 230, 269
  tax interventions, 267
  taxation, 191–192, 216, 229–231, 238–240, 249
  taxes, 211, 227, 235, 244–257, 269
  trade, 209, 271
  use, 8, 110, 191–231, 257–271

Tooth Decay, 83–84, 107
Trade Discrepancy Technique, 256
'Two Divides' in Dental Insurance Coverage, 112
Trends in Cigarette Sales, 196

U

UMI Countries, 199, 294, 302, 315–319
UMI Income Group, 310, 330
Under-Five Mortality, 398, 401
Unemployment or Unsecured Debt, 2
Unified Health System, 100
United Kingdom (*see also* UK), 32, 38, 48, 59, 62, 65–72, 97, 106–115, 124, 128, 134, 144, 179, 198, 201, 243, 373, 381, 469
United States (*see also* US), 7–19, 43, 46–50, 53, 59–72, 86, 92, 105, 124, 168, 200, 210, 238, 256, 287, 302, 338–340, 362–380
Universal Declaration of Human Rights, 439
Universal Health Coverage, 434, 438–441
Unmanufactured Tobacco Production, 208
Unmanufactured Trade Value and Balance, 272
Unprotected Sex, 411
Upper-Middle Income Countries (*see also* UMICs), 152, 165, 167, 227
Urban–Rural Inequalities, 373
U-Shaped Association, 368
US Health Care System, 96, 105, 129, 463, 483
Utility Maximizers, 463
Utility-based Health-related Quality of Life (*see also* HRQoL), 334

V

Value Added Tax (*see also* VAT), 229, 236
VAT Rates, 237
Violence against Women, 417–418
Volume Combusted Tobacco Products, 194

W

Wage Penalties, 367–370, 384
Waist Measurement, 360
Waist-to-hip Ratio, 360
Warning People on Smoking, 222
Water and Sanitation, 434, 436, 438, 452, 454
Water Fluoridation, 84, 109
Water Pipes, 193, 197
Waves of Empirical Literature, 230
WB Income Group, 272, 292–323
Weight Loss, 342, 362, 463, 476–478
Weighted Elasticities, 344
Western Pacific Region (*see also* WPR)
  cigarette excise tax rates, 246
  retail prices, 246
Whiskey Sales, 339
WHO Framework Convention on Tobacco Control (*see also* FCTC), 192, 220, 230–236, 262, 268, 271
Wine, 286, 305–349
Wine Consumption, 307, 313, 323, 331
Workers' Productivity, 369
Workforce Innovation, 111
Workforce Policies, 443–444
Work-related Stress, 22, 236
World Bank's Classification of Income, 89
World Beer Sales, 331
World Development Report, 434, 484
World No Tobacco Day 2014, 216, 250
World Values Survey, 151, 157, 161–162
WTO Agreement, 246

Y

Years Lived with Disability (*see also* YLDs), 5, 88
Years of Life Lost (*see also* YLLs), 5, 88, 337, 419

World Scientific Handbook of Global Health Economics and Public Policy

❶ The Economics of Health and Health Systems

World Scientific Series in Global Health Economics and Public Policy

ISSN: 2010-2089

Series Editor-in-Chief: Richard M Scheffler
University of California, Berkeley, USA

Published:

Vol. 1 Accountability and Responsibility in Health Care:
Issues in Addressing an Emerging Global Challenge
edited by Bruce Rosen, Avi Israeli and Stephen Shortell

Vol. 2 The Economics of Social Capital and Health:
A Conceptual and Empirical Roadmap
edited by Sherman Folland and Lorenzo Rocco

Vol. 3 World Scientific Handbook of Global Health Economics and Public Policy
edited by Richard M Scheffler

World Scientific Series in Global Health Economics and Public Policy – Vol. 3

World Scientific Handbook of Global Health Economics and Public Policy

❶ The Economics of Health and Health Systems

Edited by

Richard M. Scheffler
University of California, Berkeley, USA

World Scientific

NEW JERSEY • LONDON • SINGAPORE • BEIJING • SHANGHAI • HONG KONG • TAIPEI • CHENNAI • TOKYO

Published by

World Scientific Publishing Co. Pte. Ltd.
5 Toh Tuck Link, Singapore 596224
USA office: 27 Warren Street, Suite 401-402, Hackensack, NJ 07601
UK office: 57 Shelton Street, Covent Garden, London WC2H 9HE

Library of Congress Cataloging-in-Publication Data
Names: Scheffler, Richard M., editor.
Title: World Scientific handbook of global health economics and public policy / [edited by] Richard M. Scheffler.
Other titles: Handbook of global health economics and public policy
Description: New Jersey : World Scientific, 2016. | Includes bibliographical references and index.
Identifiers: LCCN 2015040481| ISBN 9789814612319 (set : alk. paper) | ISBN 9789814612340 (v. 1 : alk. paper) | ISBN 9789814612357 (v. 2 : alk. paper) | ISBN 9789814612364 (v. 3 : alk. paper)
Subjects: | MESH: Economics, Medical. | Delivery of Health Care. | Global Health. | Health Policy. | Quality of Health Care. | Social Determinants of Health.
Classification: LCC RA410.5 | NLM W 74.1 | DDC 338.4/73621--dc23
LC record available at http://lccn.loc.gov/2015040481

British Library Cataloguing-in-Publication Data
A catalogue record for this book is available from the British Library.

In-house Editors: Herbert Moses/Li Hongyan

Typeset by Stallion Press
Email: enquiries@stallionpress.com

Printed in Singapore

Acknowledgment

Jessica Foster was my editorial assistant and partner. She helped me in every way possible. I am very grateful to her. Kati Phillips made the handbook happen. She handled all the details and coordinated all the moving parts without missing a beat. Finally, I would like to thank Zvi Ruder. He worked hard over a long period of time to convince me that the handbook could be done. He was so right.

—Dr. Richard M. Scheffler

Contents

Acknowledgment v

About the Editor ix

List of Contributors xi

Introduction to Volume 1 xxiii
Richard M. Scheffler

Health Care Spending and Economic Growth 1
Edit V. Velenyi

Macroeconomics, Trade and Health 155
Richard Smith, Marcus Keogh-Brown, and Johanna Hanefeld

Measuring and Forecasting Global Health Expenditures 177
Thomas E. Getzen

Economics of Financing Health Care 217
Alexander S. Preker, Sherry Glied, Dov Chernichovsky, and Marisa Gil Lapetra

Alternative Financing Strategies for Universal Health Coverage 267
Joseph Kutzin, Winnie Yip, and Cheryl Cashin

Global Risk-Adjusted Payment Models 311
Camilo Cid, Randall P. Ellis, Verónica Vargas, Juergen Wasem, and Lorena Prieto

Resource Allocation and Priority Setting in Health Care Systems 363
Guillem Lopez-Casasnovas and Laura Pellise

Estimating Health Care Treatment Costs 403
Alistair McGuire and Maria Raikou

Incentivizing Health Care Utilization and Health Outcomes 421
William H. Dow, Justin S. White, and Stefano Bertozzi

Economic Evaluation of Health Care Programmes and Interventions: Applications to Low- and Middle-Income Countries 453
Paul Revill, Beth Woods, and Mark J. Sculpher

Inequalities and Inequities in Health and Health Care 489
Marisol Rodríguez and Rosa Urbanos-Garrido

Index 559

About the Editor

Richard M. Scheffler (Editor) Richard M. Scheffler is Distinguished Professor of Health Economics and Public Policy at the School of Public Health and the Goldman School of Public Policy at the University of California, Berkeley and holds the endowed Chair in Healthcare Markets and Consumer Welfare. In 2003 Dr. Scheffler served as the elected president of the International Health Economics Association. He has been a visiting professor at a number of universities including the London School of Economics, Charles University in Prague, at the Department of Economics at the University of Pompeu Fabra in Barcelona and at Carlos III University of Madrid, Spain. Dr. Scheffler has been a visiting scholar at the World Bank, the Rockefeller Foundation in Bellagio, and the Institute of Medicine at the National Academy of Sciences. He has been a consultant for the World Bank, the WHO, and the OECD. Professor Scheffler has been a Fulbright Scholar at Pontifica Universidad Catolica de Chile in Santiago, Chile, and at Charles University, Prague, Czech Republic. He was also awarded the Chair of Excellence Award at the Carlos III University of Madrid in 2013. In 2015 Dr. Scheffler was awarded the Gold Medal for Charles University in Prague for his longstanding and continued support of international scientific and educational collaboration. He earned his PhD in economics with honors at New York University.

List of Contributors

(Author bios are listed as per the Chapter order)

Edit V Velényi is a Health Economist with the Health, Nutrition, and Population (HNP) Global Practice of the World Bank, where she focuses on applied economic analysis and impact evaluation of health sector projects to improve operational and development effectiveness. Previously, she worked at the HNP Anchor, where she focused on the relationship between the macro economy and health financing. Between 2007 and 2011 she coordinated the health portfolio of the Development Impact Evaluation Initiative of the World Bank's Development Research Group. During earlier assignments with the World Bank's Africa Region and the HNP Anchor, she co-authored *Learning from Economic Downturns — How to Better Assess, Track, and Mitigate the Impact on the Health Sector* (2013); co-edited *Public Ends, Private Means — Strategic Purchasing of Health Services* (2007); and co-authored book chapters on health insurance. Edit received a PhD in Economics from the University of York, an MA from the Johns Hopkins University, School of Advanced International Studies, and an MA from the Budapest Business School.

Richard Smith is Professor of Health System Economics and Dean of the Faculty of Public Health and Policy at the London School of Hygiene & Tropical Medicine. Following undergraduate and postgraduate studies in economics at the University of York, Richard worked in Sydney, Cambridge, Bristol, Melbourne and Norwich, before joining the School in 2007. Richard has held various other appointments, including honorary posts at the Universities of Hong Kong and East Anglia, Associate Fellow at The Royal Institute of International Affairs, and editorial roles for journals including Health Economics, the Journal of Public Health and Globalization and Health. He has also acted as an expert advisor for a number of international bodies, as well as several national government departments. Richard's research has covered a number of areas of health economics, in recent years focusing upon developing the methods for macro-economic analysis of health, the economics of globalization and health, and aspects of trade in health goods, services, people and ideas. Richard has received over £30 million in grant income, published five books, more than 100 journal papers, and dozens of other works.

Marcus Keogh-Brown is Lecturer in Economic Modeling at the London School of Hygiene and Tropical Medicine. His research interests are mainly focused on the application of macroeconomic modeling to health. Previous applications of these models include infectious disease outbreaks, particularly SARS and Pandemic influenza, antibiotic resistance, dietary change, greenhouse gas reduction strategies with health co-benefits, Alzheimer's disease and malaria. In addition to various country simulations for policy analysis, Marcus has also been involved in pioneering methodological development of macroeconomic models to integrate health, demographic and epidemiological models in a single framework.

Johanna Hanefeld is Lecturer in Health Systems Economics in the department of Global Health and Development focusing on trade and health, health systems, governance, and quantitative and qualitative policy analysis mainly in low- and middle-income countries. Together with Professor Richard Smith and colleagues at the University of York, UK, she recently completed a large research project examining the impact of medical tourism on the UK NHS. She is co-editor of the forthcoming *Edward Elgar Handbook on Medical Tourism and Patient Mobility*.

Thomas E. Getzen is emeritus Professor of Risk, Insurance and Health Management at Temple University and Executive Director of iHEA, the International Health Economics Association. His textbook *Health Economics: Fundamentals and Flow of Funds* (Wiley; 5th ed., 2013) is used in graduate and undergraduate programs throughout the world and he has been visiting professor at the Woodrow Wilson School of Public Policy at Princeton University, the Wharton School of the University of Pennsylvania, the University of Toronto, and the Centre for Health Economics at the University of York. His research and consulting focus on the macroeconomics of health, forecasting medical expenditures, physician supply, price indexes, financing and public health economics. He is the editor-in-chief for the "HEN-Health Economics Network" in collaboration with SSRN and associate editor for *Health Economics*. Professor Getzen periodically updates the forecasting model of "Long Run Medical Cost Trends" for the Society of Actuaries, and served on the National Academy of Sciences IOM Committee on Public Health Strategies.

Alexander S. Preker is the President and CEO of the Health Investment & Financing Corporation in New York. He is an active investor and member of the board of several health care companies. Mr. Preker also serves as one of the Commissioners for the Global Commission on Pollution, Health and Development and as the Chair of the External Advisory Committee for the WHHSJ of the International Hospital Federation. From 2007 to 2012, Mr Preker was Head of the Health Industry Group and Investment Policy for the International Finance Corporation. Previously, he was Chief Economist for the health sector in the World Bank Group. Mr Preker has published extensively, having written many scientific articles and authored over 15 books. Mr Preker is an Executive Scholar and Adjunct Associate Professor at the Icahn School of Medicine at Mount Sinai in New York, an Adjunct Associate Professor of public policy at New York University's Robert F Wagner Graduate School of Public Policy and an Adjunct Associate Professor for Health Care Management at the Mailman School of Public Health at Columbia University. His training includes a PhD in Economics from the London School of Economics and Political Science, a Fellowship in Medicine from University College London, a Diploma in Medical Law and Ethics from King's College London, and a MD from University of British Columbia/McGill.

Sherry Glied became Dean of New York University's Robert F. Wagner Graduate School of Public Service in August 2013. From 1989–2013, she was Professor of Health Policy and Management at Columbia University's Mailman School of Public Health. She was Chair of the department from 1998–2009. On June 22, 2010, Glied was confirmed by the U.S. Senate as Assistant Secretary for Planning and Evaluation at the Department of Health and Human Services, and served in that capacity from July 2010 through August 2012. She had previously served as Senior Economist for health care and labor market policy on the President's Council of Economic Advisers in 1992–1993, under Presidents Bush and Clinton. Glied's principal areas of research are in health policy reform and mental health care policy.

Dov Chernichovsky is professor emeritus of health economics and policy of Ben-Gurion University of the Negev, Israel. He currently the Dean of the School of Health and Welafre Professions at the The Max Stern Academic College of Emek Yezreel in Israel, is a Research Associate with the National Bureau of Economic Research (NBER) in the USA, coordinates research at the Taub Center for Social Policy in Israel, and chairs the Israeli National Nutrition Security Council. Dov has been consulting for the World Bank, serves on the board of the Israeli Cancer Society, the Israeli Family Planning Association, and the Association for the Advancement of Education in Israel. Dov was a member Israeli State Commission of Inquiry into the Israeli Health Care System between 1990–1998 that led to the national health insurance legislation that was enacted in Israel in 1995. He served on other national commissions an adviser to the Israeli parliament. Dov worked for the US and German international aid agencies and the Australian government. On behalf of the World Bank, he worked in Botswana, India, Indonesia, and played roles in health system reform in Rumania, Russia, and now in Mexico, Colombia and Costa Rica.

Marisa Gil Lapetra is a Statistical Editor at OECD. Since beginning her professional career assisting the Chief Economist of the Commercial Office of the Spanish Embassy to Belgium, she has held positions as a Business Analyst at KNOEMA, as an Environmental Policy Group Communications Officer at the World Bank Family Network, and as the founder of Renewable Energy Advisory Services. Her focus is on examining social policy issues related to health and environment through an international development lens, with a mindfully incorporation of the fundamental principles and creative approach to sourcing, compiling, analyzing and displaying data to support change-agents and policymakers in their dialogue for making meaningful decisions for progress in health care access, quality and delivery for targeted populations. Marisa is a member of the National Association for Business Economics (NABE), DC. She received her Master's Degree in Econometrics and Quantitative Economics from the Universidad Complutense de Madrid and a post-graduate degree from Universite Paris X Nanterre.

Joseph Kutzin is Coordinator for Health Financing Policy at the World Health Organization, leading a team responsible for informing national policy dialog and global debates on health financing reforms to move towards Universal Health Coverage. He obtained his Master's Degree in Development Economics from Boston University, has been a visiting Fellow at Imperial College London, and in 2012 was awarded an Honorary Doctorate from Semmelweis University in Budapest, Hungary. He has 30 years' experience in health financing policy and health system reform, working in Africa, Asia, the Caribbean, Europe, and the United States. He was formerly Senior Policy Advisor to Kyrgyzstan's Ministry of Health and lead advisor on health financing for the WHO European Region, including in his role as Head of the WHO Barcelona Office for Health System Strengthening. Prior to joining WHO, he worked for both the World Bank and the Project HOPE Center for Health Affairs. He has published numerous conceptual and empirical articles on health financing and universal coverage. Highlights include his role as lead editor and main author of *Implementing Health Financing Reform: Lessons from Countries in Transition*, and as a contributor to the World Health Report 2010: *Health Financing: the Path to Universal Coverage*.

Winnie Yip is Professor of Health Policy and Economics at the Blavatnik School of Government, University of Oxford, and Senior Research Fellow of Green Templeton College, Oxford, where she co-directs the Global Health Policy Program. She is also Adjunct Professor of International Health Policy and Economics at Harvard School of Public Health. Professor Yip received her PhD in Economics from the Massachusetts Institute of Technology. Her research focuses on the design, implementation and impact evaluation of national health care systems, especially in China and Asia. Her research is funded by the National Science Foundation, Bill and Melinda Gates Foundation, the European Union Commission, the Economics and Social Science Research Council. She is a member of the Sustainable Development Solutions Network Thematic Group on Health, the Expert Group on Provider Payment of the Joint Learning Network for Universal Health Coverage, the Institute of Medicine's Standing Committee to support USAID's Engagement in Health Systems Strengthening in Response to the Economic Transition of Health and the Lancet Commission for Global Surgery. She is Associate Editor of *Health Economics*, *Journal of the Economics of Ageing*, and editorial board member of *Health Policy*, *Health Economics*, *Policy and Law*, and *Health Economics Review*.

Cheryl Cashin is Senior Program Director at Results for Development Institute (R4D) where she leads a health financing portfolio focused on global and country-level efforts to support universal health coverage in low- and middle-income countries. She received her Ph.D. in economics from the University of Washington and M.S. from Cornell University. She has worked in more than 20 countries on health financing policy development and implementation, with a particular focus on purchasing and provider payment, including capitation payment models to strengthen primary health care and improve equity within sustainable financing for UHC. She currently leads the Provider Payment Initiative of the Joint Learning Network for Universal Health Coverage (JLN). Previously, she has held academic positions at Boston University's School of Public Health and University of California, Berkeley's Nicholas C Petris Center on Health Care Markets and Consumer Welfare and has served as a health financing consultant for the World Bank, WHO, OECD and other international technical partners. She is the lead author of the recent book *Paying for performance in health care: implications for health system performance and accountability* and is a co-author of several other books and publications.

Camilo Cid is a Professor of Health Economics in the Department of Public Health of the Catholic University of Chile. Last year he was Head of the Presidential Commission for Health Insurance Reform in Chile. Currently he is on loan as the coordinator for Health Economics and Financing at the Pan American Health Organization in Washington DC. His areas of focus include health economics and public policy, financing and expenditure, health insurance and its regulation, payment mechanisms and risk adjustment. Dr Cid has served as an international advisor for several international organizations where he has worked on projects for public institutions in LAC. Previously, Dr Cid worked for over 15 years in the public sector of health, becoming the Head of the Department of Studies of the Ministry of Health of Chile. Later, he was the founder of the Department of Health Economics of the same Ministry. He was President of the Health Economics Association of Latin America and the Caribbean and is part of the Directory of the Health Economics Association of Chile. Dr Cid obtained his MA in Economics from Georgetown University and PhD in Economics from the Department of Economics of the Universität Duisburg-Essen of Germany.

Randall P. Ellis is a Professor in the Department of Economics at Boston University, with research interests in both US and international health economics topics. Dr Ellis is a past President of the American Society of Health Economists and an associate editor of both the Journal of Health Economics and the American Journal of Health Economics. Dr Ellis was one of the developers of the DCG/HCC risk adjustment models currently used by the US Medicare program for risk adjusting Part C and Part D payments, and for the Health Insurance Marketplaces. Dr Ellis serves as a consultant to Verisk Health which supports the DCG/HCC risk adjustment framework, developing models for all ages and all payer and plan types. His current and recent research is funded by the National Institute of Mental Health, The Commonwealth Fund, The Australian Research Council, and Verisk Health. This recent work focuses on risk adjustment, reimbursement systems, optimal insurance, mental health, health plan competition and in primary care payment reform.

Veronica Vargas is an economist specialized in health and has been active in global health for over 20 years. In addition to teaching Health Economics at the University Alberto Hurtado-Georgetown in Chile, Dr Vargas was an advisor to the Chilean Health Reform Commission in 2003–2004, has consulted for the World Bank, DFID, and the European Union in Latin America, the Caribbean, Asia, Africa, Eastern Europe, and the Middle East. Dr Vargas' many years of research experience have produced peer-reviewed publications on setting health priorities, payment methods for providers, risk adjustment, human resources, budgeting for results, and reproductive health and AIDS. Her other areas of expertise include health care reform, health insurance, economic evaluation, and cost of illness. Dr Vargas is an invited member of International Health Economics Association (iHEA) Scientific Committee (2009–2014).

Juergen Wasem has studied economics and political science at Pennsylvania State University, University of Sussex and Cologne University (1978–1983). He got a PhD in economics at Cologne University (1986) and a PhD in public health at Bielefeld University (1996). He has worked in the Federal Ministry of Labor and Social Politics (1985–1989). He was project leader at the Max Planck Institute for the Study of Societies (1991–1994). He was professor for health insurance at the University of Applied Sciences Cologne (1989–1991 and 1994–1997), professor for health economics in the School of Public Health at LMU Munich University (1997–1999) and professor for health care management at School of Law and Business EMAU Greifswald University (1999–2003). Since 2003 he is the Alfried Krupp von Bohlen and Halbach Foundation-Professor and director of the Institute for Health Care Management and Research at University Duisburg-Essen, Germany. He is member of the board of directors of the German Society for Health Economics, where he was president in 2013–14. His research interests are in health insurance, risk adjustment, comparative health care systems and health economic evaluation.

Lorena Prieto is an economist specialized in health economics with over 15 years' experience. She specializes in health financing and economics with research in health interventions' cost-effectiveness, evaluation of health financing reform projects, the effects of health status on labor outcomes, accessibility to health services, health care markets, health services' costing and production, and analysis of equity, efficiency, and financial sustainability. While in Boston, she worked with the Center for Multicultural Mental Health Research in two major projects dealing with cost-effectiveness of depression treatment interventions and behavioral patterns in drug abuse treatment and social services. She has been a consultant on projects in Peru, Chile, Bolivia, Suriname, Paraguay, Argentina, Guyana, Honduras, Mexico, and Guatemala for international organizations including the World Bank, Inter-American Development Bank, UNICEF, WHO, and PAHO as well as various Ministries of Health and the Brookings Institution. She is also a part-time professor at the Graduate School of the Universidad del Pacífico in Lima, Peru. Her latest publications are on out-of-pocket payments and hospital performance, with earlier publications on equity analysis.

Guillem López-Casasnovas is Professor in Economics at Pompeu Fabra University in Barcelona, Catalonia, Spain, and Member of the Directors' Board of the Bank of Spain (2005–2017). He has a degree in Economics (1978), a degree in Law (1979) from the University of Barcelona, and a D. Phil. Economics (1984) from the University of York. In addition to other many academic commitments, he is member of the Royal Academy of Medicine and Honorary Member of The

College of Economists of Catalonia, of the Advisory Council of the Spanish Health and Social Welfare Ministry and of the Advisory Council of the Catalan Health Ministry since 1984. He cofounded the Centre of Health and Economics and codirected The Executive Program on Global Health Policy Leadership with the Public Health School at the University of Berkeley and The Barcelona Graduate School of Economics. He was also President of the International Health Economics Association (2007–2013), and a Senior Advisor (2010–2012) for the WHO Group on Health Inequalities in Europe. His research interests include public finance, fiscal policy and health economics.

Laura Pellisé is Senior Researcher at the Center for Research in Economics and health (CRES) at the Department of Economics and Business at Universitat Pompeu Fabra (UPF). She has a degree in Economics from Universitat de Barcelona, holds an MSc in Health Policy and Management from Harvard University and a Ph.D. in Economics from UPF. Prior to her current position, she was professor at the Department of Economics of Universidad Carlos III of Madrid (1992–1997), joining the Spanish Ministry of Health as a technical advisor in 1997. She held, since 2001, top management positions in the largest private hospital group in Spain, USP (now Grupo Quirón Salud), and then was managing director of the Vall d'Hebron Institute of Oncology. She joined the CRES at UPF in 2011 as its Director. She is member of the group of experts appointed by the European Commission for the evaluation of SME in health care. She codirects the Master in Health Policy and Management (MADS) of UPF (Barcelona School of Management). Her research interests include health care innovation, pricing, financing and regulation in biopharmaceutical and devices industries, incentives and health care organization.

Alistair McGuire is the Professor of Health Economics at LSE Health and Social Care, within the Department of Social Policy at the London School of Economics and Political Science (LSE). Prior to this he was Professor of Economics at City University, London after being a Tutor in Economics at Pembroke College, University of Oxford. He has been a visiting Professor at Harvard University, the University of Sydney, the University of York and the Universitat Pompeu Fabra, Barcelona. He has been interested in the economics of health care for over 30 years, with extensive teaching experience and has written numerous books, articles and reports in this area on a wide range of subject matter. He has been involved in a number of major clinical trials as the lead health economist. He has also acted as an advisor to a number of governments and governmental bodies, as well as for a number of international bodies and pharmaceutical companies.

Maria Raikou is Assistant Professor at the Department of Economics, University of Piraeus, Athens, Greece. Prior to this she was a Research Fellow and Visiting Lecturer at LSE Health and Social Care, Department of Social Policy, London School of Economics and Political Science (LSE). She has a Degree in Electrical and Computer Engineering from the National Technical University of Athens (N.T.U.A.), Greece, and an MSc and PhD in Health Economics from City University, London. She has held research posts in the area of health economics at Oxford University (within the Health Economics Research Centre), City University (in the Department of Economics) and the LSE. She has published research articles in peer-reviewed journals such as Health Economics, Journal of Health Economics, British Medical Journal and economic reports, including reports for the UK Department of Health, the UK National Audit Office, and NICE, in the field of economic evaluation of health care programmes. She has also acted as a consultant to the UK Department of Health, to the UK National Audit Office, to the UK National Institute for Health and Clinical Excellence (NICE) and to a number of pharmaceutical companies.

William H. Dow is Henry J Kaiser Professor of Health Economics at the University of California–Berkeley's School of Public Health. He also is Director of the UC Berkeley Center on the Economics and Demography of Aging. In addition he is a Research Associate at the National Bureau of Economic Research, and previously served as Senior Economist at the White House Council of Economic Advisers. He received his PhD in economics from Yale University. Dow's research analyzes economic aspects of health insurance, health behaviors, and health and demographic outcomes. Honors include the John D Thompson Prize for Young Investigators awarded by the Association of University Programs in Health Administration, and the Kenneth J Arrow Award given by the International Health Economics Association.

Justin S. White is Assistant Professor of Health Economics in the UCSF School of Medicine, with joint appointments in the Philip R. Lee Institute for Health Policy Studies and the Department of Epidemiology and Biostatistics. Dr. White applies theory from health economics and behavioral economics to understand the factors that motivate individuals to adopt healthy behaviors, with special emphasis on tobacco use. In doing so, he aims to identify individuals' decision errors related to health behavior and design interventions to address these errors. He is particularly interested in the use of monetary and social incentives for changing behavior. Much of his work focuses on chronic disease prevention in low- and middle-income countries. Prior to coming to UCSF, he completed a postdoctoral fellowship in cardiovascular disease prevention at Stanford University's Prevention Research Center. He holds a PhD in health policy and MA in economics from UC Berkeley and an MSPH in health policy from UNC Chapel Hill.

Stefano Bertozzi is Dean and Professor of Health Policy and Management at the UC Berkeley School of Public Health. Previously, he directed the HIV and tuberculosis programs at the Bill and Melinda Gates Foundation. He serves on the scientific advisory boards for the President's Emergency Plan for AIDS Relief, the National Institute of Health's Office of AIDS Research, and the World Health Organization's HIV Program. Dr Bertozzi worked at the Mexican National Institute of Public Health as director of its Center for Evaluation Research and Surveys and has also held positions with UNAIDS and the World Bank. He holds a bachelor's degree in biology and a PhD in health policy and management from the Massachusetts Institute of Technology. He earned his medical degree at UC San Diego, and trained in internal medicine at UC San Francisco.

Paul Revill is a Research Fellow at the Centre for Health Economics (CHE) at the University of York. He works primarily on methodological and applied research in economic evaluation to inform resource allocation decisions in health sectors in low and middle income countries, particularly in sub-Saharan Africa and related to HIV/AIDS. He co-led reports for the HIV Modelling Consortium to directly inform the 2013 and 2015 WHO HIV Treatment Guidelines. Paul has previously worked as an economist in the Planning & Budgeting Department of the Ministry of Health in Malawi. He has a strong interest in ensuring the methods of modelling and health economics appropriately reflect the challenges and realities of resource constraints operating within programmes so that policy decisions are most likely to generate value and lead to health gains at a local level.

Beth Woods is a Research Fellow at the Centre for Health Economics, University of York. Her research interests include the application of statistical and decision analysis methods to health technology assessment and methods for prioritising health care resources and research. From 2006–2013, Beth was a Director in the Health Economics team at Oxford Outcomes, a private consulting firm, where she specialised in applied economic evaluation. During this time Beth contributed to numerous submissions to the National Institute for Health and Care Excellence and other agencies internationally. Beth holds a BA in Economics from the University of Cambridge and an MSc in Economic Evaluation in Healthcare from City University.

Mark J. Sculpher is Professor of Health Economics at the Centre for Health Economics, University of York, UK where he is Director of the Programme on Economic Evaluation and Health Technology Assessment. Mark has worked in the field of economic evaluation and health technology assessment for over 25 years. He has researched in a range of clinical areas including heart disease, cancer, diagnostics and public health. He has also contributed to methods in the field, in particular relating to decision analytic modelling and techniques to handle uncertainty, heterogeneity and generalisability. He chaired NICE's 2004 Task Group on methods guidance for economic evaluation and advised the Methods Working Party for the 2008 update of this guidance. He has over 220 peer-reviewed publications and is a co-author of two major text books in the area: *Methods for the Economic Evaluation of Health Care Programmes* (OUP, 2015 with Drummond, Claxton, Torrance and Stoddart) and *Decision Modelling for Health Economic Evaluation* (OUP, 2006 with Briggs and Claxton).

Marisol Rodríguez is Professor of Applied Economics at the School of Economics and Business of the University of Barcelona. She holds a MSc in Economics from the London School of Economics and Political Science and a Diploma in Health Systems Analysis from the School of Public Health of the Johns Hopkins University. In 1999 she was an invited fellow at the School of Public Health in the University of California, Berkeley. Between 1990 and 1998 she was the director of the Master's course in Health Economics and Health Care Management organized jointly by the University of Barcelona and the Pompeu Fabra University. She belonged to the ECuity international research group that for more than 12 years worked on successive EU projects analyzing equity in the financing and delivery of health care services in different European countries, where she was responsible for the Spanish team. She is the co-editor of the book *Social Inequalities in Health: Main Determinants and Elements for Action* [in Spanish] published by Elsevier/Masson in 2008. Recently, she has been awarded the Josep Trueta medal for her contributions to the Catalan health sector.

Rosa Urbanos-Garrido is an Associate Professor of Public Finance at the School of Economics at the University Complutense of Madrid, Spain. Her PhD was awarded with Honors (2000) and her PhD Dissertation on equity in the delivery of health care was also awarded the 2000 Prize on Public Economics by the Spanish Institute for Fiscal Studies. She has been a visiting scholar at the Department of Economics at the University Pompeu Fabra in Barcelona and the Centre for Health Economics at the University of York, UK. First Director of the Spanish Observatory of the National Health System, Dr Urbanos-Garrido has also worked as full-time advisor for the Spanish Health Minister from 2004 to 2007, and as Director General for Regional Cooperation at the Spanish Ministry for Public Administrations from 2007 to 2008. She has been a member of the Board of the Spanish Public Health and Health Care Administration Society and of the Spanish Health Economics Association. She is the co-editor of the book *Social Inequalities in Health: Main Determinants and Elements for Action* [in Spanish] published by Elsevier/Masson in 2008.

Introduction to Volume 1: The Economics of Health and Health Systems

Richard M. Scheffler
Distinguished Professor of Health Economics and Public Policy
Director of the Global Center for Health Economics and Policy Research
University of California, Berkeley

Chapters 1–3 in this volume address macroeconomic issues, which include economic growth and health care spending, the link between trade and health care, and lastly, techniques and methods for forecasting country-by-country macro health care expenditures. Chapter 1, *Health Care Spending and Economic Growth*, explores the complex relationship between health expenditures and economic growth, and demonstrates that the researchers have shifted their attention towards economic growth in a way that looks at the impact health spending on economic growth as well as its broader impact on the economy. The authors look at health investments and various health care strategies that combat epidemics such as Ebola. Chapter 2, *Macroeconomics, Trade, and Health*, looks at the interaction between health and the wider macro-economy, and analyzes the macroeconomic implications for the economy as a whole. Additionally, the authors suggest a framework for looking at and weighing the spending of health compared to other non-health expenditures. Chapter 3, *Measuring and Forecasting Global Health Expenditures*, looks at health care spending over several decades, especially the rapid growth since the middle of the 20th century. It shows that the tracking of health care expenditures as forecasting can be clearly understood by relating its growth to that of the overall economy. The chapter further examines a series of data on health care spending over multiple decades. Forecasting models are described and applied to various countries throughout the chapter. Special attention is paid to the sustainability of current spending trends and the boundaries between long-term care, retirement, and medical expenditures.

Chapters 4–9 looks at financing methods for health care (especially financing health care in a way to move us towards universal coverage), examines risk adjustment methodologies needed to implement payment and financing strategies, and the issue of priority setting in health care systems that are single payer, non-market driven systems. Chapter 4, *Economics of Financing Health Care*, uses an economic framework to explain the design of optimal financing strategies and reviews empirical evidence under different health care systems. Specifically, it looks at the impact of financing on patients, doctors, and hospitals. Applications of financing strategies are discussed in relationship to the structure of global health care financing and the role of third-party payers, both public and private. Three case studies on financing are discussed, in the U.S., The Netherlands, and Singapore. Chapter 5, *Alternative Financing Strategies for Universal Health Coverage*, takes on the critical issue of how financing impacts universal health care coverage. The chapter notes that there is no one best way to finance — in theory or in practice — but it discusses conceptual underpinnings regarding how we think about this key issue. The chapter examines the role of government and provides a synthesis of coverage in low- and middle-income countries. Chapter 6, *Global Risk-Adjusted Payment Models*, discusses the need for financing systems to risk-adjust for the underlying heterogeneity of both the patients and plans in order to reduce the incentive for risk selection. This chapter presents a practical, theoretical, and statistical set of risk adjustment models that are applied to a wide variety of countries' financing and payment systems. More than 30 countries, including those in high- and middle-income countries, are analyzed according to this risk-adjustment methodology. Chapter 7, *Resource Allocation and Priority Setting in Health Care Systems*, the authors discuss issues in single payer systems that do not use prices, and how to set priorities for pricing and spending. The chapter discusses practical problems, implications, and methodology of priority setting. Chapter 8, *Estimating Health Care Treatment Costs: Problems and Solutions*, considers the conceptual and empirical problems with estimating health care costs. The authors examine the estimation of such costs at different levels of aggregation. They argue that more attention needs to be given to this area of research because of the importance of health care cost estimation in helping to risk-adjust and predict future health care expenditure levels as well as reimbursement levels. Chapter 9, *Incentivizing Health Care Utilization and Health Outcomes*, looks at the evidence of using incentives to increase the use of health care services and improve health outcomes. In some instances, they have been a controversial tool, but there is great interest in how it can be used in an ethical and cost-effective manner. This chapter further examines these concerns as well as an important social protection program in

Mexico, but also summarizes the impact of incentives on family planning, prenatal care, immunizations, HIV and medication, and adherence to promoting non-medical behavior such as smoking cessation and STD prevention.

Chapters 10–11 in this volume look at how to evaluate interventions, and the crucial problem of inequities in the health sector. Chapter 10, *Economic Evaluation of Health Care Programmes and Interventions: Applications to Low- and Middle-Income Countries*, presents the tools of economic evaluation, such as cost-effectiveness, and shows how key policymakers have used them in economic evaluations. Specific examples are taken from the UK, Australia, and Canada, which demonstrates the usefulness of these evaluation methods. The chapter also looks at the policy challenges and evaluation methodology in low- and middle-income countries. The authors provide guidance on suitable methods that can be used to improve population health in these countries.

No issue can be more important than the inequalities in health and health care throughout the globe. Inequities and the social gradient in health persist and have widened over time. Chapter 11, *Inequalities and Inequities in Health and Health Care*, looks at socioeconomic and geographic disparities within the framework of moving towards universal coverage. It provides direction on ways of thinking about how these inequities should be addressed in economic systems and the development of health care policies.

Health Care Spending and Economic Growth

Edit V. Velenyi
Health, Nutrition & Population Global Practice, The World Bank

This chapter sets out to explore the relationship between health expenditures and economic growth, an important yet complex relationship. Understanding the evolution of health spending and economic growth nexus has been propelled by two major concerns: Spiraling expenditures and to inform health policymaking that is grounded in the broader economic and development framework.

Although per capita health expenditures have been growing, the literature and statistical analyses indicate that the growth trends have not been homogenous across regions and that the rate of growth has moderated over time. Beyond the regular checks and balances between ministries of health and finance during the budgeting process, economic crises have also played a role in 'streamlining' expenditures on health and have played a role in catalyzing structural reforms.

Policymakers and researchers have shifted attention to the health spending and growth nexus to inform national and global health policymaking in a way that connects health sector investments to the broader objective of economic growth and development. This indicates a movement toward more strategic utilization of resources, including longer time horizon for strategic planning and accentuating the bidirectional relationship between the health sector and the economy. These changes require applying a multidisciplinary research approach, going beyond the narrow boundaries of the sector. As examples of broad-based and long-term approaches, the importance of investment in system strengthening is discussed in the context of the Ebola epidemic, and the strategic management of demographic change is highlighted as a potential catalyst of sustained economic growth.

The presented evidence and the related discussions aim to contribute to identifying pragmatic approaches that could inform policymakers and technical experts regarding how more efficient and strategic spending could lead to better health outcomes, and how, in turn, improved population health status could act as an economic growth multiplier. As development through the health channel is country-specific, the chapter concludes that systematic country diagnostic is a critical input into policymaking.

The chapter concludes that health has emerged from a 'residual factor' in macroeconomic growth models into a coefficient of its own, an explanatory factor of productivity, economic growth, and poverty reduction. Yet, more research is required to guide future decisions on how to invest wisely in health and in a way that can perpetuate further growth. As the evidence base is growing but inconclusive, recommendations are made for future research.

Keywords: Health and Economic Growth; Global Health Spending Trends; Health System Vulnerability; Health Spending and Economic Crisis; Cyclicality of Health Expenditures; Health Care Financing Policy.

Introduction: Investing in Health — Investing in Growth?

The pathway from health spending to growth

- *Policymakers and development experts have long sought an answer to the question — Does investment in health help boost economic growth?*

Finding empirical evidence on the impact of health on growth and exploring the pathways through which health affects growth have been critical to inform public policy decisions, including intra- and inter-sectoral resource allocations to meet economic, development, and poverty-reduction objectives. A number of seminal reports — including the *World Development Report* (World Bank, 1993), the *Macroeconomics and Health: Investing in Health for Economic Development* (WHO, 2001), *and Health and Growth: Commission on Growth and Development* (Spence and Lewis, 2009) — have focused on the interplay between human health, health policy, and economic development[1] to better understand and provide evidence on whether, why and how spending on health can contribute to growth.

Since the release of the report by the World Health Organization's (WHO's) Commission on Macro Economics and Health in 2001 (WHO, 2001), an increasing number of papers have focused on understanding the causal pathway (and disentangling the relationships between inputs, outputs, and outcomes along the pathway) from government health expenditures (GHE) to economic growth. The report claims that:

> *"... improving the health and longevity of the poor is an end in itself, a fundamental goal of economic development. But it is also a means to achieving the other*

[1]The focus of development is not only on methods of promoting economic development, economic growth and structural change but also on improving the potential for the mass of the population, for example, through health and education and workplace conditions, whether through public or private channels (Bell, 1987). The related field, development economics, unlike in many other fields of economics, may incorporate social and political factors to devise particular plans and advise policies (Todaro and Smith, 2006).

development goals relating to poverty reduction. The linkages of health to poverty reduction and long-term economic growth are powerful, much stronger than is generally understood."

Yet, despite tacit agreement that health is an important input into development — through its effect on productivity and, more broadly, on human capital formation — there is no consensus in the empirical literature on the linkages between health and growth or even from health policies to health (Dixit, 2006; Jack and Lewis, 2009).

This arises because the causal pathway from health spending to health outcomes to economic growth is complex, which has generated a rich but unsettled body of research. This ever-growing literature aims to: (i) Estimate the magnitude of the effects between spending, health, and growth; (ii) generate more evidence, in a variety of contexts, on the direction of the relationships, using a battery of economic and econometric specifications, and also drawing on health system and health policy research tools; and (iii) identify pragmatic approaches that could inform policymakers and technical experts regarding how more efficient and/or more spending could lead to better health outcomes, and how, in turn, improved population health status could act as an economic growth multiplier.

Notwithstanding the progress in this field as a result of the increased interest (see Box 1) in the health and economic growth nexus, and the availability of more robust computational tools and advanced analytical techniques, understanding the contribution of health spending to economic growth remains unresolved. Data limitations and the limited application of more standardized techniques to make results comparable across studies — both in space and in time — continue to constrain our ability to offer resounding conclusions. Consequently, further efforts are required in: (i) Data collection; (ii) development and application of methods that help comparability; and (iii) sustained momentum by researchers to reduce the methodological challenges to establishing causality between spending — as an input into health — and health outcomes as determinants of economic growth. Beyond pushing the analytical frontiers, another challenge at the country level is (iv) to find pragmatic ways to effectively translate findings into policy response, taking into consideration overarching development goals, macro-fiscal constraints, and the political economy.

Section "Health Spending to Health Outcomes" open the discussion on the pathway from health to growth by highlighting some important findings and limitations, first with a focus on the relationship between spending and health, then turning to the nexus between health and growth (for a summary, see Table 1). Following these highlights, some of the central findings and concepts discussed in Section "Health Spending to Health Outcomes" will be further explored later in this chapter.

Box 1. The role of health in economic development — A historical perspective

The role of health in economic development has varied over time and across countries. In the 1950s and 1960s, the prevailing wisdom was that economic growth was the key to development, which has led to a strong focus on investment in physical capital and infrastructure (Ruger, 2005). Market fundamentalism under liberal economic policy emphasized that economic growth is the principal tool for economic development and considered investment in social services as 'counterproductive' (Thurow *et al.*, 1998). Neoliberal theory also held that it is growth that matters and not distribution, which was embedded in the concept of "trickle down" economic development (Srinivasan, 1994).

However, from 1960s–1980s, development theory shifted to encompass more than economic growth, embracing individuals' "basic needs" to provide the opportunity for a "full life." Academic thinking and research, which challenged the role of physical capital in economic growth, have contributed to the shift away from orthodox views of development. Research has not only found that physical capital explained a smaller share of the variation in growth, but that there was a "residual factor" in macroeconomic statistical models (Abramovitz, 1956). Among the components of the residual factor were believed to be investments in education, and later, in health (Enke, 1964). These components of "underdevelopment" were believed to be key barriers to productivity, economic growth, and poverty reduction.

Hence, development policy slowly moved from the "Washington Consensus"[2] of the 1990s, a period of market-oriented reforms, which focused on macroeconomic stability, privatization, trade liberalization, and public sector consolidation, onward to incorporating "human capital" (Grossman, 1972; 2000) and "human development" (Shultz, 1961; Srinivasan, 1994),[3] into the

(*Continued*)

[2]The term Washington Consensus was coined in 1989 by English Economist John Williamson to refer to a set of 10 relatively specific economic policy prescriptions.

[3]As Srinivasan (1994) summarizes, the first Human Development Report (HDR) defines human development as denoting "both the *process* of widening people's choices and the *level* of their achieved well-being" (United Nations Development Program, 1990, p. 9) and disarmingly admits that is notions — "the primary objective of development is to benefit people … [and] income is not the sum total of human life" — are not really new. It claims that it "differs from conventional approaches to economic growth, human capital formation, human welfare, or basic human needs" (p. 10) in viewing growth in income as being necessary but not sufficient for human development, and human beings as ends rather than means, and as participants in the development process rather than as beneficiaries. Finally, it focuses on human choices rather than on the provision of goods and services that deprived groups need. The report also introduced the Human Development Index (HDI), which it claims "captures the three essential components of human life: Longevity,

Box 1. (*Continued*)

development agenda. With the switch from the pure financial and neoliberal considerations for growth, the *bonafide* development approach engaged with social sectors. With respect to the health sector, the entry points were investments in population policies, nutrition, and prevention and treatment of communicable diseases, later followed by investments to improve health systems. For example, the *World Development Report 1993: Investing in Health* (World Bank, 1993) examines the interplay between human health, health policy, and economic development and concludes that good health is a goal itself as investing in health is one means of accelerating development. The *World Development Report 2000/2001: Attacking Poverty* (World Bank, 2001) identified good health and nutrition, effective reproductive health policies, and health services as critical for enabling countries to break the vicious circle of poverty, high fertility, poor health, and low economic growth.

Research on the relationship between health and growth gained momentum with the Millennium Development Goals (MDGs), which track changes of selected development outcomes between 2000 and 2015 and, hence, provide quantitative evidence on the success of a government's economic and development policies.

Interest has further increased with the evolving post-2015 development framework, which continues consolidating the MDG results and puts more emphasis on the multi-dimensional nature of poverty, moving toward the new goals of sustainable development (SDGs). Within the context of the health sector, the post-2015 agenda shifts the focus to non-communicable diseases (NCDs) and universal health coverage (UHC) (Vega, 2013).[4]

Prompted by the 20th Anniversary of the *1993 World Development Report: Investing in Health* (World Bank, 1993), in 2013 a Lancet Commission revisited the case for investment in health and developed a new investment framework to achieve dramatic health gains by 2035. The Commission's Report, *Global Health 2035: A World Converging within a Generation* (*The Lancet*, 2013), calls

(*Continued*)

knowledge, and basic income for decent living standards. Longevity and knowledge refer to the formation of human capabilities, and income is a proxy measure for the choices people have in putting their capabilities to use." The HDI is the equally weighted sum of the deprivation of a country with respects to the three components, measured by the proxy variables of life expectancy at birth, literacy, and real income per capita.

[4] Defined as access to needed health services and financial risk protection, UHC is a shared health policy goal, and is increasingly regarded as an overarching goal for health in the post-2015 development agenda (Vega, 2013).

Box 1. (*Continued*)

the world to begin closing the global health gap through a "grand convergence" — a bold new strategy to bring infectious, maternal and child deaths down to universally low levels within a generation; curbing NCDs and injuries; and reaching UHC through pathways that protect the poor from the outset ("progressive universalism"). Using a full income approach[5] (Summers and Jamison, 2013), the report finds that there is an enormous payoff from investing in health. While calculations show that the costs of convergence in health over the period 2015–2035 are high, the economic benefits of convergence would exceed costs by a factor of about 9 in low-income countries and around 20 in lower-middle income countries. This benefit–cost ratio makes the investment extremely attractive. The report concludes that the full income approach provides a strong rationale for allocating greater resources to the health sector and health-related sectors — and an even stronger basis for action than ever before.

Source: Author's summary based on Ruger (2005) and *Global Health 2035: A World Converging within A Generation* (Dybul, 2013; Jamison *et al.*, 2013; Summers and Jamison, 2013).

Health spending to health outcomes

With respect to the first leg of the pathway, although evidence strongly and systematically confirms that spending on health is important, the level of health expenditure has been a weak predictor of health outcomes.

For example, evidence between 1960 and 2004 indicates a global convergence in health outcomes. Exploring the evolution of the cross-country distribution of national incomes and health status between 1960 and 2004, Deaton (2006) shows that per capita incomes have steadily diverged while country-level health indicators have converged — until 1990 for life expectancy and through 2004 for the infant mortality rate. The author notes that one driver behind the slowing convergence in life expectancy was the explosion of HIV/AIDS in Sub-Saharan Africa in the 1990s (Deaton, 2006). Furthermore, an MDG-focused

[5] The full income approach combines income growth and the value of life years gained in that period. The sum of these two measures equals the change in the country's full income over a time period. In contrast with the pure GDP-based measurement of the investment value in health, the full income approach includes the valuation of life years (VLY) by the individual. The underlying argument is that if an individual lives better in Country A then in Country B because of better population-level health outcomes, then measuring the value of health investment in GDP terms only omits the value of higher quality life that is derived from better health status (Summers and Jamison, 2013).

statistical analysis highlights some important drivers that have been undermining convergence (Stuckler *et al.*, 2010). According to this study, while health expenditures have contributed to improvements in health-related MDG targets, income and health expenditure levels account for less than 1/5 of the variation in progress toward the targets. The key drivers of "unmet progress" instead are HIV and the NCD burden, followed by insufficient human resources for health. The global health policy ambition on convergence was recently laid out by *The Lancet Commission on Global Health 2035*, which presented a case for "global convergence in health within a generation," including through using fiscal policy levers to curb NCDs and embarking on progressive universalism (Jamison *et al.*, 2013). The journey toward global convergence in health, however, will require substantial investments not only in fighting diseases and strengthening health systems but by investing more resources in accompanying research to put the required additional domestic and external resources for health to good use.

The reasons why public spending on health care may not improve health may arise from market and government failures and sub-optimal technical efficacy (Filmer *et al.*, 2002). Given that health outcomes are complex products of (i) exogenous factors, for example, changes in the macroeconomic environment (see Volume 1, Chapter 2, *Macroeconomics, Trade and Health*), government priorities and policies, and the strength of institutions and governance; (ii) system characteristics; and (iii) behavioral aspects on the supply-side (provider level) and demand-side (individual and community levels), the same unit of spending can lead to a wide variation in outcomes, depending on the interplay of these factors and characteristics (see Figure 1). For example, country-level evidence shows that institutional aspects, such as increased accountability and empowerment at health care facilities and the introduction of incentives can improve value for money[6] (Lewis, 2006; Jack and Lewis, 2004; 2009). This is the central theme of the *World Development Report 2004: Making Services Work for Poor People*, (World Bank, 2003) and the health results-based financing development agenda[7] (Morgan, 2014), which aims to improve efficiency and value for money by establishing a direct link between payments and outcomes.

[6] Recent evidence suggests that inefficient incentives and lack of accountability undermine the public provision of health services, leading to underperformance and substandard care.

[7] Results-based financing for health refers to any program that transfers money or goods either to patients when they take health-related actions (such as having their children immunized) or to health care providers, when they achieve performance targets (such as immunizing a certain percentage of children in a given area). While the World Bank uses the term "results-based financing" to describe this concept, other donors call it performance-based incentives or pay for performance. But they all essentially describe the same concept of linking incentives with results.

Table 1. Highlights of health spending, health outcomes, and economic growth

Health Expenditures	**Level and Determinants of Health Spending** — The level of health expenditure is positively correlated with income. — However, income is not the only driver of health expenditure. Age, disease prevalence, technology, individual and societal factors and preferences, and demand- and supply-side health system factors jointly determine spending (Table 7). — While normative targets have been useful, it is the positivistic approach that have proven more pragmatic in terms of answering "how much a government can spend on health" and "what options it can use in the future."	**Growth in Health Spending** — To different degrees, depending on income level, health expenditure growth has been causing concerns regarding the share of the sector in the economy ("crowd out") and the fiscal sustainability of funding future health needs. This has led to the rise of cost-containment policies in developed economies. — Depending on the data type and analytical method, the literature is divided whether the income elasticity of health spending is above or below 1, and whether the rate of growth in health spending is above income growth.	**Economic Cycles and Spending** — Health expenditures respond to economic cycles. Counter-cyclical social expenditure is part of prudent fiscal and social policy (see more in Section "Is Counter Cyclicality a Feasible Future?).	**Health Spending, Growth, Poverty Reduction** — Health expenditure is an important determinant of both higher economic growth and better health status, and is therefore a key tool available to policymakers. — As improvements in health status are necessary for poverty to decrease, indirectly, spending on health contributes to poverty reduction objectives. — Postponing health spending can lead to increased financial and opportunity cost in the future.
Health Outcomes	**Health Spending and Outcomes — A Tenuous Relationship** — While spending on health is important, the level of health expenditure is a weak predictor of health outcomes. — Given that health outcomes are complex products of: (i) exogenous factors; (ii) system characteristics; and (iii) behavioral aspects, the same unit of spending can lead to wide variations in outcomes. — Health system efficiency is an important determinant of health outcomes for health spending; a driver of variation in "value for money."		**Health — A Multisectoral Outcome** — Because health outcomes are multi-sectoral in nature, complementary interventions (e.g., education or water and sanitation) are critical to improving outcomes for spending.	**Trends in Health Status** — Evidence between 1960 and 2004 indicates health outcomes are converging. — However, MDG-focused analyses show inequality in the progress in attaining the targets.

	— Strength of governance and accountability is another factor that explains variation in outcomes for spending (WDR, 2004) and the rate of progress toward health targets. For example, the strength of public sector governance and financial management proxies the extent to which governments are able to use resources efficiently and direct those to specific outcomes.			— While evidence shows that health expenditures have contributed to improvements in health-related MDG targets, income and health expenditure levels account for less than 1/5 of the variation in progress towards the targets. The key drivers of "unmet progress" are HIV and NCD burden, followed by insufficient human resources for health.
Economic Growth	**Health and Growth — A Two-Way Relationship** — Economic growth and health status are positively correlated and have a two-way relationship; better health enhances growth by improving productivity, and higher growth allows better human capital formation.	**Policy Sequencing — What comes first?** — Some results suggest that improving human development must precede or accompany rising economic growth for a country to reach sustained growth. — In terms of policy sequencing, without improvements in human development, policy that attempts to enhance economic growth is highly unlikely to lead to sustained growth.	**Macro Evidence** — While the evidence on the linkage between health and growth from macro analyses has provided argument to support calls for increased investment in health, an important limitation has been that such studies do not provide specific information as to how to invest in health to contribute to growth.	**Micro Evidence** — Evidence from micro analyses is not only more robust, but it can provide actionable information for policymakers regarding which health interventions to invest in, and how, in order to boost productivity and, therefore, contribute to economic growth. — On the other hand, a limitation associated with the micro approach is context specificity and, potentially, the limited external validity of findings.

Source: Author's summary.

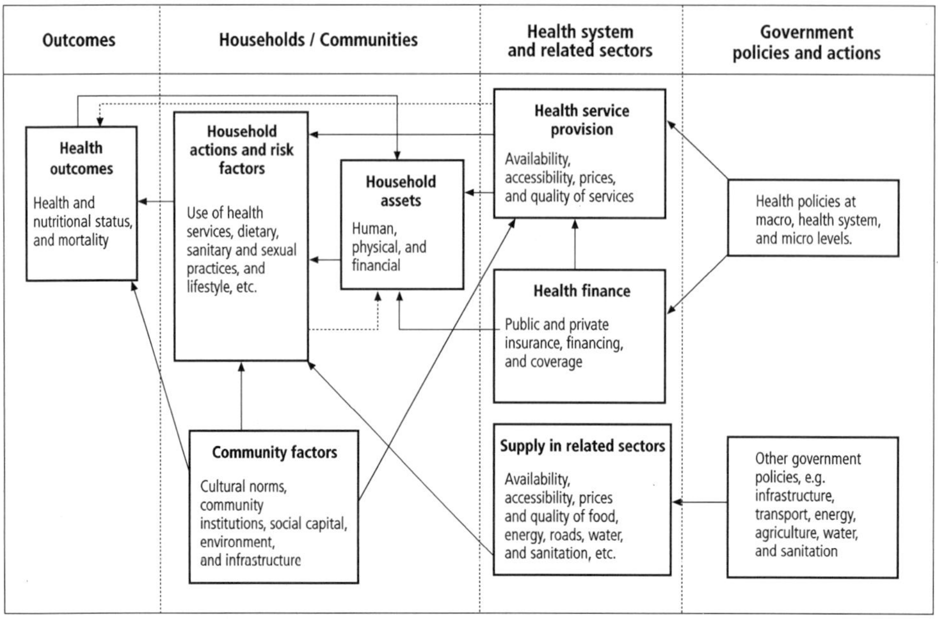

Figure 1. Determinants of health outcomes

Source: Wagstaff (2002).

Considering the tenuous relationship between health expenditure, as an input, and health outcomes, rather than focusing on the *level* of expenditure, governments, and health policy-makers must focus on how to improve the '*value for money*' associated with health spending before they argue for more resources for health. Health system efficiency has been an important determinant of health outcomes for health spending and a driver of variation in value for money.

In low-income contexts, however, efficiency gains alone are not sufficient. In 2012, the income group average of health spending per capita in low-income countries was US$38.50,[8] which is below the normative benchmarks for minimum expenditure on health per capita as set by the WHO (Sachs, 2001)(US$34 in 2001; US$40 in 2007; US$86 in 2012) and by the Taskforce on Innovative International Financing for Health Systems (US$54 in 2009).[9] Normative targets in health care

[8] Based on WHO 2013 dataset for year 2012, approximately 60% (19 out of 32) of low-income counties had less than US$40 per capita health spending.

[9] A more recent estimate by the Taskforce on Innovative International Financing for Health Systems places the number at US$54 per capita. See more on the Taskforce on Innovative International Financing for Health Systems in McCoy and Brikci (2010).

financing, such as these per capita minimum values or the Abuja target[10] — which recommends allocating 15% of government resources to the health sector — have often proven valuable in terms of international benchmarking, as policy catalysts, and may have also contributed to efforts to leverage resources. Yet, it is the positive economic approach that has proven to be more pragmatic in terms of directly informing policy processes because it focuses on understanding government behavior, posing empirical questions such as "*why existing policies are pursued … and which policies will be pursued in the future*" (Musgrave, 1959; Tandon *et al.*, 2014). Unlike the normative approach, which is grounded in theoretically ideal sets of policies, the positivistic approach focuses on what is implemented in practice, which takes into account feasibility factors, including macro-fiscal and political economy (e.g., public choice and accountability) aspects.

As noted above, beyond the level of health spending and health system efficiency, the rate of progress in improving health outcomes has also been determined by the strength of health care institutions and by public sector governance and financial management, which proxy the extent to which governments are able to use resources efficiently and target those to specific policy priorities and related outcomes. One consequence of the weak link between health expenditures, health, and growth is that beyond economic research, more investigation is required to understand the institutional context and how that influences the health-growth nexus. If institutions play a significant role in determining the magnitude of the effect of health spending on growth, then the role of health system research — as a complementary angle — gains increased importance to help explain the variation in outcomes.

Health outcomes are acknowledged to be multi-sectoral. Investments in inputs to health production are maximized only if complementary interventions, such as education, water, and sanitation are also simultaneously addressed. This raises questions about inter-sectoral resource allocation and fiscal space for health. Mainstream public finance theory holds that public resources should be utilized up to the point where the marginal benefit of an additional dollar of spending is equalized across sectors (Gillingham, 2014). However, Tandon *et al.* (2014)[11] note

[10] The Abuja Declaration, which was proposed by the African Union in 2001, is a reprioritization benchmark that sets allocations to the health sector at a minimum of 15% of government expenditures.

[11] See more, for example in a study by Tandon *et al.* (2014) on reprioritization as one source of fiscal space for health. They conclude that the operational implications of this are not easy to derive given the difficulties of estimating the costs and social benefits of public expenditure. Nevertheless, this implies that — to merit reprioritization — the health sector would need to demonstrate that the social benefits of additional public spending outlays exceed the costs of financing this increase in spending, both in terms of the additional costs of raising revenues and also in terms of foregone public spending in other sectors (something that ministries of health are often not able to articulate persuasively to ministries of finance and planning).

that, in practice, it is very difficult to address inter-sectoral prioritization questions, both because measuring the return to the marginal dollars are technically complex, and even if there is technically robust evidence, priority setting is also a product of the political economy and, therefore, investment decisions become more subjective (Hauck *et al.*, 2005). This subjective feature can be exacerbated by the long-term nature of health investments, particularly because a number of critical interventions accrue over the lifecycle and between generations — as shown for example in the early childhood development (Alderman, 2011) and maternal and child health literature (Lancet, 2008) spanning government cycles between spending on a given target and related health system strengthening, to attaining improvements in the outcome. Myopic government policies that are driven by political cycles can undermine the realization of long-term objectives in attaining population health improvement in an efficient manner because postponing essential investments in the sector today may lead to increased financial and opportunity costs in the future (Heller, 2005).

In sum, technical and policy debates regarding the role of health spending in determining health outcomes[12] and how to reduce variation in the effects of spending on outcomes (i.e., improve the efficiency of health expenditures and, therefore, value for money) are ongoing because of measurement challenges and methodological limitations, and are further catalyzed by the multidisciplinary nature of the topic, which brings about complementary views and arguments from the field of health economics, and health system and policy research.

Health outcomes and economic growth

The relationship between health and development has gradually evolved over time and by now there is a general consensus that health is a critical input into development. The (relative) importance of investing in health has increased over time (see Box 1) (Ruger, 2005; 2009).

Economic growth and health status are positively correlated and have a two-way relationship; better health enhances growth by improving productivity, and higher growth allows better human capital formation.

In general, evidence on the bidirectional relationship between human development and growth suggests that growth leads to increased investment in human development, which in turn contributes to further economic growth. This mutually reinforcing cycle means that sustained growth requires continuous investment in human development. Empirical papers also suggest that investment in human development — particularly in low-income contexts — must precede or accompany rising economic growth in order for a country to attain sustained

[12] See a review of this topic by Nixon and Ulmann (2006).

growth (Suri *et al.*, 2010; Weil, 2007). That is, human and economic development objectives and outcomes are intertwined.

Notwithstanding these general statements, the evidence base on the linkage between health and economic growth to-date is mixed. While empirical findings from macro analyses have provided arguments for global policy debates, technical discussions, and more importantly, to support calls for increased investment in health, an important limitation has been that such studies do not provide specific information as to *how* to invest in health to contribute to growth. On the other hand, evidence from micro analyses is not only more robust, but it can provide actionable information for policymakers regarding which health interventions to invest in, and how, in order to boost productivity and therefore contribute to economic growth. One limitation is, however, the context specificity of micro studies, which makes generalizability more difficult.

The ongoing debate about the nexus between health and growth — whether it is correlational or causal, and the direction[13] of the relationship — is largely due to: (i) Methodological challenges[14] (Jack and Lewis, 2009), such as measurement of health outcomes, and econometric identification problem due to endogeneity[15] and confounders (Deaton, 2006; Malaney *et al.*, 2004)[16]; (ii) differences in the analytical approaches applied across studies — macro- vs. micro-models, or growth accounting frameworks (Jack and Lewis, 2009); and (iii) the different analytical lens used by the disciplines that are interested in better understanding the health–growth link, including economics, public finance, and public health.

Overall, although the transition in research and development policy has been slow, there is an increasing body of evidence that shows health's contribution to development (see more in Box 1 and in Ruger, 2005), often with an emphasis on its potentially lagged but long-lasting implications along the lifecycle and across generations.

Objectives of the chapter

The objective of this chapter is to examine and review the relationship between health spending and economic growth, taking into account the complexity of the pathway between them and the methodological challenges that have generated

[13]The debate regarding the relationship is whether health leads to growth or growth leads to health; alternatively, if the relationship is bidirectional and the effects are mutually reinforcing.

[14]See an overview and examples in Jack and Lewis (2009).

[15]"Simple correlations of public health and economic outcomes are unlikely to measure the causal effect of health on income since public health is endogenous" (Bleakley, 2007).

[16]There may be other factors that affect both health and income (Deaton, 2006). In the context of malaria, for example, confounding factors such as climate may drive both poverty and malaria (Malaney *et al.* 2004).

debates. The review covers theory, empirical evidence, applied diagnostic tools, and policy aspects to offer multiple dimensions that are relevant to inform technical and policy decisions regarding investing in health to contribute to growth. Although the chapter discusses a broad set of issues from technical and policy perspectives, it does not aim to offer solutions as to how specifically governments should invest in health to contribute to growth. Because the literature on health spending and the nexus between health and economic growth is rich and summarized by others, (Jack and Lewis, 2009; Spence and Lewis, 2009; Gerdtham and Johnson, 2000) rather than repeating their findings, the focus here is reviewing recent literature to explore whether the findings still hold. Further, to reflect the global ambition of this publication, the chapter puts more emphasis on the developing country context and discusses applied tools and approaches that have proven useful in guiding evidence-based decisions in health policymaking. Given the more acute data limitations in low-income countries, the chapter also discusses efforts that aim to reduce knowledge gaps on the effectiveness, cost-effectiveness, equity, and sustainability of delivering health services.

In Section "Global Patterns of Health Spending — Is Health Expenditure Becoming Unsustainable?" we show the global patterns of health spending, exploring the question of whether health expenditure is becoming unsustainable. We discuss the most recent and updated time series statistics between 1995 and 2012 — for global, country income group (see more on the income group classification in Annex 3), and regional breakdowns — on (i) the level of health spending; (ii) the shares of spending on health in terms of the budget (prioritization) and the economy; and (iii) growth in health spending, including relative to economic growth ('excess growth'). Last, we discuss the drivers of health spending, with particular emphasis on income and the income elasticity of health spending, demography, and technology. Section "Health Outcomes and Economic Growth" offers an overview of the literature on health outcomes and economic growth, starting with simple correlations, and covering causal estimation and results, including Granger-type models, which test for bidirectional relationship between health and growth. This section presents findings based on macro- and micro-level data. Section "Diagnostic Tools and Government Policies to Better Invest in Health for Growth" turns to diagnostic tools and government policies to improve investment in health for growth. This includes the presentation of applied diagnostic tools, such as public expenditure review (PEP) and fiscal space analysis (FSA), and a review of areas which have been under-researched — cyclicality of health spending and health sector resilience to crises. Further, this section considers the role of long-term and multi-sectoral interventions, and the experiences and expectations arising from demographic change including its effect on health and health spending, as well as the implications for economic growth. Finally, because health and poverty are intertwined, inequality in health inputs and outcomes, and inequality of opportunities are considered as factors that can decelerate growth and attenuate the positive momentum of the human capital-growth cycle. Section "Conclusions and Recommendations for Future Research" concludes and offers thoughts for future research.

Global Patterns of Health Spending — Is Health Expenditure Becoming Unsustainable?

Health expenditure trends — Facts and myths

Globally, health policymakers and shapers of health systems, ministers of finance, private companies, and households witness the increase in health care spending with alarm. For example, one review finds that over the past 50 years, health spending in OECD countries has consistently outpaced broader economic growth, grown by 2 percentage points in excess of GDP growth (Drouin *et al.*, 2008). If such a spending pattern persisted, using historic growth projection the health expenditure forecasting (see Volume 1, Chapter 3, *Measuring and Forecasting Global Health Expenditures*) would be warning policymakers of the health sector becoming 'the largest economic sector' and, consequently, the largest economic problem.

Such expansionary trends would attracted serious interest, not only from a health care financing perspective but, more broadly, from a public finance and development perspective because an ever-increasing share of a sector means growing pressure on government budgets and may also crowd out other sectors of the economy (see more in Box 2), thereby creating inefficiencies in allocation that constrain growth and development.

The recent Global Economic Crisis (GEC) — which started as early as 2007, and has led to fiscal consolidation in a number of advanced economies — has given further momentum to investigating the relationship between health spending and the economy and to studying the implications of alternative health expenditure growth scenarios to inform policymaking.

For example, in the context of health care reform in advanced and emerging economies — which has been catalyzed by the recent economic crisis — a book published by the IMF (Clements *et al.*, 2012) reviews past health expenditure trends, studies the drivers of escalating costs, and provides projections for the increase in public expenditures for health. The analysis was provoked by the startling lack of evidence on how best to manage growing fiscal pressure in the public health sectors during economic downturns and consequent tendencies for fiscal adjustment.

A central question of the investigation was: (i) Whether and to what extent past trends would continue into the future; (ii) whether rapid spending growth that

Box 2. Myths or facts — analytical questions that help inform policymaking

At the global level, there are two related questions that have concerned policymakers with respect to the relationship between growth in health spending and economic growth.

1. Is health spending growing in a financially sustainable manner?
2. Consequently, is the sector's share of the economy growing, resulting in crowd-out of other investments and, thereby, risking other development objectives?

Financial sustainability becomes a problem when governments are unable to finance the existing level of resources because of an inability or unwillingness to generate sufficient revenues to pay for them, and when they cannot — or will not — allow any further "crowding out" of other forms of government spending (OECD, 2010).

These related questions fall under fiscal policy and can be explored through analysis of fiscal space for health (see more in Section "Diagnostic Tools and Government Policies to Better Invest in Health for Growth"). As proposed by Heller (2005), fiscal space, in general, can be defined as "*the availability of budgetary room that allows a government to provide resources for a desired purpose without any prejudice to the sustainability of a government's financial position.*" According to the author, this concept requires fiscal sustainability; the capacity of government, at least in the future, to finance its desired expenditure programs, to service any debt obligations and to ensure its solvency. Thus, any consideration of fiscal space must be made in the context of at least a medium-term expenditure framework (MTEF). Through creating fiscal space, additional resources can be made available for some form of meritorious government spending. From a public finance and development perspective, the incentive for creating fiscal space is strengthened in situations where the resulting fiscal outlays would boost medium-term growth and perhaps even pay for themselves in terms of future fiscal revenue.

The following questions have proven useful in both country-specific and cross-country investigations regarding the current role of the health sector, including its share in the budget (prioritization) and as share of the economy, as well as to inform and manage expectations regarding its future.

1. *Level of health spending — meeting essential needs, and sector and development objectives*
   - What is the trend in the level of total health expenditure per capita (at exchange rates and also in real terms)?

(*Continued*)

Box 2. (*Continued*)

- — What is the level of total health expenditure per capita relative to normative benchmarks?
- — Is the current level of per capita health expenditure aligned with sector and development objectives?
- — Is there a funding gap between available per capita resources and sector objectives?

2. *Health sector as a share of the budget and as a share of the economy*
   - — What is the sector's share of the budget — is health a government priority?
   - — What is the size of the sector as share of the economy — is health crowding out other areas/development objectives?

3. *Growth in health spending — 'Excess growth'*
   - — What is the trend in health spending per capita relative to per capita economic growth (i.e., 'excess growth')?
   - — Given the country/region/income group-specific drivers of health spending, what are the projections for health expenditure growth (historical projections and scenario analysis assuming a slow-down in growth)?
   - — Do growth projections suggest convergence or divergence for a given country or country group (income or regional)?

4. *Drivers of health spending — Decomposition of growth*
   - — What are the primary drivers of growth in health spending (total, public, and private or out-of-pocket)?
   - — What share of the variation in health spending is explained by income, and what is the income elasticity of health spending (total, public, and private)?
   - — What is the effect of demography and epidemiology on health spending?
   - — What is the effect of non-demographic factors, primarily, of technology diffusion on health spending?
   - — What are the trends in unit costs, and what are the key drivers of changes in unit costs (for selected services)?
   - — What is the effect of institutions and organizational context of the sector on health spending?
   - — What is the effect of social and behavioral factors on health spending?

Source: Author's summary.

had been observed in the past would slowdown and converge to a rate closer to economic growth.

— Regarding spending growth, using historical trends as the grounds for forecasting, the study finds that in advanced economies, public health spending is projected to increase by 3 percentage points of GDP over the next 20 years and 6.5 percentage points over the next 40 years. In emerging countries, the pressure is less severe, with a 1 percentage point projected increase in public health expenditures as share of GDP. However, more sizeble increases are projected in certain regions, such as Europe and Central Asia (ECA), and Latin America and the Caribbean (LAC). The study discusses research that combines observed past spending patterns with assumptions of decelerating future health spending (Congressional Budget Office, 2010; OECD, 2006) — motivated by the rationale that spending growth trends cannot continue at the observed rates because of long-term fiscal sustainability — and argues that imposing such assumptions about slowdown and convergence is avoidable when the objective is to forecast spending pressures to inform fiscal and health care financing policies.
— As to convergence, controlling for income and demographics, regressions indicate significantly higher spending growth for countries with below-mean spending to GDP ratio. The authors suggest that convergence to the mean within regional groups is reflective of an 'imitation' effect, mimicking features of health care systems from more advanced countries found to be appealing, such as coverage expansion and technology diffusion. However, with respect to regional break downs, the public-to-private spending ratios are substantially higher for ECA and LAC than emerging Asia, with no sign of convergence.

The debate is ongoing regarding the expected pattern of health spending and its implication on fiscal space and economic growth. Whether the growth rate of health sector expenditures should be contained, and kept inline with or below the rate of economic growth (i.e., GDP growth rate) is not an equally relevant question in all contexts. In advanced economies, where the level of expenditure is already high (see Figure 2),[17] excess[18] health spending growth poses a threat, especially

[17] Using data from WHO's National Health Account 2013, the average total health spending per capita for high income countries was US$3,292 in 2012.

[18] 'Excess health expenditure' growth is defined relative to GDP growth, calculated as the difference in the annual growth rate of health expenditure minus the growth rate of annual economic growth measured in GDP. Consequently, a positive (negative) value indicates that health expenditures are growing in excess (moderation) of economic growth. The excess growth for a period is calculated from the difference of the average growth rates of these variables. To take into account inflation and population dynamics, excess growth is calculated using growth rates based on constant per capita values.

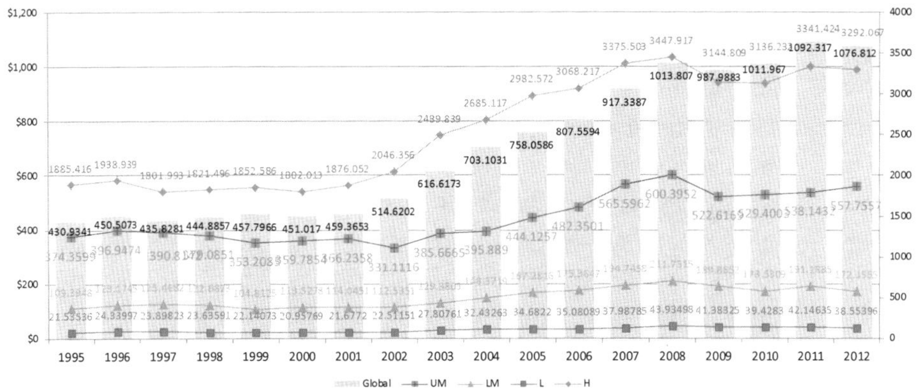

Income Group	1995	1996	1997	1998	1999	2000	2001	2002	2003	2004	2005	2006	2007	2008	2009	2010	2011	2012	Diff. 2012-1995	Growth (x)	Cum. Growth
H	1,885	1,939	1,802	1,821	1,853	1,802	1,876	2,046	2,490	2,685	2,983	3,068	3,376	3,448	3,145	3,136	3,341	3,292	$ 1,407	1.7	75%
UM	374	397	391	379	353	360	366	331	386	396	444	482	566	600	523	529	538	558	$ 183	1.5	49%
LM	109	123	125	123	105	114	114	113	129	148	167	175	195	212	190	174	191	172	$ 63	1.6	57%
L	22	24	24	24	22	21	22	23	28	32	35	35	38	44	41	39	42	39	$ 17	1.8	79%
Global	431	451	436	445	458	451	459	515	617	703	758	808	917	1,014	988	1,012	1,092	1,077	$ 646	2.5	150%

Figure 2. Total health expenditure per capita at exchange rate[19] by income group, 1995–2012

Sources: WHO NHA (2013) and WDI (2013).

Notes: Secondary right vertical axis is for the high-income group (H). Global stands for global annual average. H = high income, UM = upper-middle income, LM = lower-middle income, L = low income. The embedded table provides statistics for all income groups and the global average between 1996 and 2012, including on the difference between the end data point (2012) and the starting value (1995) (Diff. 2012–1995); the growth over the time period relative to the start value (growth *x*); and the cumulative growth between 1995 and 2012 (Cum. Growth).

where fiscal space has already become constrained, for example, due to aging, which results in a reduction in the revenue–expenditure ratio. This acute fiscal pressure can be further exacerbated by technology if unit costs further increase. On the other hand, in low-income countries, where the level of spending is not sufficient to meet coverage of essential care (see Figure 2),[20] increase in health spending and in the share of the sector in the economy (i.e., reprioritization) is often an explicit policy objective, driven by the rationale that investment in human development is a prerequisite for sustained economic growth. Yet, statistical exploration of data from WHO's National Health Accounts (NHA) (2013) reveals that, although the per capita level of health spending in low-income countries is low to start with (US$39 in 2012), not reaching the normative benchmarks discussed earlier, the average growth rate of health spending relative to economic growth in these countries is 0.78%, below

[19]The WHO's NHA database presented statistics on health expenditure at average exchange rate, which refers to current values.

[20]Using data from WHO's NHA 2013, the average total health spending per capita for low income countries was US$39 in 2012.

the other income groups calculated for the period between 1995 and 2010.[21] This implies that, although the relative weight of the sector as a share of the economy is increasing, given the low absolute values, the increase in terms of meeting health needs is justified. Another question is whether low-income countries will increasingly afford this increase and be willing to invest a higher share of their domestic resources or whether external resources for health — through budget and program support — will continue to play an important role in health financing. Overall, these stylized facts suggest that, while in high-income countries, cost containment and sector rationalization are central to the reform agenda, in developing countries, efficiency gains will not be sufficient and must be matched with increases in the level of funding, which will require increased growth of public resources for health (domestic and external) (Ooms *et al.*, 2010) or private resources (Van Der Gaag and Stimac, 2012) that meet the criteria for pooling and equitable financing.

Until around 2010, research in this field particularly focused on developed and emerging economies, where excess growth and cost containment have longer been on the agenda. The relative richness of the literature in the advanced country context is also partially due to more availability of data, including for cross-country analysis, longitudinal country-specific explorations, and panel data for cross-country studies. The evidence base has been thin in developing country contexts due to data gaps, particularly until 2010. However, recent research has increased the attention to both data collection and analytical efforts in low-income countries. Improved data and analyses are necessary to answer policy questions regarding the effectiveness and efficiency of health spending with respect to outcomes, as well as the health sector's share in the economy, its role in long-term financial sustainability, and its role in attaining development objectives. With increased emphasis on data and evidence-based policy responses, the influence of policy-relevant analysis has grown, leading to more opportunities to isolate facts from myths and to identifying pragmatic ways to trace changes and update projections to inform policy responses.

Box 2 discusses two central concerns that have troubled policymakers and researchers, and highlights questions that are used in sector reviews in preparation

---

[21] Based on calculations from WDI 2012 and WHO 2012, the average growth of the health sector in excess of GDP growth (i.e., 'excess growth') for the World Bank income groups between 1995 and 2010 was: high-income = 1.09%; upper-middle income = 0.85%; lower-middle income = 0.42%; and low-income = 0.79%. The unweighted global average was 0.79% and the weighted global average was 1.5%. The averages for the period between 1995 and 2009 are higher as this includes the GEC, which peaked between 2008 and 2009. As a result of the decrease in the denominator, even sustained per capita health expenditure — without considering countercyclical responses — leads to higher excess growth values. The corresponding average values for the income groups for the 1995–2009 period: high-income = 1.5%; upper-middle income = 1.1%; lower-middle income = 0.8%; and low-income = 0.9%. The unweighted global average was 1.1% and the weighted global average was 1.9%.

for policy formulation and in exchanges with ministries of finance (e.g., government budget planning), as well as development partners. The analytic tools that help address these questions will be discussed in Section "Retrospective and Prospective Assessment of Health Spending".

The following subsections present a brief overview of health spending patterns — level, growth, and drivers of expenditure– between 1995 and 2012. A detailed literature review and analysis of health spending is beyond the scope of this chapter. An excellent comparative review of international health expenditure trends in the OECD context is done by Gerdtham and Jönnson in the *Handbook of Health Economics* (Gerdtham and Johnson, 2000). Fleisher *et al.*, (2013) review global trends in the income elasticity of health spending; including for total, public, and out-of-pocket expenditures between 1995 and 2010.

Health expenditure trends

- *Level of health spending*

In absolute terms, global health spending has grown across all income groups and regions between 1995 and 2012. However, while during this period per capita total health spending roughly doubled at the global level, rising from US$431 in 1995 to US$1,077 in 2012, the increase has been modest for developing countries, starting from US$22 and reaching US$39 in the low-income group, and moving from US$109 to US$172 in the lower-middle-income group during the same period (see Figure 2).[22] By 2012, in the low-income group, approximately 60% of the countries had not yet reached the normative target for per capita health spending suggested by the Taskforce on Innovative International Health Financing for Health Systems (US$54), raising concerns regarding the financing of essential care for the population and attainment of health-related MDG targets.

Growth in health spending has not been unbroken. Deceleration in the growth momentum has been associated with crises, and was witnessed particularly following the GEC that exerted downward pressure on growth between 2008 and 2009, during the peak of the downturn. Although fluctuations at the lower-income level have been present, these changes have been more subtle because of the already low level of per capita health spending, which leaves less room for decline in absolute terms. Yet, the impact of the loss of a marginal dollar for health in the low-income context is much more severe compared to the effect of marginal reductions in health spending observed in higher-income groups.

[22] These statistics for health expenditures are based on current values, which in WHO's NHA database is referred to as expenditure at average exchange rate. See definitions on the WHO website at: http://www.who.int/whosis/whostat2006HealthFinancing.pdf?ua=1.

Table 2. Total average health expenditure per capita at exchange rate by region, 1995–2011

	1995	1996	1997	1998	1999	2000	2001	2002	2003	2004	2005	2006	2007	2008	2009	2010	2011
EAP	342	359	348	312	338	352	325	343	414	471	519	546	617	666	668	777	881
ECA	1,025	1,061	990	1,032	1,067	1,010	1,040	1,198	1,502	1,742	1,862	1,965	2,256	2,516	2,394	2,366	2,547
LAC	215	224	236	248	255	269	270	254	261	280	317	361	416	468	480	516	549
MENA	321	327	338	331	331	341	363	362	417	442	470	497	539	570	601	600	655
NAC	2,804	2,890	2,998	3,078	3,232	3,440	3,645	3,916	4,336	4,701	5,092	5,507	5,908	6,196	6,268	6,764	7,062
SA	28	33	37	39	40	43	42	41	46	51	56	65	75	99	98	92	116
SSF	46	48	49	47	46	43	43	46	56	69	76	84	92	108	111	123	140
Global	441	456	441	446	462	452	461	505	610	695	749	798	906	999	975	998	1,082

Source: WHO NHA 2013 by World Bank Regional Classification based on WDI 2013.
Notes: The regions are based on the World Bank classification used in 2014. The region codes in the first column of the table are: EAP = East Asia and Pacific Region; ECA = Europe and Central Asia; LAC = Latin American and the Caribbean; MENA = Middle East and North Africa; NAC = North America; SA = South Asia; and SSF = Sub-Saharan Africa.

The regional breakdown shows that the global statistic in per capita total health spending has been driven by North America (NAC)[23] and Europe and the Central Asia Region (ECA), and the regional averages were the lowest for South Asia and Sub-Saharan Africa, respectively reaching US$116 and US$140 per capital spending on health by 2011.

- *Health sector as share of the budget and share of the economy*

The normative economic question regarding health spending is that, "*Given competing and equally meritorious priorities across many sectors, how much should total government expenditure be in an economy and how public resources should be allocated across sectors?* (Tandon *et al.*, 2014).

There are associated normative benchmarks. For example, the WHO's Health Care Financing Strategy for the Asia-Pacific Region (2010–2015) proposes 4–5% for health expenditure as share of GDP. The Abuja Declaration, which was proposed by the African Union in 2001, is a reprioritization benchmark that sets allocations to the health sector at a minimum of 15% of government expenditures. Rather than assessing performance vis-à-vis arbitrary normative benchmarks, this section takes a positive and descriptive approach to discuss how countries have performed on these two variables — the share of the sector within the economy and the share of the sector within the budget — since 1995.

Share of the sector in the economy — Is there a concern for 'crowd out'?

Over the past decades, the health sector has carved out a growing share of the economy. However, the observed growth trend has been less alarming than what

[23] United States of America and Canada.

some fiscal 'doomsday' projections suggested earlier which, assuming the same historical trend to continue, forecasted that the sector's share could reach 1/5 of the economy in most OECD countries by 2050 (Drouin *et al.*, 2008). However, forecasting that was done prior to the GEC could not foresee the changes in growth patterns brought about by the downturn. Hence, because of the lack of accounting for health care financing responses due to fiscal consolidation efforts (i.e., providing an analysis of first-order effects), such estimates have an upward bias regarding the long-term perspective. In fact, if current trends are taken into account, growth in the health sector's share of the economy has moderated over time and is not distressing at the global or income group level. Calculations for the sector's share of GDP indicate approximately a global average of 7.5% by 2050, and this share for the lower-income group countries is around 5%, which is inline with the WHO's normative recommendation discussed above.

However, the variation within income groups is considerable. For example, in 2012, the sector's share within the high-income group ranged between 1.7% and 9.3%. In the upper middle-income group, the respective figures were between approximately 1% and 10.3%. In the lower-middle income group, the range was between approximately 1% and 15.4%. And, last, in the low-income group, the minimum was 1.2% and the maximum was 7%. This within-group variation partially supports the warnings that crowd-out in some countries — irrespective of the income level — is or can become an imminent concern, unless medium- to long-term sector and fiscal policies do not proactively address the question of how to maintain a healthy share that equally contributes to population health and growth objectives. There is a counter-argument, however, regarding the growth of the sector's share. Growth in the sector's share can be sustainable and even desirable. As long as (basic) needs are satisfied and the government and population are willing to spend more of their discretionary income on health, and the marginal utility of spending and extra dollar on health is positive, sector growth may not be a problem. This, however, implies sustained economic growth that can continue financing increasing demand for health.

Share of the sector in the budget — Prioritization and consolidation

The rapid expansion of public health spending in advanced economies has been a concern over the past two decades. But what has escalated the need to address the question of (un)sustainability even further was the economic crisis, a period of consolidating fiscal balances and debt levels. Policymakers have shifted more attention to how to use resources more efficiency or, if at all possible, leverage additional sources to meet the increasing demand for health care under tightening budget constraints. In the advanced country context the sense of emergency to manage the sectoral share is captured by Kotlikoff and Hagist (2007) who pointed out that:

"No country can spend an ever-rising share of its inputs on health care, indefinitely. There is a limit to how much a government can extract from the young to accommodate the old. When that limit is reached, the governments go broke."

There is no similar sense of urgency, however, in low-income countries, where — as discussed earlier — the baseline level of per capita health spending has historically been and remains low in the majority of countries. In fact, global health sector and health financing policy initiatives urge countries to spend more and increase the sector's priority on their development agenda.

A paper that discusses the determinants of reprioritization of government resources to the health sector — one of the modalities for realizing fiscal space for health — notes that countries vary widely with respect to the share of government spending on health, a metric that can serve as a proxy for the extent to which health is prioritized by governments (Tandon *et al.*, 2014). The global average for health's share of aggregate government expenditure (i.e., budget) — calculated from the WHO's National Health Account Database — was 11.6% in 2012, ranging from a low of 1.5% in Myanmar to a high of 27.7% in Costa Rica.

Inline with the literature on the drivers of health spending (see Section "Growth in Health Spending"), some of the observed variation in health's share of government spending across countries is related to differences in per capita income. Cross-country comparisons show that the share of aggregate government expenditure on health increases with income. However, in a global overview of the health's share of general government expenditures (GGE), Tandon *et al.* (2014) argue that significant variations exist in health's share of government spending, even after controlling for per capita income. The paper summarizes some of the key theoretical and empirical perspectives on why some governments spend more (or less) of public resources on health. Although empirical evidence on factors associated with government preferences for public financing of the health sector is generally scarce, the limited empirical literature that exists proposes a range of economic and noneconomic factors has been found to influence government allocations for health. Prominent among these are democracy, corruption, foreign aid, ethno-linguistic heterogeneity, and female representation in the polity of a country (Tandon *et al.*, 2014).

Another study, which draws on a panel data of 120 countries between 1995 and 2010, explores the relationship between GHE, sociopolitical risks, and international aid, while controlling for the impact of national income and fiscal capacity on health spending (Liang and Mirelman, 2014). The findings suggest that democratic accountability has a diminishing positive correlation with public health spending, and that levels of spending are higher when the government is more stable. Corruption is associated with less spending in developing countries, but with more spending in high-income countries. The analysis also finds evidence on the fungibility of development assistance for health (DAH) that is channeled through the government, and shows that the degree of fungibility of external resources increases with corruption and where ethnic tension is rife. These results suggest that reducing corruption — and hence, the role of governance and public finance management — is fundamental to improving the efficiency of public resources, as well as their level.

Global trends between 1995 and 2012 show that, on average, the health sector's share increased from 10.1% of government budget to 11.7%. The difference between the start and end data points for the sector's share of the budget was the highest for the upper middle-income country group (1.8%), followed by the low-income group (1.5%), the high-income group (1.2%), and last, by the lower middle-income group (0.4%). In 2012, high-income countries, on average, spent 13.3% of their budgets on health, with a range between 5.3% in Qatar and 20.6% in the Czech Republic. The same year, in low-income countries, the average share of the budget spent on health was 10.4%, with a low of 1.5% in Myanmar, and a high of 22.1% in Rwanda.

Although the trend for the low-income country group shows an increasing prioritization of the health sector over the period, the majority of developing countries are far from the normative benchmark set in the Abuja Declaration.[24] In fact, in 2012, globally only 42 countries spent at least 15% of their budget on health; out of which 19 were high-income countries, 10 were upper middle-income, 9 were lower middle-income, and only 4 were in the low-income country group. Reprioritization through expenditure benchmarking has been criticized because fixing the share of the budget for a specific sector and purpose does not take into account changes in the budget (e.g., as a result of economic growth or downturn) and it does not enable the government to flexibly manage resources. Generally, reprioritization through expenditure benchmarking pledges has not been successful because such pledges have not been grounded in macro-fiscal and political economic realities (Tandon *et al.*, 2014). In most countries, calls for benchmarking health shares of government expenditures have been largely aspirational.

As in the case of per capita health expenditures discussed above, the trend in the sector's share of the budget also shows fluctuations associated with economic cycles (see more in Section "Health Expenditure and the Economic Cycle"), with a noticeable drop from 2007 triggered by the GEC. However, unlike previous crises, this crisis affected high-income countries more, reflected by the mostly steady decline in the sector's share of the budget, down by a full percentage point between 2007 and 2012, from 14.3% to 13.3%. The contraction in advanced economies

[24] In April 2001, African Union countries meeting in Abuja pledged a target of allocating at least 15% of their annual government budgets to the improvement of the health sector.

also had a negative effect on aid flows, reducing fiscal space for health through external sources in low-income countries and increasing the volatility of aid flows.

Figure 5 with its embedded table illustrates that sector prioritization is a dynamic affair which takes place within the macro-fiscal context and, as such, is subject to fluctuations. Protecting the sector's share during downturns and, more importantly, the availability and quality of service delivery has been central to discussions regarding the role of countercyclical fiscal and social policies (see more in Section "Health Expenditure and the Economic Cycle").

- *Growth in health spending*

Overall, the presented trend lines for health expenditure levels and shares between 1995 and 2012 have shown steady increases, albeit with set-backs and consolidation during the GEC. Notwithstanding the downturn, the global average cumulative growth in per capita expenditures between 1995 and 2012 was 150% (see Figure 2). The sector's share of the economy grew from a global average of 3.3% in 1995 to 4.2% in 2012, which represents a cumulative growth of 27% during this period. Although the size of the health sector in the economy is the lowest in absolute terms in the low-income group (2.7%), its cumulative growth during the study period was the highest (34%), indicating convergence (see Figure 3). The sector's share of general expenditures grew from a global average of 10.1% in 1995 to 11.7% in 2012, translating into a 15% cumulative growth over time. As in the case of the sector's share of the economy, the lower income groups grew more, suggesting that the sector's priority in the budget and government development plans has been increasing (see Figure 4).

Notwithstanding the overall upward trend, statistics between 2007 and 2012 show that the growth momentum in health spending is strongly associated with economic performance. For example, during economic boom cycles, the global average growth rates for per capita total health spending were around 19.8% (2003) and 14% (2004) (Figure 6, Panels A and B with embedded table). The bust cycle, which peaked around 2008 and 2009, led to a global average of 2.5% contraction in per capita health spending in 2009.

Beyond tracking simple univariate trends over time, a variable that has attracted more attention is 'excess growth,' which incorporates into the analysis of health spending patterns the underlying growth rate in per capita income growth. The literature has focused on this variable because growth of health spending in excess of economic growth implies an increasing share of the sector over time, which is associated with risk of crowd-out, unsustainability, and distortions in the economy.

Arithmetically, 'excess growth' — as defined above — is calculated for a given year by subtracting the observed economic growth rate between t_1 and t_0 from the observed health expenditure growth rate for the same time period. For consistency, both variables are population normalized, using per capita income

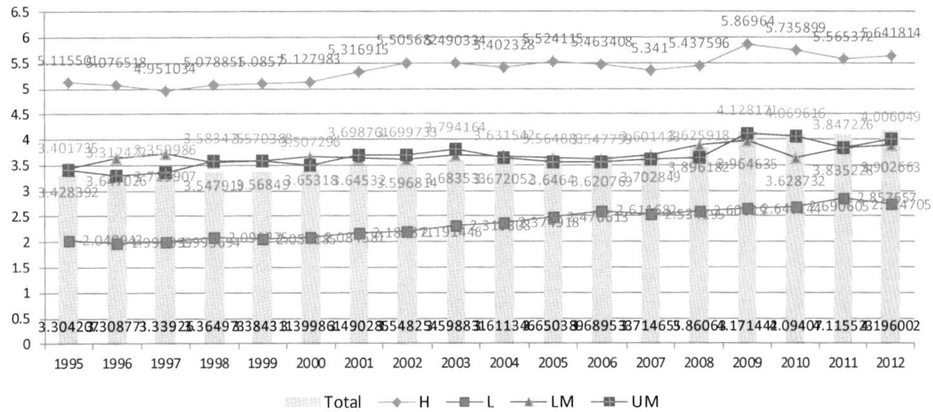

Income Group	1995	1996	1997	1998	1999	2000	2001	2002	2003	2004	2005	2006	2007	2008	2009	2010	2011	2012	Cum. Growth
H	5.1	5.1	5.0	5.1	5.1	5.1	5.3	5.5	5.5	5.4	5.5	5.5	5.3	5.4	5.9	5.7	5.6	5.6	10%
UM	3.4	3.3	3.4	3.6	3.6	3.5	3.7	3.7	3.8	3.6	3.6	3.5	3.6	3.6	4.1	4.1	3.8	4.0	18%
LM	3.4	3.6	3.7	3.5	3.6	3.7	3.6	3.6	3.7	3.7	3.6	3.6	3.7	3.9	4.0	3.6	3.8	3.9	14%
L	2.0	2.0	2.0	2.1	2.1	2.1	2.2	2.2	2.3	2.4	2.5	2.6	2.5	2.6	2.6	2.7	2.9	2.7	34%
Global	**3.3**	**3.3**	**3.3**	**3.4**	**3.4**	**3.4**	**3.5**	**3.5**	**3.6**	**3.6**	**3.7**	**3.7**	**3.7**	**3.9**	**4.2**	**4.1**	**4.1**	**4.2**	**27%**

Figure 3. Global trend in total health expenditures as share of the economy (% of GDP), by country income group

Notes: Global stands for global annual average. H = high-income; UM = upper-middle income; LM = lower-middle income; L = low-income. The embedded table provides the statistics for all income groups and the global average between 1996 and 2012. The last column shows the cumulative growth in the sector's share of the economy by income group between 1995 and 2012.
Source: WHO NHA 2013 and WDI 2013.

terms (per capita health expenditure and income).[25] Hence, if the annual rate of growth in per capita health expenditure is above the annual rate of economic growth the 'excess growth' statistics will be positive and is interpreted as the percentage by which the sector outpaced the annual growth rate of the economy. Conversely, if the 'excess growth' value is negative, it indicates that the sector has contracted relative to the annual rate of economic growth.

At the global level, Figure 7 shows that on average for the 1995–2010 period excess growth was 1.5%. During this period, excess growth had three notable peaks; one during 1998, the second between 2001 and 2003, which peaked at 7.2% in 2002; and the last at the height of the recent GEC in 2009, when the sector grew 9.7% in excess of economic growth. These peaks illustrates that 'excess growth' can have very different drivers. During 2001–2003, economic boom enabled intensified investments in health (i.e., an expansionary cycle in social expenditures). On the other hand, during the GEC the observed excess growth of

[25] For consistency, it is also important to use both values either in nominal and real terms. The statistics presented in this chapter uses nominal values from the WHO's NHA Global Database (2013).

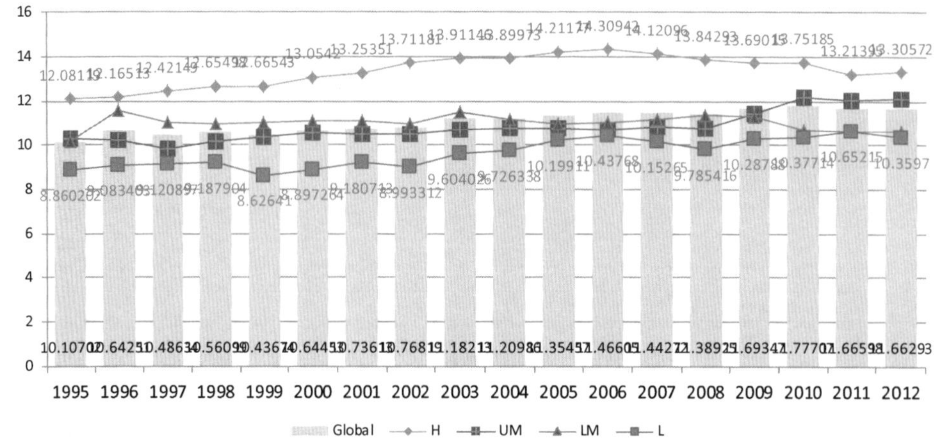

Income Group	1995	1996	1997	1998	1999	2000	2001	2002	2003	2004	2005	2006	2007	2008	2009	2010	2011	2012	Cum Growth
H	12.1	12.2	12.4	12.7	12.7	13.1	13.3	13.7	13.9	13.9	14.2	14.3	14.1	13.8	13.7	13.8	13.2	13.3	10%
UM	10.3	10.2	9.8	10.2	10.3	10.5	10.5	10.5	10.7	10.8	10.8	10.7	10.8	10.7	11.4	12.2	12.1	12.1	17%
LM	10.2	11.6	11.1	11.0	11.0	11.1	11.1	10.9	11.5	11.2	11.0	11.0	11.1	11.4	11.3	10.7	10.6	10.6	4%
L	8.9	9.1	9.1	9.2	8.6	8.9	9.2	9.0	9.6	9.7	10.2	10.4	10.2	9.8	10.3	10.4	10.7	10.4	17%
Global	**10.1**	**10.6**	**10.5**	**10.6**	**10.4**	**10.6**	**10.7**	**10.8**	**11.2**	**11.2**	**11.4**	**11.5**	**11.4**	**11.4**	**11.7**	**11.8**	**11.7**	**11.7**	**15%**

Figure 4. Trends in health expenditure as share of the government budget by income group, 1995–2012

Note: Global stands for global annual average. H = high-income; UM = upper-middle income; LM = lower-middle income; L = low-income. The embedded table provides the statistics for all income groups and the global average between 1996 and 2012. The last column shows the cumulative growth in the sector's share of the budget by income group between 1995 and 2012.
Source: WHO NHA 2013 and WDI 2013.

health expenditures was a result of declining (in some countries contracting) GDP combined with countercyclical responses in the health sector (i.e., increased GGE) to dampen the effect of the economic shock. This illustrates that growing in excess of the economy cannot be interpreted as "good" or "bad" without a deeper understanding of the context. If excess growth entails health investments that generate good returns in the short- or long-run, that qualifies as an investment that contributes to growth. If excess growth is driven by counter cyclical and targeted social policies, it would qualify as equity enhancing, which is desirable from both a humanitarian and economic perspective. Consequently, value judgments on economic growth would require a thorough understanding of the qualitative context, as well as the value-for-money dimension of the investment.

The breakdown by country income groups shows the widest fluctuation for the low-income group, which indicates that these countries are more exposed to changes in economic cycles and less accustomed to attenuating such effects through countercyclical social policies.

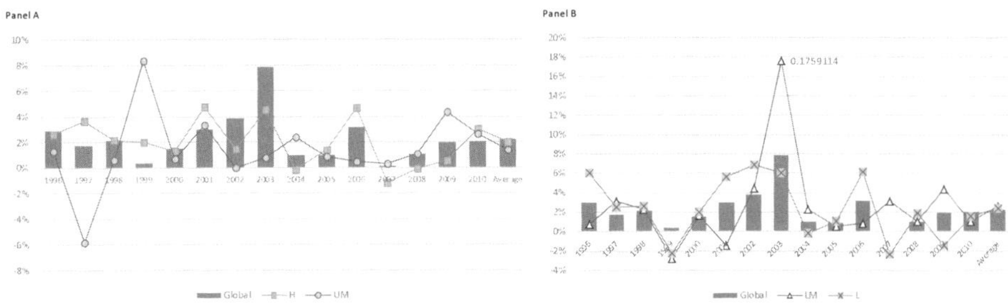

Income Group	1996	1997	1998	1999	2000	2001	2002	2003	2004	2005	2006	2007	2008	2009	2010	Average
H	2.6%	3.7%	2.2%	2.0%	1.4%	4.8%	1.4%	4.5%	-0.2%	1.4%	4.7%	-1.2%	-0.1%	0.5%	3.0%	2.0%
UM	1.3%	-5.8%	0.6%	8.4%	0.7%	3.4%	0.0%	0.7%	2.4%	0.9%	0.4%	0.3%	1.1%	4.4%	2.6%	1.4%
LM	0.8%	3.2%	2.3%	-2.7%	1.7%	-1.4%	4.5%	17.6%	2.3%	0.6%	0.9%	3.1%	1.1%	4.4%	1.1%	2.6%
L	6.0%	2.5%	2.7%	-2.2%	2.0%	5.7%	6.9%	6.1%	-0.2%	1.1%	6.1%	-2.3%	1.9%	-1.5%	1.6%	2.4%
Global	**2.9%**	**1.7%**	**2.1%**	**0.4%**	**1.5%**	**3.0%**	**3.8%**	**7.8%**	**1.0%**	**1.0%**	**3.1%**	**0.1%**	**1.0%**	**2.0%**	**2.1%**	**2.2%**

Figure 5. Growth rate in GHE as share of the budget, by income group, 1996–2010. Panel A. High and upper-middle income countries. Panel B. Lower-middle and low-income countries

Notes: Global stands for global annual average. H = high-income; UM = upper-middle income; LM = lower-middle income; L = low-income. The embedded table provides the statistics for all income groups and the global average between 1996 and 2010. The last column shows the average growth rate for the period between 1995 and 2010.
Source: WHO NHA 2013 and WDI 2013.

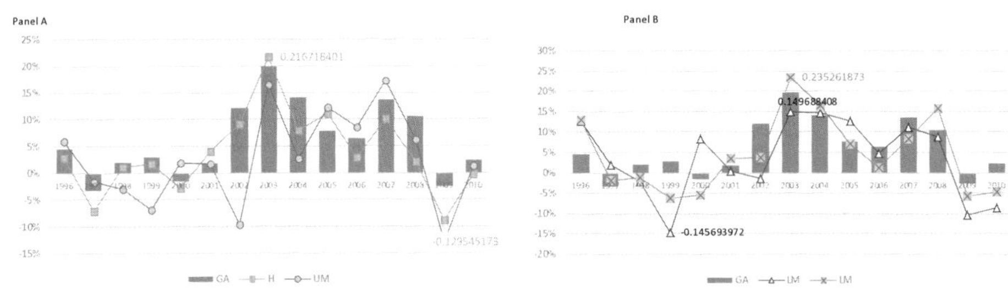

Income Group	1996	1997	1998	1999	2000	2001	2002	2003	2004	2005	2006	2007	2008	2009	2010
High Income	2.8%	-7.1%	1.1%	1.7%	-2.7%	4.1%	9.1%	21.7%	7.8%	11.1%	2.9%	10.0%	2.1%	-8.8%	-0.3%
Upper Middle	6.0%	-1.5%	-3.0%	-6.8%	1.9%	1.8%	-9.6%	16.5%	2.7%	12.2%	8.6%	17.3%	6.2%	-13.0%	1.3%
Lower Middle	12.6%	1.9%	-2.2%	-14.6%	8.3%	0.5%	-1.3%	15.0%	14.7%	12.7%	4.8%	11.1%	8.7%	-10.3%	-8.6%
Low Income	13.0%	-1.8%	-1.1%	-6.3%	-5.3%	3.4%	3.8%	23.5%	16.6%	6.9%	1.1%	8.3%	15.7%	-5.8%	-4.7%
Global Average	**4.5%**	**-3.3%**	**2.1%**	**2.9%**	**-1.5%**	**1.9%**	**12.0%**	**19.8%**	**14.0%**	**7.8%**	**6.5%**	**13.6%**	**10.5%**	**-2.5%**	**2.4%**

Figure 6. Trend in annual growth of per capita total health expenditure, by income group. Panel A. High- and upper-middle-income countries. Panel B. Lower-middle and low-income countries

Notes: Income group is based on World Bank classification. H = high-income; UM = upper-middle; income LM = lower-middle income; L = low-income; GA = global average. Figures are in percentage term representing the annual growth/decrease in total health expenditure per capita. The embedded table provides the statistics for all income groups and the global average (GA) between 1996 and 2010.
Source: Calculations based on WHO NHA 2012 and WDI 2012.

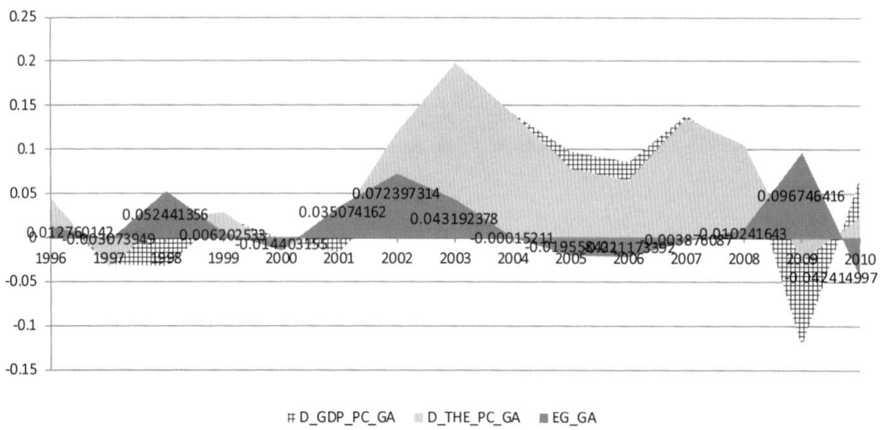

	1996	1997	1998	1999	2000	2001	2002	2003	2004	2005	2006	2007	2008	2009	2010	Average
Growth GDP_PC	3%	-3%	-3%	2%	0%	-2%	5%	16%	14%	10%	9%	14%	9%	-12%	7%	4.6%
Growth THE_CP	4.5%	-3.3%	2.1%	2.9%	-1.5%	1.9%	12.0%	19.8%	14.0%	7.8%	6.5%	13.6%	10.5%	-2.5%	2.4%	6.1%
EG_GA	1.3%	-0.3%	5.2%	0.6%	-1.4%	3.5%	7.2%	4.3%	0.0%	-2.0%	-2.1%	-0.4%	1.0%	9.7%	-4.2%	1.5%

Figure 7. Global trend in 'excess growth' (EG) of annual health expenditures over economic growth for 1995–2010

Notes: "Excess Growth" (EG) here is defined as the growth of health expenditures over economic growth measured in per capita GDP. EG_GA = EG Global Average; D_GDP_PC_GA = global average of annual growth rate of per capita GDP; D_THE_PC_GA = global average of annual growth rate of per capita total health expenditures. Figures are in percentage terms, representing the annual growth/decrease in the presented variables. The embedded table provides the statistics between 1996 and 2010, including the global average annual growth rates for health expenditure per capita, GDP per capita, and excess growth.
Source: Calculations based on WHO NHA 2012 and WDI 2012.

- *Drivers of health spending*

Since the article by Newhouse (1977), there is a growing body of economic literature that focuses on the determinants of health spending. In this formative paper, Newhouse finds that health care is a luxury good, with an income elasticity estimate above 1 (see Definition in Annex 3), and attributes 90% of the variation in health spending to income. This finding unleashed a series of analyses in various regional and institutional contexts, which applied various methodological approaches to determine whether health is indeed a luxury good and income is the dominant determinant of spending or are there other factors that are comparable in terms of their effect on health spending.

The "health as a luxury good" debate — which has been loudly seeking an answer to the question whether health expenditure will keep growing in excess of income, possibly jeopardizing the consumption of other goods and services — has been mostly framed in the context of advanced and emerging economies. In addition to rising income, which is known as the primary determinant of health spending, many of these countries have been undergoing a 'triple transition,' which has

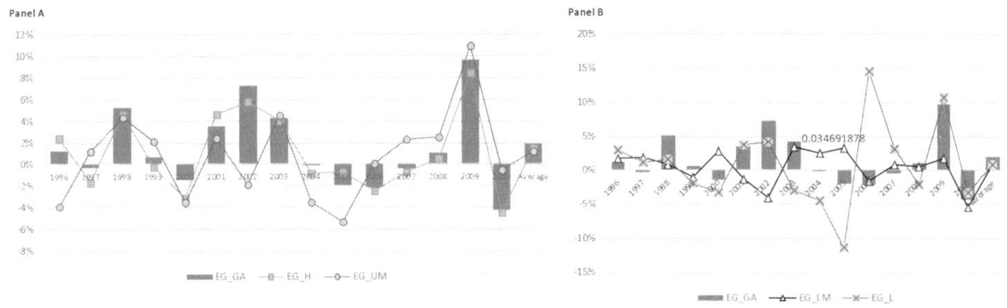

Income Group	1996	1997	1998	1999	2000	2001	2002	2003	2004	2005	2006	2007	2008	2009	2010	Average
EG_H	2.4%	-1.7%	4.7%	-0.3%	-3.1%	4.7%	5.7%	4.1%	-0.8%	-0.7%	-2.4%	-0.7%	0.6%	8.5%	-4.4%	1.5%
EG_UM	-3.9%	1.2%	4.3%	2.1%	-3.5%	2.5%	-1.9%	4.5%	-3.5%	-5.3%	0.0%	2.3%	2.5%	11.0%	-0.5%	1.1%
EG_LM	1.7%	1.9%	0.8%	-1.0%	2.9%	-1.3%	-4.0%	3.5%	2.4%	3.3%	-1.6%	0.9%	0.5%	1.8%	-5.5%	0.8%
EG_L	3.0%	1.1%	1.6%	-1.9%	-3.2%	3.8%	4.2%	-3.0%	-4.6%	-11.3%	14.6%	3.1%	-2.0%	10.7%	-3.4%	0.9%
EG_GA	**1.3%**	**-0.3%**	**5.2%**	**0.6%**	**-1.4%**	**3.5%**	**7.2%**	**4.3%**	**0.0%**	**-2.0%**	**-2.1%**	**-0.4%**	**1.0%**	**9.7%**	**-4.2%**	**1.9%**

Figure 8. Trend of excess health expenditure growth (EG) by income group, 1995–2010

Notes: "Excess Growth" (EG) here is defined as the growth of health expenditures in excess of economic growth. EG is normalized for population using per capita terms in both the health and income variables. EG_GA = EG Global Average; EG_H = EG High-Income Group; EG_L = EG Low-Income Group; EG_LM = EG Lower-Middle-Income Group; EG_UM = EG Upper-Middle-Income Group. The embedded table provides the annual statistics between 1996 and 2010 by income group, and the average excess growth for the period in the last column.
Source: Calculations based on WHO NHA 2012 and WDI 2012.

contributed to the escalation of health expenditures, including an increasing disease burden from non-communicable and chronic diseases, aging populations, and rapid technological progress. As a result of these changes, along with the fiscal tightening due to the crisis, decomposing the drivers of spending has become ever more essential to inform cost containment policies that would help keep the sector's share 'healthy' within the economy.

There is an extensive literature on the determinants of spending in the OECD context. However, as noted by some studies (Xu *et al.*, 2011; Fleisher *et al.*, 2013; Velenyi and Smitz, 2014), the evidence base has been thin in developing countries, partly due to data gaps. Approaching the MDG target date in 2015 and with the post-2015 development challenge ahead, which includes the UHC agenda, there is increasing interest in understanding the patterns and drivers of health spending in developing country contexts. This has resulted in efforts toward more and better data and analytical work to help reduce the paucity of evidence. This section will provide a brief overview of the topic, with a particular focus on recent evidence.

Income elasticity of health expenditures

An important strand of the health care financing literature discusses the relationship between income and health expenditures. Whether health is a *luxury* good — that is, economies spend more as they become richer — or a *necessity* good is extensively debated. For policy-making, the *necessity* vs. *luxury good* debate (Costa-i-Font *et al.*, 2009) is important because if elasticity (see Definition in Annex 3) is greater than one,[26] health expenditures increase faster than income, constituting an increasing share of the economy.

To date, there is no agreement in the literature either on the conclusion that "*as countries become richer, health care expenditure will account for a larger share of GDP*" or on the methodology (Dybczak and Przywara, 2010). Findings, depending on the data type and analytical approach, have been conflicting and, hence, there is no consensus that the income elasticity of health expenditures is greater than one.

For example, in his early and seminal paper, Newhouse (1977) concluded that health care is a luxury good. Fifteen years later, having found income elasticities between 0.2 and 0.4, he revised this conclusion stating that health expenditure is a necessity (Newhouse, 1992). In the last decade, the focus has shifted from economics to statistics and econometrics, arguing that variations in findings are often driven by data type, sample properties, and methodology (Gerdtham and Johnson, 2000). This finding on the data and method-driven variation in results proposed by the recent wave of more statistically and econometrically oriented literature dissents from the conclusion offered in the review of comparative health spending in advanced economies that was published in 2000, and stated that:

> "*A common and extremely robust result ... is that the effect of per capita GDP (income) on expenditure is clearly positive and significant, that the income elasticities are ... close to unity or even higher than unity. This result appears to be robust to the choice of variables included in the estimation models, data, the choice of conversion factors and the methods of estimation*" (Gerdtham and Johnson, 2000).

A systematic review of this topic is beyond the scope of this chapter. However, a brief overview of the literature between 1974 and 2013, presented in Table 3 illustrates the evolution of the methodology and the gradual shift in findings over the past 40 years.[26a] Early work in this field and estimates from cross-sectional regressions and time series for individual countries suggest that the income elasticity of health spending is above one, that is, that health is a luxury good. However, estimations for regions show below unity elasticities, notably for the Middle East, South Asia, and Sub-Saharan Africa (Van der Gaag and Stimac, 2012). Estimations based on panel data, depending on the model specification, started to empirically challenge the earlier findings and results based on cross-sectional models.[26b]

---

[26] That is health expenditure is income elastic and health is considered a luxury good.

[26a] See more on the taxonomy of previous studies on income elasticity of health care spending in Atella and Marini (2006). In the OECD context, *The 2015 Ageing Report* presents projections for health expenditures between 2013 and 2060, taking into account in the income elasticity of health expenditures and non-income drivers (European Commission, 2015).

[26b] For more on model specification see, for example, Di Matteo (2003) and Di Matteo (2004).

Table 3. Overview of estimates for income elasticity of health spending from the literature between 1974 and 2013

Methods	Sources	Findings
Cross-section Regression from OECD Countries	Kleiman (1974); Newhouse (1977); Leu (1986); Getzen (2000)	— Estimates between 1.2 and 1.5.
Aggregate Time Series Regression for Individual Countries	Xu (2011)	— Estimates of above unit elasticity, with considerable variation across countries.
Cross-section Regression — Global Data	— Musgrove *et al.* (2002) — Musgrove *et al.* (2002) — van der Gaag and Stimac (2008) — Fleisher *et al.* (2013)	— Estimates from various model specifications between 1.13 and 1.275. — Estimates of income elasticity of GHE between 1.069 and 1.194 and of OOP between 0.84 and 1.033. — Global estimate, based on a cross-section of 175 countries in 2004, is 1.09 and regional breakdown shows elasticities ranging between 0.83 in the Middle East and 1.197 in OECD countries. — Between 1995 and 2010, the global statistics for the unconditional mean nominal income elasticity of total health spending is 1.118; of government health spending is 1.152; and of OOP spending is 1.043. Elasticity estimates for total and GHE for all income groups and regions are above unity, except for in South Asia. When controlling for demography, the conditional estimates for mean elasticity are lower, at the global level 0.914, 0.933, and 0.894 for THE, GHE, and OOP respectively.

(*Continued*)

Table 3. (*Continued*)

Methods	Sources	Findings
Panel Data Methods	— Gerdtham *et al.* (1992)	— Estimates of above unit elasticity, consistent with the cross-sectional literature.
	— Hitiris and Posnett (1992)	
	— Farag *et al.* (2009)	— Income elasticity close to 1.
	— Hansen and King (1996); Blomqvist and Carter (1997); Gerdtham and Löthgren (2000); 2002); Okunade and Karakus (2001); Dreger and Reimers (2005).	— Income elasticity below 1 for low and middle-income countries, respectively 0.66 and 0.96, without taking into account non-stationarity of health and income.
		— Income elasticity is below 1, based on panel data analyses (using short panel) that study the non-stationarity and cointegration properties between health care spending and income and estimated the income elasticity of health spending controlling for non-income determinants.
	— Baltagi and Moscone (2010)	— Income elasticity of 0.87 for a group of 20 OECD countries drawing on a long panel between 1971 and 2004. The study confirms non-stationarity of health spending and most determinants and cointegration in the long run.
	— Xu *et al.* (2011)	— Elasticity, based on data from 143 countries between 1995 and 2008, is between 0.75 and 0.95 in the fixed effects model and is lower in the dynamic model.
	— Erdil and Yetkiner (2009)	— Evidence of significant bidirectional Granger-causality for 46 countries from a sample of 75 low to high-income countries between income and health expenditure.

Sources: Compilation by the author based on Xu *et al.* (2011) and Fleisher *et al.* (2013).

Table 4. Income elasticity of total health expenditure by income group, 1995–2012

Elasticity estimates for 1995–2012	Income elasticity of the	R^2	Income elasticity of GHE	R^2	Income elasticity of OOP	R^2
High-Income Countries (HIC)	1.21	0.64	1.31	0.62	0.82	0.33
Upper-Middle-Income Countries (UMIC)	0.90	0.57	0.99	0.52	0.87	0.26
Lower-Middle Income Countries (LMIC)	1.01	0.65	1.08	0.54	0.81	0.23
Low-Income Countries (LIC)	0.91	0.68	1.05	0.59	0.73	0.30
Global	**1.06**	**0.95**	**1.20**	**0.93**	**0.86**	**0.79**

Source: Author's calculations based on WHO NHA 2013 (WHO, 2013a).

Particularly models that took into account the non-stationarity and cointegration properties of health spending and its determinants found below unity elasticities. This means that, if health is a necessity good,[27] health spending does not rise faster than economic growth, rendering the concerns regarding the ever-growing share of the sector in the economy unwarranted.

Based on calculations from the WHO's NHA database (2013) (WHO, 2013a), univariate income elasticities of health expenditures (by expenditure type: total, government, or out-of-pocket) for the period between 1995 and 2012 are presented by income group in Table 4 and by region in Table 5. The R^2 statistics show the share of the variation in the respective health spending variable — total, government, or out-of-pocket — explained by income.

At the global level, the income elasticity of total health expenditures is above 1, whereby a 1% increase in income is associated with a 1.06% increase in total health spending, and income explains 95% of the variation in total health spending. However, based on these univariate statistics, it is only the high-income group where escalating health spending is a concern, with an income elasticity of total health expenditures at 1.21. Elasticities calculated for individual years show a decline during the peak of the economic crisis, which implies that expenditure increase can be contained. As expected, when the regressions are run for the income groups, within the groups less variation is explained by income, leaving a bigger room for non-income determinants of health spending, such as demography, technology, and system efficiency.

A closer examination of the income elasticities for GHE indicates that public spending on health has been driving the escalation of health expenditures, with

[27] For normal goods, when income rises, demand rises. But, increase for a necessity good is less than proportional to the rise in income, so the proportion of expenditure on these goods falls as income rises. The income elasticity of a necessity good is thus between 0 and 1.

Table 5. Income elasticity of total health expenditure by region, 1995–2012

Elasticity estimates for 1995–2012	**Income elasticity of the**	R^2	**Income elasticity of GHE**	R^2	**Income elasticity of OOP**	R^2
East Asia and the Pacific (EAP)	1.07	0.89	1.15	0.80	0.96	0.74
Eastern Europe and Central Asia (ECA)	1.11	0.98	1.25	0.96	0.83	0.86
Latin America and the Caribbean (LAC)	1.01	0.92	1.07	0.88	0.91	0.71
Middle East and North Africa (MENA)	0.89	0.89	1.03	0.91	0.63	0.62
North American Countries (NAC)	1.57	0.88	1.24	0.95	1.31	0.90
Organization of Economic Co-operation and Development (OECD)	1.23	0.96	1.29	0.94	0.99	0.75
South Asia	1.03	0.97	1.38	0.85	0.67	0.65
Sub-Saharan Africa	0.94	0.88	1.08	0.87	0.65	0.49

Sources: Author's calculations based on WHO NHA 2013. THE = *total health expenditures*; GHE = *global health expenditures*; OOP = *out-of-pocket* spending.

above unit elasticities for all income groups but the upper-middle income, where the relationship is close to unity. On the other hand, all statistics for out-of-pocket expenditures are below unity, which indicates that when it comes to private, non-pooled spending by individuals and households, health is a necessity.

Technically, the income elasticity estimates for GHE mask an important component. Because the variable for government expenditure on health in the WHO's NHA includes on-budget DAH, these elasticities by default capture some of the effect of aid channeled through the government's public financing system. Given this data limitation, the elasticity estimates absorb some of the effect of official development assistance (ODA) used for health. This means that where ODA in substantive, the estimates will be biased. For example, during economic shocks a number of low income countries have benefited from external resource flows to mitigate the adverse effects of the downturn. Under such circumstances, in the absence of aid flows health expenditures could fall more compared to the state with aid flows included, hence leading to reduced income elasticity of health expenditures. However, such empirical explorations are beyond the mandate and scope of his paper. Hence, it is acknowledged that the presented rudimentary regression estimates do not intend to isolate the effect of aid on health spending.

Related literature is discussed in Section "Retrospective and Prospective Assessment of Health Spending".

The elasticities presented in Table 5 illustrate the regional variation in the relationship between income and health spending. At the global level, the escalation in health spending over the examined period is driven by the North American Continent (NAC) and the 20 OECD countries.[28] The income elasticity of total health spending is below unity ($e < 1$) in the Middle East and North Africa and Sub-Saharan Africa. However, the income elasticity of government health spending is above unity ($e > 1$) in all regions. The elasticities for out-of-pocket (OOP) spending are the highest in the NAC and OECD zones, which indicates that higher purchasing power has been driving health spending through the private channel. The R^2 term is particularly high for NAC, where income explains 90% of the variation in OOP spending. The difference in the explanatory power of the models for income elasticity of OOP spending for the NAC ($R^2 = 0.9$) and OECD ($R^2 = 0.75$) regions implies that the modality of health system financing and the institutional context matters.

Non-income factors

In addition to the disagreement on the income elasticity of health spending, another related area with conflicting findings is the literature on the drivers of health expenditures, which aims to decompose the determinants of health spending. Compared to the early estimates by Newhouse (1977) where income accounts for 90% of the variation in per capita health spending, in a later study by Acemoglu *et al.*, 2013) — which draws on US data that covers the period between 1940 and 1990 — the share of variation in health spending explained by income is revised down to 35–70%, leaving more scope (i.e., a bigger non-income residual) for other factors such as technology and demography.

This study is particularly interesting in its methodology to establish the causal effect between income and health spending, as it harnesses exogenous shocks to address the endogeneity problem, namely, the concern that GDP and health expenditure are likely to determine each other simultaneously (Acemoglu *et al.*, 2013). In the US — where health expenditures as a share of GDP have more than tripled over the past half century — the study exploits oil price fluctuation, which affects oil producing states directly in terms of revenues and, hence, income. Using oil price as an instrument, they find an income elasticity of 0.7, which suggests that health care is a necessity. They conclude that income is unlikely to be the primary driver of the increase in the health share of GDP.

[28] The OECD grouping also includes NAC, for which separate statistics are presented. Although this may appear as double counting, to be consistent with the definition of OECD, the calculations include NAC.

Other studies also reduce the weight of income in determining health expenditures. Xu, *et al.* (2011) note that:

> *"... in determining the income elasticity of health expenditure, the identification of non-income determinants are essential for avoiding the missing variable effect. This identification may be difficult for a number of reasons, notably the limited availability of health care data at the macro as well as the micro level. The missing variable effect would induce either a downward or an upward bias depending on the sign of the correlation between the explanatory variables and the omitted variables."*

The literature has paid attention to demographic and epidemiological factors and to technology, which have been posited to be important, particularly in advanced economies, where the triple transition — aging, the growing NCD burden, and technology diffusion — have been generating increasing demand for health care, thus leading to expenditure escalation.

Demography

Traditionally, population aging has been expected to be an important driving force behind the rise in health spending. However, empirical analyses, which controlled for population age structure, countered this prior, showing that population aging is of less importance for health care expenditures than usually held and that it has a stronger impact on other aspects of the welfare state, like pension (Canadian Institute for Health Information, 2011; Di Matteo and Di Matteo, 1998; Dormont et al., 2006; McGuire *et al.*, 1993; Xu *et al.*, 2011; Zweifel and Ferrari, 1992; Zweiffel *et al.*, 1995). Although cross-sectional regressions (Fleisher *et al.*, 2013) and panel data analyses (Xu *et al.*, 2011) show that including a variable to proxy for aging attenuates the effect of income; these effects are small or insignificant, depending on the model specification. Demography has been less studied in the context of developing countries.

Technology

In advanced economies, given the availability of reliable data on how spending differs across different cohorts of the population and projections for the aging of the population, the effect of population aging on spending is well understood (Xu *et al.*, 2011).[29] What has been less clear is how non-demographic drivers of health spending, such as technological improvements[29a] in medical care and technology

---

[29] See review in Xu *et al.* (2011). In the OECD context, see more in *The 2015 Ageing Report* on the effect of demography and technology on health expenditures and budgets between 2013 and 2060 (European Commission, 2015).

[29a] Among the non-income and non-demographic drivers, the literature also discusses the Baumol effect, which may arise if labor productivity in health care grows more slowly than in the overall economy (see for example, Hartwig, 2008).

diffusion, affect spending. The growth of spending attributed to non-demographic factors has been coined "excess cost growth" (ECG) in a book on health policy reform in advanced and emerging economies (Clements *et al.*, 2012). In these countries, the authors claim, assumptions regarding ECG are the most important factor behind health care projections, particularly — as discussed above — that the effect of aging on spending increases is believed to be moderate (Smith *et al.*, 2009). Studies from OECD countries concluded that technological progress and variation in medical practice were major determinants in the level and growth of health expenditure (Newhouse, 1992).

In a systematic review of 86 studies, Sorenson *et al.* (2013) critically appraise the conjecture which claims that 'new medical technology is the key driver for burgeoning expenditures.' Their analysis suggests that the relationship between medical technology and spending is complex and often conflicting. The impact of technology on costs differed across technologies, in that some had significant financial implications, while others were cost neutral or cost saving.

They conclude that available evidence suggests new medical technology is an important determinant in rising health expenditures. Studies that quantify this relationship, mainly econometric studies, estimate that the overall impact (i.e., the proportion of the cost increase attributable to new technology) ranges from ~25–75%, averaging at about 50% (Table 6) (Sorenson *et al.*, 2013). While much of

Table 6. Literature summary of the contribution of non-income factors to increase in health spending

	Di Matteo (2005)	**Jones (2002)**	**Pricewaterhouse Coopers (2002)**	**Smith *et al* (2000)**	**Peden and Freeland (1995)**	**Cutler (1995)**	**Newhouse (1992)**
Life Expectancy/ aging	~9%	*	15%**	2%	6–7%	2%	2%
Administrative costs	*	*	15%***	3–10%	*	13%	*
Changes in financing	*	*	*	10%	4–5%	10%	10%
Personal income growth	9–20%	*	*	11–18%	14–18%	5%	<23%
Health care prices	*	*	18%	11–22%	*	19%	*
Technology	~65%	50–75%	25%	38–62%	70–75%	49%	>65%

Notes: * Not estimated; ** included aging, but also "front page treatments" (i.e., media coverage drives demand for expensive treatment), increased preventive and diagnostic activity, and consumers moving away from less expensive managed care products; *** included government mandates (including new mandated benefits) and federal and state regulatory requirements.
Source: Sorenson *et al.* (2013).

the quantitative analyses corroborate the cost-increasing effect of new technology overall, the broader spectrum of evidence, which includes cost-effectiveness studies and descriptive analyses, suggests that the relationship between technological advances and health care expenditure is not straightforward or static. Rather, it should be understood as being complex, with a wide range of potential intervening factors that change and shift the dynamic of the association, depending on the particular circumstances.

In light of these issues, the authors argue that "*decision-makers and other commentators should extend their focus beyond costs solely to include consideration of whether medical technology results in better value in health care and broader socioeconomic benefits.*"

Data limitations in developing countries have made estimation of the contribution of technology to health spending difficult. The literature is thin in this area and hence, future research should generate more evidence on the contribution of technology to spending in developing countries, and per the recommendation above, on the costs and benefits — including broader social benefits — of adapting improved technology.

Beyond the well-known forces that are associated with the increase in health spending — income, technology, demography, and epidemiology — there are a number of factors that affect growth in health expenditures. These fall under four main categories: (i) Aggregate factors; (ii) socio-economic and individual determinants; (iii) health system factors on the supply- and demand-sides, as well as public policy; and, last, (iv) market, institutional, and knowledge issues. The dynamic interaction between these factors jointly determines how health spending behaves and what implications it has on the economy. A detailed discussion on the mechanics and the magnitude of the effect of these variables on the tendency of health spending is beyond the scope of this chapter. However, an overview of the key dimensions of interest is presented in Table 7.

Health Outcomes and Economic Growth

Health outcomes

Despite the strong interest in settling the health and growth debate, technical advancements that enable complex modeling, and the growing body of methodologically well-grounded literature, the evidence base to-date is mixed and contradictory.

This section provides an overview of the evolution of the health-and-growth debate, starting with simple correlations, and turning to causal estimations, applying macro- and micro-economic approaches. For a detailed discussion of the theory of and empirical evidence on health and growth, related methodological issues, and the policy implications of findings, the reader is referred to Jack and Lewis (2009), Spence and Lewis (2009), and a more recent review, which studies the effects of health on economic development in developing economies (World Bank, 2014).

Table 7. Overview of cost drivers

Aggregate factors		Socio-economic and individual determinants		Health system and public policy factors		Market, institutional, and knowledge issues	
Macro-Fiscal		**Economic**		**Demand-Side**		**Marketplace Issues**	
— Income (GDP)	+	— Per capita income	+	— Insurance effect ("moral hazard")	+	— Absence of free-market principles driving up cost due to insurance coverage, regulation, and lack of pricing transparency.	+
— Economic growth (ΔGDP)	*	— Household-level income and distribution within household	*	— Information asymmetry	*	— Complementary private coverage, if unregulated, drives prices.	+
— Fiscal position/space	–	— Income elasticity of demand for health	–			— Market consolidation can drive prices.	+
• Debt/GDP	–						
• Primary deficit	+						
• Tax revenue/GDP	+						
• Prioritization							
Demography		**Social Environment**	–	**Supply-Side — Organizational Structure**		**Regulation**	
— Age	+	— Level and disparities in education and literacy	*	— Fragmented delivery and financing, which leads to inefficient fund use due to duplication; coordination challenges that make total cost management of care difficult; and higher administrative costs.	+	— If regulation limits market entry it may lead to increase in prices.	+
— Dependency Ratio	+	— Community/peer effects related to care seeking	*			— Regulation increases administrative costs arising from compliance.	+
— Total Fertility ratio (TFR)	+	— Norms, standards, culture				— Lack of regulation can lead to sub-standard services, which may be cheaper but utilization of such increasing long-term cost, including financial and economic.	+
Epidemiology		**Individual Characteristics and Behavioral Aspects**		**Supply-Side**		**Insufficient Evidence Base and Policy Feedback**	
— Prevalence of CDs	+	— Genetic precondition	*	— Technology development and diffusion	*	— Lack of robust evidence (e.g., causal, counterfactual analyses from field trials, *ex-ante* impact evaluation, etc.) on the effectiveness of alternative interventions.	+
— Prevalence of NCDs	+	— Life-style and behavioral aspects (risk preference)	* +	— Service capacity, provider density, and supplier-induced demand	+		
— Ratio of high-cost chronic conditions	+	— Gender gradient					

(*Continued*)

Table 7. (*Continued*)

Aggregate factors		Socio-economic and individual determinants		Health system and public policy factors		Market, institutional, and knowledge issues	
				— Mix of service providers.	*	— Lack of robust evidence on the costs and cost-effectiveness of alternative interventions (i.e., cost-effectiveness analysis of alternative interventions).	+ +
				— Provider payments can increase pressure if they reward volume rather than value for money, are biased toward relatively more expensive care, and exacerbate system fragmentation.	+ +	— Lack of robust evidence on the equity and poverty-reduction aspects of alternative interventions (i.e., targeting policies).	+
				— Unit cost in health sector relative to other sectors.		— Lack of efficient mechanisms to translate findings into policy-making and implementation at a scaled manner.	
Poverty and Inequality		**Physical Environment and Infrastructure**		**Supply- and Demand-Side**		**Malpractice Litigation**	
— Growth elasticity of poverty (GEP)[30] (Bourguignon, 2003)	+	– Environmental aspects (e.g., W&S)	+	— Over, under, and misuse arising from technical and perceived quality of care may increase costs, even in the context of underutilization as deferring care seeking leads to higher morbidity and mortality (e.g., low utilization of preventive and primary care).	+	— In developed context, malpractice litigation and related insurance coverage adds to costs due to provision of unnecessary services associated with "defensive" medicine.	+
• Poverty Headcount	*	– Public safety and violence					
• Concentration Curve[31] (Kakwani, 1977)	*						
• Concentration Index[32] (Kakwani, 1980)	*						
• Benefit Incidence	*						

Political System and Public Sector Management and Institutions — Polity or International Country Risk Guidance (ICRG) Index — Country Policy and Institutional Assessment (CPIA) Index	–	**Public Policy** — Disease promotion and prevention policy. Effective promotion and prevention can reduce treatment costs as a result of reducing incidence.	*

Note on Symbols: + indicates a positive effect of the variable of interest on health sending (increase); – indicates a negative effect on spending (reduction); * indicates an ambiguous or context-specific relationship.
Notes: The effect of some of these factors depends on the specific variable explored and the policy context. Where the factor is not amenable to easy classification into the increasing/decreasing effect on health expenditures, the start symbol is applied, for example some aspects of poverty, supply-side conditions, or the public policy context.
Sources: Author's summary based on Barros (1998); Drouin *et al.* (2008); Dybczak and Przywara (2010); Hou *et al.* (2013); Tandon *et al.* (2014); Velenyi and Smitz (2014).

[30] Growth elasticity of poverty (GEP) (Bourguignon, 2001) is the percentage reduction in poverty rates associated with a percentage change in mean per capita income. Generally, increases in per capita income tend to decrease poverty and, hence, the elasticity is positive. Standard estimates of GEP for developing countries are between 1.5 and 5, with an average estimated around 3. This means that a 1% increase in per capita income is associated with a 3% decrease in the poverty rate, the proportion of people living under the poverty threshold (e.g., $1-a-day or $1.25-a-day).

[31] The concentration curve (CC) displays the share of health accounted for by cumulative proportions of individuals in the population ranked from poorest to richest (Kakwani, 1977; Kakwani *et al.* 1997; O'Donnell *et al.* 2008; Wagstaff *et al.* 1991). The concentration curve can be used to examine inequality not just in health outcomes but in any health sector variable of interest. It can also be used to assess differences in health inequality across time and countries. When the CC lies above the line of equality (45-degree line) the variable is concentrated between the poor. For more, see O'Donnell *et al.* (2008).

[32] The concentration index (CI) (Kakwani 1977; 1980), which is directly related to the concentration curve, quantifies the degree of socioeconomic related inequality in a health variable (Kakwani, 1997; Wagstaff *et al.*, 1989). The CI equals two times the area between the line of equality (45-degree line) and the concentration curve (CC). The CI is below 0 (negative) when the variable is higher amongst poor. The CI lies in the range between –1 and 1.

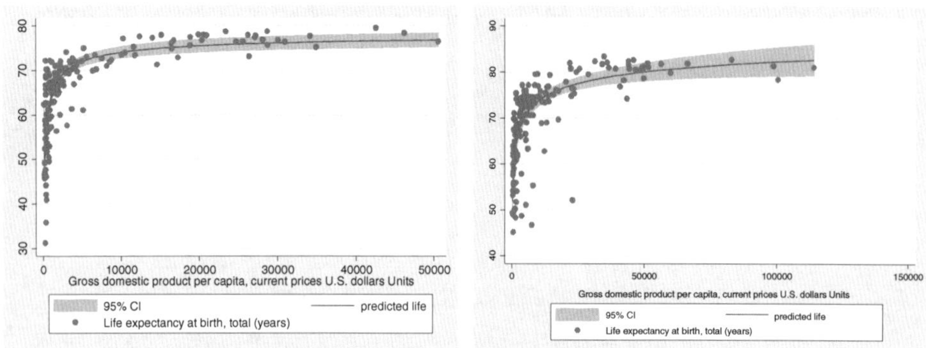

Figure 9. Preston curve with polynomial fit line using global cross section data 1995 and 2011

Sources: Authors' illustration based on data from the WHO's National Health Accounts Database (2013) and the World Bank's WDI (2013). At the global level, life expectancy moves toward and above 80 years of age in Panel B (2011) compared to Panel A (1995). The upward shift can also be observed at the lower end of the global income distribution.

- *Income and health — simple correlation*

The economic and population health disciplines were brought together only about four decades ago, in 1975, when Preston (1975) presented data on per capita income and population health status, measured in terms of life expectancy for a cross-section of countries. The concave relationship between income and life expectancy, as shown by the Preston Curve, indicates that individuals born in richer countries, on average, can expect to live longer than those born in poor countries.[33] However, the link between income and life expectancy flattens out. This means, if the relationship is interpreted as being causal, that there are diminishing returns to income in terms of life expectancy (Schultz and Strauss, 2007).[34]

Preston found that the curve has shifted upward during the 20th century, which means that life expectancy has increased in most countries, independently of changes in income. These exogenous improvements in health, measured in life expectancy, have been credited to improvements in education, better technology, vaccinations, improved provision of public health services, oral rehydration therapy, and better nutrition (Schultz and Strauss, 2007; Jack and Lewis, 2009). Overall, Preston found that improvements in health technology (the upward shifts in the curve) accounted for 75% to 90% of the increase in life expectancy, while income growth (movement along the curve) was responsible for the rest (Galea, 2007).

[33] Pritchett and Summers (1996) also corroborate that countries with higher incomes enjoy higher health.

[34] In other words, at low levels of per capita income, further increases in income are associated with large gains in life expectancy, but at high levels of income, increased income has little associated change in life expectancy.

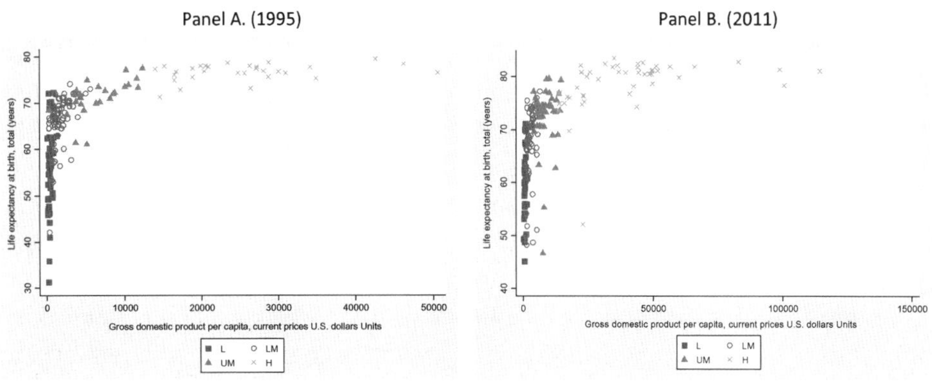

Figure 10. Preston Curve with income group markers using global cross-section data 1995 and 2011

Notes: L = low-income; LM = lower-middle income; UM = upper-middle income; H = high-income — based on the World Bank Group's income group classification.
Sources: Authors' illustration based on data from the WHO's National Health Accounts Database (2013) and the World Bank's WDI (2013).

Increases in life expectancy have been greatest in the poor countries, despite the fact that a good portion of the potential gains from better medical technology have not been realized. On the other hand, several countries in Sub-Saharan Africa have seen declines in life expectancy in the 1990s and 2000s as a result of the HIV/AIDS epidemic, even if their per capita incomes have increased during this time.

The scatter plots illustrate the change in the distribution of countries by income group classification along the Preston Curve between 1995 (Figure 10; Panel A) and 2011 (Figure 10; Panel B). An unambiguous upward movement in life expectancy, the proxy for health, can be observed at the lower end of the global income distribution, including in low- and lower-middle countries.

The policy implication of the relationship between income and health presented in the Preston Curve implies that a transfer of income from the rich to the poor would increase the average health of a society (Bloom and Canning, 2007). However, this policy prescription only holds if the relationship between income and health is causal, that is, if higher income causes longer life expectancy. If the relationship is driven by other factors, if it is spurious, or if it is reverse, meaning that health leads to higher income, then this policy measure would no longer be effective (Bloom and Canning, 2007).

The Preston Curve has been used to argue that poor countries should focus on economic growth, and that health improvements will come about spontaneously as a result of increases in income (Pritchett and Summers, 1996). Following this line of argument, according to one study, assuming that the relationship between income and health is causal, in 1990 better economic performance could have prevented more than half-a-million child deaths worldwide (Pritchett and

Summers, 1996). However, focusing on growth to improve health outcomes is in contrast with the policy implication of the finding by Preston that the upward shift of the curve has come about as a result of improved health technology rather than just increases in per capita income (Bloom and Canning, 2007; Galea, 2007). Preston did, however, acknowledge that in the poorest countries, economic growth may be necessary for improvements in health, as even the most inexpensive technologies have a cost of adoption that poor countries may not be able to afford (Deaton, 2006).

There are noted limitations of the Preston Curve, which caution policymakers against using income or macro-economic growth as the main or sole platform to improve health outcomes.

One limitation is that the Preston Curve is a relationship found in cross-country data, which holds for a sample of countries taken at a particular point in time. Research suggests that a similar relationship does not hold in time series and longitudinal data within individual countries (Spence and Lewis, 2009). As discussed earlier, exploring the evolution of the cross-country distribution of national incomes and health status between 1960 and 2004, Deaton (2006) shows that per capita incomes have steadily diverged while country-level health indicators have converged — until 1990 for life expectancy and through 2004 for the infant mortality rate. This suggests that, over time, changes in income may have diminishing returns on health investments and, hence, reducing impact on health (Deaton, 2006).

A further limitation of the Preston Curve is that it is correlational. It does not provide evidence of causality and the direction of causality; whether income leads to more health or, alternatively, whether better health, proxied by life expectancy, contributes to higher incomes (Bloom and Canning, 2007). The problem of reverse causality between health and income means that any estimate of the impact of income on life expectancy could mistakenly reflect the influence of health (e.g., measured in terms of life expectancy) on income instead. Studies that do not take into account this potential two-way causation may overestimate the importance of income for life expectancy[35] (Pritchett and Summers, 1996).

[35] In economic research, this kind of problem has traditionally been dealt with through the use of instrumental variables which allow the researcher to separate out one effect from another (Pritchett and Summers, 1996). This strategy requires identification of an "instrument" — i.e., a variable which correlates with per capita income but not with the error term in the linear regression. However, since any variable which is likely to correlate with income is also likely to correlate strongly with health and life expectancy this is a difficult task. Some research suggests that in low- and middle-income countries, the causality does indeed go from income to health, while the opposite is true for rich countries (Erdil and Yetkiner, 2009).

• *Health and growth — A causal relationship*

Correlations do not provide robust evidence for policymakers regarding the contributions of health to growth. From a pragmatic perspective, lack of robust evidence makes public expenditure choices difficult, leaving them more exposed to subjective preferences and political influences.

There are two main approaches to causal analysis to identify and estimate the direct and indirect effects of health on the selected economic variable of interest that may be used as a proxy for growth.

- Macro analysis relies on the study of the aggregate production function, where some measure of growth (dependent variable) is determined by physical capital, labor, and productivity (Jack and Lewis, 2009; World Bank, 2004). Macro analysis draws on aggregate-level data to obtain cross-country estimates on the relationship between health and growth, or explores longitudinal data to shed light on the long-run effects of health on growth.
- Micro analysis examines individual and household-level investments in health and the impact of investments on individual/household wealth (e.g., income, measured through proxy for wage, or consumption in developing country context). There is a rich literature that explores the effect of nutrition interventions, investment in early childhood development, and disease-specific interventions, such as malaria and HIV/AIDS prevention and treatment, on individual- and household-level economic well being. The advantage of this approach is that micro-level data is better suited to control for endogeneity and confounders. For example, estimates from experimental contexts — a technique that is extremely rare in macro analysis — enable researchers to be more confident in attributing causal effects. The downside of this approach is its limitation in terms of external validity; that is, that findings may not be easily applicable to other contexts, within a country or across countries. Technically, replication of results in different settings can improve external validity (Rodrik, 2008). Last, micro models do not take into account general equilibrium effects, such as the effects associated with fertility and population size, consequent behavioral choices in savings, and education.[36]

These approaches are discussed in more detail in the forthcoming section, with highlights of illustrative findings.

---

[36] This shortcoming of micro studies is technically addressed by applying a growth accounting framework, which combines macro and micro data. See studies discussed in Jack and Lewis (2009), for example, Weil (2003; 2005) and Ashraf *et al.* (2009).

Macro evidence

Macroeconomists' interest in health is based on the intuition that a healthy population is likely to be more productive than a sick one. Therefore, improving the health status of the population should foster economic growth, *ceteris paribus*.

The effect of health on growth is theoretically and empirically supported by a number of studies. For example, Fogel, a Nobel Prize winning economist, states that about one-third of the economic growth in England over the last two centuries is due to improvements in health and nutrition (Fogel, 1991; 1994; Fogel and Wimmer, 1992). Knowles and Owen (1995; 1997) include health capital in the Mankiw *et al.* (1992) augmented Solow economic growth model,[37] obtaining more significant results than for education. Applying a production function model of aggregate economic growth, which includes two fundamental components of human capital — health and work experience — Bloom *et al.* (2003c) estimate that health has a positive and statistically significant effect on growth, whereby a 1-year increase in life expectancy at the population's level contributes to a 4% increase in output.

Research also shows that, in addition to the effect of health on growth through productivity, health also affects countries' growth potential through the demographic transition (see more in Section "Riding the Demographic Waves"). For example, Bloom *et al.* (2010) explore the contribution of population health and demographic change to economic growth in China and India and find that the major drivers of the predicted take-off are improved health, increased openness to trade, and a rising labor force-to-population ratio due to fertility decline. However, earlier studies (Bloom and Canning, 2003a; Bloom *et al.*, 2003b) warn that there is nothing automatic about the effects of demographic change on population growth. For example, Bloom and Canning (2003a) contrast the experiences of East Asia and Latin America, which had "broadly similar demographic and health conditions" but while East Asia's economy grew explosively, growth in Latin America was stagnant. What set these two growth trajectories apart was the policy

---

[37]Traditionally, economic theory has given emphasis on physical capital accumulation as the most robust source of economic growth, at least in the short-run, with exogenous technical progress being the long-run determinant of growth. The exogeneity of technological progress in the neoclassical growth model and the difficulty of explaining long-term economic growth (because of diminishing returns to physical capital) have restricted the analytical capacity of the neoclassical model and its empirical verification. This problem is solved by endogenous growth models developed by Romer (1986) and Lucas (1988) giving emphasis on human capital accumulation. Human capital theory suggests that individuals and society derive economic benefits from investments in people (Sweetland, 1996). Education has consistently been emerged as the prime human capital but Becker (1993) and Schultz (1997) have argued that health and nutritional expenditure is also a part of human capital investment. This is because education is perceived to contribute to health and nutritional improvements. Education, health, nutrition, water, and sanitation complement each other, with investments in any one contributing to better outcomes in the others (World Bank, 2001).

environment, which created a favorable environment in East Asia to harness the demographic dividend. While Latin America benefited more from the first demographic dividend, East Asia excelled in consolidating the gains during the second demographic dividend[38] (Mason, 2005). For example, in the second wave, the combined effect of fewer children to support and increasing life expectancy was estimated to have led to an increase in gross national saving rates by approximately 14% points (Mason and Kinugasa, 2004) (see more on the role and effect of demography on economic growth in Section "Riding the Demographic Waves").

A number of macro studies in various regional contexts, which use long panel data, consistently find evidence of the causal relationship between health and growth. Applying growth regressions, adapted as Granger-type causality tests[39] (Granger, 1969), Mayer-Foulkes (2001a; 2001b)[40] finds strong evidence of 30-year causality from health[41] to income in 18 Latin American countries. A permanent

---

[38]As a result of the "first" demographic transition, age structures of populations become older. Economically, people often move into higher-paying jobs and countries experience higher per capita income. These social and economic changes motivate people to accumulate greater personal wealth — a process known as the "second" demographic dividend. The second dividend operates through two channels: (i) Greater accumulation of wealth, and (ii) greater investment in human capital. The extent to which a country realizes a second demographic dividend depends on how well it anticipates and organizes support for its elderly (AUC and ECA, 2013). As populations age more quickly due to lower fertility, the resources needed to support the elderly increase relative to GDP, so that families and public pension systems may experience severe strains on their resources. However, if economic policies and financial mechanisms are put in place early in the process of population aging to help workers accumulate assets — such as property, funded pensions, and personal savings — they can achieve more financial independence in old age and depend less on government and their families. In this scenario, population aging will lead to sustainable family and government support systems and boost capital, productivity, and per capita income Mason and Lee (2006). Policymakers, especially in developing countries, need to establish sound and trusted financial systems accessible so that people have the opportunity and mechanisms to accumulate wealth needed for old age (AUC and ECA, 2013). Testing for Granger causality involves econometrically testing the extent to which current and lagged values of health care expenditure (GDP) can be used to predict future values of GDP (health care spending). If both variables are found to Granger cause the other it is possible to infer bidirectional Granger causality (or 'feedback') (Devlin and Hansen, 2010).

[39]The Granger causality test is a statistical hypothesis test for determining whether one time series is useful in forecasting another, first proposed in 1969 (Granger, 1969). Ordinarily, regressions reflect "mere" correlations, but Granger argued that causality in economics could be reflected by measuring the ability of predicting the future values of a time series using past values of another time series. Since the question of "true causality" is deeply philosophical, econometricians assert that the Granger test finds only "predictive causality" (Diebold, 2001). A time series X is said to Granger-cause Y if it can be shown, usually through a series of *t*-tests and F-tests on lagged values of X (and with lagged values of Y also included), that those X values provide statistically significant information about future values of Y.

[40]For more, see PAHO (2001).

[41]The health indicator is probability of survival by age and gender groups for 1950–1990.

increment of between 0.8% and 1.5% annual income is associated with typical adult and old age health improvements. As the channels of causation are diverse — including direct productivity increases, investment in education, increased female participation in the labor force, reduced economic burden of disease — microeconometric studies can help identify the pathways of causation. In another study, Galor and Mayer-Foulkes (2004) provide evidence that human capital accumulation by the poor is only possible if a minimum level of health and well being has been attained. When families do not have enough resources to invest in the satisfaction of basic needs and health care and finance is not available for this purpose, a poverty trap exists with low health, education and income. This link between health and education contributes to explain the important, long-term effects of nutrition and health on economic growth and implies that nutrition and health play a causal role in the persistence of inequality and in the effects of inequality on growth.

Using a panel of five Asian countries,[42] Narayan *et al.* (2010) estimate that a 1% increase in health expenditure (as share of GDP) leads to at most 0.26% increase in per capita income. The same study finds no significant effect of education on growth, which was unexpected given that investments in education measured as share of GDP were higher compared to investment in health. Examining the augmented Mankiw, Romer and Weil's model (Knowles and Owen, 1995),[43] which incorporates health and education as components of human capital,[44] using panel data between 1978 and 2005 in the context of China, Li and Huang (2009) find evidence that both health and education have positive, significant effects on growth.

Numerous studies show there is a two-way relationship between human development and economic growth. On the one hand, growth allows investing in improved human development[45] (see Figure 1 for an overview of what contributes to human development).[46] On the other hand, improving the level of human development enhances an economy's growth opportunities (Duflo, 2001; Schultz, 2005).

For example, Suri *et al.* (2010) examine this feedback from human development into economic growth, which then permits further improvements in human development, allowing an economy to sustain growth and maintain improvements in human capital formation in a mutually reinforcing fashion (see Figure 1). From

[42] Five countries are India, Indonesia, Nepal, Sri Lanka, and Thailand. The period is 1974–2007. For India, using data between 1960 and 2006, Haldar and Mallik (2010) find that physical capital investment has no long-run nor short-run effect but the human capital investment has significant long-run effect on per capita GNP.

[43] The model builds on Mankiw *et al.* (1992) and Solow (1956).

[44] Knowles and Owen (1995) further extended the neoclassical growth model (Solow, 1956) to incorporate both health and education as human capital.

[45] See more on human development and its measurement in UNDP (1990), Smith (1993), McGillivray and White (1993), Srinivasan (1994), Alkire (2002), and Ravallion (2012).

[46] This draws on Strauss and Thomas (1995), Ranis *et al.* (2000), and Suri *et al.* (2010).

a panel data model, the authors find that human development plays an essential role in determining growth trajectories (using the measure of sustained growth). Not only is human development a final product in the sense that it measures basic human well-being but it is also a critical input into economic growth. Their results imply that successful policy requires an early focus on human development, not purely because of its direct impact but also because of its feedback effect on sustaining economic growth. Their results also show that human development (measured through life expectancy, infant mortality, and school enrollment) is not smoothly substitutable for other inputs in generating economic growth. The results suggest that improving human development must precede or accompany rising economic growth for a country to reach sustained growth. In terms of policy sequencing, without improvements in human development, policy that attempts to enhance economic growth is highly unlikely to lead to sustained growth.[47]

In sum, at the macro-level there has been a growing body of literature since 2001, including global, regional, and country-level studies, which provide evidence of a causal relationship between health and growth or of a bidirectional relationship between health and growth. Despite the growing evidence base on causality derived from augmented growth models, which explicitly incorporate human capital and health as part of human capital into modeling, the literature remains ambiguous regarding the impact of health on growth primarily because of the challenges of measuring health and the methodological complexity that surrounds isolating the pure effect of health on growth through various pathways.

Policy-wise, a number of papers have been influential in arguing for more investment in health on the grounds of macro evidence, raising attention to the importance of health care financing as an input/intermediary to growth, both at the global and country level (Sachs, 2001; Bloom *et al.*, 2003c). However, while the evidence obtained from macro analyses has provided an argument to support calls for increased investment in health, an important limitation has been that such studies do not provide specific information as to how to invest in health to contribute to growth. Estimates of the impact of health on growth from growth models, which use aggregate-level data, do not allow identifying the specific channels and their relative weight in contributing to economic growth. Consequently, the macro evidence base typically lacks specificity with respect to what interventions should be prioritized; it does not provide actionable answers as to *what* and *how* governments or policymakers should invest in. Notwithstanding, the macro evidence base has been critical in policy advocacy by informing discussions between policymakers

---

[47] Regarding the sequencing, for example, Weil (2007) suggests that health's positive effect on GDP is strongest in poor countries, which is also supported by the findings in Aghion *et al.* (2010). The Africa Health Brief: Health or Wealth: Which Comes First? (World Bank, 2013) also explores this question. Velenyi and Smitz (2014) explore global data to better understand the cyclical patterns between health expenditures and economic growth.

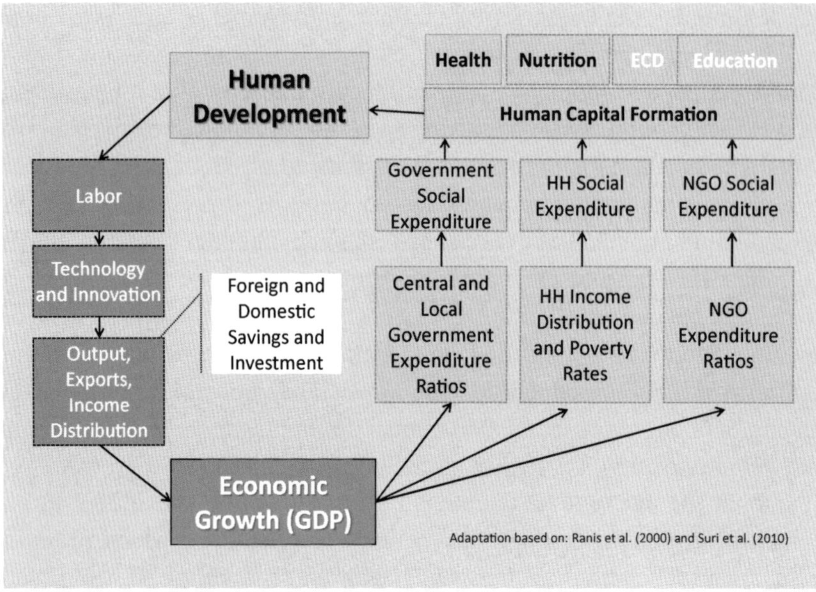

Figure 11. Two-way causality between economic growth and human development

in the health and economic development sectors; it has also been important in arguing for normative benchmarks and in providing a context and broad guidelines regarding investing in health.

Micro evidence

Given the limitations associated with the macro evidence on health and growth, the micro strand of the literature aims to minimize identification problems and to explore and estimate the causal effect between health and income at the household and individual levels, using disaggregated data and often less ambiguous measures[48] of health and income (Jack and Lewis, 2009; Spence and Lewis, 2009). From the policy perspective, the objective is to harness the power of micro analysis so that it can provide actionable information for policymakers on *which* interventions to invest in and *how* to invest in health to boost productivity and, therefore, contribute to economic growth.

Earlier studies (Jack and Lewis, 2009; Spence and Lewis, 2009) that provide a comprehensive assessment of the health and growth nexus and, as part of that, review the micro evidence, highlight areas where there is ample evidence on the

[48] For example, in the disease-specific context of malaria, infections rates and labor productivity are used as proxy measures.

effect of health on economic development through various interventions and pathways. Among these are: (i) Nutrition in the first 1000 days (Black *et al.*, 2008) and early childhood development (Alderman, 2011) which, through improved cognitive capacity, impact educational attainment and have lifetime implications on employment; (ii) maternal nutrition and health (Victora *et al.*, 2008), which determine the child's physical and mental development, and therefore the child's lifetime health status and earning potential; (iii) HIV/AIDS, which affects labor productivity and has significant intergenerational effects due to mother-to-child transmission and single-parent households or orphanage as a result of AIDS-related mortality; and (iv) malaria, which impacts labor productivity and, if severe, it leads to cognitive impairment with lifetime implications. As this literature has been extensively discussed in these comprehensive analyses, and given in the scope of this chapter, the reader is referred to these sources for further details on micro evidence.

Over the past decade, there has been an increasing interest in using impact evaluation (IE) to assess the effectiveness, cost-effectiveness, and equity implications of innovative interventions that have the promise to be scaled up at a national level or tested and applied in like contexts in other countries. The interest in using IE to learn how to improve policy implementation and development results has been growing across the development community (World Bank, 2011).[48a] Countries consider IE an important tool to inform the design and guide the implementation of their policies. As a result, there is an increasing body of micro data and economic assessment to provide robust causal evidence that can inform project design, implementation, and policymaking. A number of experimental and quasi experimental evaluations have been generating more evidence about what works, where, and how, across a variety of topics, including malaria and HIV/AIDS prevention and treatment, performance-based financing, community-based service-delivery and health insurance models. This growing body of literature aims to address particular service delivery and policy challenges with the objective of improving health system effectiveness, efficiency, and equity; that is, to provide more value for the resources in a sustainable manner. Given the pilot scale (e.g., at sub-national level) of most of these evaluations and their context specificity, there are some disadvantages to impact evaluations, including limited external validity, changing cost functions and therefore cost-effectiveness results once the interventions are

[48a] In addition to IE, which has been on the rise over the past decade to strengthen project implementation and outcomes, the Independent Evaluation Group (IEG) of the World Bank Group has been undertaking periodic assessment of the effectiveness of project supported by the health sector. Such portfolio reviews are important to assess what works and which areas require further improvement. See, for example, IEG's 2009 report on the effectiveness of health, nutrition, and population projects on health outcomes (IEG, 2009).

scaled up and, consequently, a relatively wide 'confidence interval' in terms of projecting system-wide financial sustainability and macro-level effects. Notwithstanding these limitations, impact evaluations have proven to be powerful in advising policy decisions (World Bank, 2012c). One example of a micro study that offers some contextualization of the effect at the macro-level if scaled up to the target population is an experimental evaluation of malaria prevention in agricultural workers in Nigeria. The study underscores the importance of the relationships between health care, health, productivity, macroeconomic growth, and poverty reduction. The study by Dillon *et al.* (2014) explores the effect of malarial infection on sugarcane cutters' earnings, labor supply, and productivity as they are randomly assigned malaria testing and treatment with the first-line drug. They find that both labor supply and productivity increases, which account for a 10% increase in earnings. As the authors point out, given the weight of agricultural activity in the economy and the poverty status of agricultural workers, upon scale-up, such gains could translate into macroeconomic growth,[49] and poverty reduction at the national level.[50] The fundamental insight of the study in the health and labor productivity literature is that health is a key component of human capital, and workers with superior health are more productive (Schultz, 2002).

Diagnostic Tools and Government Policies to Better Invest in Health for Growth

As the previous sections have shown, the evidence base on the health and growth nexus, although still unsettled, has been evolving to provide more and better

[49] Cross-country regressions estimate that countries with a substantial number of malaria cases grew less by between 0.55% (McCarthy *et al.* 2000) and 1.3% (Gallup and Sachs, 2001) in terms of per capita GDP. More broadly, Bloom *et al.* (2003c) estimate a production function model of aggregate economic growth including two variables that microeconomists have identified as fundamental components of human capital: Work experience and health. Their main result is that good health has a positive, sizeable, and statistically significant effect on aggregate output even when controlling for experience of the workforce. The study suggests that a 1-year improvement in a population's life expectancy contributes to an increase of 4% in output. This is a relatively large effect, indicating that increased expenditures on improving health might be justified purely on the grounds of their impact on labor productivity, quite apart from the direct effect of improved health on welfare.

[50] This is because: (i) Agricultural workers and others in physical occupations likely suffer the greatest productivity declines from malaria; (ii) malaria is the leading cause of care-seeking with 51% of individuals reporting episodes (NLSS 2003/4); (iii) the agricultural sector has the highest poverty rate (62.7%) of any occupational group in Nigeria (NLSS 2003/4); and (iv) lack of access to health care and unpredictable health expenditures have been among the leading causes of poverty and deprivation for rural and low-income households.

information for policymaking. This section focuses on analytical tools which can directly contribute to policy processes that lead to making better health investments to contribute to economic growth. Further, it discusses areas where early policy attention is required due to the time needed to harmonize across ministries/agencies, or due to the length of the time lag between the health intervention and its effect on growth and development. Specifically, the following areas will be covered:

(1) A discussion on the methods for retrospective and prospective assessment of health spending. Specifically, this section will investigate the role and benefit of health sector-specific PER and FSA for health to inform both sector expenditure and macro-fiscal policies. Under FSA for health, three modalities of fiscal space generation will be discussed, which are the most relevant from a feasibility perspective. These are: (i) Efficiency gains; (ii) DAH; and (iii) reprioritization.
(2) An exploration of how economic cycles (see Definition in Annex 3) affect health spending, with a special focus on (i) whether more countercyclical policymaking is feasible in developing countries (see Definition in Annex 3); (ii) how to prepare the health system for economic downturns and manage it through crises to attenuate the adverse effect on population health and ill-health related poverty, both of which contribute to further slackening economic growth.
(3) An investigation of the effect of demographic change on growth acceleration (or deceleration). The discussion includes examples where effective policies have enabled countries to ride the demographic waves and harness the demographic dividend, as well as counter examples where lack of strategic policy effort has resulted in a demographic break on growth (see more on the effect of demography on growth in Section "Riding the Demographic Waves" and Annex 3).
(4) Lastly, a brief entry on the relationship between health, poverty, and growth. This discussion focuses on how the distribution of health inputs and outcomes and equality of opportunity are relevant for equitable growth.

Retrospective and prospective assessment of health spending

- *A retrospective diagnostic tool: Public expenditure review* (*PER*)

The foregoing discussion regarding the tenuous relationship between health spending and health outcomes highlighted the primary reasons why investing in health may not always translate into better health outcomes. One such factor is the lack of efficiency and equity of public spending. There are a number of reasons that can explain why resources are not used efficiently, including: (i) Data and technical limitations to assess what is a "good buy" (i.e., through cost-effectiveness analysis); (ii) varying institutional and organizational context, which can make tracing funds (domestic and external) difficult across administrative levels and agencies; (iii) governance and accountability issues related to weak public finance management; and (iv) absorptive capacity at various levels as a result of administrative bottlenecks. It is these bottlenecks that a PER can help explore to provide an assessment of the most critical drivers and the specific level where they take place.

The World Bank Group has developed the PER as a core diagnostic tool to capture in a direct way the extent to which a country translates promises into an actual reality (Gaudin and Yazbeck, 2014). According to the *Core Guidance on PER in Human Development* (World Bank, 2009), the fundamental role of a sector PER[51] is to explore how well the sector spends public resources, in terms of both efficiency and equity, and whether public resources are used inline with development and policy targets. As the PER's objective is to provide policy-friendly information to governments to improve on public sector performance (Gaudin and Yazbeck, 2014), in order to be practical and actionable, a PER should "identify the sources of poor sector performance and outcomes versus spending, explore the reasons for inefficiencies and inequities," and offer policy options to address the identified bottlenecks (World Bank, 2009).

A recent systematic review (Gaudin and Yazbeck, 2014) of PERs that were carried out and published by the World Bank between 2000 and 2011 discusses the variation in the focus and policy advice of PERs by income group and region. For example, the study points out that, with increase in income at the country level, PERs move away from general public sector and multi-sectoral issues toward sector-specific challenges. A general theme across income groups is tackling inequalities. The review offers analysts resources and good practices for implementing future PERs.

PERs have been informative and instrumental in shaping public sector performance across a number of countries over the past decade. Yet, PER as a tool has its limitations and, thus, requires complementary tools to identify and address challenges more specifically and in a targeted manner. Given that PER is conducted at the macro-level and relies on aggregate data, it does not enable efficiency analysis across the service delivery network (e.g., at facility level), nor does it allow analysts to perform benefit incidence analysis of public resource use.

[51] A public expenditure review is concerned with public-based (not always government) revenues and expenditures as expressions of public policy and public involvement in the economy. Social sectors — education, health and social protection — are prime instruments of such policy and involvement.

Box 3. PER — A retrospective analytical tool to assess the efficiency and equity of public sector spending

PER is a retrospective diagnostic tool that analyzes sector expenditures at the macro-level (e.g., based on aggregate data from the national and sub-national levels), both from an efficiency and equity perspective. The sector-specific PER aims to enable policymakers to address questions regarding budgeting and the use of public funds, including the budgeting process (*de jure* and *de facto* budgeting, and changes in the locus of power over time as a result of decentralization); discrepancies between planned and executed budgets, regional variations (at the sub-national level, as well as urban and rural differentials); spending patterns by functional[52] and economic classification, and disease burden.[53] As such, a sector PER provides an analysis of the policy framework and charts institutional relations to understand public fund flows[54] and trends in flows as well as budget allocations[55] and execution at the national and sub-national levels.

Consequently, complementary analytical approaches are required at the micro level to enable assessing public resource use at the facility/provider level, including efficiency and equity aspects.

- Public Expenditure Tracking Survey (PETS) have been developed out of the observed weak association between expenditure and service delivery performance (increased resources do not translate into better outcomes), and the need to investigate the specific reasons why the resources mobilized do not impact — to the expected extent — on the health status of the intended population. PETS is a quantitative survey of the supply side of public services, which collects information on facility characteristics, financial flows, outputs (services delivered), and accountability arrangements. A PETS tracks, locates,

[52] See classification, for example: http://www1.worldbank.org/publicsector/pe/PEAMCourse04/DorotinskyBackCh3.pdf.

[53] Where relevant, as much as the data allows, PERs can explore disease-specific expenditure patterns with a focus on key burden-of-disease drivers, which are also significant in terms of financial and economic costs, for example, HIV/AIDS in countries with high prevalence of HIV/AIDS.

[54] For example, fund flow from the Ministry of Finance to the Ministry of Health and other ministries/agencies which also spend on health programs. The analysis includes development of fund flow diagrams to help identify choking points at the national and sub-national levels. Where the share of development aid is high in the sector, the expenditure review includes analysis of the role of development assistance in the sector budget.

[55] This includes discussion of the funding formula to regions, across services (preventive vs. curative), by functions (non-discretionary items, such as wages, and discretionary items, etc.), and levels of care.

and quantifies the flow of public resources across the various administrative levels of the government (Gurkan *et al.,* 2009). It aims to determine, on a sample basis, how much of the original allocations (financial, salaries, in-kind items) reach the next level of government and, ultimately, service delivery units such as health facilities. As such, PETS is a tracer survey of leakages. A major reason for undertaking a PETS is also a major challenge it faces: poor record keeping practices especially at the decentralized level of the system. Although lessons from a decade of global experience of PETS point out implementation challenges, "*PETS remains to be the most powerful tool to systematically drill down and ultimately help strengthen actual public expenditure processes for frontline service delivery impacts*" (Gurkan *et al.*, 2009).

- Quantitative Service Delivery Survey (QSDS) investigates efficiency by assessing incentives to providers and documenting outputs for comparison with expenditure data. QSDS aim at complementing the PETS studies — which focus mostly on resource flows and use — with information on the organization and provision of services within the frontline facilities and on how resource management and inefficiency impact on service delivery. This implies gathering detailed information on how services are organized, managed and provided at the facility level, and on how users benefit from these services. The complementarity between PETS and QSDS has led to several projects conducting the two approaches in combination or sequentially. Both PETS and QSDS can shed some light on the equity of resource and service use. They can be used for diagnostic purposes (identify problems), analytical (clarify or investigate the causes of the problems), or evaluation (assess the effects of a program or policy).
- The Service Delivery Indicator Survey (SDI) is a hybrid that uses modules from the PETS, QSDS, Staff Absence Survey (SAS), and observational studies. To fill data gaps in the quality of public service delivery, in 2012 the World Bank, in partnership with the African Economic Research Consortium and the African Development Bank, launched the Service Delivery Indicator (SDI) Survey, a tool that collects indicators biannually to examine the effort of health care staff ("what providers do"), the ability of health care staff ("what providers know"), and the availability of key inputs and resources ("what providers have to work with") that contribute to a functioning health facility (sdindicators.org, 2015). This tool was inspired by the *World Development Report 2004: Making Services Work for Poor People*, which proposed that health care quality is critically dependent on what service providers know and do. The SDI is a harmonized data collection and analytical effort that was designed to contribute to addressing the unfinished MDG agenda by providing information on whether public resources are turned into quality service delivery.

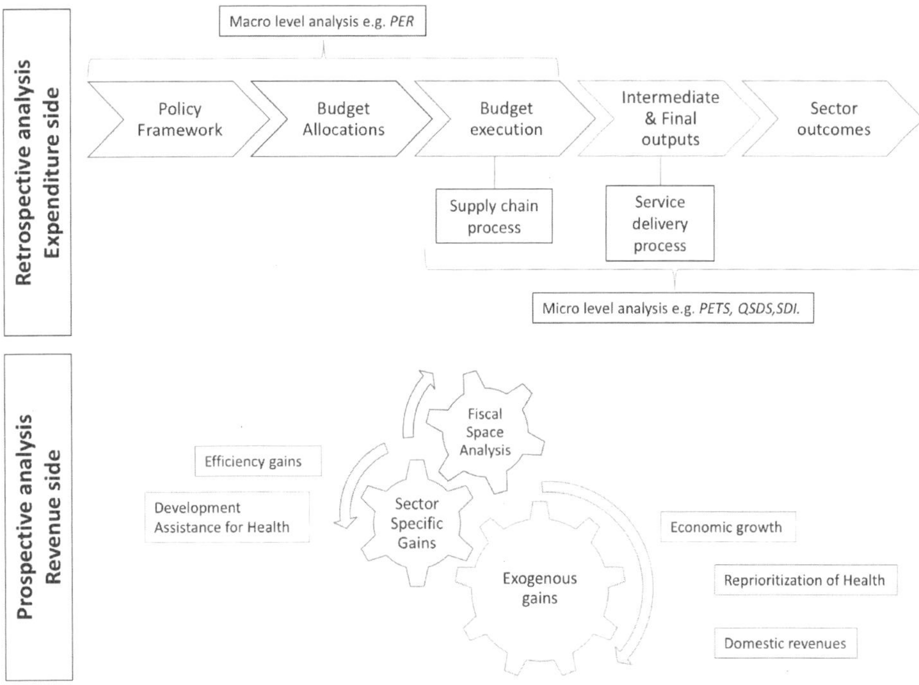

Figure 12. Diagnostic tools to improve public health spending

Source: Author.[56] Velenyi (2014) based on DFID (2010), Heller (2006), and Tandon and Cashin (2010).

Figure 12 provides an overview of the diagnostic tools discussed in this chapter to improve public health spending, including the retrospective components at the macro- and micro-levels, and the prospective tool, which is discussed in Section "A Prospective Diagnostic Tool: Fiscal Space Analysis for Health".

• *A prospective diagnostic tool: Fiscal space analysis for health*

An accompanying diagnostic tool to the PER, which focuses on the revenue side, is sector-specific FSA. Drawing on some of the points made in Heller (2005) and extending those, FSA is useful:

- To examine whether and how the government could feasibly increase its expenditure on health, consistently with revenue sources and trends, and the underlying macroeconomic framework that determines the country's fiscal envelope.

[56]The overview of the retrospective analysis is adapted from DFID (2010). Conceptually, the prospective flow draws on Heller (2006), UNICEF (2009), Tandon and Cashin (2010), Tandon *et al.* (2014).

- To provide sector-specific input into the budget process and, hence, to be used as an input into the MTEF (see more on the MTEF in Annex 3).
- To undertake projections and simulations to inform policymakers on revenue collection and resource allocation aspects with the objective of helping the government meet fiscal targets and budget predictability for the sector in the medium- to long-term.
- To inform the development of the post-2015 development agenda; which moves beyond consolidating the results of the MDG agenda toward the new goals of SDGs. In the context of the health sector, the SDGs' focus is on addressing the increasing challenge of NCD, and on systems, particularly on achieving UHC.

In sum, FSA facilitates the dialogue between ministries of health and ministries of finance and planning in developing a sector-specific financing strategy that contributes to economic growth through the channel of human capital formation. Additionally, FSA is informative for development partners in country-specific discussions and, at the global level, it informs health care financing policies and the aid architecture, for example, considerations for the creation of a "global social health protection fund," as proposed by Ooms *et al.* (2010) (see more in Annex 3).

Fiscal space for health is a dynamic concept, which requires strategic management of general government and sector-specific resources along economic cycles.[57] Further, when there are projected changes in the economy and, consequently, in the macro-fiscal environment, governments are required to manage fiscal space projections in a forward-looking manner, updating their expectations regarding the availability and management of fiscal space for health to meet sectoral and development objectives. The strategic management of government resources with economic cycles, and the forward-looking assessment of changes in the fiscal space situation — both in general and for the health sector in particular — are critical public finance management functions to get good value for public resources and to smooth financing for the sector.

[57] Business cycle (or economic cycle) refers to the economy-wide fluctuation in production, trade, and economic activity in general over several months or years (Burns and Mitchell, 1946). The term "cycle" is a misnomer, because business cycle fluctuations are neither regular nor predictable. Upward and downward movements in the cycle (expansions and contractions) can be measured by the level of gross domestic product (GDP). These fluctuations are measured relative to the economy's long-term growth trend Madhani (2010). A variable that is positively correlated with the overall state of the economy is said to be procyclical, and a variable that is negatively correlated with the overall state of the economy is said to be countercyclical.

General and sector-specific concepts of fiscal space

Fiscal policy, which covers government expenditure on health, is a key tool that governments can use to mobilize domestic resources and allocate them to achieve policy objectives. Conceptually, the general framework for fiscal space assessment was proposed by Heller (2005), who defined fiscal space as the "*availability of budgetary room that allows a government to provide resources for a desired purpose without any prejudice to the sustainability of a government's financial position*" (Heller, 2005; 2006). According to the author, this concept of fiscal space requires fiscal sustainability, that is, the capacity of the government to finance its desired expenditure programs, to service debt obligations and to ensure its future solvency. The framework emphasizes that fiscal sustainability depends on the underlying economic growth rate, which determines revenue generation and whether commitments affect fiscal space immediately or in the long run. Hence, it is argued that fiscal space assessment must be made in the context of at least a MTEF, which takes a comprehensive and forward-looking perspective of the government's budget priorities.

As a review of fiscal space for health points out (Powell-Jackson *et al.*, 2012), when applied to the health sector, the intention is to increase financial resources for health over the short- to medium-term in a way that is consistent with a country's macroeconomic fundamentals, such that the long-term solvency of the government and its economic potential is not jeopardized (Adam and Bevan, 2005).

The health sector-specific adaptation of the fiscal space concept was developed 5 years later by Tandon and Cashin (2010) who — following the general framework — proposed the definition for fiscal space for health as "*the ability of governments to increase spending for the sector without jeopardizing the government's long-term solvency or crowding out expenditure in other sectors needed to achieve other development objectives.*"

The rationale for creating fiscal space for health

In general, the objective of creating fiscal space is to generate additional resources for some meritorious government spending (or to enable tax reduction). The incentive for creating fiscal space is strengthened where the resulting fiscal outlays would boost medium-term growth and perhaps even pay for themselves in terms of future fiscal revenue (Heller, 2005; 2006).

The questions, thus, are whether creating fiscal space for health is meritorious and whether investments made using the created fiscal space can pay for themselves, for example, by increasing productivity, labor market participation, and so forth.

Heller (2005; 2006) argues that current spending on health, which adds to human capital, has valid claims on available fiscal space because such outlays can pay for themselves in the long-term, for example, through increased productivity contributing to economic growth and the revenue base. Further, he points out the inter-temporal aspect of expenditure decisions, notably, that not spending an adequate amount in a sector may weaken the sector to the extent that it would be costly and time consuming in the future to "rebuild" the sector.[58] That is, investments foregone due to cutbacks or reduced allocations to a sector could lead to an increased opportunity cost of resources because more resources would be required in the future to attain the same objective. Indeed, this aspect is discussed in the literature on crisis and health in the context of reduced fiscal space due to fiscal consolidation.

Additionally, Tandon *et al.* (2014) discuss that investment in the health sector is not a pure financial decision. There are other criteria regarding additional investment, discussed under normative mainstream economic theory, including the role of the government to offset market failures and improve equity by redistribution, and human rights perspectives. However, they point out that both the normative economic and human rights arguments apply to other sectors as well, which means that there are competing and equally meritorious priorities across many sectors (Tandon *et al.*, 2014).[59] This implies that providing financial evidence on the merit of investing in health can play a role in influencing budget allocation and overall economic development policies.

Possible and feasible sources for creating fiscal space for health

The foregoing analysis presented in this chapter so far have indicated continued increase in demand for health care and health financing, which raises questions of financial sustainability and fiscal space. Financial sustainability becomes a problem when governments are unable to finance the existing level of resources

---

[58] See connecting discussion on crisis as an opportunity in Box 5 and the case study on health system strengthening in the context of the recent Ebola epidemic in Box 15.

[59] Tandon *et al.* (2014) summarizes that mainstream public finance theory argues that public expenditures increase as long as social benefits from additional expenditures exceed the cost of raising revenues for financing and additional outlays. Regarding inter-sectoral allocations, theory holds that public resources should be utilized up to the point where marginal benefits of an additional unit of spending (e.g., dollar) is equalized across sectors (Musgrave, 1959). However, in practice, it is not easy to estimate the economic costs and social benefits of expenditure. Hence, inter-sectoral allocation decisions are often subject to preference functions and political economic factors.

Box 4. Effects of the GEC on Europe and Central Asia — Fiscal austerity and health sector reforms

Prior to the recent GEC, which started in 2007, the Europe and Central Asia (ECA) region had robust economic performance. When the crisis hit, it was expected that such a fast-growing region would have the means and tools to tackle the downturn. However, many countries in the ECA did not cope well.[60] The crisis has shown that no country is immune to external challenges. When policy controls are missing or not used efficiently, crises can reverse progress and positive performance, even in advanced economies with AAA ratings.

Given the diversity of the ECA region, the GEC did not affect all countries to the same extent. During 2003–2010, subregional breakdowns of average economic growth rates (GDP), and the consequent fiscal (GGE) and health (GHE) responses show significant variation across the region. While in all subregions, the average GDP growth rate over this period is positive, there is wide disparity between the high of 8.5% growth in the ECCU3 group (Azerbaijan, Armenia, Georgia) and the low of 0.3% growth in Southern Europe (ECCU10). The story line is similar for the growth rates in GGE and GHE. Comparatively, for most subregions — except for Russia and ECCU3 — the rate of growth in GHE is higher than fiscal growth, implying an increasing share of the health sector in the government budget during this period.

However, since these statistics are averaged for the 2003–2010 time frame, they mask the cyclical responses during the crisis. By the peak of the crisis in 2009, all but the Central Asia Subregion was in a growth contraction mode, with Central Eastern Europe undergoing the deepest GDP reduction at negative 8.7%. In 2010, most subregions had procyclical fiscal responses, except for Turkey and Northern and Western Europe, where — due to automatic stabilizers and/or fiscal stimuli — countercyclical responses are observed.

With respect to GHE, all subregions undergoing growth contraction in 2009 had a procyclical response in 2010, except for Turkey and Western Europe. As a result of the crisis, a number of countries in Europe stood on the fiscal brink. Rising debt levels, threats to fiscal sustainability, and pressures from fiscal austerity have reduced fiscal space for health. In many European countries, spending on health (Heller, 2013; WHO, 2013b) and growth rates of GHE have fallen significantly. Reduced nominal spending occurred as early as 2008–2009 in Estonia, Hungary,

(*Continued*)

[60] For more, see Chapter 5 in Hou *et al.* (2013).

Box 4. (*Continued*)

and Ireland (Burke *et al.*, 2013; Habicht, 2012; Heller, 2013). In 2009–2010, spending fell in the Czech Republic, Denmark, Estonia, Greece, Ireland, Portugal, Slovenia, and Spain (Gené-Badia, 2012; Yfantopoulos, 2013; Barros, 2013).

Concerns about sustainability of health systems in advanced economies are not new. In fact, structural or system-level aspects — such as aging, rigidities in social security systems, and technological advancements — have increasingly pressed the fiscal envelope (Heller, 2013; Hou *et al.*, 2013). The crisis has served as a catalyst for change since it has further raised the level of alert and created a more conducive environment for reforms. Crisis is an opportunity for efficiency gains. But the challenge is that, where system reforms have already squeezed efficiency, essential services can suffer (for example, loss of breadth, scope, or depth of coverage in a way that jeopardizes vulnerable groups). When system vulnerability is increasing, coordination between macro stabilization and sectoral needs also becomes more important because what might be penny-wise may well end up being pound-foolish (Gené-Badia *et al.*, 2012)[61] by undermining long-term investments in human capital.

An overview paper on the impact and policy implications of the crisis in Europe (WHO, 2013b) presents a number of illustrative examples of good and bad practices in health sector responses to the crisis and fiscal pressure. The main policy response options are summarized in Table 1 in Annex A1 and are adapted to fit the health systems vulnerability assessment framework proposed in Chapter 2 of Hou *et al.* (2013). Country cases on Greece, Ireland, and Portugal provide details on the triggers, fiscal impact, and health sector responses by these governments during the recent crisis (see Chapter 5 in Hou *et al.* (2013)). Overall, there have been clear efficiency gains across Greece, Ireland, and Portugal. However, as with all complex reforms, it is difficult to find cases of absolute success. Conflicting objectives have led some countries to backtrack on the depth, scope or breadth of coverage.

Two main conclusions can be drawn from the country cases. First, the political and economic dynamics of reform processes between the health sector and the ministry of finance, as well as within the sector, are critical. Political economy is especially important if there is not enough time for evidence-based priority setting. Second, further developing and applying country-level monitoring tools and early warning systems could help evidence-based responses (Hou *et al.*, 2013).

Notes: The analysis underlying this box applied the subregional classification for the Europe and Central Asia (ECA) Region used by the World Bank, which classifies the ECA region into 10 subgroups (ECCU1–ECCU10).
Sources: Based on Hou *et al.* (2013) and Velenyi and Smitz (2014).

[61] The Spanish crisis has raised concerns related to this very issue. Recent reforms have achieved the immediate goal of balancing annual budgets, but may prove to have negative long-term effects that may adversely impact the system.

because of an inability or unwillingness to generate sufficient revenues to pay for them, and when they cannot — or will not — allow any further "crowding out" of other forms of government spending (OECD, 2010). Achieving "value for money" in the sense of economic sustainability (Thomson *et al.*, 2009)[62] is not sufficient for the sector to operate within government budget constraints. When fiscal space is binding, the health sector must find ways to leverage new sources of finance to keep economically meritorious but financially unsustainable programs funded. This requires a thorough understanding of the general and sector-specific fiscal space contexts, as well as how macro-fiscal and sector-level objectives can be reconciled (see more in Box 4).

Box 5. The dynamics of creating fiscal space — reducing the disconnect between macro-economic and sector policymaking

Goldsbrough *et al.* (2007) notes that there is often a disconnect between macroeconomic and health sector policymaking, on the one hand, with key fiscal decisions made without understanding the potential consequences for the health sector; and on the other hand, the consequences of increasing or reallocating government spending on the country's macroeconomic and fiscal position.

A paper that discusses fiscal space for heath in the context of attaining UHC proposes some areas where clarity is required for a constructive dialogue between ministries of health, and finance and planning. The objective of a health financing policy dialogue — for example, in the context of developing a health care financing strategy or engaging in the MTEF — is to come to a common understanding between the Ministry of Health (MOH) and Ministry of Planning and Finance (MPF) about: (i) The role of the health sector in contributing to development objectives; (ii) the role the government plays in the health sector; (iii) the goals for the health sector and the resources required to achieve those goals; and (iv) how much priority will be given to health in the government budget (Cashin, 2014).

Discussions between the MPF and MOH are characterized by managing resources at the national and sector level to enable development objectives and

(*Continued*)

[62] Judging how much public resources should be spent on health care at a given point in time can depend on two different measures of "sustainability" (Thomson *et al.*, 2009): (i) Financial sustainability; (ii) economic sustainability. The latter is defined as "So long as the value produced by health care exceeds its opportunity cost, that is the value that would have been gained by spending on other areas, then growth in health spending can be said to be economically sustainable". Once this cost becomes too high, and better gains would be achieved by spending elsewhere (either in the private sector or for other components of public spending), then health spending becomes economically unsustainable.

Box 5. (***Continued***)

expectations regarding what can be attained within the given budget envelope. This common understanding should be built on a realistic picture of the country's macroeconomic and fiscal context, the constraints and competing priorities in the budget-setting process, and what the health sector needs in order to achieve the agreed upon objectives (Cashin, 2014). Thus, to enter fiscal space discussions with ministries of planning and finance, it is imperative for the health sector to have an informed view on the following central questions[63]:

- What is the current level of health spending per capita, relative to the budget, and to the economy?
- What are the main sources of health funding and do these cover current needs?
- Is the health sector spending wisely (efficiently)? If not, what are the main sources of inefficiency at macro- and micro-levels?
- How are expenditures in the sector expected to change given the medium- to long-term policy priorities and objectives, and taking into account change in the demographic and epidemiological profiles?
- Is there a funding gap to finance sector objectives?
- Can the funding gap be closed by identifying and harnessing efficiency gains?
- If efficiency gains are not sufficient or immediate, is there a way to leverage more resources?
- What are the most feasible and least disruptive ways to leverage resources — Considering timeliness of resource need and future implications of the source for the sector, as well as macro-fiscal objectives?

The framework proposed by Heller (2005; 2006) and adapted to the health sector by Tandon and Cashin (2010) identifies 5 ways to create fiscal space, including: (i) Create conducive macroeconomic conditions, particularly GDP growth and tax revenues (Heller, 2005)[64]; (ii) reprioritize health within the overall government budget; (iii) increase revenue sources for the health sector (e.g., earmarked taxes, income levy, value added tax, etc., or through borrowing from domestic or external sources); (iv) obtaining external grants, also known as DAH[65]; and (v) achieving

[63] This box is based on ongoing analytical work by the author in Botswana, Lesotho, and Mozambique which apply diagnostics such as PER, PETS/QSDS survey, and FSA.

[64] Additional revenues can be raised through tax measures or by strengthening tax administration (Heller, 2005).

[65] For more, see a discussion on making fiscal space happen in a world of scaled-up aid by Heller *et al.* (2006).

efficiency gains.[66] The general framework also discusses seigniorage; having the central bank print money in order to lend it to the government. However, this is generally not a feasible or practical option given that it undermines long-term macroeconomic stability. These sources are not independent of each other. For example, 'crowd out' — when external grants for health may encourage a government to spend less of its own resources on health — is extensively discussed in the literature (See Box 6).

Fiscal space discussions and decisions are complex — they require both technical knowledge and political and economic leverage. The sector-specific framework argues that some resources are more feasible to obtain than others, given the locus of the control levers for generating additional resources.

For example, fiscal space options that depend primarily on the macroeconomic and fiscal context and fall under the ambit of ministries of planning and finance 'fungibility' such as growth-driven fiscal expansion, domestic revenue generation through taxes, or domestic/external borrowing — are given lower probability in resulting in additional financing because these sources are beyond the sector's control (Tandon and Cashin, 2010; Tandon *et al.*, 2014). As argued in papers on fiscal space for health (Tandon and Cashin, 2010; Tandon *et al.*, 2014), the availability of such resources is typically more uncertain because the health sector competes with meritorious investment options from other sectors and, as such, the allocation decisions are a complex mix of technical and political economic considerations. Further, taxation affects demand for goods and services, as well as the labor market and, hence, competitiveness. Last, because borrowing comes at the cost of interest, it affects debt sustainability and fiscal space in the long run.

Although reprioritization[67] is also beyond the control of ministries of health, unlike taxation and borrowing, it takes advantage of existing government resources by strategically cutting lower priority expenditures in order to make room for more desirable ones, for example, within or across sectors (Heller, 2005; Tandon *et al.*, 2014). Reprioritization has become more prominent as a policy option for fiscal space. For example, Sachs (2012) argues that reprioritization combined with donor financing is necessary to address the fiscal space for health challenge, and that fiscal space contributions from other modalities — such as general revenue increase, additional borrowing, and inflationary financing — are minimal at best.

---

[66] Although in practice efficiency gains have proven to be difficult to identify and address, efficiency gains should be investigated both at the macro-level, which is done through PER (see Section "Diagnostic Tools and Government Policies to Better Invest in Health for Growth"), and at the micro-level, which is explored through facility-level data from PETS.

[67] See a thorough discussion on reprioritization by Tandon *et al.* (2014).

Box 6. Development assistance for health

The impact of development assistance on government expenditures — and whether it replaces domestic budget, hence creating a zero-sum effect — is a much studied and debated topic. Indeed, from a development effectiveness perspective, it is critical to understand how the financial support of international finance and development institutions can leverage government efforts to raise and spend more domestic resources.

Development assistance for health (Velenyi and Smitz, 2014)[68] has more than quadrupled since 1990 (Ravishankar *et al.*, 2009). However, the rate of increase in DAH appears to have slowed in recent years (IHME, 2010a, b). With respect to vulnerability and sustainability, a common concern is that DAH may crowd out public budget allocations. Until recently, the literature has been limited on the crowd-out effect of DAH on GHE and to what extent such resources are spent outside the health sector (fungibility) (Gottret and Schieber, 2006). However, given the 2008–2009 economic crisis and the consequent increased interest in changes in the pattern of aid flows, a number of papers have contributed to better understanding the dynamics of DAH on domestic spending. For example, using panel data of low-income countries for 1995–2006, Lu *et al.* find that for every US$1 of DAH given to the government, health expenditure falls between US$0.43 and US$1.14 (Lu *et al.*, 2010). However, they find that assistance given to nongovernmental organizations increases domestic resources for health from US$0.56 to US$1.72. Consistent results are found by others (IHME, 2010a, b).

Variations in methodological rigor may be behind some of the inconsistencies in findings. For example, Ooms *et al.* (2010) advise against relying too heavily on the findings by Lu *et al.* given the methodological limitations of the study, and conclude that donor policy decisions should not rely on cross-country regressions but on case-by-case analysis. In a macro analysis, Crivelli *et al.* (2012) investigate the broader question of the effect of foreign aid on government revenues. Their findings confirm that the effect of aid on the domestic budget (tax revenues) is heterogeneous, with grants creating a negative effect and loans creating a positive effect. The conclusion from these studies is that aid cannot be treated homogenously, and project-specific or budget support, grants, or loans should be treated separately.

Source: Velenyi and Smitz (2014).

[68] See Preker and Langenbrunner (2005) and Preker *et al.* (2007) for more discussion on resource allocation and purchasing.

Attaining the unfinished MDG agenda and moving toward post-2015 UHC targets despite aging populations and the increasing burden of NCDs sets a policy context that is favorable to promoting the reprioritization agenda. However, as Tandon *et al.* point out, reprioritization is a challenge for ministries of health dealing with ministries of finance and planning, especially as health is often perceived to be an "unproductive and inefficient" sector (Tandon *et al.*, 2014). Presentation of the 'health as an investment' case to get resources reallocated to the sector can also be a challenge because changes in population-level health outcomes require medium to long-term time horizons to materialize, which spans beyond government cycles. From a practical perspective, a recent review of fiscal space in health concludes that health ministries could do more to develop evidence-based, cost-effective expenditure and implementation plans, ensuring that resource allocations are fully and effectively absorbed, and providing evidence of impact of interventions on health outputs and outcomes (Powell-Jackson *et al.*, 2012). Further, health as an investment should be considered and traced across political cycles, inline with long-term development objectives.

Although the three pillars discussed above — macroeconomic conditions, increase in revenue sources, and reprioritization within the government budget — are largely exogenous to the health sector, it is critical to analyze and understand them to be able to inform and influence medium- to long-term allocation and investment decisions.

There are other sources, however, that are more relevant in the short- to medium-term and more likely to succeed, as these are within the direct control of the sector. These are efficiency gains and external financing, also known as DAH. Because raising additional resources or reallocation from other sectors is a complex process, as discussed above, the primary option to increase fiscal space for the sector lies within the sector itself.

Efficiency analysis is the starting point for identifying fiscal space (see the discussion on PER and PETS in Section "Retrospective and Prospective Assessment of Health Spending"). Indeed, it is often argued that although increased funding for the health sector may be needed, it is not an objective of health financing policy dialogue *per se*. Easing of constraints on the pooling of funds, resource allocation within the health sector, and purchasing approaches may be equally or more important for the health sector to get better value from existing funds (Kutzin *et al.* 2010).[69]

[69] See Preker and Langenbrunner (2005) and Preker *et al.* (2007) for more discussion on resource allocation and purchasing.

Consequently, efficiency analyses at the macro-[70] and micro[71]-levels are critical to inform policymakers on more accessible fiscal space options. For example, such analysis could provide estimates of the resource gaps that could be met through efficiency gains and, should a funding gap remain to obtain sector objectives, identify what portion of the funding gap could be managed through growth-induced revenue increase, increasing reliance on external resources, or reprioritization.

External assistance for health has been a significant source of funding in low-income countries. For example, in 2012 the average of external aid for health as share of total health expenditures in low-income countries was 30%, with the lowest share in Bangladesh (7.15%) and the highest in Haiti (66.9%). Although there have been more or less successful efforts to make aid flows more transparent by encouraging development partners to channel their resources to a pooled fund for sector budget support and use the government's budgeting and resource tracking system to register funds, aid poses a challenge with respect to the predictability and flexibility of resource use, which makes planning at the sectoral level difficult. It appears that aid is a viable, important, and — if resources are pre-committed and traced — perhaps it can become an increasingly more predictable source. Yet, in the medium- to long-run, it is critical to reduce aid dependency and the consequent exposure of the health sector to exogenous factors, such as economic downturns that would adversely affect aid flows and support to the sector. This is particularly, relevant for some disease-specific interventions, which are heavily tied to aid flows, such as HIV/AIDS. Another noted challenge is absorptive capacity, which can lead to unused external sources.

A review (Powell-Jackson *et al.* 2012) of the fiscal space literature concludes that few studies scratch beyond the surface in terms of understanding *how* countries have created fiscal space to attain health sector objectives. The review notes that, at the country level, most FSAs are forward-looking, and that the literature overall is skewed toward conceptual discussions rather than data-driven, rigorous examination of how fiscal space has been created, whether it has been successful and what the options are if further financing is required to meet sector objectives. There are a few analyses, however, that can provide good examples for fiscal space assessment in low-income contexts, such as the country-specific work on Indonesia

[70]These include institutional efficiency analysis, such as in fund flows across the system, across regions and levels of care. Efficiency analysis at the macro level also involves investigation of the effectiveness of the resource allocation formula in use.

[71]This includes facility-level data analysis (e.g., from PETS/QSDS types surveys, or the World Bank's new SDI survey series in Africa, which were launched in 2012). Micro analyses (e.g., cost effectiveness and data envelopment analysis) require disaggregated data on resource flows and allocation of funds by service type (preventive/treatment) and by expenditure category (wages, drugs, equipment, capital expenditures, administrative expenses, etc.), as well as output in terms of patient volumes by service type, and cost per patient using the aggregated figures.

(Tandon, 2009), Uganda (Okwero *et al.*, 2010) or Ghana (Schieber *et al.*, 2012). The authors propose that future research should place more emphasis on in-depth retrospective studies of how countries have created fiscal space, including experience in using innovative sources of financing, and cross-country analysis of how responsive health spending is to the macroeconomic environment.

Given that fiscal space assessment is not the main focus of this chapter, only one pillar is discussed below in relatively more depth, but is limited to the context of Sub-Saharan Africa. Section "One Modality of Generating Fiscal Space" offers an illustration of the importance of efficiency gains or value for money, which was identified as an entry point to identify fiscal space within the system.

One modality of generating fiscal space: Improving efficiency and value for money

In general, to attain the health targets — which are critical inputs into development — money matters; particularly in low-income contexts, where per capita spending on health is typically low. The World Health Organization (WHO) kicked off the new millennium by making a strong case for mobilizing more resources for health. The decade closed with another high-level push for "more and better resources … if the health MDGs are to be reached in 2015." (UN, 2000; TIIFHS, 2009; WHO, 2010) The first six of the 10 recommendations by the Taskforce on Innovative International Financing for Health Systems (McCoy and Brikci, 2010) aimed to raise an additional \$10 billion per year for health to reach \$60 per capita. Of this total, 60–80% of the additional funds were targeted to Sub-Saharan Africa (SSA) (Avila *et al.*, 2013).

However, increasing the level of funds in itself is not sufficient to attain sector and development objectives. Buying "value for money" — where the benefits of spending exceed the costs — is what matters. This involves: (i) A more complex assessment of the use of public funds; (ii) a thorough understanding of the health system context; and (iii) an understanding of the effects of government efficiency, governance and accountability on fund use.

In practice, it is difficult for policymakers to decide what qualifies as "good value for money" because this hinges on how benefits are defined and is further complicated by measurement challenges of benefits and costs. Given that value for money is defined as benefits exceeding costs, it could be improved by a number of changes, including (i) reducing costs through improved efficiency; (ii) improving benefits, for example, by providing enhanced quality of care; or (iii) the combination of cost reduction and benefit improvement through, for example, introducing performance-based payment for a defined volume and quality of care. Value-for-money changes correspond to the main pillars of health system objectives (OECD,

2010), including (i) access to care and financial protection;[71a] (ii) quality of care and responsiveness; (iii) sustainability of health care subject to government financial resources; and (iv) efficiency of service delivery. Briefly, in low-income contexts, this implies that value for money can be improved if access to a defined quality of essential care and financial protection is improved, and this is done in an efficient and sustainable manner, within the health sector's budget envelope and aligned with the macro-fiscal environment. There are a number of ways to improve access to quality health services at reasonable costs, including defining the benefit package based on evidence; purchasing defined volume and quality of care through pooled financing mechanisms (e.g., insurance); reforming provider payment (e.g., pay for performance), rationalizing service delivery across the levels of care and improving referral systems; use of technology to improve the efficiency of service delivery and accountability.

1. Value for Money — "Best Buys"

One pragmatic way to improve "value for money" is by targeting diseases that have proven to be both financially and economically costly given their weight in the burden of disease. Globally, in 2001, the Commission on Macroeconomics and Health (WHO, 2001) concluded that "*... extending the coverage of health services and a small number of critical interventions to the world's poor could save millions of lives, reduce poverty, spur economic development, and promote global security.*"

Consequently, targeting these conditions, which account for approximately 35% of DALYs of the total disease burden in Sub-Saharan Africa in 2010

Table 8. DALYs for 10 major cause groups, Sub-Saharan Africa, 2012

Rank	**Causes**	**DALYs (000s)**	**% DALYs**	**DALYs/100,000 population**
0	All Causes	690,532	100	75,622
1	Lower respiratory infections	69,740	10.1	7,637
2	HIV/AIDS	68,109	9.9	7,459
3	Malaria	51,326	7.4	5,621
4	Diarrheal diseases	49,280	7.1	5,397
5	Preterm birth complications	36,439	5.3	3,991
6	Birth asphyxia and birth trauma	34,166	5.0	3,742
7	Protein–energy malnutrition	20,304	2.9	2,224
8	Meningitis	19,708	2.9	2,158
9	Neonatal sepsis and infections	16,997	2.5	1,861
10	Congenital anomalies	14,437	2.1	1,581

Source: WHO (2014).

[71a]Regarding the measurement of financial protection, see, for example Wagstaff (2008) and Moreno-Serra *et al.* (2011).

(WHO, 2015) and mostly have proven cost-effective interventions to prevent and treat them, are expected to improve not only critical health outcomes but also the "value for money" proposition of public expenditures on health.

These communicable diseases pose a serious threat not only because of their direct effect on health and health expenditures, but through various pathways, on household wealth and, at the macro level, economic growth. For example, besides the human cost, HIV/AIDS is having profound effects on Africa's economic development and hence its ability to cope with the pandemic. While the impact of HIV/AIDS on people has been well documented, it has been much more difficult to observe the pandemic's effects on the African economy as a whole or to assess how it might affect Africa's future development. Cross-country regressions for the period between 1990 and 1997 suggest that HIV/AIDS has reduced the rate of growth of Africa's per capita income by 0.7 percentage points per year (Bonnel, 2000). For those African countries affected by malaria, growth was further lowered by 0.3 percentage points per year. In general, various factors related to poverty, inequality, gender inequality, labor mobility and ethnic fractionalization have facilitated the rapid spread of HIV in Sub-Saharan Africa. But what has enabled HIV/AIDS to undermine economic and social development is the erosion of some of the main determinants of economic growth such as social capital, domestic savings, and human capital. Through such channels, the HIV epidemic was transformed from a health issue into an economic disease that impairs economic and social development. Because it prevents an increasing share of the population from participating in economic growth, the HIV/AIDS epidemic increases poverty. The result is a vicious circle whereby HIV/AIDS reduces economic growth and increases poverty, which in turn accelerates the spread of HIV. Without strong and immediate action, it will prove quite difficult to overcome the cost of inaction latter on.

As the burden of disease statistics show, maternal, neonatal, and nutritional causes of death account for 17.7% of DALYs in Sub-Saharan Africa in 2010 (WHO, 2015). Hence, maternal and child health and nutrition interventions are critical to reduce the high fatality rates and morbidities arising from these conditions. There is now a clear set of globally recognized essential interventions, commodities and guidelines for reproductive, maternal, newborn, and child health (RMNCH) that have been demonstrated to achieve significant and rapid progress for RMNCH outcomes. A number of tools exist to help governments in prioritizing, costing, and phasing interventions.[72]

[72] For example, the 'List' tool facilitates comparisons between alternate investment strategies over a specified period for child survival outcomes. The 'One Health' tool enables country-level planning, costing, impact analysis, budgeting, and strategic financial planning for all major health system components. www.futuresinstitute.org/onehealth.aspx.

Maternal and childhood nutrition has substantial effect on economic growth, as underscored in the Copenhagen Consensus (2012),[73] and this is particularly relevant in low-income countries where nutrition is at the heart of economic development and poverty reduction efforts. Better nutrition increases productivity and thus economic growth through increased labor supply. The productivity losses by malnutrition occur through three pathways: Direct loss of physical productivity, indirect loss from loss in schooling and poor cognitive development, and losses from high use of health care resources. For example, evidence from Africa shows that a 1% loss in adult height as a result of child stunting is associated with a 1.4% loss in productivity. Anemia is associated with a 2.5% of reduction in wages. Productivity losses at the individual level are estimated to be more than 10% of life-time earnings, which at the macro-level can lead to a 2–3% loss in GDP. The economic benefits of improved nutrition come from reduced infant and child mortality, and reduced health care costs for sick children. Substantial benefits accrue from productivity gains due to physical stature, as well as from increased schooling performance and cognitive ability, which affects lifetime potential. Based on very high cost-effectiveness ratios, the Copenhagen Consensus concluded that out of 30 potential development investments, interventions to reduce under nutrition in preschoolers is the best way to advance global welfare.

Despite the proven effectiveness of and overwhelming evidence on the economic impact of maternal and child health and nutrition interventions, the benefits of these services do not adequately reach the target groups in the majority of low-income countries because of both supply- and demand-side constraints, which include availability and quality challenges (supply-side) and physical and financial access to care (demand-side). In the case of malnutrition, although both the private and social returns to improved nutrition are recognized and high, malnutrition has continued to persist. In fact, progress has been slow, partially because poverty imposes a constraint on households to invest more resources in children. Information asymmetry in the context of nutrition can take place either because mothers do not known when the child becomes malnourished and only start acting by the time the condition is severe, or because good nutrition practices are not known and, hence, they do not provide the right

[73] In May 2012, the third global Copenhagen Consensus was held, gathering economists to analyze the costs and benefits of different approaches to tackling the world's biggest problems. The aim was to provide an answer to the question: If you had $75 bn for worthwhile causes, where should you start? A panel including four Nobel laureates met in Copenhagen, Denmark, in May 2012. The panel's deliberations were informed by 30 new economic research papers that were written just for the project by scholars from around the world. See more online at: http://www.copenhagenconsensus.com/copenhagen-consensus-iii and https://en.wikipedia.org/wiki/Copenhagen_Consensus#cite_note-5.

nutritional mix even when they could afford it. Beyond the public good nature of nutrition interventions, which accrue benefits to the whole society, the economic impact and redistributive effects of investing in nutrition provide a clear argument for public intervention in this area.

2. Systems Approach

Attaining financing targets is not an end. Meeting sectoral and development targets requires complementary governance actions and a systems approach. As discussed above, in addition to the increased focus on what African countries can do to raise public and private resources for health (*more money for health*), there has been a growing emphasis on improving value for money of existing resources for health (*more health for money*). Following the decade of fund mobilization, particularly leveraged by the Millennium Development Goals (MDGs) which were launched in 2000, there has been increasing attention to the role of health systems and creating systems through which the population — particularly vulnerable groups such as women and children — is able to access quality health services without suffering financial hardship. Countries and their development partners (DPs) need to not only mobilize resources but also apply a systems approach to development. In the context of health financing priorities, beyond resource mobilization, this involves (i) efficient allocation of essential health services to underserved regions/populations; (ii) improved risk pooling; and (iii) strategic purchasing (see Box 7) for quality and efficiency. With UHC framing the post-2015 development agenda in health, focusing on systems to find sustainable solutions that deliver quality health care to the population has become ever more important.

However, system fragmentation remains a challenge. Fragmentation is associated with aid dependency and the complex aid architecture that governments and, in the context of the health sector, ministries of health face.

In general, the polarization between "vertical" financing (aiming for disease-specific results) and "horizontal" financing (aiming for improved health systems) of health services in developing countries is potentially destructive in that it neglects a possible "diagonal" financing (aiming for disease-specific results through improved health systems) (Jamison *et al.*, 2013). For example, in the context of HIV/AIDS, which has triggered a rapid increase of external resource flows over the past two decades, a common criticism is that, despite the great opportunities of improving health service delivery, this large-scale funding has been primarily disease-specific, neglecting other aspects of the health system. To understand this challenge, Yu *et al.* (2008) explore whether scaled-up investments in HIV/AIDS programs — driven primarily by global health partnerships — is strengthening the health systems of developing countries or whether they have unintended negative effects. They find that the evidence is mixed — mostly positive but there

Box 7. Strategic purchasing

Strategic purchasing of health services involves a continuous search for the best ways to maximize health system performance by deciding which interventions should be purchased, from whom, and how to pay for them (Preker and Langenbrunner, 2005; Langenbrunner *et al.*, 2009).

In public service delivery, the premise for shifting from passive budgeting to strategic purchasing is that it is necessary to separate the functions of financing from the production of services to improve public sector performance and accountability. The publication *Spending Wisely: Buying Health Services for the Poor* (Perker and Langenbrunner, 2005) focuses on public service delivery in the health sector, getting better value for money on health care. The authors draw on knowledge gained from experience of strategic purchasing in other sectors of the economy and extend it to the health sector in developing countries. Applying organizational and institutional economics and management science as theoretical underpinnings, the book presents arguments for a fundamental shift in the way public money is spent on health services to better serve the poor.

In the context setting the book, Preker applies agency theory to explain deviations from the optimal purchasing arrangement. The concept of 'multiplicitous agency' — when one party has to act as agent for two or more principals — can lead to irreconcilable differences for the purchaser. An example is when institutional actors in the ministry of health are more concerned about aggregate health outcomes while the ministry of finance is more concerned about the overall fiscal affordability of the health sector (Perker, 2005).

Although strategic purchasing of health care provides many advantages, the author warns too often decisions are made based on technical criteria that ignore the interest of patient and the poor. This conclusion implies that including a pro-poor focus under the strategic framework of resource allocation and purchasing is imperative. Further, assessing the performance of purchasing reforms should be explicit about the equity considerations in terms of understanding which concept and what weights are used (see more on this in Box 8 based on Hauck *et al.*, 2005).

Source: Preker and Langenbrunner (2005).

are some negative externalities. They conclude that, rather than engaging in endless debates about the comparative advantages of vertical and horizontal approaches, countries and their development partners should continue both (i) to maximize the positive synergies of investment in HIV/AIDS and other priority health programs; and (ii) to increase funding for universal primary health care.

3. Government Efficiency, Governance, and Accountability

A key message of the 2004 World Development Report, *Making Services Work for Poor People* (World Bank, 2003), which investigates how countries can accelerate progress towards the MDGs, is that success in reaching the millennium development targets, including in health, depends not just on faster economic growth and the corresponding flow of resources, but on the ability to translate those resources into basic services. The conclusion is that a substantial increase in resources must be accompanied — or, possibly, preceded — by more effective use of all resources, internal and external. An efficient government is a government that does the most with the resources it has. Government dollars are tax dollars, and the public deserves a government that spends their money as productively as possible. However, there are a number of reasons why efficiency (see more in Box 8) can falter, including weak incentives for performance, corruption, imperfect monitoring (if any), and administrative logjams. The report offers a practical framework for using resources more effectively through the 'long'[74] or 'short'[75] routes of accountability (see more in Annex 3).

Health expenditure and the economic cycle

In addition to the MDG and post-2015 development agendas (see Box 1), the question of growth and development through the health channel has also been enjoying increasing attention because of the recent GEC, which began as early as 2007. The crisis brought renewed attention to the impact of economic downturns on health sectors worldwide and revealed that no country is immune to external challenges (Hou *et al.*, 2013). One implication of the crisis was the increased vulnerability of both the health sector and individual households to fluctuations in government expenditures. Specifically, it was feared that the depth and length of the crisis may have increased the likelihood of pro-cyclical policies in public health expenditure in response to economic contraction and the subsequent increase in budget constraints (fiscal consolidation). At its extreme, it has been feared that fiscal consolidation can undermine health systems because of foregoing investments, which may lead to increased spending in the long run. Although the relationship between health spending and development in the context of economic downturns has been under-researched, countercyclical government spending has been found to be essential in fostering long-term economic and human development objectives (Brahmbhatt and Canuto, 2012; Braun and di Gresia, 2003; Darby and Melitz, 2008; Doytch *et al.*, 2010).

[74] This is also referred to as the indirect route of accountability, whereby poor people or citizens influence policymakers or politicians and then the politicians influence the providers to deliver quality care.
[75] The 'short route' stands for direct accountability between users and providers, for example where consumers and communities have a direct role in determining service delivery.

Box 8. Efficiency analysis and priority setting in health care

Diagnostics Approaches for Health Sector Efficiency Analysis

As discussed under Section "Health Outcomes and Economic Growth", globally there is significant variation in the returns on investment in health, measured in population health outcomes. One driver behind the tenuous link between health spending and health outcomes is efficiency in the sector,[76] including the efficient use of public resources to turn them into health outcomes.

Efficiency of public resource use is particularly important in resource-constrained context, where the absolute level of public expenditure on capita on health investments is typically low given the limited budget envelope. To enable improvements in population health status and, in broader terms, in human and economic development, budgets can be complemented with ODA resources. These two factors[77] motivate the diagnostic approaches discussed in Section "Retrospective and Prospective Assessment of Health Spending" (PER, PETS, and QSDS), which have been implemented in a number of countries to shed light on efficiency challenges and advise value-for-money decisions. Jointly, these approaches can be used to assess the efficiency of the sector, including allocative[78], technical, and productive efficiency.[79]

Despite their complexity and limitations, PERs, PETS, and QSDS have been instrumental in generating evidence for policy setting (Gurkan *et al.*, 2009; World Bank, 2009; Gauthier and Ahmed, 2012; Gaudin and Yazbeck, 2014; Gauthier, 2006).

- Based on a review of PERs implemented with support from the World Bank between 2000 and 2011, Gaudin and Yazbeck (2014) find that during the study period there were 70 reports across 60 countries and 4 sub-national states from all regions, with the majority of the reviews done in Africa (22), followed by Europe and Central Asia (18), and be Latin America and the

(*Continued*)

[76] See more on the measurement of efficiency in health care in Jacobs *et al.* (2006).

[77] This refers to low and inefficient public expenditures and external resources in the system/budget, which often comes with increased attention to public financial management (PFM) and accountability as part of the development effectiveness agenda.

[78] Allocative efficiency refers to the right level and combination of "factor inputs" (can be in monetized terms e.g., US$) to devote to the health system.

[79] Productive efficiency means that output cannot be produced at lower cost, that is, where the provider operates at the production possibility frontier. In practical terms, improved productive efficiency leads to increased savings.

Box 8. (***Continued***)

Caribbean Region (12) (see more Under Section "Retrospective and Prospective Assessment of Health Spending" and in Gaudin and Yazbeck, 2014). General PERs vary in terms of the depth they discuss the health sector, and the sector specific coverage also varies regarding its coverage and methodological depth, making systematic comparisons difficult. The observed variability in depth and quality of the analytical work has been calling for standard setting in PER implementation.

- As to PETS, the first tracking survey was implemented in Uganda in the education and health sectors in 1996. The hypothesis was that leakages in resource flows were behind the stagnant performance despite increasing resource flows into these sectors (Ablo and Reinikka, 1998). The tracking survey showed that from every dollar of school grant that targeted primary schools only 13 cents reached the intended beneficiaries. This finding triggered policy reforms, including an information campaign, which aimed to increase accountability by publishing in the newspapers the intergovernmental transfers of capitation grants on a monthly basis. Data from an impact evaluation PETS between 1999 and 2001 showed that as a result of the intervention the leakage reduced to 18% by 2001. The success of this first PETS, particularly the direct impact of the findings on policymaking in the education sector and the subsequent improvement in the efficiency of public resource use drew considerable attention to this newly proposed tool (Reinikka and Svenson, 2004). Tracking surveys, however, are not without challenges. Lindelow (2006) describes the conceptual and practical challenge of implementing a PETS in Mozambique, among them are system constraints to make some resources traceable (e.g., soft vs. hard budgeting, domestic vs. external resources), definitional issues and related measurement problems (e.g., what does 'leakage' mean), and data limitations. He offers three main points as conclusion. First, while tracking surveys can be useful tools for diagnosing and understanding public expenditure management issues[80] in sectors with service delivery functions, they are by no means the only tool, and in many cases may not be the best tool (Lindelow, 2006). Audits, institutional reviews, assessments of financial management procedures, and other approaches all have important roles to play. Second, when tracking surveys are driven by a

(*Continued*)

[80] These can include corruption, allocation decisions, compliance with administrative procedures, accountability arrangements.

Box 8. (***Continued***)

general question and a tight deadline the result is inevitably disappointing. He cautions regarding the design, implementation, and analysis of PETS and advises to start small and draw on qualitative assessment prior to fielding the survey. Third, due to the complexity of institutional factors, tracking surveys tend to be better at diagnosis than making inferences about the determinants of the outcomes of interest. These experiences suggest tracking surveys are valuable but require through identification, design, and implementation, as well as managing expectation on what they can and cannot address and help with.

- The first PETS and QSDS were implemented in Uganda, respectively in 1996 and 2000. For a stock-taking in a *PETS/QSDS Guidebook*, using the World Bank's web platform, Gauthier and Ahmed (2012) found more than 50 surveys implemented in more than three dozen countries between 1996 and 2009. The majority of these surveys were in the Africa Region (66%), followed by East Asia and the Pacific (14%) and the Europe and Central Asia (8%) regions. The explorations mainly focused on the health (43%) and education (42%) sectors. In sum, efforts are targeted to countries and regions where public resource flows require substantial efficiency improvements.

Economic Evaluation to Inform Priority Setting in Advanced Economies: Examples from the OECD Context

While diagnostic approaches such as PERs and PETS are useful to inform policymakers on where and how efficiency gains could be attained, they do not provide evidence on how to choose between alternative interventions or technologies that compete for scarce public resources. Priority setting, on the other hand, is a systematic approach to inform the choice between alternatives to distribute the available resources for health care optimally among competing demands subject to constraints (Hauck *et al.*, 2005). However, although there is consensus on the importance of using objective criteria for priority setting, in reality it is difficult to operationalize it. As the authors point out, the empirical application of priority setting through economic evaluation is challenged by weaknesses in the cost-effectiveness methodology, incorporating equity considerations into this approach, and the political and institutional context in which priorities are defined and implemented (Hauck *et al.*, 2005).

Economic evaluation in health care priority setting is constrained by a number of methodological barriers, which challenge the generalizability

(*Continued*)

Box 8. (*Continued*)

(external validity) and reliability of the findings. For example, cost effectiveness ranking depends on the perspective applied (provider, societal, etc.), variations in the underlying system capacity, input costs and prices, the characteristics of the target population and the epidemiology, and uncertainty in parameters required for the economic evaluation. Given these limitations, outcomes are likely not dominant.

Despite its methodological complexity, economic evaluation is useful and has been extensively applied in advanced economies. For example, in the OECD context, Pizzi and Lofland (2006) discuss the use of economic evaluation in the health sector, offering examples for the US from the United Kingdom, Canada, and Australia, including the strength and limitations of each approach. The authors note that "most developed nations have legislation, public policies, and organizations mandating the use of economic evaluation in at least one sector of the healthcare industry, most often the pharmaceutical sector."

Economic evaluation in the UK occurs within the process of Health Technology Assessment (HTA), which includes not only pharmaceutical and devices but also procedures and organizational and support systems. HTA has been applied since the early 1990s in the National Health Service (NHS) and it was institutionalized with the establishment of the National Institute for Clinical Excellence (NICE) in 1999. NICE created a formal distinction between assessment and appraisal. Assessments are objective evaluations of technologies, whereas appraisals are subjective decisions about whether to use the given technology under review. This distinction reflects on the limitations noted by Hauck *et al.* (2005); notably that despite facts based on objective assessment, governments may make priority setting decisions based on criteria other than cost-effectiveness, such as the social preference and poverty sensitivity of the government — which can be reflected through equity weights in economic evaluation — and political economic considerations. Despite the value of institutionalized economic analysis, there have been criticisms, including that the perspective taken for the economic analysis is that of the NHS' and not of the society's as a whole, that the political context may influence recommendations, and that the majority of evaluations focus on pharmaceuticals whilst in terms of sectoral share this occupies 10–15% of total health care costs. The effect of economic evaluation at the policy level, however, can vary a great deal depending on the health care system. For example, the authors contrast the UK's centralized system where recommendations are universally implemented with the complex institutional setup in the United States, which is characterized by

(*Continued*)

Box 8. (*Continued*)

multiple payers. They suggest that for economic evaluation to have similar effect in the US, where recommendations are not mandated but adapted by providers and payers, it would be required to include all stakeholders' perspective and disclose the data on which the recommendation is based.

Use of Economic Evaluation in Low Income, Low Institutional Capacity, and Low Data Availability Context

As shown above, the use of economic evaluation to inform policy processes is more widespread in developed economies. The demand for such assessments is lower in developing economies. Although one could argue that robust technical analyses would be even more relevant in severely resource constrained contexts, the political and institutional reality and data limitations can reduce the role that economic evaluation plays in priority setting in low-income and low capacity environment.

Even in areas where there is clear interest in economic assessments, cost-effectiveness for priority setting remains underutilized. As discussed in Section "Health Outcomes and Economic Growth", over the past decade, there has been an increasing momentum of exploring the effect of performance-based financing (PBF) mechanisms in developing context on provider behavior, and through that, on population health outcomes, mostly linked to the MDG health targets. Given the innovative nature of these interventions, to inform policy decisions robust impact evaluations (experimental or quasi-experimental designs) have been increasingly applied to generate estimates on effectiveness. Although the evidence base to-date is still scarce, there is a growing number of evaluations that explore the effectiveness of PBF in various contexts.

The evidence base for cost-effectiveness in the PBF evaluation context is thinner and there is less momentum and financial support to undertake such assessments. Despite its high policy relevance, cost-effectiveness has been much less thoroughly researched than the effectiveness of PBF programs. In a recent CEA study in the PBF context in Tanzania, the literature review shows that to date only 15 studies examining the cost of payment for performance (P4P) schemes have been published (Borghi *et al.*, 2015).[81] Only two of these were conducted outside of the United States and Europe. Only nine of these studies considered costs beyond the financial incentives, and only two of these studies included costs of developing and setting up the P4P scheme.

(*Continued*)

[81] In a review of the literature, Borghi *et al.* (2015) notes significant knowledge gaps in this area.

Box 8. (*Continued*)

The authors note that the costs to providers of participating in the scheme and eventual costs to patients have also been omitted from previous analyses. Outcomes, if measured, are typically restricted to changes in incentivized services, with only four studies reporting effects on outcomes and one study reporting effects on non-incentivized services. No study to date reporting on the costs or cost-effectiveness of P4P has been published from low- and lower-middle income countries.

Performing efficiency analysis (Jacobs *et al.*, 2006) and applying cost effectiveness analysis are not without challenges; these approaches face both methodological and data availability constraints and they may not be the easiest to fit into the political economic context. Nevertheless, there is increasing interest to expand economic evaluation to developing country context. Beyond the interest, however, this requires improved data availability, adapting methods to local contexts, and capacity building to apply economic evaluation to inform policy discussions.

Sources: Hauck *et al.* (2005); Pizzi and Lofland (2006); Borghi *et al.* (2015).

These intertwined themes — the cyclical nature of health spending and system vulnerability during economic crises — are explored next to raise attention to areas where further research would be beneficial to help policymakers better manage the health and growth dynamics during downturns.

- *Is counter-cyclicality a feasible future?*

The recent GEC, which started as early as 2007, has shown that no country is immune to external challenges. When policy controls are missing or not used efficiently, crises can reverse progress and positive performance even in advanced economies with AAA ratings (see Chapter 2 in Hou *et al.*, 2013; Velenyi and Smitz, 2014). The recent crisis has been unique. It emanated from advanced economies and led to prolonged stagnation and, in some cases, contraction. The depth and length of the crisis have led to fiscal turbulence that affected health sectors across a number of developed countries, requiring strategic consolidation[82] and efficiency gains to fit declining health sector budgets.

When the crisis hit, it was expected that Europe, a relatively stable and economically robust region, would have the means and tools to tackle the downturn. However, many countries did not cope well (Hou *et al.*, 2013). In the hardest

[82] High overall tax ratios in Europe put pressure for fiscal austerity on the need for spending cutbacks (Heller, 2013).

hit countries and in countries where preparedness was low, deteriorating fiscal positions have resulted in reduced fiscal space for health and, hence, procyclical policy responses (Heller, 2013; Hou *et al.*, 2013; WHO, 2013b). Such fallback into procyclical policymaking has raised concerns because, in principle, fiscal policy should avoid sudden and excessive cuts in health budgets, especially during economic shocks, when population health needs and demand for health care can rapidly increase. When demand for services increases, population coverage — particularly for essential health care and vulnerable groups — should not decline. Rather, countercyclical spending during crises is critical to protect population health and mitigate ill-health-related household financial risk. Yet, in a number of countries, obligations to meet short-term fiscal targets have compromised the government's ability to afford countercyclical responses in health (see Box 9) (Velenyi and Smitz, 2014).

Box 9. Managing the dual objectives of meeting fiscal targets and health sector objectives

Managing the dynamics or tension between fiscal discipline and consolidation and health sector objectives during crises has been a central topic for ministries of finance and health. For example, one concern expressed by Estache and Muñoz (2009) is that International Monetary Fund (IMF) conditionalities that aim at fiscal consolidation could undermine sector objectives if the focus is on short-term fiscal balance and does not include medium- to long-term growth aspects. Many analysts express concerns regarding the role of financial institutions, such as the IMF and the European Central Bank, in determining public health expenditure. In their view, conditionalities from financial institutions could lead to dismantling health systems (Baker, 2010) or chronically insufficient health budgets (Rowden, 2010). Stuckler *et al.* (2011) find that DAH is much less likely to lead to an increase in health spending in IMF-borrowing countries. They find that, on average, for each $1 of DAH, about $0.37 is added to the health system. However, evaluating IMF-borrowing vs. non-IMF-borrowing countries reveals that non-borrowers add about $0.45 whereas borrowers add less than $0.01 to the health system. This, they argue, could be because IMF macroeconomic policies specifically encourage governments to divert aid to reserves to cope with aid volatility (see more in Hudson, 2012). In addition, the Center for Global Development

(*Continued*)

Box 9. (*Continued*)

(CGD) Working Group criticizes the IMF and its programs for being too conservative by, for example, overusing wage ceilings, which could hamper sector-specific objectives.

Despite these claims and criticisms, the jury is still out on the question whether conditionalities that aim at fiscal consolidation could undermine sector objectives. Insufficient evidence and heterogeneity in methods precludes an authoritative conclusion on this matter. There is one message, however, that comes through systematically: Governments must be cautious with reform actions and go beyond planning responses for the short term. Although short-term measures to mitigate negative consequences of crises are urgent, taking a longer-term perspective that will make the health sector more resilient in the future is critical (Heller, 2013; WHO, 2009). For example, a two-wave survey of health systems in Europe (Mladovsky *et al.*, 2012; WHO, 2013b) finds that, while the majority of reforms have focused on efficiency enhancement, there have been cases that have led to a reduction in the depth, breadth, or scope of health coverage, which causes concerns not only for health outcomes but possibly also for economic growth (through the human capital channel). In the context of the recent crisis, case studies on Greece, Ireland, and Portugal (Barros, 2013; Burke *et al.*, 2013; Yfantopoulos, 2013 in Hou *et al.*, 2013) offer good illustrations of the dynamics between fiscal consolidation and health sector objectives, representing variations in country responses to the Troika's (EU–ECB–IMF) conditionalities.

Source: Velenyi and Smitz (2014).

The unexpected outcome that advanced economies have been seriously challenged by the crisis has increased concerns about the ability of governments and health sectors in low- and middle-income countries to manage the crisis and prepare for future economic downturns. Will crises reinforce the procyclical responses in developing countries, or will they be able to cope better and escape the procyclical trap (see Definitions in Box 10)? Why is countercyclical behavior important?

Countercyclical government spending has been found to be essential in fostering long-term economic and human development objectives (Brahmbhatt and Canuto, 2012; Braun and Di Gresia, 2003; Darby and Melitz, 2008; Doytch *et al.*, 2010). Standard neoclassical and Keynesian theories suggest that fiscal policy should be countercyclical, with fiscal deficits declining when the economy is expanding and increasing during downturns (Akitoby *et al.*, 2004).

Box 10. Definitions of business cycle, procyclical/countercyclical policy, and crisis typology and measurement

Business Cycle: Business cycle (or economic cycle) refers to the economy-wide fluctuation in production, trade, and economic activity in general over several months or years (Burns and Mitchell, 1946). The term "cycle" is a misnomer, because business cycle fluctuations are neither regular nor predictable. Upward and downward movements in the cycle (expansions and contractions) can be measured by the level of gross domestic product (GDP).[83] These fluctuations are measured relative to the economy's long-term growth trend (Madhani, 2010). A variable that is positively correlated with the overall state of the economy is said to be procyclical, and a variable that is negatively correlated with the overall state of the economy is said to be countercyclical.

Procyclical/Countercyclical Policy: In the context of economic policy, procyclical (countercyclical) refers to any aspect of economic policy that can magnify (attenuate) economic or financial fluctuations. Countercyclical policies cool the economy when it overheats and stimulate it when there is a downturn. Keynesian economics advocates the use of automatic and discretionary countercyclical policies to lessen the impact of the business cycle.

Defining Crisis: There is no consensus on the definitions of different types of crises despite their frequency in development economics. One of the most important common features of crises is an "abrupt" change in economic indicators. Operational definitions require an indicator and a threshold.

Crisis Typology and Indicators: In a crisis typology, Ishihara (2005) identifies seven types of crises.[84] Crisis classification matters because different types,[85] of crises affect systems and population outcomes through different pathways (see Figure A2.1 in Annex 2).

(*Continued*)

[83] In the United States, the National Bureau of Economic Research's (NBER's) seven-member Business Cycle Dating Committee examines monthly economic indicators that provide a good industry-wide economic perspective to date business cycles. They use monthly economic indicators (such as employment, real personal income, manufacturing sales, and industrial production), rather than quarterly real GDP. The monthly data allow the NBER to be more precise in setting business cycle turning points; the monthly data also typically are not subject to the same magnitude of revisions as are the quarterly GDP data (Romer, 2008).

[84] The seven types of crisis are liquidity, solvency, balance of payment, currency, external debt, growth rate, and financial.

[85] For example, Laeven and Valencia (2012) provide an update on systemic banking crises, which also explores the relationship between banking crises, currency crises, and sovereign debt crises and the likelihood and pattern of the co-occurrence of twin or triple crises.

Box 10. (*Continued*)

Measuring Crisis Depth and Length: With respect to the magnitude of crises, the literature discusses two dimensions that are relevant for quantification — depth and length. In simplified terms, a country experiences a crisis as soon as the selected crisis indicator exceeds an agreed upon threshold value (Frankel and Rose, 1996).[86] The deviation from the defined threshold, or with respect to a trend if the measurement is longitudinal, is the depth of the crisis. The start of the crisis is when the variable exceeds the threshold value, and the end of the crisis is when the indicator returns to the normal zone relative to the defined threshold. The length of the crisis is defined by the beginning and the end. In reality, it is difficult to be precise regarding the length of the crisis; hence, the need for crisis preparedness. In general, the longer the crisis is and the further away it is from the normal zone, the more severe it is. Severity can be measured, for example, in deviation from the filtered trend line in terms of standard deviation or relative to past or reference group performance in standardized *Z*-scores. These are standard metrics in the business cycle and crisis literature.

Source: Velenyi and Smitz (2014).

One component of countercyclical fiscal policy is countercyclical social policy, which includes unemployment benefits and other social transfers, as well as public expenditures on health and education (Darby and Melitz, 2008; del Granado *et al.*, 2012; Doytch *et al.*, 2010; Essama-Nssah and Moreno-Dodson, 2013; Thornton, 2008). Despite theoretical agreement on the benefits of countercyclical policies (e.g., increased cash transfers — conditional or unconditional — to the poor and vulnerable offset the effect of downturns), evidence shows that in low- and lower-middle-income countries, protecting public investments in health and maintaining public expenditures on health during crises have not been the norm (Abbas and Hiemenz, 2011; Brahmbhatt and Canuto, 2012; del Granado *et al.*, 2012; Doytch *et al.*, 2010; Lewis and Verhoeven, 2010). The consequence of procyclical behavior in less developed countries is that, rather than mitigating economic fluctuations, this behavior amplifies them, with adverse effects on government revenues, poverty levels, long-term growth, and human capital formation (Thornton, 2008).

It has been a vexing question for experts and policymakers, particularly in developing and emerging country contexts, to understand what the binding

[86] For example, negative year-on-year GDP growth; a debt-to-GDP ratio over 60%; a decrease in the value of the local currency equal to or greater than 25%, using the nominal exchange rate against the US dollar.

constraints (e.g., political economy, credit constraints, institutions, etc.) are to attaining countercyclical policymaking and, consequently, what policy options are available to break procyclical fiscal and social spending reflexes.

Notwithstanding the increased drive to understand the nature and drivers of social sector responses to economic cycles and the trend of cyclical responses over time, the empirical evidence on the relationship between business cycles and government expenditures on health is very thin (Powell-Jackson *et al.*, 2012; Velenyi and Smitz, 2014). There are only a handful of papers that explore the relationship between business cycles and social spending, and only the most recent ones have global coverage to allow for comparison across regions and income groups. From this already thin set, only a few specifically discuss the relationship between business cycles and health spending (Del Granado *et al.*, 2012; Doytch *et al.*, 2010).

Given the paucity of robust evidence on the effect of economic cycles on health spending, health economics has drawn on more established theory, empirical approaches, and findings from general fiscal policy to formulate hypotheses and guide research on the cyclicality of health spending.

The literature on cyclical policy responses to economic cycles show that, while countercyclical behavior has been primarily the privilege of advanced economies, the behavior patterns are now slowly changing. Countercyclical responses are possible, and indeed, have been observed in lower-income countries, both with respect to fiscal (Brahmbhatt and Canuto, 2012; Frankel *et al.*, 2011) and health policies (Lewis and Verhoeven, 2010; Velenyi and Smitz, 2014) — although the evidence base on the latter is in its infancy. The question, thus, remains whether the results found by Frankel and colleagues (2011) in the fiscal context — that about one-third of the developing world has been able to graduate from the procyclical trap — apply to the trend in cyclical responses of GHE to business cycles.

In the fiscal context, apart from the well-established income gradient — specifically, that poorer countries tend to be more procyclical — several factors have been found to lead to procyclical responses of fiscal policy to the business cycle, particularly in developing countries.[87] Among these, the most cited drivers of procyclical policy are political economy and constraints to accessing credit markets (Akitoby *et al.*, 2004; Calderon and Schmidt-Hebbel, 2008; Doytch *et al.*, 2010; Thornton, 2008). Therefore, studies emphasize that institutions and governance are essential companions to plain fiscal instruments, such as numerical fiscal rules or commodity stabilization funds. Hence, studies focusing on the cyclicality of health spending conjecture that the success of countercyclical response in the

[87] For more, see Thornton (2008) and references within.

health sector will also be closely related to institutional strength and governance; to the dynamics between the ministries of finance and health; and to the institutional and governance context within the sector (Velenyi and Smitz, 2014; Tandon *et al.*, 2014; Liang and Mirelman, 2014; Cashin, 2014).

Following the method presented in Frankel *et al.* (2011) in the fiscal context, one analysis (Velenyi and Smitz, 2014) that uses global data from the Fiscal Health Database[88] (World Bank, 2012a) (see more in Annex 3) investigates the relationship between business cycles and GHE by studying the change in the correlation coefficient (see more in Annex 3) for the business cycle and GHE between 1995–2002 and 2003–2010. The study had several key findings.

First, in contrast to findings in the recent wave of literature on fiscal cyclicality, which shows that an increasing share of developing countries have now become countercyclical (Brahmbhatt and Canuto, 2012; Frankel *et al.*, 2011; IMF 2009), in health expenditures there is no robust evidence to claim that developing countries have been able to escape the procyclical trap across the periods 1995–2002 and 2003–2010. While there are developing countries (LICs and LMICs) that do engage in countercyclical government health spending, the evidence on increased countercyclical behavior is robust only in the upper-middle-income (UMIC) group. Although GHE patterns during downturns are more predominantly countercyclical at the higher end of the income distribution (HICs), the recent GEC has shown that even advanced economies that have robust social safety nets can fall back into the procyclical school, especially if the crisis is deep and protracted. Going forward, if slowing growth in HICs is coupled with structural challenges (for example, demographic pressures) and rigidities of social security systems, this could put increasingly more stress on fiscal and health sector policymakers. With respect to the policy implications of such trends, in many countries, efficiency gains will need to be accompanied by structural reforms in order to avoid negative social consequences, and coordination between fiscal and social policy camps will become even more important to devising long-term economic development strategies that also take into account sector-specific needs.[89]

Second, the analysis reveals that cyclicality patterns between GHE and economic cycles are more nuanced in by-country descriptive analyses and, hence, event and case study approaches would be valuable to shed more light on the drivers of patterns and changes over time. For example, comparing the correlation coefficients

---

[88] The *Fiscal Health Database* (World Bank, 2012a) was compiled by Aaka Pande and Marc Smitz with input from Cesar Calderon, John Langenbrunner, Adam Leive, Ece Ozcelik, and Edit V. Velenyi.

[89] For example, during the drafting and negotiation of the Memorandum of Understanding for countries that engage in stabilization talks with the Troika, which consists of the European Central Bank, the European Commission, and the International Momentary Fund.

Box 11. Output gap

Output gap measures the difference between the observed value for the variable of interest and the value on the filtered trend for the given year in terms of standard deviation from the trend. Good/bad times are defined as a positive/negative output gap relative to the trend line. In terms of the measurement approach, output gap is not equivalent to growth crises measures that are provided in terms of negative GDP growth.[90] The difference is that, while growth crises are defined in terms of negative year-on-year GDP growth rate, a negative output gap does not necessarily mean that the country has a negative growth rate. For example, in the case of a slowdown of economic output in countries with high growth rates, a negative output gap simply means that, relative to the expected trend, the country's economic performance is lower than expected but not necessarily negative.

Source: Velenyi and Smitz (2014).

(see Definition and Computation in Annex 3) calculated between health expenditure and economic cycles for the 16 years of the analysis (1995–2010) with annual statistics on cycles and country-specific data, it is becomes apparent that aggregates mask significant variation both within country groups[91] and between years; hence, generalizations are not particularly useful.

Third, consistent with earlier findings regarding the asymmetry of cyclicality (see Definition in Annex 3), the study finds that at the global and aggregate levels, there is evidence that cyclical responses during "bad" and "good"[92] times differ, specifically, countercyclical responses are more likely during deep negative output gaps (see Definition in Box 11). In the income group breakdown, the averages show countercyclical coefficients between GDP and GGE for both high-income countries and middle-income countries. However, the relationship between GDP and GHE is only countercyclical for higher-income countries. As to regional vari-

[90] The National Bureau of Economic Research defines a recession in the United States as when seasonally adjusted quarterly growth rates are negative for two straight quarters. Bruno (1996) defines growth crises as at least three consecutive years of negative growth, cumulating in a drop of growth of at least 9%.

[91] See the example of Chile in Latin America in Box 18: *Illustration of Graduation to Countercyclical Spending and Fallback to Procyclical Spending.* See more in Velenyi and Smitz (2014) and references therein.

[92] "Bad" times (periods of negative output gap) and "good" times (periods of positive output gap). See Del Granado *et al.* (2012).

ation, the analysis obtains countercyclical correlation coefficients for fiscal policy during negative output gaps in East Asia and Pacific, Latin America and the Caribbean, North America, and South Asia. Yet, only two regions show consistent countercyclical patterns in government health spending during negative output gaps — Europe and Central Asia, and the Middle East and North Africa. These results imply that health sector prioritization during this 16-year period, on average, has not been successful in most regions. However, caution must be exercised when interpreting averages, since these can mask diverse responses over time.

Results from linear modeling suggest that the impact of business cycles is larger in developing countries than in advanced economies, and that the fiscal pathway is critical in determining GHE. This means that, although economic growth trajectories do matter, fiscal response from governments can outweigh or at least attenuate income effects. There are three notable macro effects that make countries' GHE more vulnerable to business cycles: (i) Deterioration in terms of trade (see Definition in Annex 3), (ii) high debt-to-GDP ratios for all income groups, and (iii) unpredictable ODA in developing countries.

Although these findings contribute to the evidence base on the cyclicality of health spending, significant knowledge gaps remain. In the descriptive statistical analysis, the correlation coefficients offer some insights into the dynamics between business cycles and fiscal and government health financing policies. Yet, these simple bivariate relationships have limitations. They show bivariate associations and not causation, and they mask a number of causal pathways that result in the observed correlation. Although the multivariate linear regression better enables exploring the drivers of cyclical responses, given the endogeneity and bidirectional properties discussed earlier, this method does not allow establishing a causal relationship between the economic cycle and health spending. Advanced multivariate panel data analysis is essential to understanding the role and weight of various dimensions shaping cyclical responses.

In a complementary overview paper, referred to earlier, Tandon *et al.* (2014) discuss the theory and limited empirical evidence behind prioritizing government spending on health, measured as the health share of aggregate government expenditure. Among the driving factors behind government prioritization of health spending, they mention democratization and lower levels of corruption. These factors are further explored through a panel data analysis of 140 countries between 1995 and 2010 (Liang and Mirelman, 2014), which explores the relationship between GHE, sociopolitical risks, and international aid, while controlling for the impact of national income and fiscal capacity on health spending. The results indicate that reducing corruption is fundamental to improve the efficiency and level of public resources for health.

Overall, as empirical evidence has evolved, data limitations and methodological challenges have hampered efforts. Because of data consistency, reliability, and frequency issues, country-specific applied analyses would be a welcome complement and validation to some of the broad, brushstroke facts that have come out of more aggregate analyses. For future research, it will be important to develop and utilize publicly available, annually updated, standardized, and reliable data; cross-country empirical modeling using panel data, possibly for longer time frames; and country-specific event analyses that incorporate more qualitative country and policy context and fine-grained data. These are essential to the evidence base evolving in this area.

- *How to manage the health sector during economic downturns*

As argued earlier, there is increased recognition that health and economic development are interconnected. Both macro and micro studies show that better health status leads to more productivity, which in turn leads to increased economic growth. Conversely, the faster the economy grows, the greater the demand for health care and health sector spending. Over the past several decades, the health sector has become an increasingly important component of the global economy, evinced by the growing portion of health expenditures as a share of gross domestic product (GDP), especially in high-income and emerging middle-income countries.

Due to the cyclical nature of economic performance, as discussed in the previous section, building health sector resilience is critical to preparing for inevitable economic downturns. The global economic crisis, which began as early as 2007, brought renewed attention to the impact of economic downturns on health sectors worldwide and revealed that no country is immune to external challenges, even those with advanced economies and AAA ratings. As the crisis deepened over time, a number of countries in Europe stood on the fiscal brink, engaging in procyclical fiscal policy. These policies have affected the health sector and resulted in reduced fiscal space for health. This dynamic is atypical as, in general, advanced economies have been known for their countercyclical behavior. However, the emerging literature shows that stereotypical cyclical behavioral patterns associated with income levels are slowly changing. There has been an observed graduation from procyclicality in lower-income countries, confirming that countercyclical responses are possible at lower income levels (Brahmbhatt and Canuto, 2012; Braun and di Gresia, 2003; Frankel *et al.*, 2011; IMF, 2009; Lewis and Vernhoven, 2010). On the other hand, there is evidence of "fallback" into procyclicality at the higher end of the income distribution, which can be associated, for example, with increased debt-to-GDP levels (Frankel *et al.*, 2011;

Box 12. Objectives proposed by the WHO to better understand and mitigate the effects of crises on health

Triggered by the GEC, which has catalyzed research to better understand the economic crises on population health, the World Health Organization (WHO) in 2009 organized a high-level consultation on "*The Financial Crisis and Global Health*." The director general of WHO, Dr. Margaret Chan, provided three objectives that the development community should aspire to attain (WHO, 2009):

(1) Build awareness of the ways in which an economic downturn may affect health spending, health services, health-seeking behavior, and health outcomes.
(2) Make the case for sustaining investments in health.
(3) Identify actions — including monitoring early warning signs — that can help mitigate the negative impact of economic downturns.

Velenyi and Smitz, 2014). In other words, advanced economies may respond in a procyclical manner, especially if the crisis is deep and protracted. Thus, lessons illustrating crisis navigation are important, regardless of where a country is on the development trajectory.

By 2009, the effects of the shock on the heath sector were indisputable, but policy reactions at the global and national levels lagged. In 2009, the World Health Organization (WHO) held high-level consultations known as "*The Financial Crisis and Global Health*" and "*Health in Times of Global Economic Crisis: Implications for the WHO Europe Region*" in an attempt to catalyze policy and technical responses. Objectives were proposed to mitigate the effect of crises on global health (see Box 12). Lewis and Verhoeven (2010) also highlight the importance of research to inform the design of social programs and sector policies that aim to reduce vulnerability to crises.

A book by Hou *et al.* (2013) aims to contribute to WHO's first and third objectives above by raising awareness of the challenges that health systems, in both developing and developed countries, face in times of economic crisis and providing a framework by which governments and policymakers can meet the critical challenge of health sector stabilization and resilience building. The expectation is, as presented in the foregoing discussion, that successful implementation of these tools can positively affect not only population health, but long-term development trajectories as well. Following the presentation of empirical evidence on the effects of crises on health and health systems (see Box 13) and the policy context, the book proposes the "ATM" framework, which stands for assessment, tracking, and mitigation of crises' effects on the health sector.

Box 13. Micro evidence on crises and health

One school of the crises-and-health literature has focused on estimating changes in final health outcomes as a result of economic crises, using micro data. Findings from applied micro studies diverge depending on whether the crisis occurs in a low-, middle-, or high-income country (Ruhm, 2000; 2012; Smith and Yazbeck, 2011). Further, even controlling for income level, there is evidence of systematic differences in the impact of crises on health as a function of the social sensitivity and preferences of the government.

In low-income countries (LICs), crises have been associated with higher infant mortality and malnutrition. The evidence indicates that malnutrition has increased in countries of South Asia (Skoufias *et al.*, 2011) and Sub-Saharan Africa (Bhalotra, 2010; Carter and Maluccio, 2003) during macroeconomic downturns. Infant mortality has been found to be countercyclical in developing countries, increasing when there are negative economic shocks (Conceição *et al.*, 2009; Mendoza and Rees, 2009; Paxson and Schady, 2004; Rukumnuaykit, 2003; Simms and Rowson, 2003). In many cases, girls are disproportionately affected by negative outcomes (Baird *et al.*, 2007; Friedman and Schady, 2009).

Evidence from high-income countries (HICs), however, suggests that economic downturns are "good for your health" (Ruhm, 2000). For example, in the United States, infant mortality is procyclical, decreasing when there are negative economic shocks. During recessions, individuals in high-income countries are more likely to exercise and less likely to smoke, drink, or engage in other health-damaging behaviors. On the other hand, Zaridze *et al.* (2009) found an increase in alcohol-related deaths in the Russian Federation during the crisis in the 1990s, as did Kwon and Jung (2009) in the developing context of Nepal and Bangladesh (Brenzel, 2012). There are fewer traffic accidents and related deaths when the economy is weak. In contrast, the sign of coefficient estimates for mental health and suicide are mostly positive during crises. The Asian economic crisis was associated with a rise in suicide mortality in Japan, Hong Kong, and the Republic of Korea in 1998. Similarly, Kentikelenis *et al.* (2012) reported a 40% increase in suicides and increases in psychiatric morbidity in Greece as a result of the GEC. However, Stuckler *et al.* (2009) showed that, despite rising unemployment during the economic crisis, suicide rates dropped in Finland and Sweden due to government commitment to social protection and use of active labor market programs.

Findings from middle-income countries (MICs) are indicate an overall negative impact of economic crises on health. However, the evidence is stronger

(*Continued*)

Box 13. (*Continued*)

on the impact of crises on intermediate indicators (government health spending and utilization of services) than on health outcomes such as the prevalence of malnutrition and infant mortality, although in cases there is evidence of the latter. Positive policy responses in Argentina and Thailand[93] (see Case Study on Thailand in Chapter 4 of Hou *et al.*, 2013) are noteworthy examples of how countries can mitigate the adverse effect of macro shocks on population health and financial protection (Gottret *et al.*, 2009; Smith and Yazbeck, 2011). As to health effects, Schady and Smitz (2010) provide country-specific estimates of the effect of macroeconomic shocks on infant mortality for a sample of mainly MICs. In most of these countries, infant mortality appears to be procyclical or acyclical. Only when shocks to GDP are very deep (15% or larger) are they consistently associated with higher infant mortality.

Source: Hou *et al.* (2013).

Assessment of health system vulnerability to crisis

The assessment chapter presented in Hou *et al.* (2013) maps out and tests a new way of assessing the vulnerability of health sectors to economic downturns. It explores thus far uncharted territory by: (i) Offering a definition of crisis-related health system vulnerability; (ii) presenting a vulnerability assessment framework to conceptualize the drivers of system vulnerability in a way that can be applied to quantitative analyses; and (iii) proposing a global vulnerability assessment tool to enable benchmarking country performance against peers and over time, help identify weak spots that reduce the country's ability to manage and mitigate crisis effects on the health sector and health outcomes, focus attention and resources, and, consequently, strengthen system resilience.

Extensive research has found that a standardized definition of economic crisis-related health system vulnerability did not exist prior to the book by Hou *et al.* (2013) (see Box 14 on the WHO's toolkit and how it differs from the ATM approach for health system vulnerability assessment proposed in Hou *et al.*, 2013). Drawing on vulnerability definitions from other areas and adapting them to this context, crisis-related vulnerability in the health system is framed as *the full range of factors that place people at risk of becoming "health insecure" and threaten universal and permanent access to quality health care services as a consequence of economic crisis.*

[93] In Thailand, public and private health expenditure fell by 36% during the Asian financial crisis of 1997–1998 (Hopkins, 2006). In response to the shock, the government had reformed its health care system to increase access and treatment for the poor. These reforms helped mitigate the effects of the East Asian financial crisis on health care utilization. Because of these reforms, Thailand was the only country in which health care utilization did not initially decline when the crisis hit.

Box 14. WHO's toolkit for assessing health system capacity for crisis management

Health crises are often unpredictable and can cause significant human suffering and loss of life and can have serious economic repercussions (WHO, 2012). The population is particularly vulnerable when national and local health systems are unable to cope with the consequences of a crisis due to a sudden increase in demand for care, which can overwhelm the institutions involved.

To make health crises more manageable, under the umbrella of health system strengthening emergency preparedness, the World Health Organization (WHO) published a toolkit for assessing health system capacity for crisis management (WHO, 2012). Until this publication, no standard formal methodology for assessing the preparedness of a health system for crises[94] has been established.

The overall goal of the WHO's emergency preparedness toolkit is to help countries minimize the impact of future health crises by assessing the capacity of their health systems to respond to various threats and identify gaps (WHO, 2012). This toolkit, which applies a health systems strengthening approach, breaks down the crisis preparedness process into manageable functions to help the ministry of health be systematic in its crisis preparedness assessment. The six functions that determine overall health systems goals and outcomes and which are under review for crisis preparedness are: (i) Leadership and governance; (ii) health workforce; (iii) medical products, vaccines and technology; (iv) health information; (v) health financing,[95] including sector-specific and multisectoral mechanisms to financing emergency preparedness and management; and (vi) service delivery.

While the WHO's health system preparedness toolkit (WHO, 2012) limits its focuses to the system level and applies a qualitative approach, the ATM (Assessment, Tracking, and Mitigation) approach proposed in Hou *et al.* (2013)

(Continued)

[94] In this document (WHO, 2012), the terms "health emergencies" and "health crises" refer to the health threats associated with new or newly emerging diseases, the accidental release or deliberate use of biological, chemical or radionuclear agents, natural disasters, human-made disasters, complex emergencies, conflicts and other events with a potentially catastrophic impact on human health, including the potential implications of climate change.

[95] Per the WHO, toolkit (WHO, 2012) on emergency preparedness in health systems, a good health-financing system ensures the availability of adequate funds for the health system, and its financial protection in case of a crisis. In addition to providing funds for essential health-sector crisis-management programs, it ensures that crisis victims have access to essential services and that health facilities and equipment are adequately insured for damage or loss.

Box 14. (*Continued*)

has a broader scope, which includes assessing the relationship between the health system and the macro economy and the impact of the crisis on the population both in terms of health outcomes and subsequent economic effects. The ATM approach relies more on quantitative assessment, including through global databases (see more in Chapter 2 in Hou *et al.*, 2013), routine health management information systems, as well as facility and household surveys (see more in Chapter 3 in Hou *et al.*, 2013).

In sum, these assessment tools are complementary, the WHO one offering a more practical instrument for MOHs to be used as a check list during preparedness assessment, and the ATM by the World Bank to establish links between the economy and health systems and offer examples of how quantitative analysis can be harnessed to inform reducing health system vulnerability and, hence, reduce the effect of shocks on the population.

This brief comparative summary was prepared on the basis of WHO (2012) and Hou et al. (2013).

The authors argue that health system vulnerability to crisis is multidimensional and, as such, requires examination of factors outside the health sector to better understand the likelihood and expected depth of vulnerability. The assessment framework captures the complex relationship between three levels: External factors, which include macro, fiscal, and demographic variables; health system-level factors, which include variables on health financing and coverage; and household-level factors. These vectors jointly determine health sector resilience and health outcomes during crisis.

The assessment framework was conceptualized to guide the development of a global vulnerability assessment tool, which relies on data from the Fiscal Space Database (World Bank, 2012a). This macro-database of 183 countries over 15 years (1995–2010) compiles a number of international data sources with the ambition to offer a synthetic data source, which, with updates, can provide continuous and standardized data for future vulnerability assessment efforts.

The proposed global health system vulnerability assessment tool will help build more awareness of the impact of economic downturns on the health sector. Further, it will provide quantitative evidence to guide decision-making and policy responses that will help mitigate the negative impacts of economic downturns. It is expected that the presented framework and global assessment tool can catalyze a process that may produce more refined instruments and increasingly more relevant data.

Despite recognized limitations and constraints, this first attempt at a vulnerability assessment tool can be used to identify: (i) Countries that have fragile macro-fiscal conditions, which make health systems more prone to contraction; (ii) how health systems perform on measures of financing and coverage; (iii) how countries perform on final outcomes measures; and (iv) where a country is placed in overall system vulnerability on the global scale.

Undoubtedly, global tools and league tables that are based on reduced dimensions of determinants to compare country performance suffer from limitations. For example, both the Human Development Index and the Doing Business Index have been heavily debated in regard to their methodological robustness and interpretation of the rankings. Such tools are not perfect, but they have been important in focusing the attention of policy makers and the development community on shortcomings in critical areas and led to the leveraging of significant resources to remedy weaknesses at the country level. Similarly, the 'policy-multiplier' effect — in terms of focusing attention and resources — of a system vulnerability assessment tool are expected to be high. Overall, the application of vulnerability assessment tools at the global and country levels could have favorable effects, both on the system and the population overall, and would require relatively small investments with potentially high human capital returns. For example, using health system vulnerability assessment tools and demanding responses where the risks are assessed to be large could have mitigated the effect of the recent Ebola outbreak (see Case Study in Box 15).

Tracking the effect of crisis on health

The experiences of the health systems in Europe and Central Asia — in particular, their limited ability to quickly track and respond to the negative impacts of economic downturns — have provided a clear signal to other countries and to development agencies that there is significant scope for health sectors to take on a more effective role in all three domains — assessment, tracking, and mitigation — to become a better steward of the health sector by understanding vulnerabilities and responding in an expeditious and targeted manner to meet the health needs of the population.[96]

Hence, to be better equipped as stewards, tracking is proposed as a diagnostic tool to check the "vital signs" (e.g., budget allocation, financial status of health insurance funds, price of imported medical goods, access and utilization statistics, etc.)

---

[96] See a review of the effect of the crisis on European health systems by Mladovsky *et al.* (2012); WHO (2013); a case study on the effect of the downturn in the Greek health care by Yfantopoulos (2013) and the case studies on Portugal and Ireland, respectively, by Barros (2013); and Burke *et al.* (2013) in Hou *et al.* (2013).

Box 15. The Ebola epidemic — Failure to invest in health systems affects economic development and regional security

As the High Level Forum on Building Resilient Systems for Health in Ebola-Affected Countries (WHO, 2014b) points out, the recent Ebola epidemic has demonstrated that investing in health systems in not simply a matter of the health sector and a concern for ministries of health. The empirical evidence gathered from the Ebola-inflicted countries since the onset of the outbreak has shown that resilient health systems are fundamentally linked to economic development. When facing epidemics, vulnerable health systems not only jeopardize the local population and economy but also risk regional stability and can trigger negative externalities globally due to the level of interconnectedness between countries today.

This recent case of the Ebola epidemic has attracted global attention to the importance of significantly under resourced and unprepared health systems (WHO, 2014b; World Bank, 2014) and, specifically, to the causal chain between investing in health system strengthening and economic development. The causal chain runs from system deficiencies, which affect behavioral responses in terms of population care seeking and, consequently, determine health outcomes, which ultimately translate into economic growth and SDGs potentials at the country and regional levels.

Health sector policymakers and health systems experts have long pointed to system-wide challenges, system fragility, particularly in low-income countries. However, system deficiencies are not quick fixes and they require significant resources. If there is one positive aspect of the recent crisis it is that the human suffering and death toll and the associated growing economic cost of the outbreak have mobilized increased attention from the broader development community, beyond the scope of the health sector. It can be argued that in the context of these countries, which is similar to a number of other countries in the Africa Region, the health sector is not merely an immediate risk to development but it poses a structural challenge to economic growth because of the demonstrated economy-wide repercussions of weak health system, which affect countries and economies on a daily basis through a number of illnesses, communicable and non-communicable.

The crisis has become an opportunity to leverage resources and steer more attention to focusing efforts on two fronts: (i) Meeting ongoing and predicable health needs to ensure access to quality essential care for the population; and (ii) building resilient health systems to withstand shocks that might arise (WHO, 2014b).

(*Continued*)

Box 15. (*Continued*)

To offer an illustration of the general discussion above, the following summary highlights the relationship between health system vulnerability and the human and economic impact of the Ebola epidemic in the three most severely affected countries: Guinea, Liberia, and Sierra Leone — referred to as "the core countries" — and also discusses the regional implications of the outbreak.

The Trajectory of the Epidemic

The Ebola epidemic started in December 2013 in Guinea, close to the borders with Liberia and Sierra Leone (WHO, 2014a). Due to poorly integrated and fragile health systems — which lack human resources, core public health capacities for surveillance, and predictable supplies — it took more than 3 months by 21 March 2014 when Ebola was identified as the causative agent of the outbreak of unprecedented proportion. By 12 April 2015, the total number of infections in the core countries reached 25,791 with a death toll of 10,689, which translates into an average death rate of 41% across the three countries (Figure 13, Panel B). However, the country-specific statistics show significant variation across the core countries both in the number of cases and the fatality rate (Figure 13, Panel B), implying different levels of health system preparedness and government responsiveness to the crisis.

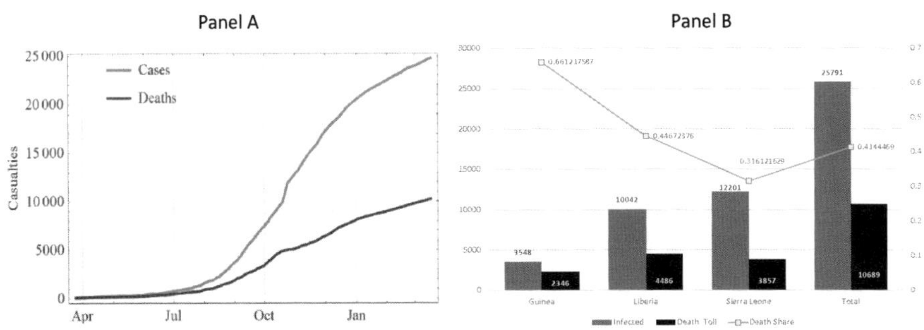

Figure 13. Panel A. Total number of infection and deaths between April 2014 and March 2015. Panel B. Number of infection and deaths, and death rate by country and total for the three core countries

Notes: Panel B: The markers on the grey line indicate the death rate for Ebola cases in the given country, for example, 66% in the case of Guinea. The right vertical axis shows the corresponding value in percentage terms. The left vertical axis shows the number of infections in numeric terms.

Sources: Panel A: Meltzer *et al.* (2014). Panel B: United Nations and WHO statistics presented in *The Economist*, 16 April 2015.

(*Continued*)

Box 15. (*Continued*)

Figure 14 offers a schematic of the main linkages within the causal chain from the health system to economic impact, which are discussed below in the context of the epidemic.

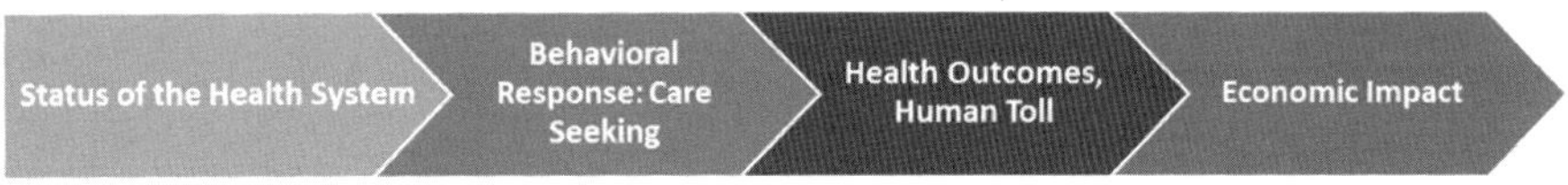

Figure 14. Schematic of the main linkages within the causal chain from the health system to economic impact of Ebola

Status of the Health System

Prior to the Ebola outbreak, weaknesses existed throughout the three countries' health systems.

- *Human Resources for Health*: A primary concern has been the lack of adequate numbers of qualified health workers, most prominently in rural areas (WHO, 2014). For example, data for 2010 from the WHO's National Health Account global database (WHO, 2013a) shows that while the income group average for low-income countries for health care personnel is 3.5 doctors per 10,000 population and 11.7 nurses per 10,000 people, the average for the three countries for these human resources in health (HRH) statistics, respectively, are 0.45 doctors and 1.61 nurses.
- Infrastructure quality, electricity, and running water have been major bottlenecks to service delivery.
- Health information, surveillance, governance and drug supply systems were weak. The number of cases can be associated with surveillance capacity. Assessments have shown that none of the three affected countries attained the minimum IHR (2005) core capacities requirements by 2012 (WHO, 2014). The Integrated Disease Surveillance and Response (IDSR) guidelines were implemented in Guinea, but only adapted for Liberia, and did not start implementation in Sierra Leone.
- *Health Care Financing*: Resources for health have been rising, reaching $67 in Guinea, $102 in Liberia, and $205 in Sierra Leone in PPP terms by 2012. However, government expenditures on health do not attain the estimated $86 per capita basic benefit package, with contribution to total health expenditures as low as $9 per capita in Guinea, $20 in Liberia, and

(*Continued*)

Box 15. (*Continued*)

$16 in Sierra Leone (WHO, 2014a; 2014b). While major investments were being made — including through DAH, which account for a large share of health expenditures particularly in Liberia — in battling specific diseases and health issues, the countries' overall health systems remained fragmented and unable to cope with unexpected challenges. The challenge in Africa and in these countries regarding health care financing is dual. On the one hand, countries need more money for health. This proposition refers to leveraging resource for health to meet the minimum benchmarks and standards. On the other hand, countries need more health for the money. This second proposition refers to buying more value for the money. For example, South Asia has a lower level of average health expenditure per capita than Sub-Saharan Africa; yet, for the level of expenditures it buys better population health outcomes. Building more robust and resilient health systems requires more funds. However, beyond focusing on the level of resources, at the same time interventions and aid must incorporate improved focus on efficiency.

Ebola Response Crowds Out Essential Care Delivery — Behavioral Response

With the onset of the outbreak existing public health services — which were already limited as discussed above — have been diverted to Ebola. The net result is that people have encountered significant barriers in accessing needed care (WHO, 2014). In some areas essential care has ceased to function, including for outcomes related to the health MDG targets, such as maternal and child health (e.g., safe delivery) and communicable diseases (e.g., malaria). Monitoring indicators show and decline in care seeking, for example, in Guinea over a year period ending in August 2014 there was a 58 percentage decline in outpatient visits, a 54% drop on hospital admissions, and 16% drop in Caesarian sections (WHO, 2014a; 2014b) . In Liberia, 62% of health facilities were closed compared to a year earlier in 2013, with immunization declined by 26% (WHO, 2014b). In Sierra Leone, while only 4% of the facilities closed during the observed critical time, service delivery for essential care suffered, showing a 39% decline in malaria treatment for children and 21% drop in immunization. Institutional deliveries declined by 11% in Guinea, 23% in Sierra Leone, and 50% in Liberia.

Health Outcomes and Human Toll

The crowd-out effects of containing Ebola on essential care could pose a risk of reversing some of the MDGs health targets; the gains made in reducing

(*Continued*)

Box 15. (*Continued*)

morbidity and mortality from HIV/AIDS, tuberculosis, malaria, and childhood diseases. Before Ebola, the countries had made significant improvements in key areas related to the health MDGs. Under-five mortality (Figure 15, Panel A) was declining and all countries had expanded coverage of basic interventions into sub-national rural districts. Skilled birth attendance was increasing and maternal mortality was declining, albeit remained at the highest level in the world (Figure 15, Panel B).

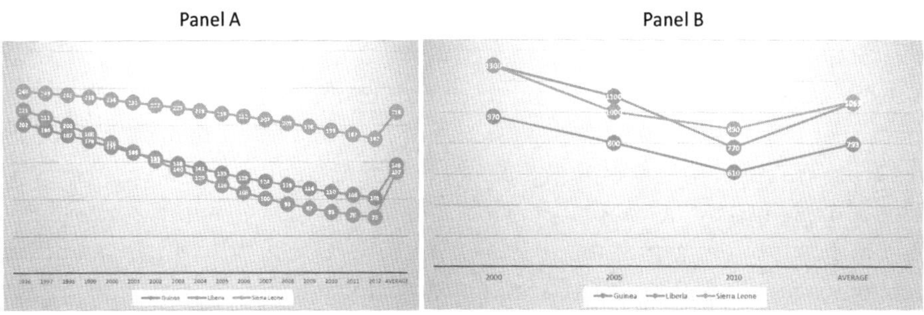

Figure 15. Panel A: Trend in under-five mortality rate for the core countries between 1995 and 2012. Panel B: Trends in maternal mortality rate in the core countries between 2000 and 2010

Source: WHO NHA Database (2014).

The human cost of the epidemic in terms of Ebola infections and human toll as of April 2015 is captured in Figure 13 (Panel B). Among the lives lost are 864 health care workers, which, as the HRH statistics above suggested, is a significant loss of human resources in the sector.

In the first phase of the epidemic, the primary focus is on containment. The estimates of immediate humanitarian costs from the World Health Organization and the United Nations have been revised upwards, from US$495 to US$600 million (World Bank, 2014).

Economic Impact

The World Health Organization focused its assessment on the relationship between health systems and Ebola, which has proven to be a bidirectional relation, health system resilience determining the ability to manage and absorb the shock, and the shock affecting health system resilience. Beyond the sector

(*Continued*)

Box 15. (*Continued*)

specific systems angle, the World Bank focused more attention on the economic impact of the epidemic and using a combination of micro and macro data estimated the short and medium-term impact of the epidemic under "low" and "high" epidemiological transmission scenarios (World Bank, 2014).

The report summarizes that beyond the human toll and suffering, the Ebola epidemic that has afflicted West Africa has had measurable economic impact in terms of forgone output; higher fiscal deficits; rising prices; lower real household incomes and greater poverty (World Bank, 2014). Factors contributing to the cost of Ebola include direct costs of the illness (government spending on health care) and indirect costs, such as lower labor productivity as a result of workers being ill, dying or caring for the sick. However, the report finds that the majority of the costs stem not from the direct and indirect costs but from the higher costs of doing business within countries or across borders. This is explained by "aversion behavior", changes in the behavior of individuals due to fear of contracting the disease (World Bank, 2014), which can affect economic activities at the local, regional, and global levels.

- According to the report, the short-term impact of the epidemic in 2014 is estimated to be $130 million in Guinea (or 2.1% drop in GDP), $66 million in Liberia (or 3.4% drop in GDP), and $163 million in Sierra Leone (or 3.3% drop in GDP), with a total loss of $359 million for the core countries. Regarding the broader impact, lost GDP for West Africa as a whole is estimated at $2.2 billion in 2014.
- In the "Low Ebola" scenario, which is closer to the observed epidemiological trajectory up to April 2015, the estimates suggest a bounce back in economic production of $43 million Guinea (or 0.7% growth in GDP), a loss of $113 million in Liberia (or 5.8% drop in GDP), and a loss of $59 million in Sierra Leone (or 1.2% drop in GDP), that is a total loss of $129 million across the three countries. Taking into account cross border and region-wide negative externalities and impact, the economic loss for West Africa is estimated for 1.6 billion in 2015.

The take-away messages from the report is that the economic impacts are already very serious in the core three countries — particularly in Liberia and Sierra Leone. Importantly, the effect is expected to be larger than the presented estimates given some limitations in the measurement of costs. Specifically, the study is focused on the short and medium-term inputs, over the next

(*Continued*)

Box 15. (*Continued*)

18 months. Hence, the analysis does not take into account the long-term impacts generated by mortality, failure to treat other health conditions due to aversion behavior and lack of supply capacity, school closings and dropouts, and other shocks to livelihoods.

The report concludes that swift policy reaction by the international community is crucial and emphasizes the connection between health systems and economic recovery and development as follows (World Bank, 2014):

> *"Starting now, the international community must learn and act on the knowledge that weak public health infrastructure, institutions, and systems in many African countries are a threat not only to their own citizens, but also to their trading partners and the world at large. The enormous economic cost of the current outbreak to the affected countries and the world could likely have been avoided by prudent ongoing investment in such health system strengthening. The Ebola outbreak has laid bare the failure of any reasoning that investments in public health infrastructure, institutions and systems can be separated from investments in economic recovery and development."*

To mitigate the medium term economic impact of the outbreak, current efforts by many partners to strengthen the health systems and fill the fiscal gaps in the core three countries are key priorities. Regarding health systems development, the WHO highlights four priority areas to improve system resilience to crisis: (i) Focus on building resilient sub-national systems; (ii) health workforce strengthening; (iii) strengthening core public health capacities for surveillance and response to fulfil obligations under the International Health Regulations (IHR) (2005); and (iv) establish predictable supplies and coordinated supply chains (WHO, 2014b). At the macroeconomic level, these efforts that aim at boosting system resilience, should be supplemented by investments in those countries and in their neighbors to renew the confidence of international tourism, travel, trade and investment partners (World Bank, 2014).

of the health system and see how an economic downturn affects system performance and health outcomes. It is argued that tracking is critical for detecting warning signals and drawing policy attention to areas that could further aggravate the effect of the crisis on the health sector and population health outcomes.

Continuous tracking and monitoring can occur at different levels, and require a variety of methods, tools, and data sources. Among the methods, tracking primarily refers to the use of contemporaneous data flows, such as administrative data from management information systems (MIS), or *ex-post* analysis of data that can be accessed with only a short lag, for example, a dedicated survey with a fast turn-around.

In contrast with the proposed global assessment tool that relies on standardized macro-data from a variety of international sources, tracking predominantly draws on micro-data collected from the system through MIS (for example, Health Insurance Fund), facility-level data, or household surveys to assess population-level effects. The global assessment tool is designed to provide information for global policy discussions, draw attention to areas of system vulnerability, and identify limitations in global data sources that can help system vulnerability assessment. Tracking, on the other hand, takes vulnerability assessment to the country level and harnesses more granular and higher frequency data. Thus, tracking is more dynamic and can more precisely inform policymaking through the identification of specific system bottlenecks. It is proposed that combining the assessment with tracking tools will provide more comprehensive data to help policymakers and governments deal with negative impacts and build health system resilience.

The author of the tracking chapter (Hou *et al.*, 2013) explores different tools (such as health management information system, health insurance fund administrator survey, labor force survey, household income and health care seeking survey) used to track the impact of the economic downturn on the health sector and, consequently, on population health and illness-related financial protection in Europe and Central Asia (ECA). The discussion focuses on both the "what" and "how" of tracking the impact of a crisis on health systems and provides illustration with selected findings[97] from a range of data collection efforts that were specifically initiated to track the short-term impact of crises, such as the effect of the GEC on the health systems and health outcomes in Europe and Central Asia, which was the most effect by the downturn compared to other regions (more than

[97] For example, coping and utilization modules of household surveys show significant reduction in food consumption or substituting toward cheaper alternatives, and reduction in medical care seeking and drug purchase. The reductions show an income gradient, with the lowest quintile foregoing the most (see Results in Chapter 3 of Hou *et al.*, 2013). Further, health insurance fund administrator surveys show reduction in the revenue bases. This, to some extent, can be offset by transfers from the general government budget (i.e., countercyclical social response). However, where government 'bailout' was not forthcoming, the revenue shortfall had a deeper impact on providers, consequently affecting service delivery (availability, quality, timeliness, and system responsiveness) (see Results in Koettl and Schneider, 2010). See more examples of crisis effect on the system, demand for health care, health spending and illness related financial protection, and on population health status in Chapter 3 of Hou *et al.* (2013).

a 10 percentage point change in growth) and the biggest deceleration in economic activity (a 6% contraction on average).

Mitigation of crisis effects

A key lesson explored under crisis effect mitigation is the important nexus between the health sector and the social protection sector, specifically through social safety net programs. Country experiences in Europe, South America, and Asia show that the most successful crisis effect mitigation programs in the health sector are those that are able to link with social safety net programs and use existing targeting instruments to scale up coverage during economic downturns (Hou *et al.*, 2013).

Significant similarities exist among different types of social programs in the delivery of services or transfers to the poor. Current technology can enable an effective management information system (MIS) to facilitate intersectoral collaboration and improve the overall governance and transparency of the system. Such integrated systems between social programs can assist all relevant programs across different aspects of operations, including eligibility assessment, beneficiary identification and registration, tracking service utilization and delivery of benefits, and facilitating coordination of different programs.

Lessons from two European Union (EU) country case studies[98] lead to two main conclusions. First, the political economic dynamics of reform processes between the health sector and the ministry of finance, as well as within the health sector are critical to ensure timely and targeted policy responses. Political economy is especially important if there is not enough time for evidence-based priority setting. Second, further developing and applying country-level monitoring tools and early warning systems could help evidence-based responses. These tools must consider changes in inputs (for example, health financing), outputs (for example, utilization), and outcomes (for example, mental health, suicide rates, chronic conditions, and so forth) to understand the effects throughout the results chain. Thus, crisis effect monitoring is not a short-term engagement. It requires a systematic and long-term impact assessment approach.

These findings lead back to the ATM framework, which may serve as a valuable tool irrespective of which income group a country is in. While advanced economies

[98] The case studies by Barros (2013) and Burke *et al.* (2013) in Chapter 5 of Hou *et al.* (2013) discuss how the crisis affected the system and population health, and how the shock was used to squeeze efficiency gains while simultaneously balancing equity considerations as fiscal space for health declined. Essentially, the message is that monitoring and early warning signals are important to enable timely responses and, therefore, effective and informed risk mitigation.

have relied more on automatic stabilizers — such as unemployment insurance and other social transfer payments — (Braun and Di Gresia, 2003; Hou *et al.*, 2013; Velenyi and Smitz, 2014) and have more developed social safety nets, the global crisis has shown that there is no place for complacency (Hou *et al.*, 2013).

The main conclusion is that the cyclical nature of economic performance makes economic downturns a recurring phenomenon. Crises vary in terms of their triggers, geographic origins and scope, length, and depth. These parameters, the extent of structural preparedness, and policy reactions by governments jointly determine the severity of outcomes and the length of the impact horizon. A global lesson from these crises is that the health sector must build systems that can effectively assess vulnerability, track system changes, and synthesize the information to improve mitigation efforts. These structural changes can and must happen and cannot come soon enough.

These last two sub-sections presented intertwined areas related to the health impacts of economic crises: The cyclical patterns of health spending and managing sector resilience during crises to mitigate the adverse effects of downturns. Based on the analysis and the evidence gap, it is proposed that descriptive diagnostic tools, such as the tools for cyclicality analysis (Velenyi and Smitz, 2014) and the global tool developed for health system vulnerability assessment (see Chapter 2 in Hou *et al.*, 2013) could be applied so that policymakers and practitioners are equipped with information on the macro-fiscal aspects of the possibility frontier, not only on system capacity and constraints. This would help in developing resilience to shocks through sectoral as well as fiscal channels. One important objective of basic diagnostic assessment would be to inform discussions on the binding constraints to countercyclical health spending during negative output gaps, to understand whether the main constraints lie within the sector or in fiscal behavior. This could then inform policy options. For example, if the binding constraint is found to be procyclical fiscal policy, then the government could improve fiscal accountability and transparency to benefit the health sector. The application of standardized tools would facilitate comparative efforts by drawing on a common framework and common measures and definitions.

Beyond tracking tools that aim to inform system management and stewardship functions, more advanced analytical work is required to isolate the drivers of cyclical responses and system vulnerability. At the macro-level, one critical constraint has been lack of standardized and comparable data that would enable cross-country and cross-time comparisons of the effect of downturns on health system performance and health outcomes. At the micro-level, more data is required both on the supply and demand sides to help establish causal relationships between crises, health system implications — including on financing and service delivery — and, ultimately, on health.

Riding the demographic waves[99]

- *Health and growth through population dynamics — The mechanics of demographic dividend*

The clearest link between health and economic growth is the documented experience of the Asian Tigers (the developed economies of Hong Kong, Singapore, South Korea, and Taiwan); what has come to be known as the 'demographic dividend' (Bloom and Williamson, 1998; Bloom *et al.*, 2000). East Asian countries achieved major improvements in health before economic take off. The demographic dividend describes the economic and social impact of the speed with which a country goes through a demographic transition (Figure 16). The leading edge of the demographic transition is the decrease in death rates, typically due to investments in life-saving interventions that sharply decrease infant and child mortality, improve nutritional status of children and mothers, and improve the overall health of the population. As families internalize the declines in infant and child mortality, they decide to have fewer children, leading to a decline in birth rates. The time gap between the decline in death and birth rates produces a natural population growth rate.

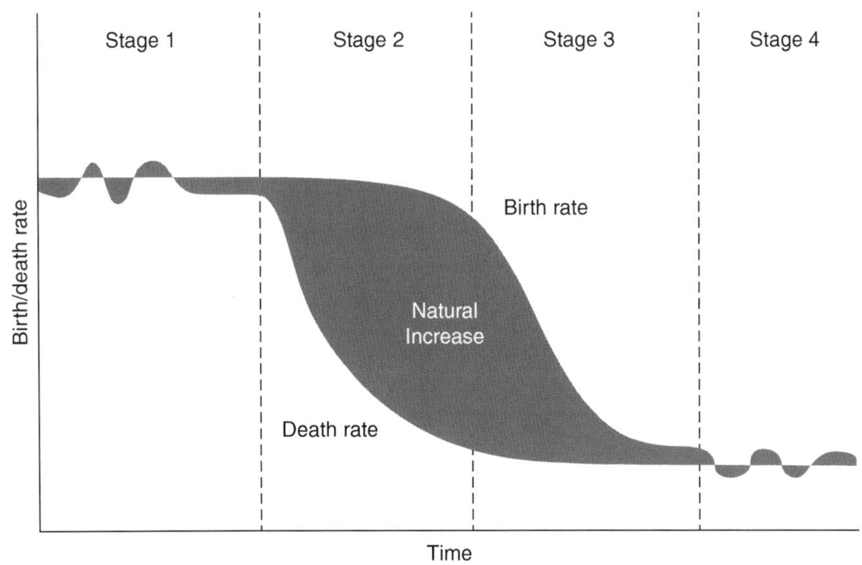

Figure 16. Demographic transition

Source: Population Reference Bureau (2006).

[99]The author is grateful to Abdo S. Yazbeck for his contribution to this section and comments.

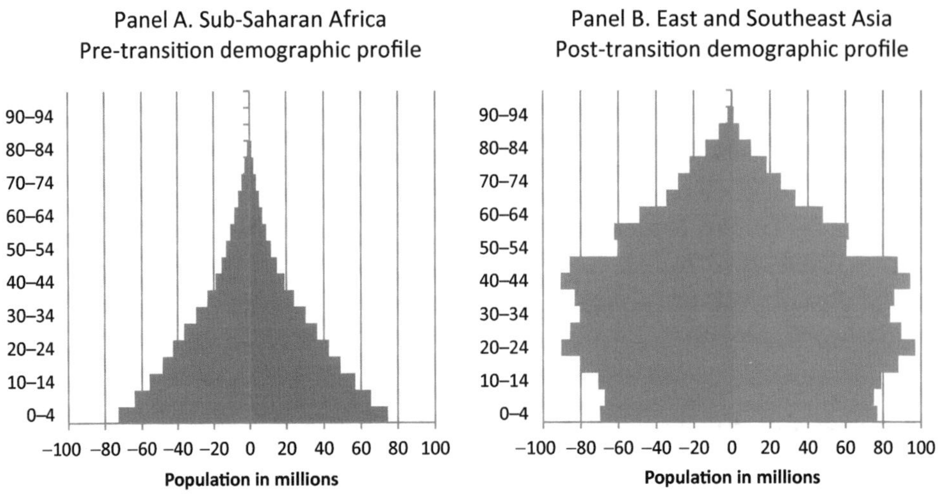

Figure 17. Population pyramids of Sub-Saharan Africa and East and Southeast Asia, 2012

Source: Raja *et al.* (2012).

This demographic transition takes place in every country and every region, but the speed with which it takes place has implications on social and economic development. The case of the East Asian Tigers best explains this link between health and wealth. The fast decline in mortality followed by a fast decline in fertility led to a dramatic change in the age structure of the countries. Figure 17 shows how a fast demographic transition has changed the age pyramid in Sub-Saharan Africa and East and Southeast Asia. On the left is what the Sub-Saharan age profile was in 2012, which is similar to what was the case in Asia pre-transition. On the right hand is the age structure for East and South East Asia in 2012 post-demographic transition. The impact of the transition is massive, with a large share of the population moving into working age, decreasing dependency and also allowing for a much larger investment in human capital for future generation.

Fertility declines have also had an impact on education investments, but this is not unique to East Asia. With fewer children, more is spent on educating each child. Recent analysis of the impact of the population dynamics in Sub-Saharan Africa confirms this link between fertility rates and education (Eloundou-Enyegue, 2013; Eloundou-Enyegue and Giroux, 2013). Figure 18 captures the percentage increase/decrease in per capita spending on education (resources per child, that is, RPC) that can be attributed to population dynamics between 1990 and 2005. Another important benefit of the fertility decline is further improvements in child health (Barker, 1990) and women's health (Finlay and Canning, 2013). Fertility declines and health improvements create a self-enforcing virtuous cycle.

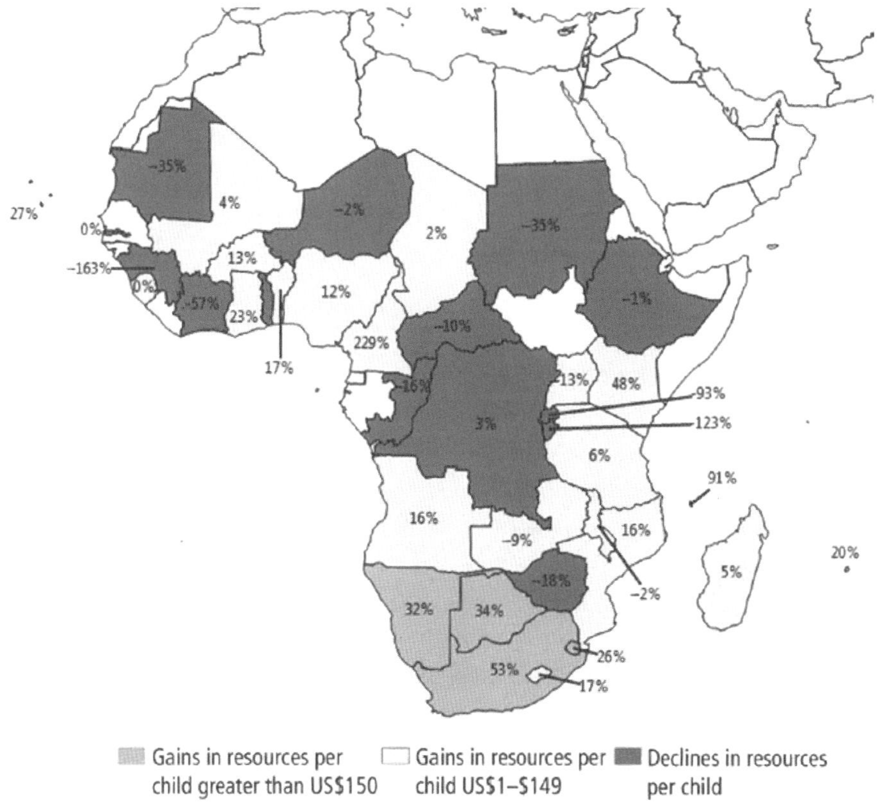

Figure 18. Contributions of age structure to recent changes in resources per child (RPC)
Source: Canning *et al.* (2015).

As noted earlier, the demographic transition not only increases investments in human capital, but it also changes the working age proportions in countries. With fewer children born, the dependency ratio declines and the share of the population that is working age increases in the medium term. Figure 19 shows the working age population ratio over time in three regions. First, each region is undergoing different stages of the demographic transition at different times, with East Asia starting the transition, followed by South Asia then Sub-Saharan Africa. Second, each region is undergoing the demographic transition at different speeds, with East Asia experiencing the fastest transition and Sub-Saharan Africa the slowest. The faster the demographic transition, the steeper the curve showing the ratio of the working age population to dependents, and the higher the peak.

The demographic dividend captures an interesting relationship between health and the potential for wealth. A fast decline in mortality triggers a fast decline in

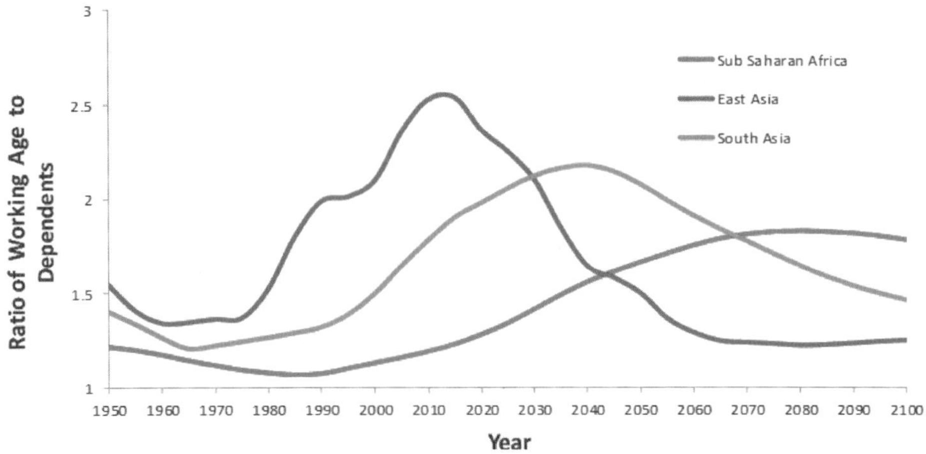

Figure 19. Ratio of working age to dependents

Source: World Bank Medium Fertility Variant.

fertility — initially leading to more children as the fertility decline is lagged — and these two factors impact human capital accumulation (through increased per capita spending on education) and a rise in the ratio of the population of working age (decrease in dependency ratio). Having smaller, healthier, and more educated families creates the potential for increased earning by a large share of the population. This potential can then be translated into increased per capita income if economies can create the demand for labor and jobs. It is estimated that in East Asia, between a quarter and third of income growth can be accounted for by this demographic dividend. A further dividend is produced if policies that encourage savings are put in place as the youth bulge moves into the productive years and starts savings that turn into investments.

• *Demographic dividend is not a destiny, it requires good policies*

Seizing the window of opportunity is a challenging task. Triggering the demographic transition by population and reproductive health policies and creating an environment that cultivates maternal and child health are a start. Yet, harnessing the demographic dividend is not automatic.

From the examples thus far, we have seen that changes in the demographic structure of a country and related social policies can lead to a dividend or drag in terms of economic development over time. The opportunity set — in terms of what a country can attain and what it should focus on — and the corresponding (sector-specific) policy set depend on where the given country is on the development and demographic trajectories. In simplified form, the demographic-related challenges and policy responses corresponding to the three development stages are as follows:

- *Low-Income Countries (LICs)*: Many low-income countries, such as in Sub-Saharan Africa, are at the early stage of the demographic transition. For these countries, increased focus on population and health policies can help trigger and accelerate the transition. Girl's education is especially important since schooling — through knowledge and long-term income effects — can change reproductive behavior.
- *Middle-Income Countries (MICs)*: Moving along the trajectory, for a number of middle-income countries, where fertility has declined, quality education and skill development are critical to prepare the youth entering the labor market. There is a gender component to skills and labor market as well. The decline in fertility rates and fewer children to care for increase female labor market participation. More skilled women are able to lock in higher wages. Increased female labor market participation coupled with higher wages increase women's contribution to economic growth.
- *High-Income Countries (HICs)*: For richer countries, where the dependency ratio and life expectancy are higher, the population's weight will be skewed to the older cohorts, which require more social expenditures. The related fiscal pressures have led to increases of retirement age and required more careful planning to secure pension and health care benefits.

To cash in the demographic dividend, governments must choose the appropriate social and economic policies. David Bloom of Harvard warns that the period of greatest potential — when the working age population is disproportionately large — in demographic terms, is a moment or two. The window of opportunity to get a country on a track toward harnessing the demographic dividend, the path traveled by East Asia, such as in South Korea, is small (see Box 16). Countries at an early stage of the demographic transition, such as in Africa (see Box 17), have a generation or two to ride the demographic waves and not be dragged under as their dependents get older. As punctuated during a panel discussion regarding the challenges and opportunities for ministers of finance and development related to the demographic transition (World Bank, 2011):

> "*Demography is not destiny. Demographic trajectories are not set in stone, nor are they implications for economic growth and development. There is huge scope that policymakers have to take advantage of these demographic and economic links.*"

Box 16. Economic growth propelled in South Korea by applying a phased, multisectoral approach to managing the demographic transition

When the demographic transition began in South Korea, mortality rates started to decline, especially for infants and children. This effectively gave rise to a baby boom, which had immediate economic consequences as children need to be fed, clothed, housed, and provided medical care and education. Since resources to support the baby boom needed to be diverted from other uses, like building up infrastructure, capital accumulation, or research and development, economic growth slowed during the initial phase, but as time went by — in a decade or two in South Korea and similarly in Thailand — three things happened. First, the baby boom ended when couples realized that they did not need to have as many children to reach their target number of children and fertility rates dropped from over 6 in 1960 to 2.4 in 1980. Second, South Korea invested very early and intensively in education. Third, the large baby boom cohorts got older, leading to a big surge in the share of the population in prime working ages, which is the prime age for savings. This represented a major expansion in the productive capacity of the South Korean economy on a per capita basis. The government also invested in job creation, ensuring that those potential workers and savers were well-equipped with capital that they needed to be productive, and took advantage of international markets to sell the goods being produced by those workers. All this gave rise to the spectacular growth of income per capita, which has been over 6% per year for decades.

Box 17. Divergence in Outcomes between East Asia and Sub-Saharan Africa

Per capita income in Sub-Saharan Africa was higher than it was in East Asia in the early 1970s, but that changed as East Asia's per capita income grew 30 times faster than that of Sub-Saharan Africa, and it did so for decades, making this a compelling story of the demographic dividend (Bloom, 2011). The fertility decline in East Asia accounts for about 2 percentage points of East Asia's growth in income per capita. The fertility decline in East Asia meant that East Asia was able to escape the burden of youth dependency, which Sub-Saharan Africa has not been able to achieve. The divergence in income growth was very closely tracked by the fertility decline in East Asia, which went down from about 6 children per woman to about 2 in the space of three decades, while in Sub-Saharan Africa it is still over 5.

Making the most of the demographic transition requires a systematic, multi-sectoral approach. It requires population, health, and nutrition policies that reduce high fertility and maternal and infant mortality. It requires education policies and programs that ensure highly skilled and productive young workers. It requires labor market policies and regulations that stimulate productive employment, maximizing economic impact. In sum, it requires long-term planning and anticipating the need to put systems in place to mitigate the negative consequences of a rapidly aging population after the demographic dividend is realized.

For many countries, including the poorest, health sector policies in population and reproductive health can encourage and subsequently reinforce the positive impact of the demographic dividend. Social protection programs, such as conditional cash transfers, can complement these policies and contribute to the productivity of the next generation. As population aging becomes imminent, policymakers can work toward expanding the coverage of financially sound pension schemes and planning for a shift in medical provision to address emerging priorities such as NCDs and chronic illnesses. These challenges are often greater in developing countries as compared to developed countries, where populations age more gradually. Most developing countries are likely to become old before they become rich.

The window of opportunity to leverage the demographic dividend is short and, hence, concrete programs and sector-specific policy actions are required to translate global knowledge into policies that incorporate the demographic aspect of growth and development to lead to population-level and economy-wide results.

The schematic in Figure 20 provides an overview matrix for social and cross cutting policies, including gender and development and macro-fiscal aspects. As the demographic transition moves along its trajectory from high to low dependency ratio and then increasing dependency because of aging, the pressure in the social delivery systems moves along depending where the bulk of the population is in its lifecycle. The simplified trajectory line, which represents the lifecycle starts with: (i) Birth and early childhood development, primarily affecting health, nutrition, and population policies; then (ii) entering youth, putting more pressure on the education sector; (iii) moving onward to working age, demanding more and better skills and labor market policies; and finally, (iv) at old age increasing demand for income protection in the form of pensions, and for chronic/geriatric care. These stages of the lifecycle — which at the aggregate level is expressed in terms of dependency ratios — crudely, correspond to the stages of economic development (LICs, MICs, and HICs). The sectoral entry points for intervention by policymakers and for technical assistance and operations, as noted earlier, includes the three sectors in human development — health, education, and social protection — and requires prudent and harmonized social policies. Further, gender and poverty reduction and economic management, including macro-fiscal

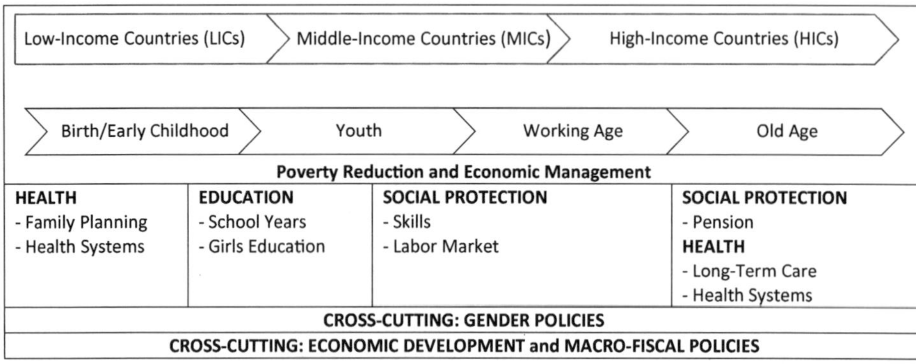

Figure 20. Planning for and managing the demographic transition — matrix for social and macro policies

Source: Author of this Chapter.

policies, are cross cutting. While, undoubtedly, there is heterogeneity within country groups and regions, this simplified graph illustrates the linkages and offers a basic conceptual guide on what it takes to harness the benefits of demographic change.

Growth, poverty and health

- *Investing in the health of the poor — More inclusive growth*

The positive relationship between economic growth and poverty reduction is well established. Yet, there is significant variation between countries in how growth reduces poverty — also known as the growth elasticity of poverty, technically defined as the percentage reduction in poverty rates associated with a percentage change increase in average per capita income (Bourguignon, 2003; Ravaillon and Chen, 1997; World Bank, 2001). Standard estimates of growth elasticity of poverty in developing countries range between 1.5 and 5, which implies that growth is fundamental to poverty reduction. However, growth in itself is not sufficient. As Bourguignon (2003) and later Iradian (2005) point out, the extent of poverty reduction depends on how the distribution of income changes with growth, on initial income inequalities, and on the sources or quality of growth.

Regarding the source of growth, for example, managing resources in natural resource-rich countries has its unique challenges[100], which can affect social expen-

[100] Complex political economy has been shown to be associated with worse performance on fiscal management (Braun and Di Gresia, 2003; Calderon and Schmidt-Hebbel 2008; Doytch *et al.*, 2010; IDB, 2009; IMF, 2009), specifically, with more propensity for fiscal profligacy. Some of the policy options recommended in the literature have been, for example, establishment of natural resource funds in resource-rich countries (Brahmbhatt and Canuto, 2012) and fiscal targets (Braun and Di

ditures, including public expenditures for health. Cyclical patterns have been claimed to be systematically different for resource-rich countries, specifically, there is more propensity for procyclical spending and more propensity for fiscal profligacy. This characteristic is relevant because complex political economy has been shown to be associated with worse performance on fiscal management (Braun and Di Gresia, 2003; Calderon and Schmidt-Hebbel, 2008; Doytch *et al.*, 2010; IDB, 2009; IMF, 2009). To attenuate procyclical fiscal responses, some of the policy options recommended in the literature have been, for example, establishment of natural resource funds in resource-rich countries (Brahmbhatt and Canuto, 2012) and fiscal targets (Braun and Di Gresia, 2003). Apart from some normative benchmarks for health expenditures as a share of government budget or as a share of the economy (see Discussion in Sections "Health Spending to Health Outcomes" and "Health Expenditure Trends"), the literature is mostly silent regarding recommendations of how to smooth social expenditures in resource-rich contexts, where procyclical responses have been more typical.

It is argued that establishing the relationship between economic growth and income distribution is critical for poverty reduction (Bourguignon, 2003; Iradian, 2005; Ravaillon and Chen, 1997; World Bank, 2001). If growth is not inclusive, inequality can further increase, which can undermine progress in human development. Fiscal policy is important not only for reducing poverty but also for improving human development and social indicators. Public spending on social sectors has a dual role — to alleviate poverty and stimulate human development. For example, in Chile (Iradian, 2005; Frankel, 2010)[101] countercyclical spending on social sectors — specifically on child and health nutrition — during fiscal adjustment helped the continued improvement of social conditions, which has contributed to sustained and more inclusive growth (see Box 18).

In the quest for attaining the MDGs, more developing countries have recognized the need for inclusive economic growth and reducing poverty and vulnerability, which has been reflected through increased budget allocation (i.e., reprioritization) to priority sectors, including health, education, and social protection, the main channels for improved human capital formation and social security.

For example, Gupta and Mitra (2004) analyze the possible links between economic growth, poverty and health, using panel data for the Indian states. Their findings indicate that, while growth tends to reduce poverty, significant improvements in health status — and, therefore, investments in health — are necessary for

---

Gresia, 2003). Cyclicality patterns have been claimed to be systematically different for resource rich countries (see more in Velenyi and Smitz, 2014).

[101] As discussed in Frankel (2010), since 2001, Chile has followed a fiscal rule that has a structural (that is, cyclically-adjusted) fiscal balance as its target. By design, such a rule ensures that temporarily high fiscal revenues are saved rather than spent.

Box 18. Illustration of graduation to countercyclical spending and fallback to procyclical spending

GDP and GHE cycles were predominantly procyclical in Latin America (LCN) during the deep and protracted crisis, which started in 2001, and did not end until at least 2005. However, there were some countercyclical responses at the peak of the crisis before the next year's budget allocation, when the increasingly constrained fiscal position bounded the health-spending frontier. These patterns are consistent with some of the observations in Braun and Di Gresia (2003), who provide more insights into the drivers of differences in cyclical responses across countries and over time. For example, they highlight prudent fiscal policies and increased fiscal transparency in Chile as possible contributors to countercyclical behavior. According to Frankel *et al.* (2011), Chile is undoubtedly the poster child of the graduation movement. But Chile is not the only country that seems to have escaped the procyclicality trap. The authors conclude that the quality of institutions (e.g., institutional strength and governance) seems to be a key determinant of a country's ability to graduate.

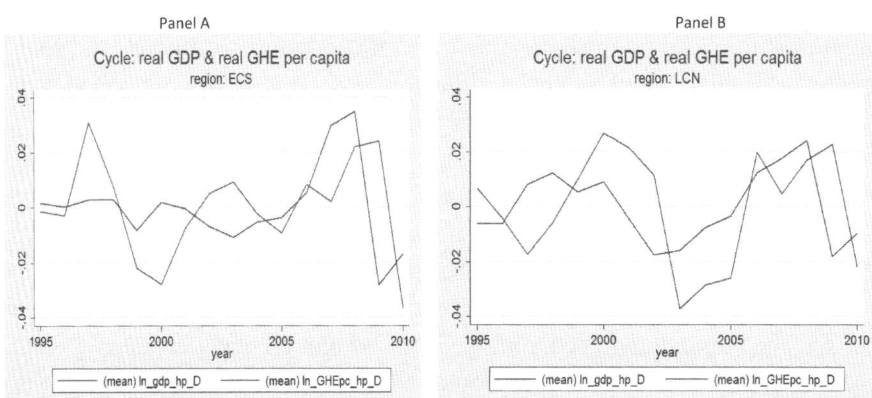

Figure 21. Cycles of GDP and GHE for Europe and Central Asia and Latin America and the Caribbean Regions, 1995–2010

Notes: Europe and Central Asia = ECS (this is an earlier code used in World Bank Databases, currently known as ECA); LCN = Latin American and the Caribbean (this is an earlier code used in World Bank Databases, currently known as LAC). Shown in blue, (mean) ln_gdp_hp_D is the cyclical component of the time series for per capita GDP growth, which is the difference between the observed value in log form (ln) and the corresponding value of the Hodrick–Prescott (HP) filtered trend line of economic growth. Shown in red, (mean) ln_GHEpc_hp_D is the cyclical component of the time series for per capita GHE growth, which is the difference between the observed value in log form (ln) and the corresponding value of the Hodrick–Prescott (HP) filtered trend line of public health expenditure growth.

Sources: Velenyi and Smitz (2014). Calculations based on data from the Fiscal Health Database 2012.

(*Continued*)

Box 18. (*Continued*)

In Figure 21, cyclical movements for GDP and GHE show a countercyclical spending pattern for Europe and Central Asia (ECA, or using the earlier region code ECS) between 2000 and 2007, with GHE declining — relative to the expected trend — when economic growth accelerates, and expanding when growth declines. However, toward the start and end points of the data series, the relationship is procyclical, especially during the global crisis — with the GDP and GHE cycles moving in the same direction. This implies that the depth and persistence of the crisis have reduced the resilience and stability of countries to an extent that GHE have declined. These patterns are empirically supported by a number of papers, including a few with regional coverage (Koettl and Schneider, 2010; WHO, 2013b), as well as country case studies (Barros, 2013; Burke *et al.*, 2013; Yfantopoulos, 2013).

poverty to decrease. Their study also provides evidence on the bidirectional relationship between growth and health, suggesting that better health enhances growth by improving productivity, and higher growth enables more investment in human capital formation. The authors conclude that health expenditure is an important determinant of both higher growth and better health status, and is therefore a key tool available to policymakers. Among other exogenous variables, literacy and industrialization seem to improve both health outcomes and growth, and reduce poverty.

In a theme paper for the *Bulletin of the World Health Organization*, Wagstaff provides an overview of poverty and health sector inequalities (Wagstaff, 2002). The author underscores that poverty and ill-health are intertwined, and this holds both across countries and within countries. He argues that, despite advanced measurement techniques and considerable evidence on the extent and drivers of inequalities in health, there is little evidence on the effectiveness of the policies that aim to combat poverty. Specifically, he points out that the failure of publicly financed health care to reach the poor is a concern for both governments and development partners. If scarce public resources are not used effectively to reach the poor with essential services, inadequate investments in human capital formation among the poor undermine both poverty reduction efforts and growth. Further, he argues that little is known about the relative importance of inequalities in the determinants of health and health service utilization. Evidence suggests that inequalities in health, and most probably in service utilization, very largely reflect inequalities in variables at the individual and household levels, such as education, income, location, and housing characteristics. This indicates that policies aimed at combating health sector inequalities should aim to reduce both inequalities on the supply side (e.g., service delivery network, quality of care, etc.) and the demand side (e.g., income, knowledge, health-specific knowledge, etc.).

The adoption of the Poverty Reduction Strategy Paper (PRSP) approach and the MDG Framework have increased the need for more systematic analysis of the poverty and social implications of reforms, including in the health sector (World Bank, 2009). Because poverty reduction has become the main goal of development, a debate has emerged over the distributional implications of reforms implemented within the pro-poor growth strategies. Consequently, the importance of equity analysis in health has increased, as shown by the establishment of health equity networks and the development of applied tools for the analysis of equity in health (O'Donnell *et al.*, 2008).

The foregoing discussion implies that investing in the health of the poor (i.e., pro-poor public health spending) is not only a distributional question within the sector, but it is a broader development objective. Improving health status and reducing illness-related catastrophic expenditures enable poor households to invest more in other essential needs, such as nutrition and education, which have lifetime and inter-generational effects on wealth.

- *Inequality of opportunity in health*[102]

Health inequalities and inequities remain high in global policy agendas. Their reduction is simultaneously perceived as a fundamental population health goal and as a key requirement for cutting back inequalities in other sectors of the economy, which, in turn, severely hold back economic development. One important challenge has been to move away from general statements, and instead adopt a rigorous evaluation of the progress made in reducing the health gap both within and between countries and of the impact of development programs on health inequities.

The *World Development Report 2006: Equity and Development* (World Bank, 2005) was an early example of moving away from such general statements by focusing on the concept of inequality of opportunity, thus making its guiding ethic concrete. The report made an unambiguous call for leveling the playing field (Roemer, 1998)[103] in human development, such that circumstances beyond the control of an individual should not pre-determine their life chances.

To advance in this field, Paes de Barros *et al.* (2009) proposed a series of practical tools for rigorously identifying, measuring and explaining inequality of

[102] The author is grateful to Pedro Rosa Dias for his comments and earlier contributions on this topic which benefited this section.

[103] Roemer introduced the concept of leveling the playing field for opportunities (Roemer, 1998).

opportunity. The authors examine the influence of a wide range of childhood circumstances on human achievement in Latin America and the Caribbean. Although the association between such factors and health outcomes is emphasized throughout the text, inequality of opportunity in health is not extensively explored. Childhood circumstances have been shown to have a strong and long-lasting effect on health later in life (Currie and Stabile, 2004; Case and Paxson, 2004, 2010). Hence, there are strong reasons to believe that a large portion of the observed health inequalities in adulthood are inequalities of opportunity; some of these may require very specific policy interventions. Yet, much of the conventional analysis of health inequalities in developing countries is focused on income- and ethnicity-related inequalities.

Rosa Dias (2009) extended the analysis of Paes de Barros *et al.* (2009) to the case of health to start bridging the gap between what we know about the early determinants of health and the analysis of health inequalities in a human development context. In a developed country context, he empirically explored inequality of opportunity in health — using Cohort data from the UK National Child Development study — and found considerable and persistent inequality of opportunity in health.

In 2010, the then Chief Economist of the World Bank (2010) noted that: "*The impacts of policies and economic changes on the poorest, once routinely neglected, are now given high priority in research. Inequality — notably inequality of opportunity — is now seen as an important problem constraining growth and poverty reduction.*" Despite such statements and the amount of resources focused on development in the health sector, there has been little empirical evidence in the developing country context on inequality of opportunity. The literature thus far — important as they are — have explored inequality of the distribution of health inputs and outcomes but less so the broader contextual setting, which is known to determine the health production function. There has also been little research on opportunities in childhood beyond the narrow definition of health inputs and the long-term implications of these into adulthood and through the lifecycle.

To reduce the knowledge gap in the developing country context, Jusot *et al.* (2014) apply an approach using the 2007 Indonesian Family Life Survey, a rich survey that includes both self-reported health outcome measures and biomarkers. Their results show large inequalities in opportunities in health compared to European countries. Concerning the transmission channels, parental — particularly maternal — health status appears to be the main channel. Compared to the findings in a developed country context, however, the effect of parental education in developing countries is smaller and more indirect. On the other hand, long-term differences in health associated with religion, language spoken, and particularly province of location suggest higher relevance for community-level variables. This finding, in contrast with earlier findings in developing countries, implies that the relevant policy response would involve addressing differentials between ethnic and religious groups and perhaps considering adjusting resource allocation patterns or development approaches across provinces.

Even though inequality of opportunity in Sub-Saharan Africa is among the world's highest, no systematic attempt has been made to measure it and unveil the network of causal effects that generate its powerful inequality traps. Paucity of good and comparable data and the lack of an adequate analytical framework partly explain this gap. Although the policy context in Sub-Saharan Africa is particularly complex, the approach proposed by Paes de Barros *et al.* (2009) is general enough to be applicable to it. For example, in the case of health, this approach would allow us to understand the circumstances that explain inequality of opportunity in health and exposure to catastrophic payments in different countries, and to analyze their evolution over time and their sensitivity to dissimilar health policy contexts. A study on inequality of opportunity in South Africa, published in 2012 (World Bank, 2012b),[104] considers the macro factors that drive growth and consequent poverty aspects. It considers opportunities among children, measured by the human opportunity index (HOI), which captures the coverage rate of basic services, adjusted for equity and differentiated by circumstances. It highlights unemployment as one of the main dimensions of inequality of opportunity. However, it does not explore the role of health contributing to inequality of opportunity in childhood and later in terms of access to jobs, compared to other middle-income countries. Given the high prevalence of HIV/AIDS and comorbidities, and known differentials in health status, which contribute to determining long-term employment opportunities, it appears that missing health is an important omission, which future research in Sub-Saharan Africa could consider. There is growing body of evidence that shows the benefits of freeing infant health from circumstantial constraints extend far beyond the associated health gains (Baird *et al.*, 2012; Miguel and Kremer, 2004). As suggested in the WDR 2006, examining inequality of opportunity in health in this region of the world would provide invaluable information on how severely it hampers human and economic development, as well as insight on what to do to reduce it.

As a result of increasing interest in evidence-based policymaking and consequent efforts to collect more and better data, an ever-growing amount of information is available from the impact evaluations of development programs that span education, health and other key areas of human opportunity.[105] The evaluation

---

[104] For a brief, see Narajan and Mahajan (2013).

[105] See, for example, the World Bank's Development Impact Evaluation Initiative (DIME), which spans all regions and various sectors (World Bank, 2015); the Health Results Innovation Trust Fund (HRITF) (Morgan, 2014), which, beyond the interventions, also funds a sizeable IE portfolio that primarily focuses on performance-based financing innovations in developing countries to improve maternal and child health and other health outcomes (see more at: https://www.rbfhealth.org/; J-PAL,

of such programs is carried out with the goal of understanding what works in development policy (accountability and effectiveness) and also the way in which programs and policies work (causal chain). Impact evaluations aim not only to measure results, but also to compare the effectiveness and cost-effectiveness of alternative interventions to help programs learn how to improve their performance over time.

However, much less emphasis has been given to determining the distributive effect of such development programs — such as by exploring quantile treatment effects during estimation (Abadie *et al.*, 2002; Frolich and Melly, 2013) — hence their potential for overall equity enhancement and levelling the playing field. For this purpose, the econometric literature is rich in methods designed for recovering such information from the available data.[106] Insights from explorations in this domain would facilitate the design and implementation of reforms, which are not only effective but also equity enhancing.

Distributional effects at the micro level and the growth elasticity of poverty (GEP — see more in Annex 3) are some key indicators to track results to better understand the medium- and long-term effects of programs. In the context of health and health care, such dimensions could be incorporated more in the battery of applied econometric techniques to further explore the wealth of information available through cross-country compilation of national survey data, tapping into the micro data collected for a large number of development programs. This would allow for deeper and valuable insights, not only into the anatomy of worldwide health inequities, but also into the largely unexplored or under-explored distributive effects of programs aimed at human opportunity and development.

In sum, such analytical work would also fit the holistic development objectives — the mandate of governments and development agencies — of poverty reduction, development, and sustained macroeconomic growth, by providing information on how policies and programs that affect human capital formation contribute to attaining these objectives.

Conclusions and Recommendations for Future Research

This chapter set out to explore the relationship between health expenditures and economic growth, an important yet complex relationship. Understanding the

the Poverty Action Lab (see more at: http://www.povertyactionlab.org/evaluations); and the International Initiative for Impact Evaluation (3IE) (see more at: http://www.3ieimpact.org/).

[106] See for example, Carneiro *et al.* (2003); Cunha *et al.* (2006); Djebbari and Smith (2008); Carneiro *et al.* (2010) and references therein; also, given that differences-in-differences are extensively used in impact evaluation programs, the *changes-in-changes* approach proposed in Athey and Imbens (2006) can be a particularly useful tool.

evolution of health spending and economic growth nexus has been propelled by two major forces: Concerns about expenditures and to inform health policymaking that is grounded in the broader economic and development framework.

On the expenditure side, concerns have been growing regarding the spiraling nature of health spending, which has been perceived as 'uncontainable' and a potential threat to crowding out resources from other sectors over time, given the continuously rising level of per capita spending on health and the sector's share of the budget and of the economy. Although per capita health expenditures have been undeniably growing, both the review of the literature and statistical analyses indicate that the growth trends have not been homogenous across regions and that the rate of growth has moderated over time. Beyond the regular checks and balances between ministries of health and finance during the budgeting process, economic crises have also played a role in 'rationalizing' or 'streamlining' expenditures on health and have played a role in catalyzing structural reforms. If trends following the GEC — which started in 2007 and peaked in 2009 — are taken into account, growth in the health sector's share of the economy has moderated over time and is not distressing at the global level. Although the findings and policy implications vary by income group,[107] there is considerable variation within groups which points out the importance of country-specific analysis and policy feedback.

More broadly, policymakers and researchers have shifted attention to the health spending and growth nexus to inform national and global health policymaking in a way that connects health sector investments to the broader objective of economic growth and development. This indicates a movement toward more strategic utilization of resources, including longer time horizon for strategic planning and accentuating the two-way relationship between the health sector and the economy. These changes, however, require applying a multidisciplinary research approach, going beyond the narrow boundaries of the sector. Long-term planning requires a strategic vision to engage in health investments that span political cycles and may not bring immediate returns. And last, such broad-based and long-term approaches require multisectoral coordination. One example, discussed in the

[107] For example, the general pattern for low-income countries is low level of health expenditures, which in the most constrained settings often couples with dependence on external resource flows for health. In such context, increasing the level of health expenditures and strategically managing donor dependency are some of the key issues for policy attention and action. On the other end of the spectrum, in advance economies structural or system-level aspects — such as aging, rigidities in social security systems, and technological advancements — have increasingly pressed the fiscal envelope. In such context, the policy focus shifts to cost containment and structural reforms to ensure the long-term operability of the system subject to budget constraints. This illustrates that the sustainability paradigms are very different at the two extremes of the development trajectory. However, in reality, there is often a blend of these challenges depending on the macro-fiscal context and system-level constraints.

chapter, where long-term planning and cross-sectoral policy coordination is required to induce growth is the strategic management of demographic change. Another example of strategic planning and spending is the case of the Ebola epidemic, which demonstrated that lack of adequate and strategic investment in health system strengthening not only undermines sector-level objectives but it can deeply affect and even reverse economic growth and development, and more broadly, has the ability to destabilize regional-level economic growth.

To update our knowledge of the health spending and economic growth dynamics, we undertook a review[108] of the relevant theoretical and empirical literature that has been generated over the past 50 years, and performed statistical analyses using publicly available global databases — such as the World Health Organization's National Health Accounts (NHA) and the World Bank's World Development Indicators (WDI) — focusing on trends over the past two decades, since 1995. The review and statistical analyses were also used to identify gaps in the literature, methodological shortcomings, and data challenges that have been hampering efforts in establishing clear causal links and estimating the magnitude of effects along the causal chain.

With respect to policy relevance, the presented evidence and the related discussions in this chapter aim to contribute to identifying pragmatic approaches that could inform policymakers and technical experts regarding how more efficient and strategic spending could lead to better health outcomes, and how, in turn, improved population health status could act as an economic growth multiplier. Although the chapter presented analytical/diagnostic tools, country examples, and discussed policy questions and options, it did not attempt to provide advice on specific 'best buy' interventions that would bring the most growth for the health dollars spent. As development through the health channel is country-specific, the chapter argued that systematic country diagnostic is a critical input into policymaking.

With the multiplicity of views presented from the vantage point of different disciplines, the chapter captured some of the dynamics that can be observed between ministries of health, ministries of finance and development, development practitioners, the broader set of actors who set the health and development policy agendas, and researchers who aim to inform decision and policy processes and the sectoral and overall development agendas.

The chapter concluded that a great deal has been accomplished over the past decades, including a growing body of evidence on the causal (or bidirectional) relationship between health and growth and on the economic returns of health investments,

---

[108] Given the depth and breadth of the literature on health spending and health outcomes and health status and growth over the past 50 years, the review focused on a selected set of formative research pieces that have shaped the discussion and agenda in a significant way. The chapter did not intend to do a systematic review of the literature as that was beyond the scope of the undertaking.

and most importantly, as a result of investments in the sector, convergence in health outcomes. In econometric terms, health has emerged from a 'residual factor' in macroeconomic growth models[109] into a coefficient of its own, an explanatory factor of productivity, economic growth, and poverty reduction. Yet, more research is required to guide future decisions on how to invest wisely in health and in a way that can perpetuate further growth. Among some of the questions where the evidence base is growing but inconclusive and not sufficiently specific are: how to manage the sector strategically through economic cycles and graduate into countercyclical policymaking; how to minimize the effect of shocks — including economic downturns, epidemics, and natural disasters — on the health system and the population; and how to plan for the long term, including through system strengthening, particularly in low-income context, and the strategic management of demographic trends.

Specifically, more attention to and investment in the following research areas would greatly contribute to the health spending and growth discourse: (i) Improved databases (including health financing, health systems, and macro-fiscal data) at the national and global level, which are more standardized, comparable, and enable replicable research; (ii) multi-disciplinary research agenda[110] as health investment decisions take place in a complex environment not in a self-contained sector-specific space; (iii) systematic sector diagnostics (e.g., PER and FSA) that is embedded in the macro-fiscal framework of the country; (iv) more focus on positive economics to understand what motivates country responses/behavior, including when they deviate from global and regional normative benchmarks; (v) more evidence on the contribution of technology to spending in developing countries, and on the costs and benefits — including broader social benefits — of adapting improved technology; (vi) further developing and applying country-level monitoring tools and early warning systems to help evidence-based responses during crises; and, finally, (vii) more robust evaluation work at the country level to continue exploring how innovative financing mechanisms perform, including their effects on the providers, the system, the population, and the economy overall.

---

[109] See more in Section Introduction: Investing in Health — Investing in Growth? and in Abramovitz (1956).

[110] For example, more development economics in health to better address the specific problems and identify evidence-based solutions in lower income countries; more investigation of the governance and public finance management aspects of the health sector to improve the effectiveness of public and external resources; more quantifiable health system science to better unpack the system-level drivers of efficiency within economic models; sustained efforts to develop health financing metrics to make the concepts, typologies, and targets more amenable for economic modeling; more applied health economics to inform systematic sector diagnostics; more applied micro-econometrics to generate evidence on effectiveness and cost-effectiveness in a variety of settings; more studies that explore the macro/fiscal dimension and use macro-econometric approaches to explore cyclical patterns, and so forth.

Annexes

Annex 1. Mitigation Options to Attenuate the Effects of Economic Crises

Table A1. Mitigation Policy Options Corresponding to the Vulnerability Assessment Framework

External Factors	System-level factors	Household-level factors
	Corresponding policy responses	
1. Fiscal responses: Maintaining public funding for the health system (a) Raising contributions and broadening the revenue base (b) Increasing transfers from government budgets (c) Automatic stabilizers: Reserves and countercyclical formulas (d) Introducing new taxes (including sin taxes) ***2. Demography*** (a) Changing cutoff age for pension (affects revenue base and social expenditures)	***1. Health system financing*** (a) Increasing user charges (b) Greater role for voluntary insurance (c) Targeting to protect people with low incomes (d) Implications for adequacy, stability, and equity ***2. Health coverage*** (a) Reducing population coverage ("breadth" of coverage) (b) Streamlining the benefits package ("scope" of coverage) ***3. Savings and structural changes*** (a) Adapting more efficient provider payment systems (b) Strengthening pharmaceutical policy (c) Strengthening primary care access (d) Restructuring or reorganizing the health system (e) Making cost-effective investments in health goods, services, technologies — more use of Health Technology Assessment for improved and evidence-based decisions	***Demand for Health Care*** Ensure continued and equitable physical and financial access to health services through: — Provision of affordable care to essential services (preventive and treatment) — Provision of safety nets (demand-side financing mechanisms, e.g., publicly subsidized schemes, targeted cash transfers or vouchers), particularly for the poor and vulnerable, to minimize the incidence of catastrophic health expenditures — Ensuring progressivity and equity of health expenditures — Behavioral change communication to reduce the risk of crisis-related health effects (e.g., nutrition, alcohol and tobacco consumption, injuries, etc.)

Notes: This table combines the health system vulnerability assessment framework proposed by Velenyi *et al.* (2013) with observed policy responses that were documented, based on key informant interviews and surveys conducted by the WHO. The mitigation options are discussed in detail in an overview paper prepared by the WHO (2013) as background material for the conference "Health Systems in Times of GEC: An Update of the Situation in the WHO European Region." This table includes minor modifications.
Source: Author based on WHO (2013) and Velenyi et al. (2013).

Annex 2. Crisis Pathways

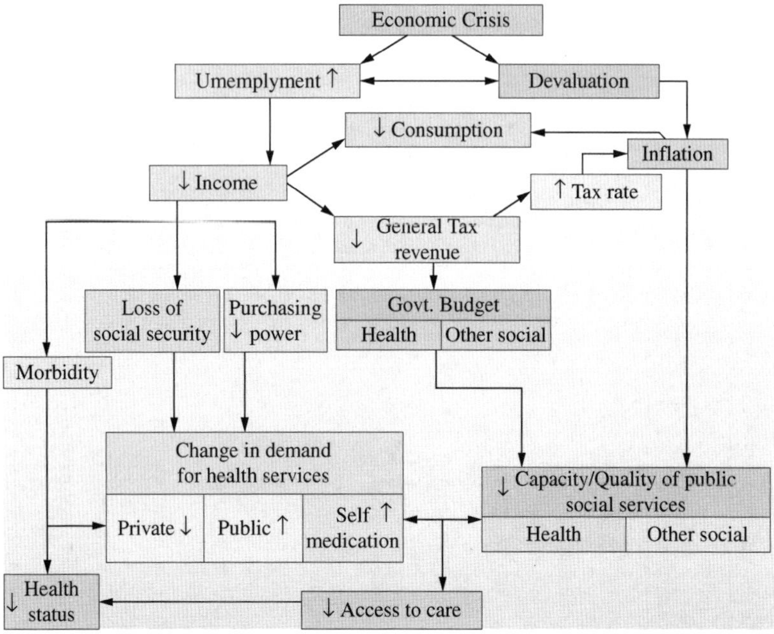

Figure A2.1. Crisis Pathways
Source: Musgrove (1987).

Annex 3. Technical Glossary and Applied Analytical Notes

Asymmetry of Spending: Del Granado *et al.* (2012) find that the cyclicality of spending is asymmetric across "good" and "bad" times, defined in terms of output gap relative to potential output. To validate this finding, we construct the variable "output gap," which measures the difference between the observed value for the variable of interest and the value on the filtered trend for the given year in terms of standard deviation from the trends (see more under ***Output Gap***). Good/bad times are defined as a positive/negative output gap relative to the trend line.

Business Cycle (or Economic Cycle) refers to the economy-wide fluctuation in production, trade, and economic activity in general over several months or years (Brahmbhatt and Canuto, 2012; Braun and Di Gresia, 2003; Darby and Melitz, 2008; Doytch *et al.*, 2010). The term "cycle" is a misnomer, because business cycle fluctuations are neither regular nor predictable. Upward and downward movements in the cycle (expansions and contractions) can be measured by the level of GDP (Darby and Melitz, 2008; Del Granado *et al.*, 2012; Doytch *et al.*, 2010; Thornton, 2008). These fluctuations are measured relative to the economy's long-term growth trend (Thornton, 2008). A variable that is positively correlated with the overall state of the economy is said to be procyclical, and a variable that is negatively correlated with the overall state of the economy is said to be countercyclical (see more under ***countercyclical** and **procyclical policy***).

Countercyclical and Procyclical Policy: In the context of economic policy, procyclical (countercyclical) refers to any aspect of economic policy that can magnify (attenuate) economic or financial fluctuations. Countercyclical policies cool the economy when it overheats and stimulate it when there is a downturn. Keynesian economics advocates the use of automatic and discretionary countercyclical policies to lessen the impact of the business cycle.

Country Income Group: The classification is based on the World Bank's income groups,[111] which is calculated using the World Bank Atlas Method.[112] The classification used is for 2012, the most recent year used in the analyses.

Correlation Coefficient: To obtain bivariate contemporaneous correlations, drawing on the calculated cyclical components for output (GDP), GGE,[113] and GHE, Velenyi and Smitz (2014) calculate the cross-correlations between the various cyclical components (see more under ***Cyclical Component***), specifically between the business and fiscal cycles (GDP and GGE), the business and government health spending cycles (GDP and GHE), and between the fiscal and government health spending cycles (GGE and GHE). These cross-correlations allow us to establish whether the relationship between business cycles, fiscal responses, and health sector responses are countercyclical or procyclical, that is, whether the cycles move in opposite directions, protecting budgets and health spending during bad times, or in the same direction, signaling increasing expenditure pressures during bad times (see more under ***Asymmetry of Spending***). A ***correlation***

---

[111] The World Bank income group classification is discussed at: http://data.worldbank.org/about/country-and-lending-groups.

[112] The Atlas Method is discussed at: http://datahelpdesk.worldbank.org/knowledgbase/articles/378832-what-is-the-world-bank-atlas-method.

[113] Ilzetzki and Végh (2008) provide a discussion on the alternative definitions of government spending measures and the trade-off between them. While the use of a general government measure is more inclusive, including both central and local governments, the use of central government spending is more in accordance with the principle of looking at social policy instruments that are directly under the control of a single social agent. Total central government spending includes more spending categories, such as government consumption, public investment, and transfers, but also interest payments, which makes this measure noisier. Much of the literature on the cyclicality of social policy has used real central government spending (for example, Kaminsky *et al.*, 2004; Alesina *et al.*, 2008), while much of the literature on the effectiveness of social policy in high-income countries has looked at government consumption or a combination of government consumption and investment (for example, Blanchard and Perotti, 2002; Perotti, 2004).

coefficient above 0 (+) implies a procyclical relationship. The higher the value[114] is between 0 and 1, the more correlated the cycles are. Conversely, a correlation coefficient below 0 (–) signals a countercyclical relationship. In this fourth step, we provide a visual overview of cyclical relationships through graphs of overlaid cycles.

Crisis: There is no consensus on the definitions of different types of crises despite their frequency in development economics. One of the most important common features of crises is an "abrupt" change in economic indicators. Operational definitions require an indicator and a threshold.

Cyclical Component of Time Series Data: The cyclical component of time series data — for example for GDP — is the difference between the observed value (typically used in log form[115] of the variable) and the corresponding value on the filtered[116] trend line). The figures obtained this way describe the cyclical behavior of the variable of interest. For example, in case of economic output (GDP), if the calculated cyclical component is positive, this means that the cycle is above the expected trend line, and if the calculated cyclical component is negative, this means that the cycle is below the expected trend line.

Demographic Transition (Demographic Dividend and Demographic Drag): The shift from high to low mortality and fertility rates results in a demographic transition, which first opens a window of opportunity for growth as dependency ratio (the ratio of non-working age population to the working age population) declines, followed by the second wave of the transition when the needs of an aging population bring major challenges for the economy generally and for social policy in particular.

- Triggered by changes in reproductive health policies that aim for lower fertility rate and improved maternal and child health, some countries (for example

[114] The standard threshold values for correlation coefficients are: (a) Weak positive (negative) linear relationship via a shaky linear rule, values between 0 and 0.3 (0 and –0.3); (b) Moderate positive (negative) linear relationship via a fuzzy-firm linear rule, values between 0.3 and 0.7 (0.3 and –0.7); and (c) Strong positive (negative) linear relationship via a firm linear rule, values between 0.7 and 1.0 (–0.7 and –1.0).

[115] This is standard procedure with data that have outliers and skewed or exponential distribution, such as income and health expenditures, to compact the dispersion of the variable. The convenience of log-transformed variables is that their difference can be interpreted in percentage change terms.

[116] Using a common practice in the business cycle literature, Velenyi and Smitz (2014) apply a linear filter to the log-transformed variables of interest to detrend the series. This is necessary because, following Lucas (1977), the business cycle component of the variable is defined as its deviation from the trend. Specifically, the Hodrick–Prescott (HP) filter is applied to extract the stationary (cyclical) component and the non-stationary (trend) component.

in Sub-Saharan Africa) are at an early stage of the demographic transition and are entering a period in which the number of workers will grow more rapidly than the population, making it possible to reap a '***Demographic Dividend***' *if* and *when* all required policies on learning and skills and labor markets are put in place.

- In other countries (which mostly fall into the middle-, upper-middle-, and high-income categories), the window for capturing the dividend is beginning to close. For example, in Europe and East Asia, the dramatic population aging that characterizes the latter part of the demographic transition requires careful planning and foresight to ensure that the population is productive, and protected in a way that is sustainable. Failing to introduce social sector policies that focus on addressing the needs of the aging population would result in a '***Demographic Drag***' that would slow economic growth.

Elasticity — See income elasticity of health expenditures.

Excess Health Expenditure Growth — also referred to as **'Excess Growth'** — is defined relative to GDP growth, calculated as the difference in the annual growth rate of health expenditure minus the growth rate of annual economic growth measured in GDP. Consequently, a positive (negative) value indicates that health expenditures are growing in excess (moderation) of economic growth. The excess growth for a period is calculated from the difference of the average growth rates of these variables. To take into account inflation and population dynamics, excess growth is calculated using growth rates based on constant per capita values.

Fiscal Policy (*Wikipedia*, 2015)[117] is the use of government revenue collection (mainly taxes) and expenditure (spending) to influence the economy (Weil, 2015). According to Keynesian economics, when the government changes the levels of taxation and government spending, it influences aggregate demand and the level of economic activity. Fiscal policy can be used to stabilize the economy over the course of the ***business cycle***. Fiscal policy, which covers government expenditure on health, is a key tool that governments can use to mobilize domestic resources and allocate them to achieve policy objectives.

Fiscal Space and Fiscal Sustainability: Conceptually, the general framework for fiscal space assessment was proposed by Heller (2005), who defined ***fiscal space*** as the "*availability of budgetary room that allows a government to provide resources for a desired purpose without any prejudice to the sustainability of a government's financial position*" (Heller, 2005, 2006). According to the author,

[117] *Wikipedia* (2015). *Fiscal Policy* [Online]. Available at: http://en.wikipedia.org/wiki/Fiscal_policy (Accessed 12 March 2015).

this concept of fiscal space requires ***fiscal sustainability***, that is, the capacity of the government to finance its desired expenditure programs, to service debt obligations and to ensure its future solvency. The framework emphasizes that fiscal sustainability depends on the underlying economic growth rate, which determines revenue generation and whether commitments affect fiscal space immediately or in the long run. Hence, it is argued that fiscal space assessment must be made in the context of at least a ***medium-term expenditure framework***, which takes a comprehensive and forward-looking perspective of the government's budget priorities. In pragmatic terms, ***fiscal sustainability*** is forward looking and is determined by dimensions such as fiscal balance, evolution of public debt, capacity of the government to finance its budget (borrowing, etc.) requirements and refinance maturing debt, assess fiscal risks, etc.; while ***fiscal space*** focuses on additional expenditure needed to promote development, stimulate growth, increase government revenue, etc. — create fiscal space to finance increasing demands (e.g., ***fiscal space for health***, etc.).

Fiscal Space for Health: The health sector-specific adaptation of the fiscal space concept was developed 5 years later by Tandon and Cashin (2010) who — following the general framework — proposed the definition for fiscal space for health as "*the ability of governments to increase spending for the sector without jeopardizing the government's long-term solvency or crowding out expenditure in other sectors needed to achieve other development objectives.*" As a review of fiscal space for health points out (Powell-Jackson *et al.*, 2012), when applied to the health sector, the intention is to increase financial resources for health over the short- to medium-term in a way that is consistent with a country's macroeconomic fundamentals, such that the long-term solvency of the government and its economic potential is not jeopardized (Adam and Bevan, 2005).

Global Health Protection Fund: Five years before the 2015 deadline of attaining the MDGs the concern was raised that the financing of the MDGs is not merely insufficient but evidence indicates that the temporary nature of the financing, as well as challenges to coordinating its delivery and directing it to the most needy recipients, hinder achievement of the goals in countries that may benefit most (Ooms *et al.*, 2010). Traditional approaches to providing DAH have not been able to address both prevalent and emergent public health challenges captured in the health MDGs. The authors suggested that these challenges demand sustained forms of financial redistribution through a coordinated mechanism. Thus, a global social health protection fund was proposed to address recurring failures in the modern aid distribution mechanism; to use established and effective strategies for aid delivery.

Growth Elasticity of Poverty (GEP): GEP (Bourguignon, 2003) is the percentage reduction in poverty rates associated with a percentage change in mean per capita income. Generally, increases in per capita income tend to decrease poverty and, hence, the elasticity is positive. Standard estimates of GEP for developing countries are between 1.5 and 5, with an average estimated around 3. This means that a 1% increase in per capita income is associated with a 3% decrease in the poverty rate, the proportion of people living under the poverty threshold (e.g., $1-a-day or $1.25-a-day).

Income Elasticity of Health Expenditures: Income elasticity of demand measures the responsiveness of the demand for a good or service to the change in the income of the people demanding the good or service. Income elasticity of health expenditures shows the change in health expenditures for a 1% increase in economic growth. Arithmetically, income elasticity of demand is calculated as the ratio of the percentage change in demand to the percentage change in income. For example: If, in response to a 10% increase in income, the demand for health services increased by 13%, the income elasticity of demand would be 13%/10% = 1.3. If, in response to a 10% increase in income, the demand for health services increased by 6.5%, the income elasticity of demand would be 6.5%/10% = 0.65. Regarding its interpretation, a positive income elasticity of demand is associated with normal goods; an increase in income will lead to a rise in demand. If income elasticity of demand of a commodity is less than 1, it is a necessity good. If the elasticity of demand is greater than 1, it is a luxury good or a superior good. A zero income elasticity of demand occurs when an increase in income is not associated with a change in the demand of a good. These would be sticky goods. A negative income elasticity of demand is associated with inferior goods; an increase in income will lead to a fall in the demand and may lead to changes to more luxurious substitutes.

Long and Short Routes of Accountability: These concepts are central in the *2004 World Development Report: Making Services Work for Poor People* (World Bank, 2003). The ***'long route' of accountability***, also referred to as the *indirect route of accountability*, is whereby poor people or citizens influence policymakers or politicians and then the politicians influence the providers to deliver quality care. The ***'short route'*** stands for direct accountability between users and providers, for example where consumers and communities have a direct role in determining service delivery.

Medium Term Expenditure Framework is a whole-of-government strategic policy and expenditure framework which balances what is affordable (in the aggregate) against policy priorities of the government. An MTEF consists of: (i) A top–down resource envelop; (ii) a bottom–up estimation of current- and medium-term (usually a 3–5 year period) costs of existing policies; (iii) matching these costs with available resources. This should take place in the context of annual budget process. As such, the MTEF shifts the psychology of budgeting from "needs" to an "availability of resources" mentality (De Silva, 2009). The MTEF is closely related to the criteria of ***fiscal sustainability*** and ***fiscal space*** (see separate entries on these above), which are better incorporated into a multi-year framework as opposed to an annual budgeting framework.

Output Gap: In terms of the measurement approach, output gap is not equivalent to growth crises measures that are provided in terms of negative GDP growth.[118] The difference is that while growth crises are defined in terms of negative year-on-year GDP growth rate, a negative output gap does not necessarily mean that the country has a negative growth rate. For example, in the case of a slowdown of economic output in countries with high growth rates, a negative output gap simply means that relative to the expected trend the country's economic performance is lower but not necessarily negative. In sum, output and GDP growth rate are different concepts. Output gap is a relative measure of the country's performance on industrial output. GDP growth rate is an absolute measure of industrial output.

Terms of Trade: The ratio between the prices of exports and imports is called the net barter terms of trade (ToT). ToT is said to be favorable when the prices of exports of a country are higher relative to the prices of its import. ToT has been found to be significant, especially for developing countries with high export shares and a high share of revenues from trade (Del Granado *et al.*, 2012; Mendoza, 1995). Mendoza (1995) finds that terms of trade are strongly procyclical, suggesting that much of the fluctuation in output in developing countries can be explained by ToT shocks. Given the definition, ToT improves if the ratio is higher. In time series analysis, ToT can be used as difference in ToT relative to the previous year. In terms of the interpretation of this proxy measure, improving ToT would increase fiscal space; however, if not used wisely, a windfall from a ToT improvement can lead to more procyclical behavior, as often observed in resource rich countries.

WHO NHA (World Health Organization's National Health Accounts) (WHO, 2014c)[119,120]: The global health expenditure database that WHO has maintained for the past 10 years provides internationally comparable statistics on national health

[118] The National Bureau of Economic Research defines a recession in the United States as when seasonally adjusted quarterly growth rates are negative for two straight quarters. Bruno (1996) defines growth crises as at least 3 consecutive years of negative growth, cumulating in a drop of growth of at least 9%.

[119] See WHO NHA Database: http://apps.who.int/nha/database. Glossary: http://apps.who.int/nha/database/DocumentationCentre/Index/en.

[120] See WHO NHA Glossary http://apps.who.int/nha/database/DocumentationCentre/Index/en.

expenditures. WHO updates the data annually, taking, adjusting and estimating the numbers based on publicly available reports (e.g., National Health Account Reports, reports from the Ministry of Finance, Central Bank, National Statistics Office, public expenditure information, and reports from the World Bank and IMF, etc.). The estimates are sent to the Ministries of Health for validation prior to publication but users are advised that country data may still differ in terms of definitions, data collection methods, population coverage, and estimation methods used. This database is source of the health expenditure tables in the World Health Statistics Report and the WHO Global Health Observatory.

References

Abadie A, Angrist J, Imbens G. 2002. Instrumental variables estimates of the effect of subsidized training on the quantiles of trainee earnings. *Econometrica* 70(1): 91–117.

Abbas F, Hiemenz U. 2011. Determinants of Public Health Expenditures in Pakistan. Discussion Papers 118422, University of Bonn, Center for Development Research (ZEF).

Abramovitz M. 1956. Resource and Output Trends in the United States since 1870. New York: National Bureau of Economic Research, Occasional Paper 52.

Acemoglu D, Finkelstein A, Notowidigdo MJ. 2013. Income and health spending: Evidence from oil price shocks. *Review of Economics and Statistics* 95(4): 1079–1095. By the President and Fellows of Harvard College and the Massachusetts Institute of Technology.

Acemoglu D, Rogoff K, Woodford M. (eds.). University of Chicago Press. ISBN: 0-226-00204-7. pp. 157–204. http://www.nber.org/chapters/c7278.

Adam CS, Bevan DL. 2005. Fiscal deficits and growth in developing countries. *Journal of Public Economics* 89(4): 571–597.

Africa Union Commission and Economic Commission for Africa. 2013. Industrialization for an Emerging Africa. Conference proceeding. 21–26 March 2013. Abidjan, Côte d'Ivoire. http://gatesinstitute.org/sites/default/files/5%20Policy%20Briefs%20on%20the%20Demographic%20Dividend_English.pdf.

Aghion P, Howitt P, Murtin F. 2010. The Relationship Between Health and Growth: When Lucas Meets Nelson-Phelps. Available at: http://scholar.harvard.edu/files/aghion/files/relationship_between_health.pdf.

Akitoby B, Clements B, Gupta S, Inchauste G. 2004. The Cyclical and Long-Term Behavior of Government Expenditures in Developing Countries. *IMF Working Paper*. WP/04/202.

Alderman H. 2011. No Small Matter. The Impact of Poverty, Shocks, and Human Capital Investments in Early Childhood Development. In: Alderman H. (ed.). The World Bank. Washington, DC.

Alesina A, Campante FR, Tabellini G. 2008. Why is fiscal policy often procyclical? *Journal of the European Economic Association* 6(5): 1006–1036.

Alkire S. 2002. Dimensions of human development. *World Development* 30(2): 181–205. Elsevier Science Ltd.

Ashraf Q, Lester A, Weil DN. 2009. When Does Improving Health Raise GDP? In: NBER Macroeconomics Annual 2008, Volume 23.

Atella V, Marini G. 2006. Is health care expenditure really a luxury good? Reassessment and new evidence based on OECD data. *Working Paper*. http://papers.ssm.com/abstract=383004.

Athey S, Imbens GW. 2006. Identification and inference in nonlinear difference-in-differences model. *Econometrica* 74(2): 431–497.

Avila C, Connor C, Amico P. 2013. Universal Coverage of Essential Health Services in Sub-Saharan Africa: Projections of Domestic Resources. August 2013. Bethesda, MD: Health Finance & Governance Project, Abt Associates Inc.

Baird S, Friedman J, Schady N. 2007. Aggregate Income Shocks and Infant Mortality in the Developing World. *Open Knowledge Repository*, World Bank, Washington, DC. https://openknowledge.worldbank.org/handle/10986/7627.

Baird S, Hicks JH, Kremer M, Miguel E. 2012. Worms at Work: Public Finance Implications of a Child Health Investment. Poverty Action Lab. First Version: October 2010. This Versions: June 2013. [Online] [Accessed: April 2015]. Available at: http://www.povertyactionlab.org/publication/worms-work-public-finance-implications-child-health-investment.

Baker B. 2010. Effect of development assistance on domestic health expenditures. *The Lancet* 376: 589–590.

Barker D. 1990. The fetal and infant origins of adult disease. *British Medical Journal* 301(6761): 1111.

Baltagi BH, Moscone F. 2010. Health care expenditure and income in the OECD reconsidered: Evidence from panel data. *Economic Modelling* 27(4): 804–811.

Barros PP. 1998. The Black Box of health care expenditure growth determinants. Economics of health care systems. *Health Economics* 7: 533–544.

Barros PP. 2013. Case Study 2: Changes in the Health Sector under Economic Crisis and Financial Rescue: Portugal. Section in Chapter 5, Lessons from the European Union. In *Learning from Economic Downturns: How to Better Assess, Track, and Mitigate the Impact on the Health Sector*. Hou X, Velenyi EV, Yazbeck AS, Iunes RF, Smith O. (eds.). The World Bank. Washington, DC.

Becker GS. 1993. The Economic Way of Looking at Life. *Coase-Sandor Institute for Law & Economics Working Paper No*. 12. Available at: http://chicagounbound.uchicago.edu/cgi/viewcontent.cgi?article=1509&context=law_and_economics.

Bell C. 1987. *Development Economics*. The New Palgrave: A Dictionary of Economics, 1: pp. 818, 825.

Bhalotra S. 2010. Fatal fluctuations? Cyclicality in infant mortality in India. *Journal of Development Economics* 93(1): 7–19.

Black RE, Allen LH, Bhutta ZA, Caulfield LE, de Onis M, Ezzati M, Mathers C, Rivera J. 2008. Maternal and child undernutrition: Global and regional exposures and health consequences. *The Lancet*. Published Online: 17 January 2008. http://www.thelancet.com/journals/lancet/article/PIIS0140-6736(07)61690-0/fulltext.

Blanchard O, Perotti R. 2002. An empirical characterization of the dynamic effects of changes in government spending. *Quarterly Journal of Economics* 117(4): 1329–1368.

Bleakley H. 2007. Disease and development: Evidence from Hookworm eradication in the American South. *Quarterly Journal of Economics* 122(1): 73–117.

Blomqvist ÅG, Carter RAL. 1997. Is health care really a luxury? *Journal of Health Economics* 16(2): 207–229.

Bloom DE, Canning D. 2003a. Contraception and the Celtic Tiger. *The Economic and Social Review* 34: 229–247.

Bloom D, Canning D. 2007. Commentary: The Preston Curve 30 years on: Still sparking fires. *International Journal of Epidemiology*. [Online] 36(3): 498–499. Available at: http://www.ncbi.nlm.nih.gov/pubmed/17550948.

Bloom DE, Canning D, Graham B. 2003b. Longevity and life-cycle savings. *Scandinavian Journal of Economics* 105(3): 319–338.

Bloom DE, Canning D, Malaney P. 2000. Demographic change and economic growth in Asia. *Population and Development Review* 26(supp): 257–290.

Bloom DE, Canning D, Hu L, Liu Y, Mahal A, Yip W. 2010.The contribution of population health and demographic change to economic growth in China and India. *Journal of Comparative Economics* 38(1): 17–33. doi: 10.1016/j.jce.2009.11.002.

Bloom DE, Canning D, Sevilla J. 2003c. The effect of health on economic growth: A production function approach. *World Development* 32(1): 1–13. Elsevier.

Bloom D, Williamson J. 1998. Demographic transitions and economic miracles in emerging Asia. *The World Bank Economic Review* 12(3): 419–455.

Bonnel R. 2000. HIV/AIDS: Does it Increase or Decrease Growth in Africa? ACTAfrica. World Bank. 6 November 2000. Available at: http://citeseerx.ist.psu.edu/viewdoc/download?doi=10.1.1.201.8357&rep=rep1&type=pdf.

Borghi J, Little R, Binyaruka P, Patouillard E, Kuwawenaruwa A. 2015. In Tanzania, The Many Costs Of Pay-For-Performance Leave Open To Debate Whether The Strategy Is Cost-Effective. *Health Affairs* 34(6). http://content.healthaffairs.org/content/34/3/406.short.

Bourguignon F. 2003. The Growth Elasticity of Poverty Reduction; Explaining Heterogeneity across Countries and Time Periods. In: Eicher T, Turnovsky S. (eds.). *Inequality and Growth*, 1st ed. Cambridge, Mass: MIT Press.

Brahmbhatt M, Canuto O. 2012. Fiscal Policy for Growth and Development. *Economic Premise 91* (October), Poverty Reduction and Economic Management Unit (PREM), World Bank, Washington, DC.

Braun M, Di Gresia L. 2003. Towards Effective Social Insurance in Latin America: The Importance of Countercyclical Fiscal Policy. Inter-American Development Bank *Working Paper* 487, Washington, DC.

Brenzel L. 2012. Literature Review on the Impact of the Global Financial Crisis on Health. Unpublished Draft. June 1, 2012.

Bruno M. 1996. Deep Crises and Reform: What Have We Learned? Washington: The World Bank.

Burke S, Barry S, Thomas S. 2013. Case Study 1: The Economic Crisis and the Irish Health System: Assessing Resilience. Section in Chapter 5, Lessons from the

European Union. In *Learning from Economic Downturns: How to Better Assess, Track, and Mitigate the Impact on the Health Sector*. Hou X, Velenyi EV, Yazbeck AS, Iunes RF, Smith O (eds.). The World Bank. Washington, DC.

Burns AF, Mitchell WC. 1946. *Measuring Business Cycles*. New York, New York: National Bureau of Economic Research.

Calderon C, Schmidt-Hebbel K. 2008. Business Cycles and Fiscal Policies: The Role of Institutions and Financial Markets. *Central Bank of Chile Working Papers* No. 481, Santiago.

Canadian Institute for Health Information. 2011. National Health Expenditure Trends, 1975–2011. Spending and Health Workforce. https://secure.cihi.ca/free_products/nhex_trends_report_2011_en.pdf.

Canning D, Raja S, Yazbeck A. (eds.) 2015. Africa's Demographic Transition: Dividend or Disaster? Forthcoming, June/July, 2015. World Bank, Washington, DC.

Carneiro P, Hansen K, Heckman J. 2003. Estimating distributions of treatment effects with an application to the returns to schooling and measurement of the effects of uncertainty on college choices. *International Economic Review* 44: 361–422.

Carneiro P. Heckman J, Vytlacil E. 2010. Evaluating Marginal Policy Changes and the Average Effect of Treatment for Individuals at the Margin. *Econometrica* 78(1).

Carter MR, Maluccio JA. 2003. Social Capital and Coping with Economic Loss: An Analysis of Stunting of South African Children. *World Development* 31(7): 1147–1163. Elsevier Science Ltd. doi: 10.1016/S0305-750X(03)00062-7.

Case A, Paxson C. 2004. Sex differences in morbidity and mortality. Center for Health and Wellbeing Discussion. Paper, Princeton University, http://www.wws.princeton.edu/chw/research/papers.php, forthcoming Demography.

Case A, Paxson C. 2010. The Long Reach of Childhood Health and Circumstance: Evidence from the Whitehall II Study. *NBER Working Papers* 15640, National Bureau of Economic Research, Inc.

Cashin C. 2014. The Macroeconomic and Fiscal Context for Health Financing Policy Informing the Dialogue Between Ministries of Health and Ministries of Finance in Support of Universal Health Coverage. Draft Paper Prepared for the Health and the Economy Program, World Bank. Also available in presentation format prepared for a Meeting on Fiscal Space, Public Finance Management, and Health Financing, Montreux, Switzerland, 9–11 December 2014. http://www.who.int/health_financing/events/2_cashin_macro_fiscal_context_for_hf_financing_policy.pdf.

Clements B, Coady D, Gupta S. 2012. *The Economics of Public Health Care Reform in Advanced and Emerging Economies* (eds.). International Monetary Fund. Washington, DC. ISBN: 978-1-61635-244-8.

Conceição P, Namsuk K, Yanchun Z. 2009. Economic Shocks and Human Development: A Review of Empirical Findings. UNDP/ODS *Working Paper*. New York, United Nations Development Program.

Congressional Budget Office (CBO) 2010. The Long-Term Budget Outlook. Washington: June, revised August.

Costa-i-Font J, Gemmil M, Rubert G. 2009. Re-visiting the health care luxury good hypothesis: Aggregation, precision and publication biases? London School of

Economics and Political Science. LSE Research [Online]. [Accessed: June 2015]. *Working paper*, Health, Econometrics and Data Group (HEDG), York, UK.http://eprints.lse.ac.uk/25303/1/Revisiting_the-health_care_luxury_good_hypothesis (LSERO).pdf.

Cunha F, Heckman J, Navarro N. 2006. Counterfactual analysis of inequality and social mobility. In: *Mobility and Inequality: Frontiers of Research in Sociology and Economics*, Morgan S, Grusky D, Fields G. (eds.). pp. 290–348.

Currie J, Stabile M. 2004. Socioeconomic status and health: Why is the relationship stronger for older children? *American Economic Review* 93(5): 1813–1823.

Cutler DM. 1995. Technology, Health Costs, and the NIH, Harvard University and the National Bureau of Economic Research. Paper prepared for the *National Institutes of Health Economics Roundtable on Biomedical Research*.

Crivelli E, Gupta S, Muthoora P, Benedek D. 2012. Foreign Aid and Revenue: Still a Crowding Out Effect? *IMF Working Papers* 12(186), p. 1.

Darby J, Melitz J. 2008. Social spending and automatic stabilizers in the OECD. *Economic Policy* 715–756.

Deaton A. 2006. Global Patterns of Income and Health: Facts, Interpretations, and Policies. *NBER Working Paper* W12735, National Bureau of Economic Research, Cambridge, MA. http://ssrn.com/abstract=948648.

del Granado JA, Gupta S, Hajdenberg A. 2012. Is social spending procyclical? Evidence for developing countries. *World Development* 42: 16–27. http://dx.doi.org/10.1016/j.worlddev.2012.07.003.

De Silva M. 2009. What is MTEF and Why It is Important? A Brief Overview. World Bank Institute. http://www.cafrad.org/Workshops/Tanger21-23_04_09/Session4_2.pdf.

Devlin N, Hansen P. 2010. Health care spending and economic output: Granger causality. *Applied Economics Letters* 2001, 8: 561–564.

Diebold FX. 2001. Elements of Forecasting (2nd ed.). Cincinnati: South Western. p. 254. ISBN 0-324-02393-6.

Dillon A, Friedman J, Serneels P. 2014. Health information, treatment, and worker productivity: Experimental evidence from malaria testing and treatment among Nigerian sugarcane cutters. *CSAE Working Paper Series* 2014-13. Centre for the Study of African Economies, University of Oxford.

Di Matteo, L. 2003. The income elasticity of health care spending. A comparison of parametric and non-parametric approaches. *European Journal of Health Economics* 4: 20–29.

Di Matteo L. 2004. What drives provincial health expenditure? *Canadian Tax Journal* 2004, 52: 1102.

Di Matteo L. 2005. The macro determinants of health expenditure in the United States and Canada: Assessing the impact of income, age distribution and time. *Health Policy* 2005, 71: 23–42.

Di Matteo L, Di Matteo R. 1998. Evidence on the determinants of Canadian provincial government health expenditures: 1965–1991. *Journal of Health Economics* 17: 211–228.

Dixit A. 2006. Evaluating Recipes for Development Success. *Policy Research Working Paper No*. 3859, World Bank, Washington, DC.

Djebbari H, Smith J. 2008. Heterogeneous Impacts in PROGRESA. IZA Discussion Paper Series. IZA DP No. 3362. February, 2008. Bonn, Germany.

Dormont B, Grignon M, Huber H. 2006. Health expenditure growth: Reassessing the threat of ageing. *Health Economics* 15(9): 947–963.

Doytch N, Hu B, Mendoza RU. 2010. Social Spending, Fiscal Space, and Governance: An Analysis of Patterns over the Business Cycle. UNICEF Policy and Practice, second draft, April.

Dreger C, Reimers HE. 2005. Health care expenditures in OECD countries: A panel unit root and cointegration analysis.

Drouin JP, Hediger V, Henke N. 2008. Health care costs: A market-based view. *The McKinsey Quarterly* September, 2008.

Duflo E. 2001. Schooling and labor market consequences of school construction in Indonesia: Evidence from an unusual policy experiment. *American Economic Review* 91(4): 795–813.

Dybczak K, Przywara B. 2010. The Role of Technology on Health Care Expenditure on the EU. *European Economy — Economic Paper 400*. Brussels, Belgium: Directorate General for Economic and Monetary Affairs, European Commission; 2010. Available from: http://ec.europa.eu/economy_finance/publications/economic_paper/2010/ecp400_en.htm.

Dybul M. 2013. A grand convergence and a historic opportunity. *The Lancet* 382(9908): e38–e39. http://www.sciencedirect.com/science/article/pii/S0140673613623442.

Eloundou-Enyegue PM. 2013. A Demographic Dividend for Africa's Schooling? Theory and Early Evidence. Background Paper for: *Africa's Demographic Transition: Dividend or Disaster?* Canning D, Raja S, Yazbeck A. (eds.). World Bank, Washington, DC. https://openknowledge.worldbank.org/bitstream/handle/10986/22036/AfrDemographicTransitionOVERVIEW.pdf.

Eloundou-Enyegue P, Giroux S. 2013. The role of fertility in achieving Africa's schooling MDGs: Early evidence for sub-Saharan Africa. *Journal of Children and Poverty* 19(1): 21–44.

Enke S. 1964. *Economics for Development.* London: Dennis Dobson.

Erdil E, Yetkiner IH. 2009. The Granger-Causality Between Health Care Expenditure and Output: A Panel Data Approach. In *Applied Economics*. Taylor and Francis, pp. 511–518.

Essama-Nssah B, Moreno-Dodson B. 2013. Fiscal Policy for Growth and Social Welfare. Chapter 1 in Moreno-Dodson, B. (ed.). Is Fiscal Policy the Answer? A Developing Country Perspective. The World Bank, Washington, DC.

Estache A, Muñoz R. 2009. Building Sector Concerns into Macroeconomic Financial Programming: Lessons from Senegal and Uganda. Africa Infrastructure Country Diagnostic, *Working Paper* 6, Africa's Infrastructure, A Time for Transition. World Bank, Washington, DC. Available at: http://infrastructureafrica.afdb.org/system/files/WP6_Finprog_Sen_Ugan_0.pdf.

European Commission. 2015. The 2015 Ageing Report. Economic and budgetary projections for the 28 EU Member States (2013–2060). EUROPEAN ECONOMY 3. 2015.

Luxembourg: Publications Office of the European Union, 2015. ISBN 978-92-79-44747-1 (print). http://ec.europa.eu/economy_finance/publications/european_economy/2015/pdf/ee3_en.pdf.

Farag M, *et al.* 2009. Does funding from donors displace government spending for health in developing countries? *Health Affairs* 28(4): 1045.

Filmer D, Hammer JS, Pritchett LH. 2002. Weak links in the chain II: A prescription for health policy in poor countries. *The World Bank Research Observer* 17(1) (Spring 2002): 47–66. The International Bank for Reconstruction and Development/The World Bank. http://www1.worldbank.org/publicsector/pe/pfma07/WeakLinkChain.pdf.

Finlay JE, Canning D. 2013. The Association of Fertility Spacing, Timing and Parity with Child Health. World Bank Background Paper.

Fleisher L, Leive A, Schieber G. 2013. Taking Stock of Fiscal Health: Recent Trends in Global, Regional, and Country Level Health Financing. *Health, Nutrition, and Population Discussion Paper*. The World Bank, Washington, DC.

Fogel RW. 1991. New Findings on Secular Trends in Nutrition and Mortality: Some Implications for Population Theory. Typescript, University of Chicago.

Fogel RW. 1994. Economic growth, population theory, and Physiology: The bearing of long-term processes on the making of economic policy. *American Economic Review* 84 (June): 369–395.

Fogel RW, Wimmer LT. 1992. Early Indicators of Later Work Levels, Disease, and Death, *NBER Historical Working Papers* 0038, National Bureau of Economic Research, Inc.

Frankel J. 2010. A solution to fiscal procyclicality: The structural budget institutions pioneered by Chile. Paper presented at the Fourteenth Annual Conference of the Central Bank of Chile.

Frankel JA, Rose AK. 1996. The Endogeneity of the Optimum Currency Area Criteria. *NBER Working Paper No.* 5700. Issued in August 1996. http://www.nber.org/papers/w5700.pdf.

Frankel J, Végh C, Vuletin G. 2011. On Graduation from Procyclicality. *NBER Working Paper* 17619, National Bureau of Economic Research. Cambridge, MA. http://www.nber.org/papers/w17619.

Friedman J, Schady N. 2009. How Many More Infants Are Likely to Die in Africa as a Result of the Global Financial Crisis? *World Bank Policy Research Working Paper* 5023, World Bank, Washington, DC.

Frölich M, Melly B. 2013. Unconditional quantile treatment effects under endogeneity. *Journal of Business & Economic Statistics* 31(3): 346–357. DOI: 10.1080/07350015.2013.803869. http://dx.doi.org/10.1080/07350015.2013.803869

Galea S. 2007. *Macrosocial Determinants of Population Health*. New York, NY: Springer. p. 175. ISBN 0-387-70811-1.

Gallup JL, Sachs J. 2001. The Economic Burden of Malaria. *American Journal of Tropical Medicine and Hygiene* 64(1,2): 85–96.

Galor O, Mayer-Foulkes D. 2004. Food for Thought: Basic Needs and Persistent Educational Inequality. *GE, Growth, Math Methods* 0410002, EconWPA. Available at: https://ideas.repec.org/p/wpa/wuwpge/0410002.html.

Gaudin, Yazbeck. 2014. Health Sector Policy Challenges in Low and Middle Income Countries: Learning from Public Expenditure Reviews. Health, Nutrition, and Population (HNP) Discussion Paper. The World Bank. Washington, DC.

Gauthier B. 2006. PETS-QSDS in sub-Saharan Africa: A stocktaking study. Report for the project "Measuring progress in public services delivery". The World Bank, 7 September 2006.

Gauthier B, Ahmed Z. 2012. Public Expenditure Tracking Surveys (PETS) and Quantitative Service Delivery Survey (QSDS) Guidebook. World Bank Poverty Reduction and Economic Management (PREM) and Human Development Network. The World Bank. Washington, DC.

Gené-Badia JJ, Gallo PP, Hernandez-Quevedo CC, Garcia-Armesto SS. 2012. Spanish health care cuts: Penny wise and pound foolish? *Health Policy* 106(1): 23–28. PMID 22494526.

Gerdtham UG, Sogaard J, *et al.* 1992. An econometric analysis of health care expenditure: A cross-section study of the OECD countries. *Journal of Health Economics* 11(1): 63–84.

Gerdtham G, Jönnson B. 2000. International Comparisons of Health Expenditures. In: Culyer A, Newhouse J. (eds.). *Handbook of Health Economics*. Volume 1A. Elsevier, North Holland.

Gerdtham UG, Löthgren M. 2000. On stationarity and cointegration of international health expenditure and GDP. *Journal of Health Economics* 19(4): 461–475.

Getzen TE. 2000. Health care is an individual necessity and a national luxury: Applying multilevel decision models to the analysis of health care expenditures. *Journal of Health Economics* 19(2): 259–270.

Gillingham R. 2014. Fiscal Policy for Health Policy Makers. *Health, Nutrition, and Population (HNP) Discussion Paper*. March, 2014. The World Bank. Washington, DC.

Goldsbrough *et al.* 2007. Does the IMF Constrain Health Spending in Poor Countries? Evidence and Agenda for Action. Center for Global Development Report of the Working Group on IMF Programs and Health Spending. Washington, DC. ISBN 1-933286-21-0. http://www.cgdev.org/files/14103_file_IMF_report.pdf

Gottret P, Gupta V, Sparkes S, Tandon A, Moran V, Berman P. 2009. Protecting pro-poor health services during financial crises: Lessons from experience. 2009. Advances in Health Economics and Health Services Research. Volume 21. Chernichovsky D, Hanson K. (eds.). *Advances in Health Economics and Health Services Research*. ISBN: 978-1-84855-664-5.

Gottret PE, Schieber G. 2006. Health Financing Revisited. A Practitioner's Guide. The World Bank. Washington, DC.

Granger CWJ. 1969. Investigating causal relations by econometric models and cross-spectral methods. *Econometrica* 37(3): 424–438. doi:10.2307/1912791. JSTOR 1912791.

Grossman M. 1972. On the concept of health capital and demand for health. *Journal of Political Economy* 80: 223–255.

Grossman, M. 2000. The Human Capital Model. In: Culyer A, Newhouse JP. (eds.). *Handbook of Health Economics*. Volume 1A. Elsevier, Amsterdam, Netherlands. http://www.sciencedirect.com/science/article/pii/S1574006400801663.

Gupta I, Mitra A. 2004. Economic growth, health and poverty: An exploratory study for India. *Development Policy Review* 22(2): 193–206.

Gurkan A, Kaiser K. Voorbraak D. 2009. Implementing Public Expenditure Tracking Surveys for Results: Lessons from a Decade of Global Experience. PREM Notes, [online] (145), pp. 1–16. Available at: http://pets.prognoz.com/prod/GetGuidlinesDocFile.ashx?data=3.

Habicht T. 2012. "Health Insurance Before, During, and After (?) Crisis. The Case of Estonia." Presented at the workshop, "Health Systems and Economic Downturns: Identifying and Managing Risks. Washington, DC, 27 September.

Haldar SK, Mallik G. 2010. Does Human Capital Cause Economic Growth? A Case Study of India. *International Journal of Business and Economic Sciences Applied Research* (IJBESAR). Eastern Macedonia and Thrace Institute of Technology (EMATTECH), Kavala, Greece, Volume 3(1), pp. 7–25, July.

Hansen P, King A. 1996. The determinants of health care expenditure: A cointegration approach. *Journal of Health Economics* 15(1): 127–137.

Hauck K, Smith PC, Goddard M. 2005. What to Buy? Revisiting Priority Setting in Health Care. Chapter 3 in Preker AS, Langenbrunner J. 2005. (eds.). *Spending Wisely: Buying Health Services for the Poor*. The World Bank. ISBN 0-8213-5918-5.

Heller PS. 2005. Understanding Fiscal Space. IMF Policy Discussion Paper. Fiscal Affairs Department. PDP/05/4. International Monetary Fund. Washington, DC.

Heller P. 2006. The prospects of creating 'fiscal space' for the health sector. *Health Policy and Planning* 21(2 January): 75–79.

Heller PS. 2013. Implications of the European Financial Crisis for Fiscal Policy and Public Financing of the Health and Social Sectors. Presentation prepared for the Conference, *Health Systems in Global Economic Crisis: An Update of the Situation in the WHO European Region*. Oslo, April 17.

Heller PS, Katz M, Debrun X, Thomas T, Koranchelian T, Adenauer I. 2006. Making Fiscal Space Happen: Making Fiscal Policy in a World of Scaled-up Aid. *IMF Working Paper*. WP/06/270. Fiscal Affairs Department. International Monetary Fund. Washington, DC.

Hitiris T, Posnett J. 1992. The determinants and effects of health expenditure in developed countries. *Journal of Health Economics* 11: 173–181.

Hopkins S. 2006. Economic Stability and Health Status: Evidence from East Asia before and after the 1990s Economic Crisis. *Health Policy* 75: 347–357.

Hou X, Velenyi E, Yazbeck A, Iunes R, Smith O. 2013. Learning from economic downturns: How to better assess, track, and mitigate the impact on the health sector. World Bank Publications. Washington, DC.

IDB (Inter-American Development Bank). 2009. *Social and Labor Market Policies for Tumultuous Times: Confronting the Global Crisis in Latin America and the Caribbean*. Report prepared for the Annual Meeting of the Board of Governors of the Inter-American Development Bank held in Medellín, Colombia, in March, 2009. Inter-American Development Bank, Washington, DC.

IEG (Independent Evaluation Group). 2009. Improving Effectiveness and Outcomes for the Poor in Health, Nutrition, and Population. An Evaluation off World Bank Group

Support since 1997. World Bank. IFC. MIGA. The International Bank for Reconstruction and Development/The World Bank. Washington, DC. http://siteresources.worldbank.org/EXTWBASSHEANUTPOP/Resources/hnp_full_eval.pdf.

IHME (Institute for Health Metrics and Evaluation). 2010a. Statistical Annex. In *Financing Global Health 2010: Development Assistance and Country Spending in Economic Uncertainty*. Seattle, WA: University of Washington.

IHME (Institute for Health Metrics and Evaluation). 2010b. Tracking Development Assistance for Health. In *Financing Global Health 2010: Development Assistance and Country Spending in Economic Uncertainty*. Chapter 1. Seattle, WA: University of Washington.

Ilzetzki E, Végh CA. 2008. Procyclical Fiscal Policy in Developing Countries: Truth or Fiction? *National Bureau of Economic Research Working Paper Series* 14191. Cambridge, MA.

IMF (International Monetary Fund). 2009. Regional Economic Outlook. Sub-Saharan Africa: Withstanding the Storm. *World Economic and Financial Surveys*. International Monetary Fund, Washington, DC.

Iradian G. 2005. Inequality, poverty, and growth: Cross-country evidence. *Working Paper* May 28. International Monetary Fund, Washington, DC, USA. http://www.imf.org/external/pubs/ft/wp/2005/wp0528.pdf.

Ishihara Y. 2005. Quantitative Analysis of Crisis: Crisis Identification and Causality. *Policy Research Working Paper* WPS3598. World Bank, Washington, DC.

Jack W, Lewis M. 2004. Falling Short of Expectations: Public Health Interventions in Developing and Transition Economies. *Social Science & Medicine* 58(2): 223–225.

Jack W, Lewis M. 2009. Health investments and economic growth: Macroeconomic evidence and microeconomic foundations. *Policy Research Working Paper Series* 4877. The World Bank. https://ideas.repec.org/p/wbk/wbrwps/4877.html.

Jacobs R, Smith PC, Street A. 2006. Measuring efficiency in health care: Analytic techniques and health policy. 2006: Cambridge University Press.

Jamison, *et al.* 2013. Global Health 2035: A world converging within a generation. Published Online. 3 December 2013. http://dx.doi.org/10.1016/S0140-6736(13)62105-4.

Jones CI. 2002. Why have Health Expenditures as a Share of GDP Risen So Much? *National Bureau of Economic Research Working Paper Series No*. 9325. Accessed March 15, 2013. Available from: http://ideas.repec.org/p/nbr/nberwo/9325.html.

Jusot F, Mage S, Menendez M. 2014. Inequality of Opportunity in Health in Indonesia. Document de Travail. UMR DIAL. DT/2014-06. May 2014. Paris.

Kakwani NC. 1977. Measurement of tax progressivity: An international comparison. *Economic Journal* 87(345): 71–80.

Kakwani N. 1980. *Income Inequality and Poverty*. New York: Published for the World Bank by Oxford University Press.

Kakwani NC, Wagstaff A, van Doorslaer E. 1997. Socioeconomic inequalities in health: Measurement, computation and statistical inference. *Journal of Econometrics* 77(1): 87–104.

Kaminsky GL, Reinhart CM, Végh CA. 2004. When it rains, it pours: Procyclical capital flows and macroeconomic policies. *NBER Working Paper 10780, National Bureau of Economic Research*. Cambridge, MA. http://www.nber.org/chapters/c6668.pdf.

Kentikelenis A, Maranikolos M, Papnicolas I, Basu S, McKee M, Stuckler D. 2012. Health and the financial crisis in Greece — Authors' reply. *The Lancet* 379(9820): 1002.

Kleiman E. 1974. The Determinants of National Outlay on Health. London: Macmillan.

Knowles, S, Owen, PD. 1995. Health capital and cross-country variation in income per capita in the Mankiw–Romer–Weil model. *Economics Letters*, Elsevier, 48(1): 99–106, April.

Knowles S, Owen PD. 1997. Education and health in an effective-labour empirical growth model. *The Economic Record. The Economic Society of Australia* 73(223): 314–328, December.

Koettl J, Schneider P. 2010. The Financial Impact of the Economic Crisis on Health Insurance Funds in Eastern Europe. World Bank, Washington, DC.

Kotlikoff L, Hagist C. 2007. Healthcare Spending: What the Future will Look Like? NCPA Policy Report. Dallas: National Center for Policy Analysis.

Kutzin J, Cashin C, Jakab M. 2010. Implementing health financing reform: Lessons from countries in transition. World Health Organisation on behalf of the European Observatory on Health Systems and Policies. Available at: http://www.euro.who.int/_data/assets/pdf_file/0014/120164/E94240.pdf?ua=1.

Kwon S, Jung Y. 2009. The impact of the global recession on the health of the people in Asia. Submitted to the Asian Development Bank and the World Health Organization.

Laeven L, Valencia F. 2012. Systemic Banking Crises Database: An Update. *International Monetary Fund Working Paper* WP/12/163. Washington, DC.

Langenbrunner JC, Cashin C, O'Dougherty S. 2009. Designing and Implementing Health Care Provider Payment Systems. How-To Manuals. The World Bank. Washington, DC. ISBN: 978-0-8213-7815-1. http://siteresources.worldbank.org/HEALTHNUTRITIONANDPOPULATION/Resources/Peer-Reviewed-Publications/ProviderPaymentHowTo.pdf

Lewis, M. 2006. Governance and Corruption in Public Health Care Systems. Center for Global Development *Working paper* 78, Center for Global Development. http://ssrn.com/abstract=984046.

Lewis M, Verhoeven M. 2010. Financial Crises and Social Spending: The Impact of the 2008–2009 Crisis. Background Paper for Global Monitoring Report 2010. World Bank, Washington, DC.

Leu RE. 1986. Public and private health services: complementarities and conflicts. In: Culyer AJ, Jönsson B. (eds.). *Public and Private Health Services: Complementarities and Conflicts*. Oxford: Blackwell.

Li H, Huang L. 2009. Health, education, and economic growth in China: Empirical findings and implications. *China Economic Review* 20(3) September 2009: 374–387.

Liang LL, Mirelman AJ. 2014. An Assessment of Sociopolitical Determinants, International Aid, and Government Health Expenditure: A Cross-country Analysis over 1995–2010.

Health, Nutrition, and Population (HNP) Discussion Paper. The World Bank, Washington, DC.

Lindelow M. 2006. Tracking Public Money in the Health Sector in Mozambique: Conceptual and Practical Challenges. Draft Paper.

Lu C, Schneider, MT, Gubbins P, Leach-Kemon K, Jamison D, Murray CJL. 2010. Public Financing of health in developing countries: A cross-national systematic analysis. *The Lancet* 375(April): 1375–1387.

Lucas RE. 1977. Understanding Business Cycles. In *Stabilization of the Domestic and International Economy*, K. Brunner and A. Meltzer (ed.). Carnegie-Rochester Conference Series on Public Policy 5: 7–29. Amsterdam.

Lucas R. 1988. On the mechanics of economic development. *Journal of Monetary Economics* 22(1): 3–42.

Madhani PM. 2010. Rebalancing fixed and variable pay in a sales organization: A business cycle perspective. *Compensation and Benefits Review* 42(3): 179–189.

Malaney P, Spielman A, Sachs J. 2004. The Malaria Gap. *American Journal of Tropical Medicine and Hygiene* 71(Suppl 2): 141–46.

Mankiw NG, Romer D, Weil DN. 1992. A contribution to the empirics of economic growth. *Quarterly Journal of Economics* 107: 407–437.

Mason A. 2005. Demographic Transition and Demographic Dividends in Developed and Developing Countries. *United Nations Expert Group Meeting on Social and Economic Implications of Changing Population Age Structures* Mexico City, 2005.

Mason A, Kinugasa T. East Asian Economic Development: Two Demographic Dividends. Conference on "Miracles and Mirages in East Asian Economic Development" (Honolulu, 2004).

Mason A, Lee R. 2006. Reform and Support Systems for the Elderly in Developing Countries: Capturing the Second Demographic Dividend. GENUS 62: 2.

Mayer-Foulkes D. 2001a. The long-term impact of health on economic growth in Latin America. *World Development* 29(6): June 2001, 1025–1033 (9).

Mayer-Foulkes D. 2001b. The long-term impact of health on economic growth in Mexico, 1950–1995. *Journal of International Development* 13(1): 123–126.

McCarthy FD, Wolf H, Wu Y. 2000. The Growth Costs of Malaria. *Working Paper No.* 7541. New York: National Bureau of Economic Research (NBER).

McCoy D, Brikci N. 2010. Taskforce on innovative international financing for health systems: What next? *Bulletin of the World Health Organization* 2010; 88: 478–480. doi: 10.2471/BLT.09.074419.

McGillivray M, White H. 1993. Measuring Development? The UNDP's Human Development Index. *Journal of International Development* 5(2): 183–192.

McGuire A, Parkin D, Hughes D, Gerard K. 1993. Econometric analyses of national health expenditures: Can positive economics help to answer normative questions? *Health Economics* 2(2): 113–126.

Meltzer M, *et al.* 2014. Estimating the Future Number of Cases in the Ebola Epidemic — Liberia and Sierra Leone, 2014–2015. Morbidity and Mortality Weekly Report (MMWR). Centers for Disease Control and Prevention before Morbidity and Mortality Weekly Report. U.S. Department of Health and Human Services. CDC.

Supplement/Vol.63/No.3. September 26, 2014. [Online]. [Accessed on: May 2015]. Av available at: http://www.cdc.gov/mmwr/preview/mmwrhtml/su6303a1.htm.

Mendoza EG. 1995. The terms of trade, the real exchange rate, and economic Fluctuations. *International Economic Review* 36(1): 101–137.

Mendoza RU, Rees N. 2009. Infant Mortality During Economic Downturns and Recovery. *Working Paper*. Available at SSRN: http://ssrn.com/abstract=1586527 or http://dx.doi.org/10.2139/ssrn.1586527

Miguel E, Kremer M. 2004. Wormed: Identifying Impacts on Education and Health in the Presence of Treatment Externalities. *Econometrica* 72(1): (January, 2004), 159–217.

Mladovsky P, Srivastava D, Cylus J, Karanikolos M, Evetovits T, Thomson S, McKee M. 2012. Policy Summary 5. Health policy response to the financial crisis in Europe. World Health Organization on behalf of the European Observatory on Health Systems and Policies 2012.

Moreno-Serra R, Millett C, Smith PC. 2011. Towards improved measurement of financial protection in health. *PLoS Med* 8(9): e1001087. doi: 10.1371/journal.pmed.1001087.

Morgan L. 2014. Results-Based Financing for Health (RBF): What's All the Fuss About? Published [Online] at http://www.rbfhealth.org/news/item/results-based-financing-health-rbf-whats-all-the-fuss. Accessed 07.12.2014.

Musgrove P, Zeramdini R, Carrin G. 2002. Basic patterns in national health expenditure. Bulletin of the World Health Organization, 80(2), pp.134–142.

Narajan A, Mahajan S. 2013. The State of Opportunities in South Africa: Inequality among Children and in the Labor Market. Inequality in Focus. Poverty Reduction and Equity Department: www.worldbank.org/poverty. Volume 2, Number 1. April 2013. The World Bank. [Online]. [Accessed: April, 2015]. Available at: http://www.worldbank.org/content/dam/Worldbank/document/Poverty%20documents/Inequality-in-Focus-April2013.pdf.

Narayan S, Narayan PK, Mishra S. 2010. Investigating the Relationship between Health and Economic Growth: Empirical Evidence from a Panel of 5 Asian Countries. *Economics Series* 2010_08, Deakin University, Faculty of Business and Law, School of Accounting, Economics and Finance.

Newhouse JP. 1977. Medical-care expenditure: a cross-national survey. *The Journal of Human Resources* 12(1): 115–125.

Newhouse JP. 1992. Medical care costs: How much welfare loss? *The Journal of Economic Perspectives* 6(3): 3–21.

Nixon J, Ulmann P. 2006. The relationship between health care spending and health outcomes: Evidence and caveats for a causal link. *The European Journal of Health Economics* 7: 7–18.

O'Donnell O, van Doorslaer E, Wagstaff A, Lindelow M. 2008. Analyzing Health Equity Using Household Survey Data. A Guide to Techniques and Their Implementation. World Bank Institute. The International Bank for Reconstruction and Development/The World Bank. Washington, DC.

Okunade AA, Karakus MC. 2001. Unit root and cointegration tests: Time series versus panel estimates for international health expenditure models. *Applied Economics* 33(9): 1131–1137.

Ooms G, Stuckler, D, Basu S, McKee M. 2010. Financing the Millennium Development Goals for health and beyond: sustaining the 'Big Push'. *Globalization and Health* 6: 17. http://www.globalizationandhealth.com/content/6/1/17.

OECD (Organisation for Economic Cooperation and Development). 2006. Projecting OECD Health and Long-Term Care Expenditures: What Are the Main Drivers? *Economics Department Working Paper* No. 447. Paris.

OECD (Organization for Economic Cooperation and Development). 2010. How Much Is Too Much? Value for Money in Health Spending. OECD Health Policy Studies — *Value for Money in Health Spending.* Chapter 1. http://www.oecd.org/berlin/46201464.pdf.

Paes de Barros R, Ferreira FHH, Molinas Vega JR, Chanduvi JS. 2009. Measuring Inequality of Opportunities in Latin America and the Caribbean. World Bank, Washington, DC.

PAHO (Pan American Health Organization) 2001. Invest in Health. Social and Economic Returns. Scientific and Technical Publication No. 582. Produced in Collaboration with The Inter-American Development Bank and The World Bank. Washington, DC. ISBN 92 75 31582 5.

Paxson C, Schady N. 2004. Child health and the 1988–92 economic crisis in Peru. *Policy Research Working Paper* Series 3260. The World Bank.

Peden EA, Freeland MS. 1995. A historical analysis of medical spending growth, 1960–1993. *Health Affairs* 14: 235–247.

Perotti R. 2004. Estimating the Effects of Social Policy in OECD Countries. *Working Paper* No. 276. Bocconi University, Milan.

Pizzi LT, Lofland J. 2006. (eds.). *Economic Evaluation In U.S. Health Care: Principles And Applications*. Jones and Bartlett Publishers, Inc. ISBN-13: 978-0-7637-2746-6.

Powell-Jackson T, Hanson K, McIntyre D. 2012. Fiscal Space for Health. A Review of the Literature. *Working Paper* 1. December, 2012. RESYST — Resilient and Responsive Health Systems. http://r4d.dfid.gov.uk/PDF/Outputs/ReSYST/Resyst-WP1.pdf.

Preker AS, Langenbrunner J. 2005. (eds.). Spending Wisely: Buying Health Services for the Poor. The World Bank. ISBN 0-8213-5918-5.

Preker AS, Liu X, Velenyi EV, Baris E. 2007. Public Ends, Private Means: Strategic Purchasing of Health Services. Washington, DC. The World Bank. https://openknowledge.worldbank.org/handle/10986/6683 License: CC BY 3.0 IGO.

Preston SH. 1975. The changing relation between mortality and level of economic development. *Population Studies* 29(2): 231–248.

PricewaterhouseCoopers. 2002. The Factors Fueling Risking Healthcare Costs. Report prepared for the American Association of Health Plans. Available from: http://heartland.org/sites/all/modules/custom/heartland_migration/files/pdfs/14621.pdf. Accessed March 15, 2013.

Pritchett L, Summers L. 1996. Wealthier is Healthier. *The Journal of Human Resources* [Online] 31(4): 841–868. http://www.jstor.org/discover/10.2307/146149?sid=21105861472341&uid=2&uid=3739936&uid=3739256&uid=4.

Raja S, Canning D, Robalino DA, Parby JI, Bakilana A. 2012. How can Africa Capture the Demographic Dividend? A Concept Note for a Regional ESW. The World Bank. 2 April 2012.

Ranis G, Stewart F, Ramirez A. 2000. Economic growth and human development. *World Development* 28(2): 197–219.

Ravallion M. 2012. Troubling tradeoffs in the human development index. *Journal of Development Economics* 99(2) November 2012: 201–209.

Ravallion M, Chen S. 1997. What Can New Survey Data Tell Us about Recent Changes in Distribution and Poverty? *World Bank Economic Review*. World Bank Group, 11(2): 357–382, May.

Ravishankar N, Gubbins P, Cooley RJ, Leach-Kemon K, Michaud CM, Jamison DT, Murray CJL. 2009. Financing of global health: Tracking development assistance for health from 1990 to 2007. *The Lancet* 373(9681): 2113–2124.

Reinikka R, Svenson J. 2004. Local Capture: Evidence From a Central Government Transfer Program in Uganda. *The Quarterly Journal of Economics* 119(2): 678–704.

Rodrik D. 2008. The New Development Economics: We Shall Experiment, but How Shall we Learn? *HKS Faculty Research Working Paper Series*. RWP08-055. John F. Kennedy School of Government. Harvard University. Revised Draft. July 2008.

Roemer J. 1998. *Equality of Opportunity*. Cambridge (Massachusetts): Harvard University Press.

Romer C. 2008. Business Cycles. In *The Concise Encyclopedia of Economics*. Second Edition. http://www.econlib.org/library/Enc/BusinessCycles.html. Accessed 1 April 2013.

Romer P. 1986. Increasing returns and long-run growth. *Journal of Political Economy* 94(5): 1002–1037.

Rosa Dias P. 2009. Inequality of opportunity in health: Evidence from a UK cohort study. *Health Economics* 18(9): 1057–1074.

Rowden R. 2010. "We've Yet to Kill Off the Washington Consensus," The UK Guardian Global, Development/Poverty Matters Blog, 24 November. http://www.guardian.co.uk/global-development/poverty-matters/2010/nov/24/washington-consensus.

Ruger JP. 2005. The Changing Role of the World Bank in Global Health. *American Journal of Public Health* January; 95(1): 60–70.

Ruhm C. 2000. Are recessions good for your health? *Quarterly Journal of Economics*. 115(2): 617–650.

Ruhm C. 2012. Sick Economies and Healthy Bodies. Presentation prepared for panel at the World Bank *Health System and Economic Downturns: Identifying and Managing the Risks*. September 27, 2012.

Rukumnuaykit P. 2003. Crises and Child Health Outcomes: The Impacts of Economic and Drought/Smoke Crises on Infant Mortality in Indonesia. Michigan State University. Michigan.

Sachs JD. 2001. Macroeconomics and health: Investing in health for economic development. *Revista Panamericana de Salud Pública* 12(2): 143–144.

Schady N, Smitz MF. 2010. Aggregate economic shocks and infant mortality: New evidence for middle-income countries. *Economics Letters* 108(2): 145–148.

Schieber G, Cashin C, Saleh K, Lavado R. 2012. Assessing the prospects for fiscal space for health in Ghana. *Health Financing in Ghana* [online]: 119–142. Available at: http://dx.doi.org/10.1596/978-0-8213-9566-0.

Schultz TP, Strauss J. 2007. *Handbook of Development Economics*. Amsterdam: North-Holland.

Schultz TP. 1997. Assessing the productive benefits of nutrition and health: An integrated human capital approach. *Journal of Econometrics* 77(1): 141–158.

Schultz TP. 2002. Wage Gains Associated with Height as a Form of Health Human Capital. *American Economic Review* 92(2): 349–353.

Schultz TP. 2005. Productive benefits of health: Evidence from low income countries. In Lopez-Casasnovas G, Rivera B, Currais L (eds.). Health and economic growth: Findings and policy implications (pp. 257–285). Cambridge, MA: MIT Press.

Shultz TW. 1961. Investment in Human Capital. *American Economic Review* 51(11) (March) 1–17.

Simms C, Rowson M. 2003. Reassessment of health effects of the Indonesian economic crisis: Donors versus the data. Viewpoint. *The Lancet* 361: 1382–1385.

Skoufias E, Tiwari S, Zaman H. 2011. Can We Rely on Cash Transfers to Protect Dietary Diversity During Food Crises? Estimates from Indonesia. *World Bank Policy Research Working Paper No*. 5548.

Smith SD, Heffler SK, Freeland MS. 2000. The Impact of Technological Change on Health Care Cost Increases: An Evaluation of the Literature. *Health Care Financing Administration Working Paper*. Available from: http://www.cms.gov/Research-Statistics-Data-and-Systems/Statistics-Trends-and-Reports/NationalHealthExpendData/downloads/tech_2000_0810.pdf.

Smith O, Yazbeck, A. 2011. Financial crisis and health in Europe and Central Asia. Presentation at the International Health Economics Association Conference. 7–11 July. Toronto, Canada.

Smith P. 1993. Measuring Human Development. *Asian Economic Journal* 7(1): 89–106, March 1993. Article first published online: 9 October 2007. DOI: 10.1111/j.1467-8381.1993.tb00103.x.

Smith S, Newhouse JP, Freeland M. 2009. Income, insurance, and technology: Why does health spending outpace economic growth? *Health Affair*s 28(5): 1276–1284.

Solow RM. 1956. A contribution to the theory of economic growth, *Quarterly Journal of Economics* 70: 65–94.

Sorenson C, Drummond M, Khan BB. 2003. Medical technology as a key driver of rising health expenditure: disentangling the relationship. *ClinicoEconomics and Outcomes Research*: *CEOR* 5: 223.

Spence M, Lewis M. 2009. Health and Growth: Commission on Growth and Development. The World Bank. Washington, DC. https://openknowledge.worldbank.org/handle/10986/2633.

Srinivasan TN. 1994. Human Development: A New Paradigm or Reinvention of the Wheel? *The American Economic Review*. Papers and Proceedings of the Hundred and Sixth Annual Meeting of the American Economic Association. May, 1994. 84(2): 238–243.

Stuckler D, Basu S, McKee M. 2010. Drivers of inequality in millennium development goal progress: A statistical analysis. *PLoS Med* 7(3): e1000241. doi:10.1371/journal.pmed.1000241.

Stuckler D, Basu S, Wang SW, McKee M. 2011. Does recession reduce global health aid? Evidence from 15 high-income countries, 1975–2007. *Bulletin of the World Health Organization* 89: 252–257.

Stuckler D, Basu S, Suhreke M, McKee M. 2009. Commentary: The health implications of financial crisis: A review of the evidence. *Ulster Medical Journal* 78(3): 142–145.

Summers L, Jamison DT. 2013. Policy Brief #2: The Returns to Investing in Health Global Health. Global Health 2035. A World Converging within a Generation. *The Lancet*. Published [Online], December 2013. [Accessed: March, 2015]. http://globalhealth2035.org/sites/default/files/policy-briefs/policy-brief-2-english.pdf.

Suri T, Boozer MA, Ranis G, Stewart F. 2010. Paths to Success: The relationship between human development and economic growth. *World Development* 39(4): 506–522, 2011. Elsevier.

Strauss J, Thomas D. 1995. Human Resources: Empirical Modeling of Household and Family Decisions. In Behrman J, Srinivasan TN (eds.). Handbook of development economics (Volume 3A, pp. 1883–2023). Amsterdam: North Holland.

Sweetland SR. 1996. Human capital theory: Foundations of a field of inquiry. *Review of Educational Research*. Fall 66(3): 341–359.

Tandon A. 2009. Giving More Weight to Health: Assessing Fiscal Space for Health in Indonesia. #46847. The World Bank. Washington, DC. Available at: http://siteresources.worldbank.org/INTHSD/Resources/topics/415176-1255443724448/FiscalSpaceforHealthIndonesia.pdf.

Tandon A, Cashin C. 2010. Assessing Public Expenditure on Health from a Fiscal Space Perspective. *Health, Nutrition, and Population (HNP) Discussion Paper*. The World Bank, Washington, DC.

Tandon A, Fleisher L, Li R, Yap WA. 2014. Re-prioritizing government spending on health: Pushing an elephant up the stairs? *Health, Nutrition, and Population (HNP) Discussion Paper*. The World Bank, Washington, DC.

Thomson S, *et al.* 2009. Addressing Financial Sustainability in Health Systems. *Policy Summary for the Czech European Union Presidency Ministerial Conference on the Financial Sustainability of Health Systems in Europe, Copenhagen.* WHO Regional Office for Europe on behalf of the European Observatory on Health Systems and Policies.

Thornton J. 2008. Explaining procyclical fiscal policy in African countries. *Journal of African Economies* 17(3): 451–464. doi: 10.1093/jae/ejm029.

Thurow L, Kapur D, Lewis J, Webb R. 1998. The world bank: Its first half century. *Foreign Policy* (110): 175.

TIIFHS (Taskforce on Innovative International Financing for Health Systems). 2009. More money for health, and more health for the money: Final report. Geneva: International Health Partnership.

Todaro M, Smith S. 2006. Economic Development. 9th Edition Addison-Wesley Series in Economics, 2006.

UN (United Nations) Millennium Development Goals. 2000. End Poverty.

Van der Gaag J, Stimac V. 2012. How can we increase resources for health care in the developing world? Is (subsidized) voluntary health insurance the answer? *Health Economics* 21: 55–61.

Van der Gaag J, Stimac V. 2008. Toward a New Paradigm for Health Sector Development. Technical Partner Paper 3. Brookings Institution and Amsterdam Institute for

International Development. The Rockefeller Foundation-Sponsored Initiative on the Role of the Private Sector in Health Systems in Developing Countries.

Vega J. 2013. Universal health coverage: The post-2015 development agenda. *Lancet* 381: 179–180.

Velenyi EV, Smitz MF. 2014. Cyclical Patterns in Government Health Expenditures between 1995 and 2010: Are Countries Graduating from the Procyclical Trap or Falling Back? *Health, Nutrition, and Population (HNP) Discussion Paper*. The World Bank, Washington, DC.

Victora CG, *et al.* 2008. Maternal and child undernutrition: consequences for adult health and human capital. *The Lancet* 371(9609), 26 January–1 February 2008: 340–357.

Wagstaff A. 2002. Poverty and health sector inequalities. Policy and practice. Theme Papers. *Bulletin of the World Health Organization* 80: 97–105.

Wagstaff A. 2008. Measuring Financial Protection in Health. *World Bank Policy Research Working Paper* No. 4554. The World Bank. Development Research Group. Human Development and Public Services Team. March, 2008.

Wagstaff A, van Doorslaer E, Paci P. 1989. Equity in the Finance and Delivery of Health Care: Some Tentative Cross-Country Comparisons. *Oxford Review of Economic Policy* 5(1): 89–112.

Wagstaff A, Paci P, van Doorslaer E. 1991. On the Measurement of Inequalities in Health. *Social Science & Medicine* 33(5): 545–557.

Weil D. 2015. *Fiscal Policy: The Concise Encyclopedia of Economics|Library of Economics and Liberty*. [Online]. Econlib.org. [Accessed: March 2015]. Available at: http://www.econlib.org/library/Enc/FiscalPolicy.html.

Weil D. 2007. Accounting for the effect of health on economic growth. *The Quarterly Journal of Economics* 122(3): 1265–1306.

World Bank. 1990. *World Development Report 1990: Poverty*. New York: Oxford University Press.

World Bank. 1993. *World Development Report 1993: Investing in Health*. New York: Oxford University Press.

World Bank. 2001. World Development Report 2000/2001: Attacking Poverty. The International Bank for Reconstruction and Development / The World Bank. Washington, DC. Oxford University Press, Inc. 200 Madison Avenue, New York, NY. 10016.

World Bank. 2003. *World Development Report 2004: Making Services Work for Poor People*. World Bank. https://openknowledge.worldbank.org/handle/10986/5986 License: CC BY 3.0 IGO.

World Bank. 2005. World Development Report 2006: Equity and Development. A Co-Publication of The World Bank and Oxford University Press. The International Bank for Reconstruction and Development/The World Bank, Washington, DC. Oxford University Press, New York, NY. http://www-wds.worldbank.org/servlet/WDSContentServer/WDSP/IB/2005/09/20/000112742_20050920110826/Rendered/PDF/322040World0Development0Report02006.pdf.

World Bank. 2009. Core Guidance: Preparing PERs for Human Development. [Online] [Accessed: May 2014]. Available at: http://siteresources.worldbank.org/EXTPERGUIDE/Resources/PER-Complete.pdf.

World Bank. 2010. Research for Development: A World Bank Perspective on Future Directions for Research. *Policy Research Working Paper*. WPS5437. Development Economics Senior Vice Presidency. September, 2010. The World Bank. Washington, DC.

World Bank. 2011. Development Impact Evaluation Initiative: A World Bank Approach to Enhance Developmental Effectiveness. Prepared by DIME and discussed by the OVPs and CODE in 2011.

World Bank. 2012a. Fiscal Health Database. Health and Economy Program, Health, Nutrition, and Population Anchor. The World Bank. Washington, DC.

World Bank. 2012b. South Africa Economic Update: Focus on Inequality of Opportunity. The World Bank Group Africa Region Poverty Reduction and Economic Management. July 2012. Issue 3. The International Bank for Reconstruction and Development/ The World Bank. Washington, DC. Available at: http://siteresources.worldbank.org/ INTAFRICA/Resources/257994-1342195607215/SAEU-July_2012_Full_Report. pdf.

World Bank. 2012c. Spotlight on Nigeria. Impact Evaluation Agenda. Motivation for Impact Evaluation. Interview with Dr. Muhammad Pate, Minister of State for Health, Federal Ministry of Health, Government of Nigeria. HRITF Impact Evaluation Toolkit. [Online] https://www.rbfhealth.org/impact. [accessed: April 2015]. Available at: http://siteresources.worldbank.org/INTIMPEVALTK/Resources/Nigeria_ Why_do_IE_Module1.pdf.

World Bank. 2014. The Economic Impact of the 2014 Ebola Epidemic: Short and Medium Term Estimates for Guinea, Liberia, and Sierra Leone. 17 September 2014.

World Bank. 2015. Development Impact Evaluation Initiative (DIME). [Online] [Accessed June 2015]. http://web.worldbank.org/WBSITE/EXTERNAL/EXTDEC/EXTDEVIM PEVAINI/0,contentMDK:23422972~pagePK:64168445~piPK:64168309~theSit ePK:3998212,00.html.

WHO (World Health Organization). 2001. *Macroeconomics and Health: Investing in Health for Economic Development* — Report of the Commission on Macroeconomics and Health. Geneva.

WHO (World Health Organization). 2009. The Financial Crisis and Global Health Report of a High-Level Consultation. WHO, Geneva, January 19. Available at: http://www. who.int/mediacentre/events/meetings/2009_financial_crisis_report_en_.pdf.

WHO (World Health Organization). 2010. The World Health Report. Health Systems Financing. The Path to Universal Coverage. Switzerland. ISBN 978 92 4 156402 1.

WHO (World Health Organization). 2012. Strengthening Health-System Emergency Preparedness. Toolkit for Assessing Health-System Capacity for Crisis Management. WHO Regional Office for Europe. Copenhagen, Denmark.

WHO (World Health Organization). 2013a. National Health Expenditure [Online] Database. [Accessed 2013]. Downloaded from: http://apps.who.int/nha/database.

WHO (World Health Organization). 2013b. Summary: Health, Health Systems, and Economic Crisis in Europe: Impact and Policy Implications. Draft for review by WHO and European Observatory on Health Systems and Policies.

WHO (World Health Organization). 2014a. Health Systems Situation in Guinea, Liberia, and Sierra Leone. Ebola and Health Systems Meeting. 10–11 December 2014.

WHO (World Health Organization). 2014b. High Level Meeting on Building Resilient Systems for Health in Ebola-Affected Countries. 10–11 December 2014. Geneva, Switzerland.

WHO (World Health Organization). 2014c. National Health Account. [Online] Database. [Accessed 2014]. Available: http://apps.who.int/nha/database.

Xu K, Saksena P, Holly A. 2011. The Determinants of Health Expenditure. A Country-Level Panel Data Analysis. Results for Development. World Health Organization. *Working Paper*. December 2011. http://www.who.int/health_financing/documents/cov-report_e_11-deter-he/en/.

Yu D, Souteyrand Y, Banda MA, Kaufman J, Perriëns JH. 2008. Investment in HIV/AIDS programs: Does it help strengthen health systems in developing countries? *Globalization and Health* 4: 8. Debate. Open Access. Biomed Central. http://www.globalizationandhealth.com/content/4/1/8. doi:10.1186/1744-8603-4-8.

Yfantopoulos J. 2013. Coping with Crisis: The Impact of the Economic Downturn on the Health Systems of Greece. Unpublished draft prepared for *Learning from Economic Downturns: How to Better Assess, Track, and Mitigate the Impact on the Health Sector*. In Hou X, Velenyi EV, Yazbeck AS, Iunes RF, Smith O. (eds.). The World Bank. Washington, DC.

Zaridze D, Brennan P, Boreham J, Boroda A, Karpov R, Lazarev A, Konobeevskaya I, Igitov V, Terechova T, Boffetta, P, Peto R. 2009. Alcohol and cause-specific mortality in Russia: A Retrospective case-control study of 48,557 adult deaths. *Lancet* 373(9682): 2201–2214.

Zweifel P, Ferrari M. Is there a Sisyphus syndrome in health care? In: Zweifel P, Frech II HE. (eds.). *Health Economics Worldwide.* Dordrecht: Kluwer Academic Publishers, 1992.

Zweifel P, Felder S, Meier M. 1995. Ageing of population and health care expenditure: A red herring? *Health Economics* 8(6): 485–496.

Macroeconomics, Trade and Health

Richard Smith, Marcus Keogh-Brown, and Johanna Hanefeld
London School of Hygiene & Tropical Medicine

Health and economics have a symbiotic relationship. Although this is often examined at the individual level, it is less often examined at the more macro-level. Yet, the health sector itself is a major economic sector, in terms of employment for instance. It is linked to other sectors of the economy, in terms of the consumption of intermediate goods and services, and is integrated within the global market for goods, services and people that are subject to considerable international trade. This chapter considers these wider links, exploring the evidence for economic interactions between health and the wider macroeconomy, and considers the issues of trade and health in some detail. The chapter also introduces some macro-economic approaches that have been used in health, such as Computable General Equilibrium (CGE) modeling, before presenting some specific examples and results. Capturing the macroeconomic implications of health policies on other sectors and the wider economy is essential if health policies are to be considered and weighed against non-health policies. Macroeconomic modeling provides an even playing field for policy assessments and a medium through which health and non-health policy implications can be jointly assessed using the same framework.

Keywords: Globalization; Trade; Macro-Economics; World Trade Organization; GATS; TRIPS; Computable General Equilibrium.

Introduction

Health and economics have a symbiotic relationship. It is well known that the health of an individual determines their productivity and ability to work, and that having greater access to resources enables better nutrition and access to health care. Yet, often within health economics, these broader relationships are ignored, or if they are recognized, are analyzed at the individual level within microeconomic analysis, such as that typified by the 'cost of illness' approach, where the time which a patient is absent from work is estimated as the wages they would have earned for working during that time, together with the costs of travel to obtain treatment. At the other end of the spectrum, there are macroeconomic assessments that consider health as a factor associated with economic growth, with a proxy measure — such as life expectancy or DALYs — seen as an independent variable in growth models.

Both of these forms of analyses are, of course, valid in their own right and in the specific context of the analysis being conducted. However, there is a growing recognition of a wider set of interactions between health and the macroeconomy. The health sector itself is not an isolated market but: (i) is linked to other sectors of the economy in terms of the consumption of intermediate goods and services (electricity, utilities, technology, construction, pharmaceuticals) and it is a major economic player in terms of employment, the financial industry and private health care provision; and (ii) is not just domestic, but integrated within a global market for goods, services and people that are subject to considerable international trade.

This chapter considers these wider links, exploring the evidence for economic interactions between health and the wider macroeconomy, and considers the issues of trade and health in some detail. The chapter also introduces some macroeconomic approaches that have been used in health before presenting some specific examples and results in the penultimate section.

Evidence of Links between *Health* and the Wider Economy

The relationship between health and the wider economy, and the role of trade within this, is not a new phenomenon. As Liverani and Coker (2012) outline, the rapid spread of cholera associated with increased global trade in the 19th century, and multiple pandemics, led to a considerable death toll. While governments imposed containment measures to control the disease, the economic interests of the mercantile elite suffered as these measures slowed the circulation of people and goods which was so crucial to commercial profit. A desire to temper health concerns with economic interests was soon evident. An assembly of 12 governments thus met in Paris in 1851 to establish a basis for common agreements on quarantine and the containment of cholera, leading eventually to the first International Sanitary Convention in 1892 and other international treaties in the following decades (Howard-Jones, 1975), which ultimately led to the International Health Regulations and, following the outbreak of Severe Acute Respiratory Syndrome in 2003, the Revised International Health Regulations in 2005 which are intended "to prevent, protect against, control and provide a public health response to the international spread of disease in ways that are commensurate with and restricted to public health risks, and which *avoid unnecessary interference with international traffic and trade*" (WHO, 2005 — emphasis added).

As alluded to earlier, there is considerable literature on the role of health in economic growth including not just health in general and growth (Daron Acemoglu and Simon Johnson, 2007) but also HIV and growth (Lovász and Schipp, 2009; McDonald and Roberts, 2006) and malaria and growth, for example (Gallup and Sachs, 2001). Beyond the confines of economic growth, however, there is clear evidence of the impact which health-related events can have on the wider economy, not just directly on the productivity and ability of people to work, but also on other sectors, for example animal-related sectors and their impacts to production, consumption and trade. This is especially the case for communicable disease, although increasingly is being seen with respect to non-communicable diseases (NCDs). For instance, with respect to communicable disease, some studies have retrospectively estimated that individuals who were *in utero* during the 1918 Spanish influenza pandemic were up to 15% less likely to graduate from high school, wages of men were 5–9% lower, socioeconomic status was substantially reduced and the likelihood of being poor rose as much as 15% (Almond, 2006). There is also evidence of some positive economic effects from this pandemic, with the total mortality rate significantly and positively correlated to the growth in income per capita from 1919 to 1930 across US states (Brainerd and Siegler, 2003), which may be attributable to a return to trend following the temporary disruption caused by the flu pandemic. However, it illustrates the complexity concerned in assessing the full economic picture of a health issue and policies that may be associated with tackling them, as we indicate later in this chapter.

More recently, the Severe Acute Respiratory Syndrome (SARS) outbreak of 2002–2003 provides an interesting example, as the health effect was relatively moderate in comparison to the significant economic effect. The outbreak began in late 2002 in the Guangdong province of China and spread rapidly, reaching its peak in the second quarter of 2003. By July 2003 the outbreak was declared over, having affected nearly 30 countries, infecting approximately 10,000 individuals, of which 10% died. The cumulative health impacts of SARS were much smaller than had been anticipated, but globalization played a key role in determining the impacts on the wider economy. The economic effects resulting from changes in behavior, especially tourism and travel, were notable. The Canadian Public Health Agency (Canada, 2003) suggested SARS costs of $350 million to tourism, $220 million in reduced airport activity, and $380 million in non-tourism retail sales. Overall estimates of the direct and indirect costs of SARS were placed at up to $2 billion. Keogh-Brown and Smith (2008) suggest that SARS caused losses to Hong Kong GDP of approximately US$3.7 billion (approximately 2.3%) and a 3% loss in China's GDP, even where only <0.03% of Hong Kong and around <0.0004% of China's population were actually infected with SARS.

The economic impact of NCDs is increasingly documented. For example, a recent study estimated that 5–10% of overall US health care expenditure was due to NCD-related health effects of being obese or overweight (Tsai *et al.*, 2011). In the UK, the annual cost of obesity to the UK economy including lost productivity was estimated at £15.8 billion per year in 2007.[1] Other studies, such as Butcher and Park (2008) and Lakdawalla *et al.* (2004), suggest that some increases in unemployment rates in the US in the face of overall improvements in population health may be attributed to obesity. Similarly, while their results may reflect associations rather than causal effects, Lindeboom *et al.* (2009) present evidence of the existence of differences in employment probabilities between obese and non-obese men and women which do not disappear when controlling for many potentially important factors. Carter *et al.* (2013) show that health shocks, such as cancer registration, result in a significantly increased risk of subsequent non-participation in the labor force.

There is also a burgeoning literature on the converse relationship of how wider economic forces are impacting health. A significant example here concerns tobacco. Trade and regulation of intellectual property in trade agreements relevant to health have included aspects of tobacco control, including restrictions around advertising for tobacco. Consumption of cigarettes and other tobacco products and exposure to tobacco smoke collectively constitute the world's leading preventable cause of deaths in adults (Holford *et al.*, 2014). The production of cigarettes is controlled by a small number of large transnational companies. As ownership and manufacturing is concentrated, trade of cigarettes and tobacco is particularly important. Tobacco companies have sought to use provisions within trade agreements to fight national tobacco control policies. An example of this has been the use of intellectual property rights relating to trademarks to contest plain packaging for cigarettes, for example in Australia (Thomas and Gostin, 2013; Gleeson and Friel, 2013). Here, trade agreements provide the opportunity for companies to contest the issues in national court. Another avenue is to contest public health regulation through trade agreements and to report countries to the World Trade Organization (WTO) dispute settlement mechanism or to bilaterally threaten or impose sanctions. Again, these mechanisms have been employed by transnational tobacco companies (Alemanno and Bonadio, 2011).

Although tobacco is a relatively clear cut issue for many, when it comes to other areas associated with trade, such as those concerning nutrition, the issues are more complex. A recent review of literature on trade and nutrition identified three pathways through which trade impact is associated with nutrition and health (Walls *et al.*, submitted 2014). The first pathway is through the price and

---

[1]Public Health England, http://www.noo.org.uk/NOO_about_obesity/obesity_and_health.

availability of food: an example of this is how international trade policy can affect availability and price of fruit in importing and exporting countries. This can have both positive and negative impacts on health through the types and quantities of food consumed, which in turn determines the nutritional status within a population. In exporting countries where fruit provides a major source of income, the domestic price may be prohibitive or availability low as consumers there may have to compete with international markets. Equally, where trade agreements and regulations have limited or abolished tariffs on imports, often processed food produced by large transnational companies has become cheaper than domestically produced primary produce. The second pathway through which trade agreements impact nutrition and health is through the increase in income generated by trade. While the effects of trade on poverty reduction and health have been subject to extensive debate (e.g., Dollar, 2001), there is strong evidence that highlights the clear link between trade and growth in GDP and a linked increase in health. A third pathway through which trade impacts health and nutrition is through government revenue: Through taxes on goods, through the increased income generated by trade, and through tariffs where these remain. These mark significant sources of revenue for governments, which in turn may then be invested in the provision of health care and social services improving population health.

Evidence of Links between *Health Care* and the Wider Economy

There is a significant global trade element to all domestic health systems. This has historically been most readily apparent with respect to the trade of goods, especially medicines, medical devices and technologies. Access to medicines is largely determined by trade, as manufacturing capacity for pharmaceuticals is highly concentrated with patents for many medicines held by a comparatively small number of companies. Table 1 shows the top ten pharmaceutical companies

Table 1. Top ten pharmaceutical companies by sales value, 2012

Corporation	Rank	Headquarters	Sales value (US$ million)
Novartis	1	Switzerland	50,761
Pfizer	2	US	46,930
Merck & Co	3	US	40,115
Sanofi	4	France	37,780
Roche	5	Switzerland	35,069
GlaxoSmithKline	6	Britain	32,714
AstraZeneca	7	Britain	31,893
Johnson & Johnson	8	US	27,933
Abbott	9	US	26,715
Teva	10	Israel	24,846

Source: IMS Health (2013).

by sales value in 2012. Their headquarters are located in the US, Switzerland, Britain, France, and Israel (see Table 1). Over the past decades, a growing industry for generic manufacturing has developed in India and a small number of other low- and middle-income countries. This concentration of manufacturing capacity in a small number of countries has made trade in pharmaceuticals a key issue for global health (Mullard, 2014).

Trade in medicines has not in all instances led to an increase in access to medication. Rather, many have argued that trade and the conditions relating to trade and specifically intellectual property rights enshrined in trade agreements have had severe effects on the availability and affordability of medicines in many low-income countries. Specifically, the agreement on Trade Related Intellectual Property Rights (TRIPS) adopted by the WTO in 1995 has received attention in this regard. TRIPS requires WTO member states to respect and grant patents for a period of 20 years, or face sanctions. The TRIPS agreement became a focus of international attention in relation to access to anti-retroviral treatment for HIV and AIDS. The annual cost for treatment with life-saving medication at the beginning of the 2000s was around US$12,000 per year, putting it beyond the reach of most public health systems and patients in low- and middle-income countries where the greatest burden of HIV is found (Roemer-Mahler, 2010). At the same time, the patent provisions within TRIPS initially prevented the export and use of generic, cheaper versions of such intellectual property to be imported from India where the largest capacity for generic manufacturing exists. Dramatically, even in countries where domestic manufacturing capacity existed, notably in South Africa, drug companies initially sought the protection of their intellectual property by taking the government to court in 1998. However, following national and international protest, the drug companies withdrew from the court case (Berger and Kapczynski, 2009). In part due to the awareness raised through the South African court case, including strong advocacy from civil society organizations such as the Treatment Action Campaign, Member States at the WTO agreed on the Doha Declaration TRIPS and Public Health, which allows countries to break a patent guaranteed under WTO regulation if it declares a national public health emergency. Where an emergency is declared, countries can then manufacture a generic version of the medication or import it where manufacturing capacity is lacking. While implementation of TRIPS provisions themselves varied, following the DOHA Declaration, the price of antiretroviral treatment per person per year fell to US$300 initially in large part due to the availability of generic medication. The price drop in treatment for HIV has demonstrated the relationship between price of medication and intellectual property regulation (Roemer-Mahler, 2010).

Following the Doha Declaration, further trade agreements have been passed which have affected intellectual property and, by extension, the availability and price of medicines. Many regional and bilateral trade agreements passed between the US and the EU and other countries have included so-called 'TRIPS plus' provisions, where countries commit to stronger patent protections than those set out in the DOHA protocol; an example of this is the Central American Free Trade Agreement (Sell, 2007). The example of intellectual property and the TRIPS agreement in relation to medication for HIV highlights the influence that trade and the regulations set out in trade agreements have on access and affordability of medicines.

Trade in services

However, trade does not only affect health care through goods traded but increasingly through the trade of services, sometimes referred to as invisibles. While trade historically has been in primary and in manufactured products, increasingly services, such as telecommunications and electricity, and also health and finance, are traded across borders (Reisman, 2014). Acknowledging this trend in 1995, the WTO created the General Agreement on Trade in Health Services (GATS), which explicitly covers trade in services. GATS defines the different modes of services traded and provides a framework for such trade to happen between countries under the umbrella of the WTO. This includes important provisions such as non-discrimination of foreign investors and providers.

Trade in health services covers several activities defined primarily under four modes of provision. GATS Mode 1 refers to the cross-border provision of medical services. This is primarily telemedicine, where diagnosis or expertise is provided by, for example, a physician in a different country, or where medical records are transcribed by a service provider in another country (Smith *et al.*, 2009a). A recent review of telemedicine found that examples documented in the literature mainly relate to telepathology, telesurgery, emergency and trauma telemedicine and teleradiology, and that exchanges across borders were mainly between physicians consulting on patient cases, rather than between patient and physician (Saliba *et al.*, 2012). It identified cross-border supply of health services as driven by the need to address shortages in expertise predominately in low- and middle-income countries, highlighting the positive potential of this form of trade.

GATS Mode 2 is defined as the consumption of health services abroad and commonly referred to as medical travel or medical tourism, where a patient leaves his or her country of residence to travel abroad with the explicit purpose of accessing treatment (Smith *et al.*, 2009a). A growing academic literature has focused on medical tourism in recent years (see also chapter by Hanefeld *et al.* later in this volume), yet the absence of robust data sets on the volume of tourists traveling remains a challenge to comprehensively understanding impact and scope of medical travel (Hanefeld *et al.*, forthcoming 2014). Despite data limitations, the impact of medical tourism on the health of patients and populations is beginning to emerge. Researchers have noted a lack of regulation (Whittaker, 2011). As most medical tourism takes place in the private sector and is organized by individual patients, providers or facilitators, it holds risks for patients, including limited mechanisms for redress where complications may have occurred (Lunt and Carrera, 2010; Vick, 2012). There is also a lack of clear information and guidance for patients on what to look for when choosing a provider abroad, potentially adding to the risk of complications (Horsfall *et al.*, 2013).

Research has also highlighted the risks arising from transmission of infectious disease as a result of medical tourism. While there are reports of such cases, including an outbreak of NDM1 in the UK (Chan *et al.*, 2011) and reports of a medical tourism-related case of disease in Singapore, these appear to have been relatively isolated cases. A further focus of research assessing the impact of medical tourism on health has been on the health systems impact in originating and recipient countries. Here again, evidence suggests a complex impact that is not uniform. Researchers have identified that incoming medical tourism may lead to movement of public sector workers to the private sector in recipient countries, adding to internal inequities in human resources (NaRanong and NaRanong, 2011). Research focused on fertility tourists and on organ donations has also highlighted the potentially negative impact of medical tourism on equity in recipient countries, where medical tourists with greater financial resources use scare services or donations that as a result may be unavailable to the domestic population (Whittaker and Speier, 2010). Yet, where quantitative analysis of national level impact has been conducted, the evidence generally suggests that medical tourism has an overall positive effect on national income for the recipient country (NaRanong and NaRanong, 2011; Lautier, 2008; Siddiqi *et al.*, 2010).

Recent research focused on the UK has also indicated that incoming medical tourists may be particularly lucrative private patients as their average spending on medical procedures was higher when compared to domestic private patients (Hanefeld *et al.*, 2013). Originating health systems may benefit financially from patients' travel where these represent a saving on services that would have otherwise been provided to the patient within the public system and where costs of future health services can be avoided. On the other hand, patients returning with complications from treatment abroad may represent a cost to health services in originating countries (Miyagi *et al.*, 2012). In sum, the impact of medical travel on health systems and on individual patients' health is complex and varied. There are clear benefits to health systems which appear not to have been fully explored so far. Significant risk to the individual patient in absence of regulation remains.

A further aspect of trade in health services — GATS Mode 3 — relates to the commercial presence of health investors from one country in another country

(Smith, 2004; Smith *et al.*, 2009a). Such investment generally takes the form of either a portfolio investment where investors buy shares of companies, or of foreign direct investment, such as through the purchase and investment in hospital and health care providers (Reisman, 2014). Both types of commercial presence in health appear to be increasing, as private provision of health care and commercialization increase even within public health systems such as the UK National Health Service (NHS). There are concerns about the for-profit motive of foreign investors who may repatriate profits made, rather than provide tax revenue or reinvestment in a country, and relating to volatility of funding for health services. However, foreign commercial presence allows for new resources where these may sometimes be limited. In practice, foreign direct investment has in some instances been tied to other modes of trade in health services, for example, where foreign investors may fund a health care facility aimed at medical tourists. Internationally famous 'health care brands', such as the Mayo Clinic based in the US or the Indian Apollo hospital chain based in India, have expanded to hospitals abroad, providing not only investment but also technology, knowledge, and quality assurances. As in the other GATS modes, evidence of commercial presence specifically in the health sectors of low- and middle-income countries is still limited (Smith *et al.*, 2009a).

Finally, GATS Mode 4 covers the movement of human resources for health between countries, including for training and employment (Connell, 2013). This aspect has received comparatively greater attention within global health, as many low- and middle-income countries report increasing shortages in human resources for health and health workers moving to positions in high-income countries, pointing to a highly inequitable impact of this mode of service trade (Aluttis *et al.*, 2014). Further attention has been on the link between Mode 2 (the consumption of services abroad) and human resources, as health workers in low-income countries may move to the private sector to cater to incoming medical tourists rather than provide services in the public sector (NaRanong and NaRanong, 2011).

Discussion of the evidence base on trade in health services, therefore, highlights negative and positive impacts. A common thread across the different types of trade is that impact of health services trade has so far only been explored to a limited extent and health considerations within trade policy have been largely neglected.

Trade agreements

Evident from the examples about linkages between trade, health, and health care is the central role of trade agreements and the regulations set out within these. The example of the TRIPS agreement and its impact on access to medicines has highlighted the immediate and far reaching effect of intellectual property regulation on the availability and price of medicines. The more recent examples of trade agreements and their impact on health relate to the extent to which provisions for trade and 'national treatment' or protections of investors within trade agreements may be in conflict with national public health regulations or the ability of governments to regulate marketing, availability and prices of goods traded. Tobacco companies using trade agreements to seek circumventing plain packing (meaning using standardized, non-branded packing) regulation of cigarettes is one example of this (Gleeson and Friel, 2013).

Further concerns relate to trade agreements currently in negotiation, such as the Trans Pacific Partnership Agreement, which are expected to have even stronger industry and investor protections (Friel *et al.*, 2013). These may limit countries' ability to regulate, for example, specific food content or marketing of foods in specific areas such as targeting high-sugar food advertisements to children.

In addition to concerns regarding the potentially negative consequences for health resulting from the provisions set out within agreements governing trade, limited or no attention has been awarded to examining potentially positive health effects of these agreements on health. Fostering trade or strategic marketing of specific 'healthy' goods may make these more accessible and available to consumers. Similarly, strategically planning for trade in health services to address gaps within services, utilize excess capacity or save costs may help alleviate challenges and restrictions faced by health systems. To foster and harness such positive potential will require further research to inform policies and regulations governing trade.

Macroeconomic Approach to Health Economic Analysis

Assessing wider implications and relationships of the sorts outlined thus far may often require a different form of analysis than that familiar to most economists working within health and health care. Different approaches have been used to specifically assess the macroeconomic impacts related to health. These models may be econometric, especially those concerned with estimating the effect of health on growth, or more usually, mathematical models of economic behavior. Growth models stem from the work by Solow (1956) on economic growth. Solow used the fact that saving and population growth rates vary across countries and demonstrated that these two factors can be used to explain how different countries reach different levels of steady-state income per capita. Mankiw and Weil (1992) extended this model to show the importance of capturing human capital and later studies have extended this to capture health more explicitly using growth models or regressions including, for example, growth models of HIV (Roe and Smith, 2008) which incorporate epidemiological projections of mortality and morbidity into a multi-sector growth model. Growth models have, at their heart, neoclassical production functions and are used to explain economic growth in terms of labor growth, capital accumulation and increases in productivity. Changes in the health status of a population affect labor and thus economic growth. While these models are able to consider aggregate economic effects, they lack the detail of some of the more modern macroeconomic simulation approaches where more detailed economic behaviors are specified and where some models are able to capture supply and demand effects with sectoral detail.

The Computable General Equilibrium modeling (CGE) approach has become one of the macroeconomic simulation models more recently used. This uses microeconomic theory to capture the behavior of different agents in the economy (government, consumers, producers, rest of the world), and parameters are calibrated based on a social accounting matrix (SAM) for a particular year. CGE models are based on neoclassical economic theory and capture both supply and demand constraints and decisions. They are able to simultaneously capture both the demand-side effects on a health system and the supply-side effects from health-related changes in the available labor force of an economy. The CGE approach has been recognized and recommended by the World Health Organization as a tool for health policy analysis for several years (World Health Organization, 2009) and has been applied in multiple areas including foot and mouth disease (Blanke *et al.*, 2001; Australian Productivity Commission, 2002); influenza pandemics (Smith *et al.*, 2009b; Keogh-Brown *et al.*, 2010a; Dixon *et al.*, 2010; Smith and Keogh-Brown, 2013; Chant, 2009); non-communicable disease (Lock *et al.*, 2010; Jensen *et al.*, 2013); antimicrobial resistance (Smith *et al.*, 2005; 2006); and HIV (Bell *et al.*, 2003; Boucekkine *et al.*, 2009; Corrigan *et al.*, 2005).

Examples of CGE Modeling Health

Pandemic influenza

Using the CGE modeling approach, several studies have attempted to analyze direct illness effects of influenza pandemics by modeling the production effects of changes in labor supply (Smith *et al.*, 2011; Keogh-Brown *et al.*, 2010a). These suggest that the direct estimates of the GDP loss from labor supply reductions due to influenza-related morbidity and mortality vary between approximately 0.2% for milder outbreaks (similar to the 1959/68 flu pandemics), up to 1.6% for severe outbreaks (similar to 1918 Spanish flu) which suggests that, even for significant outbreaks, the direct health-related economic effects may be relatively small. Smith *et al.* (2009b) modeled an extreme disease scenario for the UK which estimated the economic effect of 14% GDP loss due to labor supply reductions, but this scenario combined an extreme clinical attack rate with SARS-like mortality.

In an article by Smith and Keogh-Brown (2013), estimates are presented of the macroeconomic impact of an H1N1 (Swine Flu) pandemic from 2009 on the economies of South Africa, Thailand, and Uganda. Estimates suggest that the direct illness effects of such a pandemic are less than 0.5% loss of GDP but that the relative impacts on different economies will vary. Ugandan impacts were relatively larger than those for South Africa and both countries' estimates were 50% to 100% larger than those for Thailand.

Keogh-Brown *et al.* (2010a) compared the impacts of potential flu pandemics in four European countries: the UK, France, Belgium, and the Netherlands. Economic impacts for mild disease were projected to be approximately 0.5% GDP loss and more severe pandemics were estimated to impose direct illness effects of around 2% GDP loss, but there were variations within countries. The UK's labor-intensive service sectors resulted in the largest projected impact being for the UK. France and Belgium exhibited similar relative impacts and the Netherlands suffered the smallest losses in this hypothetical modeling exercise.

Behavioral change

While many of the direct illness effects estimated for communicable disease outbreaks are relatively small, the CGE analyses of influenza pandemics also capture the potential indirect effects on the economies concerned. For example, the effects of school closure and prophylactic absence from work. In Smith *et al.* (2009b), prophylactic absence from work was modeled as an effect triggered in an individual by the knowledge that someone in their social network has died from the disease. The authors estimated the size of the average social network to be approximately 300 people and, by modeling disease scenarios of differing severity and including potential interventions (vaccination) of differing efficacy, they were able to highlight the potentially much greater economic impact of a fear-induced response to avoid work compared with the disease-only effect. The scenarios modeled showed that if a behavioral response that prompts individuals to refrain from work can be avoided, then the potential value of interventions to prevent a harmful economic response might be greater than the value of preventing negative health effects alone. In addition, should fear be the driver of behavioral change, the mortality rate of an outbreak might have a more significant effect than the number of people infected. The validity of these conclusions are clearly dependent on the assumptions made in scenario design, but the model results capture interaction effects which could not be captured from a microeconomic approach focused on health alone. The other pandemic modeling studies by Keogh-Brown *et al.* (2010b) and Smith *et al.* (2011) found similar behavioral change effects where prophylactic absence and school closure effects outweigh the economic impacts of the disease itself.

Non-communicable disease (NCD) and public health impacts

CGE models have also been used to assess the impacts of non-communicable disease on the economy. As well as the health-related macroeconomic impacts, the wider macroeconomic impacts of both health-focused interventions and non-health focused interventions with health-related externalities have been assessed.

In the paper by Lock *et al.* (2010), an assessment is made of the macroeconomic impacts of healthier eating as a result of reductions in consumption of meat and dairy products in the UK and Brazil. Non-communicable disease reductions, specifically ischaemic heart disease, were used to estimate the health effects. The authors suggest that, while reductions in consumption of unhealthy goods can generate positive health-related macroeconomic effects, the substitution effects from reduced consumption are key drivers of both the health and economic impact. For example, if reducing consumption of meat and dairy products leads to increased consumption of other unhealthy food goods, it will reduce the health benefits. In addition, the ease with which other sectors can expand in response to reduced consumption of unhealthy products will also drive the economic impacts. The authors also highlight that countries, like Brazil, which are dependent on international trade in meat products may suffer economically if their trade partners reduce consumption of meat. Such countries will also suffer in terms of adverse health effects if reductions in trade lead to increased availability of unhealthy goods on the domestic market.

In an article by Jensen *et al.* (2013), a CGE model is used to assess the health and macroeconomic effects of interventions designed to meet sector-specific UK greenhouse gas emissions reduction targets over the period 2010–2030. This paper provided an innovative extension from previous health-focused CGE studies, as it not only captured the health and wider macroeconomic effects of interventions, but also captured demographic, social security and age-specific health and macroeconomic impacts. Three interventions were modeled, each of which involved a greenhouse gas reduction strategy with associated estimates of health co-benefits, health harms and health care expenditure effects. Health co-benefits are collateral benefits for health that result indirectly from the greenhouse gas reduction strategies. An active travel scenario targeted UK transport sector emissions by reducing urban motorized transport and assumed health co-benefits and harms of a complementary increase in walking and cycling. The road pricing tax, health effects, and efficiency gains from reduced congestion resulted in an almost GDP-neutral impact by 2030 (−£169 m), suggesting that, based on the model assumptions, the combined goals of health gains and greenhouse gas reductions can be met at (almost) no cost.

A second intervention, 'Healthy Diet,' targeted agricultural emissions and used a fat tax charged on high-fat products to accomplish a UK-wide 30% reduction in consumption of dietary saturated fat and to achieve corresponding health benefits. Considerable health benefits (£4.7 billion) were insufficient to counter the fat tax losses of (£100 billion) over the 20-year period of the model, yielding an overall loss to UK GDP of £96 billion. The magnitude of this loss is attributed to the distortionary effect of the tax imposed on saturated fat and the absence of any efficiency improvements from the tax policy. A third intervention targeted greenhouse gas emission reductions in the household energy sector by investing in UK-wide improvements in home insulation and ventilation control with associated health co-benefits and harms. Health co-benefits yielded economic gains of £450m but the investment in home insulation imposed costs of £49 billion, which were partially countered by home energy efficiency savings of £24 billion. This intervention, in particular, highlights the additional value of a macroeconomic approach to analysis since, when viewed from the partial equilibrium perspective, the cost of investment would be almost compensated for by the efficiency savings. Several specific health co-benefits and harms were considered in this study. In summary, the largest savings to health care expenditure resulted from reductions in disease burdens from Diabetes, Ischaemic Heart Disease (IHD), and Depression. IHD, together with Cerebrovascular disease and Depression, also made the largest contributions to the health-related expansion of the labor force, while reductions in IHD and Cerebrovascular disease burdens amongst older people result had the largest impact on increasing social security costs due to increased survival in old age. The model not only revealed a notable difference between the full and partial equilibrium impact of the interventions for all three applications, but the introduction of demographics highlighted that many of the health benefits from reduced NCDs occur in older age groups rather than working population individuals and yielded negative GDP per capita effects for some scenarios and timescales. The extension of the CGE approach to incorporate demographic and other measures within the modeling framework is another reason why the CGE approach is an ideal tool for holistic analysis of both health- and non-health-related policy implications. The integration of CGE models with other models is a valuable methodological extension in which health-focused CGE modelers are making important headway.

Integrative approaches

The combination of economic models with other kinds of mathematical models has been used in the environmental sciences for several years. These models are known as Integrated Assessment Models (IAMs) and are multi-equation mathematical models, designed either in the natural science or engineering sciences to make future projections of the earth system or from an economic perspective to focus on the human system and its effects on, for example, land use and greenhouse gas emissions. In the economic context, IAMs combine models which describe the physical processes of climate change (General Circulation Models or GCMs) with economic models in order to find optimum policies (minimize environmental and/or economic cost) (Parson and Fisher-Vanden, 1995). These models have grown in popularity to inform the debate over the economic feasibility of some climate change policies. Examples of these models include the DICE model (Nordhaus and Radetzki, 1994), the RICE model (Nordhaus, 2010), the FUND model[2] and the PAGE model (Hope, 2006).

The RICE model is an extended and updated version of the DICE model. It is based on the Ramsey growth theory model whereby the capital stock in the 12 region, single sector economic model is extended to allow investment in natural capital (the environment). The model is able to capture the effects of reducing current consumption in order to prevent potentially harmful economic effects of climate change in the future and the production function of the model determines output using capital, labor, and carbon-energy as inputs. The integrated model also includes population demographics and a geophysical component to capture and link CO_2 emissions, a carbon cycle, radiative forcings, a simple climate model, and regional climate–damage relationships. The model also has an additional module to generate estimates of sea-level rise (SLR). The Climate Framework for Uncertainty, Negotiation and Distribution (FUND) integrated assessment model is a dynamic model of climate change. It is a combination of several linked models including demographics, technology, economics, emissions, atmospheric chemistry, climate, sea level, and impacts covering 15 regions and dynamic single year time steps from 1950 to 2300. The PAGE model is a probabilistic integrated assessment model that is intended to be relatively simple and is designed to approximate results from more complex scientific and economic models to form both regional and global impacts of climate change, and social costs of different greenhouse gases. The model produces estimates for eight world regions, ten time periods to the year 2200 for the impact measurements which include sea level, economic and non-economic measures. The probabilistic model is based on uncertainty and uses probability distributions and multiple simulations to build up full probability distributions of the scientific and economic results, which include the global mean temperature, the net present value of impacts and the SC CO_2. However, these integrated assessment models do not capture the sectoral detail of CGE models nor do they contain the same level of detail in terms of demand and

[2]http://www.fund-model.org/.

supply relationships and constraints. They also omit the potentially important health-related impacts of climatic change.

However, recent developments in health-focused CGE models have sought to fully integrate health, demographic and economic models in a single framework in the context of malaria elimination (Jensen *et al.*, 2014). By fully integrating these models, the resulting model framework is able to capture the feedback effects of, for example, (i) changes in malaria prevalence on the economy and demographics (survival), (ii) changes in the economy on demographics (urbanization) and malaria (malaria and public health interventions) and (iii) changes in demographics on malaria (urban/rural location) and the economy (skill and location of the workforce). These health-focused integrated frameworks are also being extended to be applied in the context of non-communicable disease such that policy assessments can be made that account for not only the whole-economy impact of health effects but also the wider interactions between health, health-related policies and the economy, non-health interventions and health-related externalities, and demographics.

Conclusion

While the influences of health on the macroeconomy and vice-versa have long been established, the comparatively rare use of macroeconomic approaches in health effect estimation and the disregard of health effects in many macroeconomic policy applications reveals that much still needs to be done in order to enable holistic policy analysis that correctly values the health effects and health implications of those policies. Key among these are policies relating to trade and agreements governing trade between countries. While liberalization of economies and trade is advancing the understanding of health effects associated with economic changes, these are only understood to a limited degree. Specifically, the extent to which better understanding of the health effects of trade could be used to harness health through trade has not been explored.

Detailed, sector-specific health economic analysis has an important role to play in capturing individual-level costs and health sector implications of health policies and disease burdens, without which budgeting decisions and treatment recommendations cannot be made. However, the macroeconomic implications and methods for macroeconomic analyses of health are currently under-researched and under-utilized.

A partial equilibrium approach to health economic evaluation is not able to adequately estimate the magnitude of the wider economic implications or the potentially catastrophic welfare implications of health-focused policies which impose significant demand or production constraints, either directly through behavioral change. As some of the studies mentioned in this chapter show, policies which have positive health effects can have significant wider economic costs. While these costs should not necessarily preclude policy implementation, taking a partial perspective to analysis by which only positive health and economic benefits are declared, does not provide a sufficient evidence base and thus many health policies are not calculated to minimize the impact on the wider economy and livelihoods.

Simultaneous capture of the macroeconomic implications of health policies on other sectors and the wider economy is essential if health policies are to be considered and weighed against environmental, trade and agricultural policies. Similarly, the potentially significant health effects and externalities of non-health focused policies should also be captured and considered as their contribution may be relevant to policy optimization decisions, as the example of trade agreements highlights. Macroeconomic modeling provides an even playing field for policy assessments from both health and non-health perspectives and a medium through which health and non-health policy implications can be jointly assessed using the same framework. In addition, while macroeconomic modeling of health is a relatively new discipline, recent methodological developments show that health-focused CGE models are not just utilizing existing state-of-the-art methodologies but also in extending them.

In summary, there is a need for health economists and health policymakers to adopt a combined approach to economic policy analysis by utilizing both micro- and macroeconomic approaches. This will help facilitate better understanding of macroeconomic policy, including trade policy, on health. By increasing the use and popularity of approaches such as CGE modeling in the health field, the importance of capturing health-related macroeconomic effects will be highlighted and dialogue will be facilitated across disciplines to enable optimum policy decisions which account for both the health benefits and overall economic implications of policies, while also accounting for important demographic, welfare, environmental, trade, and agricultural implications.

References

Alemanno A, Bonadio E. 2011. Do you mind my smoking? Plain packaging of cigarettes under the TRIPS agreement. *John Marshall Review of Intellectual Property Law* 10.

Almond D. 2006. Is the 1918 Influenza pandemic over? Long-term effects of in utero influenza exposure in the post 1940 U.S. Population. *Journal of Political Economy* 114: 672–712.

Aluttis C, Bishaw T, Frank MW. 2014. The workforce for health in a globalized context — Global shortages and international migration. *Global Health Action* 7: 23611.

Australian Productivity Commission. 2002. Impact of a foot and mouth disease outbreak on Australia. *Research Report Series, Melbourne. Distributed by Ausinfo, Canberra;* p. xxxii.

Bell C, Devajaran S, Gersbach H. 2003. The long-run economic costs of AIDS: With an application to South Africa. *Unpublished Manuscript.*

Berger J, Kapczynski A. 2009. The Story of the TAC Case: The Potential and Limits of Socio-Economic Rights Litigation in South Africa. *Human Rights Advocacy Stories.*

Blanke A, Sinclair T, Sugiyarto G. 2001. The Economy-Wide Effects of Foot and Mouth Disease in the UK Economy. *Third Annual Conference European Trade Study Group.* Brussels, Belgium.

Boucekkine R, Desbordes R, Latzer H. 2009. How do epidemics induce behavioral changes? *Journal of Economic Growth* 14.

Brainerd E, Siegler MV. 2003. The Economic Effects of the 1918 Influenza Epidemic. *CEPR Discussion Paper No. 3791* [Online].

Butcher KF, Park K-H. 2008. Obesity, disability, and the labor force. *Economic Perspectives*, XXXII.

Canada PHAO. 2003. Learing from SARS. Renewal of Public Health in Canada. *A Report of the National Advisory Committee on SARS and Public Health* [Online].

Carter KN, Gunasekara FI, Blakely T, Richardson K. 2013. Health shocks adversely impact participation in the labour force in a working age population: A longitudinal analysis. *Australian and New Zealand Journal of Public Health* 37: 257–263.

Chan HL, Poon LM, Chan SG, Teo JW. 2011. The perils of medical tourism: NDM-1-positive *Escherichia coli* causing febrile neutropenia in a medical tourist. *Singapore Medical Journal* 52: 299–302.

Chant L. 2009. *The Macroeconomic Impact of HIV/AIDS in South Africa.* University of Sussex.

Connell J. 2013. Contemporary medical tourism: Conceptualisation, culture and commodification. *Tourism Management* 34: 1–13.

Corrigan P, Glomm G, Mendez F. 2005. AIDS crisis and growth. *Journal of Development Economics* 77.

Daron Acemoglu, Simon Johnson. 2007. Disease and development: The effect of life expectancy on economic growth. *Journal of Political Economy* 115: 925–985.

Dixon PB, Lee B, Muehlenbeck T, Rimmer MT, Rose AZ, Verikios G. 2010. Effects on the U.S. of an H1N1 epidemic: Analysis with a quarterly CGE model. *Centre of Policy Studies/IMPACT Centre Working Papers g-202* [Online].

Dollar D. 2001. Is globalization good for your health? *Bulletin of the World Health Organization* 79: 827–833.

Friel S, Gleeson D, Thow A-M, Labonte R, Stuckler D, Kay A, Snowdon W. 2013. A new generation of trade policy: Potential risks to diet-related health from the trans pacific partnership agreement. *Globalization and Health* 9: 46.

Gallup J, Sachs J. 2001. The Economic burden of malaria. *American Journal of Tropical Medicine & Hygiene* 64: 85–96.

Gleeson D, Friel S. 2013. Emerging threats to public health from regional trade agreements. *The Lancet* 381: 1507–1509.

Hanefeld J, Horsfall D, Lunt N, Smith R. 2013. Medical tourism: A cost or benefit to the NHS? *PLoS One* 8: e70406.

Hanefeld J, Smith DR, Lunt N, Horsfall D. forthcoming 2014. What do we know about medical tourism — A review of the literature with discussion of its implications for the UK NHS as an example of a public health care system. *Journal of Medical Travel* In Press.

Holford TR, Meza R, Warner KE, Meernik C, Jeon J, Moolgavkar SH, Levy DT. 2014. Tobacco control and the reduction in smoking-related premature deaths in the United States, 1964–2012. *Journal of the American Medical Association* 311: 164–171.

Hope C. 2006. The marginal impact of CO_2 from PAGE2002: An integrated assessment model incorporating the IPCC's five reasons for concern. *Integrated Assessment Journal* 6: 19–56.

Horsfall DG, Lunt N, King H, Hanefeld J, Smith RD. 2013. The impact of the internet on medical tourism. In Botterill D, Pennings G. (eds.). *Medical Tourism and Transnational Health Care.* London: Palgrave Macmillan.

Howard-Jones N. 1975. *The Scientific Background of the International Sanitary Conferences, 1851–1938.* Geneva: World Health Organization [Online].

Jensen H, Keogh-Brown M, Smith R, Chalabi Z, Dangour A, Davies M, Edwards P, Garnett T, Givoni M, Griffiths U, Hamilton I, Jarrett J, Roberts I, Wilkinson P, Woodcock J, Haines A. 2013. The importance of health co-benefits in macroeconomic assessments of UK Greenhouse Gas emission reduction strategies. *Climatic Change* 121: 223–237.

Jensen HT, Keogh-Brown M, Smith R, Bretcher M, Chico M, Drakely C. 2014. Malaria in Ghana: Integrated macroeconomic and epidemiological-demographic impact assessment. *Health Economics Study Group.* Sheffield, 2014.

Keogh-Brown MR, Smith RD. 2008. The economic impact of SARS: How does the reality match the predictions? *Health Policy* 88: 110–120.

Keogh-Brown MR, Smith RD, Edmunds JW, Beutels P. 2010a. The macroeconomic impact of pandemic influenza: Estimates from models of the United Kingdom, France, Belgium and The Netherlands. *European Journal of Health Economics* 11: 543–554.

Keogh-Brown MR, Wren-Lewis S, Edmunds WJ, Beutels P, Smith RD. 2010b. The possible macroeconomic impact on the UK of an influenza pandemic. *Health Economics* 19: 1345–1360.

Lakdawalla DN, Bhattacharya J, Goldman DP. 2004. Are the young becoming more disabled? *Health Affairs* 23: 168–176.

Lautier, M. 2008. Export of health services from developing countries: The case of Tunisia. *Social Science & Medicine* 67: 101–110.

Lindeboom M, Lundborg P, Van Der Klaauw B. 2009. Obesity and Labor Market Outcomes: Evidence from the British NCDS. *IZA Discussion Paper No. 4099.*

Liverani M, Coker R. 2012. Protecting Europe from diseases: from the international sanitary conferences to the ECDC. *Journal of Health Politics, Policy and Law* 37: 915–934.

Lock K, Smith RD, Dangour AD, Keogh-Brown M, Pigatto G, Hawkes C, Fisberg RM, Chalabi Z. 2010. Health, agricultural, and economic effects of adoption of healthy diet recommendations. *The Lancet* 376: 1699–1709.

Lovász E, Schipp B. 2009. The impact of HIV/AIDS on economic growth in Sub-Saharan Africa. *South African Journal of Economics* 77: 245–256.

Lunt N, Carrera P. 2010. Medical tourism: assessing the evidence on treatment abroad. *Maturitas* 66: 27–32.

Mankiw R, Weil 1992, A contribution to the empirics of economic growth. *Quarterly Journal of Economics* 107(2).

McDonald S, Roberts J. 2006. AIDS and economic growth: A human capital approach. *Journal of Development Economics* 80: 228–250.

Miyagi K, Auberson D, Patel AJ, Malata CM. 2012. The unwritten price of cosmetic tourism: An observational study and cost analysis. *Journal of Plastic, Reconstrucitve Aesthetic Surgery* 65: 22–28.

Mullard A. 2014. Large drug firms narrow their therapeutic interests. *The Lancet* 383: 1873.

NaRanong A, NaRanong V. 2011. The effects of medical tourism: Thailand's experience. *Bulletin of the World Health Organization* 89: 336–344.

Nordhaus WD. Economic aspects of global warming in a post-Copenhagen environment. *Proceeding of the National Academy of Sciences of the USA 2010.*

Nordhaus WD, Radetzki M. 1994. *Managing the Global Commons: The Economics of Climate Change.* Cambridge, MA, MIT Press.

Parson EA, Fisher-Vanden K. Searching for Integrated Assessment: A Preliminary Investigation of Methods, Models, and Projects in the Integrated Assessment of Global Climatic Change. Consortium for International Earth Science Information Network (CIESIN). University Center, Michigan 1995.

Reisman D. 2014. *Trade in Health. Economics, Ethics and Public Policy.* Cheltenham, Edward Elgar.

Roemer-Mahler A. 2010. Business strategy and access to medicines in developing countries. *Global Health Governance* IV.

Roe, Smith. 2008. Disease dynamics and economic growth. *Journal of Policy Modeling* 30(1).

Saliba V, Legido-Quigley H, Hallik R, Aaviksoo A, Car J, Mckee M. 2012. Telemedicine across borders: A systematic review of factors that hinder or support implementation. *International Journal of Medical Informatics* 81: 793–809.

Sell S. 2007. TRIPS-Plus free trade agreements and access to medicines. *Liverpool Law Review* 28: 41–75.

Siddiqi S, Shennawy A, Mirza Z, Drager N, Sabri B. 2010. Assessing trade in health services in countries of the Eastern Mediterranean from a public health perspective. *International Journal of Health Planning & Management* 25: 231–250.

Solow RM. 1956. A contribution to the theory of economic growth. *Quarterly Journal of Economics* LXX: 65–94.

Smith RD. 2004. Foreign direct investment and trade in health services: A review of the literature. *Social Science & Medicine* 59: 2313–2323.

Smith RD, Chanda R, Tangcharoensathien V. 2009a. Trade in health-related services. *Lancet* 373: 593–601.

Smith RD, Keogh-Brown MR. 2013. Macroeconomic impact of a mild influenza pandemic and associated policies in Thailand, South Africa and Uganda: A computable general equilibrium analysis. *Influenza and Other Respiratory Viruses* 7: 1400–1408.

Smith RD, Keogh-Brown MR, Barnett T. 2011. Estimating the economic impact of pandemic influenza: An application of the computable general equilibrium model to the U.K. *Social Science Medicine* 73: 235–244.

Smith RD, Keogh-Brown MR, Barnett T, Tait J. 2009b. The economy-wide impact of pandemic influenza on the UK: A computable general equilibrium modelling experiment. *British Medical Journal* 339: b4571.

Smith RD, Yago M, Millar M, Coast J. 2005. Assessing the macroeconomic impact of a healthcare problem: The application of computable general equilibrium analysis to antimicrobial resistance. *Journal of Health Economics* 24: 1055–1075.

Smith RD, Yago M, Millar M, Coast J. 2006. A macroeconomic approach to evaluating policies to contain antimicrobial resistance: A case study of methicillin-resistant *Staphylococcus aureus* (MRSA). *Applied Health Economics Health Policy* 5: 55–65.

Thomas BP, Gostin LO. 2013. Tobacco endgam strategies: Challenges in ethics and law. *Tobacco Control* 22: i55–i57.

Tsai AG, Williamson DF, Glick HA. 2011. Direct medical cost of overweight and obesity in the USA: A quantitative systematic review. *Obesity Reviews* 12: 50–61.

Vick L. 2012. The perils of cosmetic surgery/medical tourism. *Clinical Risk* 18: 106–109.

Walls HL, Cornelsen L, Friel S, Smith RD. Submitted 2014. The impact of international food-related trade policy on nutrition and health: A Systematic Review.

Whittaker A. 2011. Cross-border assisted reproduction care in Asia: Implications for access, equity and regulations. *Reproductive Health Matters* 19: 107–116.

Whittaker A, Speier A. 2010. "Cycling overseas": Care, commodification, and stratification in cross-border reproductive travel. *Medical Anthropology* 29: 363–383.

WHO 2005. International Health Regulations. In WHO (ed.). Geneva.

World Health Organization 2009. WHO Guide to Identifying the Economic Consequences of Disease and Injury. World Health Organization, Geneva.

Measuring and Forecasting Global Health Expenditures

Thomas E. Getzen
iHEA and Temple University
getzen@temple.edu

Section "Introduction and Historical Background" of this chapter briefly reviews the literature on medical spending, which suggests that health expenditures began small but steadily increased throughout history (from 1% to 4% of GDP), then began to increase rapidly among wealthier developed countries after 1950. Section "Measurement: Temporal, Spatial and Administrative Units of Observation" examines temporal and spatial dimensions of measurement, which suggest that the evolution of global health expenditures may be best observed by tracking health expenditures as a share of GDP over decades. Nominal and real per capita amounts are subject to distortions created by lags and currency valuation. Months and years are too short a span, while persons, households and provinces are too small. Section "Lags, Business Cycles, and Growth Trends" covers growth in the components of health expenditures (population, income, inflation, excess due to technology and other factors). A model of national health expenditure decisions over time is presented and used to explain empirical findings of varying distributed lag responses to macroeconomic growth and development. Section "Forecasting National and Global Health Expenditure Trends" considers the methods and accuracy of national health expenditure forecasting. Section "Aging, Health Expenditures and Fiscal Burdens" addresses some problems of variable identification, with specific applications to population aging and the aggregate fiscal burden of care for the elderly. Section "Global Health Spending Patterns 1850–1955 and 1960–2075" discusses the sustainability of current trends and the boundaries between long-term care, retirement and medical expenditures. It concludes by proposing that rising longevity and medical costs are best viewed as aspects of a process of economic and human development transforming the 20th and 21st centuries, rather than as isolated phenomena. The six sections each conclude with a discussion of policy implications, even the most technical sections regarding measurement, aggregation and lags, where the policy implications may not be immediately apparent. While nominal policies are publicly stated, it is often these "technical details" regarding boundary definition, timing and measurement that show how policy actually operates, that shape public opinion, and that drive future financial decisions.

Keywords: Forecasting; Trends; Lags; Health Spending; Excess Cost Growth; Business Cycles; Aging.

Introduction and Historical Background

Medical Spending: The first 5,000 years

For as long as there has been money to spend, there have been health expenditures. The earliest financial records are those inscribed in Sumerian cuneiform tablets *circa* 5000 BC. Listed there are prices for medical treatment; ½ mina of silver for a slave, 1 mina for a worker in the household, and 2 minas for a member of the family (Pritchard, 1958). The Code of Hammurabi (*circa* 1772 BC) spells out fines for different types of medical malpractice (botched surgery, substitution of inferior drugs). Later, the Hippocratic Oath refers explicitly to payments from patients and the conditions for free care. The conclusion that medical care has been an economic activity with market prices (and subsidized government care or free care through religious institutions) throughout human history is inescapable. A quick review of economic history indicates that medical care was a steady but relatively small part (1%–4%) of total market activity until about 1950. However, it is difficult to compare Sumerian silver minas to millions of euros, or even the "Geary-Khamis" dollars in the Maddison estimates of historical global economic output (Maddison Project, 2014). It could be questioned whether it is even possible to estimate comprehensive measures of "health expenditures" prior to the construction of national income and product accounts in the 20th century.

Prior literature

Seminal publications on health expenditures include the 36-volume *Report of the Committee on the Costs of Medical Care* 1932, the 1956 *Guillebaud Report* on the costs of health care in the UK, Jean-Pierre Poullier's 1977 OECD publication *Public Expenditures on Health*, and Robert Fogel's *The Escape from Hunger and Death, 1700–2100*: *Europe, America and the Third World*. Archival information exists allowing estimation of health spending in absolute and relative terms using methods familiar to cliometricians. On the production side, the fraction of labor devoted to medical work yields a rough estimate of the health share of total economic output when combined with some reasonable assumptions about wages and non-labor inputs. On the demand side, the fraction of household spending devoted to health is used as a starting point, keeping in mind the importance of non-private funding and the difference between these "typical" families and a true national average.

The first comprehensive and rigorous estimate of total national expenditures on health was made by the researchers in the United States under the Committee on the Costs of Medical Care (CCMC, 1932).[1] Their estimate of 3.5% for the year 1929 is still taken as having established a standard for this era and is incorporated into the official national health expenditure accounts maintained by the Office of the Actuary and reported to the Organisation for Economic Co-Operation and Development (OECD, 2000). Nothing comparable was done until Brian Abel-Smith and Richard Titmuss produced the Guillebaud Report on the costs of the National Health Service (NHS) in the United Kingdom in 1952 (Abel-Smith and Titmuss, 1956). A decade later, Abel-Smith organized the available international data on expenditure in a report for the World Health Organization (WHO), an exercise repeated in 1968 (Abel-Smith, 1963; 1967). Similar data was used by Joseph Newhouse to analyze the determinants of national health expenditure in 1977, reporting that after per capita income is accounted for as a determinant of health expenditures, "there is little left to be said," a result confirmed by a number of others over the next 30 years (Gerdtham *et al.,* 1992; Getzen, 1990; Maxwell, 1981; Newhouse, 1977; 2014).

The OECD health data set providing comparative annual health expenditure estimates for most developed nations from 1960 to the present has now become familiar to most health economists. Organizing, collating and harmonizing data from many sources and different periods was a tremendous advancement in methodology, carried out almost single-handedly by Jean-Pierre Poullier during the 1970s and 1980s (OECD, 1977; Poullier, 1986). After he regularized this effort within the OECD structure, it was passed on to a group of economists who now perform annual updates and periodic benchmark revisions. The solid line in Figure 1 uses this OECD dataset to

[1]There is an estimate of 2.5% of GDP given in a 1928 compendium of works by the insurance executive and health economists Louis I Dublin (1928), but it does not indicate the basis or methodology of the estimate, or the precise year and scope. Studies of health expenditures were carried out at various times by the Social Security Administration until the 1960s, but they were much more comprehensive with regard to public than private expenditures, and are not entirely consistent.

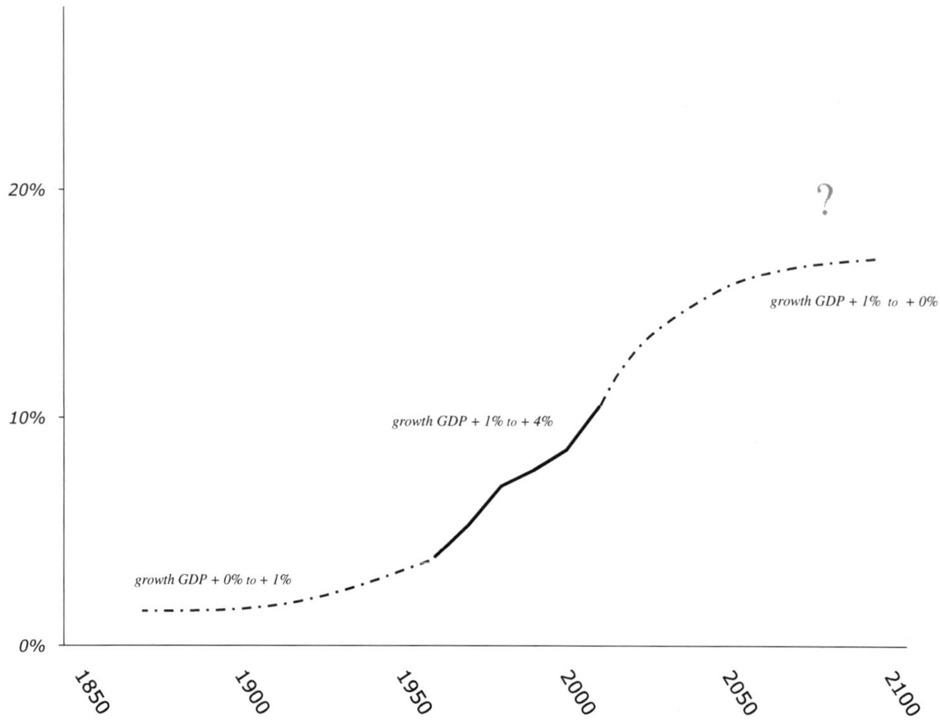

Figure 1. Health share of GDP

Source: OECD Health Data 2014 and author calculations.

graph the average rate of growth in the health share of Gross Domestic Product (GDP) among selected countries since 1960. The dotted line before 1960 represents a reasonable set of estimates for growth prior to the postwar surge in spending that will be discussed in Section "Global Health Spending Patterns 1850–1955 and 1960–2075". The dotted line after 2015 represents a forecast indicating that growth is expected to moderate over the coming decades, as will be discussed in Section "Forecasting National and Global Health Expenditure Trends".

With detailed data available for the past 50 years, empirical research has been able to determine that national health spending is highly related to a country's state of economic development and per capita GDP, as well as to some specific elements of the medical workforce and organization, but is not determined or is only weakly affected by life expectancy, morbidity, population aging, the division between public and private financing, or available measures of per unit medical prices. The more limited historical records available for previous millennia cannot be reviewed in detail here, but indicate an average health expenditure within a range of 0.5%–5% of total spending, which grew more slowly than in recent decades and differed widely across locations and between urban and rural areas, and would also support the following generalizations.

Historical generalizations for medical expenditures in prior millennia (5000 BC to 1960)

- Medical expenditures were small but significant since the start of history.
- Expenditures were concentrated on drugs and procedures, not "care."
- The transformation to modern scientific medicine with rapid increases in spending during the 20th century was preceded by and dependent upon the industrial revolutions of the 19th century, as well as the demographic transition that began in the 18th century.
- Expenditures varied widely by the type of health system and the patients they served (for example, urban vs. rural; India vs. Europe; poor vs. rich; or factory worker vs. farmer). There were a multiplicity of "systems" within each nation, and price discrimination was used inside and between systems.
- Medical leadership in research and innovation shifted from France to Germany, then to the UK, then to the US, and is now drifting toward India and China.
- Pharmaceutical firms have been the most international and future-oriented segment of the health care industry.
- Academic medical centers with expensive research programs, while nascent in the 19th century and earlier, started to become dominant around 1960.
- Health expenditures had begun to rise rapidly in many developed countries by 1960.

Generalizations for modern health expenditures (1960–2015)

- Increased spending reflects economic growth.
- Health care spending responds slowly and with a lag to major macroeconomic shifts.
- Population aging has been concurrent with but not a major cause of the rise in health expenditures.
- Twenty years is not long enough to judge historical trends.

Policy Implications. The premise of this chapter is that lessons gleaned from the study of health expenditure growth across countries over long periods of time growth will help to make policies more effective and reduce the number of times that failed policies are retried. The most important lesson is that the major health policy objective of the 20th century was reached — science advanced extending the lives of people across the world as the ravages of disease were reduced. However, there have been unintended consequences, mostly notably the continued and unsustainable increase in costs. Long-range planning and management of systems has become a critical necessity as longevity of 75 or 100 years becomes widespread. Workers currently entering the labor force will not retire until 2050 or later, yet retiree health benefits already impose a heavy fiscal burden on governments. Research to find out why expenditures move up or down over time (or why they do not) and how long it takes to know the difference, may or may not make cost cutting less painful, but it may well make the process of managing expenditures more rational and accurate. It might also stop the false demonization of some purported "causes" of expenditure increases (e.g., longevity, drug abuse, obesity and pollution) and prevent the application of policies that have repeatedly failed in the past. Better analysis of the past 150 years will create better public understanding of the extent to which excess growth has already moderated and perhaps reduce the panic response that engenders bad policy. "Technical" refinements in methodology, such as better measurement of trends and variance, will enable more distinctions between good and bad policy to be made on the basis of evidence rather than ideology, bias, or advantage to a particular interest group.

Measurement: Temporal, Spatial and Administrative Units of Observation

Data is sometimes analyzed because, like Mount Everest, "it is there." The availability of administrative data is no substitute for careful thinking about what units of observation would be best suited to the study of a particular subject of interest, or how different geographic and temporal spans of observation may make some phenomena very prominent while hiding or obscuring others. The unit of observation should be matched to the span of the phenomena that is to be observed (usually somewhere between 0.1 times and 10 times the length). It is not helpful to study global warming with daily temperature observations, much less hourly or second-by-second observations, since the signal would be overwhelmed by noise. Conversely, the dynamics of a lighting bolt from the clouds cannot be observed with annual or monthly observations, but in this case photographs taken every second are useful and multiple observations over a fraction of a second even more so. The choice of spatial units poses similar issues (see Getzen, 2000a; 2006).

Employment offers a useful starting point for studying health system change because it is not subject to many of the problems inherent in financial measures (such as adjustments for inflation, taxation, exchange rates, timing of payments, or the border-crossing funding flows that occur when local expenditures are covered by NGOs, federal insurance plans, or other payments originating from out-of-area). The health shares of labor can sometimes even be calculated for pre-market agricultural economies. Furthermore, a wide range of temporal units are available (by month, year, decade, or century) for different geographic units

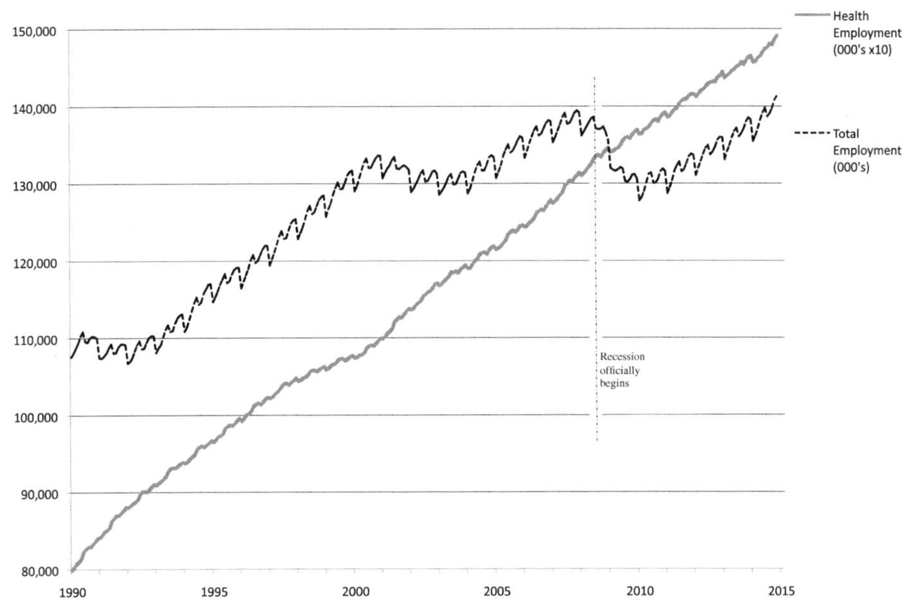

Figure 2. Employment in health and total employment: US 1990–2014

Source: BLS Data 2014 and author calculations.

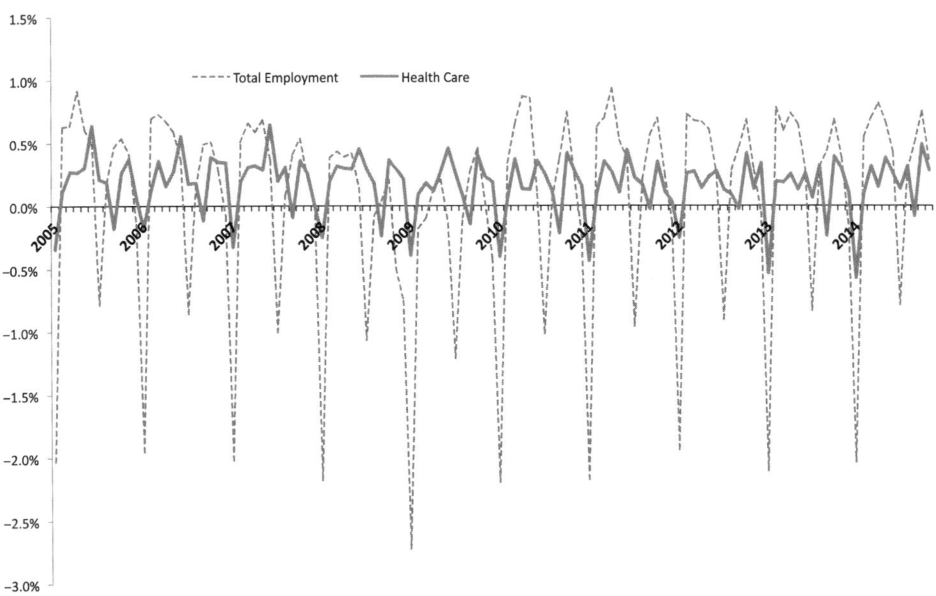

Figure 3. Monthly % change in employment, health and total: US 2005–2014

Source: BLS Data 2014 and author calculations.

(precincts, towns, cities, provinces, nations). Figure 2 plots total employment and health employment for the US from 1990 to 2014. It is evident that health employment is growing more rapidly and is much less variable. The difference in variance is even more apparent in Figure 3 showing the month-to-month

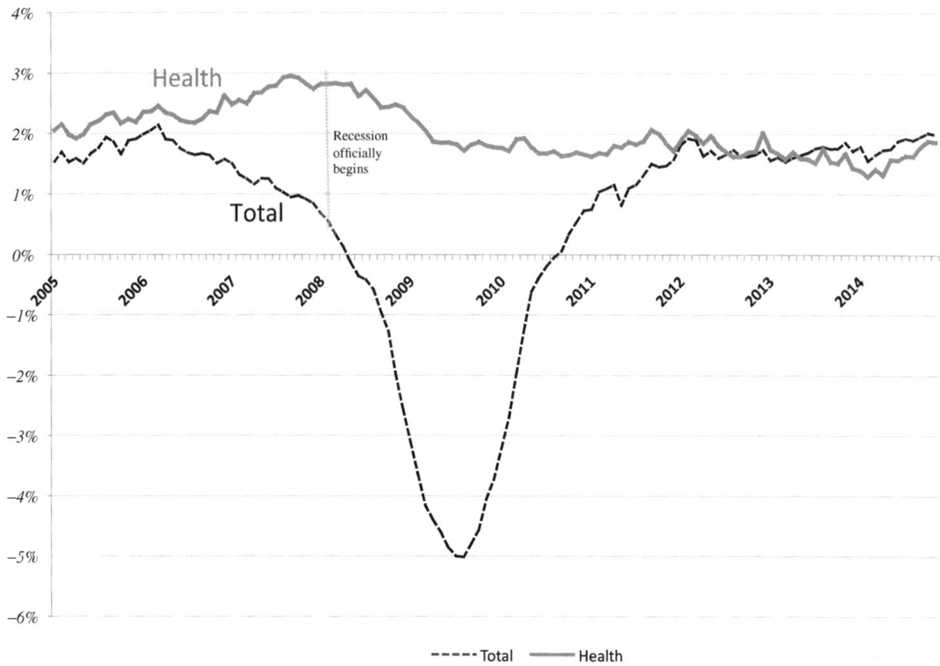

Figure 4. 12-Month change in employment: US 2005–2014
Source: BLS Data 2014 and author calculations.

change. Figure 4 graphs the percentage change over the preceding 12 month span, removing seasonal variation and smoothing the series.

Technological Dynamism and Fiscal Inertia

Medical knowledge changes quite rapidly, but changing the organization and systems of payment is a slow and drawn-out process. Coordinating thousands of patients, doctors, hospitals and payers is time-consuming. Hence, the response to any sudden change in the environment (such as a recession) tends to be delayed and extended. The public and political consensus required to restructure medicine cannot be formed very quickly.

Investments in physical and human capital build delays into the structure of medicine. Hospitals take years to construct, and the education of doctors and other health professionals place them into occupational categories that remain rigid for decades. Figure 2 indicates how inertial the modern medical system has become. The sluggish response to changes in the macroeconomic environment are also clear in Figure 5a, which shows how health spending in Finland declined in response to that country's sharp recession in 1991, but only after a lapse of 2 years. The response to inflationary shocks is similarly slow and delayed, as can be seen in Table 1, presenting Canadian data around the time of the OPEC (Organization of the Petroleum Exporting Countries) oil embargo and attendant spike in prices.

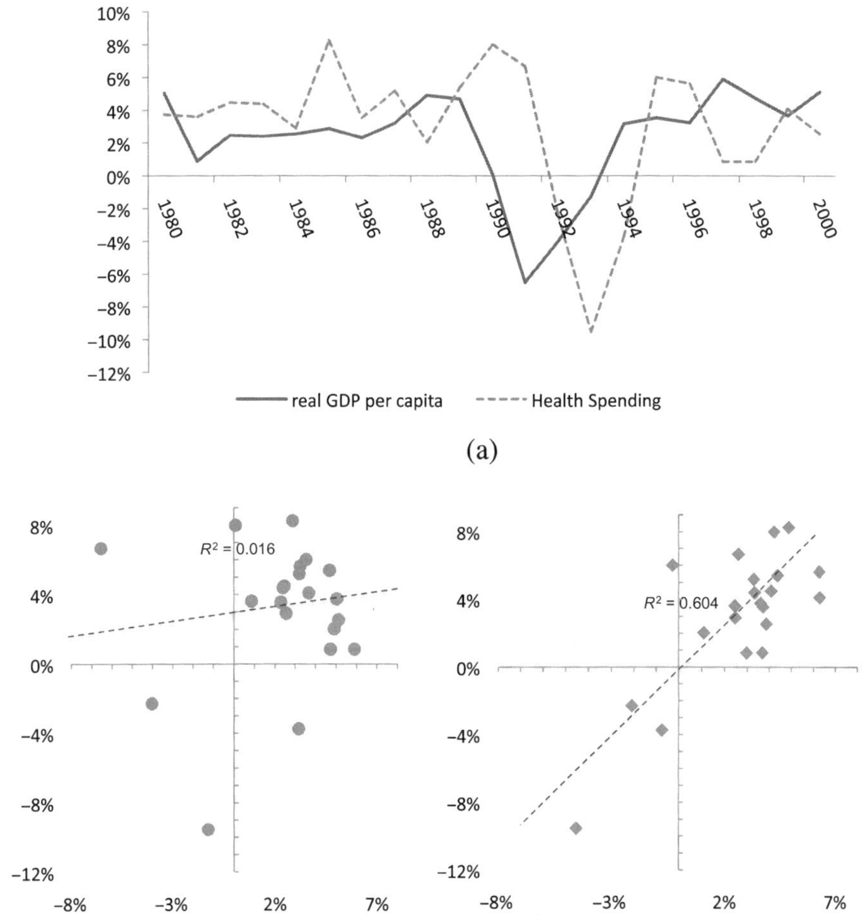

(b) (c)

Figure 5. Finland 1980–2000 (a) Annual % growth in real GDP and health spending. (b) Correlation with current growth. (c) Correlation with lagged growth

Source: OECD Health Data 2014 and author calculations.

Table 1. Inflation and health employment in Canada

Canada	Inflation (%)	Employment: Nurses	Employment: Total	Ratio	Health Share % of GDP
1972	5.6	152,005	8,447,000	0.0180	7.3
1973	8.9	159,274	8,860,000	0.0180	7.0
1974	14.4	168,530	9,220,000	0.0183	6.9
1975	9.8	177,182	9,364,000	0.0189	7.4

Notes: How the financial measure of health share is distorted by delayed adjustment to the 1974 spike in inflation.

Source: OECD (1990). *Health Care in Transition*. OECD: Paris.

Decomposition: Inflation, Population, GDP and Excess Growth

Reports on spending typically make the distinction between total and per capita amounts and separate the growth rates into real and inflation components. Comparisons of health expenditures over time are often expressed in terms of the share of GDP or fraction of total wages. Decomposition shows that growth in the share is computationally identical to the excess growth in health spending (as compared to growth in GDP or wages). Let:

Y = nominal GDP
  g = growth in nominal GDP
  r = growth in real GDP
  d = inflation rate (GDP deflator)
H = nominal health spending
  h = growth in nominal health spending
  x = "excess" growth ($h-g$)
S = health share of GDP (H/Y)
  s = growth rate of health share.

Health spending is decomposed as:

Growth in health spending = inflation + real GDP growth + excess growth.

Taking account of compounding:

$$h = (1 + d) \times (1 + r)(1 + x) - 1.$$

Then s, the growth rate in the health share of GDP, is readily seen as simply equal to x, the excess growth rate in health spending.

$$s = (\mathrm{H} \times (1 + d) \times (1 + r)(1 + x)/\mathrm{Y} \times (1 + d) \times (1 + r))/(\mathrm{H}/\mathrm{Y}) - 1 = x.$$

Since the percentage growth in share is identical to excess growth, the two terms will be used interchangeably here. Graphs of shares are often more intuitive and quickly grasped than plots of nominal spending or excess growth rates since they are comparable across time periods, regions, countries and groups without regard to population, price levels, exchange rates or other factors that would require adjustment. Share estimates tend to be more reliable and available than spending estimates for historical periods and organizational subgroups, and illustrate:

- Spending relative to total resources available (budget constraint) at each point in time.
- Where growth is equal to GDP + 0% (curve is flat and horizontal).
- The rate of excess growth (slope is steeper where excess growth is larger).
- The point of maximum excess growth (located at the inflection point of the curve).

Excess growth is the best general measure for comparing health spending across time and place, but care must be taken since share is calculated as a *Health*: *Total* ratio, and hence any mismatch between numerator and denominator in definition or boundary will distort the ratio. Most importantly, the lags between a rise (or fall) in GDP mean that most of the month-to-month and year-to-year variation in growth rates are due to temporary changes in GDP rather than changes in the long run trend of health spending (which are inertial and occur much more slowly). Table 1 illustrated how a measure of physical resource use (labor) can avoid the distortions arising from delayed adjustment to price levels. However, the delays in labor adjustments due to shifts in real GDP growth remain. Researchers intend to determine how health consumption changes in response to permanent income changes, but current data correlations show primarily the response to transitory income changes (Friedman, 1957; Getzen, 2014).[2] This mismatch in timing can be reduced econometrically by using a smoothed version of GDP that more closely approximates the "true" rate of income growth as perceived by the public and policymakers. A moving average of growth over the preceding years appears to remove most, but not all, of the distortions caused by transitory GDP fluctuations, and is discussed in greater detail later in Section "Lags, Business Cycles and Growth Trends".

A Model of Health Spending: Decisions and Transactions

Spending occurs when a transaction takes place. Sometimes, a transaction is as simple as the exchange of money for services at a point in time, but most medical transactions are embedded in a complex web, with most cash flows determined by private and government insurance contracts with agreements, rules and specifications that may run for many years. Only a small portion of medical exchanges are as simple as buying a bottle of aspirin or paying $1,200 to have a tooth capped. A skeletal description of the complex medical care spending process can be modeled as follows. Let:

i = individuals	N = Nations
y = individual income	Y = National Income
ψ = individual decisions	Ψ = National Decision
h = individual medical spending	H = National Medical Spending

M = Medical System
δ = tax rate
t = time (in years).

[2]The classic presentation of the "permanent income" hypothesis is that in Milton Friedman's Theory of the Consumption Function (Friedman, 1957). More specific application to the estimation of national health expenditures is provided by Getzen (2013, Chapter 13, 299–306; 2014).

Although individuals and nations must make expenditures from current income (supplemented by savings or debt), those decisions are usually based on their expectations of long-run permanent income, denoted by $ɏ_t$ for individuals and $Ɏ_t$ for the nation as a whole.

Expected Permanent Income: $ɏ_t = f(y_t, y_{t-1}, y_{t-2}, \ldots, y_{t-n}, z)$,
$Ɏ_t = f(Y_t, Y_{t-1}, Y_{t-2}, \ldots, Y_{t-n}, Z)$.

National health expenditures are a combination of government and private spending. The government budget is a fraction of total current national income, determined by the tax rate δ. Individual budgets are determined by earnings less taxes. However, government strongly influences individual spending through the regulation of medical care and insurance. Most individual spending is a residual response to collective rules, subsidies and risk-pooling, rather than a personal expenditure commensurate with their own personal assessment of the value of treatment (i.e., premiums, co-payments, mandates, inflation). Individual citizens have some power over how the national budget is spent, but only through the political process.

Government Budget: $\delta Y_t = \delta \Sigma y_{it}$.
Individual Budgets: $(1 - \delta)\, y_t$.

The medical care system (M) at a point in time (t) is determined by the individual and national decisions made in prior years and also by some exogenous parameters (Z), such as technology, biology, historical accidents, trade, and so on. Decisions are made atomistically by individuals (ψ_i) and politically by nations (Ψ) in each year. An individual making a decision at a point in time y_{it} does so based on the medical care system as it then exists (M_t), their estimated permanent income at that time (ψ_{it}), the decisions they have made in prior years, and other factors such as tastes, preferences, and health status. National decisions are made each year (ψ_t) and the budget is allocated with the goal of optimizing current and future states of the medical care system balanced against other goals and objectives (defense, education, debt, etc.). Similar to individuals, the nation must take the current overall state of the medical system as a given, but it is also attempting to optimize based on the nation's estimate of how those decisions will affect the system in future years M̶ ($\text{M̶}_{t+1}, \text{M̶}_{t+2}, \ldots, \text{M̶}_{t+n,}$). The estimated future state of medicine in each future year is indicated by a single strike as M_{t+n}. The rolling cumulative estimate of the path of medical care over all future years is indicated by double-strike as M̶.

$$h_{it} = f(\psi_{\mathrm{it}}, \{1-\delta\}\mathrm{y}_t, \mathrm{M}_t, \not{y}_{\mathrm{t}}, z),$$
$$\mathrm{M}_t = f(\mathrm{M}_{t-1}, \Psi_t, d\not{\mathrm{Y}}_{\mathrm{t}}, \mathrm{Y}_{\mathrm{t}}, \mathrm{Z}),$$
$$\mathrm{H}_t = f(\delta\mathrm{Y}_{\mathrm{t}}, \Psi_t, \mathrm{M}_t, \not{\mathrm{Y}}_t, \not{\mathrm{M}}, \mathrm{Z}) + \sum h_{it}.$$

Thus, individual health spending (h_{it}) depends on a set of individual decisions, disposable income, the state of medical organization/technology, and other factors (including health status). The current state of medicine (M_t) depends of the state of medical organization/technology inherited from the prior year, supplemented by new decisions and financed with current (and future) national budgets. The nation's health spending (H_t) is determined by its current and permanent income, the current state of medicine, as well the expected effect of the decisions taken on future states of medical care, with a stub added to account for individual health spending.

These equations are largely recursive and cannot be solved — medical spending depends on a medical care system that is a complex function of prior and expected future states, which are themselves determined by decisions affecting organization and technology that are only intermittently and incompletely observable, and virtually never quantifiable. What these equations can do is to isolate those variables that are observable, and provide some insights into a temporal structure that must then be estimated.

The state of the medical care system (M_t), is a convenient construct, but not observable or quantifiable. Decisions (Ψ_t) are only occasionally visible, and have effects that may only become apparent with the passage of time. The two variables within the model that are observable and measurable are income and health spending. Everything else resides within a black box. Thus, the only reduced form that can actually be estimated is:

$$\mathrm{H}_t = f(\mathrm{Y}_t, \mathrm{Y}_{t-1}, \mathrm{Y}_{t-2}, \ldots, \mathrm{Y}_{t-n}, \mathrm{Z}).$$

Even though most of the internal structure is unobservable, the model does suggest why the health care system has such a long memory and where that memory resides — in the structure of the medical care system itself. It takes a long time to craft and implement major changes. Once established, the residual effects of a major policy shift will linger for decades. The fiscal impact will eventually decline, but a pattern of delays or lingering effects is itself evidence that the change was structural. Empirical estimates of such delays and interactions may provide insights into the interior workings of the health care system that are hidden behind the details available on the surface. This model does not provide much additional empirical content, but it does provide a way to conceptualize how change occurs and how it is (or is not) reflected in measures of total health expenditure. It provides a means for understanding why the patterns of spending resulting from business cycles would not be the same as those resulting from productivity shocks, and why patterns will differ across countries whose medical organization differs, or across categories of spending for which the transactions are very different (for example, contracts for hospital construction compared to out-of-pocket (OOP) spending for drugs).

Aggregation, Cross-Sections, Time Series and Uncertainty

The creation of double-entry National Income and Product Accounts (NIPA) was a major accomplishment, part of the work for which Simon Kuznets and Richard Stone were awarded Nobel prizes. It rests on a fundamental accounting identity: *Income = Consumption + Investment* (with relevant supplemental additions and subtractions for taxation and government expenditure, foreign trade, and so on). Empirical analysis of macroeconomic phenomena and trends, a topic made critical by the great depression in the 1930s, blossomed with the availability of data on GDP, price levels, productivity, and other variables that were comparable over time and across countries. Similarly comparable data series for health care were generally lacking until recently, and are still less regular and homogeneous. Hence, the OECD health data set constructed by Poullier was also major achievement in this regard, even though it does not begin until 1960 and still has a number of gaps and discontinuities. Collating and harmonizing information from so many disparate sources is difficult. National statistical agencies must rely on reports from hospitals, physicians or insurance plans to supplement any direct observations on patients, which are often limited to queries regarding illness episodes or OOP payments. Definitions, nomenclature, categories, organizational and geographical boundaries, even the dating of a fiscal year, may all be different from one country to the next, and usually change over time. Many adjustments and judgment calls are required to collate and harmonize datasets, as well as significant effort and hard choices between conflicting estimates.

Most expenditure measurements in health economics come from administrative records or surveys rather than experiments or field trials. Observations are often bounded by the vagaries of regulatory procedures, functional limitations, managerial goals or historical precedent rather than designed to match the expected span of impact or the phenomenon of interest to the researcher. The level of temporal and spatial aggregation must be chosen carefully to avoid misleading results. Time series and cross-sectional analyses each have strengths and weaknesses, but the combination in panel data is more technically challenging, more prone to misinterpretation and error. Aggregation and extrapolation from a limited number of observations to make a national estimate is difficult; to make such data internationally consistent across a number of years is a heroic effort. However, once the OECD health data set was created, it was easy to use and there was no way to forestall casual analysis by researchers with little understanding of the assumptions, caveats and limitations inherent in the data.

The lack of long time series data and the number of gaps and discontinuities has sometimes forced health economists to use local or provincial data to estimate the effects of health policies. Two conceptual errors may plague such analyses. The first is the use of cross-sectional results to make inferences across time. While it is certainly true that 2001 will become 2002, and in turn become 2003 and so on, Spain will never become Sweden, nor will Mississippi become Massachusetts. Health and policy change over time, not place. The second is a failure to appreciate the econometric implications of accounting identities and how a fixed budget implies errors that are not independent, but are forced to sum *exactly* to 0. Whatever deviations are made in one area or category *must* be offset by deviations in the opposite direction in other areas or categories. In practice, most budgets are slightly porous so that the sums are not exact: Borrowing, saving, deficits and "creative accounting" can ease the rigidity of financial constraints — but only for a while, and usually with increasing difficulty as gaps become wider. Similarly, definitions of households or of categories such as health, housing, food and transportation may have blurred boundaries that creates inconsistencies leading to double- or under-counting. It is the work of NIPA and the system of health accounts (SHA) to reduce or eliminate such inconsistencies, yet "discrepancy" amounts of varying magnitudes are always used to make the calculations balance (OECD, 2000; WHO, 2011). A series of research attempts to reconcile national health expenditure estimates constructed by US Office of the Actuary with those found during large scale patient surveys (namely, the Medical Expenditure Panel Survey, which surveys of families, individuals, providers, and employers across the US) show disparities of 5% to 30% between the two estimates (Sing *et al.*, 2006).

Policy Implications. Using excess growth in health care (i.e., percentage increase in share) as the core measure of health expenditures is not just a technical decision, it forces attention on the central cost problem: health expenditures rising faster than the ability to pay for them. Focusing instead on the raw amounts or even real adjusted growth rates would divert attention toward prices, utilization, illness categories, and other intermediates or peripheral issues, rather than the gap between expenditures and ability to pay. The core issue, however, is the gap. Only by earning more or spending less can a country bring finances back into balance. Losing weight, shortening the length of hospital stays, limiting price increases or closing clinics will not accomplish this end (although all such remedies have been tried, often repeatedly). Control comes from staying within a budget. Apparently, "technical" concerns regarding the matching of temporal and spatial units actually reflect major policy concerns: since any change in an inertial health care system will only be revealed slowly, monthly and annual observations are too short, and observations on precincts, cities, provinces, regions and other sub-national units are too small. Only by observing the changing health share of GDP over many years can the effects of national policies on medical professions and health financing be seen. The external cross-currents and random noise that obscure the dynamics of health spending growth must be smoothed over or filtered out. The fact that spending is usually lower on Sundays or in the middle of winter may be true but not very meaningful. Much more important are the developments in medical science and technology occurring over decades or centuries.

Observations of households or local firms providing health insurance do not change fact that aggregates and per capita average payments are mostly determined by workforce regulations, standards of care, regulations, tax policies and subsidies that are national in scope. Some trends may even be influenced by forces that are trans-national or global. Awareness of problems in aggregation and the temporal and spatial units of observation suggest that short-, medium- and long-run forecasts of health spending may require different methods, as does the study of per personal spending by individuals or groups (see Section "Aging, Health Expenditures and Fiscal Burdens").

Lags, Business Cycles and Growth Trends

Year-to-year variation in health spending is most strongly affected by a delayed response to business cycles, the vagaries of rising and falling incomes, and inflation. Observed variation over any span shorter than a year is plagued by seasonal fluctuations, timing and measurement errors, arbitrary allocations (e.g., how much less depreciation for February since it has only 28 days, how much more for a month with 3 biweekly pay-periods rather than two?) and so on, so that such fluctuations have to be treated primarily as noise. This noise, and even the business cycle fluctuations, tend to average out over longer spans of observation so that the underlying growth trends are revealed. From this broader perspective it appears that, although growth in health costs has seemed inexorable since 1960, it was actually rather flat or only modestly rising during the decades and centuries prior. Closer analysis indicates that after surging during the 1960s and 1970s, excess cost growth in the health sector began to fall, and is now just 1% above the rate of GDP growth or less in many countries.

The techniques developed to measure economic growth with the system of national accounts can be extended to analyze the growth in the health sector. Health expenditure in Canada and US grew from $2 billion in 1960 to $135 billion in

Table 2. Growth components, OECD countries 1960–2005

	Annual % growth in total NHE (in %)	Population growth (in %)	Increase in price level (in %)	Real GDP per capita (in %)	Share (excess) growth (in %)	Health share of GDP 2005 (in %)
Canada	9.7	1.3	4.3	2.4	1.3	**0.099**
France	10.8	0.6	5.0	2.6	2.3	**0.111**
Germany	7.8	0.9	3.1	2.0	1.6	**0.107**
Japan	10.4	0.7	3.2	3.8	2.3	**0.082**
Netherlands	9.5	0.8	4.1	2.3	2.1	**0.098**
Spain	17.0	0.8	8.2	3.3	3.9	**0.083**
Sweden	10.0	0.4	5.4	2.2	1.6	**0.092**
Switzerland	7.6	0.7	3.3	1.5	1.9	**0.112**
UK	10.8	0.3	6.3	2.2	1.7	**0.083**
USA	10.0	1.1	4.0	2.1	2.5	**0.154**

Source: OECD Health Data 2012, author calculations.

2005, an average growth rate of 9.7% per year. Table 2 presents the total health expenditure increase from 1960 to 2005 for several OECD countries decomposed as population growth, price growth, real per capita GDP growth, and excess growth (the percentage increase in health share of GDP).[3]

Growth accounting decompositions similar to the one above can be made for most countries, revealing broad similarities (such as growing populations, rising percapita incomes, substantial inflation) but also significant differences for sub-periods and within particular countries (for example, rapid population growth with little income growth in much of Africa, deflation and population shrinkage in Japan since 1990, global inflation spiking during the 1970s, recession and recovery cycles, or growth spurts in Spain and Ireland). One purpose such component analyses is to separate out general macroeconomic trends so as to more clearly reveal the growth pattern for a specific sector, such as health, where rising costs are of particular concern to policymakers.

The sources and patterns of variation in measured growth differ according to the frequency of observation (Table 3). High frequency measurement (minutes, hours, days) captures mostly transitory noise that is irrelevant in the long run. The ordinary mid-range troughs and peaks of the business cycle are best seen in observations of quarters or years. In order to reveal long-run growth trends and to

[3]The standard growth decomposition procedure is to first to calculate the rate of "excess growth" by the percentage increase in share (equivalent to the percentage rate of growth in health expenditures net of the rate of growth in nominal GDP). GDP is then similarly decomposed into the growth in population and price inflation, designating the remainder as "real growth in per capita income" and typically attributed to technology or productivity.

Table 3. Focal point by frequency (*temporal spans of observation*)

(*Span*)	**Focus on Variation due to**
Days, Months	**Transitory noise**
Quarters, Years	**Business cycles**
Decades, Centuries	**Long-run growth trends**

see what caused health expenditures to take even larger shares of GDP, patterns of growth across decades or centuries must be examined.

Health is inertial. Like other major categories of pooled public spending (education, defense, pensions), it responds more slowly to change than finance, housing, commodities and other sectors of the economy. Hence, it is not surprising that hourly, daily, or monthly observations are dominated by noise. Even the quarterly observations exploited to define the beginning and end of recessions are of little use. It will be necessary to extend the span of observation to encompass more than five decades to understand the causes of spending that has raised the health share of GDP from less than 4% to more than 10% in many developed countries.

Business Cycles and Variable Lags

Because health care is inertial, the rates of growth in health spending in 1995 may carry more information about 1994, 1993, 1992, 1991 or even prior to 1990 than it does about current conditions. Figure 5b has the same data as Figure 5a in Section II, showing GDP growth and annual health spending for Finland 1980–2000. In 5b, the data is presented in a scatterplot (rather than a time series as in 5a). Without temporal ordering, there appears to be almost no correlation between contemporaneous GDP and health spending. A data transformation using a lagged 3-year moving average of GDP as in Figure 5c reveals some of the correlation. The dynamics of the process and the strength of the income–expenditure relationship over time are much more fully revealed by regular time series, as originally presented in Figure 5a. In other words, timing matters. A researcher looking only at contemporaneous correlations, or just one or two lags, could seriously underestimate the strength of the relationship between spending and the business cycle, or even conclude that there was no relationship. The lag transformation smoothes the GDP curve and shifts it in time to show more of the relationship. In Finland, the lag between the 1994 recession and the corresponding decline in health expenditure growth was about 3 years. The structure of lags seems to vary between countries and by the particular type of spending (e.g., hospital construction, diagnostic testing, drugs). Analysis of data for the US shows relatively long average lags, with peak response to shifts in GDP coming after 4 years. Regressions for total national health expenditures (NHE) and various categories of spending are shown in Table 4.

Table 4. *Regression*: Growth in real health expenditures (%) US 1960–2009

		Real per capita GDP growth						*Deflator*			
	Constant	Year 0	Year 1	Year 2	Year 3	Year 4	Year 5	Year 0	Year 1	Time	R^2
US – Total NHE	0.046	**0.17**	**0.07**	**0.04**	**0.19**	**0.29**	**0.23**	*−0.28*	*−0.12*	−0.0006	**0.702**
Hospital	0.068	**−0.17**	**0.06**	**0.06**	**0.14**	**0.39**	**0.24**	*−0.15*	*0.25*	−0.0011	**0.705**
Physician	0.044	**0.03**	**0.36**	**0.14**	**0.13**	**0.37**	**0.03**	*−0.52*	*−0.69*	−0.0006	**0.312**
Dental	0.009	**0.36**	**0.16**	**0.22**	**0.18**	**0.22**	**0.32**	*−0.41*	*0.07*	−0.0002	**0.311**
Pharmaceutical	−0.071	**0.73**	**0.34**	**0.70**	**0.71**	**0.09**	**0.15**	*−1.04*	*−0.95*	0.0016	**0.457**
LTC	0.058	**0.22**	**0.65**	**0.45**	**0.18**	**0.54**	**0.35**	*−0.67*	*0.03*	−0.0013	**0.662**
Insurance Admin	0.064	**0.17**	**0.44**	**0.26**	**0.34**	**0.57**	**0.49**	*−0.57*	*0.12*	−0.0013	**0.470**
OOP	−0.006	**0.43**	**0.26**	**0.13**	**0.11**	**0.26**	**0.00**	*−0.57*	*−0.53*	−0.0001	**0.245**

Source: www.cms.gov/nationalhealthexpenddata 22 May 2011.

ARIMA (autoregressive integrated moving average) analysis confirms most of these results, but even 50 years is an insufficient number of observations to provide much certainty about the standard error of the coefficients. Aggregation provides data with an "average lag" that is a composite of many different processes of varying lengths. Most of the residual, however, is white noise, so that smoothed long-run graphs (i.e., observation frequencies of 6 to 10 years or more with repeated observations) yield a good representation of the underlying trends. Most of the random annual errors and business cycle effects can be filtered out by comparing health expenditures to a "smoothed" version of real per capita income (6-year moving average (MA) for GDP, 3-year MA for deflator) as shown in Figures 6a and 6b.

Once fluctuations due to business cycles and random errors have been filtered out and spending is smoothed with a 10- or 20-year moving average, the underlying "excess growth" trend that has been raising the health sector's share of GDP becomes more clearly visible. The annual percentage growth rate of per capita income in the US, although variable (SD = 2.1%), appears to be stationary and integrated of order 1.[4] Indeed, despite two world wars and a great depression, real per capita growth in each 20-year period throughout the entire 20th century stayed close to 2%. Most other countries in the OECD since 1960 show similar stationarity. However, national health spending is not integrated to the same degree but trends downward, and thus would appear to require further differencing in order to become stationary. This poses a number of econometric problems. Is it appropriate to measure variability relative to a simple mean, (4.5%), or should it be relative to a trend-line stretching down from 7% to 2%? How many times should the health series be differenced in order to become stationary for an ARIMA analysis? Can the two series be treated as co-integrated? Decomposition clarifies and resolves a number of these problems. It indicates that excess growth has slowed dramatically from 1970 to 1990. However, that slowing itself poses additional questions, questions that cannot be answered until the span of observation is expanded beyond 50 years.

Long-Run Trends and Growth Surges

Estimates of health expenditures prior to 1960 become increasingly irregular the farther back one goes. Edouard Ducpetiax, William Playfair, and others carried out small surveys of household consumption in Europe during the 19th century (Stigler, 1954). In the US, Carroll Wright carried out massive surveys of household spending among thousands of industrial workers in Massachusetts, and subsequently in several other states, between 1880 and 1910. These and the reports published by the International Labor Organization (ILO) on France, Germany, Norway, Sweden, and the UK yield results indicative of health spending in the range of 2%–5% of total

[4]That is, the percentage growth rate does not itself trend up or down or display regular patterns of variability, more or less stable with a random walk around the mean of 2.1% per year.

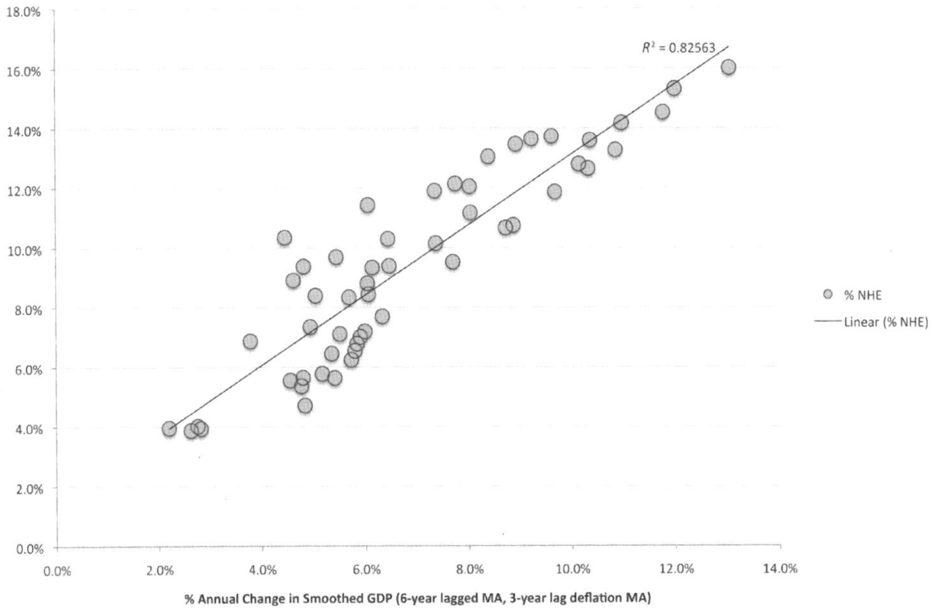

Figure 6a. Growth in US NHE and smoothed GDP (regression scatterplot 1960–2012)

Source: OACT (2014) National Health Expenditures and author calculations (Getzen, 2014).

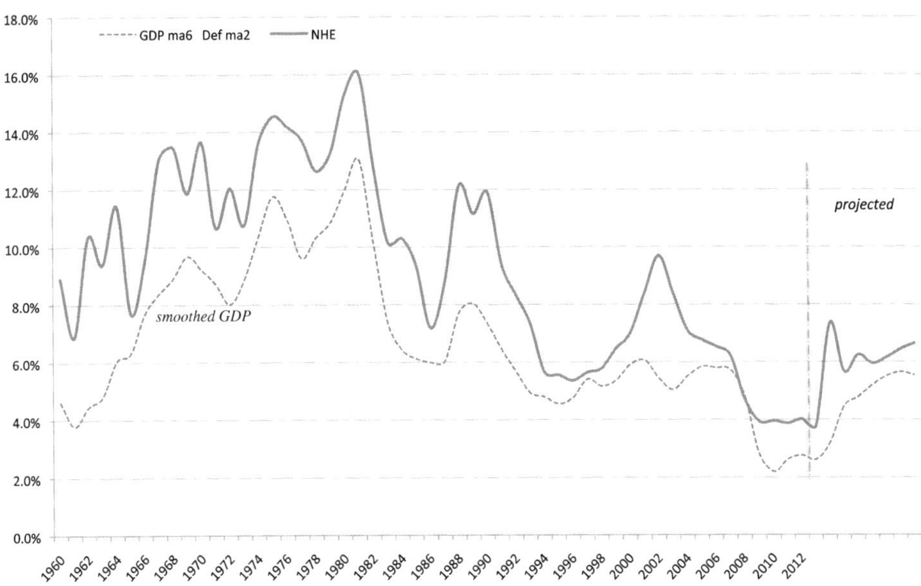

Figure 6b. Growth in US NHE and GDP (smoothed): Time series graph 1960–2012

Source: OACT (2014) National Health Expenditures and author calculations (Getzen, 2014).

household consumption. The frequently cited estimates of the Committee on the Costs of Medical Care (CCMC) of 3.7% of GDP in 1929 fall within this range, as does an earlier estimate by Louis Dublin, an insurance executive who wrote and lectured extensively about health economics during the 1920s (see Footnote 1).

Alternate estimates for growth of the health sector can be obtained from the production side, measuring health labor relative to total employment. Data from the decennial census in the US indicates that health occupations accounted for 11% of total labor in 2010 compared to the 18% of GDP accounted for by health spending (Table 5). The ratio of spending share to labor share is greater than one (1.7:1) because the earnings of health workers are above average. This ratio was similar in 1960. Since the ratio has been relatively stable, between 1.7:1 and 2.0:1 during each of the last 6 decennial census years, extrapolation back to early census years may not be unreasonable. In 1930, health labor was 1.8% of GDP and expenditures 3.5%. In 1900, health labor was of the 1.2% of GDP, and in 1850, it was 0.9%. There were about 12 ancillary workers for every physician in 2010, compared to only 7 in 1960 and less than 1 prior to 1900. Since ancillaries earn less than physicians, the relative shares of expenditure:labor used for extrapolations to the 19th century should be higher, perhaps 2 or 3:1. In 1850, there were

Table 5. Decennial employment and expenditures, 1850–2010

									Growth Rate	
				Physicians Per million		**Ancillaries Per Physician**	**Health % of Labor**	**GDP**	***Labor Share (in %)***	***GDP Share (in %)***
	Population	**Employees**	**Health**							
1850	23,192	5,372	**46**	41	*176*	*1.1*	**0.8**	—	—	—
1860*	31,443	8,595	**61**	55	*175*	*1.1*	**0.7**	—	***−1.8***	—
1870	39,818	12,925	**103**	64	*162*	*1.6*	**0.8**	—	***1.2***	—
1880	50,156	17,392	**114**	86	*171*	*1.3*	**0.7**	—	***−1.9***	—
1890	62,948	23,318	**170**	105	*166*	*1.6*	**0.7**	—	***1.1***	—
1900	75,995	29,073	**346**	131	*173*	*2.6*	**1.2**	—	***5.0***	—
1910	91,972	37,371	**486**	152	*166*	*3.2*	**1.3**	—	***0.9***	—
1920	105,711	42,434	**634**	151	*143*	*4.2*	**1.5**	—	***1.4***	—
1930*	122,775	48,830	**900**	163	*133*	*5.5*	**1.8**	3.5	***2.1***	—
1940	131,669	51,742	**1,020**	175	*133*	*5.8*	**2.0**	3.9	***0.7***	*1.1*
1950	150,697	59,230	**1,450**	198	*131*	*7.3*	**2.4**	4.3	***2.2***	*0.9*
1960	180,671	67,990	**2,064**	234	*129*	*8.8*	**3.0**	5.2	***2.2***	*1.8*
1970	205,052	79,802	**3,277**	297	*145*	*11.0*	**4.1**	7.2	***3.1***	*3.4*
1980	227,726	104,058	**5,403**	433	*190*	*12.5*	**5.2**	9.2	***2.4***	*2.4*
1990	250,132	123,473	**7,580**	587	*235*	*12.9*	**6.1**	12.5	***1.7***	*3.1*
2000	282,172	131,720	**10,103**	772	*274*	*13.1*	**7.7**	13.8	***2.3***	*1.0*
2010*	310,233	130,275	**13,777**	935	*301*	*14.7*	**10.6**	17.9	***3.3***	*2.6*

Source: US Bureau of the Census, Historical Statistics of the United States: Colonial times to 970 (1975); Bureau of Labor Statistics, annual employment data tables. Employment and population stated as millions of persons.
Notes: *1860 total civilian employment extrapolated.

about 18 physicians for every 10,000 population, a physician:population ratio that stayed almost constant before falling to just 13 in 1930, although these physician were more educated and by then assisted by more than three nurses and other ancillary workers apiece. The physician:population ratio did not begin to rise significantly until 1970, but then grew rapidly, almost doubling over the next 30 years. Although extrapolating from sparse occupational data to estimate national health expenditures is a stretch, it is not unreasonable to consider that, since the health share of employment did not increase between 1850 and 1890, the health share of GDP probably also grew very little during that period. There clearly was growth from 1900 to 1929 (when the first verifiable estimate of 3.5% of GDP was made) since, even though physician supply grew slightly less than population, the number of ancillaries per physicians increased from just 1 to more than 3.

In what may have been the first modern study of the national health expenditure trends, J.R. Seale, a physician and travelling fellow from Oxford studying at Harvard, examined US government and private data for the period 1929–1956. In *The Lancet*, he observed that ***"the proportion of the gross national product devoted to medical care tends to remain constant"*** (emphasis in the original). He went on to add that it "rises during national economic depressions and it falls during wars. A persistent rise in real per capita gross national product will tend to result in a very gradual increase in the proportion (Seale, 1959) (Figure 7)." Like Malthus,[5] Seale had the misfortune of making a generalization just before a major change that reshaped economic behavior occurred: 20 years later, rising costs were being deemed a "crisis" and "unsustainable" in most OECD countries (Getzen, 2013; Hanes and Prescott, 2002).

Estimates for the years before 1960 are spotty and less consistent, yet they allow two empirical generalizations to be stated with some confidence: Health expenditures were lower before 1950 than afterward, and were rising much more slowly. Spending relative to per capita income rose slowly if at all in most countries during many of ten prior decades (Getzen, 2014).

The Surge in Health Spending: 1960–2006

In 1960, the average expenditure share of GDP among developed countries was near 4%. Those at the higher end (the US at 5.1%, Germany at 5.2%, and Canada

[5] Thomas Malthus' 1798 classic *Essay on the Principle of Population* led to the term "Malthusian" being applied to a subsistence economy where gains in productivity are soon dissipated by "more mouths to feed." Unfortunately, the industrial revolution took hold soon after, as did significant reductions in birth rates, so that increasing economic productivity greatly raised per capita income (and not just population) during the ensuing decades. For a more extended discussion, see the article by Hansen and Prescott (2002) in the *American Economic Review* or Chapter 15 in the Getzen (2013) text.

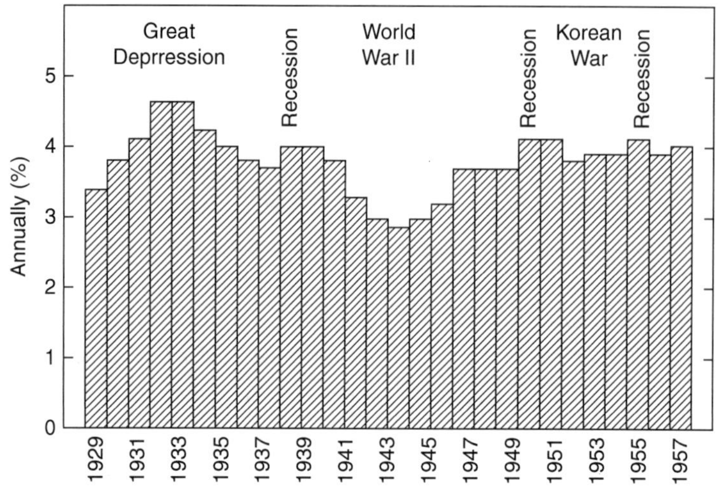

Figure 7. Seale (1959): US health expenditure relative to GDP 1929–1956

at 5.4%) were not very far out of line, nor were those at the lower end (Norway at 2.9%, Iceland and Japan at 3.0%, and Belgium at 3.4%), except for Spain (at 1.5%), which was arguably still emerging as a modern economy. Health shares more than doubled for almost all of these countries before the end of the century, implying excess growth rates on the order of GDP+2% or more. Something had changed to radically accelerate spending by 1960.

In 1850, the share of household consumption among early industrial workers devoted to health was more than 2%. A century later it had grown, but still accounted for only about 4% of earnings. Since the share had not yet doubled during this span of 100 years, the average rate of excess growth was less than 1% annually, and was probably more on the order of 0.25–2.5%. Rapidly rising per capita incomes pushed medical spending to rise rapidly as well, but not nearly as rapidly as they did in the decades after 1960.

Since the global recession began in 2007, the health share of GDP has risen very little in most countries, and clearly fell during 2010 (Morgan and Astolfi, 2014) (Figure 8). Whether or not the recent slowdown marks the end of a 50-year surge in spending is still unclear. What is clear from the data is that most countries experience a period of rapid expansion in the health sector once economic development passes a certain point, and that the rate of excess growth, after surging to GDP+3% or GDP+5%, begins to moderate in the following decades, falling to GDP+1% or lower.

The path of growth in Spain provides an illuminating example, albeit somewhat extreme. Starting from a low base in 1960, the health share more than doubled

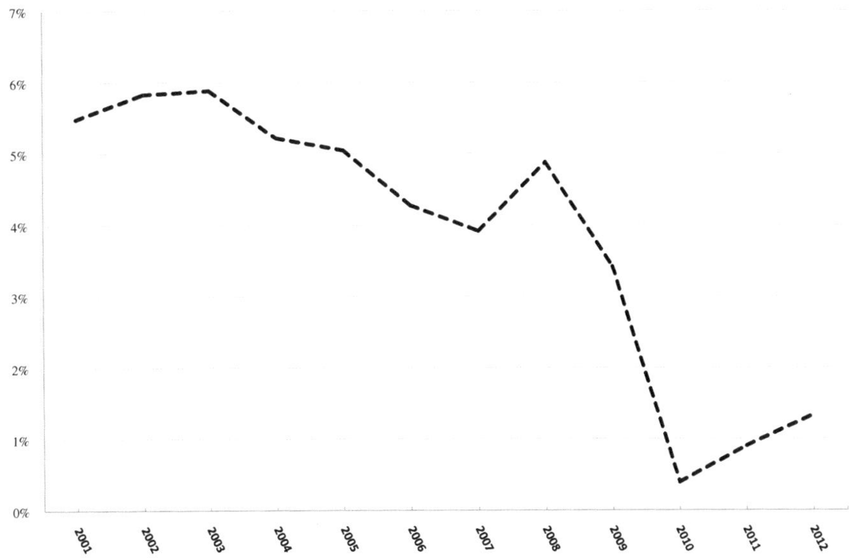

Figure 8. OECD Health Expenditure Growth Rates 2000–2010

Source: OECD Health Data 2014 and author calculations.

within the next 10 years. Although still below the OECD average, it continued to grow more rapidly, doubling again over the next 30 years. By 2010, the differential between Spain and the OECD average was less than 1% of GDP (9.6% for Spain vs. 10.5% OECD average). Although the path of health expenditures in Spain and among the other developed countries over the next 30 years is still unclear, projections of future excess growth of GDP+0 to 1% are not unreasonable.

Policy Implications. Stepping back from this dense and detailed discussion of historical data, several implications for policymakers become clear. First, economic growth is the main driver of health spending. Second, change occurs only slowly and within the heavily regulated and professionally ossified health sector, so that any shock or sudden shift in GDP or inflation is passed through only slowly. Third, in order to see the effects of prior policies or workforce disruptions, these lagging macroeconomic effects must be filtered out. Otherwise, each year's fluctuation will be over-interpreted as the result of some policy or external cause rather than more appropriately seen as reflecting the turbulent flow and eddies of the macroeconomy. Finally, it should be noted that, however challenging the rise in health care costs since 1960 has been, it clearly has begun to moderate sometime during the past 25 years. The recent, sharp drop in response to the great recession may not mean that expenditures will no longer rise faster than GDP, yet it is likely to be counted as part of a period of very restrained growth.

Forecasting National and Global Health Expenditure Trends

Forecasts of what medical expenditures will be over the next year or two must take account of hundreds or thousands of factors: emerging diseases; new drug launches and patent expirations; insurance regulations; OOP payments; aging, childbirth and other changes in demographic group composition; advances in diagnostic imaging; physician workforce; hospital construction, and so on. There are many commercial and government forecasters in each country diligently striving to make such forecasts using the best available information. A consensus average of the available reports is usually able to predict medical cost growth to within one or 2% for the next 1 or 2 years. However, many of these factors will average out over the next 10 years and are unknown or impossible to predict much farther into the future. Long-run forecasts fruitfully ignore most of the detail that occupies short-run forecasters, concentrating on a few key elements, with the underlying trend in excess health expenditure growth being foremost among them.

Short-, medium- and long-run forecasts use different methods and have different purposes (Getzen, 2000b). Annual budgets and health insurance premiums are set using short-run forecasts, so these estimates are best expressed in nominal currency amounts, as these are the terms in which budgets are cast. Medium-range forecasts of 3 to 10 years are better stated as real inflation-adjusted per capita expenditures to allow for comparisons over time and place, and to indicate the change in resources required to meet expected cost increases. Annual fluctuations over the next 5 or more years are dominated by the business cycles and the delayed adjustment of the health care system to macroeconomic shocks. Most of these cyclical disturbances will pass within a decade and hence can be ignored for forecasts extending beyond that span. Long-run forecasts of 20–75 years are mostly used for projecting government obligations and retiree health liabilities. Nominal dollar statements are almost useless. (What would it mean to say that Germany will spend 34.27 trillion deutschmarks in 2050? How much inflation will there be before a child born today will retire?) Such forecasts are much better expressed as a share of GDP or as a percentage of wages.

Expressing long-run projections as percentage growth in share, or equivalently as *excess growth* of GDP+x%, focuses attention specifically on *health spending* rather than general inflation or wage increases. Statements regarding amounts spent, even real per capita amounts, confound the health forecast with the GDP forecast. They give little insight into whether the burden of payment for care will be larger or smaller relative to the ability to pay, and it is this fiscal gap that is the major concern of policymakers — not the nominal amount or per capita insurance premiums. It is growth in the health share that should be the target of health forecasters — not inflation or per capita income, which are better left to macroeconomic forecasters.

The literature on long-run health forecasts is fairly thin, especially when compared to the voluminous literature assessing macroeconomic forecasts (Getzen 1992b). The only regular sources of forecasts are national statistical agencies, the OECD, the World Bank, and WHO. Even these sources tend to make their forecasts available at irregular intervals and use different boundaries, definitions and methodologies so that results are hard to compare over time, and almost never go back after the fact to assess the accuracy of forecasts made in prior years. Evaluating a single forecast made by an independent researcher at one point in time and never followed up is even more difficult and less valuable. For the most part, healthcare forecasting models have only been evaluated with respect to old data already recorded before the forecast was made. Such backcasting exercises are of limited use in assessing future results.

Accuracy

Any single forecast can happen to be almost correct, or not, by chance. Assessment of accuracy requires a series of forecasts that are published in advance and then compared to sequent outcomes. Macroeconomic forecasts start with a basic standard: The "naïve" forecast that the level (or growth) this period will be the same as it was last period. The results of the forecast made by the model are then compared, after the fact, to a naïve forecast. Other common standards for comparison are a moving average over the past Y years, an exponential smooth, or an average of published forecasts. It is surprisingly hard for experts to consistently improve on a naïve forecast. The number of professionals outmatching common formulas that can be programmed into a spreadsheet is, of course, even smaller. Expert judgment rarely beats a technical forecast made carefully by fitting a very simple model onto prior data.

One of the few studies comparing prospective forecasts to actual spending data was done by the US Office of the Actuary to examine the predictive performance of their projections for 1997 to 2009. They found that they tended to overestimate the rate of spending growth, with an accuracy of about ±1% each year. However, it is possible that positive and negative errors might offset each other. To assess long-run trend accuracy, it is necessary to measure the cumulative growth over a longer time span and compare forecast to actual. Getzen later examined all of the Medicare Office of Actuary (OACT) projections from 1986 to 2002 at 1-, 2-, 5-, and 10-year spans, finding that cumulative annualized errors were about 1% (e.g., 10.46% over 10 years) (Getzen, 2015).

The shorter-term ups and downs of employment, inflation and stock indexes are often of greater interest to market analysts than the long-run trend, making mean absolute percentage error (MAPE) a preferred measure of accuracy in most market applications. However, the issues are rather different in national health expenditure forecasting. Actuaries making 10- or 20-year budget projections are more concerned with getting the long-run trend right than with the ups and downs of monthly or yearly fluctuations, making cumulative error a more relevant measure of accuracy.

Once cyclical macroeconomic fluctuations are filtered out by using moving averages to smooth inflation and real GDP growth, there is very little additional information that can be added to improve a forecast of the excess health spending growth trend over time. Although we know that there will be technological advances, we do not know exactly what they will be, how long it will take to implement them, or how much they will influence spending. In effect, there are just part of the trend. The same limitations apply to future changes in obesity, infectious disease incidence, disability, mortality or a host of other factors. What is required for long-run national health expenditure forecasts are data series long enough to show how the rate of share growth has surged and subsided over time, such as that provided in Figure 9 for the US. Excess growth was around 1% above GDP for several decades before 1955, probably back into the 19th century. Sometime after 1955, excess growth accelerated, surging above +4% during the late 1960's. Recessions and a variety of administrative efforts slowly reduced excess growth down toward GDP+0%, eventually holding health spending steady at 13.5% of GDP from 1993 to 2000. Renewed growth took the health share above 17% by 2010, when the great recession and new administrative control again restrained growth. Projections by the OACT, Congressional Budget Office, and the Society of

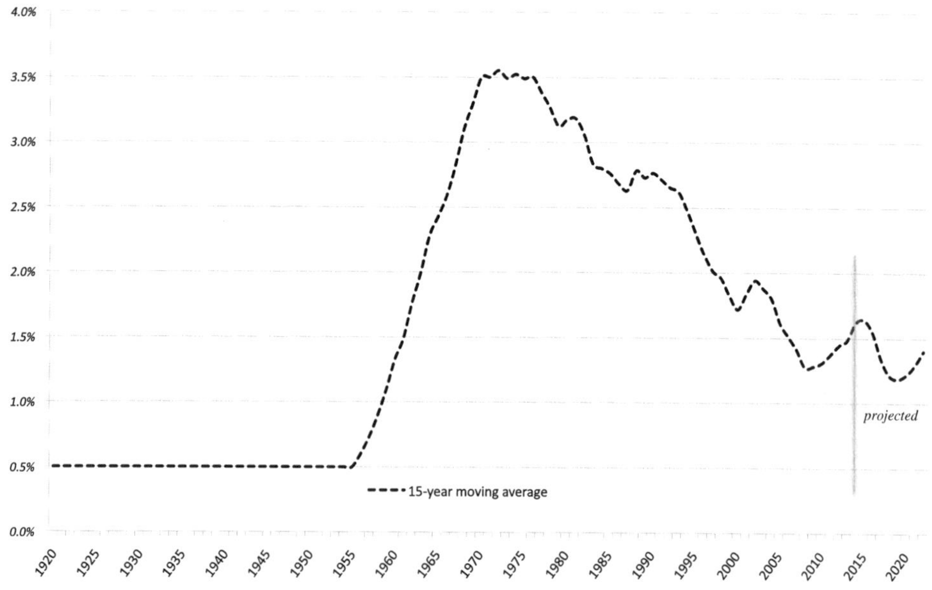

Figure 9. Excess medical cost growth rate in the US 1930–2020 (smoothed)

Sources: OACT 2014, Historical statistics of the US 2006, and author calculations.

Actuaries are consistent, forecasting long-run future excess growth of 0.5%–1.5% for the US. The OECD health data and current projections for many nations look similar but with smaller surges consistent with their current health shares, closer to 10%. Additional cliometric effort is needed to extend the data series for most countries back into the decades prior to 1960.

Focusing on the excess growth rate that pushes the health share upward, and removing monthly and annual fluctuations, makes the task of forecasting vastly easier, effectively narrowing it to a single parameter. *Health expenditures are projected to increase at a rate of GDP+*x*%, and the share of the economy consumed in the health sector will rise from its current level by* x*% a year.* The task is made computationally simple, yet still subject to residual uncertainty. Forecasting research indicates that this level of uncertainty could be the limit for accuracy with current data and methods. Plus or minus 1% is the most that can be said. The range may be narrowed as methods and data improve, yet the persistence of uncertainty in macroeconomic forecasts of monetary supply, exchange rates, inflation, trade, GDP, unemployment and other variables, after decades of diligent efforts by the leading statistical agencies of the world, suggest that further improvements in accuracy may not come easily or quickly.

Policy Implications. The starting point for policymakers is understanding that data on spending must be collected, refined and analyzed to reduce the welter of detail and complexity. Having done so, legislators today must accept that an unsustainable burden of excess cost growth accumulated in prior decades. Rather like overweight patients who continue carbohydrate loading after outgrowing youthful sports, national health systems must now control consumption and work off some organizational fat so that excess is not accumulated again. The task of health policymakers is as simple, and as difficult, as that.

Aging, Health Expenditures and Fiscal Burdens

The difference in phenomena observed at different organizational (micro and macro) and temporal (short and long) scales is well illustrated by comparing individual and population aging. The observation that medical spending increases with a person's age is well known. Yet, just because each individual's medical expenses are increasing does not mean that the average expense per person for the national health system as a whole must increase. Doctors and their patients, who tend to age together, must ignore or reframe their daily experiences in order to see a bigger picture. From a macro perspective, as in Figure 10a, it becomes apparent that there was only a weak correlation between each nation's spending per capita and population age across the OECD in 1975. Figure 10b shows that the rate of increase in the percentage of population above age 65 over the ensuing 25 years was not at all correlated with increases

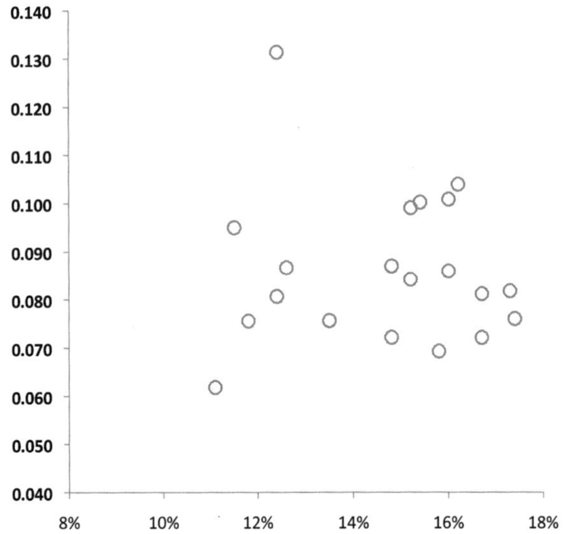

(a)

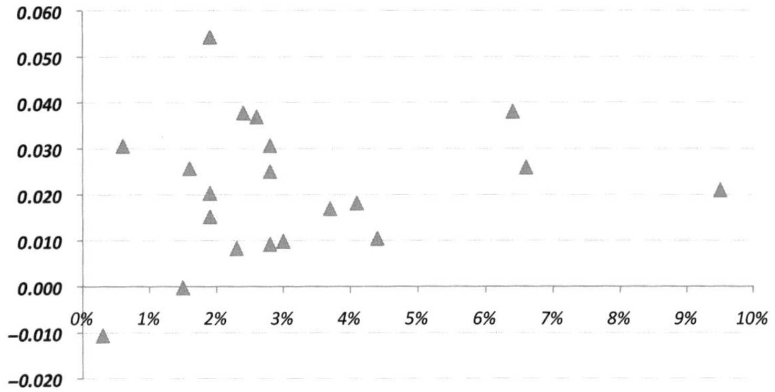

(b)

Figures 10. Population aging correlation with health spending growth

Source: OECD Health Data 2014 and author calculations.

in the health share of GDP. Using "share of GDP" normalizes the data to adjust for exchange rates and the unitary elasticity of incomes and wages, removing several sources of spurious correlation that tend to plague multivariate regressions, especially those that include variables already strongly correlated with income such as education and longevity. The weak correlation at a point in time is mostly secondary rather than causal. More developed countries have more wealth and more old people, and also spend more on medical care. These countries also have higher rates of urbanization, literacy, automobile ownership, and financial services; and lower rates of fertility, infant mortality, civil unrest, and transactions costs.

One reason for the persistence of the idea that aging has caused the rapid rise of health care costs may have been that it was so obviously true at the individual level that "common sense" generalizes that it should also hold for the national average. The atomistic fallacy that what is true for the individual must be true for the group was reinforced by the simultaneous incidence of increasing longevity and increasing costs. They rise together because both are being pushed upward by the same underlying factor (economic development), yet one does not cause the other, or vice-versa, in any simplistic way. The mounting stack of empirical studies showing that most medical cost growth was caused by factors other than population aging, and the lack of cross-national time-varying correlation between national health costs and the age of national populations confirms the hypothesis that they are co-determined rather than causally related. However, even though aging *per se* is not a major cause of the rise in average medical costs, longevity *is* financially burdensome for both households and governments, with increasing medical costs being a major element.

Spending on the Elderly is Not Constant

Medical expenditures on elderly patients have increased rapidly during the 20th century, primarily because spending on patients of all ages has increased rapidly. Even the relative spending on old persons relative to the young is not a constant, but shifting over time, as shown in Table 6.

A different pattern might have emerged in these data from the US without the creation of universal health insurance for those over age 65 and the poor (but not working people), in 1965. The constraints that kept spending below 200% of the mean in the 1950s were already eroding in the early 1960s. After the passage of Medicare and Medicaid, spending on the old quickly soared to 500% of that for the young. Since 1990, the exuberant generosity toward the medical care of the old has dissipated. In 2013, Medicare spending actually declined in both real and nominal dollars, despite the movement of an increasing number of baby boomers into coverage. While unlikely to ever again dip to the miserly levels of the 1950s,

Table 6. US spending per person by age category

	1953	1963	1970	1977	1987	1996	2000	2004	2010
All persons*	$69	143	291	616	1,664	3,153	3,803	5,276	7,097
Under age 65*	$65	127	234	452	1,088	2,115	2,650	3,953	5,392
Age 65 and older*	$109	299	809	1,962	5,830	10,285	11,778	14,797	18,425
**in nominal dollars*									
Ratio: Over age 65/ under age 65	**1.7**	**2.4**	**3.5**	**4.3**	**5.4**	**4.9**	**4.4**	**3.7**	**3.4**

Sources: Cutler and Meara (1997); Meara *et al* (2004); Hartman *et al.* (2008); Getzen (2013, Chapter 10); Lassman (2014).

the ratio of spending for medical care among those over age 65 is likely to hover closer to 3 times that of the young rather than the 1987 peak of 5.4 times. Other OECD countries usually have ratios in the range of 2.5–4.5, but much work still remains to trace how the path of the old:young spending ratio has evolved over time in each country.

Policy Implications. Any forecast of future health spending for the elderly depends heavily on two distributional parameters: (1) What share of total economic resources should be spent on health (*health share of GDP*) and (2) how much more should be spent on the care for the elderly relative to the young (old:young spending ratio). Both are determined primarily by politics and social choice rather than demographics or biology. The most important conclusion from the empirical studies reviewed above is that spending on medical care for the elderly is not driven by illness, but by policies, even if many of those policies are embedded in administrative decisions and not publicly articulated, since coming out in favor of cutting benefits to the old, or the young, is generally viewed as self-destructive behavior by politicians — however, having physicians and health services managers make decisions that stay within a fixed budget is not. A corollary is that innovation in medical technology is a result of increased spending, as well as a cause of increased spending. There is reflexive feedback between health policy and expenditures: A rise (or fall) in spending will create pressure for a change in health policy, and any significant change in health policy will tend to force expenditure growth up (or down). Health policy and health spending must always be considered interdependent and endogenous to a greater or lesser degree.

Population aging gathered a great deal of attention during the 1960s and 1970s and was often blamed for the sudden rise in national health spending. At the time, life expectancy and medical costs were both growing rapidly, and it seemed natural to assume that the relationship was causal. "Demographic" models were constructed that projected future health expenditures using a linear matrix that mimicked the format used for projections of future pension payouts (the "c" are "age–sex" "categories" or "age–sex–disease/disability" categories if more detail is desired).

$$\text{Total Cost} = \sum \text{cost}_c \times \text{pop}_c \times (\text{Total Population Growth} \times \text{Other Cost Growth}).$$

Projections made with such demographic/disease models worked very well in forecasting medical costs for a particular group of insured persons for the next year or two, but failed when extended to aggregate national cost trends over 5, 10 or 50 years. Among the first analyses of total cost trends and population aging was that carried out by Barer and Evans for British Columbia in the late 1980s (Barer *et al.*, 1989). They found that demographic/disease changes for persons age 65+ accounted for only a small fraction of overall aggregate health spending increases, and were overwhelmed by underlying medical costs increases (increases in price and utilization driven by income and policy, not attributable to increased illness or disability). The finding that most medical cost increases were driven by factors other than aging was confirmed repeatedly in many subsequent studies (Getzen, 1992a; Gerdtham *et al.*, 1992; Steinman *et al.*, 2007; Zweifel *et al.*, 2004). Why then was the erroneous perception that aging caused cost increases so persistent? Because it made sense based on the immediate experience of both patients and physicians, and because the two trends came to prominence at the same time. The temporal association was not coincidental, as both increased longevity and increased medical costs were being driven by the same force: The rapid modern development of post-industrial economies after World War II. This coincidence, while not in itself indicative of causality, does point to the underlying cause.

Global Health Spending Patterns 1850–1955 and 1960–2075

The discussion in this final section centers on how and why health spending rose so rapidly after 1950, after having been steady or only slowly rising for many previous decades, and what the pattern of growth is likely to be from now until 2075. Prior to 1850, medical care was not very scientific or useful. The most common therapeutic intervention in Western medicine during the 19th century was the use of a lancet to open a vein, even though it soon became common knowledge among physicians that bleeding did little to cure diseases. Medical care was often limited to sage advice, the laying on of hands, and attempts at prognosis. Healing usually occurred because most people naturally got better as they were fed and rested. Expenditures rose as per capita incomes rose, but there was little excess growth because there was little extra benefit.

The leading centers of medical science and pharmaceutical innovation were in Europe. Rapid advances were made in the fields of bacteriology, pathology and diagnostic testing. Germany excelled in the production of chemicals and drugs, and in 1883 had created the first broad national health insurance program. Collective financing elsewhere was mostly limited to charity, guilds and friendly societies. The practice of medicine took time to catch up to the new scientific advances, and was little changed in the first decades of the new century. Medical nihilism was still prevalent among practitioners and there was little reason for patients to choose and pay for a university-educated physician over an herbalist, homeopath, mystic, or Christian Science reader.

By the 1920s, the practice, organization, and financing of medicine had begun to undergo a virtual revolution, incorporating science into a number of new and effective treatments. By 1960, research was carried out in huge academic medical centers and pharmaceutical companies on a scale that just 50 years earlier had been unknown, and indeed unthinkable. The developments over this span are ably reviewed in Robert Fogel's (2004) *The Escape from Hunger and Premature Death, 1700–2100*, Roy Porter's *The Greatest Benefit to Mankind (1999),* and the edited volume on *The Therapeutic Revolution* by Morris Vogel and Charles Rosenberg (1979).

In 1960, the year the OECD health dataset begins, expenditures across the developed countries averaged about 4% of GDP, little different from the estimated level of medical spending relative to incomes of industrial workers or the urban middle and upper classes in 1850 or 1920 (although rural farmers still relied mostly on home remedies and spent little on professional care back then). Antibiotics and advanced surgical techniques had brought about a medical revolution, but costs had not yet exploded. The US became the world's largest economy, and medical leadership had followed riches to reside in Boston, Baltimore, Chicago, New York, and San Francisco. However, it was the European countries that first established truly national health financing systems that paid for health care for all (or almost all) citizens. The surge in spending that started around 1960 was led by the US, and spending grew most rapidly in that country for the next 50 years, eventually exceeding 15% of GDP and still headed higher. Expenditures also rose in almost every wealthy developed country, sometimes later and more slowly, but most approached 10% by 2015.

Amongst this wealth of detail and statistics, a common pattern can be discerned. Medicine underwent a transformation akin to the demographic transition and industrial revolution. Massive population growth began during the 18th century for many of the OECD countries, while urbanization and the industrial revolution came afterward and significant growth in per capita incomes for the masses usually only arrived in the late 19th century. It is not yet clear why it took a century more for the transformation of health care. Perhaps sudden premature mortality had to fall and incomes rise to make-to-make ameliorating disease and lengthening lifespan worthwhile, or the congregation of people into larger cities sufficient to generate knowledge, or enough wealth accumulated to fund research that took decades to yield practical results. Whatever the cause, it is clear that developmental transformation of the health sector came after many decades after the advances in population, agriculture and trade.

Some trends for the next hundred years are already evident. The rise in population due to demographic transition has already ended in many developed countries, and appears be slowing across the globe. The health sector has already climbed above 4% in South Korea, Brazil, Eastern Europe, and Turkey as middle class consumption swells. Europe was the dominant medical market in the 19th century, and the US in the 20th century, but by the end of the 21st century, both India and China will each have health expenditures larger than Europe or the US.

Development, not disease, drives spending on health. Yet while the trends in longevity may be fairly clear, and some aspects of disability tentatively projected, the scope and magnitude of development over the next century and any possible future transitions (or stagnations or reversals) is cloudy. Will advances in technology lengthen lifespan and rectangularize morbidity and mortality to such an extent that curative medicine is cheap or irrelevant? Will industrial technology advance to yield nearly infinite clean energy so that cost is no longer a concern to policymakers and possessions no longer accepted as measures of development? More prosaically, will the surge in costs that followed the medical revolution eventually subside like the population surge of the demographic transition, bringing an end to excess health cost growth?

Two major economic uncertainties — income distribution and productivity growth — may have significant influence over the future path of income growth. Broad national financing of medicine has pulled the spending of all citizens within each country up toward the levels of a favored urban and industrial minority and hence raised the level of expenditure as a share of GDP. It may not be coincidental that the "middle classing" of an economy has often coincided with the transformation of medical practice and financing. Political support for broadly equal health financing is placed under strain as poor or median households, who gain from distributive equity, fall farther and farther behind the income groups at the top 10% or 1%. Less developed countries often have great disparities, with a few at the top obtaining world-class medical care while the masses crowd into under-staffed clinics. In the US, the Medicaid program for the poor often uses restricted provider networks that serve relatively few middle-class or wealthy patients. Even in Norway, eminently wealthy and egalitarian, top earners tend to buy preferential access. Increasing inequalities of income and wealth since 1980 have already put stress on the financing systems for health care in almost every developed country. Extreme inequality could fragment a health system into disparate tiers, with those at the bottom having only limited access to the most modern medicine.

Conflict over income inequality will be exacerbated if the long-run trend of per capita income growth starts to slow or stagnate. The ability of modern economies to maintain 2% to 3% annual productivity increases as they did in the 20th century has recently come into question (Gordon, 2014). Catch-up growth will keep emerging economies well above that rate, but may do little for the citizens of developed countries that may already be entering a more mature and slower stage of growth. Furthermore, barring catastrophic interruption of current trends, almost every country in the world is likely to have achieved development by the end of the 21st century.

Since, historically, the rate of excess health cost growth among developed nations usually surged to GDP+3% or more before decelerating to +1% or less over the next 20 to 50 years, it is likely that the emerging economies will follow this pattern, but do so more rapidly. Eventually, all countries will reach a higher plateau with a constant health share (sustainable growth near GDP+0% or less). Whether that will take a few decades or a few centuries is an open question (i.e., it could reach that plateau after the health share grows to 20%, or not until it approaches 50% of GDP). Some factors suggesting higher growth are the increasing value of life and health relative to other goods and services as per capita incomes surpass 10 times or 100 times subsistence levels. With a lifespan of 120 years, even middle-aged workers have many years to save for retirement and the long-term care that is the greatest financial risk toward the end of life. On the other hand, technological advances continually commodify medicine. Treatments and vaccines for tuberculosis have become cheap, and soon hepatitis, HIV/AIDS will experience similar price reductions. Patent expirations have already slowed the growth of pharmaceutical spending. Robotic surgery may do the same for that field. Since both upward and downward forces are likely, the path of expenditure growth may well depend on the relative balance.

Policy Implications. The most important insight to be gained is the ability to see the "medical transformation" and surge of health financing as a developmental stage, like the demographic transition or the industrial revolution. It was successful, wildly so, far beyond the expectations of the public or politicians. Dealing with success, and costs, of this magnitude is hard. No one in 1960 anticipated today's pension crises or the need for housing for millions of disabled elders. Other policy lessons are more prosaic. Periodic measurement of costs can help a nation maintain a sustainable level of medical costs, but analysts should not fail to adjust for lags or pay too much attention to temporary fluctuations lest they be distracted by all the noise. Medical technology will undergo major advances, yet since we do not know what they are or the magnitude of their financial effects, a long-run forecast incorporates technological growth in the underlying secular trend. The effects of legislation and organizational reforms are similarly endogenous.

Changes in trend are more apt to result from invisible shifts in administrative procedures and political will than public rhetoric or votes in Parliament. Microsimulation models using age/sex/disease projections are necessary to estimate the presumptive budgetary impact of policy proposals but are rarely as accurate at forecasting actual growth rates as the macro models that usually ignore the particularities of legislation and technology. Despite that, it is helpful to consider the mounting evidence that all health costs, and especially costs of the elderly relative to the mean, are determined by the political process that shapes the health care system of each nation, and not by demography or disease.

References

Abel-Smith B. 1963. *Paying for Health Services*. WHO Public Health Papers No. 17, World Health Organization: Geneva.

Abel-Smith B. 1967. *An International Study of Health Expenditure*. WHO Public Health Papers No. 32, World Health Organization: Geneva.

Abel-Smith B, Titmuss R. (Guillebaud Report) 1956. *The Cost of the National Health Service in England and Wales*. Cambridge University Press: Cambridge.

Barer M, Pulchins I, Evans R, Hertzman C, Lomas J, Anderson G. 1989. Trends in the use of medical services by the elderly in British Columbia. *Canadian Medical Association Journal* 141: 39–45.

Bureau of Labor Statistics (BLS). Employment, Hours and Earnings — National, www.bls.gov (10 December 2014).

Committee on the Costs of Medical Care. 1932. *Medical Care for the American People* (26 Volumes). University of Chicago Press: Chicago.

Cutler, David and Ellen Meara. 1997. The Medical Costs of the Young and Old: A Forty-Year Perspective. *NBER Working Paper* #6114. Accessed at www.NBER.org.

Dublin LI. 1928. *Health and Wealth, a Survey of the Economics of World Health*. Harper: New York.

Fogel R. 2004. *The Escape from Hunger and Premature Death, 1700–2100: Europe, America and the Third World*. Cambridge University Press: Cambridge.

Friedman M. 1957. *A Theory of the Consumption Function*. University of Chicago Press: Chicago.

Gerdtham U, Sogaard J, Andersson F, Jonsson B. 1992. An econometric analysis of health care expenditure: A cross section study of the OECD countries. *Journal of Health Economics* 11(1): 63–84.

Getzen T. 1990. Macro forecasting of national health expenditures. In Rossiter L, Scheffler R (eds.). *Advances in Health Economics and Health Services Research* 11: 27–48.

Getzen T. 1992a. Population aging and the growth of health expenditures. *Journal of Gerontology: Social Sciences* 47(3): S98–S104, 1992.30

Getzen T. 1992b. International health spending forecasts: Concepts and evaluation. *Social Science & Medicine* 34(9): 1057–1068.

Getzen T. 2000a. Health care is an individual necessity and a national luxury: Applying multilevel decision models to analysis of health care expenditures. *Journal of Health Economics* 19: 259–270.

Getzen T. 2000b. Forecasting health expenditures: Short, medium and long (long) term. *Journal of Health Care Finance* 26: 56–72.

Getzen T. 2006. Aggregation and the measurement of health care costs. *HSR: Health Services Research* 41(5): 1938–1954.

Getzen T. 2013. *Health Economics and Financing*, 5th edn. New York: Wiley: New York.

Getzen T. 2014. Macroeconomic dynamics of health: Lags and variability in mortality, employment and spending. In Culyer AJ (ed.). *Encyclopedia of Health Economics* (2): 165–176. Elsevier: San Diego.

Getzen T. 2015. Accuracy of long-run actuarial projections of medical costs. *Working Paper* #2213648. www.ssrn.com (2 January 2015).

Gordon R. 2014. The Demise of U.S. Economic Growth. *NBER Working Paper* #19895.

Hansen G, Prescott E. 2002. Malthus to Solow. *American Economic Review* 92(4): 1205–1217.

Hartman, M, *et al.* 2008. US health spending by age, selected years through 2004. *Health Affairs* 27(1): w1–w12.

Historical Statistics of the United States. 2006. In Carter SB *et al.* (eds.). New York, Cambridge University of Press.

Lassman, David *et al.* 2014. US health spending trends by age and gender: Selected years 2002–2010. *Health Affairs* 33(5): 815–822.

Maddison Project. www.ggdc.not/maddison/maddison-project/home.htm [15 November 2014].

Maxwell R. 1981. *Health and Wealth.* Lexington Books: Lexington Mass.

Meara, Ellen, Chapin White and David M. Cutler. 2004. Trends in medical spending by age, 1963–2000. *Health Affairs* 23(4): 176–183.

Morgan D, Astolfi R. 2014. *Health Spending Continues to Stagnate in Many OECD Countries. OECD Health Working Papers* #68. OECD: Paris.

Newhouse J. 1977. Medical care expenditure: A cross-national survey. *Journal of Human Resources* 12: 115–125.

OACT. 2014. NHE Projections. www.cms.gov/Research-Statistics-Data-and-Systems/Statistics-Trends-and-Reports/NationalHealthExpendData/NationalHealthAccounts Projected.html [10 November 2014].

OECD. 1977. *Public Expenditure on Health.* Organisation for Economic Cooperation and Development: Paris.

OECD. 2000. *A System of Health Accounts*, Version 1.0, Paris, 2000.

OECD. 2014. OECD Health Data, downloaded 10 October 2014 from http://www.oecd.org/els/health-systems/health-statistics.htm.

Porter R. 1999. *The Greatest Benefit to Mankind: A Medical History of Humanity.* Norton: New York.

Poullier JP. 1986. Levels and Trends. In Culyer AJ, Jonsson B. (eds.). *Public and Private Health Services.* Blackwell: London, pp. 11–41

Pritchard JB. 1958. *The Ancient Near East.* Princeton University Press: Princeton.

Seale, JR. 1959. A general theory of national expenditure on Medical Care. *The Lancet* 7(102): 555–559, October 10.

Sing M, Banthin J, Selden T, Cowan C, Keehan S. 2006. Reconciling medical expenditure estimates from the MEPS and NHEA. *Health Care Financing Review* 28(1): 25–40.

Steinman L, Telser H, Zweifel P. 2007. Aging and future healthcare expenditure. *Forum for Health Economics & Policy* 10(2).

Stigler GJ. 1954. The early history of empirical studies of consumer behavior. *Journal of Political Economy* 42(2): 95–113.

Vogel M, Rosenberg M. 1979. The Therapeutic Revolution: Essays in the Social History of American Medicine. University Penn Press: Philadelphia.

WHO 2011. *System of Health Accounts (SHA).* www.who.int/health-accounts/methodology/en/ [14 December 2014].

Zweifel P, Felder S, Meier M. 2004. Population ageing and health care expenditure. *Geneva Papers on Risk and Insurance* 29(4): 652–666.

Economics of Financing Health Care

Alexander S. Preker
Columbia University/Health Investment & Financing

Sherry Glied
New York University

Dov Chernichovsky
Ben-Gurion University

Marisa Gil Lapetra
OECD

Good practices in health care financing are an application of useful economic theories, models, and empirical evidence about what does and does not work under different circumstances. It underpins the behavior of patients, doctors, and hospitals, as well as the analytical techniques developed to facilitate resource allocation decisions related to health care. This chapter explores the underlying economic principles of financing health care. We cover the importance of understanding the economics behind health care financing; the global health care spending structure; economic variations in health care financing at the national level; the origins of third-party payments in health care; the economics of health insurance and government interventions; and major controversies related to the economics of health care financing. Three illustrative case studies are provided as examples of health care financing principles in the US, Netherlands, and Singapore.

Keywords: Health Insurance; Health Financing; Health Care Funding; Health Care Payment; Universal Health Care; Financial Risk in Health Care.

Introduction

This chapter looks at the economics of financing health care. The chapter distinguishes between the financing of health care — prevention, cure, rehabilitation and palliative or extended care — and the financing of the determinants of better health (Jacobs and Rapoport, 2002). The latter refers to the economic and financial mechanisms that influence economic growth, individual socioeconomic status, education (especially in the case of women during childbearing age and children), nutrition, and investments in health-promoting environmental conditions such as better housing, water, sanitation systems, roads, infrastructure, and a number of other major determinants of good health outcomes.

Both health care and other health determinants influence health outcomes. During the 20th century, the most powerful determinant of health outcomes was a country's wealth in terms of GDP. This correlation appears to be present throughout this 100-year time period, independent of the specific year (World Bank, 1993).

Significant economic growth over the past 20 years throughout the world has translated into significant improvements in health outcomes for billions of people throughout the world. This can be seen by comparing the health status of the global population in 1990 and 2012 (The Lancet Commission on Investing in Health, 2013). See Figure 1.

The major advances that have taken place in the development of knowledge of disease origins, ways to maintain good health, and scientific approaches to prevention (including the intersectoral determinants of illness), treatment, rehabilitation and long-term care have led to remarkable improvements in health status over the past century (Rockefeller Foundation, 2014).

The economics of better health therefore goes well beyond the economics of better health care. The omission of other topics from this chapter should not be an indication that the authors do not consider these topics important, but rather that they are not within our scope and will be dealt with in other chapters of the handbook.

Instead, the chapter focuses on the underlying economic principles of financing health care and provides three illustrative case studies as examples of the application of those principles in the US, Netherlands, and Singapore.

Importance of Understanding the Economics of Health Care Financing

Understanding the economics of health care is important for a number of reasons. First, health is important to both individuals and society, and health care is one (though not the only) way of modifying the incidence and impact of ill health and disease. The availability of health care can determine an individual's quality of life and the prospect for survival. Economic analysis of health care financing offers a unique and systematic intellectual framework for analyzing important issues in health care and for identifying solutions to common problems.

Second, the economics of health care financing is a matter of life and death in that people with serious illness who cannot pay for known and affordable interventions

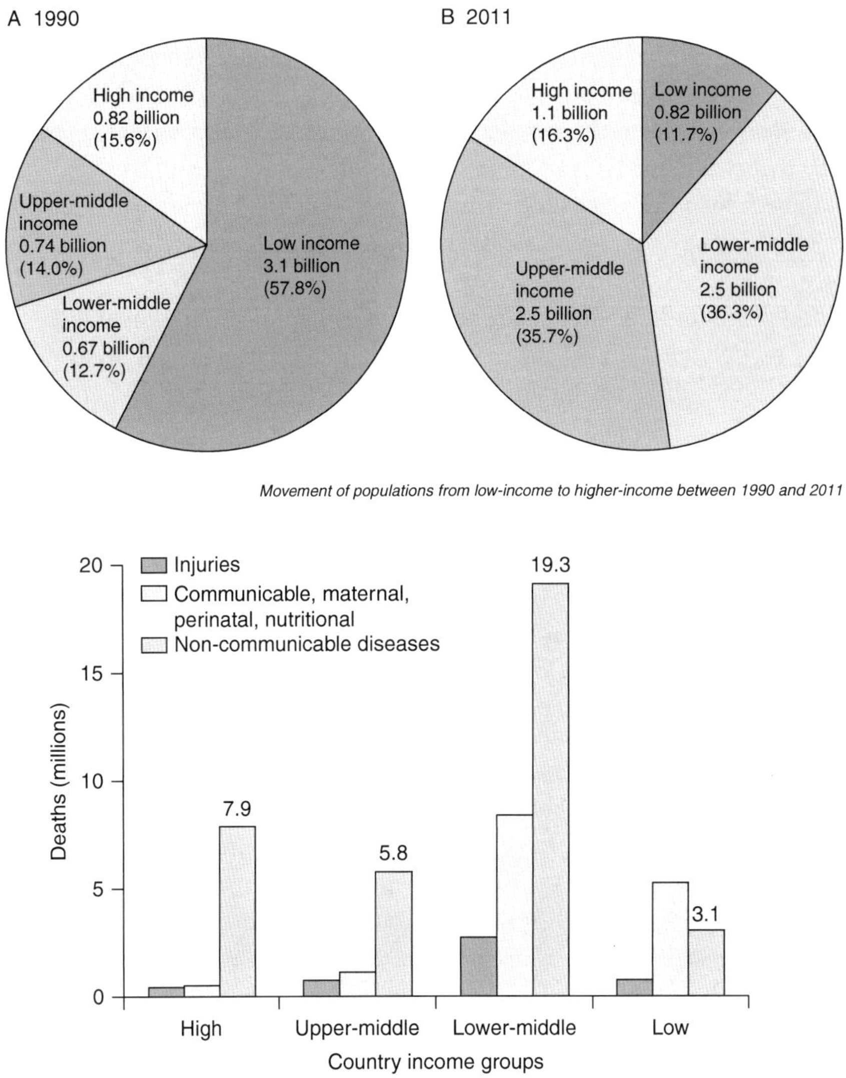

Figure 1. Major shift in disease patterns over past 20 years

Source: Preker — adapted from the Lancet Commission on Investing in Health, 2013.

will simply recover naturally or die. This has been experienced by millions of people and was a main driving force for the recent reforms in the US (Preker *et al.*, 2013).

Third, the health care sector is very large. Health care is a major component of spending, investment, and employment in every developed country; thus, the economic performance of the health care system is crucially linked to the overall economic well-being of a country and its citizens (Reinhardt *et al.*, 2002; 2004; Fuchs, 2005).

Fourth, decisions about how health care is funded, provided, and distributed are strongly influenced by the economic environment and economic constraints. Global, national, and local policy responses to health issues are a central part of how societies deal with their citizens. For those working in health services, familiarity with the theory and methods of the economics of financing health care is essential, both to understand the context of a medical practice, and because evidence on productivity, efficiency, and value for/of money are an increasingly important part of the norm in modern health care systems (Hsiao and Stason, 1979).

Good practices in health care financing are an application of useful economic theories, models, and empirical evidence about what works and what does not work well under different circumstances. It underpins the behavior of patients, doctors, and hospitals, and analytical techniques developed to facilitate resource allocation decisions related to health care. Health financing has evolved into a highly specialized field, drawing on related disciplines including epidemiology, statistics, psychology, sociology, operations research, mathematics, statistics, and actuarial science.

The Structure of Global Spending on Health Care in 2012

In 2012, global GDP was about US$70 trillion, spending on health care was about US$7 trillion, and spending in low- and middle-income countries was about 10% of total spending, or US$770 billion (WHO, 2012).

Regional spending patterns on health care vary greatly across the world (Gottret and Schieber, 2006). Low- and middle-income countries that bear the highest burden of disease still spend the least in both absolute and relative terms on health care. See Figure 2.

In 2012, only some 10% of US$7 trillion was spent in low- and middle-income countries which have the highest burden of disease.

Funding channeled through risk-pooling mechanisms is lowest in low-income countries that often need such protection the most. As much as 80% of total spending in low-income countries is from out-of-pocket payments by consumers of care — the most inequitable type of financing because it hits the poor hardest and denies all individuals the financial protection from catastrophic illness that public and private insurance mechanisms provide. In middle-income countries, the percentage of out-of-pocket spending ranges from 40% to 60%, while the range of out-of-pocket spending in higher-income countries is much lower, at 20 to 40%.

Relative to GDP, many low-income countries spend less than 5% of GDP on health care, while most upper-income countries spend between 10 and 18% on GDP. On a per capita basis, the individual disparity between low- and higher-income countries is very large.

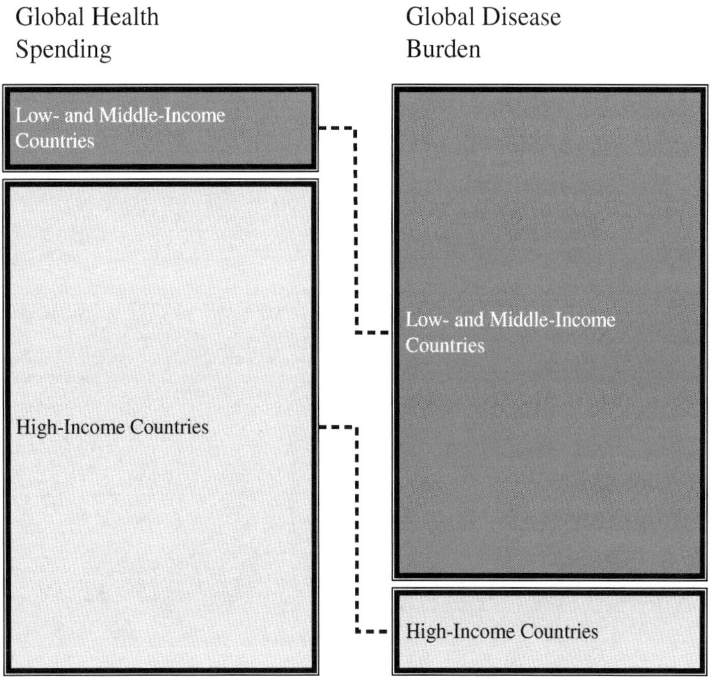

Figure 2. Low- and middle-income countries are not spending enough

Source: Preker — adapted from Gottret and Schieber, 2006.

External sources of funding can account for as much as 60% of total health spending in some low-income countries but much less in middle-income countries. Overall, donors provide 16% of health care funding in low-income countries.

Economics of Variations in Health Care Financing at the National Level

Often the economics of health care financing is equated with the economics of private health insurance markets. Although private health insurance is an important part of health care financing, the economics of health care financing is much broader and more complex than health insurance.

A good starting point for understanding the economics of health care financing is to look at the flow of funds through the health care system (Preker *et al.*, 2010; Preker *et al.*, 2007b). See Figure 3.

Figure 3 emphasizes three major aspects of the economics of health care financing: (a) Recurrent funding of operating expenses; (b) capital expenditure on investments; and (c) external donor funding (mainly relevant in low- and middle-income countries). We will describe each of these in turn.

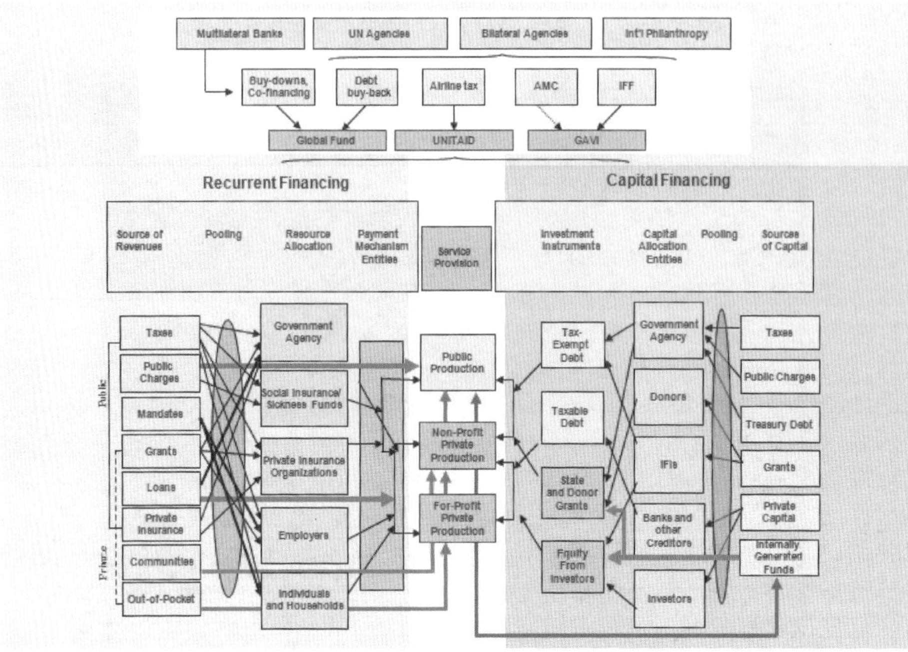

Figure 3. Consumers, governments and donors must all play a role

Source: Preker.

Recurrent funding for operating expenditures. Under recurrent financing (left side of Figure 3), financial resources are collected from a variety of sources. Once collected, they are pooled (or mixed in some way) as they are channeled through some form of administrative agency before being allocated to providers using different types of payment systems. Money may come from a variety of sources, such as taxes, insurance premiums (public or private), grants, loans, community pools or household pocket money. The funds that are collected from these sources are then pooled and passed to various administrative organizations such as a government department in the ministry of health (MOH) or social welfare, public health insurance fund, private health insurance fund or some form of self-administered household program like a medical savings account. These administrative agencies usually keep the money in commercial banks or government treasuries until the money is paid to health care providers, using familiar funding mechanisms such as fees-for-service, capitation payments or global budgets.

Out-of-pocket spending by households may bypass both the pooling and the agency part of this diagram when patients pay providers directly at the time that they seek care. Patients may also pay providers directly when the insurance system is set up to reimburse the patient for expenses incurred rather than paying providers directly for the services that they would otherwise bill to the health insurance program.

All countries in the world use a mix of these different types of recurrent funding mechanisms. No country in the world relies only on one source of funding or a single funding agency. The great variety of health care funding mechanisms seen in different parts of the world reflects the almost infinite variations in which these aspects of recurrent funding can be combined.

The policy options for funding health care are, however, often stereotyped as belonging to either a UK-style National Health Service model (with tax funding dominating), German-style "sickness fund" model (with government or social insurance dominating), or US-style private health insurance model (with private insurance dominating). This oversimplified portrayal of health care financing ignores the reality of a rich range of choices that underlie the recurrent funding of health care as seen in Figure 3. It also ignores the significant out-of-pocket spending in most low- and middle-income countries.

Capital expenditure on investments. The capital expenditure story (right side of Figure 3), mirrors the flow of funds seen under recurrent financing already described. Money may come from a variety of sources such as taxes, a component of insurance premiums (public or private), grants, loans, community pools and individual private investments. An additional source of capital investment funding is through internally generated funds. This is not seen in recurrent expenditure flows. As in the case of recurrent funding, capital funds are then channeled though some form of administrative agency (government agency, banks, and a variety of different investment instruments) before being allocated to providers.

At this point, however, the nomenclature of capital funding departs from the familiar terms used in recurrent financing. In the case of capital funding, the instruments tend to fall into two categories — debt and equity — which may be either public or private. Unfortunately, there are a number of confusing terminologies in capital finance, such as public and private equity, which do not correspond to the same notion in recurrent funding, in that public equity means shares that are issued on a stock market rather than government sources of capital funding. This chapter focuses mostly on the economics of recurrent funding, so we are introducing the notion of capital funding merely to show the parallelism and also to emphasize that it is important to understand both sides of the equation.

There is a great deal of controversy, globally, about the role of the public and private sectors in capital funding. We will deal with some of this controversy in the section below on policy debates.

External donor funding. External donor funding belongs to either the recurring or capital side, or both. It is therefore not a separate topic. It has no real application in most mature market settings, but it is a significant source of recurrent funding in many developing countries and may be the only source of capital funding in many low-income countries. Once again, the money which comes from a variety of sovereign, non-profit and private for-profit entities, is often pooled and channeled through some form of administrative agency that then disburses the funds according to its mandate to cover recurrent or capital expenditures. Different organizations follow different rules in the allocation of donor funding, which can cause great distortion and confusion in countries where such funds are a significant part of the overall health care budget.

Recent studies indicate that external donor assistance has a limited direct impact on health outcomes. Development assistance for health has a direct impact on mortality under age 5, after controlling for volatility (Gottrett and Schieber, 2006). But it does not affect maternal mortality directly — it does so only indirectly, through its effect on government health spending, which translates into employment of more staff and general hospitals that may include maternal care. This outcome is not surprising given donor assistance's fungibility (aid substituting for domestic sources of funding), volatility (aid flows varying from year to year) and crowding out (aid money displacing private funding), as well as the off-budget nature of a significant amount of aid (World Bank, 2014).

Unfortunately, much of donor aid is actually used to service existing debt, leaving many countries with little additionality[1] from the donor assistance they receive (World Bank, 2014). At the same time, low- and middle-income countries often find it very difficult keeping track of the multiple off-budget funding tracks and often conflicting incentives introduced through the strings that donors attach to the spending of their money. To overcome this problem, there has been a recent trend for donors to give their funds to a common pool that is easier for countries to manage. Most developed countries do not face these problems in health care financing so we will not go into all the variation about these arrangements in donor funding mechanisms in this chapter.

Economics of Health Insurance and Government Interventions

Having moved from direct payment at the point of consumption of health care to some form of third-party-payment system leads to economic behavior in the health sector that is very different from the classic supply, demand, price equilibrium seen in the case of ordinary consumption of goods and services.

In this section, we will look in more detail at the economics of several aspects of recurrent funding related to: (1) Health insurance markets, (2) government subsidies and (3) direct consumer purchasing of health care from providers, which are the three main pillars of health care financing in most countries. In most countries,

---

[1] Additionality refers to the financial impact of donor aid. For example, when donors contribute \$1, countries may lower the amount they spend by \$0.80. Here, the additionality is 20% of \$1.

these three funding mechanisms coexist in different proportions. In each case, it is useful to discuss the economic characteristics under the headings described earlier (collecting revenues, managing risks, and paying providers) and summarized as follows (Preker *et al.*, 2013):

a. Collecting revenues
   i. Recurrent and capital funding models.
   ii. Monetary and non-monetary incentives.
b. Managing risks
   i. Insurable and non-insurable risks.
   ii. Insurance, re-insurance and stop loss measures.
c. Paying providers
   i. Performance incentives.
   ii. Administrative capacity.

We will not describe in detail the full range of topics related to paying providers since this is the subject of other chapters in the Handbook. (For example, see Volume 1, Chapter 6, *Global Risk-Adjusted Payment Models*, and Volume 3, Chapter 7, *Pay for Performance in Health Systems: Theory, Evidence and Case Studies*.) Nor will we delve into all the details on capital finance. We will only refer in passing to these topics in this chapter and refer the reader other sources for a more detailed discussion on this subject (Preker and Langenbrunner, 2005).

Economics of health insurance

Health insurance systems distribute money, *ex-post*, from healthy to sick people, from rich to poor people and from people engaged in the labor market to people that are not currently employed, including the unemployed, children and the elderly. This pools the financial risks associated with illness and injury. This pooling can occur in a private, voluntary system (Pauly *et al.*, 2006) or in systems with public fiscal or regulatory intervention. Universal national health insurance or national health service systems pool risk by paying for coverage and care through income taxes or other broad-based taxes. Mandated models pool risk by requiring that certain groups participate in arrangements that cross-subsidize the costs of health insurance among groups with varying income or health status. In general, mandated insurance models accomplish this cross-subsidization through mandatory payroll taxes or workplace-based premium payments.

The first large-scale health insurance system, which was developed by German Chancellor Otto von Bismarck beginning in 1883, used a social insurance model. Originally, workers and their employers in certain industries were required to contribute to health insurance pools, which at first paid claims only for earnings lost due to illness. Next, medical care was provided as a service through the community. Only later, in a third phase did the insurance funds become a third party insurance payment system for health care. In Germany, this system has evolved into a nearly universal program that includes workers, retirees, dependents, and non-workers. Many other developed and developing country health insurance programs also incorporate such transfers from those that have to those that need under various types of social contracts.

Several developing countries have mandated health insurance programs, usually covering public employees and sometimes certain other formal sector employees (Hsiao and Shaw, 2007). In Africa, social health insurance programs have been established in Ghana and Kenya (Hsiao and Shaw, 2007). The main financing for these programs comes from payroll taxes or workplace-based premiums, but most also rely on substantial infusions of general revenues. General revenue financing is a necessary element of these systems if they are intended to cross-subsidize people based on their income as well as on their health status, as discussed below.

Economists are divided in their views about the advantages and disadvantages of policy financed or mandated health.

Some of the benefits are described as follows:

Buying insurance to cover medical care costs instead of paying for them out of pocket serves two important purposes. First, it pools risks across people. Because the direct costs of medical care when ill are extremely high, but few people get very ill, individuals may buy insurance as a way of pooling resources. From this pool, the high cost of care can be covered for the unfortunate few who get extremely ill. Health insurance, transferring income from the healthy to the unexpectedly sick, is valuable because in most circumstances, the marginal utility of income when sick is greater than the marginal utility of income when healthy.

The second important role that insurance can play is allowing individuals to smooth their expected consumption by purchasing insurance. Thus, instead of facing low health care costs when healthy, high costs when sick, and constant uncertainty about whether their health costs will be high or low, individuals can buy insurance such that the costs of medical care can be constant regardless of their actual health status. An important assumption behind this rationale for insurance (beyond that individuals can afford to pay for health care if they fall sick) is that individuals are risk averse and therefore prefer to pay a set amount with certainty against the risk of having to pay a large amount for health care when needed.

These general benefits of insurance arise in both private and public insurance arrangements. Public insurance may generate additional benefits by overcoming the problem of adverse selection, which can lead to the failure of private insurance markets.

Adverse selection occurs when people incorporate knowledge of their own poor health status into their decisions about insurance coverage. People who expect to use health services that cost more than the price of insurance in the coming year usually buy coverage. People who are healthy and have a low probability of using health care services place a lesser value on health insurance, even if they are risk averse, and this group may not be better off purchasing insurance. Therefore, whatever the health insurance costs, individuals who expect to spend more than its price on health care services will buy, and individuals who expect to spend less may not buy. Even when everyone buys coverage, adverse selection leads healthier people to choose less-comprehensive health plans than they might otherwise buy in order to signal their healthy status.

This process of self-selection can ultimately cause the insurance market to collapse (as occurred in voluntary fraternal health insurance in the US in 1920s). In the developing-country context, selection effects (and the fear of such effects) may also confound efforts to establish new private insurance plans. By mandating that both healthy and sick people buy the same health plans, publicly financed or regulated insurance can eliminate the efficiency losses due to adverse selection. Requiring participation in the same health plans also generates long-term risk pooling. In that way, people are assured of obtaining health insurance at reasonable prices in the future, even if they subsequently develop chronic health conditions.

Public health insurance markets may have other advantages over private insurance. In many situations, these markets operate at lower administrative cost than do private insurers because they can use existing revenue-collection arrangements and do not need to take steps to address adverse selection. When providers exert some monopoly power, large public insurers can serve as an effective countervailing force. When insurance markets do not yet exist, public insurers may be better able to overcome the legitimacy and credibility problems that make it difficult to establish a new private insurer. In some developing countries, however, governments have less legitimacy and credibility than private actors, suggesting that arrangements that rely on private insurance markets (with mandatory side payments) may be more desirable.

Most importantly, public health insurance arrangements can be a vehicle for redistributing income within the population, from higher-income people to lower-income people and from healthier people to sicker people. In this role, public insurance systems combine an insurance function with a redistributive function.

Yet publicly financed or mandated health insurance also generates inefficiencies for several reasons. First, mandates and taxes on labor alter the marginal gains from employment. This change in incentives usually leads to changes in the supply of or demand for labor and consequent deadweight losses. Second, the provision of free or subsidized health insurance effectively increases people's income even if they do not work. This income effect weakens the incentive to participate in the labor market. Third, the governance of public insurance is subject to the usual political economy problems of government.

The first two of these inefficiencies of public financing and mandates occur because people's contributions to the system are typically disconnected from the benefits they receive from the system. This disconnect occurs whenever redistribution is an important element of the public insurance arrangement.

It is avoidable, however, in the case of non-universal, non-redistributive mandatory health insurance when the beneficiaries fully value the benefits they receive (Summers, 1989; Preker and Carrin, 2004), as described in the forthcoming section.

- *Non-universal social insurance*

Consider a situation in which employees in one sector of the economy value health insurance at its full cost. Private insurance plans do not arise, however, because of the above-mentioned problems of selection, legitimacy, and so forth.

Now suppose that all employees in this sector are mandated to contribute to and participate in a single health insurance plan, but those outside this sector do not participate in the plan. In this case, employees do not perceive the mandatory premium as a tax. They are willing to accept a decrement in wages equal to the full cost of the health insurance plan, since they desire health insurance and can obtain it only by working in this sector. The mandatory payment buys equally valuable services and therefore does not alter the marginal gains from employment. Workers may even be willing to give up more than the cost of insurance in wages, if desirable health insurance is efficiently provided through the mandatory workplace program. This implies that there are no deadweight losses from the mandate and that revenues associated with the mandatory program do not detract from fiscal space. In this scenario, mandatory health insurance generates a Pareto improvement (see figure 4).

This favorable situation exists only as long as workers value the health insurance package (at least) at its full cost. If health insurance is available to non-workers at a lower cost (for example, through a publicly financed program), workers will not be willing to trade wages for mandatory health insurance benefits 1:1 and there will be deadweight losses. If worker premium payments are used to finance benefits for non-workers (such as the unemployed), these additional payments will be perceived as taxes. The payments will alter the marginal benefit of working, generating deadweight losses and reducing fiscal space.

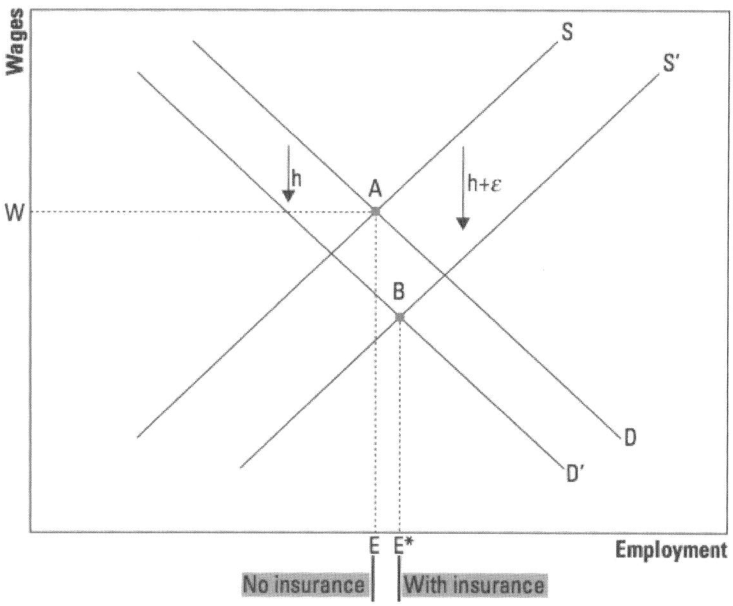

Figure 4. Labor market effects of mandated health insurance

Notes: Point A = no health insurance; point B = nonuniverseal social health insurance; h = the cost of benefits; ε = the amount that workers value benefit in excess of cost.
Source: Glied and Preker — adapted from Preker *et al.* (2013).

- *Labor market effects*

While non-universal social insurance programs limit deadweight losses, they may generate distortions within the labor market. First, if the provision of insurance is less costly under the mandatory program than otherwise, the existence of the mandate will reduce the total cost of labor in the covered sectors. Some workers will be willing to accept reductions in wages greater than the cost of coverage in order to obtain access to health insurance. The mandate may artificially induce growth of the formal sector.

Second, the opportunity to obtain insurance through the mandatory program may make jobs in the covered sectors particularly attractive to workers who value health insurance more than average. Workers who value coverage highly may make job choices based on coverage and not productivity. As a result, worker mobility may decrease, leading to labor market inefficiencies.

- *Summary*

As the above discussion suggests, there is an inherent tension in the design of a social insurance program. Mandatory insurance programs that are narrow in scope and cover only one economic sector can, at least in principle, generate Pareto improvements for the limited population they serve. Narrowing the program can, however, generate distortions in favor of the covered sector and reduce worker mobility. Moreover, narrow programs do not address the widespread need for health care financing and do not generate redistribution. Efforts to expand the comprehensiveness of services and populations covered in these programs can, however, generate deadweight losses and consume fiscal space. A "social insurance" Program that covers the entire population and the full scope of services is simply a National Health Insurance (or National Health Service) Program financed through a payroll tax.

Following are some of the major market imperfections that have been observed in both public and private health insurance markets that governments try to address through various forms of regulation or by bypassing insurance mechanisms altogether and engaging instead in the direct financing of health services (see Glossary of Terms):

d. Information asymmetry.
e. Cream skimming.
f. Moral hazard.
g. Adverse selection.
h. Insurance death spirals.
i. Under and over insurance.
j. Problems related to technical and allocative efficiency.
k. Labor market and other adverse macro effects.

The role of government interventions and subsidies

Because of the many institutional factors described above, health insurance markets are imperfect and do not follow the usual principles of supply, demand, price equilibrium, etc., that would be observed in other parts of the economy and other parts of the health sector.

To address these problems, governments often intervene in insurance markets, using a range of instruments ranging from just providing consumers with reliable information so that they can make informed choices, or regulation to protect consumer interests, or more intrusive interventions such as mandates, establishing public insurance programs and directly funding health care without insurance, like in the UK, Canada, and many other OECD countries.

Europeans, Canadians, Australians, and many others who live in countries where universal coverage was achieved many years ago, watched with bewilderment the debates in the US Congress and Senate. How could anyone be opposed, they asked, to reforms aimed at securing access to affordable health insurance for the currently unprotected in the world's richest country? What argument, they asked, could anyone possibly give to oppose a reform that would extend protection to those vulnerable segments of the population?

Yet, it is precisely the same type of debate — often fueled by ideologically oriented stakeholders and donors — heard in India, Kenya, Pakistan, Senegal, Uganda, and many other countries struggling themselves to introduce health insurance reforms.

Well intended as these interventions may be, and with notable successes in terms of providing comprehensive coverage against the financial risk of illness through publicly subsidized social health insurance or state-funded health care, even in some of the most successful programs, government intervention in health care financing is often associated with:

a. Market distortion in the supply, demand, and price of health insurance.
b. Collection of rents and other forms of corruption.
c. Price fixing with underfunding and restrictions in choice.
d. Unfunded mandates and fiscal space limitations.

Major Controversies Related to the Economics of Health Care Financing

The key issues that will be discussed in this section include:

a. Pooled sources of funding versus out-of-pocket spending.
b. Core government budgets versus insurance based funding approaches.
c. Public mandatory insurance versus private voluntary insurance.
d Supply-versus demand-side subsidies.
e. Political promises versus fiscal constraints.
f. Universal coverage versus target approaches.
g. Subsidies for infrequent catastrophic risks versus frequent low-cost Care.
h. Insurable versus non-insurable risks.
i. Multipillar versus monolythic systems.

Pooled sources of funding versus out-of-pocket spending (the 20/80 to 80/20 rule)

Low-income countries often rely heavily on government funding and out-of-pocket payments for financing health care. At an early stage of economic development, a country's ratio of prepaid to out-of-pocket sources of financing is often as low as 20:80. In countries with higher income levels, this ratio is reversed: Prepaid sources make up 80% of financing sources. Countries on an optimal development path will progress from the 20:80 to 80:20 (see Figure 5). But many of the fragile

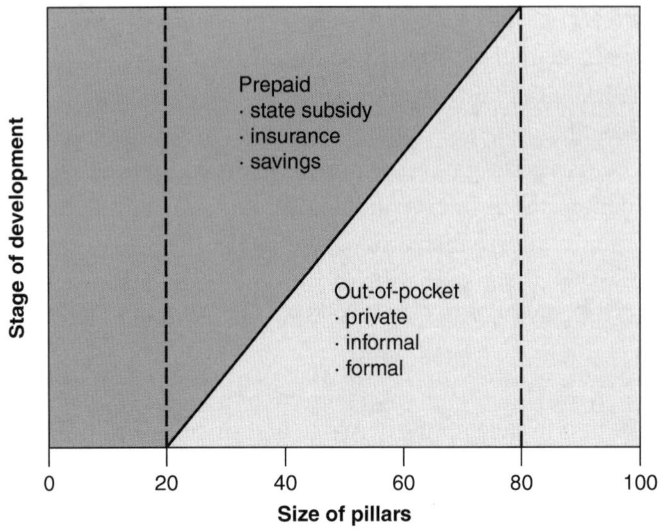

Figure 5. The Rule of 20:80 and 80:20 in financing health care

Source: Preker — adapted from Preker *et al.* (2013).

low-income countries are on a slower and suboptimal development path toward a 40:60. Without a significant shift in policy direction and implementation, out-of-pocket spending will continue to represent a large share of total health care expenditure, leaving many households exposed to financial hardship or impoverishment, despite significant government spending on health care.

This development process can take decades. Some estimate that it took 180 years of slow progress before Germany reached universal coverage from the time of the early "Krankeakssen" (German Sickness Funds) to the modern German system. More recently, the Affordable Care Act signed into law in 2010 was landmark health reform legislation in the US after more than 100 years of slow progress toward expanding coverage (see Box 1). Attempts to leapfrog this long development process — admirable as it may be in terms of objectives — often fail to be effective at improving the out-of-pocket spending ratio during implementation.

Core government budgets versus insurance-based funding approaches

As countries move up the development path from low-income levels to higher income levels, they are faced with some important choices in terms of the funding of health care.

Box 1. 130 Years of slow progress towards universal health care in the OECD

At the end of the 19th Century, most western countries relied mainly on direct out-of-pocket payment and unregulated markets to finance and provide health care. In 1938, New Zealand became the first country with a market economy to introduce compulsory participation and universal entitlement to a comprehensive range of health services, financed largely through the public sector (the UK followed a similar path when — 10 years later — it established the National Health Services (NHS) in 1948). Universal access to health care in many eastern European countries — Albania, Bulgaria, the Czech Republic, Slovakia, Hungary, Poland, Romania, and the USSR — was achieved through similar legislative reforms. A number of other middle- and low-income countries have followed a similar path.

Today, the population in most OECD countries (with the exception of Mexico, Turkey, and the US) enjoy universal access to a comprehensive range of health services that are financed through a combination of general revenues, social insurance, private insurance, and user charges. In 13 of the OECD countries, universal access was achieved through landmark legislative reforms that guaranteed their population such benefits (Australia, Canada, Denmark, Finland, Greece, Iceland, Italy, New Zealand, Norway Portugal Spain, Sweden, and UK), while most other OECD countries achieved similar coverage through voluntary and regulatory mechanisms like the recent Affordable Health Care Act in the US. The latter brought the US closer to the universal coverage

The OECD experience in introducing universal health care can be regarded as taking place in two phases: (a) A policy formulation phase; and (b) an implementation phase.

During the policy formulation phase, the design of the reform needs to consider both the financing and service delivery aspects. Without access to health services, legislation that mandates universal financing is little more than a paper law.

After the design of a successful system of financing universal access, a major stumbling block in most countries has been the political economy of policy formulation and dealing with various stakeholders with vested interests that may resist such reforms for a variety of reasons that will be discussed later.

But in reality the real work starts when all of the policy design and political processes have finished. The heavy lifting really starts during implementation. This includes *inter alia* determination of entitlement, identification and registration of members, collection of contributions, setting up actuarial risk sharing mechanism, designing and implementing payment systems, monitoring

(*Continued*)

Box 1. (*Continued*)

and evaluation, control for fraud and abuse, as well as a myriad of other administrative processes.

Many well intended and well designed health insurance reforms around the world have failed over and over again not because of lack of money or political opposition but rather because of poorly conceived and executed implementation.

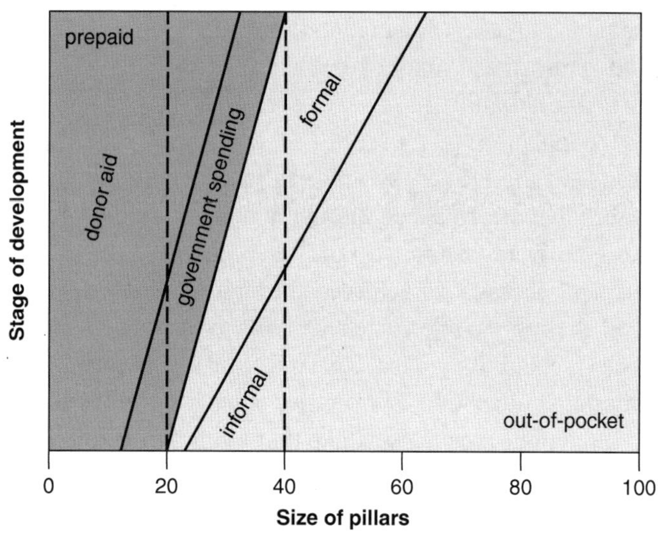

Figure 6. Sub optimal development path in financing health care
Source: Preker — adapted from Preker *et al.* (2013).

At very low-income levels, a large share of government funding may come from donors rather than domestic sources of financing (Figure 6). Although donor assistance may be critical to the development of the health system in these countries, the health sector often becomes vulnerable to donor dependence, volatility in financial flows, and fungibility (Gottrett and Schieber, 2006). In many of the countries that choose this donor-reliant development path, a large share of the out-of-pocket expenditure continues to be informal payments in the public sector and on private sector spending, exposing households to whatever cost the local market can bear. So even though in theory they are covered through public provision of services or some form of public insurance, in reality they are still making payments for health care, with its associated negative impact on low-income groups.

One of the first choices countries face in improving funding for health care is whether to rely on public, tax-based funding or introduce a contributor health insurance system (public or private). Over the past 50 years, many countries have tried to fund health care through core government funding, like the British National Health Services where there is no insurance (see Figure 7). The advantages of such direct government funding are that funding for health care can be aligned with other public policies, use the existing taxation system to collect needed funds and ensure that equity objectives, such as coverage of the poor and other vulnerable groups, are included in covered population.

Central government funding of health care in countries that have weak taxation capacity and public sector corruption, however, often leads to many problems, including under-funding and significant government failure in funding health care.

As an alternative, countries can use insurance-based approaches (see Figure 8) instead of core government funding. We will discuss the advantages and disadvantages of these two forms of health care financing — dominant reliance on government subsidies and dominant reliance on health insurance based approaches — in the forthcoming sections.

High out-of-pocket expenditure by low-income households in most developing countries, and also by low-income households in higher-income countries including Europe and the US, provides a "prima facie" case that insurance is both desirable and affordable — if it can be offered with relatively moderate loading costs (e.g., administrative costs, losses due to fraud and abuse, profits, and transaction costs associated with meeting regulatory requirements). Figure 9 shows that the share of out-of-pocket spending on health care is greater at low-income levels in every part of the world.

First, analysis of household survey data indicates that both the willingness and ability to pay for health care — even among the poor — are far greater than the government's capacity to mobilize revenues through formal taxation mechanisms. In much of Sub-Saharan Africa and South Asia, the relative share of health expenditures financed directly through households is as high as 80% of total expenditures.

Second, reviews of community participation in micro-insurance programs in low-income countries indicate that households — even poor ones — are insurable. Often they already benefit from micro loans and savings, crop insurance, burial insurance, and community health insurance. Health insurance involves some transfer of resources from rich to poor, healthy to sick, and gainfully employed to inactive. Households in low-income settings understand the nature of such transfers and are willing to contribute to them, proving they believe that outlays today will lead to benefits tomorrow. Too often, however, governments and national insurance programs break such trust by collecting contributions under one set of

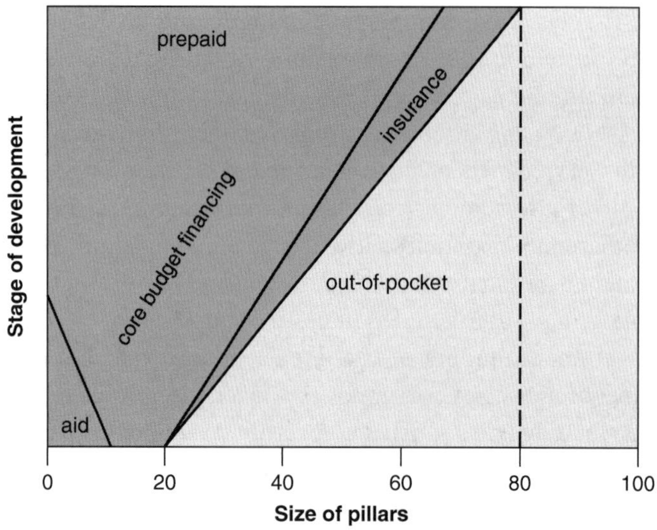

Figure 7. Progress toward subsidy based financing of health care

Source: Preker — adapted from Preker *et al.* (2013).

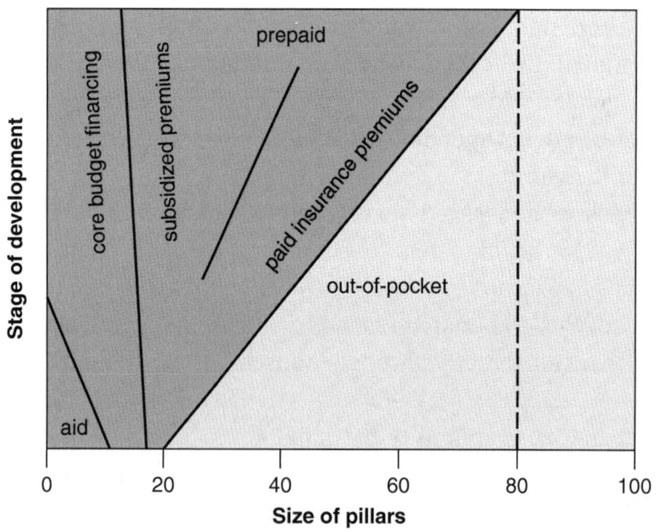

Figure 8. Progress towards insurance based financing of health care

Source: Preker — adapted from Preker *et al.* (2013).

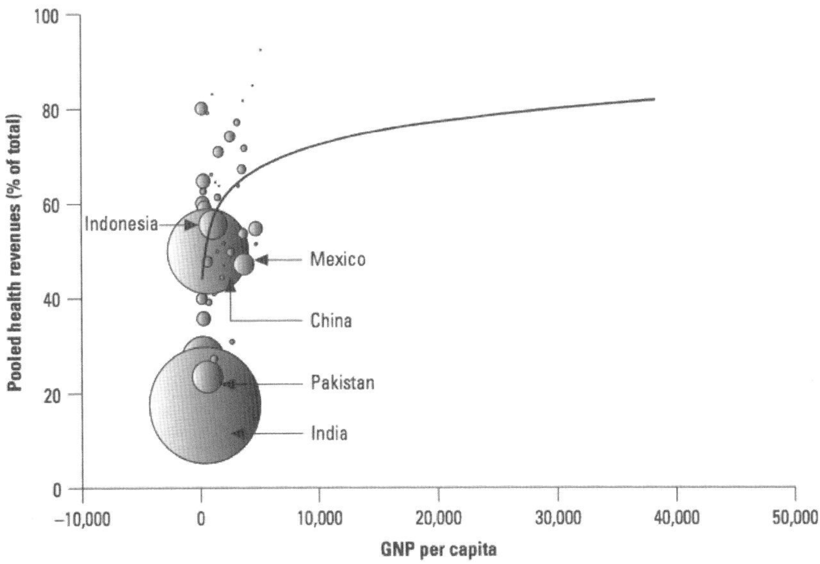

Figure 9. Out-of-pocket spending highest in low-income countries

Note: The share of the world's 1.3 billion people living on less than US$1 a day is indicated by the size of the bubble.
Source:Preker — adapted from Preker *et al.* (2013).

conditions and then changing the rules of entitlement. Micro-insurance is unlikely to be a viable solution in middle and high-income level settings because the premiums and benefit programs would be below what most members would expect as their insurance coverage. Such programs are therefore more relevant in low-income, resource-constrained environments.

Public mandatory insurance vs. private voluntary insurance

Two alternative approaches have been the focus of recent efforts to expand coverage through insurance-based mechanisms.

Public Mandatory Insurance. The first approach is some form of mandatory public national or subnational health insurance program. The second approach is a voluntary private health insurance program.

The arguments in favor of and against a mandatory public national health insurance are similar to those for core government funding. Policy oversight over coverage and benefit packages and simplicity in administration remain significant positive elements. Weak execution capacity and the bureaucratic policy present in this approach remain some of the negative aspects.

Private Voluntary Insurance. Voluntary private health insurance can also play a useful role in complementing other financing mechanisms such as core government funding, subsidies, mandatory public insurance, savings, and user fees to achieve the objectives of equity, risk management, and household-income smoothing. For example, there could be a basic mandatory public program that provides coverage for most conditions that are considered at a given country income level but some population groups would like to provide additional benefits to their members. This is how employment-based insurance programs often started. The argument against this approach is that the better-off part of the population would have more comprehensive coverage than poorer parts of the population. The acceptability of this approach depends of the social views of the society in the country where it would be implemented.

Demand for private voluntary health insurance is not concentrated only in the highest-income groups, but extends to lower-income groups as well (Pauly *et al.*, 2008). Demand for health insurance among lower-income groups appears to exist for two reasons: First, the risk (even if small) of being exposed to high out-of-pocket payment poses a considerable threat to many households; second, the variance of potential out-of-pocket spending is sufficiently large that many households would be willing to pay more than the expected value of the benefits to avoid exposure to the upper extreme in expenditures. Insurance plans should therefore be able to charge premiums that would cover the cost of expected benefits and the loading cost.

In most countries, low-income populations account for the greatest share of out-of-pocket expenditure in the aggregate. But at the individual level, because the expected out-of-pocket expense varies with income, making such insurance affordable to low-income populations in a voluntary market will require market segmentation. In this way, lower-income people could have their premiums adjusted based on their below-average spending and setting premiums in relation to average expense across all other income groups.

As an indicator of the feasibility of introducing such insurance in low- and middle-income contexts, Pauly *et al.* (2008) suggest using the amount people would be willing to pay for insurance beyond the expected value of benefits and comparing this “risk premium” (as part of the total premium) with the administrative expense share of insurance premiums. In many countries, this risk premium (expressed as a percentage of expected benefits for full coverage insurance) was in the range of the expected administrative expense that markets could generate. This formula is especially relevant in comparing the viability of insurance that would pay for some care (such as hospitalization only or drugs only insurance policies) and comprehensive insurance covering hospital, physician, and drug expenses. The authors found that the risk premium for stand-alone drug insurance is relatively low, even though spending on drugs constitutes a large share of total out-of-pocket spending. These findings suggest that comprehensive insurance (rather than a hospitalization-only or a drugs-only policy) might be the most feasible way of achieving good financial protection.

Based on this research, it can be predicted that risk-averse households will voluntarily purchase health insurance if the associated expenses are smaller than the "risk premium" they would be willing to pay. That risk premium depends on the variance of the losses the insurance will cover and on the extent of a household's risk aversion. If the loading cost is low, households are more willing to contribute to an insurance program.

Supply- vs. demand-side subsidies

In terms of subsidies, governments can either spend their funds by paying providers directly or indirectly through some form of third party payments system (or some mix of the two types of subsidy channels. At the risk of oversimplification, the first system is generally financed through taxation. The second system is often financed through voluntary or mandatory health insurance payments. Citizen demand for risk protection is a common motivation for both. Demand for public insurance may also be motivated by externalities such as care for contagious diseases or the altruistic and paternalistic ones that reflect consensus about the health and health care of fellow citizens.

The use of the tax system generates economic distortion or "excess burden" compared with private voluntary health insurance. This observation may be especially relevant for developing countries with poorly administered tax systems or small shares of the economy in the formal sector. The reason for economic distortion is both that incomes are low and that tax-collected funds are costly and therefore scarce. In this sense, private voluntary health insurance, which will generate less distortion, is less costly. The emergence of private voluntary health insurance is therefore not only a desirable alternative to public provision but also an unavoidable one. Private voluntary health insurance may be the desirable instrument when public insurance is too costly to be efficient.

Employment-based insurance chosen voluntarily responds to worker perception of coverage and cost savings associated with group insurance. Compared with public provision or group insurance, individual insurance can allow each person to get exactly the insurance he or she demands, but the administrative cost will be high. In contrast, group insurance will generally have lower administrative cost and less adverse selection but less perfect tailoring to individual desires. The relative costs and benefits of each of these alternatives determine which system is more viable in a given context.

As described above, the alternative to full public provision is some form of subsidization of insurance premiums (public or private). This strategy can tap private willingness to pay and still achieve equity and efficiency goals if coupled with appropriate premium subsidies for the poor and measures to avoid known effects of insurance failure. Because people value insurance, they are willing to make at least a small private payment that can be matched with a public subsidy. These household contributions lower the needed level of public subsidies, which can then be spread more widely.

Two approaches underpin recent efforts to expand coverage through insurance-based mechanisms (Pauly, 2007) (see Figure 10). The first approach uses supply-side subsidies paid by the government to health care providers, to compensate them for services provided to target populations. Under this approach, health insurance is introduced for a small part of the population that can afford to pay for it and from whom employers can easily collect payroll taxes — usually civil servants and formal sector workers. Meanwhile, the poor and low-income informal sector workers continue to get health care from government-subsidized public hospitals and ambulatory clinics. Although at first sight, this policy option would appear to be pro-rich because only the formally employed who can afford to pay can join the insurance program, in reality it frees up public money that would otherwise be spent on people who have the means to pay for their

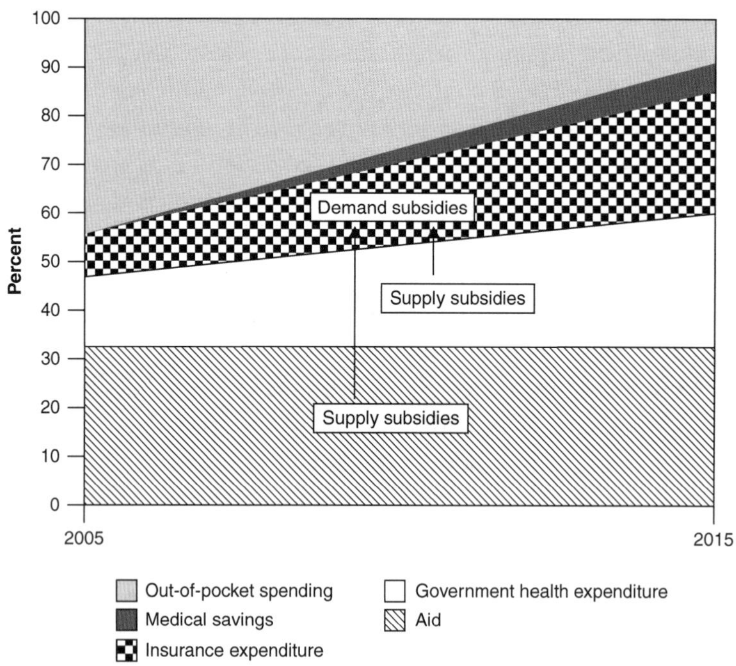

Figure 10. Shift from supply- to demand-side subsidies

Source: Preker.

insurance premiums. These funds can then be used to subsidize care for the poor and informal sector workers who may not have the means to pay for it themselves. It allows health ministries to use their limited government finances to target subsidies to pay for the contribution of poor members rather than for everyone.

The second approach uses demand-side subsidies paid by the government to certain target populations, to help pay the cost of insurance. Under this approach, health insurance is introduced for a broader segment of the population by applying a demand-driven approach, involving paying for or subsidizing premiums for the poor and low-income informal sector workers (patient-based subsidization). This allows a more rapid expansion of coverage, by using resources collected from the contributing part of the population to subsidize the premiums of the poor and low-income informal sector workers, rather than subsidizing their service providers (Figure 10). This approach offers the advantage of allowing more direct targeting of poor households than the supply-side subsidies described in the previous example (Schellekens *et al.*, 2007).

There is now good evidence that if subsidies were given to poor households rather than to providers, this would ensure that the subsidies are actually used on health services received by the poor rather than by the rich. Such subsidy transfers could take the form of vouchers to buy care directly or premium subsidies so that the poor can have access to the same type of health insurance as the rich. A viable health insurance program requires that everyone pay an actuarially sound premium (Cichon *et al.*, 1999). This does not necessarily exclude the poor if there is a partial or full subsidy for their premiums. The advantage of this approach is that the poor can then choose the services they feel meet their needs, and service providers will be paid accordingly, thereby achieving both equity and efficiency objectives.

In summary, it is important to emphasize that households — even the poor — are insurable. Health insurance involves some transfer of resources from rich to poor, healthy to sick, and gainfully employed to inactive. Households in low-income settings understand the nature of such transfers and are willing to contribute small amounts of money today if it secures benefits needed tomorrow. Current systems for financing health care beyond the basic public services in most low- and middle-income countries deprive the poor of such financial protection against the cost of illness beyond those basic public services provided under insurance. Under such financing arrangements, the subsidies would be used to pay for insurance to cover health risks beyond such a minimal package of services.

Political promises versus fiscal constraints

Ideally, everyone would have access to a full range of health services at the time they need health care, without distinctions in the type of illness or their ability to pay. In reality, even in the richest countries in the world the sky is not the limit. There are

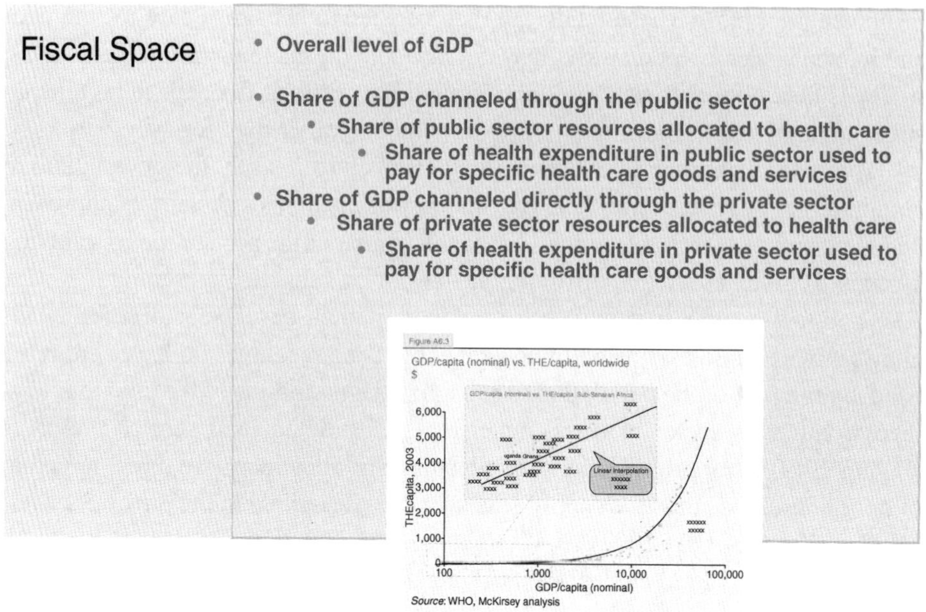

Figure 11. Fiscal constraints on health care spending

limits to what each society can afford to pay and what governments are able to subsidize. As more advanced and expensive treatments and technologies become available even rich countries cannot afford to pay for all available interventions.

The overall fiscal envelope that can be devoted to health care has an absolute limit in that it is a percentage of the country's GDP. Richer countries have both a higher absolute spending on health care in terms of dollars spent per capita and higher relative spending on health care in terms of the percentage of GDP spent on health care (both private and public). Although some countries try to push this limit by deficit spending, in the medium-term, the size of the GDP places boundaries on the amount of spending that is feasible in each society (see Figure 11).

Universal coverage versus targeting

Even with donor funding, poor countries ultimately spend less on health care than rich countries. This leads to important trade-offs that must be made between the breadth of population coverage and the depth/quality of the services provided. Low- and middle-income countries that try to leapfrog the 20:80 to 80:20 development path by introducing legislation to force universal coverage through either

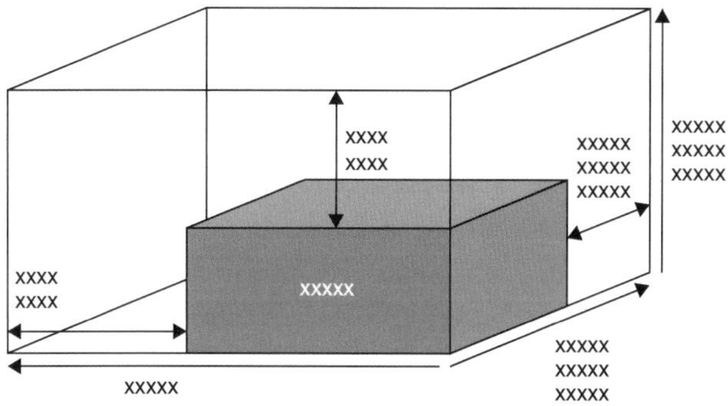

Figure 12. Trade-offs between population coverage, cost and quality

Source: Preker — adapted from the Lancet Commission on Investing in Health, 2013.

health insurance or direct government funding end up having to provide very limited benefit coverage and compromising on the quality of the services they provide or cover (see Figure 12).

Subsidies for infrequent catastrophic risks versus frequent low-cost care

Insurance gives providers a more sustainable source of funding and protects households from economic shocks at the time of illness. Insurance helps channel household expenditure on health care through a more efficient and effective financing mechanism than direct out-of-pocket payments. It may also increase the total funding envelope allocated to health care through an insurance effect (meaning that households paying for insurance will still buy some services directly and pay for them fully out of pocket due to limits on what is covered in their benefits package; this tendency may lead to higher overall health care spending). In low-income countries, there will still not be enough resources to go around even with insurance. Difficult decisions therefore need to be made about which benefits to include and which not to include under health insurance.

One way to look at this challenge is to reexamine the frequency and cost of treating medical events. One approach is to cover high-frequency events associated with relatively low-cost interventions (basic package). In recent years, many low- and middle-income countries have introduced publicly financed health care systems that offer the whole population such benefits through public providers.

Under this approach, everyone has access in principle to what is considered an essential package of basic services. The resulting services are often underfunded when offered to the whole population, and less frequent but more expensive or life-threatening conditions have to be excluded from the basic package. Therefore

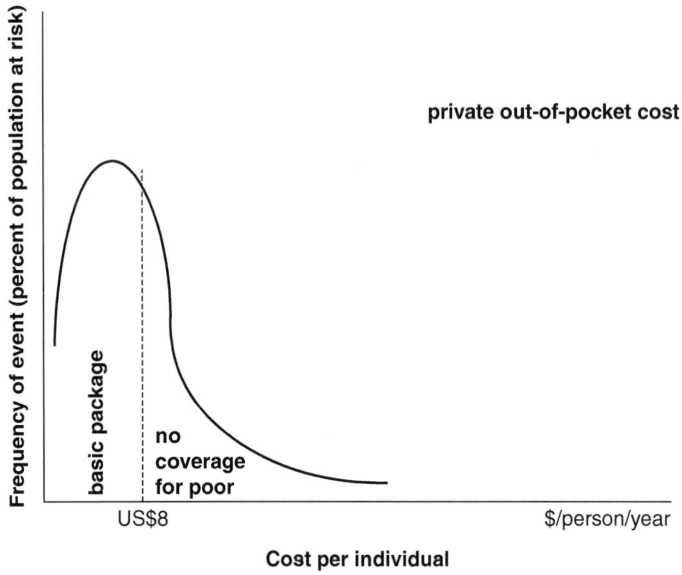

Figure 13. Subsidizing basic care

Source: Preker — adapted from Preker *et al.* (2007a, 2010).

in reality, under this approach, the population including the poor still end up paying out-of-pocket for a large share of their health care, even though in principle they are offered universal access to care (see Figure 13).

The alternative approach, as suggested above, is to let households that can afford it cover the high-frequency and low-cost interventions themselves. This frees up significant public and donor funds that can then be used to subsidize the premium of risk-sharing mechanisms, especially in the case of the poor and vulnerable populations. This allows poor people to access care beyond the base minimum under such subsidzed insurance. People's willingness and ability to pay for health care — even among the poor — is far greater than their governments' capacity to mobilize revenues through formal taxation mechanisms. In much of Sub-Saharan Africa and Asia, the relative share of health expenditures financed directly through households already runs as high as 80% of total expenditure, so such a policy shift by governments would only confirm what is already happening on the ground.

Scarce households are already paying for their health care under the existing system through informal user fees. Therefore, instead of tying up public resources on care that households are both willing and able to pay for themselves, scarce public funds could be used on public health interventions with large externalities and on health insurance premiums for the poor to give them access to more expensive, unaffordable care? (see Figure 14).

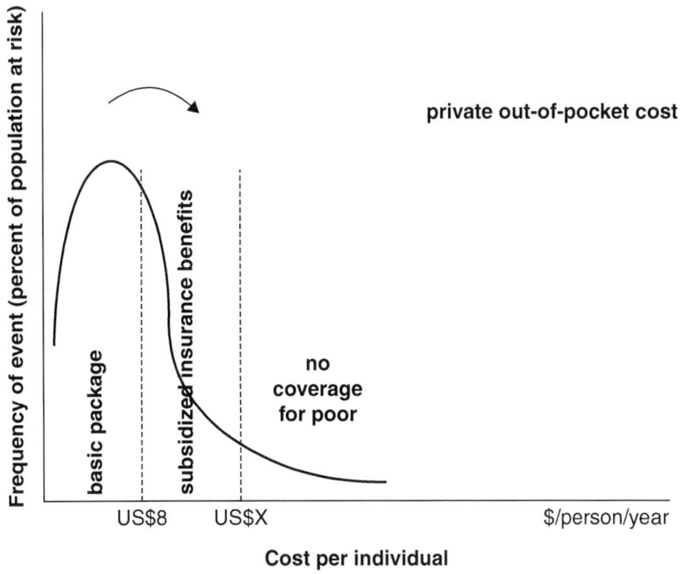

Figure 14. Subsidizing post basic care

Source: Preker — adapted from Preker *et al.* (2007a, 2010).

Some very expensive care, such as treatments for HIV/AIDS or expensive treatment for malaria and other priority public health programs, are too costly to include in the expanded insurance benefits under such a system without additional subsidies. The current approach for dealing with this problem is to leave it to governments and the international donor community to cover the costs of this expensive care through direct supply-side subsidies that finance free public services for the poor or expensive vertical parallel programs (Smith *et al.*, 2005) such as HIV/AIDS, malaria and other priority public health programs in low-income countries.

Another approach to covering less frequent, high-cost medical conditions and events is for donors and governments to channel these additional earmarked resources through health insurance programs that would cover the tail end of the distribution. Under this approach, these programs could benefit from risk-mitigation mechanisms such a re-insurance or targeted subsidies and be better integrated into the overall health system. Funding for the current vertical programs could be integrated under health insurance schemes in an actuarially sound manner as a supplemental or reinsurance pillar (Preker *et al.*, 2013).

This approach would allow the donor agencies to continue to earmark their funding for the targeted programs for which their constituents have given their money, while benefiting from a more refined spending mechanism and targeting of the poor rather than the current direct supply-side subsidies to providers. It also

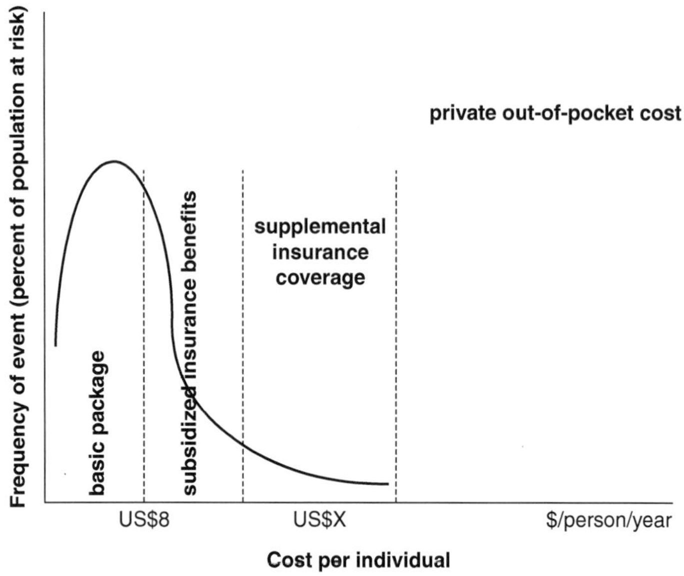

Figure 15. Subsidizing supplemental insurance coverage for high costs
Source: Preker — adapted from Preker *et al.* (2007a, 2010).

has the added benefit of allowing better integration of care and more comprehensive quality assurance and care management, thus contributing to a general strengthening of the health system. See Figure 15.

By including prevention and health promotion activities under the insurance package and by becoming much more active in quality assurance and care management. Members of such insurance programs will also be more willing to contribute to a scheme that provides such benefits. See Figure 16.

Insurable versus non-insurable risks

Looked at in a different way, health insurance programs designed in this way will allow a better matching of risk with appropriate financing instruments. High-frequency conditions associated with low-cost interventions — considered non-insurable risks in technical terms — can be financed through direct household contributions or a demand-side subsidy from governments and donors. Less-frequent conditions associated with higher-cost interventions — considered insurable risks in technical terms — can be covered by insurance and reinsurance (or supplemental insurance) with governments and donors channeling a premium subsidy through existing insurance programs. See Figure 17.

The Dutch health care system has moved from reliance on a mix of insurable and non-insurable risks to a more direct targeting of insurable risks using risk-rated health insurance, with premium subsidies made available to individuals

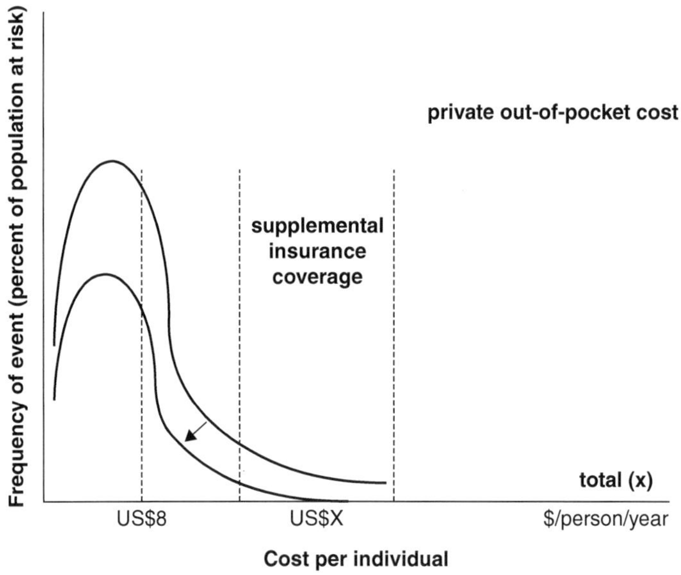

Figure 16. Subsidizing preventive care that reduces the cost curve
Source: Preker — adapted from Preker *et al.* (2007a, 2010).

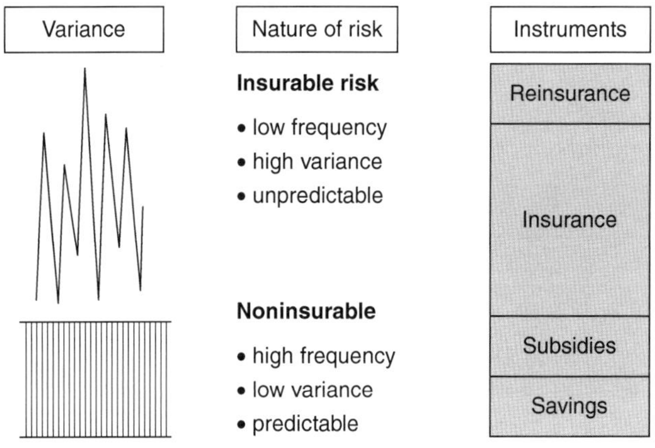

Figure 17. Insurable versus non-insurable risks
Source: Preker — adapted from Preker *et al.* (2010).

based on their risk profile rather than on their means to pay for services. By doing this, income distribution issues have been removed from the health care financing equation and have been replaced by a more traditional risk-management approach that focuses on ensuring that health insurance mechanisms are used to manage risk, not achieve other social objectives which can be handled better through other instruments. See Box 2.

Box 2. The Dutch risk-rated health insurance system

The Dutch health insurance systems provides a fascinating example of a system of health insurance that provides excellent access to high quality care at an affordable cost by using available funds efficiently.

In the 1980s, Dutch policymakers became aware that their health care system lacked these incentives to achieve the above objectives. The Dekker Commission noted that on the supply side, heavy involvement by the government in determining the price and volume in the delivery of health care services made the system both inflexible and fragmented.

On the supply side, the funding systems prevented substitution of cheaper outpatient care for expensive institutional care. There were spending ceilings. Service capacity and prices were regulated centrally. The sickness funds were little more than bookkeepers. They bore no financial risk because the government reimbursed all the costs of the insured.

On the demand side, the lack of cost-sharing and other methods to deal with moral hazard meant there were few, if any, incentives to reduce consumption of health services.

Competition. Under the Health Insurance Act of 2006, the sickness insurance funds were abolished and Dutch citizens were required to purchase their health insurance from profit-making private health insurers, which prior to 2006 insured only the wealthiest third of the population. The new private health insurers negotiate on behalf of their members with care providers, such as hospitals, general practitioners and pharmacies the scale, quality and price of services charged their members. The insured now 'vote with their feet.' They may change their health insurer once a year if the premium is too high, or the quality of care, bought on their behalf, is too low. This incentivizes both health care providers and health insurers to be efficient in the delivery (providers) and purchase (insurers) of health care.

Risk Adjustment. In many countries, prohibition of premium differentiation and the establishment of a uniform basic set of benefits, give health insurers strong incentives to insure only those persons with good health risks and shun those with poor health risks (preferred risk selection) in order to guarantee a profit. Insurers with a relatively sick portfolio of insured persons would be obliged to charge all their members higher flat-rate premiums in order to remain profitable. This would create incentives for the healthier members of the group to find a different insurer with a lower premium at their next annual election. As

(*Continued*)

Box 2. (*Continued*)

only the sickest remain in the original plan, the premium would have to be raised again. Eventually the premium would be so high and the plan membership so small, the insurance plan would become unviable and withdraw from the market. This is what insurers call the "death spiral" for an insurance plan.

Under the new health insurance rules in the Netherlands, the above problems are addressed through risk adjustments. Health insurers receive financial compensation for insured persons with an unfavorable risk profile (like the elderly, chronically ill and people who are incapacitated and have higher health costs). Each year all health insurers receive from the Health Insurance Fund a financial contribution known as the risk adjusted contribution. The size of the contribution depends on the composition of their insured populations. Health insurers with a relatively large number of insured persons with an unfavorable risk profile (older and sicker individuals) receive a higher contribution than those with a relatively large number of insured persons with a favorable risk profile (younger and healthier individuals).

Ideally, when the risk adjustment works properly, the health insurer no longer has an incentive to select a young and healthy membership. Those that are able to manage their expenditure well, will even have an incentive to cover older and sicker populations because of the higher risk adjustment that they will receive. Insurers are encouraged to cover individuals who need insurance. Such risk adjustment creates a level playing field for health insurers, regardless of the composition of their insured populations. Health insurers are encouraged to direct their effort and resources to achieving more efficiency in the delivery of care, rather than in acquiring or shedding certain groups of insured persons. Health insurers that operate less efficiently (i.e., by purchasing services at a higher price or by organizing care less efficiently) than the average health insurer, will eventually not be able to remain in business.

A number of other countries use an *ex-ante* risk adjustment system for health insurers. They include Belgium, Germany, the United States (Medicare program), Ireland, the Czech Republic, Switzerland, and Israel. Although the Dutch health insurance reform is still "work in progress" there are already good indications that the intended incentives are working and that there has been a dramatic change in the insurance landscape since introduction of the Health Insurance Act of 2006. In the near future this could have a dramatic impact on other countries adopting a similar model.

Multi-pillar versus monolithic systems

The literature on health care financing is marred by definitional problems that have led to a great deal of confusion and have contributed to futile ideological arguments. Although health systems have been stereotyped as belonging to either an UK-style National Health Service model, German-style "sickness fund" model, or US-style private health insurance model, this portrayal of health care financing is an oversimplification of the trade-off between competition and solidarity-based approaches (Chinitz *et al.*, 1997). Notions of solidarity, social health insurance, social protection and universality, and other values-laden terms will be avoided.

In reality, most countries use a combination of voluntary and mandatory mechanisms through both public and private financing agents (see Figure 18). Under such a multi-pillar system, different mechanisms can be used to address different policy objectives.

As is evident from the high reliance on out-of-pocket expenditure, most donor- and government-funded programs in low- and middle-income countries have failed to achieve risk-management and income-smoothing objectives through any single mechanism alone. As a result, almost all of them already rely on a *multi-pillar* system for financing health care. Under a multi-pillar system, donor and government funding tend to be spent on mandatory programs whereas the direct household and savings components tend to be voluntary. Insurance falls somewhere in between. The general trend observed in most low- and middle-income countries is to increase government spending and/or insurance coverage over parallel to a reduction in the relative share of out-of-pocket spending.

Singapore is an excellent example of a country that uses a highly effective multi-pillar health care system that costs much less than any of the health care systems in the OECD and yet health outcomes are much higher across a wide range of indictors, including mortality, morbidity, efficiency, effectiveness of care and consumer satisfaction. See Box 3.

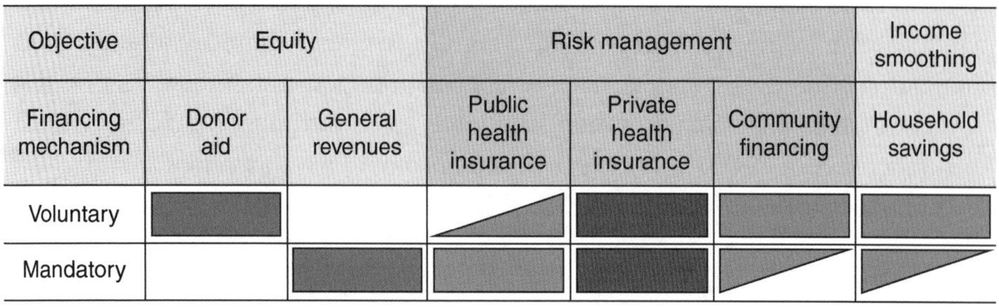

Figure 18. Multi-pillar approach to financing health care

Source: Preker — adapted from Preker *et al.* (2010).

Box 3. The Singapore comprehensive multi-pillar health insurance

Singapore is the country par excellence that has introduced a multi-tier health financing system that combines a different instrument for many of the major financial risk categories across both groups of illnesses and across the lifecycle.

The underlying philosophy is to combine personal responsibility of individuals and household, with the protection against risk that can be offered through health insurance and subsidies from the state. In practical terms, this translates into affordable copayments for individuals and household, spreading of risks by insurance programs and subsidies by the state to cover the cost of care that is not affordable to some income groups.

The following summary of the historical evolution of the Singapore health care system demonstrates how over time Singapore added pillars to it health care system, ending up with a very sophisticated multi-pillar system

1983 National Health Plan
1984 Medisave
1985 Hospital Restructuring
1990 Medishield
1993 Medifund
1993 White Paper-Affordable Health Care
2000 Clustering/ElderCare fund
2002 ElderShield

Under the combined

MEDISAVE is a compulsory savings plan. Contributions from individuals are matched by employers and deposited in a personal savings account. The contributions are tax exempted and the savings accounts carry interest. It is compulsory for working individuals. When someone gets sick, the first dollar is a copayment. After that there is a withdrawal from the savings account up a limit that protects the value of the account.

MEDISHIELD is a catastrophic insurance plan. Individuals also contribute to a national health insurance program called Medishield. After copayments and some expenses have been covered through Medisafe, for more serious and expensive care, Medishield provides more traditional health insurance coverage.

(*Continued*)

Box 3. (*Continued*)

MEDIFUND is a health endowment fund. The state also has a providence fund that is financed through the government to cover subsidies for poor people. This protects the actuarial balance of Medishield so that it can be operated as a real insurance program not a mixed insurance and subsidy program like the national insurance programs in many countries.

ElderShield is a disability insurance program. A national severe disability insurance program was also introduced deal with special home care or health care needs in nursing homes of people who are disabled. This allows a better match between insurance instruments and long-term costs associated with known disabilities.

ElderCare Fund is a long term care program. Finally, to deal with the special custodial problems of the ageing of the population, an interest bearing fund was established to cover operating subsidies to voluntary nursing homes for elderly and other step-down care services. This operates as a hybrid between a pensions program and a long term care subsidy program by getting individuals to contribute towards their long term care cost throughout their working career.

Although this may seem like a gold-plated health insurance program, in reality it is one of the cheapest programs among developed countries. And despite low spending on health care, Singapore has better health outcomes than many countries that spend three or four times as much per capita on health care.

The Agency Role of Health Insurance as Payers

Before the 20th century, knowledge about the origins of poor health and effective interventions was limited. Most people approached health care as they did the consumption of other goods and services in the economy (see Figure 19). There was no expensive technology, and most serious conditions led to death. Loss of employment and burial costs were the most expensive part of illness. The economics of financing of health care was the same as the economics of most other consumer goods and services (Preker *et al.*, 2007a).

Industrialization and the scientific revolution changed all of this. As understanding about the causes, prevention, and treatment of illness deepened, interventions become more complex and expensive. Health care was no longer the exclusive domain of traditional healers. Other actors become involved. These included policymakers, specialized institutions involved in regulation and finance, complex organizations specialized in delivery of services (hospitals, clinics, diagnostics),

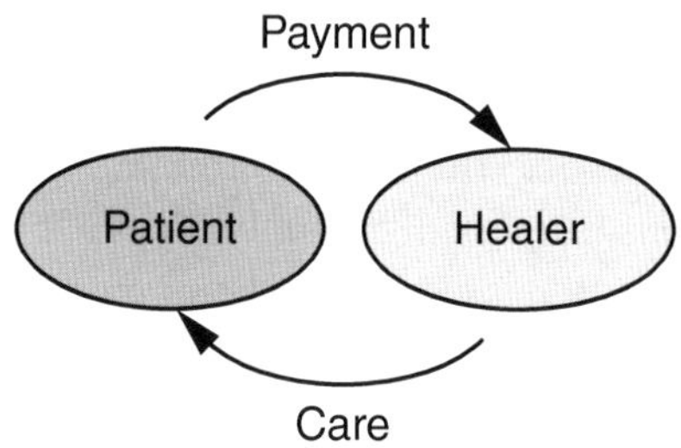

Figure 19. The principal and agent relationship between patients and healers

Source: Preker — adapted from Preker and Langenbrunner (2005).

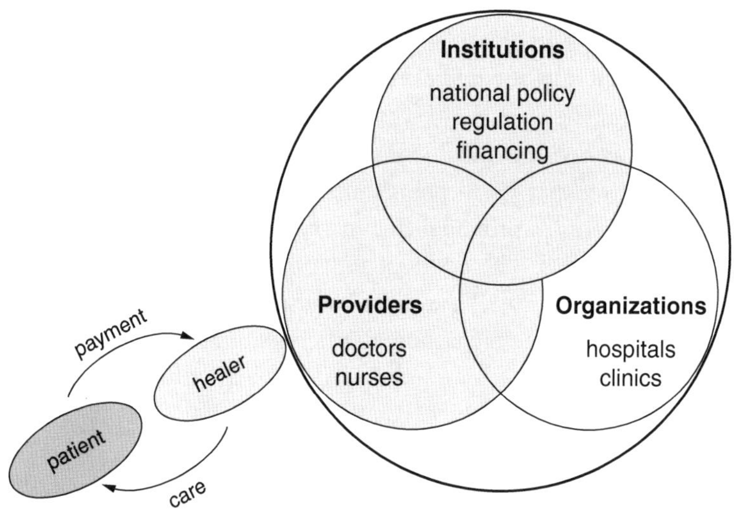

Figure 20. Functional differentiation

Source: Preker — adapted from Preker and Langenbrunner (2005).

and a range of specialized providers (doctors, nurses, pharmacists, dentists, allied health workers). Through this process, the health system slowly became differentiated beyond the simple patient–healer relationship (see Figure 20).

Can an individual not just buy health services in the same way he or she would go to the local market to buy bread, milk, or fruit? The answer is both yes and no. Much of the time, consuming health care is no different from consuming other goods and services. Patients have to inform themselves about their health problems and learn about which part of the health care system can help them. In doing this, they may ask for help when the problem is complex, just as the average consumer needs help when the TV, computer, or car breaks down. Modern technology forces people to become increasingly interdependent. Health care is not unique in this respect.

But in other respects, health care is very different. The fear of pain, disability, and death is different from the fear of living without a TV or computer for a few days. Asymmetry in information is often great between patients and their health care provider about both the causes and likely effectiveness of treatment. The cost can be catastrophic, often a third party — the government or an insurer — pays the bill. This can make individuals and households make decisions they would not make when consuming other goods and services. They usually need help from both a health care provider who can advise them what to do and from organizations that handle the dual complexities of financing and delivering high-level care.

By controlling the "purse strings," health insurance organizations are in a powerful position to create the needed incentives for providers to behave in ways that would secure not only the highest quality of care but also be responsive to the needs of the patients they serve. So why does this so often not happen?

Agency theory provides valuable insights into this question, highlighting both the strengths and weaknesses of health insurance organizations (Stiglitz, 1989). According to this theory, a principal (the hirer) contracts with an agent (the hired) to perform certain duties. The contract must be attractive to both principal and agent. From the agent's point of view, the contract must be at least as attractive as alternative available contracts (participation constraint) (Arrow, 1986). From the principal's point of view, the contract must be structured in such a way and have incentives to ensure that the agent will act in the principal's best interest (incentive compatibility constraint) (MacDonald, 1984).

Agency theory has been used extensively to examine the function of insurance as an intermediary (Eisenhardt, 1989; Bergen *et al.*, 1992). In theory, the principal–agent relationships work best when several preexisting conditions are met:

- Both the principal and the agent try to maximize their utility independently.
- Agents must try to maximize income but minimize effort.
- Pay must be correlated with outcomes and with effort by the agent.
- The principal must have perfect information about the agent's activities.
- The principal and the agent must enter voluntarily into a contract.

When the above conditions hold, the principal cannot exploit the agent because the contract is voluntary. And the agent cannot shirk or cheat if his pay is related to effort and outcomes. A well-designed contract maximizes the utility of this relationship for both the principal and the agent.

In practice, several constraints to agency theory are notable (Fama, 1980): Uncertainty of outcomes, information asymmetry, moral hazard, and adverse selection. Most outcomes depend on factors other than a single agent's actions. The effectiveness of any agent is often codependent on the action of others (Holmstrom, 1982). Success in terms of outcomes cannot be fully attributed to any single agent. In fact, outcomes often depend on the aggregate effort of a team, making it equally difficult to blame any one agent for failure. Because successful outcomes are difficult to attribute to any given action and sometimes difficult to observe, agents are often paid according to inputs (effort or time spent) or output (units of production) rather than true outcomes or results in terms of better health or financial protection against illness. However, in most instances, outcomes are not perfectly correlated with inputs or outputs, but instead result from both effort and some other unobservable variables (Stiglitz, 1989). Due to information asymmetry (one party knowing more about a given situation than the other party), principals often do not have full knowledge about the action that agents should or did take on their behalf (Arrow, 1986). For instance, when individuals use insurance to pay for risk-related events, special incentives are needed to ensure that the purchasing agents address: (1) Adverse selection problems that can arise by charging high-risk individuals higher subscription rates than low-risk individuals, and (2) moral hazard problems, in which an individual, once insured, increases risky behavior (Pauly, 1968). In both cases, the purchaser who is paid on the basis of input or output volumes rather than outcomes, has little incentive to execute policies that limit unnecessary utilization of services. Since the principal cannot observe an agent's every action, it is easy for the agent to use this information asymmetry to his advantage. Designing payment systems that share such risk in a balanced way between the principal and agent is, therefore, crucial to the success of contracting arrangements (Stiglitz, 1974; Shavell, 1979).

The most frequently described agency relationship in the health sector is the interaction between the patient and his or her doctor. Patient advocacy and ethical confidentiality dimensions are the most frequent focus of this type of agency relationship. Special agency issues arise when patients are not fully competent to make decisions about their own health care, as is the case of children, the mentally ill, or the physically impaired (Zweifel, 1994). Related issues arise when dealing with poor or disenfranchised population groups that financial or social constraints may prevent from exercising full autonomy.

In addition to the doctor–patient relationship, agency and contract theory have been extensively applied to the purchasing and contracting of health services (Evans, 1984; Dranove and White, 1985; McGuire *et al.*, 1988; Ryan, 1992a; 1992b; Mooney and Ryan, 1993; Propper, 1995; Levaggi, 1996). As agents, purchasers of health care confront many of the same problems of adverse selection, moral hazard, and information asymmetry that plague the insurance industry in general (Outreville, 1998; Dionne, 2000) and health insurance more specifically (Enthoven, 1988; Newhouse, 1993; Cutler and Zeckhauser, 2000). Similar observations have been made in low-income countries (Musgrove, 1996; Schieber, 1996; Preker *et al.*, 2001; Dror and Preker, 2002).

But under whose instructions should the people and organizations act in an agency role? How do they behave in reality? Do they really follow the orders they are given? When do they merely execute decisions made elsewhere and when do they exercise decision rights of their own? And when they exercise such decision rights, in whose interest do they act — for the individual patient, the population at large, politicians, health care professionals, or bureaucrats with their own vested interests? Answers to these questions provide insights into the role that health insurance programs may play as agents of public policy, health care providers and consumers of health care, as well as insights into the policies that must be put in place to make health insurance programs responsive to the needs of people who need health care and protection against the cost of illness.

At a deeper level lies a more basic question: Who should decide on what to spend resources when there are not enough for everyone and on what basis should such decisions be made? Patients, households, health care workers, health insurance agencies, civil society, and governments all have legitimate — but often conflicting — claims. The interest of the principal(s) involved and the extent of decision rights given to the health insurance agency can have a profound impact on the way priorities are set and executed, who benefits from collective purchasing arrangements, which providers are used, the payment mechanism, and the price paid for the resulting services. The impact on the health and human welfare of people affected by such decisions can be dramatic. These decisions often determine who lives or who dies.

In the health sector, health insurance agencies usually serve as agents for several powerful principals other than individual patients. Three important agency relationships are predominant. They are: (1) The relationship between health insurance agencies and individual health care providers (doctors, nurses, allied health care workers); (2) the relationship between health insurance agencies and various institutional actors (policymakers, regulators, insurers, and other funding agencies); and (3) the relationship between health insurance agencies and health care organizations (hospitals, clinics, ambulatory services). In reality, there are more than three agency relationships because the stakeholders under each of these three major categories all exert some influence over the health insurance agents. Policymakers, regulators, and funding agencies often have very different interests. Hospitals, clinics, and ambulatory services expect different services from health insurance agencies. While private (self-employed) doctors often have direct contact with health insurance agencies, nurses and other health care professionals do not. Their expectations will be different.

The greater the overlap in interest among the various powerful stakeholders, the more likely it is that the health insurance agencies will have a coherent authorizing environment that will coincide with the interest of the patients that they should also serve (Moore, 1995) and achieve optimal social welfare outcomes in health insurance (Mirrlees, 1974). When the overlap between stakeholders is small, there is a risk of poor performance by the agent and dissatisfaction on the part of the principals.

The objectives of the three organizational principals described above are often very different. Institutional-level actors are often closely aligned with the current political agenda, while health care organizations are more likely to be aligned with the bureaucratic interests of civil servants and the staff running them. Individual health care providers are usually aligned with the underlying social values of the society in which they work and professional concerns. These differences in perspective cause serious problems for all parties — for the principal, who does not have the undivided attention of a loyal agent (Ross, 1973), for the agent who has to serve several masters, and for the patient who is often left out of the discussion (see Figure 21).

Tensions often arise between health care providers who act on behalf of individual patients and policymakers and institutions that focus more on national and population-level issues. The purchaser is often pressured by individual health

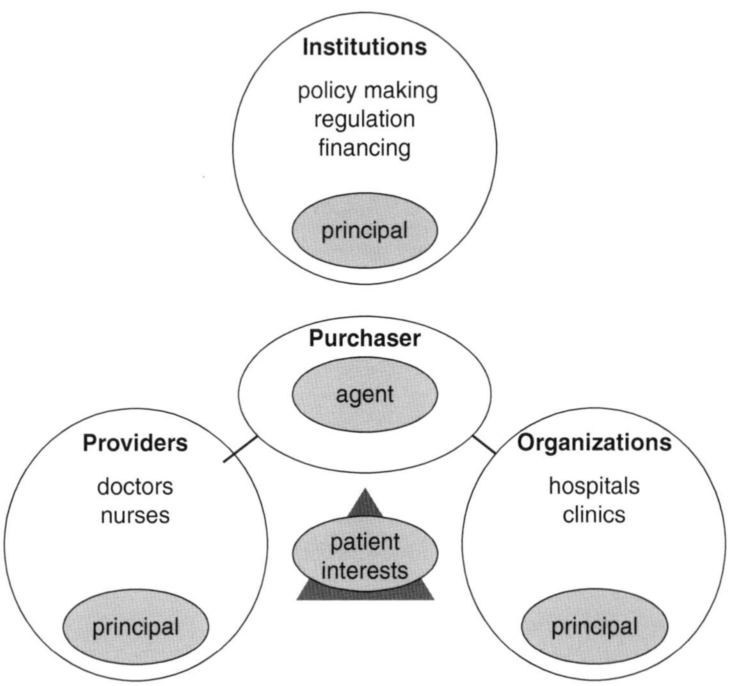

Figure 21. The multiplicitous agency relationship of health insurance

Source: Preker — adapted from Preker and Langenbrunner (2005).

care providers to finance the most recent and best quality of care for his or her patient. At the same time, the institutional actors in the MOH are often concerned about aggregate health outcomes and those in the ministry of finance (MOF) are concerned about the overall fiscal affordability of such care. This leads to an irreconcilable situation for the purchaser who has to act as an agent on behalf of two or more principals, each with a very different agenda.

Conclusions

The 20th century was an amazing period for financing health care, which gave billions of people throughout the world better financial protection against the impoverishing effects of illness and access to affordable health care. New funding mechanisms were introduced that allowed greater accountability and efficiency in the uses of scare resources.

At the same time, health-financing reforms become a trigger for disputes over ideological positions, tension between social classes and political vested interest groups. Health financing reforms were often a central part of political platforms, with governments winning and losing elections based on their support or opposition to such reforms.

Although a technically well-designed program may be superior to a poorly designed program, often political acceptability was more important to the final success of a health financing reform than its technical design and contents. Equally important is the implementation. There have been many examples of well-designed and politically successful health financing reforms that failed spectacularly due to poor implementation. The lessons learned during implementation, while beyond the scope this chapter, are critical and should be considered by countries intending to institute health care financing reforms.

Glossary

Ability to pay (ATP). A subjective social judgment usually based on a comparison of a proposed payment amount and a household's income or wealth. ATP for health insurance must be considered in the context of copayments and transaction costs. Reflects a value judgment about whether the household can obtain socially acceptable levels of other goods after paying for care or insurance. This concept of fairness may be an important consideration in designing a micro-insurance scheme and setting premiums.

Actual premium. The premium arrived at by estimating the average benefit payout, insurer administrative expenses, a safety margin for contingencies, and profits. If profits are at the competitive level the actual premium will be the lowest premium sustainable in the long run.

Adverse selection. Also called *antiselection.* Occurs when insurers are unable or are not permitted to charge premiums based on risk levels known to buyers of insurance; can arise either from asymmetric information (buyer knows risk and insurer does not) or regulation (buyer is not allowed to use information it knows in setting premiums). Adverse selection disturbs the operation of the insurance market. The lower-risk insured, knowing the likelihood of events but facing a price higher than that which reflects that risk, chooses not to insure; high risks facing a premium lower than one which reflects risk choose to overinsure. The insurer, having less information, accepts a contract that does not include premiums for low-risk events. Insured temporarily gain from the insurer's inability to distinguish "good" and "bad" risks. In the longer run, adverse selection results in low risks' exiting the insurance market. Providing asymmetric information incentivizes only people who expect to use above-average amounts of care.

Asymmetrical information. Parties to a transaction have uneven access to relevant information that governs an informed choice. Such asymmetry can result in an inequitable transaction in favor of the party with the most information, or it can result in the abandonment of the exchange.

Benefits package. A list of specific benefits agreed upon in the health insurance contract. While private insurance typically offers modules of benefits from which to choose, microinsurers may offer a standard package for simplicity and fairness.

Community rating. A method for determining insurance rates on the basis of the average cost across all insured regardless of risk level for providing health services in a specific geographic area. This method ignores the individual's medical history or the likelihood of the individual's using the services. All members of a community pay the same premium without considering individual health status or other determinants of expected demand. *Modified* or *adjusted community rating* allows premiums to vary with some characteristics relevant to risk (like age, gender, price levels in the locality, or family size) but not with health indicators or any other characteristics that affect demand.

Copayment. An insurance policy provision requiring the insured to pay a fixed monetary amount per unit of service of the type of care insured (e.g., $20 per doctor office visit).

Cream skimming (preferred risk selection). An exercise whereby an insurer charging identical premiums to different risks which it can identify selects only a part of a larger heterogeneous risk group ("preferred risks"). When the insurer reduces its loss ratio but continues to charge the same premium as when higher risks were covered, the insurer can retain a profit from cream skimming. This profit depends on the insurer's ability to distinguish several subgroups with different expected costs within the larger group and to predict the (lower) future health care expenditure of individuals in the preferred group. Basing insurance premiums on risk prevents cream skimming.

Cross-subsidies. Amounts effectively paid when some insurance buyers pay more than others relative to expected benefits. The wealthy members may pay higher premiums than the poor, but not use higher benefits, or the healthy may pay the same as the sick for lower expected benefits. The poor and the sick are said to receive cross-subsidies from the wealthy and the healthy.

Deductible. A provision requiring the insured to pay part of the loss before the insurer makes any payment under the terms of the policy. Deductibles typically are found in property, health, and automobile insurance contracts. The purpose of establishing deductibles is to eliminate small claims and reduce the average pure premium and administrative costs associated with claims handling. Deductibles can also reduce moral hazard by encouraging persons to be more careful with respect to the protection of their property and prevention of loss. Annual deductibles and waiting periods are the most common forms of deductibles in health insurance contracts.

Defined benefit pension. The amount, usually formula-based, guaranteed to each person who meets defined entitlement conditions. The formula usually takes into account the individual number of contribution or insurance years and the individual amount of earnings during the same period.

Delphi method or nominal group technique. A method of business forecasting that consists of panels of experts expressing their opinions on the future and then revising them in light of their colleagues' views so that bias and extreme opinions can be eliminated.

Demand. The amounts of a good or service that consumers seek to buy at different prices. *Solvent demand* implies the ability to pay (socially determined sufficient resources left over after payment for the good in question) as well as the willingness to pay. *Elasticity of demand* is a measure of the responsiveness of quantity demanded of a particular good or service to a change in its price. *Elastic demand* implies that as the price goes up the total expenditure falls. *Inelastic demand* implies that as the price goes up total expenditure also goes up. Necessities typically have inelastic demand (given an adequate income base). For example, the imperative to have an aching tooth removed means that the dentist is in a position of power to charge a high price; such dental services have inelastic demand, and it is unlikely that a lower price would attract people not suffering from toothache to have a tooth removed. The concept of "necessity" and therefore of what has an inelastic demand is cultural. In some cultures pre-natal care may not be considered a necessity. Demand for some procedures may be truncated in poor communities. *Truncated demand* means that, although the demand for surgery (for example) is inelastic and does not change with price, above a certain price it becomes zero. As half an operation is not an option, the demand is truncated because of poverty.

Experience rating. A system in which the insurance company evaluates the risk of individuals or groups by examining their health history and past claims experience when setting premium rates. *Modified experience rating* places limits on the extent to which rates may vary based on claims experience or health status.

Externalities. Benefits or costs with an impact beyond the parties to a transaction. That impact is not considered in the buy/sell decision and so is not reflected in the price. Pollution is an example of an external cost; safe waste disposal has external benefits.

Free-riding. Exists in health care when persons can benefit from a health care system without contributing to the system.

Managed care plan. A scheme that pools risks and directly provides or arranges for health care services. Use is controlled by mechanisms other than patient cost sharing.

Market failure. A condition in which a market does not efficiently allocate resources to achieve the greatest possible consumer and producer welfare. The four main market failures are public good, market control, externality, and imperfect information. In each case, a market acting without any government- imposed direction does not direct an efficient amount of resources into the production, distribution, or consumption of the good.

Medical underwriting. A process of detailed medical scrutiny of health status, medical history, and other information used by insurers to counter adverse selection and accomplish four specific goals: Ascertain the level of risk associated with the person or group applying for insurance, decide if a policy should be sold, decide the terms of the policy, and decide the premium level for the policy.

Moral hazard. An insurance-prompted change in behavior that affects the probability of a loss-producing event or the amount of benefits conditional on occurrence of an event. For example, an insured's demanding tests that would not be demanded in the absence of insurance (demand-side moral hazard). Provider-induced moral hazards include over-servicing (supply-side moral hazard).

Pay-as-you-go. Refers to a system of insurance financing under which total expenditure (benefit expenditure plus administrative expenditure) in a given period is met by income (contributions and other sources) from the same period. Pay-as-you-go financed insurance schemes do not accumulate reserves, except contingency reserves; surpluses and deficits translate into increases or decreases in the premium.

Premium. Fee paid by an insured to an insurance company in return for specified benefits. Under social insurance the premium is called *contribution.* See also *Contribution.*

Public goods. There are two aspects to public goods: It is difficult to prevent non-payers from consuming them (non-excludable), and their consumption by one party does not affect their consumption by others (non-rival). Vaccination is an example — those who do not pay and are not vaccinated cannot be excluded from enjoying the lower prevalence of disease; and the fact that they are healthy as a result does not affect another's ability to be healthier as a result of the program. Government usually provides public goods, because private businesses do so profitably.

Reinsurance. The transfer of liability from the primary insurer, the company that issued the contract, to another insurer, the reinsurance company. This mechanism allows a diversification of the risk and enlarges the risk-pooling base, thereby reducing the risk of insolvency for the reinsuring firm. However, reinsurance extends only to risk defined in the cession contract (called *treaty*). For example, a treaty to cede fluctuations in payouts will not cover the primary insurer against the financial risk of insolvency, for example, because of poorly run or unviable insurance.

Reserves. Funds set aside to meet unforeseeable liabilities (i.e., obligations that have not yet materialized) or statutory requirements, and stemming either from shareholders' capital or, in the case of mutuals, members' contributions and from accumulated surplus. Reserves are part of the own funds (in contrast to provisions that support liabilities to parties other than shareholders or other owners). A major financial management goal is to minimize reserves and thus maximize funds available for current use.

Risk. The probability or likelihood that a specified health event (for example, the occurrence of a disease or death) will occur to an individual or population group within a specific period of time.

Risk equalization. Provisions under which insurers with higher risk profiles receive a transfer of funds from insurers with lower risk profiles. Used in many countries with community rating schemes.

Risk pooling. A health system function in which collected health revenues are transferred to purchasing organizations, and the pooled risk of bearing the financial burden of future unexpected health services is shared and dispersed over large numbers of heterogeneous contributors. Insurers pool risk through reinsurance.

Risk rating. Calculation of health insurance premiums based on the risk of each client. When the premium is calculated based on the risk not of a single individual but of a group, this is called *community rating* or *group rating*. When the premium is set in relation to the client's income, this is called *income rating*.

Risk segregation. Each individual or member of an individual risk class faces a premium based only on that risk class and is not averaged with other distinctive risk classes.

Risk selection. A practice of excluding those who may present a higher risk for the insurer by making more, or more costly, claims.

Risk sharing. Individuals agree to split the cost of future risky events. Insurers share risk through reciprocal relationships and reinsurance. Loan guarantees and insurance are among the many ways of sharing risks.

Self insurance. A group pays all claims out of its own resources without sharing risk with an outside insurer. For example, a large employer providing coverage to workers under an arrangement in which it pays total claims regardless of their magnitude is self-insuring.

Social insurance. A compulsory insurance program that is shaped by broader collectively chosen objectives than just interest of each individual principal or agent, while retaining insurance principles that persons are insured against a definite risk.

Supplementary private health insurance. Provides coverage for health services that are not fully covered by a public program, such as luxury care, elective care, long-term care, dental care, pharmaceuticals, rehabilitation, alternative or complementary medicine, or superior amenity services in the hospital (differs per country).

Underwriting. The process by which the insurer decides what risks to cover and what premiums to charge. The profit objectives may conflict with what some regard as social obligation. For the reinsurer, underwriting considerations determine the risks of the primary insurer that can be accepted for reinsurance, and which the insurer will retain.

Waiting period. A mechanism that protects the insurer against adverse selection by delaying the period before an individual will be covered for any services he or she receives after the effective date of coverage. Access is restricted during the period of delay but not afterward. Policy premiums are still paid during this time.

Willingness to pay (*WTP*). Willingness to pay for health care or health insurance is affected by a household's income, tastes, and culture and measures the perceived benefit from the good or service. It differs from "ability to pay." There are commonly two ways to estimate WTP.

References

Arrow KJ. 1986. Agency and the Market. In *Handbook of Mathematical Economics* (eds.). Arrow KJ and Intriligator MD, Vol. 3, North-Holland: Amsterdam.

Bergen MS, Dutta Walker OC. 1992. Agency relationship in marketing: A review of the implications and applications of agency and related theories. *Journal of Marketing* 56(3): 1–24.

Chinitz D, Wasem J, Preker AS. 1997. Balancing Competition and Solidarity in Health Care Financing. In (ed.) Saltman RB, Figueras J, Sakallarides C. *Critical Challenges for Health Care Reform in Europe,* pp. 55–77. Copenhagen: World Health Organization/ European Observatory on Health Care Reform.

Cichon M, Newbrander W, Yamabana H, Weber A, Normand C, Dror DM, Preker, AS. 1999. *Modelling in Health Care Finance: A Compendium of Quantitative Techniques for Health Care Financing.* Geneva: International Labour Office /ISSA.

Dionne G. 2000. *Handbook of Insurance*. Boston, MA: Kluwer.

Dranove D, White, WD. 1985. Agency theory: New insight into the health care industry. *Journal of Medical Practice Management* 4(3): 165–169.

Dror D, Preker AS. (eds.). 2002. *Social Re-Insurance: A New Approach to Sustainable Community Health Financing.* Washington, DC: World Bank/International Labour Organisation.

Eisenhardt KM. 1989. Agency theory: An assessment and review. *Academy Management Review* 14(2): 57–74.

Enthoven AC. 1988. *Theory and Practice of Managed Competition in Health Care Finance*. Amsterdam: North Holland.

Evans RG. 1984. *Strained Mercy: The Economics of Canadian Health Care.* Toronto: Butterworth's.

Fama EF. 1980. Agency problems and the theory of the firm. *Journal of Political Economy* 88(2): 288–307.

Fuchs VR. 2005. Healthcare spending reexamined. *Annals of Internal Medicine* 143: 76–78.

Gottret P, Schieber GJ. 2006. *Health Financing Revisited: A Practitioner's Guide*. Washington, DC: World Bank.

Holmstrom, B. 1982. Moral hazard in teams. *Bell Journal of Economics* 13(2): 324–340.

Hsiao WC, Stason WB. 1979. Toward developing a relative value scale for medical and surgical services. *Health Care Financing Review* 1: 23–39.

Hsiao WC, Shaw RP. 2007. *Social Health Insurance for Developing Nations*. Washington, DC: World Bank.

Jacobs P, Rapoport J. 2002. *The Economics of Health and Medical Care,* 5th ed. Sudbury, MA: Jones and Bartlett Publishers.

Levaggi R. 1996. NHS contracts: An agency approach. *Health Economics* 5: 341–352.

MacDonald GM. 1984. New directions in the economic theory of agency. *Canadian Journal of Economics* 17(3): 415–440.

McGuire A, Henderson J, Mooney G. 1988. *The Economics of Health Care: An Introductory Text.* London and New York, NY: Routledge Kegan Paul.

Mirrlees J. 1974. "Notes on Welfare Economics, Information, and Uncertainty." In *Contribution to Economic Analysis* Balch, MS *et al.* (ed.). Amsterdam: North-Holland.

Mooney G, Ryan M. 1993. Agency in health care: Getting beyond first principals. *Journal of Health Economics* 37(12): 125–135.

Moore M. 1995. *Creating Public Value*. Boston, Mass.: Harvard University Press.

Musgrove P. 1996. *Public and Private Roles in Health: Theory and Financing Patterns*. Washington, DC: World Bank.

Newhouse JP. 1993. "*Free for All?: Lessons from the Rand Health Insurance Experiment.*" *Rand Corporation. Insurance Experiment Group*. Boston: Harvard University Press.

Outreville JF. 1998. *Theory and Practice of Insurance*. Boston, Mass.: Kluwer.

Pauly MV. 2007. Insights on Demand for Private Voluntary Health Insurance in Less Developed Countries. In (ed.). Preker AS, Scheffler RM, Bassett MC. *Private Voluntary Health Insurance in Development: Friend or Foe,* pp. 23–54. Washington, DC: World Bank.

Pauly MV. 1968. The economics of moral hazard: Comment. *The American Economic Review* 58(3) Part 1: 531–537.

Pauly MV, Blavin FE, Meghan, S. 2008. "Is There a Market for Voluntary Health Insurance in Developing Countries?" *NBER Working Paper No.* W14095, National Bureau for Economic Research (NBER), Cambridge, MA.

Pauly MV, Zweifel P, Scheffler RM, Preker AS, Bassett MC. 2006. Private health insurance in developing countries. *Health Affairs* 25(2): 369–379.

Preker AS, Lindner E, Chernichovsky D, Schellekens OP. 2013. *Scaling Up Affordable Health Insurance: Staying the Course*. Washington, DC: World Bank.

Preker A, Langenbrunner JC (ed.). 2005. *Spending Wisely: Buying Health Services for the Poor*. Washington, DC: World Bank.

Preker AS, Carrin G. (eds.). 2004. *Health Financing for Poor People: Resource Mobilization and Risk Sharing*. Health, Nutrition and Population Series. Washington, DC: World Bank/International Labour Organisation.

Preker AS, Liu X, Velenyi E, Baris E. (eds.). 2007a. *Public Ends, Private Means: Strategic Purchasing of Health Services*. Washington, DC: World Bank.

Preker AS, Zweifel P, Schellekens O. (eds.). 2010. *Global Marketplace for Private Health Insurance: Strength in Numbers*. Washington, DC: World Bank.

Preker AS, Scheffler R, Schellekens O. (2007b). *Private Voluntary Health Insurance in Development: Friend or Foe*? Washington, DC: World Bank.

Propper C. 1995. Agency and incentive in the NHS internal market. *Social Science & Medicine* 40(12): 1683–1690.

Reinhardt UE, Hussey PJ, Anderson GF. 2004. U.S. healthcare spending in an international context. *Health Affairs* 23: 10–25.

Rockefeller Foundation. 2014. *Health & Well-Being: Science, Medical Education and Public Health.* The Rockefeller Foundation Centennial Series. New York: Rockefeller Foundation.

Ross S. 1973. The economic theory of agency: The principal's problem. *American Economic Review* 63(2): 134–139.

Ryan M. 1992a. *The Economic Theory of Agency in Health Care: Lessons from Non-economists for Economists.* Discussion Paper No 03/92. Aberdeen, UK: University of Aberdeen, Health Economic Research Unit.

Ryan M. 1992b. *The Agency Relationship in Health Care: Identifying Areas for Future Research.* Discussion Paper No 02/92. Aberdeen, UK: University of Aberdeen, Health Economic Research Unit.

Schellekens OP, Lindner ME, Lange JMA, Van der Gaag J. 2007. *A New Paradigm for Increased Access to Healthcare in Africa.* Issues Brief, International Finance Corporation (IFC), Washington, DC.

Schieber G. (ed.). 1996. *Innovations in Health Financing.* Washington, DC: World Bank.

Shavell S. 1979. "Risk sharing and incentives in the principal and agent relationship. *Bell Journal of Economics* 10: 5–73.

Smith PC, Preker AS, Light DW, Richards S. 2005. Role of Markets and Competition. In (ed.). Figueras J, Robinson R, Jakubowski E. *Purchasing to Improve Health Systems Performance,* 102–121. Buckingham, UK: Open University Press.

Stiglitz JE. 1974. Incentives and risk sharing in sharecropping. *Review of Economic Studies* 41(2): 219–255.

Stiglitz JE. 1989. Principal and Agent. In (ed.). Eat-well J. *Allocation, Information and Markets,* London: Macmillan.

The Lancet Commission on Investing in Health. 2013. Global health 2035: A world converging within a generation. *The Lancet.* Special Issue: 2013.

WHO. 2012. *World Health Report 2012.* Geneva: WHO.

World Bank. 1993. *The World Development Report: Investing in Health.* Washington: World Bank.

World Bank. 2014. *World Bank Group Support to Health Financing.* Washington: World Bank.

Zweifel P. 1994. Agency relationship in psychotherapy: An economic analysis. *Social Science & Medicine* 39(5): 621–628.

Alternative Financing Strategies for Universal Health Coverage

Joseph Kutzin

Coordinator, Health Financing Policy
Department of Health Systems Governance and Financing
World Health Organization, 20 Avenue Appia, 1211 Geneva 27
Switzerland

Winnie Yip

Professor of Health Policy and Economics
Blavatnik School of Government
10 Merton Street, Oxford OX1 4JJ
United Kingdom

Cheryl Cashin

Senior Program Director
Results for Development Institute
1111 19th Street, NW, Suite 700
Washington, DC 20036, USA

Many countries have identified Universal Health Coverage (UHC) as the goal for their health systems, and health financing reforms are at the core of strategies to move in this direction. While there is no one "best" financing strategy that applies in every context, this chapter synthesizes both theory and practice into principles that can be used to guide country progress with their financing reforms, while also highlighting pitfalls to avoid on the path to UHC. It begins with the conceptual underpinnings of both UHC and health financing policy, arguing that the emergence of UHC after the Second World War had profound implications for public policy on health coverage, particularly with regard to the role of general government revenues and the weakening of contributory-based entitlement. This is followed by a synthesis of lessons with a particular focus on low- and middle-income countries (LMICs), including the importance of increasing reliance on compulsory revenue sources raised through diverse mechanisms, reducing fragmentation in pooling arrangements and addressing inefficiencies through strategic purchasing and effective provider payment methods (PPMs). We then address a key challenge facing LMICs — extending effective access and financial protection to the informal sector who comprise the majority of the population.

Keywords: Universal Health Coverage; Health Financing.

Introduction/Overview of Chapter

Background

Universal Health Coverage (UHC) has gained great attention among policymakers and academics since the publication of the World Health Organization's (WHO) World Health Report in 2010 (WHO, 2010a). Health system reform plans from Indonesia to Mexico to Nigeria to Thailand have used UHC as a justification, often grounding this in constitutional or legal guarantees that have long gone unfulfilled. However, the specific health financing approaches used or proposed as part of these plans vary greatly across countries. While this is consistent with the idea that there is no blueprint strategy that applies to all countries, it is a concern where the label of "UHC" is applied but the proposed strategy is not consistent with the concept of UHC or fails to incorporate core lessons from experience. For purposes of this chapter, we use a definition of financing for UHC derived from the World Health Report (WHO, 2010, p. 6):

"Financing systems need to be specifically designed to:

- Provide all people with access to needed health services (including prevention, promotion, treatment and rehabilitation) of sufficient quality to be effective;
- Ensure that the use of these services does not expose the user to financial hardship."

Taken literally, these conditions cannot be fully achieved anywhere. Even where all people are protected from financial risk, there is always some gap between the need for and use of services, and quality often varies. To transform UHC from a mere aspiration to a practical concept requires identifying the specific goals embedded within the definition and orienting policy toward *progress* on these goals. Hence, we reframe the goal as *moving toward UHC*, meaning taking actions to reduce the gap between the need for and use of services, improve quality and improve financial protection. Further, UHC implies that these goals be assessed at the level of the entire system or population rather than within specific financing schemes (Kutzin, 2013).

The agenda of health system reform to progress toward UHC extends beyond health financing. For example, while health financing actions directly affect financial protection, so do actions to improve the availability and price of medicines.

Similarly, many parts of the system (service delivery, human resources, medicines, technologies, financing) influence equity in service use relative to need. And financing is typically only a complementary instrument for influencing quality — reforms in service delivery, human resources/medical education, medicines, technology and information play the leading role. The focus of this chapter is on financing reforms, but key linkages between financing and other aspects of the system, particularly service delivery, will be noted as relevant throughout the chapter.

Key messages

It is not relevant to define a single, "best" model of health financing for UHC because systems are dynamic and path-dependent.[1] Thus, the best option for a country in a given circumstance may not be relevant for another country. The issue is not what specific strategy is best in an abstract sense, but rather, given where a country is today, what are promising directions to take to enable progress on the UHC goals. That being said, however, there are important lessons learned from both theory and practice that provide useful principles to guide progress and avoid well-known pitfalls in health financing policy. These lessons are reflected throughout the chapter, but we note them here in brief:

- Countries should seek to move toward predominant reliance on compulsory funding sources (general tax revenues, earmarked payroll taxes, or a combination), as voluntary mechanisms suffer from serious shortcomings. Indeed, no country has attained universal population coverage based on a system organized around voluntary prepayment. Moving toward compulsory sources is a major challenge for fiscally constrained countries that are typified by large shares of the population who are not in regular salaried employment. We address this context head-on in the chapter, with particular attention to policy options for countries in such contexts.
- Countries that have made significant progress toward UHC have had the benefit of a strong political commitment to UHC, reflected in the prioritization of health in their national budgets. All potential government revenue sources for the health sector have potential consequences for other sectors in the broader economy, however. The efficiency and equity impacts of alternative tax instruments (e.g., income tax, corporate tax, value-added tax) are highly context-specific and arise from the combined impact of all tax measures. In turn, their implications for

[1] In this context, "path dependent" means that each country already has its health financing arrangements that have developed and changed over a period of years. When embarking on a new reform agenda, such as one explicitly oriented to UHC, these arrangements provide the unique "starting point" for the reforms, with decisions on what to do next contingent, at least in part, on what is already in place.

social welfare need to be considered in concert with the level and distribution of benefits made available through the spending they finance.

- There is a general trend toward greater diversification of revenue sources, including a diminishing role for payroll tax funding. This is a practical consequence of the "ideology" of UHC. With the move toward UHC, entitlement to health coverage is being delinked from employment, and from direct contributions more generally. On the practical side, wage-linked contributions cannot generate a sufficient revenue base, both in high-income countries (because of aging populations and macroeconomic concerns regarding increasing wage-based taxation) and also in low- and middle-income countries (LMICs) (because of low participation rates in formal sector employment).
- Whatever the level of prepaid funds, countries should seek to maximize the redistributive capacity of these funds by reducing or eliminating fragmentation in pooling arrangements to the extent possible.
- Countries cannot simply spend their way to UHC; the way the funds flow through the system and whether spending can be matched to priority programs, populations, and services also matters. Attention to addressing inefficiencies is essential to sustain progress, with purchasing/provider payment the central instrument in the health financing armamentarium to achieve this purpose.
- Effective reform requires policy coherence, meaning a focus on alignment of policy measures across the financing system as well as alignment with the rest of the health system A narrow focus on single-instrument "magic bullets" (such as social health insurance, user fee introduction or elimination, results-based financing (RBF), diagnosis-related groups (DRGs), insurance competition, etc.) will be inadequate and may do more harm than good.

Overview of chapter

Following this introduction, Section "Core concepts and the implications of UHC for health financing policy" provides a deeper exploration of the underlying concepts of UHC and health financing policy, as well as the implications of UHC for public policies on health coverage. Section "Health financing for UHC: Lessons learned and core challenges synthesizes lessons learned and core challenges" in health financing for UHC based on global experience. This is followed by a systematic exploration in Section "Alternative approaches to financing for UHC in the context of high informality" of financing options for UHC in the context of high labor force informality, distinguishing alternatives broadly by the basis for entitlement (contributory vs. non-contributory) and defining specific choices within these categories based on empirical experience. We conclude in Section "Conclusions" with a derivation of adaptable principles to guide financing reforms, pitfalls to avoid, and core public policy questions that need to be addressed.

Core Concepts and the Implications of UHC for Health Financing Policy

Health financing policy and UHC: Conceptual approach

Health financing policy and related reforms are best understood in terms of specific functions and policies, rather than by historical labels (e.g., Beveridge, Bismarck) that are largely linked to the main source of funds (Kutzin, 2001). Regardless of the labels attached to them, health financing arrangements in all countries include:

- Revenue raising — Sources of funds, contribution methods used, and mechanisms for their collection.
- Pooling — Arrangements for the accumulation of prepaid funds on behalf of a population within the system.
- Purchasing — Transfer of funds to providers on behalf of a population, incorporating both provider payment mechanisms and the organizational/institutional structure of purchasers.
- Benefit design and rationing policies — Entitlements and obligations of the population with regard to health services, including measures such as patient cost sharing (user fees/copayments), service exclusions and waiting lists, which countries use to ration access.
- Stewardship of the financing system — Government's role in orchestrating the financing arrangements, including governance of health financing agencies, regulation of markets and information provision.

The WHO definition of UHC noted above embodies three specific goals: Equity in service use, sufficient quality, and financial protection. The aim of financing (and other system) reforms is thus to move systems toward these goals[2] by considering the ways that reforms can *influence* progress. Based on the health financing functions, this has led (Kutzin, 2013) to the specification of intermediate objectives of financing for UHC:

- Equity in the distribution of health system resources.
- Efficiency in system organization, service delivery, and administrative arrangements.
- Transparency and accountability of the system to the population.

---

[2]While it is not the purpose of this chapter to justify UHC as a goal, we note that this specification is consistent within a wider framework on health systems performance in which financial protection is an overall goal of health systems, and equity in use and quality are intermediate objectives with regard to the goals of improving health (overall level and equity in health) and responsiveness (WHO, 2000; 2007; Murray and Frenk, 2000).

A detailed functional analysis of a country's health financing system is needed to provide a sound basis for understanding how it is organized and how it functions, which in turn can support a diagnosis of the ways in which it may be contributing to under-performance relative to the UHC goals and intermediate objectives. This requires not only exploring the organization of each "sub-function" but also their alignment/misalignment with each other as well as across a range of different financing schemes that might exist in a given country.

Foundations for public policy on health coverage: From Bismarck to UHC

UHC is not a new concept. In many ways, it emerged after the Second World War, underpinned in many countries by a broad value consensus such as *social cohesion* in European countries (Figueras *et al.*, 2012) and *human security* in Japan (Reich *et al.*, 2011). A *right* to health or health care is reflected in the text of the WHO Constitution (WHO, 1948) and the Universal Declaration of Human Rights (United Nations, 1948). It is also reflected in many national constitutions, for example the constitutions of South Africa (1996) and Mexico (2013) declare that everyone has the right to access to health care services.

The advent of UHC has marked a change in the underlying rationale for public policy on health service coverage. Prior to this, beginning in 1883 with Bismarck in Germany, followed by several other European countries and Japan over the next 40 years, the motivation was different. These countries sought to support industrial development through a healthier workforce with a concern to mitigate growing political pressures from labor unions (Saltman and Dubois, 2004; Ikegami *et al.*, 2011). The coverage policies introduced — health insurance for workers in the formal sector of the economy funded by mandatory contributions of employers and employees — were consistent with these underlying motivations. It meant, however, that large shares of the population, particularly those working in agriculture or otherwise outside of the formal/industrial economy, did not have any explicit form of entitlement.

The shift from "workers" to "people" as those entitled to coverage after the Second World War had important implications for health financing policy.[3] In particular, it meant that there had to be a shift away from a purely contributory

[3] In fact, some countries moved in this direction earlier. In Hungary in 1920 and the USSR in 1937, health services were made available to the entire population, financed either wholly from general tax revenues or a combination of these with social insurance contributions. New Zealand took similar measures between 1939 and 1941 to extend service coverage to its entire population (Abel-Smith, 1987).

funding mechanism and basis for entitlement. More specifically, the use of revenues from general public budgets were needed to provide all or nearly all of the funds, as is the case in the British NHS established in 1946 (Abel-Smith, 1987), or to supplement compulsory health insurance contributions to ensure coverage for the poor and others outside of the formal sector of the economy, as in Japan, which achieved universal population affiliation with its health insurance system in 1951 (Ikegami *et al.*, 2011).

Much of the advice provided to LMICs in the 1980s and 1990s on health financing encouraged them to initiate compulsory health insurance for formal sector workers. Such recommendations (e.g., Akin *et al.*, 1987; Griffin and Shaw, 1995) were implicitly based on (or at least consistent with) the pre-war rationale for public policy on health coverage, combined with a politically hopeful (or naïve) expectation that such coverage programs would be fully self-funding and thus enable public subsidies for health services to be captured by the poor. Unfortunately, this approach tended to concentrate even greater shares of public subsidies on the formal sector population. In 1992 in Thailand, for example, public spending per person covered was 916 baht in the civil servants scheme, 480 baht in the scheme for private sector workers, and only 214 baht in the scheme for low-income persons (Hsiao, 1993).

Such recommendations were also consistent with the view that the way coverage had expanded in currently high-income countries, starting with the formal sector and then gradually expanding, was "the way," and that LMICs should proceed down this path. In retrospect, this approach not only neglected the change in the underlying public policy rationale motivating action on health coverage, it also failed to account for another contextual shift: the development and diffusion of medical technology. In 1900 in Europe, governments were simply not faced with life-or-death choices as to which population groups would have preferred access to the latest medications. But by the 1990s if not before, the health Minister of every country in the world, including LMICs, had to confront this. By initiating explicit coverage with the formal sector, LMIC governments provided privileged access to such technologies to a relatively small part of their populations that were both economically advantaged and well organized. As a result, those initially covered pushed for more subsidies and benefits, not for the extension of the same entitlements to the rest of the population. This different medical context meant that the political response to following the historical (pre-war) pattern of European health coverage expansion in the post-war setting of today's LMICs exacerbated rather than compensated for underlying social inequalities with regard to health and health service use (Savedoff, 2004; Kutzin, 1997; González-Rossetti, 2002). Such approaches tended to segment health financing and often service delivery systems by social class and have proven very resistant to change, as evidenced by the inability of countries such as Mexico (Knaul *et al.*, 2012) and Thailand (Prakongsai *et al.*, 2009) to unify their systems. But at least in these two countries, if not others as well, such explicit inequalities proved politically unsustainable, stimulating UHC-oriented reform agendas that began to delink entitlement from contribution (and labor force status) and rely predominantly on general government budget revenues as the main source of funds for coverage expansion.

Health Financing for UHC: Lessons Learned and Core Challenges

An adaptable approach to health financing policy

In addition to the specification of goals and intermediate objectives, as well as the functional approach to understanding health financing arrangements in any country, policy analyses and recommendations need to be guided by an approach to applying these concepts. For this, three factors need to be considered that, broadly, address the following questions:

(1) Where are we going?
(2) From where are we starting?
(3) How far and how fast can we go?

The first issue is to orient the direction of reforms to specific policy objectives. For these, countries can be guided by the broad UHC goals and intermediate objectives, tailoring these to their specific circumstances (for example, how do problems of equity in service use, inefficiency, or transparency manifest themselves in the country?). The second question is grounded in a fundamental policy reality: the starting point for any reform is the system that currently exists in the country. Understanding this requires a detailed functional analysis of the country's health financing arrangements. Combining these first two questions can lead to conclusions (or plausible hypotheses) with regard to how the current organization and operation of health financing in the country is contributing to performance shortcomings with regard to the UHC goals and intermediate objectives. In addition to these analyses, the third question speaks to the context — the factors largely outside the control of health policymakers — that have implications for both what can be implemented and what can be attained in terms of progress towards UHC. While many of these are country-specific, two critical contextual factors are relevant in all countries: The country's fiscal capacity (in particular, its ability to generate tax revenues) and the structure of its public administration (Kutzin, 2008).

This approach leads to the conclusion that the question of whether or not there is a "best model" for health financing is not particularly relevant. Even though the UHC goals and intermediate objectives are broadly shared, the starting point and context for health financing is unique to each country. In addition, the specific ways that performance problems manifest themselves also vary across countries. The "right reforms" for any country to move towards UHC depend critically on these factors. This recognition led the authors of the World Health Report to write that "Health financing strategy needs to be home-grown — pushing in the direction of universal coverage out of the existing terrain." (WHO, 2010, pp. 90–91). However, this conclusion does not mean that every country is on its own, with little of value to be gleaned from experience elsewhere. In fact, there are important lessons from experience that can help one country avoid the mistakes of others, and that can provide principles to guide the policies and actions that aim to reform and align health financing sub-functions to support progress toward UHC (Kutzin, 2012).

Lessons from experience: Revenue raising, pooling, purchasing and benefits

- *Compulsion, subsidization, and adverse selection*

All countries that are recognized to have made substantial progress toward UHC — where the entire population is able to use publicly guaranteed services with high degrees of financial protection — rely predominantly on compulsory funding sources. While not a perfect reflection of this, Figure 1 shows the general pattern, which is that where governments spend more on health, people have less need to pay out-of-pocket at the time of use. It is well known that high levels of out-of-pocket payment are associated with higher risk of catastrophic and impoverishing health payments, and that the need to pay at the point of use exacerbates inequalities in service use.

Similarly, relatively few countries rely on voluntary prepayment to provide significant resources for their health systems. Figure 2 shows that in only five countries in 2012, voluntary health insurance (VHI)[4] accounted for more than 20% of total health spending. Among high-income countries other than the USA, VHI plays a negligible role with the exceptions being where it provides an explicitly complementary function (covering patient cost sharing in the statutory system, as in France and Slovenia) or where it offers supplemental benefits beyond those in

[4]VHI means that the decision to become insured is not mandated by government but is a choice made by an individual or an entity on behalf of that individual (e.g., an employer). VHI can be managed by private commercial companies, NGOs, "communities," and even governments.

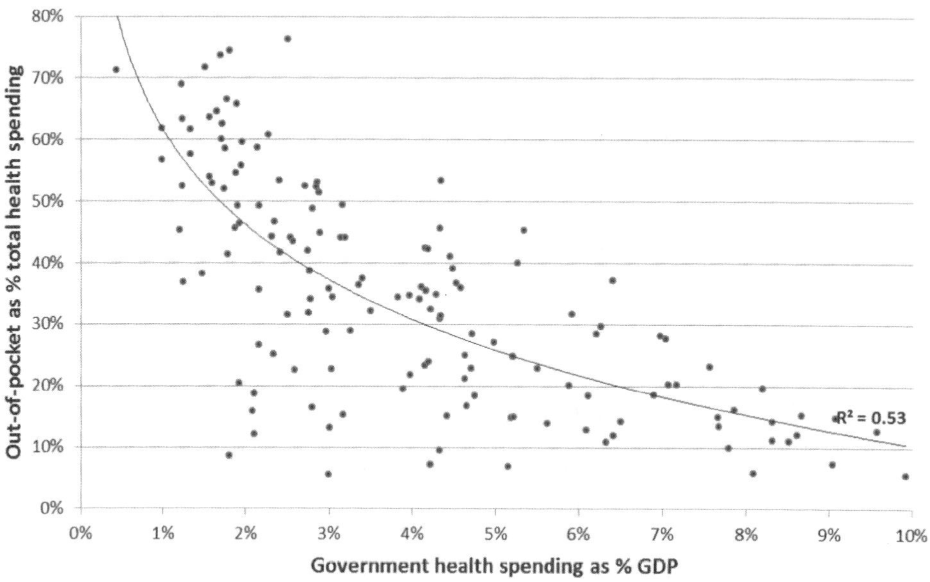

Figure 1. Relation between levels of government and out-of-pocket health spending, 2012

Source: WHO (2014). Excludes countries with population less than 600,000. Also excludes 10 countries where external funds accounted for more than 40% of estimated total health spending.

the main compulsory system (such as covering private "amenity beds" in hospitals in Ireland and Germany) (Mossialos and Thomson, 2004).

The minimal role for voluntary prepayment is not an accident; it reflects both theory and experience with regard to the shortcomings of voluntary approaches. All forms of VHI suffer from *adverse selection* (Cutler and Zeckhauser, 1998). Individuals who know they have worse health status are more likely to enroll, and so over time this makes health insurance more expensive than the average actuarial cost of a premium across the entire population. Insurers respond by raising premiums, driving more people out of the market. Ultimately, those who need the coverage most are least able to afford it. This runs counter to the objective of pooling, which is to maximize the redistributive capacity of prepaid funds from the healthy to the sick.

Writing in the aftermath of the failed effort in the USA to pass legislation to create universal insurance coverage in the mid-1990s, Victor Fuchs wrote that:

> "No nation achieves universal coverage without subsidization and compulsion. Both elements are essential. Subsidies without compulsion will not work; indeed, they could make matters worse since the healthy flee from the subsidized common pool, only to return when they expect to use a great deal of care. Compulsion without

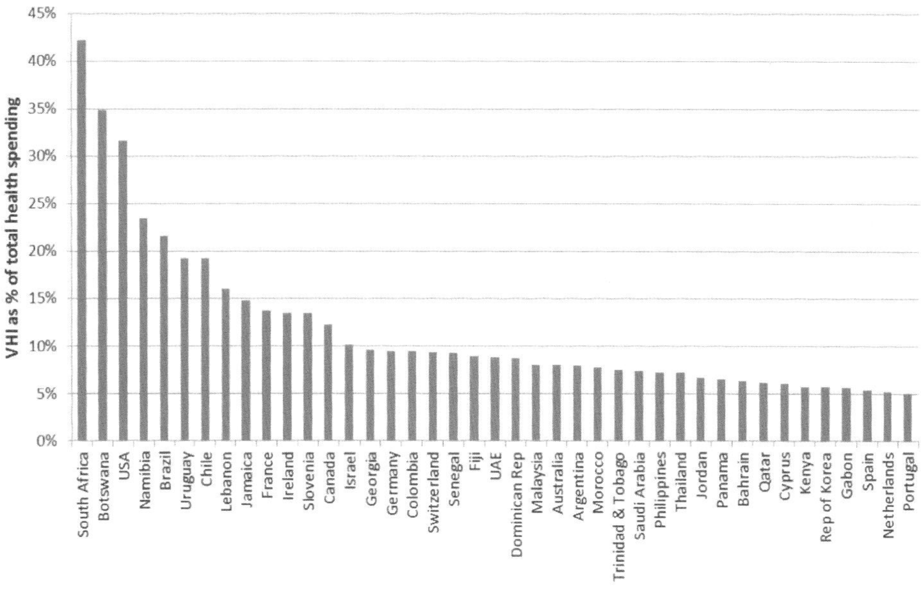

Figure 2. Countries in which VHI accounted for more than 5% of total health spending, 2012
Source: WHO (2014). Excludes countries with population less than 600,000.

subsidies would be a cruel hoax for the millions of poor and sick who cannot afford health insurance." (Fuchs, 1996, pp. 188–189).

This phenomenon has been observed around the world, independent of a country's level of income, or whether the ownership of the insurance is commercial, not-for-profit, "community," government, or where, for example, people outside of formal employment are allowed to voluntarily prepay into a national social health insurance (SHI) scheme (Bitran, 2014; Baeza and Packard, 2006). It is simply the nature of a VHI market.

The lesson is both simple and clear: moving toward fulfillment of the "Fuchs conditions" (compulsion and subsidization) in health financing is a guiding principle for health financing policy oriented toward UHC. It is also the fundamental reason why many fiscally constrained LMICs face such difficulties in making progress. Current fiscal challenges, however, should not lead countries or analysts to believe in magic, however, such as expecting that because a VHI program is owned by a not-for-profit entity such as a local community, it will achieve high rates of coverage. Both theory and evidence (see, for example, Acharya *et al.*, 2012) are consistent on this reality. Thus, moving towards UHC in many countries must include strategies to increase the share of total health spending coming from compulsory (i.e., taxes, whether direct or indirect) sources.

- *Delinking entitlement from contribution and the critical role of general budget revenues*

While it is commonly assumed that in countries where entitlement to health coverage has been linked to employment, wage-based contributions (payroll taxes) many of these countries combine these with general budget funding, and several have increased reliance on the latter in recent years (Busse *et al.*, 2004; Sheiman *et al.*, 2010). As noted previously, this has been driven in part by the shift toward UHC as the underlying rationale for public policy on health coverage, with entitlement for each person in society rather than only for those in the labor force, and in part by the practical realities of different tax instruments in each country. Broadly, high-income countries are facing the demographic challenge of aging populations, with a shrinking share of working-age adults to provide a base for employment-linked contributions. In lower-income countries, the small share of employment in the formal sector from which payroll taxes feasibly can be collected does not provide a sufficient revenue base. Hence, moving toward predominant reliance on compulsory sources requires a focus on general budget revenues in most countries.

In France, for example, until the end of the 1990s, funding for the statutory health system depended almost exclusively on payroll contributions from employers (63%) and employees (32%). Since 1998, most of the employee payroll contribution has been substituted by an earmarked tax, the General Social Contribution (CSG), which is levied not only on wage income but also income from financial assets and investments, pensions, unemployment benefits, disability benefits and gambling. The CSG is now one of the main sources of funding for the insurance system (37%). In addition, specific taxes on tobacco and alcohol consumption and on the pharmaceutical industry complement the revenue base. However, while this change has widened the revenue base for health coverage, it has not increased the actual amount of revenue collected (Chevreul *et al.*, 2010).

In Japan, universal coverage is 49% financed by social insurance contributions, 37% by general taxes (25% national, 12% local), and 14% by out-of-pocket contributions (Ikegami and Maeda, 2014). In Ghana, although government sources only contribute about 53% of total health spending, the sources are diversified and mostly from general revenue. In addition to supply-side subsidies from general budget funding, Ghana's National Health Insurance Scheme is funded by an earmarked portion of the value-added tax (VAT) (more than 75% of the revenues of the scheme), social security contributions (18%), as well as grants, investment income, and premiums paid by non-exempt individuals such as self-employed and informal sector workers (NHIA, 2012). Similarly, the financing reforms in Mexico and Thailand introduced during the 2000s were entirely funded from general budget revenues, with entitlement made available to all individuals who were not already affiliated with one of the contributory social security schemes for formal sector workers (Prakongsai *et al.*, 2009; Knaul *et al.*, 2012). A review of reforms in 9 LMICs also pointed to the increased reliance on general tax revenues to fund coverage expansions (Lagomarsino *et al.*, 2012).

Priority for health in the government budget using the (context-specific) right mix of sources

Figure 1 showed that the dependence of systems on out-of-pocket spending (OOPS) falls as the level of public spending on health (as a share of GDP) increases. More specifically, where public spending on health is less than 4% (or even 5%) of GDP, very few countries depend on OOPS for less than 20% of total health spending, a threshold below which the risk of catastrophic spending is generally small.[5] In an accounting sense, public spending on health is a product of two factors, as shown in this simple equation:

$$\frac{\text{GGHE}}{\text{GDP}} = \frac{\text{GGE}}{\text{GDP}} * \frac{\text{GGHE}}{\text{GGE}}$$

GGHE = general government health expenditure
GGE = general government expenditure
GDP = gross domestic product

Put another way, in any year, the level of public spending on health is the product of a country's fiscal capacity (proxied by GGE/GDP) and the priority it gives to health in public resource allocation (GGHE/GGE).[6] So to move in the direction of greater reliance on compulsory sources of funds for the health system, both fiscal context and government priorities matter. And in fact, most countries that have made significant progress toward UHC have had both the benefit of strong macroeconomic conditions and commitment to priority for health in the budget. That being said, macroeconomic conditions are outside the scope of influence of the health sector, and even the government may have limited scope to substantially increase overall tax revenues in the short run. Policy priorities are

[5] A cross-country analysis has suggested that once OOPS are reduced to below 15% of total health spending in a country, very few households experience catastrophic expenditures, as measured using a threshold of 40% of non-subsistence household consumption (Xu *et al.*, 2003). Hence, a 20% OOPS share of total health spending is a more generous threshold (though more realistic for most countries) for increased risk of catastrophic costs.

[6] In the calculation of GGHE and GGE, compulsory social insurance contributions (and expenditures from these) are included as part of government, in line with public finance logic that recognizes such contributions as a form of direct taxation.

less subject to these contextual factors and indeed vary greatly across countries. In 2012, for example, the average share of public spending devoted to health was 11.5%, but ranged from 1.5% in the lowest (Myanmar) to 28% in the highest (Costa Rica). Within this range were low-income countries that have very high priority to health (e.g., Rwanda, Liberia and Malawi allocated more than 17% of public spending to health) and some high-income countries with the reverse (e.g., Qatar and Cyprus devoted less than 7%) (WHO, 2014).[7]

A review of experience with reforms for UHC in 11 countries (Maeda *et al.*, 2014) found that the priority for health in the government budget has been maintained or increased in those countries that have made progress expanding coverage. The scope for increasing the share of the total budget allocated to health will be limited in part by the share of the budget that is actually discretionary, or not already accounted for by earmarks, other legislated expenditures, and debt payments. Civil servant wage spending in particular has been treated as a nondiscretionary expenditure, often crowding out government spending in other priority areas. Public debt and debt servicing (interest payments) are also major constraints. Debt relief initiatives, such as the Highly Indebted Poor Countries (HIPC) Initiative of the IMF and World Bank, which reduce the volume of debt payments a government makes and thus reduce nondiscretionary expenditures, provide an important opportunity to create room for more health spending.

To secure priority for health in the budget, some countries have dedicated a specific tax or a share of government revenue to be earmarked for health, such as Ghana's earmarked of the revenue from the VAT to fund the National Health Insurance Scheme or the earmarking of taxes on alcohol and/or tobacco consumption ("sin taxes"). Increasing budget allocations have been achieved in some countries without specific financial commitments (e.g., earmarks), however, and earmarking and budget targets do not always ensure overall health funding is protected (Maeda *et al.*, 2014). Earmarked payroll taxes are considered to introduce inefficiencies in the economy by distorting labor market decisions, and other earmarking is considered to impose constraints on fiscal policy, which reduce flexibility and possibly allocative efficiency (Tandon and Cashin, 2010). In practice, the effectiveness of earmarking taxes or revenue for health appears to be mixed in terms of increasing overall funding or improving its stability. In some countries, the earmarked allocations for health have been offset by reductions in other parts of the health budget (Sheiman *et al.*, 2010). On the other hand, the extent to which earmarking for health creates inefficiencies in budget allocations has not been studied. One study of 11 countries committed to UHC found that only three (Brazil, France, and Ghana) have some form of explicit budget earmarks.

---

[7]The calculations exclude countries with population less than 600,000 people.

Other countries that have made significant progress toward UHC have done so without such earmarks, but have consistently kept their budgetary allocation to health relatively high (Maeda *et al.*, 2014). In Japan, for example, the Ministry of Finance and the Ministry of Health, Labor and Welfare negotiate to set the fiscal subsidy each year, and the fee schedule and payment systems are adjusted every two years to meet the changing fiscal envelope (Ikegami and Maeda, 2014). In Vietnam, there is no specific earmark, but legislation does specify that health expenditure must increase as a share of the total government budget. In Thailand, the lack of a specific earmarked revenue source for its "Universal Coverage Scheme" was not an impediment to scaling up public funding to ensure the entire population was covered (Maeda *et al.*, 2014).

All of the potential government revenue sources for the health sector involve some trade-offs for the broader economy. Evidence from high-income countries shows that property taxes are least distorting and damaging for growth, followed by consumption taxes, the personal income tax, and the corporate income tax (IMF, 2011). Taxation of capital income has a potentially strong impact on investment. Similar evidence is not available for lower-income countries, however, and the efficiency impact of different types of taxes is likely to be highly context-specific depending on composition of the economic activity and the strength of the institutions. The equity impact of taxes also may not be obvious, since the impact of a tax cannot be determined in isolation. "A regressive tax may be the only way to finance strongly progressive public expenditure (IMF, 2011)." On the other hand, the merit of the spending that is financed by new or increased taxes may not justify a disproportionate burden on lower income groups or distortions in the economy they create.

For the health sector, additional criteria that matter for assessing revenue options are whether sources of funds are in alignment with the other health financing functions of pooling and purchasing, and whether the sources provide a stable and predictable revenue base. For example, several LMICs have opted to introduce earmarked payroll taxes as a source of new revenue for the health sector because they could be collected in off-budget funds and avoid the restrictions in the public budget systems that limit the effectiveness of pooling and purchasing (Kutzin *et al.*, 2010b). What matters is the combined impact of all tax measures as well as the magnitude and distribution of the benefits from the spending they finance.

- *Enhance redistributive capacity of prepaid funds*

While increasing the overall share of spending from compulsory sources is important for progress towards UHC, the way these prepaid funds are organized also matters, and changes in these *pooling arrangements* have been at the core of financing reforms for UHC in many countries. A given level of funding organized into fewer pools has more redistributive capacity than the same level of funding organized into more pools. Even in settings where the scope for increasing tax revenues for health is greatly constrained, by reducing fragmentation in pooling (i.e., barriers to redistribution arising from the organization of fund pools) it is possible to increase redistributive capacity (WHO, 2010b).

In addition to the structure of pooling arrangements, the *composition* of funding pools also matters. Simply put, in order to enhance redistribution from the healthy to the sick, pools must be comprised of both healthy and sick people. So for example, to the extent that poorer people have greater health service needs, schemes that only serve the poor (as in the US Medicaid program, for example) will have limited scope for redistribution within the pool and hence will require a larger budget per capita than would a similarly sized pool serving a more diverse risk mix.

Fragmentation is pervasive and takes many forms. One of the most common manifestations found in LMICs is the existence of separate pools for separate population groups linked to employment status. This is the pattern found in many Latin American countries in which there is a contributory (though often subsidized) SHI scheme for the population working in the formal sector, and a budget-funded public system for the rest of the population (Londoño and Frenk, 1997; Frenk, 1995). As described previously, this situation is a consequence of the approach of starting explicit coverage programs for the relatively well-off, best-organized part of the population. The consequence is typically both inequities as the formal sector captures a disproportionate share of subsidies and services, as well as inefficiency arising from the duplication of functional responsibilities (including sometimes separate service delivery arrangements) for health financing in the same geographic area.

But there are many other forms of fragmentation. The ex-USSR countries inherited systems of integrated financing and delivery that were administratively decentralized — each level of government budgeted and operated its own system, and once budgets were allocated there was no scope for redistribution across these boundaries. This also had severe efficiency consequences because the system was organized by level of government rather than geography, so within the capital city of any region there were financing and delivery arrangements for the city and the provincial (oblast) levels of the system (Kutzin *et al.*, 2010a). More generally, fiscal decentralization is a common source of fragmentation, particularly where revenue raising-responsibility is delegated to lower levels of government.

Fragmentation between public and voluntary/private pooling is a major source of inequity in South Africa, which is the country with the world's highest share of total health spending coming from VHI (see Figure 2), more than 42% in 2012. Yet this level of spending serves only about 16% of the population, resulting in huge inequalities between the relatively well off and the rest of the population (Health Economics Unit, 2010). There are also other problematic forms of fragmentation, such as multiple small-scale insurance funds, competing insurers in a compulsory insurance market without adequate risk equalization mechanisms to serve as a virtual pool among them, geographically overlapping but non-competing statutory insurance funds, and many others.

There is no blueprint for a policy response, but experience demonstrates that countries can take action to enhance redistributive capacity by either reducing fragmentation or mitigating its consequences. For example, in Thailand and Mexico, where there were existing SHI schemes covering the formal sector, it was not possible to create a single unified national scheme. Their governments compensated by creating budget-funded, non-contributory schemes for the rest (majority) of the population and gradually increasing its level of subsidy so that funding levels were nearly equalized (Prakongsai *et al.*, 2009; Knaul *et al.*, 2012). In Ghana, the legislation that established the National Health Insurance Scheme included strong incentives for small-scale (village level) schemes to aggregate into one district-level mutual health insurance scheme and linked each of these to the national scheme (Agyepong and Adjei, 2008; WHO, 2013a). Rwanda's system similarly combines top–down funding flows from general tax and external sources with some bottom–up contributions from the population, and there are funding flows that enable redistribution across schemes within a district, across districts, and up to the national level (Makaka, 2012). In Kyrgyzstan and Moldova, the response to the fragmented budgetary system inherited from the USSR was to create a "single payer" National Health Insurance Fund, sourced from (mainly) general tax revenues supplemented with payroll tax. A unified national pool covers both formal and informal sector populations in both countries (Kutzin *et al.*, 2009). And even in the United States under the Patient Protection and Affordable Care Act (ACA),[8] the state of Arkansas agreed to accept Medicaid

[8]The ACA was adopted in 2010 and has numerous features aimed at reducing the number of American citizens who do not have public or private insurance. The main features of the ACA are summarized in Kaiser Family Foundation (2013). In a global context, what is important to note is that the reform aims to address core problems in pooling in the US health system, particularly coverage shortfalls in the private health insurance market for individuals and small groups, and uneven coverage by the publicly-funded insurance program for the poor, Medicaid. In each state, the reform has established an insurance market "exchange" to help individuals choose among insurance plans that meet standards defined in the ACA. Insurers are not allowed to exclude persons with pre-existing conditions, and all individuals are required to become insured or face a federal tax penalty. There are also income-related subsidies available to support the purchase of insurance on the exchanges. Premiums on the exchange are community-rated rather than individually-rated, and the

expansion but largely eliminated as a separate pool, instead enabling beneficiaries to buy coverage on the state health insurance exchange in the same manner as other residents who do not have employment-based coverage. This approach, if implemented as planned, would end the segregation of much of the state's poor population into the Medicaid pool and instead merge them with non-poor persons, thus increasing the ability of the system to redistribute in relation to the health service needs of the population (Allison, 2014).

Overall, by moving to both increase the relative size of compulsory prepaid pools, increase the diversity of the health risks covered in these pools, and reduce fragmentation in the overall structure of pooling, these reforms have enabled increases in the redistributive capacity of their health financing systems.

- *Strategic purchasing for efficiency and results*

While mobilizing sufficient public resources and organizing pooling to maximize redistributive capacity are essential for achieving equitable and affordable health care access for all, it is of equal importance that collected resources be efficiently used in order to maximize and sustain the provision of benefits for the population. Strategic use of the purchasing function is the key health financing instrument for this purpose.

Historically in many LMICs, the government directly funds government-run/owned health facilities by paying for their *inputs* such as personnel, medicines, supplies and equipment through line-item budgets, often reflecting bureaucratic inertia. Little attention is given to how financial incentives or other mechanisms might be used to motivate providers to improve quality or efficiency, as their accountability is for inputs, not for delivering specific outputs or outcomes. In contrast, strategic purchasing involves proactive and explicit selection of predefined outputs and outcomes based on some combination of demand and population need, linking payment to information provided on the delivery of

exchange creates a pool among those who obtain coverage through this route. This is meant to reduce the problems associated with the very small pools that existed in the individual and small business market. The ACA also expanded Medicaid coverage by increasing eligibility to all persons with incomes below 133% of the Federal poverty line. In the US federal system, Medicaid is run and partially funded by the states, but under the ACA, states which accepted the Medicaid expansion would have this 100% funded by the central government for the first 3 years (2014–2016), with this share gradually declining to 90% by 2020 and thereafter. Apart from the Arkansas plan, Medicaid remains a separate pool. This is an important difference from other high-income countries with mandatory contributory health insurance arrangements, such as Germany, Japan, the Netherlands, and Switzerland. Those countries also subsidize lower income persons from general budget revenues to ensure that everyone is covered, but none of those countries have a separate health insurance pool for the poor.

these pre-defined products and, where choices of providers exist, selecting the most qualified and efficient to purchase from. In doing so, the purchaser seeks to improve efficient allocation of resources and effective service delivery in order to maximize population health and reduce financial risk (Figueras *et al.*, 2005). Critical factors that influence the effectiveness of purchasing as a policy instrument include: (1) PPMs and (2) organizational structure of purchasers.

A PPM is the mechanism through which funds are transferred from the purchaser to the provider of health services, and each PPM embodies specific incentives which influence provider's behavior in treatment decisions, and thus quality and efficiency of service provision. In designing payment systems, key considerations include: (1) Whether payment is made prospectively or retrospectively; (2) the unit of payment; and (3) the level of payment. Together, they determine the amount of risk borne by the providers versus the purchaser. Any provision of service involves some level of uncertainty in costs. The more risk is borne by the provider, the greater incentive there will be for the provider to reduce costs — especially if the provider is able to retain savings, but it can also create incentives for reducing necessary care and thus compromise quality. In general, the more prospective a PPM and the more aggregate the unit of payment is, the greater risk is borne by the provider (Ellis and McGuire, 1990; Ellis and Miller, 2008; Roberts *et al.*, 2002, Chapter 9).

International experience with PPMs suggests some generalizable lessons. For example, fee-for-service (FFS) reimbursement of activities reported by provider is inflationary. When FFS is combined with expansion of service coverage, it can lead to rapid health expenditure growth and threaten the sustainability of financing. China's recent expansion of health insurance coverage coupled with FFS speaks to this point. Despite the increase in population covered by China's SHI and in the rates of insurance reimbursement, the financial burden on households has not reduced and in some cases, increased, because health expenditure has grown at an even faster rate under FFS (Meng *et al.*, 2012; Wagstaff and Lindelow, 2008). In countries where services are underprovided, FFS can be used in the initial phase to incentivize providers to provide more services, and many countries (e.g., Ghana, Indonesia) have initiated payment reforms with this mechanism as a way to get buy-in from providers and boost utilization (Maeda *et al.*, 2014). However, efforts should be made from the earliest stages to plan for a transition to methods that operate within an overall budget cap, in order to avoid entrenched provider behavior in over-provision. These include prospective payment methods such as capitation and global budgets, or methods such as case-based payment (typically based on DRGs) as a basis for determining the size of hospital budgets or as a reimbursement mechanism that is combined with volume caps or adjustment factors that limit overall expenditure growth beyond a pre-determined limit.

At the other extreme, input-based payment tends to incentivize providers to increase inputs according to the actual basis for budgeting (e.g., beds or staff), but provides no incentives to improve efficiency or quality, or to respond to patients' needs. The global trend shows that more countries are moving away from pure FFS or input-based PPM, towards more aggregated and output based PPM such as global budget, capitation and case-based payment, in particular, the DRGs payment system (Langenbrunner *et al.*, 2005; Charlesworth *et al.*, 2012). Each has its pros and cons, and no single PPM is perfect. In short, PPMs that have the highest incentives for cost savings and efficiency improvement also have the greatest risk of selecting against more severe patients and under-providing in terms of quality and quantity.

There are important interactions between how PPMs are designed and the incentives they provide to facilitate integrated delivery, rather than further fragmenting service delivery, which is the dominant situation in most LMICs. For example, under a capitation payment system, providers are paid a fixed amount per person registered with the provider, or reside in a catchment area for a given period of time, usually a year. Depending on the scope of services included in the capitation payment rate, the incentives embodied in a capitation payment method vary. If only outpatient services are included in the capitation rate, providers have incentives to refer patients to inpatient facilities. Whereas if the capitation rate includes a population-based scope of services, providers have incentives to treat patients at the lowest cost settings, invest in prevention and coordinate care with other providers. Similarly, if global budgets are paid for each facility separately, each facility has incentives to refer out the sickest patients, which could lead to poor care coordination, risk selection and more expensive care.

As a result, governments are progressively moving towards blended or mixed payment regimes that capitalize on the benefits of various schemes. For instance, pay-for-performance (P4P), often used interchangeably with terms such as "performance-based funding" (PBF), "paying for results," or RBF, has dominated the literature on strategic purchasing as increasingly decision-makers seek to refine traditional PPMs. P4P programs link payment of individual providers or institutions to predefined outcome or output/activities that have established evidence of being cost-effective in improving health outcomes (Peabody *et al.*, 2011; Sutton *et al.*, 2012; Witter *et al.*, 2012; Yip *et al.*, 2014). Typically, P4P elements are combined with traditional payment methods such as capitation or global budget and give health care providers a bonus payment rewarding them for meeting or exceeding agreed-upon performance targets. Should providers fail to meet those targets or underperform, payment could also be held back. The most commonly chosen performance targets are output or process indicators that are easily measurable, verifiable and where well-established evidence enables them to be linked to good outcomes. Examples include the Quality and Outcomes Framework (QOF) in the UK for primary health care services and a number of maternal and child health focused programs in LMICs (Basinga *et al.*, 2011; Morgan *et al.*, 2011; Cashin *et al.*, 2014).

The organizational structure of purchasing is closely linked with that of pooling, and has implications for the incentive environment facing providers and hence the effectiveness of purchasing as an instrument. Fragmentation in pooling necessarily implies fragmentation in purchasing, limiting the effectiveness of each individual purchaser. As providers are faced with multiple purchasing arrangements, the leverage each purchaser on the provider is reduced to the share of revenue or population it represents for a provider. As seen in the US, fragmentation in purchasing also leads to problems of cost shifting, that is, when a purchaser exerts cost control on the provider, the provider shifts its cost over to the other purchasers with more generous contractual terms. This poses potential barriers to controlling overall health system costs (Wu, 2010; Frakt, 2011; Robinson, 2011).

Effective purchasing is dependent on having an effective purchaser. The primary responsibility of the purchaser is to purchase on behalf of the people or enrolled population. Because of asymmetry of information in the health care sector, individuals do not possess the knowledge and information to be an effective purchaser. An entity should therefore have explicit responsibility for purchasing. More specifically, this entity should be empowered to make evidence-based decisions on (1) what services to purchase, (2) which providers to purchase from and (3) how to purchase. Such entities can take a variety of organizational forms and ownership — for example, government health ministries, local health authorities, public autonomous agencies, private health insurers (whether commercial or not-for-profit) or non-governmental organizations (NGOs). In some countries in which governments do not have the capability to take on this role within their core line ministries or government departments (either due to lack of relevant skills, the rigidity of public finance systems that do not allow movement away from rigid line-item budgets, or a combination), they have either established public autonomous agencies (e.g., Moldova's National Health Insurance Company, Ghana's National Health Insurance Agency) or have contracted out the purchasing function to NGOs or private insurance companies (e.g., India's RSBY government-sponsored health insurance scheme for persons below the poverty line). In either case, it is essential to strengthen government capacity to ensure that purchasing practices are aligned with policy priorities, either to manage the contracts with external purchasers or to take on this role within some form of public agency.

The mere establishment or contracting of an agency to take on this role does not guarantee that purchasing will be strategic. Many such organizations focus largely on financial concerns only — balancing their books and reducing cost outlays — and pay little attention to quality of care. This was a concern in the early years of India's RSBY program, for example. Conversely, Thailand established the National Health Security Office (NHSO), a quasi-public organization, as the purchaser, with a board chaired by the Minister of Public Health and comprised of key stakeholders including members of local government, civic society groups, professional bodies and technical experts. The board is responsible for setting the benefits provided by the Universal Coverage Scheme, making the policy rules and guidelines that govern the NHSO, and determining providers' reimbursement mechanism. In this way, it has the capacity to ensure that the NHSO aligns with government objectives. More generally, the lesson is that the incentives and accountabilities of purchasing agencies need to be aligned with public policy objectives as part of the process of moving toward more strategic purchasing in the health system as a key instrument for sustaining progress toward UHC.

Alternative Approaches to Financing for UHC in the Context of High Informality

Why labor force informality is a core challenge

As noted above, it is necessary to meet the Fuchs conditions (compulsion and subsidization) for a financing system to make rapid progress toward UHC. More broadly, we summarize attributes of the various health financing functions and policies that are important for making and sustaining progress towards UHC in Table 1.

Table 1. Directions for reform in health financing functions and policies

Health financing element	**Desirable attributes/directions for reform**
Revenue sources and contribution mechanisms	Moving toward predominant reliance on compulsory sources of funds (i.e., various forms of direct and indirect taxation) — the enabling factor to meet the Fuchs conditions
Pooling	Reducing barriers to redistribution, increasing diversity of health risks within pools
Purchasing	Establishing and strengthening incentives for efficiency and quality in purchasing mechanisms
Benefits and rationing measures	Promoting use of cost-effective services and limiting out-of-pocket burden, especially for the poor, in the design of policies on benefits and rationing (and their alignment with purchasing)
Stewardship of financing	Unified, coherent, goal-driven, and evidence-informed governance arrangements in the financing system

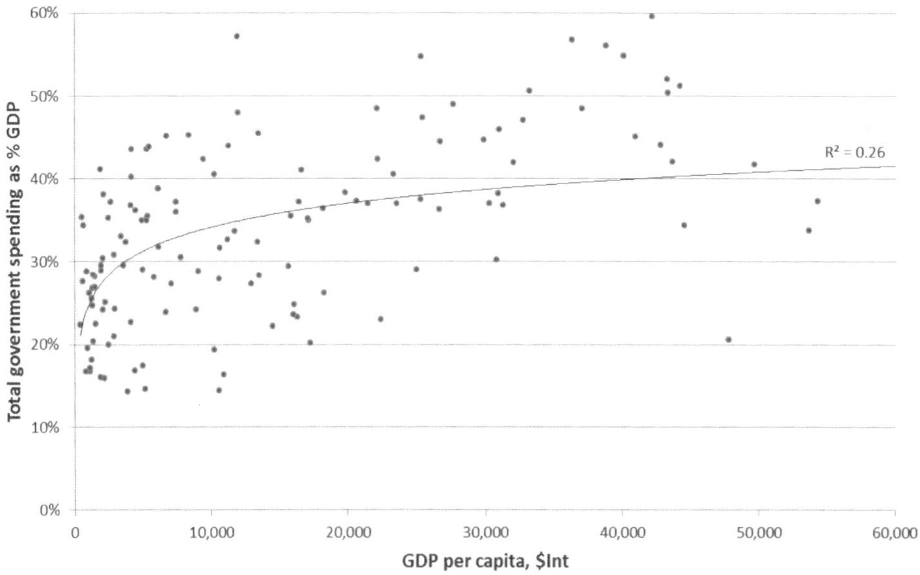

Figure 3. Relation between country income and overall public spending, 2012

Source: WHO (2014). Excludes countries with population less than 600,000.

From a health financing perspective, the extent of informality reflects the size of the population that is not in receipt of predictable salaries or wages. As such, this is a population that is difficult to tax, and this challenge is greater in LMICs because they tend to have larger shares of the population in the informal economy than high-income countries (ILO, 2014). Lower tax revenues mean lower capacity for public spending, including on health. The link between GDP per capita, the extent of informality, and public spending is supported by the data in Figure 3. Several authors (Schieber and Maeda, 1997; Gottret and Schieber, 2006; Kutzin and Jakab, 2010) have also pointed to this as one of the main reasons why LMICs are more dependent on non-government (mainly out-of-pocket) funding sources. And indeed, the data are consistent with this interpretation, as reflected in Table 2. Overall, governments in richer countries spend more not only in total but as a share of their economies, and this translates into less dependence on household spending. The situation is reversed for low-income countries, which suffer the greatest burden of OOPS. While this broad pattern emerges from the data, it is also not strictly deterministic. There is considerable variation around the trend shown in Figure 3, revealing both countries with similar income levels but very different fiscal capacity, as well as countries with different income levels but similar fiscal levels. For any specific country, therefore, the extent of both informality and implications for the mix and level of public revenues needs to be understood.

Table 2. Fiscal capacity and dependence on OOPS by country income group, 2012

Country income group	Total government spending as a % of GDP	Out-of-pocket as a % of total health spending
High	41	21
Middle	33	37
Low	25	43

Source: WHO (2014). Excludes countries with population less than 600,000.

While informality is a major challenge for meeting the Fuchs conditions, the implications for the other desirable features of health financing (Table 1) are not inherently problematic. However, many policy decisions countries already made have actually caused problems related to informality. With regard to pooling, for example, the exclusion of persons outside the formal sector from explicit forms of coverage, or the establishment of entirely separate schemes for the poor have created fragmentation along labor market or income dimensions. As a consequence of having established separate pools in this way, the reform process in many countries has also created differences in purchasing mechanisms along these dimensions. For example, where SHI schemes have been established for formal sector employees, one consequence has been the concentration of scarce skills for health service purchasing on behalf of a relatively small and privileged part of the population (Kutzin, 1997). And similarly, formal sector SHI schemes have tended to have an explicit, funded entitlement, while the rest of the population often suffers from vague and poorly funded entitlements that are difficult to enforce at the point of service. This was the case, historically, in Mexico and Thailand, where the informal sector population was disadvantaged by lower levels of public funding per capita than formal sector workers (Prakongsai *et al.*, 2009; Knaul *et al.*, 2012).

Thus, from a health financing policy perspective, the "problem of informality" is mainly an issue of fiscal capacity, with informality constraining the ability of countries to generate enough public revenues, particularly from direct taxation, to ensure that most funding for health comes from public sources. In looking to policy responses in any country, it is important to separate the clear issue of the fiscal implications of informality from past policy choices that can be addressed through a reform agenda. Indeed, inequalities that were caused by past policy choices (again, most obviously the decision to initiate explicit coverage programs for the formal sector, as in Mexico and Thailand, or historically inherited patterns of inequality, as in South Africa) have been key political drivers of the UHC reform agenda over the past decade.

Health financing reform options to move toward UHC in a context of high informality

Here we apply the functional approach to establish a categorization of options that countries have used in their health financing strategies aimed at progressing toward UHC. As with all such frameworks, there is some over-simplification, and it remains important to understand the nuances in each particular case rather than fall into the trap of thinking in terms of overall models of financing. Keeping this in mind, the two broad categories of options are defined in terms of the *basis for entitlement*, and in particular, whether this is *contributory* or *non-contributory*.[9] According to the System of Health Accounts (OECD *et al.*, 2011), one of the key criteria for distinguishing between types of financing schemes is whether, under a particular scheme, entitlement to benefit derives from a specific contribution made by or on behalf of an individual (contributory-based entitlement), or whether entitlement derives from some other factor, such as citizenship, residence, poverty status, etc. (non-contributory entitlement). This is a useful distinction from a policy perspective and not merely for accounting purposes. Within these two broad categories, we identify a set of options that different countries have applied.[10] These are summarized in Table 3, and are reviewed in more detail in the remainder of this section.

- *Non-contributory options*

A1. Universal, budget-funded, population-based systems

This approach is used in several high-income countries, such as the United Kingdom, Spain, and the Nordic countries. In these countries, entitlement is not linked to any specific contribution or labor force status, and they have also been fairly successful at promoting equity in financial access and financial protection for their populations. Many LMICs have, historically, tried to do the same, but most have fallen short for a variety of reasons. A universal, fully budget-funded system requires substantial public revenues, and for many LMICs in which adequate funds were not forthcoming, there have been mismatches between what was publicly promised (e.g., free service in government facilities) and what was

[9] It is worth emphasizing that having a non-contributory basis for entitlement does not imply that beneficiaries do not financially contribute. Indeed, in countries that rely predominantly on indirect taxation for public revenues, anyone who purchases a product subject to tax is contributing. The distinction here — and countries vary in the choices they make with regard to this — is whether or not entitlement to health benefits actually derives from a specific contribution made for that purpose.

[10] Some countries also use a mix of contributory and non-contributory approaches.

Table 3. Categorization of financing reform options to move towards UHC despite high informality

Non-contributory-based entitlement options	Contributory-based entitlement options
A1. Universal, budget-funded, population-based systems	
A2. Budget-funded program for all persons not already covered by an explicit social security mechanism	B1. Compulsory SHI for the formal sector, and a largely unsubsidized informal sector who must prepay directly for their coverage (often combined with non-contributory funded coverage for the poor or otherwise vulnerable)
A3. Entitlement for some population groups to a range of services	
A4. Universal population guarantees for a set of specifically defined services	B2. Compulsory SHI for the formal sector, fully funded coverage for the poor, and heavily subsidized coverage for the informal "middle"

realized in practice (e.g., shortages of key inputs, informal payments). In some countries, this approach was connected to non-strategic "passive" PPMs reflected in historical, input-based supply-side budgeting practices,[11] although this is by no means inherent (as reflected in the experience of the UK and many of the other countries noted here).

An exception to this pattern has been Sri Lanka, although it differs from the high-income examples because the budget-funded public system coexists with high levels of OOPS. However, because there is good physical access to free government outpatient and inpatient health facilities combined with a private outpatient service sector that offers greater amenities, the use of public facilities is strongly pro-poor while private use is pro-rich, and hence the OOPS is heavily concentrated among the rich for ambulatory services and medicines. As a result, it has achieved good indicators of both service coverage and financial protection, despite having a low overall level of public spending on health (less than 2% of GDP) and relying on passive budgeting of government health facilities (Rannan-Eliya and Sikurajapathy, 2008).

---

[11] *Passive provider payment* is the opposite of strategic or active purchasing. *Input-based historical supply-side budgeting* refers to when the budget for a year is effectively based on the previous year's budget, plus/minus a%, and typically justified according to inputs such as the number of beds or staff.

A2. Budget-funded, explicit coverage program for persons not covered by existing social security health insurance schemes for the formal sector

This is the approach reflected by the reforms in Mexico and Thailand. In Mexico, the *Seguro Popular* (Popular Health Insurance) is open to anyone not enrolled in the social security system. While initially planned with a beneficiary contribution, this has been largely dropped because it was found to be both administratively costly and a barrier to affiliation. While called "insurance," it is mainly a revision to the inter-governmental resource allocation formula in Mexico's federal system. Under the *Seguro Popular*, transfers from central to state governments for health are driven by the enrollment of the non-salaried population in the program, with the overall level of the transfers greatly increased as well. The program also included legislation to ensure beneficiaries have access to a comprehensive package of essential services, as well as to an explicit set of costly, specialized interventions. For these latter services, a "Fund for Protection against Catastrophic Health Expenditures" was established, which essentially functions as a centralized purchasing/contracting agency. Overall, the government's commitment to redress past inequalities through this program was reflected in a much higher rate of growth in the Ministry of Health's budget (which included the *Seguro Popular*) than in the existing social security schemes, such that public spending per beneficiary in the social security schemes was 2.1 times that of the rest of the population in 2000 but fell to only 1.2 times by 2010 (Knaul *et al.*, 2012).

Thailand's approach to coverage was similar, although reform there did not have to address the challenge of operating within a federal budget system. The Universal Coverage Scheme (UCS) began with the plan to include a small contribution, but then dropped this, similar to the *Seguro Popular*. It combined several previous coverage programs — one for the low-income population, a subsidized VHI program, and a scheme for the elderly — into one and merged the funding for this with previous supply-side budgets. A new pooling and purchasing entity was established as an independent public agency with a representative board — the NHSO. In the UCS, the NHSO enters into contracts with providers and pays using closed-end mechanisms (capitation and DRGs within an overall budget cap). Since its introduction in 2002, coverage has grown rapidly, and impressive results in financial protection and access to services have been documented (Prakongsai *et al.*, 2009; Evans *et al.*, 2011). And similar to Mexico, the government's commitment to the UCS has greatly narrowed the gap in public funding per capita with the existing social security scheme for private sector workers (though a budget-funded scheme for civil servants remains funded at much higher levels).

This approach has much to commend it. Unable to merge with existing, entrenched schemes for the formal sector, but with the political support to mitigate the inequitable consequences of this, they each established a parallel scheme, funded entirely from general budget revenues, but with explicit commitments to deliver on benefits for the population. By opening coverage to everyone not enrolled in social security, the schemes avoided costs and complications related to targeting, and they also created pools with more socio-economic diversity than would have been the case with a targeted scheme for the poor.

The real challenge for countries considering moving in this direction, as with the broader universal non-contributory approach, is fiscal capacity and the ability to manage expenditure growth. Mexico and Thailand had both the fiscal capacity and the political commitment to raise public spending for this purpose. In Thailand, for example, health represented about 10% of total public spending in 2002, the year the UCS was introduced. It rose quickly to over 14% in 2007 and has stayed in the 14–15% range ever since. Despite its relatively low fiscal capacity, this share has enabled it to ensure that public spending on health remains at around 3% of GDP (WHO, 2014). This level of spending is quite low by international standards in terms of achieving low dependence on OOPS (see Figure 1), but combined with the strong attention to efficiency and cost control reflected in the PPMs used, it has been enough to sustain progress. Other countries considering this approach need to incorporate a realistic sense of what can be provided from general budget revenues as well as learning from the approaches used to get the most from pooling and purchasing arrangements.

A risk of going with this approach is that it can reinforce fragmentation. In both the Thai and Mexican cases, the reforms were a response to an already fragmented system, and at least in the Thai case, the aim was to merge with the schemes for civil servants and private sector workers (but they have been unable to do so). As noted above, the starting point matters, so this option needs to be considered carefully as one way to compensate for fragmentation that may already exist, while ensuring that it does not introduce fragmentation into a system that does not have this particular manifestation of the problem.

A3. Entitlement for some population groups to a range of services, funded from general revenues

This approach may be relevant for highly constrained fiscal contexts, and includes measures such as exemptions from user fees/copayments or budget-funded insurance coverage for the poor. While targeting brings costs and complexity, these can be mitigated if the health sector takes advantage of existing mechanisms (e.g., for food or cash assistance) rather than creating its own.

Within this broad option are examples that involve an explicit split between purchase and provision for the covered services or population groups, and other approaches that do not. The beneficiaries of Cambodia's Health Equity Funds (HEFs), for example, are identified through a proxy means test[12] implemented by the Ministry of Planning. These identified poor persons qualify for free services in government health facilities. The HEFs receive donor and government budget revenues and use these to pay the user fees in these facilities on behalf of their beneficiaries. In other words, the HEFs support means-tested user fee exemptions with a purchasing mechanism to enable the promise of free services to be realized, and indeed, positive effects on both equity in service use and financial protection for the poor have been documented, although the targeting mechanism was not perfect (Annear *et al.*, 2013).

This approach contrasts with the generally poor performance of simple exemptions from user fees for certain categories of the population (McPake *et al.*, 2011), which is another variant of this option. Without the link to an explicit purchasing mechanism, it tends to result in an unfunded mandate, relying entirely on decisions made by health workers at the point of service. This highlights the importance of alignment of different elements of financing policy — in this case the alignment of purchasing methods with defined benefits, and both of these with service delivery arrangements — in order to ensure that the desired results are achieved. It also suggests implementation prerequisites, namely the existence of some type of targeting mechanism that pre-identifies those who are entitled, and the administrative capacity to link the results of this targeting to beneficiary identification at the level of the purchaser and the provider (and the beneficiary as well).

These prerequisites are reflected in another variant of this approach, targeted subsidies for health insurance coverage, as in the RSBY and several state-budget-funded insurance programs in India. In these schemes, all persons who have a card showing that they are below the poverty line are entitled to join, and the schemes pay for hospital services up to an annual financial limit per person. As in Cambodia, entitlement depends on the results of a proxy means test implemented by government for other purposes (e.g., food subsidies) but used to determine beneficiary status for health coverage. There are important variants within India, however. Under RSBY, those entitled to join still have to pay a (very) small annual registration fee. Conversely in the scheme sponsored by the state government of

---

[12]The aim of means testing is to identify and distinguish those families or individuals that have the capacity to pay something for health services from those which are too poor and cannot. However, it is difficult and costly to implement an administrative mechanism for this purpose, and hence some countries including Cambodia rely on "proxies" that are relatively easy to identify and are well-correlated with household income. For more on this, see Qingyue *et al.* (2010).

Andhra Pradesh, those who qualify (under a more generous definition of the poverty line that includes about 80% of the population) are automatically enrolled (La Forgia and Nagpal, 2012).

While the implementation details vary considerably within the bounds of this approach, several features emerge as important. In contrast to the Mexican and Thai examples, it relies on targeting, which is both costly and subject to errors of inclusion and exclusion. But it is the incremental rather than the absolute costs that matter, and in India and Cambodia, for example, the health reform simply uses the results of existing targeting mechanisms implemented by government. It is hard to imagine circumstances in which it would be advisable for the health sector to undertake its own, parallel program of means testing. Still, the results of the means tests have to be linked to the health system at both the purchaser and provider levels (and updated periodically), and this does impose additional costs. So for fiscally-constrained countries considering this approach as compared to the untargeted option, these incremental administrative costs have to be taken into account to ensure it is worth going this route.

A4. Universal population guarantees for specific services

In a sense, this approach involves targeting specific services rather than population groups as the means for coverage expansion. Examples would be untargeted free care initiatives such as the blanket elimination of user fees for maternal and child health services, as in several African countries in recent years (Meessen *et al.*, 2011). It also includes approaches used in very different contexts. In Moldova, for example, about 20% of the population was uninsured under the national health insurance program, despite various efforts made over the years. In 2009, the government passed legislation that extended primary care coverage to all persons irrespective of their insurance status (Shishkin and Jowett, 2012). Similarly in Chile, the reform known as Universal Access with Explicit Guarantees (AUGE is the Spanish acronym) defined a set of specific treatments (initially 56, then 69, and then 80) guaranteed[13] to all citizens regardless of their insurance affiliation, funded by a 1% increase in the VAT (Bitran, 2013).

What has made these initiatives different from simple declarations of free or guaranteed services has been the connection of these promises to provider accountability for delivery, and to a funding source, often supported by a specific

[13] In fact, the "guarantees" under the AUGE program include not only the right to these specific services but also guarantees with regard to quality (definition and adherence to treatment protocols for these services), maximum waiting times, and limits to patient cost-sharing for these services (Bitran, 2013).

provider payment mechanism that links the funding to the promised entitlement. Perhaps most notable among these developments has been the link between selective user fee removal and RBF. The link between the defined entitlement and the payment mechanism is similar to the Cambodian HEF approach described above, with the key difference being that the HEF is targeted according to population characteristics (poverty status) but not according to the type of service. Conversely in Burundi, for example, implementation of a Presidential decision to eliminate user fees for maternal and child health services involved replacing the lost fee revenue with an RBF mechanism to give providers an incentive to treat pregnant women and children while simultaneously eliminating the demand-side financial barrier of the fees (WHO, 2013b).

As shown here, expanding specific services for everyone (or for all in defined groups such as pregnant women and children) is an approach that has been applied in countries of various income levels. It can be coordinated with any other financing scheme that may exist in a country, or it may be implemented independently. As with many of the other reforms described, effective implementation requires combining the expanded entitlement with a funding mechanism and especially a PPM targeted to the expanded services. It is notable because this option is a means to expand coverage that does not involvement enrollment in an "insurance scheme". Further, because entitlement is related to the specific populations who are potential beneficiaries of the incentivized services on a non-contributory basis, employment status is irrelevant to coverage. While avoiding the costs and complexity associated with a contributory approach, it does require strong capacities for service purchasing and a willingness to set explicit priorities.

- *Contributory options*

B1. Unsubsidized coverage for the non-poor informal sector

This is perhaps the option that is considered most frequently by LMIC governments seeking to expand coverage. It involves some effort to differentiate within the informal sector between those who are poor and thus unable to contribute, and those who are not poor but are not captured by the country's tax system. Thus, implementation of this approach requires that government has the administrative capacity to implement some type of targeting mechanism, as well as the fiscal capacity and willingness to fund coverage for the poor. Persons in the informal sector who are not deemed to be poor may be either required or asked to prepay for their health coverage, though in countries with limited tax collection capacity, such contributions tend to be de facto voluntary.

In theory, this approach offers several advantages, as it would be equitable relative to the ability of people to contribute. In practice however, it does not work (despite its popularity). Most fundamentally, the non-poor informal sector tend to remain uncovered if they do not benefit from substantial subsidies (Acharya *et al.*, 2012). This is the core problem of adverse selection in VHI markets described above, and it applies regardless of whether the insurance is managed by a commercial company, a "community", or the government. Beyond the problem of these markets, there are other barriers to participation. One may be the desire of some persons in the informal sector to avoid paying income tax, and related to this, fear that if they register for health insurance they will be more easily "captured" by the tax system. Another may arise in single-pool contexts that bundle together the health insurance contribution with other elements of social security, thereby raising the price of enrollment (Baeza and Packard, 2006). For this combination of reasons, this approach tends to result in a "missing middle" problem in terms of population coverage: The "top" covered by formal social security health insurance, the "bottom" covered from targeted budget funds, but the middle (non-poor informal sector) remains at potentially great financial risk for health care costs.

B2. Heavily subsidized coverage for the informal sector population

This approach aims to balance recognition of the limits of contributory-based entitlement with the retention of that aspect of "personal responsibility" for providing for one's coverage, as well as a concern with the fiscal implications of going for a fully non-contributory approach. Even in high-income countries with contributory systems, there is an explicit role for budget subsidies to both fully subsidize for those deemed unable to do so, and partially subsidize those outside of regular salaried employment. They recognize that this is the only way to attain 100% population coverage in their context. In Japan for example, 25% of the revenues of the health insurance system come from general budget transfers (Ikegami *et al.*, 2011). In Hungary, such transfers account for about 60% of health insurance fund revenues (Szigeti *et al.*, 2012).

In most LMICs that provide some subsidies (or lower contribution rates) for the non-poor informal sector, success with this approach has proven more challenging. As with the first option, there tends to be low participation. Retention is also a problem; there is a high dropout rate the year after acute health events. With this approach, it remains an administrative challenge to determine the boundary between who should be fully subsidized and who only partially subsidized. Two countries, however, have had much greater success (90% or more) in contributory population affiliation to their health insurance programs — China's New Cooperative Medical Scheme (NCMS) and Rwanda's Community Based Health Insurance (CBHI). Their experiences have several implementation features in common that are likely to have contributed to this and may be relevant elsewhere (Hou *et al.*, 2012; Yip *et al.*, 2012; Musango *et al.*, 2013). Beyond this, at least in the Rwandan case, these reforms have been linked to important gains in financial access, financial protection, and increased use of priority services (Sekabaraga *et al.*, 2011).

The first common element has been the magnitude of the subsidies, which enables the expected cost of the "premium" to the population to be much less than the perceived value of the benefit. The magnitude of this "contribution–entitlement gap" (Baeza and Packard, 2006) is a key factor in stimulating demand. In both countries, budget subsidies flow to both the supply side (e.g., direct salary payments) and the demand side (or perhaps more accurately, the "purchaser" side, i.e., subsidies flowing to the insurance fund), while the benefit package for the subsidized population is the same as that of everyone else. Contributions are not based on an actuarial calculation but rather on what is deemed to be affordable for the population taking into account the government's ability to afford the subsidies.

In China's NCMS, there is an explicit link between public and private contributions that may be particularly interesting for countries in which part of the challenge is concern from finance ministries that they do not know where the money given to the health sector is going. In this program, when an individual makes his/her prepayment for coverage, it triggers a contribution from local and central governments that is four times (on average) the amount of the individual's prepayment.[14] Thus, it is very explicit that the finance authorities are "buying health insurance" for the population, and moreover, that with their subsidy policy, they are leveraging prepayment from the population. From the individual's perspective, their relatively small contribution leverages a large contribution from the state on their behalf. So this funding model provides an excellent example of complementarity between public and private funding sources.

In Rwanda, the subsidy policy is slightly less explicit, but significant. It relies to a greater extent than China on supply-side subsidies for salaries and some other costs of the health system. The government also fully subsidizes the contributions for about 25% of population that are deemed to be unable to contribute (based on each community's own assessment). For the rest, there are two contribution rates linked to income (Republic of Rwanda, 2010; Musango *et al.*, 2013). The supply-side subsidies and the full subsidies for the poor mean that these contribution rates are in fact not set on a full actuarial basis but instead create an affordable mechanism to bring more household prepayment into the common pool.

The second common element is the role played by local government officials as active intermediaries in the enrollment process. Both countries use a

[14] And for those individuals deemed to be extremely poor, the Ministry of Civil Affairs pays the entire contribution on their behalf.

well-organized system of incentives or targets for local officials to enroll eligible populations into the coverage program. In China, leaders of local governments (usually the deputy mayor in charge of health) were given explicit enrollment targets to reach, and together with a set of other performance targets, they form the basis of local government leaders' promotion. They, in turn, instruct NCMS office staff to find the most effective ways to enroll people, including going door-to-door, taking advantage of other collective activity, for example, immunization days, driving around vans with slogans on the benefits of NCMS. In Rwanda, part of each district mayor's pay depends on getting their population enrolled in the local Community-Based Health Insurance scheme. Behind these policies is a political reality that is less easily replicated; both countries have very strong central governments with an ability to instruct, guide or otherwise organize local government actions. The extent to which these two countries' abilities to achieve high enrollment are dependent on this government structure has not been systematically studied, and thus it is premature to draw strong conclusions. Applied research is needed to explore how some aspects of the approaches used by these two countries — particularly the role and magnitude of subsidies and the engagement of local government as active intermediaries — are applied in different political contexts.

Conclusions

UHC is more than an aspirational goal: It embodies widely shared health policy objectives on which all countries seek to make progress — equity in service use, quality and financial protection. The emergence of UHC after World War II marked a change in the underlying rationale for public policy on health coverage, from a focus on workers and labor productivity, to a right (often constitutional) of citizenship. This shift had important implications for health financing policy, as it meant that entitlement to benefits could no longer be solely based on a specific contribution made for that purpose. If 100% of the population is to have a funded entitlement, then some of the funding must come from general budget revenues to ensure that those unable (due to their incomes) or unwilling (due to adverse selection) are included. However, much of the health financing advice coming to LMICs since the 1980s was implicitly based on copying the historical patterns of development that began around the start of the 20th century, specifically the contributory approaches focused initially on the formal sector workforce. As the shortcomings of this approach — particularly the exacerbation of inequalities — relative to UHC have become more widely recognized, and especially as several countries have taken alternative pathways and have documented successes, it has become clear that alternatives to those historical models are needed.

The search for a "best model" of health financing is not a relevant undertaking because the "right next steps" for any country depend critically on the starting point: Their existing arrangements for health financing and the wider health system, specific aspects of context such as fiscal capacity and the structure of public administration, and a range of other factors that require a tailored, country-specific policy response. This reality does not mean, however, that there is little to be gained from international experience. Much is known about what works and what does not, and this knowledge should not be ignored. In this chapter we have identified lessons from both theory and practice that can be crystallized as a set of principles — not specific reforms — that offer promising directions for progress as well as guarding against pitfalls to avoid.

By looking at financing reforms from a functional perspective, and informing our analysis with both country experience and some of the core foundations of health economics (particularly the economics of VHI markets), we have identified desirable directions for change (Table 1), building on the essential features identified by Fuchs (compulsion and subsidization). The context of low formal workforce participation found in most LMICs poses a particular challenge for meeting the "Fuchs conditions" because of the difficulty of generating revenues from direct taxes. And going the route that many are taking, expecting that a large percentage of persons in the informal sector can be made to contribute most of the premium for their coverage, is a pitfall that flies in the face of both theory and evidence. Thus, taking into account both the need to meet the Fuchs conditions with the fiscal context associated with high informality, leads to the conclusion that for most LMICs, financing reforms to move towards UHC will require greater reliance on general revenues sourced from indirect taxes. An additional important lesson from the reform experience highlighted here and elsewhere (Kutzin *et al.*, 2010b) is that, irrespective of whether new revenues are generated or needed, *changing how existing budget revenues are used* is key to successful reform.

The reform experiences of Thailand, Mexico, Burundi, Rwanda, China, Cambodia, Kyrgyzstan, and other countries illustrate the importance of changing how existing budget revenues are used — whether the reform involved changes in the level, flow and flexibility of budget funds alone, or whether it involved a combination new revenues and changes in the use of budget funds. While, of course, more funding can enable greater progress toward UHC goals, what has marked relatively successful reform experiences is an increase in the flexibility in the use of these revenues, in particular allowing for strategic purchasing techniques to be applied to revenues from the public budget.

The importance of changing how general budget revenues can be used to transform health systems points to a key public policy question: How has it been possible to do this, given that most public financial management (PFM) systems are quite rigid when it comes to the planning and use of revenues that come out of the annual budget process? There seem to be two broad approaches, and further analysis of these is central to the "financing for UHC" reform agenda in the future. One option is to modify the existing PFM systems to accommodate this flexibility, such that within routine processes it will be allowed to match some budget revenues to either specific populations or specific services (rather than buildings and inputs) and make payments to the providers accordingly. The other, which may be more frequent, involves "going around" the core PFM system by channeling general revenues to new purchasing entities (as with the Thai NHSO, Kyrgyz or Moldovan national health insurance funds, or Cambodian HEFs, for example). Regardless of the approach chosen, there is clearly a need for more intensive engagement with a country's finance and budget authorities to reach understanding on the need for flexibility in the use of funds in the health sector, and combining this with an approach to demonstrate new and better ways that health authorities can be held accountable for the use of public funds.

There are also important policy questions related to pooling. Both theory and evidence suggest that countries should seek to avoid creating separate pools for different population groups, such as the poor, formal sector and informal sector. In order to maximize the redistributive capacity of prepaid funds, countries should seek to both reduce barriers (fragmentation) between pools and to increase diversity of health risks within pools. The challenge is how to do this in the context of path-dependent structural arrangements for pooling that exist in many health systems. This is another example of why searching for a "best" might be irrelevant. Instead, what would be potentially useful for decision-making is to understand how different countries have been able to enhance pooling within the constraints of their historical arrangements, political economy, and system of public administration.

Another set of important policy questions for which further applied research is needed relates to the need to align different aspects of health financing (such as purchasing and benefits) as well as the alignment with service delivery. While alignment makes sense, it is not always the case that all aspects of reform can or should proceed simultaneously. Sequencing matters, but there has not been much knowledge generated from reform experience on this issue. It would appear obvious, for example, that a country should not proceed with a purchasing reform or new benefit package if the service delivery arrangements are not in place. But how to put them in place is an issue, especially if financial mechanisms are part of the means of doing so. Related to this is another key issue: Thinking through the appropriate mix of supply-side funding vs. the types of "purchaser-side" funding flows that have been a part of many of the reforms described in this chapter. The case for supply-side budgeting would seem to involve the scaling-up agenda: Investment in new capacity to extend service coverage. But again, there has been inadequate analysis of country experience with regard to the supply-side and purchaser-side flows. And if the evidence leads, as it likely would, to something other than an "all or nothing" conclusion, it will be essential to synthesize the types of factors that call for greater focus on one type of funding flow than another, and also to consider how to combine these in a coherent way. Countries are certainly using both approaches now, but policy makers need guidance on how these can be better aligned.

References

Abel-Smith B. 1987. Social Security. *Encyclopædia Britannica*. http://www.britannica.com/EBchecked/topic/551402/social-security/38961/National-health-schemes.

Acharya A, Vellakkal S, Taylor F, Masset E, Satija A, Burke M, Ebrahim S. 2012. The impact of health insurance schemes for the informal sector in low- and middle-income countries: A systematic review. *World Bank Research Observer* 28(2): 236–266.

Agyepong IA, Adjei S. 2008. Public social policy development and implementation: A case study of the Ghana National Health Insurance scheme. *Health Policy and Planning* 23: 150–160.

Akin J, Birdsall N, de Ferranti D. 1987. Financing health services in developing countries: An agenda for reform. Washington, DC: The World Bank.

Allison A. 2014. Arkansas's alternative to Medicaid expansion raises important questions about how HHS will implement new ACA waiver authority in 2017. *Journal of Health Policy, Politics and Law* 39(5): 1089–1098.

Annear PL, Ahmed S, Ros CE, Ir P. 2013. Strengthening institutional and organizational capacity for social health protection of the informal sector in lesser-developed countries: A study of policy barriers and opportunities in Cambodia. *Social Science & Medicine* 96: 223–231.

Baeza CC, Packard TG. 2006. *Beyond Survival: Protecting Households from Health Shocks in Latin America*. Washington, DC and Palo Alto, California: The World Bank and Stanford University Press.

Basinga P, Gertler PJ, Binagwaho A, Soucat ALB, Sturdy J, Vermeersch CMJ. 2011. Effect on maternal and child health services in Rwanda of payment to primary health-care providers for performance: An impact evaluation. *Lancet* 377(9775): 1421–1428.

Bitran R. 2013. Explicit Health Guarantees for Chileans: The AUGE Benefits Package. UNICO Studies Series 21. Washington, DC: The World Bank.

Bitran R. 2014. Universal Health Coverage and the Challenge of Informal Employment: Lessons from Developing Countries. HNP Discussion Paper. Washington, DC: The World Bank.

Busse R, Saltman RB, Dubois HFW. 2004. Organization and financing of social health insurance systems: Current status and recent policy developments. In Saltman RB, Busse R, Figueras J (eds.). Social Health Insurance Systems in Western Europe. World Health Organization on Behalf of the European Observatory on Health Systems and Policies. Berkshire, England: Open University Press.

Cashin C, Chi Y-L, Borowitz M, Smith P, Thompson S (eds.). 2014. *Pay for Performance in Health Care: Implications for Health System Performance and Accountability.* Open University Press.

Charlesworth A, Davies A, Dixon J. 2012. Reforming Payment for Health Care in Europe to Achieve Better Value. The Nuffield Trust: UK.

Chevreul K, Durand-Zaleski I, Bahrami S, Hernandez-Quevedo C, Mladovsky P. 2010. *France: Health System Review.* European Observatory on Health Systems and Policies.

Cutler DM, Zeckhauser RJ. (1998). Adverse selection in health insurance. In Garber A (ed.). *Frontiers in Health Policy Research, Volume 1.* Cambridge: MIT Press.

Ellis RP, McGuire TG. 1990. Optimal payment systems for health services. *Journal of Health Economics* 9(4): 375–396.

Ellis RP, Miller MM. 2008. Provider payment and provider incentives. In Heggenhougen, K and Carrin G (eds.). *Encyclopedia of Public Health.* New York: Elsevier.

Evans TG, Chowdhury MR, Evans D, Fidler AH, Lindelow M, Mills A, Scheil-Adlung X. 2011. Thailand's Universal Coverage Scheme: Achievements and Challenges. An independent assessment of the first 10 years (2001–2010), Synthesis Report.

Figueras J, Lessof S, McKee M, Durán A, Menabde N. 2012. Health systems, health, wealth and societal well-being: An introduction. In Figueras J, McKee M (eds.). *Health Systems, Health, Wealth and Societal Well-being: Assessing the Case for Investing in Health Systems.* World Health Organization Regional Office for Europe and the European Observatory on Health Systems and Policies. Berkshire, England: Open University Press.

Figueras J, Robinson R, Jakubowski E. 2005. Purchasing to improve health system performance: Drawing the lessons. In Figueras J, Robinson R, Jakubowski E (eds.). *Purchasing to Improve Health Systems Performance.* European Observatory on Health Care Systems. Buckingham, England: Open University Press.

Frakt AB. 2011. How much do hospitals cost shift? A review of the evidence. *Milbank Quarterly* 89(1): 90–130.

Frenk J. 1995. Comprehensive policy analysis for health system reform. *Health Policy* 32: 257–77.

Fuchs VR. 1996. What every philosopher should know about health economics. *Proceedings of the American Philosophical Society* 140(2): 186–96.

González-Rossetti A. 2002. Social health insurance in Latin America. Background paper. In: *DFID Health Insurance Workshop, London, 9–10 April 2002.* London, Institute for Health Sector Development.

Gottret P, Schieber G. 2006. *Health Financing Revisited: A Practitioner's Guide.* Washington, DC: The World Bank.

Griffin CC, Shaw RP. 1995. Health insurance in sub-Saharan Africa: Aims, findings, policy implications. In Shaw RP, Ainsworth M (eds.). *Financing Health Services through*

User Fees and Insurance: Case Studies from Sub-Saharan Africa. World Bank Discussion Paper 294. Washington, DC: The World Bank.

Health Economics Unit. 2010. Who benefits from health care in South Africa? HEU Information Sheet No. 5. Cape Town: School of Public Health and Family Medicine, University of Cape Town. http://uct-heu.s3.amazonaws.com/wp-content/uploads/2010/02/IS5_heu_WhoBenefitsFromHealthCare.pdf.

Hou Z, Van de Poel E, Van Doorslaer E, Yu B, Meng Q. 2012. Effect of NCMS coverage on access to care and financial protection in China. Tinbergen Institute Discussion Paper TI 2012-039/3, and *Working Paper* 09, Health Equity and Financial Protection in Asia Project. http://www.bmg.eur.nl/fileadmin/ASSETS/bmg/english/HEFPA/Publications/Working_Papers/HEFPA_WP_09.pdf.

Hsiao WC. 1993. Health Care Financing in Thailand: Challenges for the Future. In Health Financing in Thailand: Proceeding of a National Workshop. 11–13 November: Petchaburi Province, Thailand.

Ikegami N, Maeda A. 2014. Overview. In Ikegami N (ed.). *Universal Health Coverage for Inclusive and Sustainable Development: Lessons from Japan*. Washington, DC: World Bank. http://www-wds.worldbank.org/external/default/WDSContentServer/WDSP/IB/2014/10/10/000442464_20141010104230/Rendered/PDF/911630PUB0Box30see0also0888620Sep25.pdf.

Ikegami N, Yoo, B-K, Hashimoto H, Matsumoto M, Ogata H, Babazono A, Watanabe R, Shibuya K, Yang, B-M, Reich MR, Kobayashi Y. 2011. Japanese universal health coverage: Evolution, achievements, and challenges. *The Lancet* 378(9796): 1106–1115.

ILO (International Labour Organization). 2014. *Global Employment Trends 2014: Risk of a Jobless Recovery?* Geneva: International Labour Organization.

IMF (International Monetary Fund). 2011. *Revenue Mobilization in Developing Countries*. Washington, DC: International Monetary Fund.

Kaiser Family Foundation. 2013. Summary of the Affordable Care Act. Publication #8061-02. Menlo Park, California: The Henry J. Kaiser Family Foundation. https://kaiserfamilyfoundation.files.wordpress.com/2011/04/8061-021.pdf.

Knaul FM, González-Pier E, Gómez-Dantés O, García-Junco D, Arreola-Ornelas H, Barraza-Lloréns M, Sandoval R, Caballero F, Hernández-Avila M, Juan M, Kershenobich D, Nigenda G, Ruelas E, Sepúlveda J, Tapia R, Soberón G, Chertorivski S, Frenk J. 2012. The quest for universal health coverage: Achieving social protection for all in Mexico. *The Lancet* 380(9849): 1259–1279.

Kutzin J. 1997. Health insurance for the formal sector in Africa: 'yes, but...' *Current Concerns* series, ARA Paper number 14. WHO/ARA/CC/97.4. Geneva: World Health Organization, Division of Analysis, Research and Assessment. Also available, under the same title. In: Beattie A, Doherty J, Gilson L, Lambo E, Shaw RP (eds.). 1998. *Sustainable Health Care Financing in Southern Africa: Papers from an EDI Health Policy Seminar Held in Johannesburg, South Africa, June 1996*. Washington, DC: World Bank, Economic Development Institute.

Kutzin J. 2001. A descriptive framework for country-level analysis of health care financing arrangements. *Health Policy* 56(3): 171–204.

Kutzin J. 2008. Health financing policy: A guide for decision-makers. Health Financing Policy Paper 2008/1. Copenhagen, Denmark: World Health Organization, Regional Office for Europe, Division of Country Health Systems. http://www.euro.who.int/_data/assets/pdf_file/0004/78871/E91422.pdf.

Kutzin J. 2012 Anything goes on the path to universal health coverage? No. *Bulletin of the World Health Organization* 90: 867–868.

Kutzin J. 2013. Health financing for universal coverage and health system performance: Concepts and implications for policy. *Bulletin of the World Health Organization* 91(8): 602–611.

Kutzin J, Jakab M. 2010. Fiscal context and health expenditure patterns. In Kutzin J, Cashin C, Jakab M (eds.). 2010. *Implementing Health Financing Reform: Lessons from Countries in Transition*. Copenhagen, Denmark: World Health Organization, on behalf of the European Observatory on Health Systems and Policies.

Kutzin J, Cashin C, Jakab M, Fidler A, Menabde N. 2010b. Implementing health financing reform in CE/EECCA countries: Synthesis and lessons learned. In Kutzin J, Cashin C, Jakab M (eds.). 2010. *Implementing Health Financing Reform: Lessons from Countries in Transition*. Copenhagen, Denmark: World Health Organization, on behalf of the European Observatory on Health Systems and Policies.

Kutzin J, Jakab M, Shishkin S. 2009. From scheme to system: Social health insurance funds and the transformation of health financing in Kyrgyzstan and Moldova. In Chernichovsky D, Hanson, K (eds.). *Innovations in Health System Finance in Developing and Transitional Economies*. Advances in Health Economics and Health Services Research, Volume 21, pp. 291–312. Bingley, UK: Emerald Group Publishing.

Kutzin J, Shishkin S, Bryndová L, Schneider P, Hroboň. 2010a. Reforms in the pooling of funds. In Kutzin J, Cashin C, Jakab M (eds.). 2010. *Implementing Health Financing Reform: Lessons from Countries in Transition*. Copenhagen, Denmark: World Health Organization, on behalf of the European Observatory on Health Systems and Policies.

La Forgia G, Nagpal S. 2012. *Government-sponsored Health Insurance in India: Are You Covered?* Directions in Development series. Washington, DC: The World Bank.

Lagomarsino G, Garabrant A, Adyas A, Muga R, Otoo N. 2012. Moving towards universal health coverage: Health insurance reforms in nine developing countries in Africa and Asia. *The Lancet* 380: 933–943.

Langenbrunner J, Orosz E, Kutzin J, Wiley M. 2005. Purchasing and paying providers. In Figueras J, Robinson R, Jakubowski E (eds.). *Purchasing to Improve Health Systems Performance*. European Observatory on Health Care Systems. Buckingham, England: Open University Press.

Londoño JL, Frenk J. 1997. Structured pluralism: Towards an innovative model for health system reform in Latin America. *Health Policy* 41(1): 1–36.

Maeda A, Araujo E, Cashin C, Harris J, Ikegami N, Reich M. 2014. Universal Health Coverage for Inclusive and Sustainable Development: A Synthesis of 11 Country Case Studies. Washington, DC: The World Bank.

Makaka A. 2012. Role of government stewardship and leadership in SHP. Presentation to Regional Conference on Social Health Protection in East African Community.

11 September, Kigali, Rwanda. http://moh.gov.rw/english/wp-content/uploads/2012/09/Presentation-on-Governance-in-Rwanda-CBHI_-Makaka.pptx.

McPake B, Brikci N, Cometto G, Schmidt A, Araujo E. 2011. Removing user fees: Learning from international experience to support the process. *Health Policy and Planning* 26(Suppl 2): Ii104–ii117.

Meessen B, Hercot D, Noirhomme M, Ridde V, Tibouti A, Tashobya CK, Gilson L. 2011. Removing user fees in the health sector: A review of policy processes in six sub-Saharan African countries. *Health Policy and Planning* 26(Suppl 2): Ii164–ii29.

Meng Q, Xu L, Zhang Y, Qian J, Cai M, Xin Y, Gao J, Xu K, Boerma JT, Barber SL. 2012. Trends in access to health services and financial protection in China between 2003 and 2011: A cross-sectional study. *Lancet* 379(9818): 805–14.

Mexico 2013. Political Constitution of the United Mexican States http://www.globalhealthrights.org/wp-content/uploads/2013/10/Mexico-Constitution-En.pdf.

Morgan L, Beith A, Eichler R. 2011. In Brief: Performance Incentives for Improved Maternal Health: Taking Stock of Current Programs and Future Potentials. Health System 2020 Report. Bethesda, Maryland: Abt Associates, Inc. http://www.healthsystems2020.org/content/resource/detail/85773/.

Mossialos E, and Thomson S. 2004. *Voluntary health insurance in the European Union*. Copenhagen: World Health Organization on behalf of the European Observatory on Health Systems and Policies.

Murray CJL, Frenk J. 2000. A framework for assessing the performance of health systems. *Bulletin of the World Health Organization* 78(6): 717–731.

Musango L, Makaka A, Muhongerwa D, Kalisa IR, Elovainio R. 2013. Strategies towards universal health coverage in Rwanda: Lessons learned from extending coverage through mutual health organizations. *The African Health Monitor* 17: 6–10.

OECD, Eurostat WHO. 2011. *A System of Health Accounts*. Paris: OECD Publishing.

Peabody J, Shimkhada R, Quimbo S, Florentino J, Bacate M, McCulloch CE, *et al.* 2011. Financial incentives and measurement improved physicians' quality of care in the Philippines. *Health Affairs* 30(4): 773–781.

Prakongsai P, Limwattananon S, Tangcharoensathien V. 2009. The equity impact of the universal coverage policy: Lessons from Thailand. In Chernichovsky D, Hanson K (eds.). *Innovations in Health System Finance in Developing and Transitional Economies*. Advances in Health Economics and Health Services Research, Volume 21, pp. 291–312. Bingley, UK: Emerald Group Publishing.

Qingyue M, Beibei Y, Liying J. 2010. Means Testing for Targeting the People in Health Programs: A Systematic Review. Geneva: Alliance for Health Policy and Systems Research. http://www.who.int/alliance-hpsr/projects/alliancehpsr_meanstesting_systematicreviewshandong.pdf.

Rannan-Eliya RP, Sikurajapathy L. 2008. Sri Lanka: "Good Practice" in expanding health care coverage. In Gottret P, Schieber GJ, Waters HR (eds.). *Good Practices in Health Financing: Lessons from Reforms in Low- and Middle-Income Countries*. Washington, DC: The World Bank.

Reich MR, Ikegami N, Shibuya K, Takemi K. 2011. 50 years of pursuing a healthy society in Japan. *The Lancet* 378(9796): 1051–1053.

Republic of Rwanda 2010. Rwanda National Health Insurance Policy. Kigali, Rwanda: Ministry of Health.

Roberts MJ, Hsiao W, Berman P, Reich M. 2002. *Getting Health Reform Right: A Guide to Improving Performance and Equity*. Oxford, England: Oxford University Press.

Robinson J. 2011. Hospitals respond to Medicare payment shortfalls by both shifting costs and cutting them, based on market concentration. *Health Affairs* 30(7): 1265–1271.

Saltman RB, Dubois HFW. 2004. The historical and social base of social health insurance systems. In Saltman RB, Busse R, Figueras J (eds.). *Social Health Insurance Systems in Western Europe*. World Health Organization on behalf of the European Observatory on Health Systems and Policies. Berkshire, England: Open University Press.

Savedoff WD. 2004. Is there a case for social insurance? *Health Policy and Planning* 19(3): 183–184.

Schieber G, Maeda A. 1997. A curmudgeon's guide to financing health care in developing countries. In: Schieber G (ed.). *Innovations in health care financing: Proceedings of a World Bank Conference, 10–11 March 1997*. Discussion Paper No. 365, Washington, DC: The World Bank.

Sekabaraga C, Diop F, Soucat A. 2011. Can innovative health financing policies increase access to MDG-related services? Evidence from Rwanda. *Health Policy and Planning* 26(Suppl. 2): Ii52–ii62.

Sheiman I, Langenbrunner J, Kehler J, Cashin C, Kutzin J. 2010. Sources of funds and revenue collection: Reforms and challenges. In Kutzin J, Cashin C, Jakab M (eds.). 2010. *Implementing Health Financing Reform: Lessons from Countries in Transition*. Copenhagen, Denmark: World Health Organization, on behalf of the European Observatory on Health Systems and Policies.

Shishkin S, Jowett M. 2012. A review of health financing reforms in the Republic of Moldova. Health Financing Policy Paper 2012/1. Copenhagen: World Health Organization, Regional Office for Europe. http://www.euro.who.int/_data/assets/pdf_file/0009/166788/E96542.pdf.

South Africa. 1996. Constitution of the Republic of South Africa, 1996. http://www.globalhealthrights.org/wp-content/uploads/2013/10/South-Africa-Constitution-1996.pdf.

Sutton M, Nikolova S, Boaden R, Lester H, McDonald R, Roland M. 2012. Reduced mortality with hospital pay for performance in England. *New England Journal of Medicine* 367(19): 1821–1828.

Szigeti S, Evetovits T, Gaál P. 2012. How does the increasing reliance of the Hungarian social health insurance fund on tax revenues affect the sustainability of the health sector? An analysis based on the 2011 edition of the system of health accounts. Budapest: World Health Organization, Regional Office for Europe (draft).

Tandon A, Cashin C. 2010. Assessing public expenditure on health from a fiscal space perspective. Washington, DC: The World Bank.

United Nations. 1948. Universal Declaration of Human Rights. http://www.un.org/en/documents/udhr/index.shtml.

Wagstaff A, Lindelow M. 2008. Can insurance increase financial risk? The curious case of health insurance in China. *Journal of Health Economics* 27(4): 990–1005.
WHO (World Health Organization). 1948. Constitution of the World Health Organization. http://apps.who.int/gb/bd/PDF/bd47/EN/constitution-en.pdf?ua=1.
WHO (World Health Organization). 2000. *The World Health Report. Health Systems: Improving Performance.* Geneva: World Health Organization.
WHO (World Health Organization). 2007. *Everybody's business: Strengthening health systems to improve health outcomes. WHO's framework for action.* Geneva: World Health Organization. http://www.who.int/entity/healthsystems/strategy/everybodys_business.pdf.
WHO (World Health Organization). 2010a. *The World Health Report — Health Systems Financing: The Path to Universal Coverage.* Geneva: World Health Organization.
WHO (World Health Organization). 2010b. *Fragmentation in pooling arrangements.* Technical Brief No. 5. Geneva: World Health Organization. http://www.who.int/healthsystems/topics/financing/healthreport/FragmentationTBNo5.pdf?ua=1.
WHO (World Health Organization). 2013a. *Ghana: Coverage Expansion Through Political Commitment and Innovative Policy Choices.* Success Stories series, Providing for Health (P4H) network. http://www.who.int/providingforhealth/PH4_Ghana_success_story.pdf.
WHO (World Health Organization). 2013b. Burundi: Adoption of Performance Based-Finance to Fund Fee-Exempt Health Services. Success Stories series, Providing for Health (P4H) network. http://www.who.int/providingforhealth/PH4_Burundi_success_story.pdf.
WHO (World Health Organization). 2014. Global Health Expenditure Database. http://apps.who.int/nha/database.
Witter S, Fretheim A, Kessy FL, Lindahl AK. 2012. Paying for performance to improve the delivery of health interventions in low- and middle-income countries. *Cochrane Database Systematic Review* 2: CD007899.
Wu V. 2010. Hospital cost shifting revisited: New evidence from the balanced budget act of 1997. *International Journal of Health Care Finance and Economics* 10(1): 61–83.
Xu K, Evans D, Kawabata K, Zeramdini R, Klavus J, Murray C. 2003. Household catastrophic health expenditure: A multicountry analysis. *Lancet* 362: 111–117.
Yip WC, Hsiao WC, Chen W, Hu S, Ma J, Maynard A. 2012. Early appraisal of China's huge and complex health-care reforms. *Lancet* 379: 833–842.
Yip W, Powell-Jackson T, Chen W, Hu M, Fe E, Hu M, Jian W, Lu M, Han W, Hsiao WC. 2014. Capitation with pay-for-performance improves primary care providers' antibiotic prescribing practices in rural China. *Health Affairs* 33(3): 502–510.

Global Risk-Adjusted Payment Models

Camilo Cid
Universidad Católica de Chile

Randall P. Ellis
Boston University

Verónica Vargas
World Bank

Juergen Wasem
Universität Duisburg-Essen

Lorena Prieto
Universidad del Pacífico, Lima

Global health care payment systems reflect enormous differences in provider characteristics, health systems, and development levels. Risk adjustment is used for payment and performance measurement to correct for demand heterogeneity and incentives for plans and providers to prefer healthy, low-cost patients. This chapter reviews the practical, theoretical, and statistical aspects of risk adjustment models, which use socio-demographic variables and more recently morbidity and pharmaceuticals, to predict outcomes. Diverse uses of risk adjustment include geographical budget allocations, health plan premium equalization, pay for performance, primary care provider payment, integrated provider networks, and rewards for good doctor performance. Settings in more than 30 countries are examined, which include high-, middle- and low-income countries, competitive health plans and single-payer systems, integrated provider networks, clinics, and solo practice primary care doctors. Recent concepts in health economics are highlighted that hold potential for improving efficiency and equitable patient access to health care.

Keywords: Healthcare Payments Systems; Risk Adjustment; Risk-Adjusted Payments.

Introduction

Every health care payment system must make payments to a diverse set of health plans, hospitals, clinics, physicians, laboratories, pharmacies, and other types of health care providers. Some health care systems rely on competition among multiple health plans[1] ("multiple payers") to generate funds and pay providers. In other "single payer" health care systems, payment allocation decisions are made centrally by a single government entity; or funds are allocated geographically to regions, states, counties or cities within a single payer structure. A related challenge is that within a health plan, a provider network, or even a clinic or hospital, there will be variation in the cost, utilization level, and health status of patients seen, and it is therefore useful to control for this patient heterogeneity within a provider group when distributing payments. Risk adjustment is a tool that is useful for correcting or controlling for this heterogeneity in all of these payment settings.

The problem of heterogeneity is that the cost of treating patients is never randomly distributed across different groups, whether those groups be insurance plan enrollees, residents in a given state or other geographic region, or users seen by a given hospital, clinic, pharmacy, or individual provider. Nonrandom cost variation introduces efficiency problems (e.g., inadequate resources for certain health plans, regions or providers, leading to undertreatment) as well as fairness problems (e.g., overpaying for some groups, underpaying for others). Parallel concerns about efficiency and fairness across groups also arise when identifying high- or low-quality health plans, regions, or providers.

Risk adjustment is a technique used to calculate the expected cost (or quality, or utilization) of treating a specific group using information about the members of that group. In many cases, risk adjustment is used to allocate funds between different groups, or at least to develop norms against which actual funding levels can be compared. Often, the goal is to "level the playing field" to ensure that a plan/region/provider group that attracts a sicker-than-average set of enrollees will receive greater resources, or be recognized for achieving higher quality or lower quantity than expected when assessing performance.

The remainder of this chapter describes more carefully why risk adjustment is done and how it is done. After defining risk adjustment, Section "Payment Systems in Health- and Risk-Adjustment" characterizes the problems that risk adjustment intends to solve. It then turns to describing the types of information that can be used for risk adjustment as well as alternative estimation methods. Also discussed is the distinction between *conventional risk adjustment*, in which

[1]Health plans refer to entities that pay providers of health care services. When health plans pool resources and bear risk, they are also referred to as insurance plans or insurers. Not all health plans bear risk or provide insurance. When provider networks receive per capita payments, then they bear risk and become the insurer.

existing payment patterns are captured in the risk adjustment formula, and *optimal risk adjustment*, where risk adjustment prices are viewed as tools for correcting underlying distortions. Section "Risk adjustment classification systems" presents commonly used classification systems, their limitations and a comparison of the predictive power of models. Sections "Risk Adjustment with Competing Health Plans and "Risk Adjustment in Single Payer Systems" discuss how risk adjustment is used in various countries, contrasting uses in countries that have competing health plans with countries that have single-payer systems. Section "Risk Adjusted Payments to Individual Providers" discusses risk-adjusted payments to individual providers and country examples. Section "Discussion: Risk-Adjusted Payments and Improving Efficiency and Equity" summarizes the key lessons in the risk adjustment experience, policy concerns and issues that are still being discussed and that need to be addressed in future studies or applications.

Payment Systems in Health- and Risk-Adjustment

Payment systems

Health care markets are characterized by problems that differentiate them from other markets: large information asymmetries (which lead to risk selection and moral hazard); externalities; imperfect competition; heterogeneity on both the demand and supply sides; and substantial uncertainty that creates a demand for insurance. Insurance in particular distorts consumer choices and conceals consumers' willingness to pay. Thus, market prices of individual services (often called "fee-for-service" (FFS) prices), which typically balance willingness to pay with the marginal cost, lose this key role in most health care markets. When the public sector makes regulations, sponsors insurance, or delivers health care, these decisions further disturb normal market performance, especially in the case of payments.

Pricing problems are particularly severe in public health care systems, where in most cases the funder or payer (the government) is the residual creditor for payments, which creates incentives for overpricing and oversupply that work against efficiency (Ortún *et al.*, 2001). Even if market-driven prices for each service are replaced by fixed rates set by a regulator, service-level pricing will rarely reach a desirable result, since generously insured consumers will tend to demand and receive too many services (demand-side moral hazard). Regulated service prices also tend to affect markets through their effect on providers (supply-side moral hazard). If the price of a given service is set above its marginal cost, then providers will tend to oversupply that service. Problems are even worse when prices are not cost-related, which routinely happens when a government does not have information on actual costs or their dynamics over time (Newhouse *et al.*, 1989). Given this, health systems in many countries are implementing alternative payment systems that place less reliance on FFS pricing and change the incentives facing consumers and suppliers (Paris *et al.*, 2010; Ellis and Miller, 2008).

Most health care payment systems can be classified into four types. The first type is a cost-based reimbursement system that retrospectively pays for the care provided, often in the form of FFS. Under this type of system, providers choose the number, type and quality of service, without much concern for the financial consequences because they are fully reimbursed for expenses incurred. The second type of system is a bundled payment system, in which payments are based on a predetermined contract that establishes conditions between the payer and the provider and does not directly compensate for increases in care provided. Bundled payments can either be based on predetermined information, in which case it is called a prospective payment system, or the bundled payment can be based on information that emerges during the payment period (such as the number and types of diagnoses) in which is it can be called either a concurrent or retrospective payment system. Bundled payments can either be for a period of time such as a year ("capitation") or for event such as an episode of treatment (e.g., hospital payment for "diagnosis related groups"). The third type of payment system is a budgeted system that relies on an integrated estimate of costs between the funder and the provider. How incentives work in a budgeted system depends on how these budgets are negotiated and updated. For example, in budgeting for results, the objective is to transform financial resources into outputs and outcomes, which is a multistep process. The budgeting process includes quantification of intermediate objectives, description of interventions, as well as the activities and their associated financial resources. Finally, the fourth type of payment system — considered to be the state-of-the-art mechanism in countries more developed in this area of payment methodologies — are mixed payment systems, also called risk-sharing plans, which combine prospective and retrospective features to balance the tradeoff between efficiency and selection (Newhouse, 1996).

Both fully retrospective and mixed payment systems rely on "bundled payments" for all or part of their payments. Prospective payments — whether per person-month, or per event — can promote efficiency because they reduce the financial incentive on the margin to oversupply services, because these payments do not depend on provider-level health spending. Indeed, when marginal payments are below marginal costs, providers may undersupply some services: The theory is that bundled payments give incentives for providers to make the right decisions about which services to provide, given their competition for patients, altruism and concerns about reputation ensuring adequate supply. The central challenge with bundled payment is that it creates incentives for selection, in which providers or health plans try to avoid treating or enrolling patients that are expected to be unprofitable. (How this selection occurs is discussed further below.) In general, retrospective payments may minimize risk selection problems, but worsen efficiency through overprovision. Balancing these two goals — minimizing risk selection and improving efficiency — is an argument for using mixed payment systems, where some but not all costs are shared (Newhouse, 1996).

Definition of risk adjustment and uses for payment

In their classic study, van de Ven and Ellis (2000) define risk adjustment as using available information to calculate the expected costs or health of individuals or groups of patients for a fixed time period (usually one year). When used for payments to health plans, this implies the need for subsidies for individuals or health plans with higher risks, in order to improve both efficiency and equity in the health system. More recent discussions of risk adjustment generally include its use for controlling for variables while measuring utilization (e.g., numbers of emergency room visits or admissions), quality, or performance measures. This section focuses on the use of risk adjustment for payment purposes.

Every modern health care system can be thought of as having four groups of agents: consumers who receive health care services; providers who provide it; a sponsor who gathers revenue in a wide range of ways, to be used for insurance purposes; and one or more health plans responsible for paying providers. The boundaries between health plans and providers can be blurry in some health care systems, where the health plan owns or directly controls the providers. Two examples of this are managed care plans in competitive systems or single-payer plans with public ownership of facilities. In these cases, as in vertically integrated firms, provider payment decisions are made internally within the health plan-provider groups (Ellis and Fernandez, 2013).

Premium-based risk adjustment systems rely on interactions between the sponsor and the health plan(s). The sponsor pools resources, whether premiums or income-based contributions from diverse enrollees, and then uses a risk adjustment payment formula to calculate per capita payments that go to the health plan. Both the specific institutions used and the structure of payment flows can vary by country, but a common system is that consumers pay a premium (in Europe, called their solidarity contribution), which may be either fixed or, more commonly, calculated as a fraction of their income, to government agency that in turn pays a risk-adjusted per capita amount to the corresponding health plan (Cid, 2011).

A risk-adjusted premium payment system enables the contribution of an individual or worker enrolling in a health plan to differ from the revenue received by their health plan for their care. In this scenario, payments to health plans reflect each individual's expected cost of health services utilization, regardless of whether it is more or less than the amount the individual contributed. An ideal risk-adjustment formula levels the playing field, so that a health plan is indifferent between accepting healthy or sick, young or old, or rich or poor enrollees, because they are paid based on the enrollees' expected risk. Most analytical models of risk adjustment suggest that such a perfect system creates strong incentives for efficiency. Unfortunately, no empirical risk adjustment model can ever be perfect in calculating risk. There will always be incomplete information available to the regulator calculating risk adjustment payments, or political or ethical constraints may prohibit the use of certain types of information. Even when health plans and the sponsor have the same information, consumers will generally have private information which may lead to selection problems. This could, in turn, lead to problems of inefficiency, low quality and poor access for high-risk groups.

Risk adjustment can be done at the individual or group level. For example, the costs of treating a city, county, state or region can be aggregated, or the characteristics of a health plan can be used instead of individual-level characteristics. Most risk adjustment frameworks calculate risk adjusted payments for each individual in a population, and then sum up these predictions to the group level. Results from the UK (Rice and Smith, 2001) and the US (Ash *et al.*, 2000) show that individual-level information is much more predictive than aggregate information. Individual-level information should ideally include demographics, health status, socioeconomic characteristics and expenditure data for each health service received. But this level of disaggregation is not easily available. For instance, a health care system may not be able to assign health care expenditures to specific individuals in a health care plan or provider system. Even if only group-level information is available, aggregate models may still be useful in reducing the risk for the provider and improving provider efficiency. Risk adjusted, pooled payments still tend to promote efficiency, because the provider group or region internalizes the cost burden: If the group overspends on some patients or services, it must save on other patients or services to avoid losing money. Risk adjustment based on population characteristics may also improve the equity of payments and promote access to care, but, as mentioned above, if consumers can actively choose what plan or group to be in, then incentives for risk selection will persist.

Why Use Risk Adjustment in Payment Systems?

The primary motivation for risk adjustment is risk selection — the tendency in insurance markets for nonrandom sorting between alternative health plans. Risk selection can arise from a variety of processes, for example an individual may have more information about her health status than the health provider or health plan, or the provider may have better information about the a patients expected cost. These information asymmetries lead to both demand- and supply-side selection incentives

(Newhouse, 1996). On the demand side, individuals may use their private information towards adverse selection — with higher-cost consumers disproportionately enrolling in more generous or better quality health plans. Risk selection can also result in a favorable selection problem on the supply side when health plans or providers distort the service levels they offer so as to try to attract profitable enrollees (Glazer and McGuire, 2000). Depending on the market and the payment system, either adverse or favorable selection can result (Newhouse, 1996).

The preceding discussion assumes that selection is made in insurance markets that insure individuals for a fixed unit of time, such as a year. But selection can also occur whenever bundled payments create sorting incentives in other settings, such as per hospital day, per admission, per activity, per episode of treatment, or per bundle of provider services. The choice of the unit of payment affects both the risk selection incentives and the riskiness of the payment system to providers. Risk adjustment can be used to control for observable variables that affect cost, utilization or quality measures for any of these various units of payment although the terminology of severity adjustment is often used in such settings.

Risk selection exists because health care spending varies widely across individuals both for random and systematic reasons. This variation is called risk. Risk pooling — insuring large groups of enrollees — is effective at averaging out variation that is random and unpredictable, although if health care providers or insurers serve only modest numbers of enrollees (e.g., less than 10,000), then even random risk can remain important. More problematic is variation that is predictable and systematic. Agents bearing systematic risk face incentives to attract profitable enrollees, who are usually low-cost, healthy enrollees or patients.

Risk selection is affected by regulations and the structure of the entire health care payment system. For example, regulators may restrict plan benefits or plan behavior intended to attract healthy enrollees, or regulators may restrict who or how often consumers get to change plans. The structure of premiums as well as reinsurance and provider payment systems also affect risk selection, as well as risk bearing and care incentives. Unlike these other features, which may also address fairness or efficiency concerns, risk adjustment has as its primary purpose the reduction of risk selection. As mentioned above, providers may risk select to avoid unprofitable, usually sicker patients or reduce spending, saving at least a portion of the fixed payment received. One direct consequence may be a reduction in service quality for a proportion of the population (and in an extreme case, being denied insurance or access to care). This emphasizes the importance of the information used by risk adjusters: A good expenditure prediction is one that adjusts the fixed payment to the estimate made by the provider. Risk adjustment models that use only age and sex as adjusters, while better than no risk adjustment, leave significant risk selection incentives (Ash *et al.*, 1989; Pope *et al.*, 2000; Rice and Smith, 2001).

Optimal risk adjustment is a concept used to describe a payment model in which both the demand-side and supply-side selection incentives mentioned above are addressed, given allowed payment systems (Glazer and McGuire, 2000). A related term is "perfect risk adjustment" (van Barneveld *et al.*, 2001), which fully compensates providers for all the predictable expenses for each individual, and solves efficiency and selection problems (van de Ven and Ellis, 2000). The key concept in optimal risk adjustment is to use risk adjustment not only to pay plans (or providers) the predicted cost of services provided, but also to correct any undesirable incentives for over or under provision of services. In the presence of imperfect risk adjustment signals, this may require biased rather than unbiased payments for signals. For example, if only half of the patients with an expensive condition in a plan are actually observed to have this condition, then one may need to (substantially) overpay the plan for each observed signal of this condition (or provider's panel of patients) and underpay for those without this signal. This insight is in Glazer and McGuire (2000).

Alternative information to use for risk adjusted payment models

- *Prospective vs. retrospective information*

Before discussing the different types of information that can be used for risk adjustment, it is worth highlighting that two fundamental approaches are distinct. This section focuses initially on models that predict spending in a fixed period of time, usually a year, which is called the prediction period. Prospective (or *ex ante*) models use only information that exists prior to the beginning of the prediction period for which spending is being modeled; while retrospective (or *ex post*) models use information that may not be known until the end of the year (Table 1). While in principle retrospective models can use information even for multiple periods prior to the base period, such as from period $t - 1$, in practice this is rarely

Table 1. Prospective and retrospective payment

Model	$t-1$	t	$t+1$
Prospective	Base period = Source of RA information	Prediction period Final payments made using information from period $t-1$	Not needed
Retrospective	Not needed	Prediction period = Base period = Source of RA information	Final payments for period t are calculated and made using information from period t

Note: RA: Risk adjustment.
Source: Authors, adapted from Cid (2011).

done, since it increases the challenge of what to do when such long periods of prior information are not available.

Age and gender are generally known at the beginning of the year, although newborn and deaths are exceptions. Early risk adjustment models all adopted a prospective framework whereas a retrospective approach, using conditions observed during the prediction period, are increasingly becoming more popular. Retrospective (concurrent) models[2] generally have much higher predictive power than prospective models, and hence it is important to keep this in mind when comparing different information sets.

The above discussion focuses on predictions for a fixed period of time. For prediction of other periods, such as hospital episodes or outpatient episodes, the norm is to use diagnoses that occur during the episode itself, which is a retrospective framework. But since bad things sometimes happen to patients during a hospital stay, (e.g., an infection, injury or heart attack due to poor quality care) it is common practice to use only some, but not all information that arises during a hospital stay or other episode of treatment. In the US, hospital DRG payments are often called a form of "prospective payment" in that the "principal diagnosis" hospitals are supposed to use is the diagnosis recorded at time of discharge that was the principal reason for the patient's admission. By this criterion, a patient admitted with a broken arm who subsequently had a heart attack (AMI) while in the hospital should be recorded as admitted for a broken arm, not as for an AMI. Moreover, recently in the US hospitals are being denied payment for expensive patients where outcomes or diagnoses signal unsafe or poor quality care (e.g., bed sores). Obviously this use of information is difficult to audit and controversial, but the concept is that it is the prospective cause of the admission, not the retrospective treatment that is supposed to be used. Because procedure information is also used in the US DRGs, they are *de facto* in part a cost-based retrospective reimbursement system.

- *Demographic only models*

The first risk adjustment models were introduced in the US in the 1980s for Medicare managed care plans. Their earliest payment formulas used only age, gender, whether the patient was in a nursing home, and disability status to predict annual health care spending. The model also included geographic adjustment at the county level to capture cost of living and practice style variation (García Goñi, 2006). This demographic-only model had low predictive power: Pope *et al.* (2000)

[2] Many risk adjustment modelers prefer to use the term concurrent rather than retrospective risk adjustment since in principle truly retrospective models can also be estimated that use information from time extending beyond the prediction period. This distinction becomes particularly important when only a single month of spending is being predicted.

estimated that a demographic risk adjustment model only explained 1.5% of spending variability for the Medicare population in a prospective regression model; Ash *et al.* (2000) predicted 2% in a similar model using privately insured, Medicaid, and Medicare samples. Models using only age and gender as adjusters typically explain about 3–4% of the variation in total annual health spending when the full age distribution is included (van de Ven and Ellis, 2000).

Demographic models use actuarial cells, where each cell represents the expected cost of a previously defined risk group. Until 2009, the German risk equalization model basically used socio-demographic variables and included over 700 cells or risk groups, as is the case with Swiss and Israeli models (van de Ven *et al.*, 2007). The Chilean model adjusts the AUGE benefit basket expenditures between ISAPRES (private insurers) using 36 cells defined by gender and age groups (Cid *et al.*, 2006).[3]

- *Diagnoses-based models*

To improve prediction, risk adjustment models started including diagnoses based on two lines of research. The work of Weiner *et al.* (1996) at Johns Hopkins University introduced the Adjusted Clinical Groups (ACG) grading system that initially only allowed the use of outpatient diagnoses, but later evolved to add all types of care. A second line of research has its origins at Boston University, and its most representative works are Ash *et al.* (1989), Ellis *et al.* (1996) and Pope *et al.* (2000). The Diagnostic Cost Group (DCG) classification system initially used only data from the principal diagnoses of hospitalized patients, but was later expanded to include diagnoses from all sources, including outpatient care and was renamed as the Hierarchical Condition Category (HCC) model. Diagnostic classification systems have also evolved in Europe through the work of van Vliet and van de Ven (1993); Lamers and van Vliet (1996) in the Netherlands; Wasem *et al.* (2006) in Germany.

The underlying assumption of diagnosis-based risk adjustment is that diagnoses are an unbiased measure of each enrollee's true health status. This may not be true if diagnoses are either unreliable because of incomplete coding, or distorted by strategic up coding by providers or health plans to increase payments. Every system that has started requiring diagnoses on claims for payment or monitoring

[3] Chile's health sector reform was implemented in 2005 and it is known as AUGE Reform. It defined a basic package to cover selected health problems, with guarantees that began with 26 health problems and was since expanded twice and now includes 80 health problems. The basket defines interventions and guarantees. All sectors must comply with this basket, but it is considered "basic" since the public insurer (FONASA) and the private insurers (ISAPRES) provide coverage for other health problems than the ones in the basic basket.

finds that, initially, the quality of diagnostic coding is highly incomplete, and needs to be audited.

- *Pharmaceutical prescription-based models*

Pharmaceutical prescriptions are also a potential source for variables to predict costs, given that the use of certain medications can infer the existence of certain chronic diseases. Although the explanatory power of prescriptions is similar to that obtained from robust diagnoses-based models, the major concern is that these models may promote perverse incentives for efficiency, as in the case of models based on historical spending (García Goñi, 2006). Higher expenditures in the last year or greater use of high-cost pharmaceuticals are rewarded with increased reimbursement for the following year.

The Netherlands introduced the use of Pharmacy-based Cost Groups (PCGs) in 2002 and added inpatient diagnostic cost groups in 2004 (Lamers *et al.*, 2003; van de Ven *et al.*, 2007). The Dutch system's focus on a narrow set of originally 12 (now 17) PCGs was intended to capture chronic conditions.

- *Survey-based models*

Health surveys, e.g., SF-36 and EQ5D, contain other explanatory variables that can be included in a linear regression model to explain health expenditures. In a survey, patients can express their self-perceived health status, quality of life, health care received, etc. The predictive power of these models is not superior to those based on diagnoses, and difficulties in collecting the survey data and the unreliability of some answers make diagnoses-based models preferable to survey-based models (García Goñi, 2006).

Pope *et al.* (1998) is a popular paper because it explores survey-based risk adjustment for the US population. It presents a simulation with the short version SF-36, along with eight other types of surveys or self-reports and compares it with an early diagnosis-based model (the CMS-HCC model). Pope *et al.* (1998) find that the explanatory power is relatively low. Self-reported functional status gave an adjusted-R^2 of 2.52%, self-reported chronic conditions was 2.74%, self-reported health was 3.11%, SF-36 was 4.05%, and for a comprehensive survey it was 4.18%. In contrast, a diagnosis-only model using prospective HCCs almost doubled the predictive power, explaining 7.27% of the variation. Combining diagnostic information and survey data performed only somewhat better at 7.85%. All models used US prospective data (Pope *et al.*, 1998). More recent work done in the UK and Australia has confirmed that once diagnostic information is present, survey information adds relatively little to the predictive power of a risk adjustment model, both in a retrospective and prospective framework. More recently,

Gravelle *et al.* (2011) and Ellis *et al.* (2013) explore the incremental information that can be acquired in using surveys in addition to diagnostic information.

- *Income, need, and other demographic adjusters*

Income, poverty, housing characteristics, unemployment, and other socioeconomic information is often used to allocate funds geographically to provider groups or regional authorities in many public, single-payer systems, although in many countries such information is transitioning to using individual-level information. A good example of this is in the UK, where it has gradually evolved from using aggregated information about geographic areas to using individual-level information to allocate budgets for hospital and community care. The UK evolved from allocating funds to 14 resource allocation-working areas to using a person-based approach. Gravelle *et al.* (2011) demonstrated that morbidity markers based on diagnoses largely eliminated the usefulness of most attributed need and supply-side variables for hospital budgets, while Dixon *et al.* (2011) found similar results for primary care trusts.

Methods for calculating risk adjustment

In general, there are basically three ways to adjust for risk: Synthetic indices methods; actuarial cells formulas; and regression formulas. In the latter field, despite extensive research, including econometric research of predictive models, the simplest and most applicable models are linear regression models, which can be classified into different types depending on the explanatory variables used (Ellis, 2008).

- *Synthetic indices method*

The English (and UK) per capita allocation is known as the "synthetic indices" method. It weighs population using aggregated geographic area medical need information. This method takes into consideration the simultaneity of supply and demand forces in determining health care use and expenditure, as well as the accepted definition of health care. The formula Resource Allocation Working Part (RAWP) and its adaptation for Scotland (Share model), Wales, and North Ireland employs the concept of normative utilization, defined as the expected use of services in each geographic area if the responsiveness to the needs of the population were equal to the national average. In practice, this normative utilization estimation requires excluding the part of demand that is induced by the supply.[4]

[4]The best risk adjustment systems attempt to separate the non-legitimate factors, unrelated to the purpose for which funding is postulated, from legitimate factors as the observed differences in health spending.

The adjusted per capita system has been used in England since 1970 and is the fundamental resource allocation system in the country. The formula has been extensively studied and has had significant variations over time, where the more important changes occurred in 1976, 1989, 1994–1995, and 1999–2000. The initial formula separated operational expenditures from investment expenditures, since these expenditures are planned for differently, and only operational expenditures were included in the adjusted per capita payment. By 1999–2000, the risk adjustment formula converged both types of expenditure into a single formula that considered demographic, additional health needs and health service provision cost variations.

Similar models are used in Spain, Italy, and Canada among others. Spain adjusts its per capita by population, past health expenditures, and health service utilization. Italy uses a budget ceiling for each region based on an adjusted per capita (Lo Scalzo *et al.*, 2009). Between 1978 and 1997, the formula used in Italy changed many times, and since then, it has considered health service demand, age structure, and population health status (mortality). In Canada, some provinces have used regional adjustment based on age, gender, and socioeconomic status since 1994 (Ellis, 2008).

- *Actuarial cells models*

The matrix or actuarial cell method creates an array where the value of each cell represents the expected expenditure for a person who is characterized by certain variables (e.g., the cell may be at the intersection of sex and age). This method is limited by the availability of information at the individual level, despite being a more suitable method, in comparison to an aggregate data method.

Individual records must include expenditure or utilization information, as well as other variables to measure health needs and therefore costs. The ACG approach is an example of a cell-based model, using diagnostic information and aggregating it into clusters (see below).

- *Regression models*

Regression models that create predictions using multivariate models are the most common form of estimation. These can be estimated using either individual-level data (which is generally preferred) or aggregate data, using geographic averages. Regression models using aggregate data were used in Belgium until 2006 and still underlie the UK budget allocation formulas. These models use population-level data series and they have been criticized for their inaccuracy and the arbitrariness of the variables included. Aggregate risk adjustment models are better than no risk adjustment, but leave significant incentives for selection at the individual level.

- *Differences between rate cell and regression approaches*

There are important differences between the two risk-approximation models discussed above (cell and regression models). In rate cell models, each patient is classified uniquely into a single group choosing the most useful for determining severity or patient costs. Patients are typically allocated based on a complex algorithm in which the more complex or more costly, are allocated first. A Clinical Risk Group (CRG) is one of these models. The advantage of these models is that they are simple to construct and the disadvantage is that they are less predictive than regression models, since the latter can capture a large variety of types of patients, and cell models are limited to the array of cases built (Ellis, 2008). Another important difference is that there are models that require not only diagnoses but also procedure information (such as CRGs) while others do not (like DxCG and ACG). Finally, the models differ in the types of disease classification used (ICD-9 or ICD-10) and in their design. Although usually all patients are allocated into a group, because models have translation systems, they are not perfect and there is always a remnant of loss of information in the translation process.

- *Linear vs. nonlinear specifications*

Early models of individual-level health care spending most preferred nonlinear prediction models that either model the log of spending or decompose spending into a probability of use and level of use models. Such models can generate errors which tend to be close to normality, but create problems in predicting spending levels in the presence of heteroskedasticity. More recently, the preference has been to use linear risk adjustment models, which is to say that the dependent variable is left in its natural, untransformed state, and explanatory variables enter in additively on the right side. Some explanatory variables may themselves be interactions of other variables, including diagnostic conditions and demographic information. The standard estimation approach (Ellis *et al.*, 1996) adopted in the US and Germany is to model spending per month, or equivalently, "annualized spending" as the dependent variable which is spending divided by the fraction of the year each enrollee is eligible, and to weight each observation by the fraction of the year eligible. This is exactly equivalent to using "spending per month" as the dependent variable, and weighting each observation by the number of months a person is eligible for coverage. To accommodate newborns, deaths, and people who move into and out of health plans or regions, models that can accommodate partial year eligibility are important.

A substantial literature, including work by top econometricians, has validated that with very large samples (exceeding a million observations) linear regression models dominate nonlinear models in generating unbiased predictions. Noted econometrician Andrew Jones (2011) summarizes: "It is notable that the simple linear model, estimated by OLS, performs quite well across all of the criteria, a finding that has been reinforced for larger datasets than the one used here." Nonlinear models may be superior when the goal is hypothesis testing, but for payment purposes, OLS generates better predictions (Dixon *et al.*, 2011; Gravelle *et al.*, 2011; Ellis *et al.*, 2013).

- *Recalibration methods*

For any given classification system or modeling framework, a user from a different country using a different subset of consumers from the population has a variety of choices of how to reestimate or recalibrate a model to fit. If the sample is large enough, then reestimation of the entire model (with perhaps 500 or 1,000 parameters) on the new sample is the preferred approach. The current, most highly refined models (CMS-HCC, HHS-HCC, DxCG, ACG, CRG from the US, and the German and Netherlands models) require sample sizes of more than one million person years to avoid overfitting problems of more than 0.01 in the R^2 in prospective and retrospective models. Given this, many users use simplified classification systems with a smaller subset of diagnoses. Researchers in Australia used a coarser classification system with only 127 condition categories to model their sample of 800,000 person years (Ellis *et al.*, 2013). An approach that can be used on even smaller sample sizes (10,000 to 200,000) is to use lightly recalibrated models in which regressions use risk scores calibrated on other samples or other countries. This can be done with a single right hand variable, such as $Y = \alpha + \beta * RRS$ or simple splines can be used. For example, a three step spline model would use $Y = \alpha + \beta 1 * RRS + \beta 2 * (\max(RRS-1.0, 0.0) + \beta 3 * (\max(RRS-2.0, 0.0)$. While this approach does not allow for variation in treatment practices for specific illnesses, empirically it will generally achieve R^2 that is within 90% or better of the R^2 achieved with full recalibration (Winkelman and Mehmud, 2007). Even across different countries, relative risk scores are highly correlated (Ellis *et al.*, 2013).

Measures used to compare and evaluate risk adjustment models

Risk adjustment models are typically evaluated using five metrics of predictive power. First, the conventional R^2 — which measures the fraction of total variation in the dependent variable explained by the model — is by far the most common means of comparison. Closely related is the root mean squared error — the square root of the average of the squared error — which for a given dataset will generally give the same ranking as the R^2. A third metric is the Mean Absolute Prediction Error, (MAPE), $\sum_{i=1}^{n}\left(\left|Y_i - \hat{Y}_i\right|\right)/n$. A fourth metric is the closely related Cummings

Prediction Measure (CPM) which expresses the MAPE in relation to the mean absolute deviations around the sample average. Both the MAPE and CPM are popular because they do not square outliers, which can give a significantly different rating of models and ends up attaching equal importance to deviations at all levels of the distribution rather than focusing on predictions of the largest outliers. Finally, it is common to also evaluate models in terms of predictive ratios — which can be calculated as ratios of actual spending to predicted spending — for various subgroups of the sample about which one is particularly concerned about selection incentives. High-cost groups, groups with certain chronic conditions, low-income households, and geographically remote areas are examples of groups for which undertreatment is a common concern, and predictive ratios, which are ideally close to one for all subsets, provide a useful measure.

As discussed in van de Ven and Ellis (2000) there are a number of adjustments to the dependent variable or sample that can greatly affect all measures of model performance. All of the following measures can change the R^2 by more than a few percentage points, making it hard to compare results across studies: using retrospective (concurrent) rather than prospective diagnoses, excluding or top coding outliers, focusing on subsets of the total population, using only within-rather than out-of-sample goodness of fit measures, overfitting the models on samples that are too small, and failing to adequately distinguish between "out of the box" model performance, where coefficients are taken as given, and recalibrated models in which all of the model parameters are reestimated on a new sample. For a good discussion of these issues, see Winkelman and Mehmud (2007) which was prepared for the US Society of Actuaries.

Sample calculations for a risk adjustment system

All risk adjustment systems start by estimating — either through regressions or cell average — models that predict total spending using variables that capture disease and demographic information. The dependent variable in this model could be total spending, or any of a large number of other performance measures. Although estimated in levels, the standard practice with risk adjustment is to express the predictions from the model in terms of relative risk scores (RRS), which show individual *i* costs (or utilization or anything) called Y_i, divided by the sample mean, $\bar{Y}$. Table 2 provides an example of how the RRS would be calculated for a 25-year-old male using the US Health Insurance Marketplace system (Kautter *et al.*, 2014b).

This person is predicted by the model to have costs that are 4.098 times the average cost of the full sample if in a Gold plan, which is projected by actuaries to cover between 80% and 90% of total health care spending.

Table 2. Calculation of RRS for a male with the given characteristics in a Marketplace Gold Plan

Information	Risk score weight
Male, age 25	0.223
Diabetes with acute complications	1.199
Major Depressive and Bipolar Disorders	1.698
Asthma	0.978
RRS	4.098

Note: The RRS for an individual is the sum of the risk score weights associated with all variables by that individual.
Source: Risk score weights are from Kautter *et al.* (2014b) for the US Health Insurance Marketplace.

Once risk scores are assigned to each person, the information can be used together with premium and enrollment information. The following information illustrates how information is used within a given rating area in the US Health Insurance Marketplace for a simplified case where there is only one plan metal level. (In reality, there are five metal levels — Platinum, Gold, Silver, Bronze, and Catastrophic — that vary in the generosity of benefits, and consumers in the actual market will make adjustment for plan generosity.) All calculations are usefully done using the month rather than the year as the unit of analysis, to accommodate individuals who are enrolled in plans for less than a full year (as well as births and deaths). Ignoring subsidies, each plan would receive premium revenue that depends primarily on enrollee age and number of enrollees. In this example with four plans, total premium revenue is $100 million for 250,000 eligible months, implying a mean premium revenue of $400 per month. Plans may differ in their premiums, enrollments, and RRSs. After calculating the average RRS of 1.030, the overall average risk adjusted premium is $388.35. This can be used to calculate the risk adjusted revenue that each plan receives. The final column shows the net transfers into each plan. Although the first two plans have identical premiums and enrollments, Plan A ends up making large net transfers into the program because of its very healthy, low risk score population, while Plan B is a net recipient of funds. Plan C, even though it has the smallest enrollment and highest premium, is the largest net recipient because of its extremely high average risk score.

Health information system a major limitation

Estimation of individual-level risk adjustment places a number of requirements on the health information system which are often a challenge. For one thing, it is important to be able to uniquely identify individuals — patient confidentiality and

Table 3. Risk adjustment sample calculations

Health Plan	Total premium revenue ($)	Number of eligible months	Average premium per month ($)	Average RRS	Risk adjusted average premium ($)	Risk Adjusted total revenue ($)	Net transfers into plan ($)
	A	B	C = A/B	D	E = C/D	F = B*D* (Mean of E)	G = F – A
A	20,000,000	50,000	400	0.900	444.44	17,475,728	–2,524,272
B	20,000,000	50,000	400	1.100	363.64	21,359,223	1,359,223
C	15,000,000	30,000	500	1.450	344.83	16,893,204	1,893,204
D	45,000,000	120,000	375	0.950	394.74	44,271,845	–728,155
Totals	*100,000,000*	*250,000*				*100,000,000*	*0*
Means (per month)			*400*	*1.030*	*388.35*		

Source: Authors.

the lack of standardized identifiers across the insurance system are common barriers to this. Second, in many health care systems used to working on a budgeted system (e.g., where hospitals get a fixed budget for providing care to virtually anyone who shows up), it is challenging to attribute services to specific individuals. Similar problems were present in the US when it implemented its DRG payment systems in the 1980s, and more recently in Australia and Germany as they have developed case-based payment systems and risk adjustment models. A third problem is that many information systems do not yet require or keep track of diagnoses for each patient visit. Although requiring diagnoses for hospital reimbursement and monitoring has become fairly routine in most countries, requiring office-based physicians to record diagnoses remains a challenge in many countries. A related problem is that diagnoses recorded by some providers (nurses, home health workers, ambulance paramedics) may be unreliable for use in risk-adjusted payments. Providers who record diagnosis may not be properly trained or they may not have the required information, which could translate into errors in the reporting. So screens on which diagnoses are to be used for risk adjustment (as are applied in the US and Germany) can be challenging to develop and incorporate. Cost information for calculating per person costs, even under a fee-based payment system, can be remarkably difficult to sum up, with the large number of duplicate claims and claims adjustments that are common. Finally, the ability of modern health IT systems to over- or under-record and misreport diagnostic information presents a challenge. Once health plan or provider revenue is based on recorded diagnoses, then there are incentives for coding creep (upcoding to increase reimbursement) by interested parties. In health equalization fund settings, which are zero sum payment adjustments, coding intensity creep may jeopardize fairness but not necessarily increase public or private costs.

Risk adjustment and performance-based payments

Performance-based payment is a new funding mechanism which may be understood as complementary to the risk-adjusted capitation systems. Current international trends in payment methods include paying for results, where incentives are grouped into two categories: first, fixing productivity to the achievement of quality objectives, also known as pay-for-performance (P4P); and second, compensating primary care health workers so that they receive payment comparable to that of hospital health care workers (Palomo *et al.*, 2011). Payment of financial incentives as a method for increasing the quality of care (P4P) has been increasing in recent years in a number of countries, as have related studies. However, according to Eira and Ortún (2012), the authors do not support the use of the P4P nor do the financial incentives improve health outcomes. Countries like Australia, Belgium, Czech Republic, Hungary, Italy, Japan, New Zealand, Portugal, Spain, and UK, already include bonuses for primary care physicians in the context of P4P (Paris *et al.*, 2010).

According to Scheffler (2010), under P4P the payment structure is based on quality and efficiency measures associated with rewarding the achievement of goals while controlling for case mix differences or morbidity. The rewards are financial and can also be associated with reputation via the publication of measurements and rankings. In OECD countries in 2008–2009, there were 13 countries using primary care bonus payments for physicians in P4P schemes, 9 of them using bonus payments for specialists, 7 using bonus payments for hospitals, and 16 using incentives to comply with guidelines or treatment protocols. Countries like Hungary, Italy, New Zealand, and Portugal only used them for APS physicians. The Czech Republic, Poland, and Spain, also used bonus payments for specialists. Belgium, Japan, Turkey, the UK, and the US all used bonus payments for the full range of providers, i.e., PCPs (primary care practitioners), specialists and hospitals. Thus, P4P programs were reported in a total of 19 OECD countries, using bonuses to incent PCPs, specialists or hospitals (or some combination of these). The majority of the P4P programs used quality objectives related to preventive health care and chronic disease management (Scheffler *et al.*, 2012). In any case, even performance bonuses need to be risk adjusted because otherwise they may create perverse incentives to avoid the sickest patients, since positive performance measures are more easily obtained with healthier populations.

A recent work by Ash and Ellis (Ash and Ellis, (2012); Ellis and Ash (2012)) illustrates the use of risk adjustment models to calculate payments for primary care practices and reward good provider performance. The model simulates the risk adjusted per capita payment for primary care providers using a sample of private insurance beneficiaries, including Medicare beneficiaries. They simulate using a regression model on age, sex, and 394 DxCG HCCs in a retrospective (concurrent) model that uses diagnoses from the same year as the prediction year. This is a refinement of the model currently used for Medicare capitation payments to health plans (although the Medicare Model is prospective and not concurrent). The Ash and Ellis model prospectively defines and places a monetary value on the set of activities for comprehensive primary care: The PCAL (primary care activity level). The PCAL model explains 67% of cost variation capturing primary care burdens at the individual patient level. The PCAL model also achieves an R^2 of 52% for total expenses and 32% for predicting payment to PCPs (physicians). In the same study, Ash and Ellis explore the use of risk adjustment to calculate risk adjusted performance measures, predicting emergency room use and use of high-cost or low-effectiveness antibiotics. Vats *et al.* (2013) describe the implementation of the PCAL model at four primary practices.

Risk Adjustment Classification Systems

The US Centers for Medicare and Medicaid Services (CMS) Hierarchical Condition Category (HCC) models

The diagnostic classification system that has received the greatest attention is the CMS–HCC classification system, which is used for risk adjustment by the US Medicare program, for private insurance exchanges, and by Medicaid plans. It starts by mapping each of the 15,000 ICD-9 diagnoses into approximately 80 Condition Categories (CCs). A given individual can have any combination of the CCs, allowing considerable flexibility in capturing diverse combinations of diseases. Hierarchies are then imposed on these CCs (and hence they become Hierarchical Condition Categories or HCCs) so that each person only gets credit for prediction for the most serious HCC within a broad bodily system or associated with a particular disease. For instance, a person with the HCC for metastatic cancer does not also get credit for the HCC of the location of cancer in each body organ, and a person with lung cancer HCC does not get credit for a cough (minor signs and symptoms HCC). Imposing these hierarchies improves clinical coherence and reduces model sensitivity to coding intensity but has very little impact on model predictive power. The most recent major revision of the CMS model is described in Pope *et al.* (2011). The CMS–HCC model is used to pay for non-drug medical costs of Medicare enrollees who choose not to enroll in the traditional Medicare plan, but instead choose Medicare Advantage Plans that are typically managed care options with reduced cost sharing in exchange for reduced choice of providers and tighter utilization review.

The CMS–HCC classification system is also used to risk-adjusted payment for the US Medicare Part D prescription drug benefit program (Kautter *et al.*, 2012). For that program, predictions are made about prescription drug spending only, rather than total medical spending. The size of the transfers in the Part D program, unlike the Part C program just described, are determined in part through a one-time auction simultaneous bidding process (Decarolis, 2015).

In 2014, the US Department of Health and Human Services (HHS) introduced a further revised HCC system for use in redistributing funds among the competing health plans in the new Health Insurance Marketplace (originally called an Exchange) set up in each US state (Kautter *et al.*, 2014a; 2014b). That formula started with 264 HCCs and, after applying principles for simplification that drop discretionary, vague and common low-cost HCCs, ends up with 127 HHS–HCCs in the final, preferred model. The approach uses conventional weighted least squares algorithms with no attempt to correct for behavioral responses to the payment system (Glazer and McGuire, 2000; Glazer *et al.*, 2014).

An important innovation of the HHS–HCC approach is that it reallocates premium revenue among competing health plans within a rating area as zero sum transfers, similar to how it is done in Germany and Switzerland (Pope *et al.*, 2014). A stylized example of the process is discussed in Section "Diagnostic Cost Group (DxCG) System". One challenge of doing this in the US is accommodating the substantial variation in plan generosity that is allowed in the Marketplace, unlike the European funds.

Diagnostic Cost Group (DxCG) System

The DxCG classification system is a private proprietary system licensed by Verisk Health of Waltham Massachusetts, US, which builds upon the classification system developed for Medicare. The diagnostic classification starts by grouping diagnoses coded in the International Classification of Diseases (ICD) system into clinically homogeneous groups, called DxGroups. (Both ICD-9 and ICD-10 versions are available.) The most recent DxCG models classify all 15,000+ diagnoses into 1,010 DxGroups based solely on clinical similarity. These DxGroups are then further collapsed into 394 condition categories (CCs) based on both major disease types and similarity of costs. Most but not all DxGroups map to a CC. Hierarchies are imposed on the CCs to create Hierarchical Condition Categories (HCCs), which identify the most costly manifestation of each disease. Since CCs are not mutually exclusive, a single person may be classified into several categories. CCs can also be further aggregated in to 127 Related Condition Categories (RCCs), and 31 Aggregated Condition Categories (ACCs).

The DxCG HCC classification system was modified to accept ICD-10 diagnoses and implemented in Germany (where the 80 selected HCCs are called Hierarchical Morbidity Groups (HMGs)) for allocating funds between a large number of competing sickness funds (health plans) starting in 2009 (Buchner *et al.*, 2013). DxCG models have also been evaluated in Canada, Chile, Spain, the UK, and Australia (see Table 4).

Table 4. Predictive risk adjustment models results from selected models

Data's place and year	Type of risk adjustment	Prospective R^2 (%)	Retrospective R^2 (%)
Canada–Alberta 1998–1900	ADG	7	25
	CRG	5	31
	DCG/HCC	9	47
Canada–Ontario 1988–1900	Age–sex	2	2
	ADG	6	21
	CRG	6	31
	DCG/HCC	8	37
Canada–Quebec 1988–1900	Age–sex	4	4
	ADG	8	22
	CRG	12	43
	DCG/HCC	12	33
Germany 2001–2002	Demographic RSA	6	7
	ACG	9	14
	ACG+PM	12	21
	CDPS	12	19
	DCG/HCC	15	26
	PCG+DCG	15	30
	RxGroups+IPHCC	24	48
US 1998–1999	ACG	9.9	28.2
	CDPS	14.9	35.5
	DCG/HCC	15.4	46.6
	Medical RX	11.9	24.4
	RxGroups	13.2	27.9
	RxRisk	11.1	21.3
	ERG	14.8	34.7
Spain (Cataluña) 2006–2007	CRGs		38.2
Chile 2001, 2007, 2008	DxCG with 2001 data		36.1
	RxGroups		74.4
	DxCG with 2007 data		40.0

Sources: Ellis (2008) (Canada, Germany and US); Cid (2011); Cid and Salazar. (2010); Ibern *et al.* (2008) (Chile); Coderch *et al.* (2014) (Spain).

Adjusted Clinical Groups (ACG)

The Adjusted Clinical Groups (ACG) system is a proprietary system developed and currently licensed by researchers at Johns Hopkins University. The original system used a rate cell approach that allocates all diagnoses codes into 32 diagnostic groups, known as Aggregated Diagnostic Groups (ADGs). Classification is based on four clinical dimensions: Duration, severity, diagnostic certainty, and specialization of care. All diseases, including those newly discovered, can be classified according to these dimensions and categorized into one of these 32 groups. The system uses a branching algorithm to place people into one of 93 discrete ACG mutually exclusive categories, based on the particular combination of ADGs of each individual, as well as age and gender. Predictive models are based on linear regression models.

This system has been used in the US and in several other countries. It is generally used in studies that assess its possible inclusion in the countries' or regions' risk-adjustment methodology as in Canada, Taiwan, Spain, South Korea, and Sweden. Recently, there has been an ACG pilot in Chile at the primary health care (PHC) level (see Table 4).

Episode Treatment Groups (ETGs) and Episode Risk Groups (ERGs)

Episode Treatment Groups (ETGs)® are a proprietary classification system licensed by Optum Inc. of the US that groups medical and pharmacy claims into episodes of care. It was first described in the literature in 1996. Unlike other groupers considered here, its primary focus is on creating clusters of services, possibly overlapping in time, into episodes of care, separated by clean periods in which there are no services provided. Procedure, diagnostic, and time information as well as provider type are all used in the process of creating episodes. Episode Risk Groups (ERGs) combine information from different episodes during a year to predict annual health care spending at the individual level (Dang *et al.*, 1996a; 1996b).

Clinical Risk Groups (CRGs)

Clinical Risk Groups (CRGs) were first marketed in 1999 by the US company 3M (who also licenses Diagnosis Related Group (DRG) groupers and other classification systems worldwide) and are used to classify people into mutually exclusive clinical categories, based on the information generated by their contact with the health care system. It requires a patient database for all activity in all areas or levels of care and interventions coded in ICD-9-CM. The CRG classification system uses age, gender, diagnoses, procedures, and dates of service information, which differentiates it from other classification systems that avoid procedure and date information. van de Ven and Ellis (2000), among others, would argue that using procedure information in a risk adjustment model for payment weakens cost containment incentives, similar to cost-based reimbursement.

The CRG method emphasizes chronic diseases through various types of breakdowns of 1,099 CRGs, 441 ACRG1, 176 ACRG2 and 46 ACRG3 into clearly identifiable categories from the clinical point of view, and because they are mutually exclusive, it facilitates the analysis (Inoriza *et al.*, 2009). CRGs differ from other grouping systems in that they use a rate cell approach rather than a linear regression model to make predictions: Each individual is ultimately classified into a single CRG that predicts their annual cost.

Baixa Emborda county in Catalonia has been using CRGs since 2002 (Inoriza *et al.*, 2009; Orueta *et al.*, 2006). Inoriza *et al.* (2009) present a description of morbidity for the period 2002–2005. CRG exercises have also been studied for the population of Quebec in Canada (Berlinguet *et al.*, 2005). The latter study compares the three main models (DxCGs, ACGs and CRGs) and found similar predictive power among the three but argues that the CRG worked better on clinical relevance, resource forecasting and transparency, ease of use and simplicity (Berlinguet *et al.*, 2005).

RxGroups (of DxCG Inc.) and Pharmacy-based Cost Groups (PCGs)

RxGroups are clusters of medically similar drugs that can be used for risk adjustment. The DxCG RxGroup classification system groups more than 100,000 National Drug Codes (NDCs) into one of 155 RxGroups, which in this case are mutually exclusive (unlike the DxGroups which in some cases a person could be in two CCs). RxGroups are based on the therapeutic indication of pharmaceuticals and does not attempt to cluster these classes by disease. The latest version supports the use of ATC codes,[5] and this allows it to be used outside of the US.

The Chilean Ministry of Health studied the use of pharmacy information using an RxGroup framework for a regional health service's per capita allocation in 2009 (Ibern *et al.*, 2008a).

Since 2002, the Netherlands' system has used pharmacy information intended to capture the costs of selected chronic conditions (van de Ven *et al.*, 2007).

[5] ATC refers to the Anatomical Therapeutic Chemical Classification System.

Other classification systems

In addition to the classification and predictive frameworks already described, several other approaches are commonly used. The Chronic Disability Payment System (CDPS) was developed by Richard Kronick and colleagues and is used in several US states to make capitation payments to Medicaid managed care plans (Kronick *et al.*, 1996). Charlson *et al.* (1987) Comorbidity Index (with 17 disease categories) and the Elixhauser (1998) system (with 33 disease categories) are diagnosis-based classification system in which weight on each component were based on clinical judgment rather than regression coefficients. For a recent application and comparison, see Bing *et al.* (2008). A third, more elaborate system called the Clinical Classification System (CCS) is documented and evaluated in Radley *et al.* (2008), and builds upon the Agency for HealthCare Research and Quality (AHRQ) disease classification system, with 259 conditions. An advantage of each these four systems is that the coding of the diagnostic classification systems are free and in the public domain, although the disadvantages include that they are not automatically updated, and do not use hierarchies to reduce the sensitivity of the models to coding intensity. None of these systems include software that generates risk scores, but rather they create predictive variables that can be used to create customized risk adjustment models.

The US Society of Actuaries has also evaluated artificial intelligence algorithms that can be used to predict spending, however this modeling approach leads to customized predictive models that are not easily transferred to new datasets and time periods, and have been criticized for not revealing clinically coherent classification systems (Winkelman and Mehmud, 2007).

Predictive power comparisons

At the individual level, demographic models predict no more than 2.5% to 3.0% of the expenditure variance. When used in combination with other diagnostic and sociodemographic variables, which may include age and sex, these models can increase their predictive power by about 10 times or more (Cid, 2011). However, a comparison of diagnoses models shows differences in predictive power, and studies related to populations from different countries, analyzed mostly by Ellis (2008), show significant differences. Models that combine information such as CRG, RxGroups, and the ERG tend to be better predictors than those using only one type of information. Retrospective models predict much better than prospective models, because retrospective models use information of the year being predicted. RxGroups is the prospective model that has the best predictive results, for example, in Germany (24%) and the Netherlands, although it is not the most studied. The most studied models are those that incorporate diagnostic codes, such as DxCG, ACG, CRG, and the ones that fit best are the DxCG/HCC models.

Retrospective (concurrent) models are generally used as an assessment tool or to make payment simulations. Examples are RxGroups in Germany, DxCG/HCC, and CRG in Canada–Quebec (43%), and DxCG in Chile (36.1%) (Cid, 2011).

In the case of Chile, Table 4 includes several different studies: Cid (2011) examines risk adjustment between public and private health plans, (FONASA and ISAPREs, respectively) using DxCG; Cid and Salazar (2010) evaluate risk adjustment models to reallocate funds both among ISAPREs and also between ISAPREs and FONASA plans using data from 2007 using DxCG; Ibern *et al.* (2008a) study a public sector population to consider risk adjusted per capita payment models using RxGroups for setting a budgetary ceiling for public health care services.

It should be noted that these studies refer to different populations and contexts. In the German case, it uses the entire social health insurance population and compensates risk between health plans; in the case of the US, it is used for allocations by Medicare, Medicaid, and the privately insured population. In Canada, they use territorial allocations for province health authorities' populations and eventually PHC physicians.

Risk Adjustment with Competing Health Plans

In some countries where social security prevails over the national health system, risk adjustment is used in some level or phase of resource allocation. In some cases, countries use a per capita payment as a risk-adjusted subsidized premium allocated to the sickness fund or health plan, or as a way to allocate resources or global budgets for health provision between regions of countries or territories.

Risk adjustment in social health insurance programs

• *Risk adjusted payments in risk equalization systems in Europe*

During the 1990s, a number of European countries introduced or enforced competition between different social health insurance plans by abolishing regional monopolies of the plans and introducing or expanding plan choice for the insured. These countries accompanied the introduction of competition with mandatory open enrollment and with the implementation of risk adjustment (van de Ven *et al.*, 2003).

With regard to the financial flow, two types of systems in which the risk adjustment mechanism is embedded can be observed: In the Netherlands, Belgium, and Israel, a central health fund is established. In these countries, the insured pay solidarity contributions to the central health fund, the insurers receive risk adjusted capitation payments from the fund, and (in the Netherlands and Belgium), the insured pay sickness-fund-specific additional nominal premiums to their health insurer (Lamers *et al.*, 2003; Schokkaert and van de Voorde, 2003); in Israel, no additional premium is allowed, so the health plans have tight budgets imposed through the risk adjusted capitation payments (Shmueli *et al.*, 2003). This model is called "external" risk adjustment in the terminology of van den Ven and Ellis (2000). On the other hand, in Switzerland, the insured pay the solidarity contribution to their sickness fund, and risk adjustment occurs between these insurers: Payments flow from those with above average good risks (healthier enrollees) to those with above average bad risks (sicker enrollees) (Beck *et al.*, 2003). This model is called "internal" risk adjustment, as the risk-adjusted payments are within the health insurance system and not from a central fund "outside." Germany in 2009 has switched from the internal to the external model (Göpffarth and Henke, 2013).

In all of these countries, risk adjustment started with age and gender as risk adjusters. Germany added an invalidity marker beginning in 1994, followed in 2001 by a variable for being registered in a disease management program as a proxy for morbidity (Buchner and Wasem, 2003); finally, in 2009, a model adding the use of diagnoses (based on the DCG model) and to a limited extent pharmacodes was implemented (Buchner *et al.*, 2013). The Netherlands started risk adjustment in 1993, added region and source of income as variables in 1995, pharmacy-based cost groups and diagnostic based cost-groups in 2002 and 2004 (Lamers *et al.*, 2003; van de Ven *et al.*, 2007). They had further developments later on, among them making use of multiple-year high-cost groups since 2012, thus implementing a variable referring to the actual costs of the individual insured (van Kleef and van Vliet, 2012). Belgium started risk adjustment with, in addition to age and gender, a set of socioeconomic variables like unemployment, mortality or urbanization — until 2002, these variables were used on the aggregate level of local sickness funds. However, since then, individual data became available and started being used (Schokkaert and van de Voorde, 2003). In 2006, Belgium added health status data, based on inpatient diagnoses and outpatient pharmacy prescriptions (van de Ven *et al.*, 2007). Switzerland, until 2011, only used age and gender as variables, then they added information about whether the insured was hospitalized the year before (van de Ven *et al.*, 2013). From 2016 onwards, a health status indicator based on past high expenditures for drugs will be added to the Swiss Model. Israel has basically remained with its model in which only age and gender are used as risk adjusters; however, a variable for remoteness for those living in remote areas has been introduced in the meantime.

In the Netherlands and Germany, introduction of risk adjustment went along with an increase in the financial responsibility of the health plan. In the Netherlands, health plans traditionally were not risk-bearing entities, as differences between revenues and expenditures were financed from the outside through *ex post* compensation. In Germany, before the introduction of risk adjustment all expenditures for seniors were pooled and financed through *ex post* compensation. Today, in both countries, health plans have to carry their marginal costs when increasing expenditures. In contrast, in Belgium still today 92% of the differences between risk adjusted payments to health plans and their actual expenditures are compensated *ex post* (van de Ven *et al.*, 2013). However in Switzerland, even before the introduction of risk adjustment, health plans had to carry full financial risk (Beck *et al.*, 2003).

Also, in some countries of Eastern Europe, multi-payer systems have been established after the breakdown of the socialist systems. In the Czech Republic as well as in Slovakia, insured can choose between various health plans, and there is a risk adjustment mechanism implemented between the funds, adjusting for the different age structures of the plans' memberships.

- *Risk adjustment in Latin America*

In Latin America, there are some countries that explicitly use risk adjustment for resource allocation in a health coverage program. In Chile, there is a very small fund between ISAPREs for the Guarantee Scheme (GES). Cid *et al.* (2010) assessed that the fund is insufficient for risk adjustment because of the legal rigidity of certain parameters — used to determine its size and level of risk adjustment — and the small use of GES among ISAPREs. Hence, in the eight years this fund has existed, it has actually only worked as a pilot of risk adjusted payments by sex and age (Cid *et al.*, 2010). In Colombia, risk-adjusted capitation — using sex and age — has been in place for 20 years to finance the *Entidad Promotora de Salud* (EPS) and *Administradora del Regimen Subsidiado* (ARS) (Ministry of Social Protection, 2011). Yet, the system has been criticized because of the differences between the subsidized and contributory schemes plans, benefits, per capitas and their adjustment that has only recently been equaled (Giedion and Cañón, 2014). It is argued that the differences in plans, when compared with European models with multiple health plans, generated greater segmentation in the system.

Recently, the Uruguayan health system has increasingly used risk adjustment to allocate FONASA's resources to "*mutuas*" (HMO-type entities). The Uruguayan reform created a fund to which workers, enterprises and the state contribute, in order to pay providers on an adjusted per capita basis (using age and sex). Its implementation has been gradual since 2008. The health system has had favorable results related to the reform, which include increasing population covered, lowering the burden of out-of-pocket costs (giving Uruguay the lowest out-of-pocket expenditure in Latin America), and significantly increasing public spending in health (which reached 6% of GDP in 2012) (Oreggioni, 2013). These results place Uruguay as one of the few countries that are achieving WHO recommendations for middle-income countries to increase public expenditure in health and decrease out-of-pocket expenditure as part of the efforts towards universal coverage (WHO, 2010).

Risk adjustment in the secondary private insurance markets: The experience of Australia, Ireland, and South Africa

A large number of countries use or are contemplating the use of risk adjustment for equalizing payments among competing private health insurance funds, notably in settings where the public sector is the primary insurer and private insurance is secondary to this public sector. Because the secondary private insurance is voluntary, selection issues are potentially serious. In Australia, risk selection into the private insurance markets is countered by open enrollment, penalties for delaying purchase, and retrospective risk equalization between voluntary secondary insurance plans, which is based on the proportion of the population over age 65 and the percent of claimants with high costs in the previous four quarters (Milliman, 2015).

In Ireland, risk selection is countered by open enrollment, lifetime coverage, community rating and minimum benefits. Only age is currently used for risk equalization, although recent proposals suggest expansion to include gender and prospective, diagnosis-based health status measures (Milliman, 2015).

In South Africa, where risk selection is regulated via open enrollment, community rating, and prescribed minimum benefits for specific diseases, risk adjustment mechanisms for equalizing revenues have been explored using data from 2005, but not implemented (Milliman, 2015).

Risk adjustment in the US Medicare advantage program and the health insurance marketplace

The US Medicare program, which is a national program that insures the elderly (over age 65) and disabled populations, was the earliest adoption of risk adjusted capitation payments in the US. The risk adjustment formulas, first started in 1972, have been updated approximately every 4 years. The earliest formula used age, gender, whether or not an individual was institutionalized (in a nursing home or long-term care facility), and whether the person was also eligible for Medicaid coverage due to having a low income or medical need. In 2000, Medicare implemented a prospective risk adjustment formula that used only the principal diagnoses from inpatient hospital stays during the prior year (Pope *et al.*, 2000). This risk adjustment formula was modified in 2004 to start using diagnoses from all types of medical encounters, as long as the diagnoses are coded by clinicians (Pope *et al.*, 2004). Both the transition from the demographic only model and from the inpatient diagnosis only models were phased in gradually over time, with payments during the transition periods (3 years each) being a weighted average of the two risk adjustment formulas.

As discussed above in the classification systems section, in 2014 the US Department of Health and Human Services (HHS) introduced a further revised HCC system for use in redistributing funds among the competing health plans in the new Health Insurance Marketplace set up in each US state (Kautter *et al.*, 2014a; 2014b). This program had enrolled more than 8 million Americans as of the end of 2014, and is being used to reallocate funds within each of 501 geographically defined risk rating areas. Since the program is using a retrospective payment approach, the results of this application are not yet available.

Risk Adjustment in Single Payer Systems

Many countries use per capita resource allocation in the health sector, with models that seek equity in the distribution of financial resources, such as the British Resource Allocation Working Party (RAWP), which was practiced until 1989 and still is the most paradigmatic example of such an allocation formula. It was adapted for Scotland (Model Share Scotland), Wales, and Northern Ireland. It also serves as the framework for payment allocation models in Canadian provinces, in Spain, Italy, and elsewhere, and is most commonly associated with the actuarial cells method.

National Health Service (NHS) or National Health Insurance System (NHIS) payments

In general, discussions of payment mechanisms refer to the payment distributed to a single and isolated provider, while payment systems usually refer to a network or Organized Delivery System (ODS), like NHS and NHIS.[6] Health care provision

[6] A National Health Service (NHS) system is one where the provision is public — there is no insurer or pooling of resources — and it's financed based on general taxes. The resources collected and allocated to health are assigned to subnational levels — health authorities in charge of a pre-defined population — through distribution formulas based on health needs. Health coverage is universal and therefore there is a single national pool that distributes risks. Health service provision may be public or private (for-profit or not-for-profit), although it is more common for them to be public, while the private sector takes a more complementary role. A National Health Insurance System (NHIS) is a single fund pooling resources from social security contributions and general taxes and is also a single-payer. As in a national health system, health coverage is universal with a single national pool that distributes risks with solidarity in the funding and that reduces discrimination based on health risks. The provision of health services can be public and/or private, and for-profit or not-for-profit.

happens in an environment of multiple providers that must act in coordination with each other. In this context, the system of incentives must take into account that health services are provided at different levels of care and that the level where services are performed should be the one with the greatest expected health gains (Shortell, 1996; 2000). This type of payment system considers costs, access and quality of care provided at the appropriate level.

Health care coordination is defined as the coordination of health care interventions that are necessary for the patient, regardless of the provider, in order to reach a common goal. Health care coordination is focused on the interaction between providers, and when it reaches the highest level of coordination, it is considered integrated (Vázquez *et al.*, 2012).

Health systems' complexity has increased as a result of the increase in the number of available health care services due to a high level of specialization and ambulatory-based care. This has been a consequence of the technological change in health care and an increasing population with complex chronic diseases and co-morbidities, which is in turn linked to an aging population. These are issues that contribute to difficulty in coordinating care. To achieve coordination and combat fragmentation in health systems, many policies emphasize collaboration between providers instead of promoting direct competition — for example, the promotion and development of health service networks that include different types of providers and different levels of care in a specific area, so that access is hierarchical; that provide coordinated care across a continuum of services to a defined population; and that are responsible for patients' costs and health outcomes. The main goals of such policies are to improve the overall efficiency and continuity of care in the health system, by way of an intermediate objective: Improving the care coordination or achieving clinical integration.

A per capita payment system promotes coordination between different levels of care and decentralization with appropriate risk transfer. The risk transfer will be appropriate to the extent that the per capita payment is available for the network of providers and for all levels and according to its characteristics (for example, whether it is risk-adjusted). Different payment mechanisms can coexist in an ODS: Global budget, FFS, wages, per capita, etc. However, risk-adjusted per capita financing is one of the most powerful regulatory tools to promote integration across providers.

An adjusted per capita payment is considered a mixed payment system. It considers risk adjustment as a prospective characteristic based on past morbidity (and/or any other risk-adjusted) and recognizes retrospective cost structures or fixed costs that must be covered, as well as the effects in the current period of health planning in these structures. This is a payment mechanism that recognizes both what the provider "is" (the retrospective component associated with the planned costs of installed capacity) and what the provider "does" (the prospective component associated with interventions and risk).

Globally, there are per capita systems where the allocation of resources is defined based on areas, regions, authorities or health services that are associated with populations. It is defined as the amount of resources allocated for a person to receive health care at any necessary level for a specific period. The goal is to provide the necessary financing and resources to areas and health providers based on social determinants of health and the degree of inequality in the area in which they are located (Hernández-Aguado *et al.*, 2012).

Many countries use per capita resource allocation in health, using models that seek equity in the distribution of financial resources, such as the British Resource Allocation Working Party (RAWP) which was practiced until 1989. Today, the UK uses a number of different formulas to allocate funds for hospitals, pharmaceuticals, and office-based care, and is seeking to balance existing expenditure patterns with needs arising especially from inequalities. Buck and Dixon (2013) provide a useful discussion of changes in the allocation formula over time, while Monitor and National Health Service (2014) describes the detailed new payment systems.

Table 5. Risk adjuster for per capita payments used in countries with health systems similar to NHS or NHIS

Country	**Type of system***	**Risk adjusters**
Australia	NHIS	Age, gender, ethnical group, indigence, mortality, education level, geographic area (rural/urban)
Canada	NHIS	Age, gender, socioeconomic status, ethnicity, distance
Denmark	NHS	Age, number of children in single-parent families, number of apartments rented, unemployment, education, immigration status, social status, elderly living alone
England	NHS	Age, mortality, morbidity, unemployment, elderly living alone, ethnicity, socioeconomic status
Finland	NHS	Age, disability, morbidity, archipelago, distance
Italy	NHIS	Age, gender, mortality, morbidity, utilization
New Zealand	NHIS	Age, gender, welfare status, ethnicity, rural/urban
Norway	NHS	Age, gender, mortality, elderly living alone, civil status
Portugal	NHS	Mainly based on historical precedents; age, relative burden of disease (diabetes, hypertension, tuberculosis, AIDS)
Spain	NHS	Percent of population over 65 years of age, insularity (region = islands)
Sweden	NHS	Age, gender, civil status, employment status, occupation, house ownership, high use

Notes: *Classification based on Böhm *et al.* (2012).
Sources: Adapted from Cid (2011), Ellis (2008), París *et al.* (2010) and Böhm *et al.* (2012).

Payments in segmented systems: The case of FONASA Chile

In segmented health systems — where different types of systems exist for different population groups — the public segment can usually be associated with an NHS- or NHIS-type system. This is the case in Chile's health system, where the public sector is hierarchically organized, according to geographical areas and populations, into 29 "health services" (regional health authorities) that include the hospitals and primary care providers of the municipalities that are under their umbrella. The Fondo Nacional de Salud (FONASA) in Chile is the public insurer.

In Chile, the public health sector uses different payment mechanisms. Hospital care receives activity payments that use different levels of aggregation of activities. Primary care receives a per-capita payment. Also, all levels of care receive an important portion of their resources from historical budgets. The activity payments are specified through the Valued Services Program (PPV, per its name in Spanish) of the budget, which is composed of tariff-based packages of interventions, including some PPV that address the health problems prioritized by the AUGE Reform. Currently, the PPV represents 50% of total hospital expenditure and, because PPV tariffs are higher than the rest, there are incentives to increase the use of PPV in resource allocation.

Table 6. FONASA's main payment system components

Budget component	**Level of care**	**Purchasing mechanism**	**Payment mechanism**
Primary health care (APS)	Primary	APS agreement	Per capita
		Programs	Budget
Institutional Care Modality (*Modalidad de Atención Institucional*, MAI)	Secondary y Tertiary	Valued Services Program (*Programa Prestaciones Valoradas*, PPV) agreement	Diagnosis-based payment (*Pago Asociado a Diagnóstico*, PAD) Valued services payment (*Pago por Prestaciones Valoradas*, PPV)
		Institutional Services Program (*Programa Prestaciones Institucionales*, PPI)	Fee-for-service (*Pago por Prestación*, PPP) Budget
Free Choice Modality (*Modalidad de Libre Elección*, MLE)	Any	MLE* agreement	Diagnosis-based payment (*Pago Asociado a Diagnóstico*, PAD) Fee-for-service (*Pago por Prestación*, PPP)

Notes: *In the MLE, the beneficiary purchases a coupon to seek care from a provider of her choice, generally from the private sector. Through this mechanism, FONASA beneficiaries can access care outside the public provider network by making a predetermined copayment.

Source: Authors, based on FONASA information.

The FONASA payment system has been studied; some authors propose that it does not ensure the promotion of greater equity and cost containment in the health system and that there are areas where the system's sustainability is at stake. It is a system that tends to unbalance the allocation of resources, and there are incentives for providers to increase their allocation through a specific payment mechanism (PPV) trading off another (PPI). In a sector where there are multiple necessary health services and a payment system that is biased toward a specific type of mechanism, most efforts will be directed towards the favored services and payments, putting the remaining services at risk of underutilization (Castro *et al.*, 2006). Therefore, studies recommend moving the existing payment system toward a more comprehensive system that encourages the elimination of waiting lists and introduces incentives for better health outcomes through integration between levels of care. A recommended payment system would take into account the different levels of care, based on complexity-adjusted costs and within the budget ceiling computed based on a risk-adjusted per capita (Cid and Ibern, 2008).

Risk Adjusted Payments to Individual Providers

This section discusses risk adjusted payments from health plans or sponsors to providers — which we refer to here as "individual providers" — which is different than paying providers in a network.

Main characteristics of individual provider payment methods

There are many ways that individual health care providers can be paid. Payments can be based on provider characteristics. Or, payments can be based on quantities of services provided or on patients' individual characteristics or population characteristics. Payments can also be based on hybrids of these characteristics. Each method creates provider incentives that affect the quantity and quality of health care services provided. The performance of each payment method depends on whether the explicit or implicit incentives shape providers' behavior as desired and expected.

Many countries are moving away from salary and fixed budget systems, which only consider provider characteristics, toward service-based and patient-based payment systems, including payment for results (PFR). This path shifts the financial risk progressively from the payer to the provider and strengthens efficiency incentives to keep services and costs to a minimum, while reaching the desired quality and health outcome goals. Shifting risk to the provider is often a reason for applying some variant of PFR at the margin, which does not base a provider's entire revenue or income on results.

Table 7. Selected *PPMs* by main focus of incentive design

Payment locus	**Individual provider (physicians, psychologist, nurses)**	**Primary health facility (group, health center, health post)**	**Hospital**
Provider	Salary by specialty and experience	Flat capitation based population in catchment area	Fixed budget Block grant Global budget
Services	Fee schedule Pay-for-performance	Fee schedule Fee-condition-on-quality	Cost based payment (staff salaries, lab material, and drugs) Fee schedule Fix payment per procedure Per diem rate Per admission
Individual patient	Health-based risk-adjusted capitation Bonus per treated case	Per-member-per-month rate Per-member rate risk-adjusted Bonus per treated case Bonus per target	Case-based payment DRG Inpatient DCG Protocols compliance
Population		Per-member-per-month rate Per-member-per-month rate risk-adjusted Budgeting for results Bonus per coverage Bonus per target	Diagnostic Cost Group

Sources: Adapted from Ellis and Miller (2008) and Musgrove (2011).

- *Providers' characteristics and incentives*

Payments to providers may depend on the provider's own characteristics. For example, doctors can be paid a salary according to their experience and specialty, regardless (at least from a short-term perspective) of how many or which patients they see and regardless of what services they provide. Similarly, in many countries hospitals receive "block grants." Block grants are budgets based on hospital size or type without explicit regard to the number or type of patients seen or the services provided. Many public hospitals around the world receive annual budgets adjusted for the number of beds, with again no direct relationship to the number or type of patients. Some of the incentives associated with annual budgets include risk selecting patients, under providing care, and even reducing quality of care to reduce costs.

- *Quantity of services and incentives*

Payments for specific services or procedures — such as a patient consultations, immunizations, or surgical procedures — are issued retrospectively, after the services are provided, and are paid according to the quantity of services given. These FFS payment systems can either allow the provider or the payer to set fee levels. Fee schedules set by the payer are the most common form of reimbursement for doctors. Under this system, if a health facility is responsible for purchasing the inputs (e.g., staff salaries, lab materials and drugs) and the fee for an additional service exceeds the marginal cost of delivery, then providers face a financial incentive to deliver as many services as possible.

On the other hand, there are some innovative modifications of FFS aimed at linking these incentives to results and reining in overutilization. For example, some FFS payments are conditional on quality of care, that is, health care providers are paid for delivering services that follow explicit protocols and conform to specific quality norms, with a system of inspection and auditing to assure compliance and to raise quality where necessary. This type of payment is known as results-based financing (RBF) (Musgrove, 2011). Another example is the CMS Physician Feedback/Value-Based Payment Modifier Program that gathers comparative performance information for adjusting the Medicare FFS physician fee.

- *Patients' characteristics, risk adjustment and incentives*

Another option is that provider payments can be designed based on patient characteristics. Patient characteristics might refer to a simple count of the number of beneficiaries, to patient demographic characteristics, to socioeconomic status, or to the patient's health conditions. Diagnostic related groups (DRGs) are one example of a payment system mostly defined by patient characteristics, in this case the patient's diagnosis.

If a provider assumes responsibility for all the care a patient may need during an interval of time, ranging from a month to a year, even for several health conditions, and is paid a fixed amount for providing that care, then the payment method is called capitation. The Oregon Alternative Payment Methodology (APM) demonstration project in the US is one example of a capitated payment methodology, where participating community health centers (CHCs) no longer earned revenue based on the number of individual patients seen, but instead received a monthly payment based on the size and composition of their patient populations (Hostetler *et al.*, 2015). Also, general practitioners in a number of countries (e.g., the Netherlands and England) are primarily paid by risk-adjusted capitation for registered patients. Ultimately, the capitation fee may be risk-adjusted for the health conditions of a patient or other patient characteristics. This means that the provider will receive a higher-than-average capitation for a sicker patient than for a healthier one. Under this scenario, a physician's gross income depends upon both the total number of patients and the characteristics of the patients he cares for. The physician's income does not depend on the type of provider administering the service, nor on the type or the quantity of services provided. As in the previous case, the incentives of flat capitation systems are to reduce costs per patient, risk select patients, overuse referrals, and on the positive side increase preventive care.

- *Patients' characteristics, risk adjustment and pay-for-performance (P4P)*

Rewarding providers for high performance is another payment approach for aligning provider incentives with patient and population welfare. These payment mechanisms potentially include performance bonuses to providers for extending service to additional beneficiaries. P4P payments could also incentivize increasing certain types of services (e.g., preventive care, immunizations, etc.) if these are linked to higher payments. They can also incentivize either process outcomes (i.e., adherence to evidence-based protocols), and/or health outcomes (i.e., decreasing maternal mortality). Meaningful and verifiable measures of results are an essential component of this method of payment. Many arrangements are possible. The ideal is perhaps for verification to be undertaken by a neutral third party, even if the principal pays the corresponding costs. Another important component is "attributional validity" — the evidence that observed outcome differences relate directly to quality of provider's care rather than to other contributing factors not under the control of health care providers. To maximize the fairness of P4P measures, risk adjustment may need to be considered (Iezzoni, 2009; Iezzoni, 2013). (See also Volume 3, Chapter 4 of this Handbook, *Pay for Performance in Health Systems: Theory, Evidence and Case Studies*.)

- *Refining incentives and hybrid payments*

Since no single form of health care payment is without drawbacks, and there is always a possibility for perverse incentives (overproduction or underproduction of services), mixed payment systems are nearly always a superior method (Ellis and Miller, 2008). Over the past two decades, payment mechanisms that combine provider, service, and patient characteristics have been developed. Payment systems combining all three of these dimensions are, for example, some of the Diagnostic Related Grouping (DRG) payment systems adopted in many countries. Some DRG payments are a fixed price per admission, with the payments reflecting patient characteristics (their diagnoses and age), health services provided (procedure codes), and provider characteristics (type of hospital) (Ibern *et al.*, 2008b).

Another example is the German system for paying ambulatory physicians, which currently has features that combine both FFS and salary payments. Physicians receive a FFS reimbursement, but the total of all such payments is subject to a cap, which varies by provider specialty. The payment caps work much like a salary, while the fee schedule is based on services actually provided. Another method is paying providers partly by FFS, on top of salary or whatever payment system is already in place. These methods are an improvement from only paying for inputs and base the incentive on outputs or results. Payment contracts under capitation may also specify particular outputs that providers must deliver, like for example improving coverage for key patient and services attributes.

Risk-adjusted capitation payments and Primary Health Care (PHC)

Financing systems of PHC are mostly based on capitation and/or combinations of capitation with other systems, especially FFS. In general, the recommendation is to use these types of systems in PHC and to avoid a FFS-only mechanism. However, FFS combined with salaries are also very common, especially at the level of GPs (general practitioners) or primary care physicians, whether working individually or in groups. In countries like Australia, Belgium, Canada, France, Germany, Ireland, and Japan, among others, the FFS system predominates, whereas salaries are paid to PHC physicians in Greece, Iceland, Mexico, Portugal, and Sweden. In contrast, other countries, such as Hungary, Italy, Poland, and Slovakia, among others, pay physicians on a capitation basis (Paris *et al.*, 2010).

In general, countries with a social security health system, financed by social security premiums or contributions from salaries and employers, also structure their payments to PHC doctors with FFS. Countries with national health systems, financed by general taxation, tend to arrange financing of PHC physicians in per capita payments, with exceptions in both cases (Holland and Australia, respectively). This may be because national health systems are generally Organized Delivery Systems, where capitation is naturally a more convenient mechanism. Social security systems, on the other hand, are commonly less hierarchically organized and therefore less associated with territories and populations, which may explain the tendency toward FFS (Böhm *et al.*, 2012).

It is also important to note that medical practice in PHC can vary between countries. In many countries, PHC is a private practice, individual or collective; in other countries, public sector physicians are paid practice-related salaries. The medical practice structure also determines whether per capita payment systems reach the physician or not.

Table 8. PHC payment systems in selected OECD countries

Countries	PHC provider (physicians) payment system	Type of medical practice (primary and secondary)	Geographical/provider per capita payment system*?
		NHS or NHIS	
Australia	FFS	Private group	Yes. 17 health areas
Canada	FFS	Private group, Private individual	Yes. Varies by province. Alberta has 17 Regional Health Authorities
New Zealand	Capitation + FFS	Private group	Yes. 4 health regions
Denmark	Capitation + FFS	Private group	Yes. 4 health regions
Finland	Salary, capitation + FFS	Public centers, Private group	Yes. 452 municipalities
Italy	Capitation + FFS	Public centers	Yes. 21 regional governments
Norway	Salary, capitation + FFS	Private individual	Yes. 19 regional governments
Portugal	Salary, budget	Public centers	Yes. By region/sector
Spain	Salary + per capita proportion (15%)	Public centers	Yes. By region/sector (CCAA)
Sweden	Salary	Public centers	Yes. Different health services by region/sector
United Kingdom	Capitation + allocation + FFS	Private group	Yes. Different health services by region/sector: 303 PHC Trusts
Ireland	Capitation	Private individual	No. Historic cost by heath area
		Health Social Security Systems	
Czech Republic	Capitation + FFS (before FFS)	Private individual	
Hungary	Capitation	Private individual	
Japan	FFS	Private clinics	
Korea	FFS	Private individual	
Mexico	Budgets	Public centers	Yes. Health areas
Poland	Capitation	Private clinics	Yes. Different health services by region/sector

(Continued)

Table 8. (*Continued*)

Countries	PHC provider (physicians) payment system	Type of medical practice (primary and secondary)	Geographical/provider per capita payment system*?
		Health Social Security System	
Turkey	Salary	Public centers	
Greece	FFS	Private individual	
Austria	Capitation +FFS	Private individual	
Belgium	FFS	Private individual	
France	Capitation +FFS	Private individual	Yes. 25 regions
Germany	Capitation	Private individual	
The Netherlands	Capitation	Private group	
Switzerland	FFS	Private individual	
Chile	Salary	Public centers	Yes. 320 municipalities

Note: *In practically all of these cases, per capita payments are adjusted.
Source: Adapted based on Wagstaff (2009), Vargas and Wasem (2006), Cid (2011), Paris *et al.* (2010).

Some countries have risk-adjusted capitation payment systems for geographical areas and the populations of these areas, whether these are PHC centers, Health Regional Offices or Local Offices. These risk-adjusted capitation models exist in virtually all countries with national health systems (Australia, Canada, New Zealand, Denmark, Finland, Italy, Norway, Portugal, Spain, Sweden, and the UK) and in some of the social security systems as well (Mexico, Poland and France).

Risk-adjusted payments in low- and middle-income countries

In low- and middle-income countries, adjusting payments for risk factors occurs mostly in a framework of public and community health plans, as contracts are set between insurers and health providers. In this context, capitated payments, adjusted by demographic variables, such as age and sex, are common. Payment methods can affect provider satisfaction with a health plan. For example, payment methods may affect population enrollment in a voluntary health plan through their impact on the quantity and quality of health care services. It is also plausible that payment methods influence the extent to which direct providers encourage people in their communities to join the plan (Robyn *et al.*, 2012).

Table 9 presents examples of public and community health plans' use of demographic risk adjustment in combination with P4P.

- *Argentina*

Argentina's *Plan Nacer*, launched in 2004, provides public health insurance to uncovered pregnant women and children under the age of six, who are not covered

Table 9. Selected examples of risk adjustment and health insurance in LMIC

Country	Scheme	Payment type	Risk adjusters	Payment recipient	Format
Argentina	Provincial Maternal and Child Health Insurance	Capitation and payment for performance	Age/sex groups — pregnant women and children under 5 — and relative strength of provincial health system	Provincial government and health care providers	MoH transfers 60% per capita for children upon verification of enrolment and 40% in performance fees. Targets are negotiated with each province
Chile	National Primary Health Care Program	Capitation and salaries	Age, urban/rural, and socioeconomic variables	Municipality and public health centers	FONASA transfer 60% per capita upon verification of enrolment
China	New Cooperative Scheme, Linyi County, Shandong Province	Capitation and payment for performance	Population size, age, outpatient visit, cost per visit, geographic differences, and satisfaction of enrollees	Village clinics and health centers	80% of per capita payment are monthly and remaining 20% at the end of the year
Rwanda	Community-based health insurance established in 1999	Some providers are paid monthly capitation and P4P	Pregnant women, children, and HIV/AIDS patients	Facilities receive funding and have discretion over its use	Capitation payments are monthly. Facilities allocates 77% of the PBF funds to personnel amounting to a 38% increase in staff salaries

Source: Authors.

under any insurance (The World Bank, 2013). *Plan Nacer* uses an innovative combination of capitated assignment and pay-for-performance. Risk adjustment is based on age and gender groups and the relative strength of the provincial health system. Target indicators for performance are negotiated annually; this is a crucial feature of the program because it allows a province with a weaker health system to aim for a lower target than better-off provinces. The funds flow from the provinces to the contracted health care providers (public or private), and up to half can be used to pay incentives to staff. The progress of the program is monitored by internal audits that verify the work performed and by independent auditors who submit regular reports to the National Ministry of Health (IEG, 2011)

- *Chile*

In 1995, the Ministry of Health of Chile introduced capitation at the PHC level. The Ministry of Health allocates a prospective capitation rate for all registered beneficiaries. The rate covers the administrative costs, pharmaceuticals and salaries for the health care personnel. The formula includes an age adjustor, as well as socioeconomic adjustors (geographic location of the health centers and income level of the municipality). An example of age, location, and socioeconomic adjusters would be a health center located in a rural area receiving an upward adjustment of 20% and a poor municipality an upward adjustment of 18% (Vargas and Wasem, 2006). The per capita covers, on average, 70% of expenditures, and the remainder is covered by budgets of specific programs.

- *China*

The New Rural Cooperative Medical Scheme (NRCMS) has been providing basic health security for rural residents in China since 2003. The central government encourages city and local governments to design their own schemes and pilot programs. Meanwhile, in the primary care sector of China, experiments are in progress in which capitation, global budget, or salary are combined with pay-for-performance to improve quality and to encourage providers to practice prevention and management of chronic illnesses. During 2006–2009, Qianjiang Province introduced capitation and pay-for-performance. The reform was expected to eliminate incentives for overprescribing and prescribing expensive medicine, and thus to help contain surging medical costs. Yip *et al.* (2010), in collaboration with the government of Ningxia Province, a predominantly rural area in northwest China, conducted a matched-pair cluster-randomized experiment between 2009 and 2012. The aim of the study was to evaluate the effects of capitation with pay-for-performance on primary care providers' antibiotic prescribing practices, health spending, outpatient visit volume, and patient satisfaction. Some evidence was found that certain types of provider payment (capitation, salary plus performance bonus) can lead to efficiency gains and can contribute to improved community-based insurance performance in developing countries.

- *Rwanda*

Rwanda's community-based health insurance program was established by the government and pays a monthly capitation amount to partner health centers based on the number of registered insured. Additionally, providers are rewarded for providing services to pregnant women and children, such as prenatal care visits, immunizations for children and pregnant women, institutional deliveries, and HIV testing. Incentive payments are offered for each of these services provided and are weighted using overall quality scores. This set of incentives motivated providers to increase delivery of contracted services. Researchers found that the program increased institutional delivery rates by 23% and preventive service use among children under age 4 by 25–50% (Basinga *et al.*, 2011).

Discussion: Risk-Adjusted Payments and Improving Efficiency and Equity

Health care insurance and provider payment systems are constantly changing, and they vary across countries and scenarios, but they share the same goal of trying to increase efficiency, improve fairness and promote high quality, cost effective health care. Unfortunately, as Joseph Newhouse (1996) has identified, plan and provider payment systems that create attractive incentives for efficient production may create incentives for risk selection that create new problems for efficiency, access and quality. Risk adjustment is an important tool for offsetting risk selection, but it remains imperfect and in need of further refinement and research.

A central theme of this article is the tradeoff between selection and incentives. Just because cost-based reimbursement and retrospective payments often create too little incentive for cost containment does not mean that one should go to the other extreme and use a fully prospective payment system. It can be attractive to aim instead for a mixed system that includes retrospective and prospective factors. Retrospective characteristics address the risk selection problem while prospective characteristics provide incentives for efficiency. The best combination of both will depend on specific contexts. An important part of the context is whether health care provision is based on provider networks designed to cover certain populations. A new concern and goal is that the payment system achieves planned or desired health outcomes.

The optimal risk adjustment is one that reflects the expected costs of the provider for the health care needs of the population so that incentives are aligned properly to reach desired levels of quality in health services, efficiency and to avoid risk selection. The ability to more closely predict providers' expected costs is linked to having the relevant morbidity information for patients served. The increasing use of morbidity information has taken sponsor estimates closer to providers' expected costs, significantly improving incentives and outcomes as a result.

Health economics has adapted microeconomic tools that are applied in the development of risk-adjustment methodologies. Although there is still a long way to go, there have been important milestones in the evolution of payment systems, with the central design for these systems aimed at responding to populations' health needs.

Specific discussions

- *Using need rather than illness-based indicators*

Risk adjustment payment models traditionally focus on payments that reflect health status variation, but demographic factors such as education, income and access can also affect health care needs. More problematic is that supply-side availability also affects utilization, while many feel that increased supply should not automatically enable increased payments. A major problem of measuring health needs is the difficulty obtaining direct measures of the need for care. This is generally done using utilization as an indirect measurement. However, this utilization depends on the available level of supply. For example, if there is oversupply, there is induced demand regardless of actual health needs. The opposite may also be true where demand is limited by a lack of existing supply creating access problems. The latter is very common in developing countries. Differences in provider policies may also affect the level of use, which may lead to an incorrect perception of differences in need. When the efficient levels are unknown, this can often be problematic. In some settings, satisfied demand is the closest concept to health need that can be estimated using available data.

- *Using past expenditures*

Health expenditures in a year are often highly correlated with spending in the previous year. Therefore, it is common to use lagged spending to predict future spending, and even to use this as a payment model. Some budgeted systems increase future spending nearly in proportion to the magnitude of lagged amount. If the incremental revenue from spending money in a year has too much effect on future revenue, it can generate perverse incentives that work against efficiency and cost containment. It can also be unfair, if differences in health spending between two providers or regions are due not only to differences in health status and illness but also due to different medical practices. Thus, if two providers treat people of similar severity with different procedures, using payments based on past expenditures tends to reward the provider who spends more and punish the provider that is most efficient. Basing payments in part on some lagged spending measure is a very simple way to implement a desirable mixed payment system, but bundled payments using something other than lagged spending is needed to avoid perverse incentives.

• *Conventional vs. optimal risk adjustment*

Glazer and McGuire, since 2000, have developed an alternative framework to conventional risk adjustment that is only just beginning to be incorporated in international payment systems. In their framework, conventional retrospective and prospective risk adjustment models do not completely solve the risk selection problem, because they remain imperfect, and selection problems can still be serious. They propose a framework for implementing optimal risk adjustment formulas, in which, despite only using prospective information, the weight given to each explanatory variable is not determined by regression analysis, but instead is chosen to maximize efficiency and quality in the provision of services. In order to maximize efficiency, the weights are selected to minimize the variance between premiums and expected costs (in a context of competing health plans). Further elaboration of optimal risk adjustment is found in Breyer *et al.* (2011). The access problem to health plans created by risk selection is minimized once it has guaranteed an efficient level of quality in service provision (García Goñi, 2006). The criticism of conventional risk adjustment, and cell and regression models in particular, is that they do not base calculations on previously established parameters to reach optimal situations.

Concluding thoughts and remaining challenges

As mentioned in the introduction, two key health policy concerns are efficiency and equity. The efficient allocation of resources in health optimally distributes resources within health care systems maximizing gains in social welfare and health status improvements (reduction in morbidity and mortality). An equitable allocation reduces differences in health care access, utilization, and ultimately of health status, across groups or regions, for example, by allocating more resources where there are greater health needs, in order to increase the availability of services and quality of care. Hereby, the payment system plays an important role in the goal of achieving greater efficiency, and to the extent it also considers health care needs, it may also achieve greater equity. The policy questions that this chapter addresses are: Which are the payment mechanisms used in different countries and health systems? What are the alternative risk adjustment tools and how do they vary between the different health care systems? Does risk adjustment account for the differences across regions, demography, epidemiology, socioeconomic variables, health status, etc. between groups? What variables are being used to make these adjustments?

The overview presented in this chapter has tried to summarize both the theory and the practice of risk adjustment payment methods. This has required a broad view, considering not only risk adjusted capitation payments between competing health plans, but also risk adjustment as a budget allocation tool for regional budgeting in single payer systems. Bundled payment can be used not only to allocate funds between health plans, but also to pay providers, such as hospitals and primary care practices. Both prospective and retrospective prediction models are currently being used, and yet comprehensive research evaluating their advantages and disadvantages is still lacking. The review of how risk adjustment can be used in practice is only of many possible ways that payment calculations can be made, and further work is needed to evaluate alternative approaches, both for their statistical fit as well as for their incentive properties. Risk adjustment is only one tool for combating risk selection, and other mechanisms — such as premium structures, reinsurance, and provider risk sharing are further alternatives that deserve greater attention.

This chapter has briefly reviewed both developed and developing countries in its analysis. The rich set of payment innovations implemented in middle and lower income countries appears not to have been systematically reviewed previously from the perspective of risk adjustment, but calls out for further examination and study. The cost savings and quality consequences of different payment systems and risk adjustment methods also could benefit from further study. Many different types of information are being used, and there are growing concerns about some of this information being gameable, or readily manipulated to the advantage of the fund recipients. This is another example of an area deserving of further research. Finally, this chapter has not concentrated the analysis on issues of fairness and equity, which are an important motivation for risk adjusted payments in many settings. Further developments in this direction are also very important.

References

Ash AS, Ellis RP. 2012. Risk-adjusted payment and performance assessment for primary care. *Medical Care* 50(8): 643–653.

Ash AS, Ellis RP, Pope GC, Ayanian JZ, Bates DW, Burstin H, Iezzoni LI, McKay EM, Yu W. 2000. Using diagnoses to describe populations and predict costs. *Health Care Financing Review* 21(3): 7–28.

Ash AS, Porell FW, Gruenberg L, *et al.* 1989. Adjusting Medicare capitation payments using prior hospitalization data. *Health Care Financing Review* 10: 17–29.

Basinga P, Gertler PJ, Binagwaho A, Soucat A, Sturdy J, Vermeersch CMJ. 2011. Effect on maternal and child health services in Rwanda of payment to primary health-care providers for performance: An impact evaluation. *The Lancet* 377(9775): 1421–1428.

Beck K, Spycher S, Holly A, Gardiol L. 2003. Risk adjustment in Switzerland. *Health Policy* 65(1): 63–74.

Berlinguet M, Preyra C, Dean S. 2005. Comparing the value of three main diagnosis based risk adjustment systems (DBRAS). Canadian Health Services Research Foundation (CHSRF) Report.

Bing L, Evans D, Faris P, Dean S, Quan H. 2008. Risk adjustment performance of Charlson and Elixhauser comorbidities in ICD-9 and ICD-10 administrative databases. *BMC Health Services Research* 8: 12.

Böhm K, Schmid A, Götze R, Landwehr C, Rothgang H. 2012. Classifying OECD Healthcare Systems: A Deductive Approach (*TranState Working Papers*, 165) Bremen: Sfb 597, Staatlichkeit im Wandel", 2012 ISSN 1861–176.

Breyer F, Bundorf KM, Pauly MV. 2011. Health Care Spending Risk, Health Insurance, and Payment to Health Plans. In: Pauly M, McGuire T, Barros P (eds.). 1st ed. Amsterdam: North Holland, Elsevier, 691–762.

Buchner F, Wasem J. 2003. Needs for further improvement: Risk adjustment in the German health insurance system. *Health Policy* 65(1): 21–35.

Buchner F, Göpffarth D, Wasem J. 2013. The new risk adjustment formula in Germany: Implementation and first experiences. *Health Policy* 109(3): 253–262.

Buck D, Dixon A. 2013. Improving the allocation of health resources in England. The Kings Fund.

Castro R, Cid C, Román A, Butala N. 2006. Changing health care provider incentives to promote prevention: The Chilean case. *Harvard Health Policy Review* 7(2): 102–112.

Charlson ME, Pompei Peter, Ales KL, MacKenzie CR. 1987. A new method of classifying prognostic comorbidity in longitudinal studies: Development and validation. *Journal of Chronic Diseases* 40(5): 373–383.

Cid C. 2011. "Diagnoses-Based Risk Adjusted Capitation Payments for Improving Solidarity and Efficiency in the Chilean Health Care System: Evaluation and Comparison with a Demographic Model". Department of Economics, Institute of Business and Economics Studies, Institute for Health Care Management, University of Duisburg Essen, Germany. http://duepublico.uni-duisburg-essen.de/servlets/DocumentServlet?id=25690.

Cid C, PIbern. 2008. "Regulación del financiamiento a Hospitales: 'yardstick competition' aplicada a los hospitales públicos en Chile". Cuadernos Médicos-Sociales (Santiago de Chile) 48(3): 155–164.

Cid C, Muñoz A, Sánchez M, Tegtmeier R. 2006. "Fondo de ajuste de riesgo en el sistema isapre". Superintendencia de salud, 2006. http://www.supersalud.gob.cl/documentacion/569/articles-3902_recurso_1.pdf.

Cid C, Salazar E. 2010. Ajuste de riesgos usando los DxCG: Algunas alternativas para mejorar el diseño de un Fondo de Compensación Solidario entre Isapres. Documento de trabajo del Departamento de estudios y desarrollo de la Superintendencia de Salud, Febrero de 2010. http://www.supersalud.gob.cl/documentacion/569/articles-5765_recurso_1.pdf.

Coderch J, Sánchez-Pérez I, Ibern P, Carreras M, Pérez-Berruezo X, Inoriza JM. 2014. Predicción del riesgo individual de alto coste sanitario para la identificación de pacientes crónicos complejos. *Gaceta Sanitaria* 28(4): 292–300.

Dang DK, Pont JM, Portnoy MA. 1996a. Episode treatment groups: An illness classification and episode building system — Part I. *Medical Interface* 9: 118–122.

Dang DK, Pont JM, Portmoy MA. 1996b. Episode treatment groups: An illness classification and episode building system — Part II. *Medical Interface* 9: 122–128.

Decarolis F. 2015. Medicare Part D: Are insurers gaming the low income subsidy Design? *The American Economics Review* 2015; 105: 1–35.

Dixon J, Smith P, Gravelle HSE, Martin S, Bardsley M, Rice N, Georghiou T, Dusheiko MA, Billings J, Lorenzo M, Sanderson C. 2011. A person based formula for allocating commissioning funds to general practices in England: Development of a statistical model. *British Medical Journal*, 343(7833): 1–16. doi:10.1136/bmj.d6608.

Eira C, Ortún V. 2012. Incentivos financieros en la mejora de la calidad asistencial". Informe SESPAS 2012. *Gaceta Sanitaria* 2012. doi:10.1016/j.gaceta.2011.11.006.

Elixhauser A, Steiner C, Harris DR, Coffey RM. 1998. Comorbidity measures for use with administrative data. *Medical Care* 36: 8–27. doi: 10.1097/00005650-199801000-00004.

Ellis RP, Miller MM. 2008. Provider payment methods and incentives. In: Heggenhougen K (ed.). *Encyclopedia of Public Health*, 1st ed. San Diego: Academic Press, pp. 322–329.

Ellis RP. 2008. Risk adjustment in health care markets: Concepts and applications. In: Lu M. Jonnson E. (eds.). *Financing Health Care: New Ideas for a Changing Society*, 1st ed. Weinheim, Germany: Wiley-VCH.

Ellis RP, Ash AS. 2012. Payments in support of effective primary care for chronic conditions. *Nordic Economic Policy Review* 2: 191–210.

Ellis RP, Fernandez JG. 2013. Risk selection, risk adjustment and choice: Concepts and Lessons from the Americas. *IJERPH* 10(11): 5299–5332.

Ellis RP, Fiebig DG, Johar M, Jones G, Savage E. 2013. Explaining health care expenditure variation: Large-sample evidence using linked survey and health administrative data. *Health Economics* 22(9): 1093–1110.

Ellis RP, Pope GC, Iezzoni LI, Ayanian JZ, Bates DW, Burstin H, Ash AS. 1996. Diagnosis-based risk adjustment for medicare capitation payments. *Health Care Financing Review* 12(3): 101–128.

García Goñi M. 2006. Ajuste de riesgo en los mercados sanitarios. En: Ibern P, editor. Integración asistencial: Fundamentos, experiencias y vías de avance. Barcelona: Masson; 2006. pp. 187–208.

Giedion U, Cañón O. 2014. Colombia: El Plan Obligatorio de Salud. En: Giedion U, Bitrán R, Tristao L, Editores. Planes de Beneficios de Salud en América Latina. Una comparación regional. BID, Washington DC, mayo 2014.

Glazer J, McGuire TG. 2000. Optimal risk adjustment in markets with adverse selection: An application to managed care. *American Economic Review* 90(4): 1055–1071.

Glazer J, McGuire TG, Shi J. 2014. Risk Adjustment of Health Plan Payments to Correct Inefficient Plan Choice from Adverse Selection. *National Bureau of Economic Research Working Paper No. 19998.*

Göpffarth D, Henke KD. 2013. The German Central Health Fund — Recent developments in health care financing in Germany. *Health Policy* 109(3): 246–252.

Gravelle H, Dusheiko M, Martin S, Smith P, Rice N, Dixon J. 2011. Modeling Individual Patient Hospital Expenditures for General Practice Budgets. CHE Reseach Paper 73.

Hernández-Aguado, Santaolaya M, Campos P. 2012. "Las desigualdades sociales en salud y la atención primaria". Informe SESPAS, 2012. *Gaceta Sanitaria* 2012. doi:10.1016/j.gaceta.2011.09.03.

Hostetler C, Sisulak L, Cottrell E, Arkind J, Likumahuwa S. 2015. *Origins In Oregon: The Alternative Payment Methodology Project.* [online] Health Affairs Blog. Available at:

http://healthaffairs.org/blog/2014/04/14/origins-in-oregon-the-alternative-payment-methodology-project/ [Accessed 25 January 2015].

Ibern P, Ortún V, Meneu R, García-Goñi M. 2008a. "Sistema de asignación poblacional de recursos. Informe para MINSAL–FONASA". Centre de Recerca en Economia i Salut, Universitat Pompeu Fabra.

Ibern P, Ortún V, Meneu R, García-Goñi M. 2008b "Sistema de pago de los egresos hospitalarios". Informe para FONASA–MINSAL. Centre de Recerca en Economia i Salut, Universitat Pompeu Fabra.

Iezzoni LI. 2009. Performance measurement for health system improvement: Experiences, challenges and prospects. In: Smith P (ed.). Risk adjustment for performance measurement, 1st ed. Cambridge: Cambridge University Press, pp. 251–285.

Iezzoni LI, ed. 2013. Risk adjustment for measuring healthcare outcomes, Fourth edition. Ann Arbor, Michigan: Health Administration Press.

Independent Evaluation Group (IEG) 2011. Results-Based Health Programs in Argentina and Brazil: Performance Assessment Report, IEG Public Sector Evaluation, Report No.: 62571, The World Bank Group: Washington.

Inoriza JM, Coderch J, Carreras M, Vall-llosera L, García-Goñi M, Lisbona JM, Ibern P. 2009. La medidad de la morbilidad atendida en una organización sanitaria integrada. *Gaceta Sanitaria* 23(1): 29–37.

Jones AM. 2011. Models for health care. In *Oxford Handbook of Economic Forecasting*. Clements MP, Hendry DF (eds.). Oxford University Press, New York.

Kautter J, Ingber M, Pope GC, Freeman S. 2012. Improvements in Medicare part D risk Adjustment. *Medical Care* 50(12): 1102–1108.

Kautter J, Pope GC, Keenan P. 2014a. Affordable care act risk adjustment: Overview, context, and challenges. *MMRR* 4(3): E1–E11.

Kautter J, Pope GC, Freeman S, Patterson L, Cohen M, Keenan P. 2014b. The HHS–HCC risk adjustment model for individual and small group markets under the affordable care act. *MMRR* 4(3): E1–E46.

Kronick R, Dreyfus T, Lee L, Zhou Z. 1996. Diagnostic risk adjustment for Medicaid: The disability payment system. *Health Care Financing Review* 17(3): 7–33

Lamers LM, van Vliet RCJA. 1996. Multiyear diagnostic information from prior hospitalization as a risk-adjuster for capitation payments. *Medical Care* 34(6): 549–561.

Lamers L, van Vliet RC, van de Ven WPMM. 2003. Risk adjusted premium subsidies and risk sharing: Key elements of the competitive sickness fund market in the Netherlands. *Health Policy* 65(1): 49–62.

Lo Scalzo A, Donatini A, Orzella L, Cicchetti A, Profili S, Maresso A. 2009. Italy: Health system review. *Health Systems in Transition* 11(6): 1–216.

Milliman. 2015. Medical underwriting and risk adjustment practices in 8 countries around the world. Downloaded on 26 March 2015 from http://www.milliman.com/insight/health/Medical-underwriting-and-risk-adjustment-practices-in-8-countries-around-the-world/.

Ministerio de la Protección Social. República de Colombia. 2011. Estudio de la suficiencia y de los mecanismos de ajuste de riesgo para el cálculo de la Unidad de Pago por

Capitación para garantizar el Plan Obligatorio de Salud en el Año 2008, Colección Estudios de Suficiencia UCP-POS. Bogotá Colombia, Septiembre 2011. ISBN Colección: 978-958-8717-25-8, ISBN: 978-958-817-28-9.

Monitor and National Health Service 2014. The NHS payment system: Documents and guidance. https://www.gov.uk/government/collections/the-nhs-payment-system-regulating-prices-for-nhs-funded-healthcare May.

Musgrove P. 2011. Financial and other rewards for good performance or results: A guide tour of concepts and terms and a short glossary. World Bank; Washington DC; May 2011.

Newhouse JP, *et al.* 1989. Adjusting capitation rates using objective health measures and prior utilization. *Health Care Financing Review* 10: 41–54.

Newhouse JP. 1996. Reimbursing health plans and health providers: Selection versus efficiency in production. *Journal of Economic Literature* 34: 1236–1263.

Oreggioni I. 2013. Equidad, Gasto público, mancomunación de fondos y protección financiera en el Sistema Nacional Integrado de Salud de Uruguay. División Economía de la Salud Dirección General del Sistema Nacional Integrado de Salud. IV ENCUENTRO DE UNIDADES DE ECONOMÍA DE LA SALUD. 7–8 de Noviembre, 2013 — Santiago, Chile.

Ortún V, López G, Puig J, Sabés R. 2001. El sistema de financiación capitativo: Posibilidades y limitaciones. Fulls Economics del Sistema sanitario N°35, marzo 2001, 8–16, 45.

Orueta JF, Urraca J, Berraondo I, *et al.* 2006. Adjusted Clinical Groups (ACGs) explain the utilization of primary care in Spain based on information registered in the medical records: A cross-sectional study. *Health Policy* 76: 38–48.

Palomo L, Gené-Badia J, Rodríguez-Sendín J. 2011. "La reforma de la atención primaria, entre el refugio del pasado y la aventura de la innovación". Informe SESPAS 2012. *Gaceta Sanitaria* doi:10.1016/j. gaceta.2011.06.010.

Paris V, Devaux M, Wei L. 2010. Health Systems Institutional Characteristics: A Survey of 29 OECD Countries, *OECD Health Working Papers*, No. 50.

Pope GC, Kautter J, Ingber MJ, Freeman S, Sekar R, Newhart C. 2011. Evaluation of the CMS-HCC Risk Adjustment Model Final Report. Centers for Medicare & Medicaid Services Website. https://www.cms.gov/MedicareAdvtgSpecRateStats/downloads/Evaluation_Risk_Adj_Model_2011.pdf. Published March 2011.

Pope GC, Adamache KW, Walsh EG, Khandker RK. 1998. Evaluating alternative risk adjusters for Medicare. *Health Care Financing Review* 20(2): 109–129.

Pope GC, Bachofer H, Pearlman A, Kautter J, Hunter E, Miller D, Keenan P. 2014. Risk transfer formula for individual and small group markets under the affordable care act. *Medicare & Medicaid Research Review* 4(3): E1–E23.

Pope GC, Ellis RP, Ash AS. 2000. Principal inpatient diagnostic cost group models for Medicare risk adjustment. *Health Care Financing Review* 21(3): 93–118.

Pope GC, Kautter J, Ellis RP, Ash AS, Ayanian JZ, Iezzoni LI, Ingber MJ, Levy J, Robst J. 2004. Risk adjustment of Medicare capitation payments using the CMS–HCC model. *Health Care Financing Review* 25(4): 119–141.

Radley DC Gottlieb DJ, Fisher ES, Tosteson ANA. 2008 Comorbidity risk-adjustment strategies are comparable among persons with hip fracture. *Journal of Clinical Epidemiology* 61(6): 580–587.

Rice N, Smith PC. 2001. Capitation and risk adjustment in health care financing: An international progress report. *Milbank Quarterly* 79(1): 81–113.

Robyn PJ, Sauerborn R, Barnighausen T. 2012. Provider payment in community-based health insurance schemes in developing countries: A systematic review. *Health Policy and Planning* 28(2): 111–122.

Scheffler RM, Fulton BD, Cashin C. 2012. Provider Pay for Performance Programs in Health: Key Factors and Selected Country Case Studies. Draft. http://ghlf.berkeley.edu/Prereadings/LondonGHLF/Speakers%20-%20Prereadings/Scheffler%20-%20P4P%20Programs%20in%20the%20OECD.pdf.

Scheffler RM. 2010. "Pay For Performance (P4P) Programs in Health Services: What is the Evidence?" World Health Report 2010 Background Paper, 31. http://www.who.int/healthsystems/topics/financing/healthreport/P4PWHR2010ShefflerFINAL.pdf.

Schokkaert E, Van de Voorde C. 2003. Belgium: Risk adjustment and financial responsibility in a centralised system. *Health Policy* 65(1): 5–19.

Shortell SM, Gillies RR, Anderson DA, Erickson KM, Mitchell JB. 1996. Remaking health care in America. *Hospitals & Health Networks* 70(6): 43–44.

Shortell SM, Gillies RR, Anderson DA, Erickson KM, Mitchell JB. 2000. Remaking health care in America: The Evolution of Organized Delivery Systems. 2nd ed. San Francisco: Jossey-Bass.

Shmueli A, Chernichovsky D, Zmora I. 2003. Risk adjustment and risk sharing: The Israeli experience. *Health Policy* 65(1): 37–48.

The World Bank. 2011. Financial and other rewards for good performance or results: A guided tour of concepts and terms and a short glossary. Washington DC: World Bank.

The World Bank. 2013. Argentina — Increasing utilization of health care services among the uninsured population: The Plan Nacer program.

van Barneveld, EM, Lamers LM, van Vliet RCJA, van de Ven WPMM. 2001. Risk sharing as a supplement to imperfect capitation in health insurance: A tradeoff between selection and efficiency. *Journal of Health Economics* 20: 147–168

van de Ven WPMM, Ellis RP. 2000. Risk adjustment in competitive health plan markets. In: Culyer A, Newhouse J (eds.). *Handbook in Health Economics*, 1st ed. Amsterdam: North-Holland/Elsevier, pp. 755–845.

van de Ven WPMM, Beck K, Buchner F, Chernichovsky D, Gardiol L, Holly A, Lamers LM, Schokkaert E, Shmueli A, Spycher S, Van de Voorde C, van Vliet RCJA, Wasem J, Zmora I. 2003. Risk adjustment and risk selection on the sickness fund insurance market in five European countries. *Health Policy* 65(1): 75–98.

van de Ven WPMM, Beck K, Buchner F, Schokkaert E, Schut FT, Shmueli A, Wasem J. 2013. Preconditions for efficiency and affordability in competitive healthcare markets: Are they fulfilled in Belgium, Germany, Israel, the Netherlands and Switzerland? *Health Policy* 109(3): 226–245.

van de Ven, WPMM, Beck, K, Van de Voorde, C, Wasem, J, Zmora, I. 2007. Risk adjustment and risk selection in Europe: 6 years later. *Health Policy* 83(2–3): 162–179.

van Kleef RC, van Vliet RCJA. 2012. Improving risk equalization using multiple-year high cost as a health indicator. *Medical Care* 50(2): 140–144.

van Vliet RCJA, van de Ven WPMM. 1993. Capitation payments based on prior hospitalization. *Health Economics* 2: 177–188.

Vargas V, Wasem J. 2006. Risk adjustment and primary health care in Chile. *Croatian Medical Journal* 47(3): 459–468.

Vats S, Ash A, Ellis R. 2013. Bending the cost curve? Results from a comprehensive primary care payment pilot. *Medical Care* 51(11): 964–969.

Vázquez ML, Vargas I, Nuño R, Toro N. 2012. "Organizaciones sanitarias integradas y otros ejemplos de colaboración entre proveedores". Informe SESPAS 2012 *Gaceta Sanitaria* doi:10.1016/j. gaceta.2011.11.006.

Wagstaff, A. 2009. Social health insurance vs. Tax-financed health systems- Evidence from the OECD. *Policy Research Working Paper* 4821 Development Research Group, The World Bank, Washington DC, USA, January 2009.

Wasem J, Lauterbach LM, Schrader WF. 2006. Klassifikationsmodelle für Versicherte im morbiditätsorientierten Risikostructurausgleich (Clasificación de modelos de ajuste de riesgos para compensación estructural de riesgos basada en morbilidad). Wissenschaftliches Institut der AOK 2006

Weiner JP, Dobson A, Maxwell SL, Coleman K, Starfield B, Anderson GF. 1996. Risk-adjusted Medicare capitation rates using ambulatory and inpatient diagnoses. *Health Care Financing Review* 17(3): 77–99.

Winkelman R., Mehmud S. 2007. A comparative analysis of claims-based tools for health risk assessment. Schaumburg, Ill.: Society of Actuaries.

World Health Organization (WHO) 2010. Health Systems Financing: The path to universal coverage. The World Health Report: Geneva.

Yip WCM, Hsiao W, Meng Q, Chen W, Sun X. 2010. Realignment of incentives for health-care providers in China. *The Lancet* 375(9720): 1120–1130.

Resource Allocation and Priority Setting in Health Care Systems

Guillem Lopez-Casasnovas and Laura Pellise
Universitat Pompeu Fabra (Barcelona)

The combination of constrained resources and increasing demands in health care is making priority setting a crucial factor for health policy, and as choices about the allocation of resources are required to be increasingly explicit, priority setting and rationing drift away from a straightforward process. This chapter aims to review the main challenges regarding prioritization. Section "Concepts Regarding Priority Setting" describes the concepts and normative economic grounds of priority setting. Section "Institutions for Priority Setting in Health Care" maps out a review of sound practical experiences with priority setting. Section "Final Thoughts" provides thoughts on the development of prioritization mechanisms and the policy implications and limitations of these mechanisms, as well as the potential use of priority-setting concepts for allocating resources and for informing decisions about issues such as coverage and cost sharing.

Keywords: Resource Allocation; Health Care Financing; Priority Setting; Insurance Coverage; Innovation; Sustainability.

Introduction

From many points of view, health care systems are improving their capacities to heal and to extend lives. Innovation and improvements in health care systems, together with many other factors, have helped improve health indicators worldwide. However, health care expenditures are under increasing pressure. Governments are struggling to keep health care budgets under control, especially in some developed countries, as health care budgets are often increasingly restricted by economic downturn and the costs associated with aging populations. Moreover, in all countries, the gap between technological innovation and health care expenditure capacity is likely to remain or increase in the future.

Thus, in most of the Organisation for Economic Co-Operation and Development (OECD) public health care systems since the 1980s, there has been a need to ensure that any additional resource spent on health care is worth it. It is not just an issue of cost minimization, but of making choices between alternatives, which is what economics is about. Outputs, throughputs and outcomes are the focus as well as the key to the efficiency goal. Defining these parameters becomes the most relevant challenge for priority setting in health care systems.

This chapter aims to review the core concepts behind priority setting. The first section describes the concepts and normative economic grounds of priority setting. The second section maps out a review of sound practical experiences with priority setting. The third section provides thoughts on the development of prioritization mechanisms and the policy implications and limitations of these mechanisms, as well as the potential use of priority-setting concepts for allocating resources and for informing decisions about issues such as coverage and cost sharing.

Concepts Regarding Priority Setting

Rationing, priority setting and economic evaluation

There are several key concepts and terms that should be defined in our discussion of priority setting: rationing, economic evaluation and cost-effectiveness. Rationing (the action) and priority setting (the tool), are terms that are quite close and even sometimes used interchangeably. However, rationing usually implies the withholding of resources from individual patients, whereas priority setting has a less negative connotation, referring more to populations than to individuals (Dickinson *et al.*, 2011), and to a means for rationing. Although strictly speaking, these two terms have different meanings, they are closely related in terms of their policy implications. For that reason, they will be used in this chapter to refer to the process by which resource allocation decisions are both made and implemented in health care systems.

Economic evaluation, which is defined as "the comparative analysis of alternative courses of action in terms of both their costs and their consequences" (Torrance and Drummond, 2005), when applied to the health sector, provides a systematic framework to assess the relative costs and benefits of alternative health care interventions. A health care intervention that is "cost-effective" is one in which additional health benefits have been leveraged against their additional costs, resulting in a more efficient health care provision. Economic evaluation is hence used to inform resource allocation decisions.

Economic evaluation can be applied at different levels in the decision-making structure of health care organizations. At an aggregate level, economic evaluation may be applied to assess the relative value of building additional capacity into the system (health care service facilities), promoting health actions among alternatives (either from inside or outside of the health care sector) or even the allocation of funds to sectors other than health care (such as education or income support). On a lower level, once an initial health care spending capacity has been determined, we can implement economic evaluation to choose among more disaggregated health care areas such as procedures or types of services or among different beneficiaries. This is often made on an isolated or marginal basis, despite the need to recognize the existence of intersections among alternatives.

When used to determine a package of services and procedures to be covered under an insurance policy, whether public or private, the typology of the selected treatments and services may be of two types: (i) those included in a "basic package" (guaranteeing "right to access"), usually with the filter of a medical agent, perhaps some "enforceable" rules (legal entitlements or citizens' charts), or (ii) those considered beyond the basic package, under the constraints of either "hard" or "soft" rationing, dependent upon the role of the public regulator for private complementary care (community premiums, tax deductibility, etc.).

Applying economic evaluation to health care rationing is not exempt from controversy. As an example, controversy may arise on the question of including a certain treatment in the covered package of treatments and the consequent need to replace that new treatment with another previously covered due to budget constraints (investing and disinvesting), or increasing the extent of currently funded treatments (by adding to the covered package specific indications that were not previously considered). We will later discuss the extent of these controversies in health policy.

Economic evaluation is nowadays used not only for rationing health care coverage but also for measuring the performance of a whole health care system relative to other countries' or regions' health care systems. These measurements may be a means to attract more or less resources to the sector. In such analyses, the most common measures of output are mortality and morbidity, such as life expectancy, and impairment-free life expectancy (Field and Gold, 1998), or even improved versions of the Quality Adjusted Life-Year (QALY) by incorporating data on health-related quality of life to produce estimates of Quality Adjusted Life Expectancy (QALE). An interesting example of economic evaluation applied to international measures of performance is Bloomberg's ranking of countries based on the efficiency of their health-care systems.[1] Each country[2] has been ranked on three criteria: Life expectancy (weighted 60%), relative per capita cost of health care (30%), and absolute per capita cost of health care (10%). Countries were scored on each criterion and the scores were weighted and summed to obtain their efficiency scores. Relative cost is health cost per capita as a percentage of GDP

---

[1] See results at this link: http://www.bloomberg.com/visual-data/best-and-worst/most-efficient-health-care-2014-countries.

[2] Included were countries with populations of at least 5 million, GDP per capita of at least $5,000, and life expectancy of at least 70 years.

per capita. Absolute cost is total health expenditure, which covers preventive and curative health services, family planning, nutrition activities and emergency aid. Finally, economic evaluation is used to estimate the cost of illness or burden of disease, with the aim of assessing the overall scale of one specific health problem compared with other health problems (Mooney and Wiseman, 2000). Disability Adjusted Life Years (DALYs) have been extensively used in economic evaluations to monitor the burden of disease in both developed and developing countries (Lopez and Murray, 1998). However, such a use of economic evaluation is considered to be useful to size the problem associated with a disease, but does not provide any recommendation as to how many resources (including a measure of the opportunity costs) are worth being invested to fix it.

Welfarism and extra-welfarism in economics

A common fallacy in health and health care is that if universal access to health care, or low financial barriers to health care, can be achieved, then fairness can be reached by using patient needs as the main driver of resource allocation (Culyer, 2010a). However, to the extent that budgets are binding, adopting a new intervention that "works" (cost-effective) and is needed will necessarily entail reallocating resources, leaving other needs unsatisfied. That loss is the opportunity cost of the adopted intervention — that is, what is foregone by making one decision rather than another in the allocation of resources. In order to minimize opportunity costs, interventions that work better than others need to be identified. That is, evaluative techniques need to be applied for setting priorities. When opportunity costs are taken into account, an extra-welfarism approach is adopted, where decisions take a community perspective, allowing comparison of relative effectiveness among different interventions. It can even enable tradeoffs to be made, for example, by comparing the welfare losses from taxation to the benefits from increased public revenues and expenditures.

However, this is a less straightforward exercise than in a welfarist approach (Culyer, 2012). Indeed, a welfarist approach builds on individual preferences of the members of society, where actors are rewarded for arrangements they dislike and are willing to pay for things they want. Economic transactions between parties would, by these means, be reached on Pareto criteria, and willingness to pay (WTP) would be used as the main criteria for allocating resources in the health care arena (Musgrove, 1999). In an extra-welfarism approach, economic evaluation becomes the main tool to assist decisions regarding which interventions are preferred for the community in terms of health, given both the scarcity of resources and the need to make choices among alternative initiatives. For further reading, the book by Culyer (2012) is a perfect introduction to these concepts.

Uncertainty and decision-making in practice

There are, as just mentioned, many difficulties in decision-making that arise from the evidence of relative effectiveness or value under an extra-welfarism approach. For instance, one difficulty arises from the existence of uncertainty in the decision-making process. It is, in spite of increased evidence, still an unavoidable component of decision-making. Indeed, the British Medical Journal *Clinical Evidence*, calling on the knowledge of information specialists, editors, peer reviewers, and expert authors, highlights how evidence-based treatments are, for certain indications, based on randomized controlled trials. They find that more than 50% of the treatments have an unknown effectiveness, and an additional 15% have harmful or unlikely benefits at all. Only 11% of the treatments have a beneficial effect and 23% are likely to be beneficial.[3] Figure 1 illustrates the results.

Comparable results have been found in the US (Poonacha and Go, 2011). The National Comprehensive Cancer Network (NCCN), a not-for-profit alliance of 21 comprehensive cancer centers designated by the US National Cancer Institute and dedicated to improving the quality and effectiveness of care provided to patients with cancer, categorized evidence from I (highest degree of evidence, with

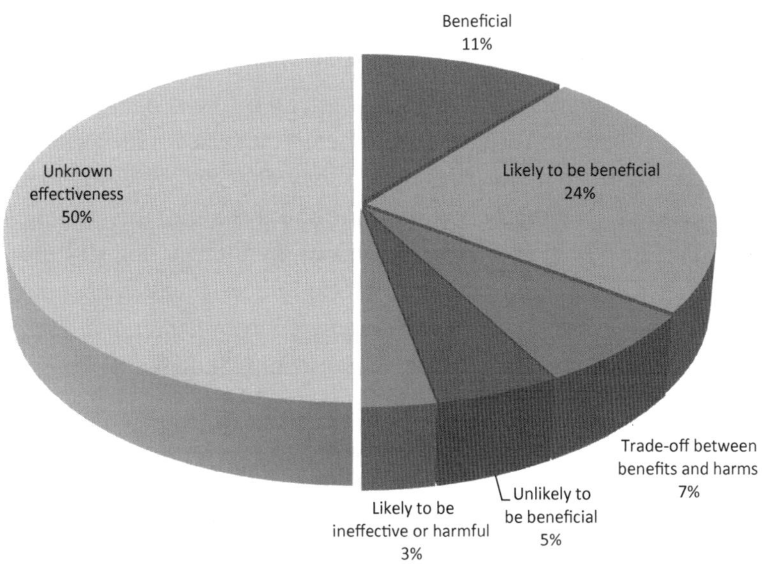

Figure 1. Categorization of the effectiveness of treatments
Source: *Clinical Evidence* (BMJ), 2011.

[3]As noted by the authors, "these data reflect how different treatments stand up in light of evidence-based medicine and are not an audit of the extent to which treatments are used in practice or for other indications not assessed in *Clinical Evidence*."

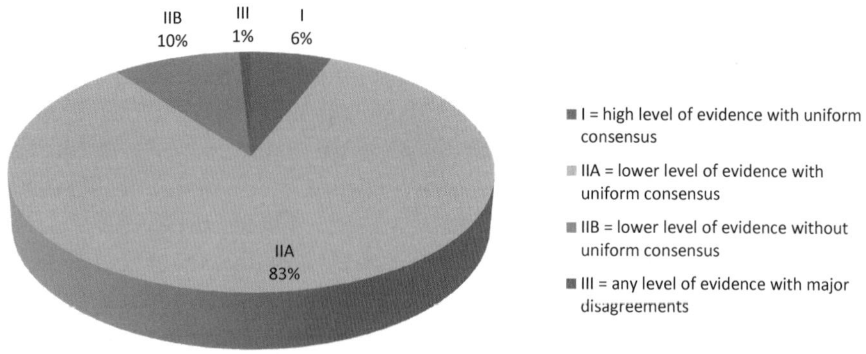

Figure 2. Distribution of categories of evidence and consensus for all guidelines in oncology, according to the NCCN

Source: National Comprehensive Cancer Network.

consensus) to III (lowest level of evidence).[4] They found that the majority of the recommendations (83%) were based on category IIA and a minority (6%) were based on Category I (the highest level of evidence with uniform consensus), as illustrated in Figure 2.

As a result of unavoidable uncertainty in decision processes, the alternative of doing nothing is often considered the baseline case, converting the analysis of decisions into an analysis of incremental costs and consequences of any action. Being that uncertainty is an inherent ingredient in these analyses, the central question becomes how much uncertainty there is and how much can a decision process bear. In some circumstances, technology changes are worth their cost, in spite of the fact that they might be expensive and in spite of uncertainties. Cutler and McClellan (2001) report on the benefits of technology changes produced in the treatment of heart disease, low-birth weight infants, breast cancer, depression, and cataracts. As illustrated in Figure 3, extracted from Cutler and McClellan, in all of these cases but breast cancer, benefits from technological changes are so large that they dwarf all of the uncertainties one may think of in such analyses.

Priority setting and fairness

Priority setting is not exempt from controversy since there is no single, generally accepted way of undertaking it. Priority setting may be done on an efficiency basis (as a "health maximand" function), but other criteria could also be used for

[4]The NCCN definitions for Evidence and Consensus are as follows: Category I, high level of evidence with uniform consensus; Category IIA, lower level of evidence with uniform consensus; Category IIB, lower level of evidence without a uniform consensus but with no major disagreement; and Category III, any level of evidence but with major disagreement.

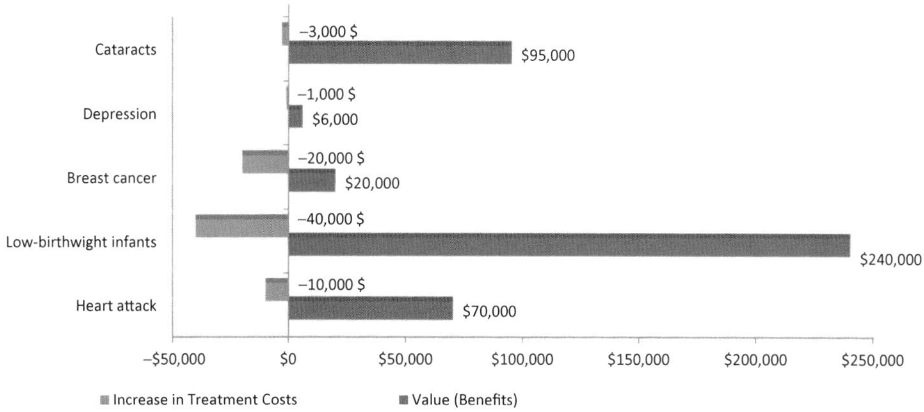

Figure 3. Medical innovation: Value and costs

Source: Authors' elaboration based on Cutler and McClellan (2001).

priority-setting purposes. For instance, the degree of the negative externality that a health care condition may cause on the patient's relatives or caregivers could be considered as a criteria for priority setting. The existence of significant catastrophic costs associated with treating a disease may also count as a criteria for priority setting (Musgrove, 1999). Adding social and equity concerns (that is, looking for a "fair" distribution of health); taking categorical constraints into account (by defining, for example, a threshold of minimum entitlements per individual); or considering criteria to be used on a case-by-case basis for a limited number of cases where a trade-off exists (for instance, across treatments for a common illness) are frequent additional considerations and criteria used for priority setting in practice.

In order to evaluate progress toward presumed social goals in allocating resources under explicit priority setting principles, it is important to know who accrues these social benefits and under what distributional weights. Using cost-effectiveness and QALYs for priority setting implicitly compares the value gains of alternatives irrespective of other characteristics (unless otherwise specified), such as the nature of the disease, beneficiary characteristics or social implications. No equity concerns are explicitly taken into account, but rather, all QALYs are considered equal. However, maximizing population health (efficiency) may not yield equitable solutions (distributive fairness), neither in the horizontal sense (that is, equal treatment of people in equal situation), nor in the vertical sense (unequal treatment of those unequal). There is no consensus about what "treatment" or "situation" may implicitly be taken into account for equity purposes (Culyer and Wagstaff, 1993).

There are, however, a variety of proposals on the table regarding equity concerns. Some authors link equity to morbidity or mortality, which are the closest concepts to medical "need" (or need understood as absence of health) (Williams, 1962). However, *health* absence and *health care* absence are sometimes confounded: much health care may have low productivity or effectiveness to achieve better health conditions. Health indicators may signal a lack of health care resources and/or many other flaws the health care sector cannot fix. The only health care that might be "needed" is that which is effective.

For some others, equity is regarded as equal "capacity to benefit" from a health care intervention (i.e., the difference between a person's predicted health with and without health care). However, this criterion for measuring equity does not take into account the starting point, that is, current health differences among people. Indeed, individuals who are initially relatively healthy might benefit more than those in poor health, even though the latter might be those with higher health care deficits. So, this criterion might eventually increase differences.

Despite these nuances, in practice, allocative targets usually consist of maximizing total outcomes, with or without accounting for initial health endowments and with or without accounting for an individual's capability to benefit from health care, which affects their relative maximum benefit achievable (Culyer and Wagstaff, 1993). The approach adopted will affect the precise amount of resources to be allocated, either in terms of equal resources (input values, expenditure levels) for equal access, equal consumption, or in order to achieve equal health.

Besides the set of economic criteria involved in economic evaluation, one may find other ways of rationing based on some concept of need, such as the Rescue Principle (McKie and Richardson, 2003). These alternative criteria do not include any economic rationale, since they do not account for the relative effectiveness of the intervention nor for its costs. Implicitly, there are logical inconsistencies. For example, the Rescue Principle assumes somehow that death might be avoided, not just postponed, as a consequence of health care interventions. Something similar can be concluded from a Needs Assessment, a kind of analysis consisting of prioritizing health care services on the basis of need in such a way that it can clearly lead to an inefficient use of resources, because it overlooks the potential for patients to benefit from health care interventions and ignores the costs of interventions. In summary, it does not offer a realistic mechanism for trading off different alternatives in a binding budget context.

The critical role of economic evaluation and its different forms

As mentioned before, economic evaluation in health provides a systematic framework to assess the relative costs and benefits of alternative health care interventions. By choosing to provide interventions that are deemed cost-effective, health care provision should be made more efficient while health benefits could either remain the same or increase.

There are three main forms of economic evaluation. Cost-effectiveness analysis (CEA) focuses on the consequences of an intervention as measured in terms of natural units on a one-dimensional scale: That is, *effectiveness* in terms of mortality rate decreases or some other measure of results expressed in natural (nonmonetary) units. Cost–Utility Analysis (CUA) applies when consequences of an intervention are measured as units of a cardinal utility function that maps the multi-dimensional concept of health onto a scalar index. QALY is the most frequently used measure of utility used in such analyses. Finally, Cost–Benefit Analysis (CBA) is used when *monetary units* prevail as the unit of measurement and evaluation technique for both the costs and benefits of an intervention.

There are, additionally, partial evaluation methods that are worth mentioning. Firstly, *cost-description analysis or cost-of-illness studies.* These generally rely on the estimation of the economic burden of a specific disease to society (for example, to the health care system, government, or employer) and allow attention to be drawn to particularly high-cost disease areas. They inform decision-makers on the absolute and relative magnitude of the burden of a disease and offer an indication of the amount of resources that could be saved if the disease were eradicated. They are hence useful for guiding future research that aims to stimulate better utilization of health care resources. However, a clear limitation of cost-of-illness studies is that they say nothing about outcomes or efficiency, and, consequently, different alternatives cannot be really compared.

Secondly, *cost-minimization analysis* is a partial approach to economic evaluation and is used in circumstances where there is already good existing evidence to suggest that the interventions under consideration are equally effective. Given equal outcomes, the evaluation involves the comparison of costs alone to determine the lowest-cost alternative. In other words, the aim is to minimize the cost of producing a certain level of outcome, with the cheapest option being the most efficient.

Specific developments on the methodologies for economic evaluation have reached a high level of sophistication. Very recently, the Consolidated Health Economic Evaluation Reporting Standards (CHEERS) statement (Husereau *et al.*, 2013) was developed by a task force supported by ISPOR (International Society for Pharmacoeconomics and Outcomes Research), as part of a broader initiative to facilitate and encourage the exchange of expert knowledge and develop best practices. The statement is an attempt to consolidate and update previous health economic evaluation guidelines into a single document for researchers reporting the outcomes of economic evaluations and editors and peer reviewers assessing them for publication.

Table 1 summarizes the CHEERS statement and the variety of recognized evaluation options (Husereau *et al.*, 2013). In spite of such a varied menu of options, many academics still believe that full economic evaluation analysis for

Table 1. Forms of economic evaluation, according to the CHEERS committee

Approaches	**Definition**
Cost-consequences analysis	Examines costs anf consequences without attempting to isolate a single consequence or aggregate consequences into a single measure.
Cost-minimization analysis (CMA)	The consequences of compared interventions are required to be equivalent, and only relatives costs are compared.
Cost-effectiveness analysis (CEA)	Measures consequences in natural units, such as life years gained, disability days avoided, or cases detected. In variant of CEA, often **cost–utility analysis (CUA)**, consequences are measured in terms of preference-based measures of health, such as QALYs or DALYs.
Cost–benefit analysis	Consequences are valued in monetary units.

Notes: Specific forms of analysis reflect different approaches to evaluating the consequences of health interventions. Health consequences may be estimated from a single analytical (experimental or non-experimental) study, a synthesis of studies, mathematical modeling, or a combination of modeling and study information.
Source: Husereau *et al.* (2013).

priority-setting purposes must be done through one of the three methods: *Cost-Effectiveness Analysis* (CEA), *Cost–Utility Analysis* (CUA) or *Cost–Benefit Analysis* (CBA).

It is worth noting that, besides identifying and defining the various forms of economic evaluation, the aim of the CHEERS Committee was to provide recommendations, in the form of a checklist, to optimize reporting of health economic evaluations. Their checklist of items to include when reporting economic evaluations of health interventions has been published in more than 10 scientific journals, becoming an unavoidable international reference for professionals in this field.

- *Cost-effectiveness analysis (CEA) insights*

Returning to the main evaluation method, CEA, the outcome of interest is health or health-related quality of life. CEA measures outcomes in natural (physical) units which are often disease specific (e.g., infections or cancers prevented, lives saved, cases detected, patients correctly treated, or life-years gained). CEA always compares two or more interventions (not a stand-alone analysis). Health is sometimes compared to an alternative average situation, and the resulting difference between these two situations yields an average cost-effectiveness ratio (ACER); for example, if effectiveness is measured as length of life, ACER would give a measure of increased costs, in units of money, against benefits in life-years gained.

If two alternative interventions are compared and are mutually exclusive, however, the resulting comparative index will be the so-called incremental cost-effectiveness ratio (ICER). The ICER of an intervention is defined as the ratio of incremental costs and incremental benefits compared to the next most effective intervention; that is, to compare additional costs to additional benefits in natural units.

CEA puts interventions side-by-side on the basis of their cost for each unit of outcome. It is hence a method of comparing the opportunity costs of alternative interventions which have a common desired benefit or outcome (Torrance and Drummond, 2005). Although the health outcome measured in a CEA makes this analysis different from CBA — which measures outcomes in monetary units — according to Culyer (2010b), the monetary value of a CEA's outcome measure is left implicit and, "in a budget-constrained system motivated by health maximization, it is the shadow price of the budget, or incremental cost-effectiveness ratio (ICER)."

All in all, on the one hand, CEA is a helpful analytic tool when outcomes are difficult to value monetarily, when those that are measurable are not commensurable, or when the objectives are set in terms of health itself. On the other hand, however, CEA has some important limitations.

Firstly, CEA fails to account for non-health outcomes. Additional analysis, sometimes called cost-consequence analysis, where aspects other than health outcomes are also taken into account, is required, or CBA may be a solution.

Secondly, an important limitation of CEA arises when one needs to compare interventions across different medical conditions, because CEA addresses only a single dimension of disease-specific outcome. Moreover, it may be difficult to capture all possible effects of an intervention on a single outcome, as in the case of life extension when the quality of the life changes together with other side effects. CEA is more useful when effectiveness has a single dimension of interest. Some of the measures may be soundly different, as for instance the increase in Forced Expiratory Volume in sprirometry, the number of cases hospitalized for a specific diagnosis, the number of symptom-free days, the number of fractures prevented, cardiovascular events avoided, pain-free days, life-years gained, disability-days saved, percentage of vision gained, and so on. CEA becomes useful when consequences can be captured in a single measure of outcome and the decision concerns how to achieve that particular outcome. It then allows for alternative interventions or actions to be sorted out in relative, not absolute, terms.

Thirdly, CEA deals with intermediate output data that cannot be directly compared across different areas of health care (e.g., detection of allergies vs. mammography) or between different moments in time (whether an individual's health has improved or declined), and this information is necessary in order to be able to compare changes in health.

Finally, CEA deals with health indicators without taking into account individuals' or patients' preferences in health states, even though preferences in health states may differ greatly across patients.

Consequently, CEA appears to be useful only under restricted circumstances. Some of these problems are tackled with another evaluation methodology, CUA.

- *CUA insights*

In CUA, the outcome measure is utility instead of a natural measure of health. That utility indicator may be used to measure a single effect or multiple effects. CUA is more demanding from a methodological point of view, but a more valuable technique, with a common numerator to match up several alternatives by healthy years or, more typically, measured as quality adjusted life-years (known as QALY's). The QALY is a measure of overall health calibrated over one year. More specifically, it represents one year of life, adjusted for health-related quality of life. It incorporates both length of life and health-related quality of life into a single index (Williams, 1995). The QALY accounts for both changes in the number of years lived (mortality) and the changes in quality of those years (how well). By using QALYs, we identify health state outcomes. They are described as the number of years alive (T) of each individual, weighted by a valuation of that health (W). The quality adjustment to life is made by assigning a value of 1 to "full health," and a value of 0 to the state of "death." Intermediate values represent intermediate states. And then we can calculate average outcomes (W.T) and differences before and after interventions.

All methods for obtaining quality weights start with a health state description (e.g., a general health state, or a condition-specific description). Note that these descriptions involve judgments about the important characteristics of different health states, but they tell us nothing about how different states are valued. The quality adjustment is a proxy for satisfaction/well-being. It reflects consumers' judgement about what they consider good and bad in relation to their health. They are necessarily subjective: They elicit an individual's preferences for, or value of, one or more health states. Nonetheless, there is some confusion about the term utility, which has, for some, a materialistic connotation, given the use of this term in other areas of economics. Culyer states that, regarding CUA, "modern confusion" about the 'utility' of health-related quality of life has arisen because it is entirely appropriate to use the theory of utility measurement also to measure other entities such as health. But that does not mean that what is being measured is a *utility*, at least not in the usual sense of an indicator of the strength of a preference …

It is a pity that the term "cost–utility analysis" ever came to replace the much more neutral "cost-effectiveness analysis" (Culyer, 2010b).

The most delicate part of computing QALYs is quantifying the above-mentioned adjustment to life years. This requires measurement of an individual's health-related quality of life for a period of time and giving it a quality of life score on the ratio scale mentioned previously, with 1 representing full health and 0 representing the state of death. Data from individuals is hence an input of the QALY. The most popular survey-based methods are Visual Analog Scale, Time Trade-Off, and Standard Gamble. The resulting value of the adjustment may vary according to the method used. For instance, the Time Trade-Off method asks individuals how many years of life are they willing to give up in order to enjoy full health rather than remaining in their current ill-health state, which can be a challenging question to answer. In a pilot study (Dolan, 1997), it was found that respondents cannot be expected to compare a large number of health states using that method. When direct interview methods such as these are not available or complete, indirect methodologies can be used, which are based on mapping procedures, expert judgment, and regression methods to estimate lacking information.

QALY arithmetic is based on three simplifying assumptions: (i) The value of life years is assumed to be linear, a convenient simplification; (ii) a multiplicative combination of life duration and health adjustment is postulated; and (iii) for non-chronic health states, values of different periods with different health states are just added up. The first of the assumptions on linearity is sometimes relaxed by introducing discounting possibilities or risk aversion. Other limitations of QALYs are frequently mentioned (Culyer, 2012). Firstly, it is only a measure of health outcomes. It does not reflect the potential social outcomes of an intervention that are not taken into account in the questionnaires nor in the increase in years lived). It also does not reflect the processes (the means) related to the intervention. Too much emphasis is sometimes allegedly placed on the results of the health intervention under analysis. Secondly, the dependence on human inputs to get answers to the questionnaire may make some groups' answers less reliable, such as young children and the mentally ill. Their preferences are consequently less well reflected.

QALYs fit into an extra-welfarist approach, or the so-called "societal decision-making view." This approach takes as exogenously defined a societal objective and a given budget constraint for health care. It then considers CUA as a technical tool to solve a constrained optimization problem. This is, however, a much more complex exercise due to the required specification of an objective (QALY maximization) and the means to measure the achievements (under QALY assumptions). When used for priority setting, the aggregate QALY value obtained, as a result of either a linear or weighted process, is not universally accepted.

Moreover, the conversion of the cost per QALY as a tool for setting priorities among services or indications, given a binding budget, requires an explicit decision on a threshold that is critical for the process. All these aspects clearly need the strong external legitimacy of public representatives in order to award them with a normative content. The deliberation process becomes even more important than the parameters and the goals to be achieved.

In contrast, CBA stays in the field of traditional welfarism, where health care interventions are to be judged in the same way as any other proposed welfare component. That is, according to whether they represent a potential Pareto improvement[5] (as measured by a compensation test), and not just according to whether they improve health outcomes or preferences. On the other hand, for most developed countries' health systems, there is a clear reluctance regarding the prescriptions of the welfare theory to health care. The conditions of rationality and consistency required of individuals with respect to maximizing their utility have shown to be repeatedly transgressed, and the acceptance of the current distribution of income as the starting point of a WTP method is widely rejected.

Social value judgments and ethical dilemmas

As mentioned previously in this chapter, rationalizing health care, by whatever means including a rigorous explicit system of priority setting, results in some form of rationing which, in its most negative sense, implies exclusion or rejection of some procedures, services or technologies. These rationing decisions might be very difficult to take and to be accepted by beneficiaries. For that reason, decisions need to be grounded on sound and explicit ethical principles. Otherwise, a lack of legitimacy of the decisions is bound to become the Achilles' heel of the whole priority system.

The deliberative process, defined as the process by which conclusions are reached and recommendations are made, is a key component (Shah *et al.*, 2013) of success. Basically, this process must, firstly, be accountable with regard to beneficiaries involved in the health care initiative under evaluation and, secondly, preserve individual freedom and autonomy so that excluded health care procedures or devices from the benefits' package should not be prohibited. Individuals should be given the option of acquiring any rejected intervention that is deemed effective, under their individual responsibility. Thirdly, processes and criteria are to be explicit and clear. In addition, need (in the sense of fairness as perceived by

---

[5]Pareto optimality is a state of allocation of resources in which it is impossible to make any one individual better off without making at least one individual worse off.

the community) is a value to be held, as it opens the participation process to the community from a social perspective, with priorities based on common good and not on individual wants.

Although legitimacy is a crucial aspect of rationing processes, an adequate process does not preclude decision-makers from facing more fundamental judgements involved in priority setting, such as whether more health is always better, or whether public preferences violate monotonicity. In standard social welfare functions, a gain in efficiency should always overcome any loss due to potential increases in inequality. How efficiency and equity are leveraged depends very much on the distribution and on the extent of social aversion to health inequalities.

Priority setting is not just about applying a methodology. It needs to be anchored in a given social context, and this context is a determinant for the process. In fact, the results of the process and the decisions made depend very much on the social context. In other words, social costs are reflected not only by the additional costs held in public budgets when an intervention is selected to be covered by the public benefits package. An intervention may alternatively be covered through specific regulation, copayments and complementary community premiums, and produce other kinds of social costs. For example, an excluded treatment due to a poor cost effectiveness ratio is equivalent to a covered treatment with a "one hundred per cent copayment," in which case, social costs are appear at the individual level. Fiscal expenditures (tax deductions) are a form of copayment too, and charging a mandatory premium on employers is also a form of tax. All these alternatives, however, show different political strands, social culture, and a different tolerance of disparities between or within cohorts, ordered either by income, age or type of illness.

In summary, the issues at stake in priority setting are, firstly, the value given to health — that is, whether we are getting aggregate good value for money in health care. Secondly, one should consider how value differences that may arise within sub-groups of individuals should be addressed, and how these differences affect results in delivering and financing health care. Thirdly, it must be determined where the threshold should be for an intervention to be publicly covered. That is, what magnitude of incremental cost-effectiveness (cost increase per each health outcome or QALY gained) is excessive to justify the inclusion of a treatment or intervention into the benefits package? Is the £30.000 per QALY gained, as defined by the NICE in England, an optimal threshold? Finally, explicit decisions should be made regarding equity. There needs to be consensus on the desired distributional effects of the interventions, that is, consensus on either setting equal weighting of benefits or some other form of categorical equity concept.

The difficulty in dealing with these issues from the pure political arena has led some countries to delegate priority-setting processes to independent agencies. These independent agencies have relieved policymakers from the suspicion of political bias in the priority-setting process, and, at the same time, from implementing unpopular cost reduction decisions or disinvesting from new or existing procedures. We shall, in the next section, explain how specific agencies that are considered to be references worldwide are addressing priority-setting processes.

Institutions for Priority Setting in Health Care

Here, we review the realities of priority setting processes in six different countries, four of which are known for being precursors for establishing explicit priority setting mechanisms. Table 2 summarizes the study cases and their main characteristics.

United States: Comparative effectiveness research

Among all the countries chosen for analysis, the US is the country where private insurance and welfarism approaches are more dominant in the health care system.

Comparative Effectiveness Research (CER) became a focal issue in the US during the 2009–2010 health reform debate (Luce *et al.*, 2010) as a means for priority setting. In its hope to expand coverage while limiting use of treatments that did not work well, the Obama Administration decided to invest $1.1 billion on CER, portraying it as the first step to government rationing. The Institute of Medicine (IOM), an independent, non-profit organization that works outside of government, to provide advice to decision-makers and health care stakeholders, defined and endorsed CER as follows: “CER is the generation and synthesis of evidence that compares the benefits and harms of alternative methods to prevent, diagnose, treat and monitor a clinical condition, or to improve the delivery of care. The purpose of CER is to assist consumers, clinicians, purchasers, and policymakers to make informed decisions that will improve health care at both the individual and population levels” (IOM, 2009). CER is a different term from CEA. An important component of CER is the concept of Pragmatic Trials. These clinical research trials measure effectiveness (the benefit the treatment produces in routine clinical practice). This is different from regular clinical trials, which measure efficacy (whether the treatment works or not). CER is closer to Health Services Research techniques and does not necessarily include economic evaluation. CER was not meant for decision-making, but as an input for Health Technology Assessment Analysis (Luce *et al.*, 2010).

Table 2. Summary of case studies: Health technology assessment (HTA) agencies and their basic characteristics

	Health care system	Independent agency	Role	Method for priority setting
(a) US[6]	Private providers and Obamacare	The Institute of Medicine	Advice	CER (Comparative Effectiveness Research)
	Medicaid (Federal and state coverage)	The Oregon Health Services Commission	Responsibilities on the package definition	Some form of CEA
(b) England & Wales	Tax-financed	NICE — National Institute for Health and Care Excellence (publicly funded)	Clear responsibilities linked to decisions on pricing and coverage	Economic evaluation
(c) Germany	Social Insurance with competing companies	IQWUIG — Institute for Quality and Efficiency in Health Care (paid by sickness funds)	Advice to the Federal Joint Committee	Efficiency frontiers
(d) France	Social Insurance with competing companies	HAS — *Haute autorité de santé* (publicly funded)	Advice	Economic evaluation
(e) Sweden	Tax-financed	SBU — swedish Council on Health Technology Assessment (fees from the industry)	Do or explain why not to do it	Economic evaluation
(f) Netherlands	Social Insurance with competing companies	CVZ — National Health Care Institute (publicly funded)	Clear responsibilities linked to decisions on pricing and coverage	Economic Evaluation

[6]The US offers a large set of examples regarding HTA initiatives. The CER is illustrative of a very idiosyncratic and innovative view which is worth analyzing, for the sake of its influence on other health care systems. Although only two initiatives have been described in this chapter, the CMS (Centers for Medicare and Medicaid Services) experience could have also been added, as an example of a government agency with more similarities to European experiences. For those interested in the CMS experience, see the information at these links: http://www.cms.gov/Regulations-and-Guidance/Legislation/CFCsAndCoPs/index.html?redirect=/cfcsandcops/16_asc.asp; https://www.healthcare.gov/glossary/minimum-essential-coverage/.

The US Congress, in the American Recovery and Reinvestment Act (ARRA) of 2009, tasked the IOM to recommend national priorities for research questions to be addressed by CER and supported by ARRA funds. In its 2009 Report (IOM, 2009), the authoring committee established a working definition of CER, developed a priority list of research topics, and identified the necessary requirements to support a robust and sustainable CER enterprise.

It is a limited version of other countries' agencies. It is grounded on research that evaluates and compares health outcomes and the clinical effectiveness, risks and benefits of two or more medical treatments, services or related items. The IOM "identifies what works best for which patients under what circumstances. And provides doctors and patients with the information they need to make the best medical decisions" (IOM, 2009). However, "implementation of CER must preserve patient access to a wide array of medicines, rather than limiting choice by using the resulting data to mandate coverage or payment levels" (IOM, 2011). The Director of Public Health Systems, Finance, and Quality Program in the Department of Health and Human Services explains, "The social budget is limited — we have a limited resource pool. It makes terribly good sense to at least know the price of an added benefit, and at some point we might say nationally, regionally, or locally that we wish we could afford it, but we can't" (Honoré *et al.*, 2011).

CER has some limitations as a priority-setting tool. It does not consider costs, nor does it consider concerns about efficiency. CER analysis is affected by issues such as the heterogeneity in the patient effects of treatments (like pain, nausea, incontinence) that cannot make for a single outcome index. Moreover, these effects are sometimes exogenous (gene type, at the static level, or gene mutation at the dynamic one); sometimes, they are endogenous (spillovers from other treatments, user behavior, heterogeneous provider skills and know-how, scale economies). This is certainly a common problem to all economic evaluation but it reminds us that CER is less than perfect, too.

Finally, according to the IOM (2011), "if cost considerations were added, the endogeneity of prices for alternative treatments should be accounted for, and CER would resemble economic evaluation tools to a greater degree." In any case, CER, especially in the context of the Patient Protection and Affordable Care Act (ACA), signed into law on 23 March 2010, certainly opened a door to assign a role for public subsidies and copayments based on comparative effectiveness, perhaps for some variation in the treatment effects on the supply-side, or on the patient benefits on the demand-side, and more controversially, on how the benefits are valued by patients.

Indeed, the ACA stipulated that a set of qualified health plans (QHPs) would cover an "essential health benefit" package, to be defined by the Secretary of Health and Human Services (HHS) based on the scope of benefits offered by a typical employer plan. At the request of HHS, the IOM undertook a study to make recommendations on the criteria and methods for determining and updating the essential health benefits (EHB) package. The committee was not to specify the details of the package. The IOM report was issued by the end of 2011 (IOM, 2012). The IOM saw two main questions: (1) How to determine the initial EHB package and (2) how to update the EHB package.

In considering how to determine the initial EHB package, the IOM committee "was struck by two compelling facts: (1) If the purpose of the PPACA is to provide access to health insurance coverage, then that coverage has to be affordable; and (2) the more expansive the benefit package is, the more it will likely cost and the less affordable it will be. How to balance the competing goals of comprehensiveness of coverage and affordability was key."

The committee concluded that it was best to begin simply by defining the EHB package as reflecting the scope and design of packages offered by small employers. The committee considered four policy domains — economics, ethics, population-based health, and evidence-based practice — in determining the EHB package in general. From these policy foundations, the committee recommended criteria to guide the aggregate EHB package.

Benefits mandated for insurance coverage by individual states should be subject to the same review and criteria. Products and services that do not meet the criteria should not be included, according to the report. The report also described specific criteria to guide methods for updating the EHB, for inclusions and exclusions. It recommended that HHS officials should gauge potential services and products against a set of criteria including medical effectiveness, a good evidence base, safety, improved outcomes, and cost-effectiveness.

Besides the IOM recommendations based on CER, the experience of priority setting in Oregon's Medicaid program starting in the early 1990's represents the most explicit, as well as one of the most controversial, and innovative at that time, examples of priority setting in health care (Ham, 1998). The goal of the program was to limit coverage to a bundle of services according to a cost-effectiveness ranking. A Quality-of-Well-Being Scale was first obtained, which had to be abandoned due to criticisms on the methodology, and substituted by another where expert knowledge and intuitive judgments about appropriateness were added. Since then, the Oregon system keeps updating the methodology. It represents an example of the potential difficulties of implementing explicit priority setting mechanisms in a context like the US (Sabik and Lie, 2008).

England and Wales: The NICE

The National Institute for Health and Care Excellence (NICE) is a non-departmental public entity of the Department of Health in the United Kingdom, serving both the

English NHS and the Welsh NHS. It was established in 1999, redesigned in 2005 (NICE, 2005), and finally renamed the National Institute for Health and Care Excellence in April 2013 (The Health Service in England, 2012), as a result of its new responsibilities on social care. It also changed from a special health authority to a non-departmental public body. As such, NICE is "accountable to our sponsor department, the Department of Health, but operationally independent of government. Its guidance and other recommendations are made by independent committees" (NICE, 2008).

The standard approach of NICE to technology appraisals takes one of two forms: A single technology appraisal (STA) which covers a single technology for a single indication, or a multiple technology appraisal (MTA) which normally covers more than one technology, or one technology for more than one indication. MTAs are very common and take 54 weeks from the initiation of the process to issuing guidance. STA is a faster process. As proof of its relevant activity, until the February 2014, NICE Guidelines amounted to 413 regarding interventional procedures, 303 on technology appraisals, 184 on clinical guidelines, and 49 on public health. Among similar organizations elsewhere, NICE is unusual in that it publishes details of evidence and reasoning.

From a methodological point of view, the ICER from CUA plays a crucial role in helping NICE to reach a recommendation. NICE makes recommendations regarding the adoption of new health technologies by reviewing evidence on clinical effectiveness and cost-effectiveness. Each technology appraisal may contain more than one recommendation. Recommendations are classified into 4 categories: recommended, optimised, only in research, and not recommended. If NICE recommends adoption, clinical commissioning groups (CCG) [previously, Primary Care Trusts (PCTs)[7]] are expected to make the treatment available. If NICE does not make a positive recommendation, the CCGs are less likely to commission the treatment.

NICE defines an ICER threshold as the cost per QALY above which a product or a service is recommended not to be publicly funded. The threshold limit has been at the heart of many debates. One suggestion is to set the threshold to "optimally exhaust" (in maximizing the health gain) a fixed budget. However, NICE does not use a precise ICER threshold that automatically defines a technology's cost effectiveness (Towse and Pritchard, 2002). Cost per QALY gained

[7]**A primary care trust** (PCT) was part of the National Health Service in England from 2001 to 2013. PCTs were largely administrative bodies, responsible for commissioning primary, community and secondary health services from providers. Until 31 May 2011, they also provided community health services directly. Collectively, PCTs were responsible for spending around 80% of the total NHS budget. PCTs were abolished on 31 March 2013 as part of the Health and Social Care Act 2012, with their work taken over by CCG.

ranges commonly from £20,000 to £30,000 per QALY. Below £20,000, usually the treatment is recommended; above £20,000 the decision would not be taken exclusively on the grounds of cost-effectiveness but could be accepted for a "particular feature of the condition and the population using the technology," that is, for example, for an innovation that changes QALYs, in such a way that it has not been appropriately captured in the QALY measure. Above a most plausible ICER of £30,000 per QALY gained, the benefits would need to be identified as an increasingly stronger case.

The guidance within NICE's first edition *Guide to the Methods of Technology Appraisal* (NICE, 2003) established that "... an additional QALY is of equal value regardless of other characteristics of the individual such as their socio-demographic details, or their pre- or post-treatment level of health." However, this was in fact a reflection of the absence of a consensus on how to deal with differences that were explicitly recognized by NICE (Shah *et al.*, 2013). A period of research on how to deal with different weight considerations yielded a second edition of the *Guide to the Methods of Technology Appraisal* (NICE, 2008) so that, "The Institute considers equity in terms of how the effects of a health technology may deliver differential benefits across the population." In January 2009, supplementary guidance was issued and NICE was instructed to give special weighting to the health gains of individuals in the later stages of terminal illness. Between January and April that year, nine technologies were considered that fit into this context (Longson and Littlejohns, 2009). Three criteria are required in order to qualify for this exception: (i) The treatment is indicated for patients with a short life expectancy, normally less than 24 months; (ii) there is sufficient evidence to indicate that the treatment offers an extension to life, normally of at least an additional 3 months, compared to current NHS treatment; and finally (iii) the treatment is licensed or otherwise indicated for small patient populations. This is equivalent, in practice, to a threshold increase.

Given the ethical issues involved in priority setting, the aim of NICE is to make criteria publicly accessible, reasonable (applying relevant principles) and challengeable through appeal. The threshold works at any rate as a numerical line which allows for comparisons across treatments. It avoids accepting unfavorable cost-effectiveness ratios in some areas simply because existing alternatives (the "going rate") are relatively inefficient, as in comparative effectiveness. But from an ethical perspective, there remains the question of whether a "QALY is really a QALY," or if more weight should be given to QALYs accruing to patients with relatively severe illnesses or which impose a relatively high burden of disease; patients in the later stages of disease with a short life expectancy (less than 2 years); or additionally whether more weight should be given to treatments to be licensed for small patient populations and to treatments for which no alternative treatment with comparable benefits is available through NHS. In these circumstances, the rescue principle is a powerful human impulse.

The principles are explicit, but there are plenty of caveats. For instance, NICE cannot in principle discriminate according to the cause of illness or how "deserving" of a treatment the individual may be. This includes even those conditions that may have been contracted or exacerbated due to the individual's lifestyle or occupation. However, if the behavior is likely to continue and can make a treatment less cost-effective or clinically less effective, then it may be appropriate to take into account those features for treatment differentiation. Notice that it is often impossible on an individual basis to determine whether a condition may be fully dependent on a person's own individual behavior.

The 2010 Equality Act (Equality Act, 2010), a Parliament Act to require Ministers, when making strategic decisions, to have regard for the desirability of reducing socio-economic inequalities, is another caveat. It urged NICE to actively extend health equality efforts regarding sex, age, race, disability, and socioeconomic status, despite the fact that NICE was not initially expected to make recommendations on the basis of individuals' income, social class or position in life. Nor were individuals' social roles at different ages expected to affect the decisions about cost effectiveness. Indeed, NICE has been very reluctant to depart from the criterion of "a QALY is a QALY." It is legitimated to increase overall population health, regardless of whether differences among groups remain the same or increase. According to a utilitarian approach, the overall increase in health may cause deterioration in terms of its distribution, meaning potential for greater disparities between groups. But now NICE may take these distribution effects into consideration, on a case-by-case basis and make decisions that produce overall health improvement — focusing on all levels of the health and socioeconomic gradient — and a targeted focus on the most disadvantaged. These hybrid decisions, despite being more difficult to achieve, depart from a "QALY is a QALY" policy.

In addition, weighting health gains for severely ill patients implies that fewer resources will ultimately reach preventive and public health programs which are meant to favor the healthiest groups. The justification to apply smaller weights to potential health gains among more economically advanced populations is, however, far from obvious from a universal perspective.

The cost-effectiveness (C-E) threshold in itself is an estimate of health forgone, as other NHS activities are displaced to accommodate the additional costs of those technologies recommended by NICE. It will change as circumstances and the NHS change. It represents the implicit values from past NICE decisions. It does not necessarily reflect society's WTP for health improvements. The overall threshold will, in reality, depend on the programs of care where disinvestment takes place or how expenditure on particular programs change with the overall budget; a sort of average marginal elasticity of spending with respect to income. Changes in budgets are, in practice, incremental and it may be the case that the elasticities of program expenditure in time of budgetary increase (when new initiatives are added) are not the same as in times of budgetary decrease (when the focus is on disinvestment). Estimates of the cost per life-year gained when disease-specific mortality changes were transformed into life-year gains were (for the years 2006/2007) £15.837 for cancer; £9.974 for circulatory problems; £5.425 pounds for respiratory problems; £21.538 for gastro-intestinal and £26.428 pounds for diabetes (Dakin *et al.*, 2013).

On the cost side of the ICER, there are also important methodological challenges. Indeed, there is a variety of methodological options in the economic evaluation process, such as parsing out the pecuniary vs. non-pecuniary costs as well as the direct vs. indirect, tangible vs. intangible, medical and non-medical, related and unrelated, and present vs. future costs. Non-pecuniary costs and benefits are those such as an earlier return to work after healing, which increase well-being to society; pecuniary costs and benefits are those such as the cost of drugs substituting for inpatient care treatments. They cannot be considered, out of their net difference, since otherwise it is a purely redistributive effect; opportunity costs such as days lost after being treated (if they would have been lost anyway being untreated) should not be accounted for either. Direct costs are viewed as those "ingredients in a recipe" while indirect costs refer to secondary costs related to other productive activities. Different time horizons imply the need to use some given discounting factors; and indications must be provided on how to offset resources when they approach average or marginal costs, with full capacity, in the short- or long-term.

NICE Guidelines (NICE, 2008) offer indications regarding these methodological issues:

(1) The analysis has to be made from the NHS perspective, that is, the implication of an innovation on other aspects of society are ignored; in principle, neither production nor consumption-related costs are included.
(2) Relevance first: Aspects regarding treatability, progression, duration, incidence, prevalence, and budget impact need to be explained.
(3) The analysis is to capture direct medical-related costs. Preventing adverse effects and avoidable admissions are considered to be direct effects.
(4) Adopt unit (full) costs (training costs included).
(5) The time horizon is in the range of 3–5 years.
(6) The appraisal should include some sensitivity analysis, searching for robustness, if possible.
(7) "Double counting" is to be avoided, regarding some aspects of costs and benefits already measured into QALYs.

The most controversial issue remains the need for increased government accountability to Parliament through tighter monitoring of the threshold application. There is still little acceptance among medical professionals and patients that health care resources are limited (Drummond *et al.*, 2013). As a consequence, rationing and the NICE lack popularity, and separate budget funds have started to emerge where ICER criteria are not required to the same extent as in the general NHS budget, as in the case cancer and musculoskeletal diseases.

Germany: The IQWIG

The *Institut für Qualität und Wirtschaftlichkeit im Gesundheitswesen* (IQWIG), the Institute for Quality and Efficiency in Health Care, was created in 2004. IQWIG is the German agency responsible for assessing the quality and efficiency of medical treatments, including drugs, non-drug interventions (e.g., surgical procedures), diagnostic and screening methods, and treatment and disease management (IQWIG, 2014). IQWIG also supplies health information to patients and the general community. The organization is independent of private industry, contracted solely by the Federal Ministry of Health and the German Joint Federal Committee.

The design and methodology used by the IQWIG was designed by an external panel of international experts (IQWIG, 2009). One of the stated pillars was that: "IQWIG should only address the determination of a ceiling price at which a superior health technology in a given therapeutic area should be continued to be reimbursed." Comparisons across diseases were to be avoided and this, as will be detailed later, brought the need to implement the "efficiency frontier approach." An important reason for focusing on a single therapy was, according to the commissioned experts (Caro *et al.*, 2010), that the German health care system, based on social insurance, is not bound to a fixed national budget and therefore need not consider funding priorities across therapeutic areas, but should instead make sure that the system offers a portfolio of health care benefits that maximize health outcomes for a given level of invested resources. This characteristic made the IQWIG significantly different from other similar institutions worldwide, and has received strong criticism among academics (Brouwer and Rutten, 2010), some of whom consider this to open the door to inefficient interventions and to accepting unfair situations produced by the use of different thresholds across interventions or cases (Drummond and Rutten, 2008).

Unlike NICE, the IQWIG methodology is not based on CUA nor ICER, but on *the efficiency frontier approach* and on the establishment of price ceilings. The methodology consists of a comparison of benefits and costs among different alternatives. On the benefits side, evidence-based clinical measures are used.

The advantage of this source of information is that clinicians are familiarized with it (Caro *et al.*, 2010). The disadvantage is the limitations in successfully obtaining good metrics out of these measures, especially within the constraints imposed by IQWIG: They need to be cardinal and aligned with the prerequisites of clinical trials (with a time horizon, end-point, etc.) (Drummond and Rutten, 2008).

Costs are assessed primarily from the perspective of the insured individuals, and out-of-pocket costs must be included. Total net expenditure is the measure of interest: Therefore, any savings produced by the intervention should be considered too. The no-intervention alternative is rarely expected to have a total net expenditure of zero. The time horizon under examination has to be sufficiently long to cover all the significant costs and not necessarily those included in the clinical trial periods, and the production gains and consumption effects should be subtracted from the costs of extending survival.

Benefits and costs combined yield the efficiency frontier representing the trade-off between costs and benefits and identifying the interventions that provide the most value for any given level of investment Caro *et al.* (2010) display this trade-off graphically (see Figure 4) by plotting the interventions at their estimated net cost (horizontal axis) and benefits (vertical axis) and drawing line segments linking the options that are dominant.

IQWIG's concept of efficiency involves not only health-related morbidity and mortality and quality of life, but also time and effort invested and patients' treatment satisfaction. This may go into a single scale (i.e., experience utility), including a unique cost per outcome threshold. For this purpose, a relative efficiency frontier

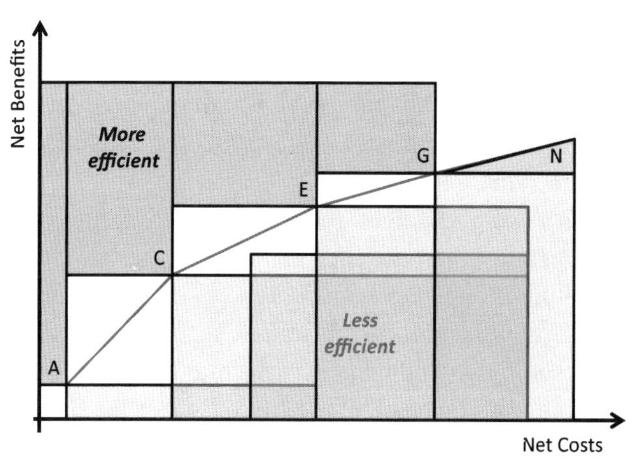

Figure 4. The efficiency frontier approach to economic evaluation of health care interventions

Source: Reproduced from Caro *et al.* (2010).

may be considered as the information basis along with the value of the benefits and total net costs, the estimated budget impact and the uncertainty around all the estimates. The aim is then to approach quality and efficiency. IQWIG's conclusions can be used by the German sickness funds to cut reimbursement for drugs declared to be ineffective. However, it is a requirement that no patients should be excluded on cost grounds alone.

IQWIG's responsibilities were expanded in two health care reforms in 2007 and 2010. With the 2007 Act to promote competition of statutory health insurance, the IQWIG was commissioned to weigh the costs of drug therapies against the benefits previously determined. Prior to that, the assessment of drugs was restricted to health care beneficial effects (i.e., to the evaluation of benefits and harms of drug interventions). With the 2010 Law on the Reorganization of the Pharmaceutical Market, it became the responsibility of the Federal Joint Committee to assess the effects of newly approved drugs. If a health improvement had been established, the price of the new medicine needed to be negotiated between the Central Federal Association of the Health Insurance Funds and the company concerned. The assessment is performed on the basis of information the manufacturers are obliged to submit to the Federal Joint Committee, which then generally commissions IQWIG with the assessment of the dossiers.

IQWIG reports on specific topics as requested by the Federal Joint Committee or the Federal Ministry of Health, following the principles of evidence-based medicine. IQWIG also undertakes projects and research on its own initiative. The work of its staff is supplemented by projects which are contracted externally, and these projects are advertised publicly. Work on these projects must be conducted according to IQWIG's current methods.[8] Stakeholders and the interested public can also get involved in IQWIG's work. IQWIG publishes all of its results online, and interested persons and parties may submit written comments on report plans (protocols) and on preliminary reports. Comments are considered and may even lead to changes in the final report.

IQWIG provides support rather than making decisions. It follows Health Services Research techniques, those used for evidence-based health care, focusing on specific therapeutic groups. As a result, funding priorities make sense among alternatives that fall within one therapeutic area, in contrast to a more global analysis of priority setting, intending to set priorities across very different types of therapies and innovations. The result of the analysis takes the form of a "maximum reimbursement" for specific treatments that are found to be better than existing treatments from the insurance company perspective.

---

[8]https://www.iqwig.de/index.925.en.html.

France: La Haute Autorité de Santé

The Haute Autorité de Santé (HAS) — or French National Authority for Health — was set up in August 2004 with the aim of "improving the quality of patient care and guaranteeing equity within the health care system." The HAS performs a wide range of activities including assessment of drugs, medical devices, and procedures; publication of guidelines; accreditation of health care organizations; and certification of doctors. The HAS is an independent public body with financial autonomy. It is mandated by law to carry out specific missions on which it reports to the government and the Parliament. It liaises closely with government health agencies, national health insurance funds, research organizations, unions of health care professionals, and patients' representatives.

Its scope includes assessing health care technologies (including drugs, devices, and diagnostic and interventional procedures) for pricing and reimbursement, developing clinical guidelines and public health guidance, performing hospital accreditation, accrediting patient information websites, creating disease management models, continuous professional education, and developing guidance and recommendations on the most effective health care strategies.

Technology assessment reports regarding an innovative initiative in health care, at HAS, include a comparison with other medical and non-medical strategies. They address clinical and community benefits measured in terms of medical effectiveness (real-life), health economics (efficiency), impact on the organization of care, and some aspects of social choice and other relevant ethical issues. HAS follows a multidisciplinary approach that includes members from the fields of economics, ethics/philosophy, and social sciences, as well as patient associations, general practitioners and specialists, and it adopts a societal perspective.

Since the constitution of the *Commission d'Évaluation Économique et de Santé Publique* (CEESP), in July 2008 (Lise Rochaix and Xerri, 2009), HAS has also addressed the assessment of risks due to inappropriate decisions taken in the health care system, due to excessively delaying market access of innovations or due to introducing technologies that turn out to be inefficient, not cost-effective or with a low benefit–risk ratio.

All new drugs must be assessed by HAS before inclusion in the compulsory benefits package, called *Service Médical Rendu* (*SMR*). Once considered to be a reimbursable drug, regulated prices are set following a separate negotiation, by the Economic Committee for Health Care Products (CEPS). HAS' technical report on the clinical value-added of a drug is a fundamental ingredient in the price determination. To determine the price, they primarily take into account the clinical added value of the medicine, the prices of other medicines serving the same therapeutic purpose, the forecast or recorded sales volumes of the new drug, and the actual and foreseeable uses of the new drug.

The HAS reports on incremental effectiveness, and reimbursement recommendations may be positive or negative opinions with full or restricted indications for certain situations or subpopulations. Drugs are compared to existing therapies, and recommendations depend on the clinical added value or ASMR (*Amélioration du SMR*): Major clinical improvement (ASMR I), important clinical improvement (ASMR II), moderate clinical improvement (ASMR III), minor clinical improvement (ASMR IV), with ASMR V for no clinical improvement. According to ASMRs' categorization, reimbursement decisions are taken: (i) Level V is only reimbursable if it is cost saving; (ii) Most innovative drugs Levels I, II and III are eligible for faster access at a European price (price notification instead of negotiation). On the assessment of added value, the question to be answered is what is the added value and for what population. This leads to a target population and recommendations for use in clinical practice. Uncertainty may force the HAS to ask for additional data collection and studies.

Currently, *SMR* only considers efficacy and safety to define a relative position of a new drug with respect to other available therapies, taking into account the severity of the condition the drug is indicated for, whether the drug prevents, cures or relieves symptoms, and the benefit the product may have for public health. For the future, a relative therapeutic index is expected to be implemented, and pharmaceutical companies will have to put more emphasis on portraying the total economic benefit of a drug, not just its clinical superiority, or ASMR.

Sweden: The Swedish Council on Technology Assessment in Health Care (SBU)

In 1987, the Minister of Health formally established and funded the Swedish Council on Technology Assessment in Health Care (Statens Beredning for Utvärdering av Medicinsk Teknologi, SBU). The Government's instructions to SBU in 1987 were as follows: The agency must provide evidence-based information on matters of health technology to advise health policy and practice and to inform the general public, without regulatory functions (Jonsson, 2009). The SBU reviews the benefits, risks and costs of methods used in health care delivery, with the aim of identifying which method is the most appropriate for treating a specific disease and patient group, but also to determine which methods are ineffective or not cost-effective, so that they can be avoided. The SBU also identifies important knowledge gaps, that is, areas in which further research is urgently needed (Anell *et al.*, 2012). The Government's instructions to SBU are not much different today: "SBU is mandated to make scientific assessments of new and established health technologies from a medical, economic, societal, and ethical perspective."

The SBU has no regulatory power, and its first challenges were to "establish proper incentives to make clinicians use the findings from the SBU, to build a strong collaboration with the medical profession, and to develop a level of trust in SBU that its findings would be viewed as an integral and fundamental part of professional practice" (Jonsson, 2009).

SBU assessments include a systematic review based on protocols for inclusion and exclusion criteria and for grading evidence presented in all relevant studies in the international literature (i.e., clinical studies, economic evaluations, and studies addressing other issues on subjects such as nursing, ethical, and social aspects). The assessments also include a synthesis with recommendations for health policy and practice. Assessment of pharmaceuticals has not been a priority at SBU, because the Medical Products Agency in Sweden has a mandate to assess the safety, efficacy, and effectiveness of drugs. However, an important issue for HTA generally is the appropriate indications for use. Although SBU has focused its assessments on that issue in a few projects on pharmaceuticals, it may want to consider further efforts in this regard.

During the major economic downturn of the Swedish economy at the beginning of the 1990s, an important priority agenda was established in the Parliament regarding most areas of policymaking. A Priority Setting Commission was appointed in 1992 comprised of members of Parliament and expert advisers. The Commission accomplished its task in the health care arena by 1995 and published a report entitled "Priorities in Health Care — Ethics, Economy, Implementation" (Swedish Government, 1995). The key components of the Commission's proposals were: (i) A so-called "ethical platform" and (ii) practical advice for priority setting in the form of two lists, one for political and administrative priority setting and another for clinical priority setting.

The ethical platform sets forth the principles that should form the basis of medical prioritization:

(i) Human dignity — all humans beings have equal dignity and the same rights, regardless of their personal characteristics and their functions in the community.
(ii) The principle of need and solidarity — with need meaning that resources should be committed to fields where needs are greatest, and solidarity meaning paying attention to the needs of groups less able or inclined to exercise their rights.
(iii) The cost-efficiency principle, which is that one should aim for a reasonable relation between cost and effect, measured in terms of improved health and improved quality of life. The cost-efficiency principle should only be applied in comparisons of methods for treating the same disease, since where different diseases are involved, a fair comparison of the effect is impossible.

Priority setting was defined as dealing with (i) The treatment of life threatening, acute diseases and diseases which, if left untreated, would lead to permanent disability or premature death; (ii) the treatment of severe chronic diseases, palliative terminal care and care of people with reduced autonomy; and (iii) prevention, with a documented benefit for habilitation/rehabilitation as defined in the *Swedish Health and Medical Services Act*.

A National Board of Health and Welfare (the NBHW) was then appointed by the Parliament to develop guidelines in accordance to that framework. The guidelines are produced in collaboration with other actors, such as the SBU or the TLV (regarding pharmaceutical and dentistry products and services). The NBHW developed a national model for explicit priority setting. (See Table 3, where the first row shows analytical categories and the second row shows measures used.) The model is based on the ethical framework, with the ultimate outcome in the form of a ranking ranging from 1 to 10, where 1 is the highest and most prioritized and 10 is the lowest and least prioritized. In addition, instead of a rank, the labels "don't do" or "do" can be assigned in cases where there is no proof of benefit or harm or when something needs to be further evaluated (Waldau, 2010). To simplify the list, the rank order can be divided into three larger groups, where rank 1–3 represents what needs be done and is considered to form part of the core activities of the health care system, rank 4–6 is what ought be done and is perceived as expected services, and rank 7–10 is what could be done if economic circumstances allow.

This model is designed to work in most cases of vertical prioritization regarding treatment alternatives on the bsasis of clinical evidence (need), but when and how it should be carried out is left to local and regional authorities. In February 2011, the NBHW announced a working process to revise the national model. Recently, the NBHW started to use the model to develop national guidelines for all levels of health care decision-making and prioritization. Guidelines are being developed for use in resource-demanding areas, for example, for large patient groups with chronic diseases, such as breast, colorectal and prostate cancer; dementia; depression and anxiety disorders; and diabetes. The guidelines are based on thorough literature reviews and health economic calculations. But a bit of imprecision exists regarding the treatment of less severe acute and chronic diseases and care related to cases other than treating a disease or curing an injury.

The extended time it takes for SBU to complete its assessments, sometimes reaching a period of 2 to 3 years, is a source of concern and critique. Indeed, in 1996, SBU developed a special program called Alert to rapidly (usually within 6 to 12 months) assess specific, mostly new, innovations in health care. Except for the Alert program, SBU generally does not assess a single technology at a time, but all technologies surrounding a specific health problem — often including

Table 3. The prioritization model in Sweden

Health condition/ intervention	Severity level of health condition	Patient benefit effects of intervention	Evidence of effect	Cost per life years gained/QALY	Health economic evidence	Rank order
Condition and actual state/Action or intervention	Level of severity: Very high, high, moderate or low	Benefit/effect: Very high, moderate or low	Evidence grades 1–4, or: Very good to insufficient scientific evidence or standard clinical practice	Low, moderate, high, very high or cannot be appraised	Good, some calculated or estimated	1–10 "do not do" R&D[a]

Notes: [a]*1 is the highest, 10 is the lowest priority rank. "Do not do" = "no medical benefit or harmful". The "R&D" label was used for interventions of unknown benefit and in need of evaluation.*
Source: Waldau (2010).

prevention, diagnosis, and treatment and always including both established and new technologies, which is much more time-consuming.

The situation today (Waldau, 2010) regarding priority setting is such that the National Parliament keeps an authority to define a "framework" through legislation, based on the interpretation of the "ethical platform," and further developments or more concrete priority setting decisions, with actual priority setting in practice, in hands of the County Councils at a more decentralized level. Several County Councils have developed their own specific models for priority setting within the framework set by the National Parliament. The National Priority Commission is in charge of disseminating information on Parliament's priority-setting decisions, developing methods to promote implementation of those decisions, monitoring and evaluating the effects of the decisions, and comparing the Swedish situation with international experience. The Commission holds meetings with local groups on ethical matters within County Councils or Municipalities.

Netherlands: The Dunning Report

Since the 1980s, priority setting has become a key issue in making choices in health care in the Netherlands. The 1991 Dunning Report, in order to give a response to the political concern on what the health care system should cover in the Netherlands, established four criteria for the definition of the Dutch basic health insurance package: Necessary care (a purely political criteria), effectiveness (more technical criteria), efficiency (measured in terms of cost-effectiveness), and individual responsibility (leaving room for individual responsibility to pay for some benefits, again a political criteria). These priority-setting criteria could result in an exclusion of medical treatments from compulsory health insurance coverage and/or in the development of protocols and guidelines for inclusion and the selection of patients by health professionals. The discussion on the introduction of *in vitro* fertilization (IVF) into the basic health insurance package and the exclusion of dental care for adults has shown that, on the basis of the Dunning criteria, it is not easy to leave services out of the basic health insurance package. The second strategy — the application of the Dunning Committee's criteria by the use of protocols, guidelines, and budget restrictions — seems to be even more difficult to realize. More patients assert their right to health care benefits before courts. The courts' decisions have shown that it is difficult to prove that government is responsible for non-delivery due to *force majeur*. Courts attach much importance to the Dunning criteria and, in particular, the criterion of necessity.

The Dunning criteria received support (and still do) for necessary care under three alternatives: (i) If individual necessity equals individual demand; (ii) under a medical approach with doctors establishing necessity of care; and (iii) under a

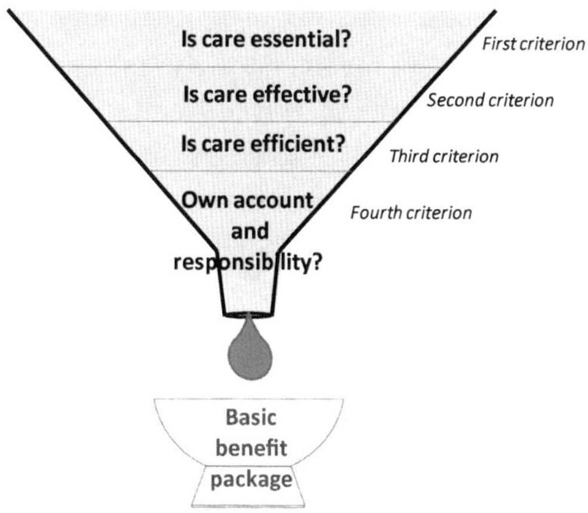

Figure 5. The Dunning's funnel[9]
Source: Reproduced from Schäfer *et al.* (2010)

community approach, meaning care necessity established from the point of view of the community.

The Central Government makes decisions on the basic health insurance package relying on advice from the Health Care Insurance Board (CVZ). Ministerial proposals for changing the benefit package have to be approved by Parliament. Decisions about the composition of the benefit package are guided by an algorithm, which is known as the "Dunning's Funnel," represented in Figure 5 (Schäfer *et al.*, 2010).[9]

The Committee indeed defined four cumulative criteria: (1) Services should be essential, (2) effective, (3) cost effective and (4) unaffordable for individuals. "Essential" refers to the capacity to prevent loss of quality of life or to treat life-threatening conditions. The affordability criteria is political and open, and states that some services might not need to be included in the basic package in case they are considered to be affordable for individual citizens and for which they can take responsibility.

Although the Funnel was a step forward, in practice, the criteria are not always easy to apply. For instance, what constitutes "essential care" is arguable, and decisions can be hampered by lack of information on the efficiency of a service. Other problems may arise with regard to treatments of diseases resulting

[9]In practice, an example of the decision rationale for excluding a service from the basic package could be, for IVF: (1) Regarding "necessity" from a community point of view, likely exclusion, and from a professional and individual's point of view, likely inclusion. (2) On the "effectiveness" criterion, inclusion. (3) On the "efficiency" criterion, the cost would need to be calculated and leveraged against effectiveness. (4) On the "individual responsibility" criterion, inclusion. Therefore, as a result of combining the four criteria, IVF would be left out of the basic package.

from unhealthy behavior or when pharmaceuticals covered by basic health insurance are used by those other than the intended patient groups. Critics of the process say that the criteria are too general. It is difficult to determine which benefits are or are not essential and hence would be excluded from the basic package; affordability for individual patients differs from case to case and cannot therefore be readily determined at the macro level; and only a few services can be said to be entirely ineffective or inefficient, since effectiveness and efficiency depend on the medical indication, which again cannot be properly determined at macro level (Linander, 2011).

A Dunning's Funnel effort was made to remove the contraceptive pill from the basic benefit package and failed. The same happened for IVF treatments, long-term psychotherapy, transportation by taxi, speech therapy and home-help, dentistry for adults, long-term physiotherapy, incontinence pads, colostomy bags, and hearing aids. Today, the basic package is very comprehensive, including 95% of present health care services. Indeed, it proves difficult to eliminate existing services from the basic package on the basis of the Dunning Committee criteria. Instead, an alternative way to constrain the basic package is often to curtail the treatment to specific cases, instead of just eliminating it. Yet despite its limitations, the Dunning's Funnel process has been generally accepted.

Final Thoughts

High-income countries are struggling with the question of how to cope with the growing pressure of health care expenditures as a result of a combination of budget constraints and advances in technology. We have reviewed a number of approaches developed and tried in a variety of countries, but there is no clear hegemonic system. There is no single best way to allocate resources nor is there a sole way to set priorities. Rather, it varies from country to country.

Priority setting is the process by which health care decision-makers make choices about competing expenditure alternatives within a budget constraint. Hence, all forms of priority setting create rationing and, consequently, an exclusion. In the case of allocating public resources under budget constraints, this exclusion (the opportunity cost) needs to be more explicit. Although in the academic literature, there are clear methodological limitations for making opportunity costs explicit (Birch and Gafni, 2003), in a public policy arena, individuals or patients who lose resources are likely to step forward, and political controversy is likely to arise from the inclusion of new technologies and the exclusion of others. How these challenging aspects of priority setting processes are successfully handled depends on many factors, such as the context (Culyer, 2010b), the culture, the deliberative process (Shah *et al.*, 2013), the level at which the decisions are made (Tso *et al.*, 2011), leadership (Dickinson *et al.*, 2011), and other contextual factors. At the end of the day, similar methodologies may yield different prioritization results.

Besides the context, economic evaluation (specifically, cost–utility or cost-effectiveness analysis), are at the root of priority setting in all the experiences reviewed. Economic evaluation, however, has important limitations regarding both the economic methodologies and their applications in real-world circumstances. One limitation of economic evaluation has to do with its tight-fitting application to trade-offs concerning health care services and lack of comparability of utility measures regarding health care versus other public services competing for funding. Moreover, CEA is based on the assumption of perfect divisibility and comparable size programs. This means that no economies of scale or differences in size are ignored in such kinds of analysis (Birch and Gafni, 2003), and decision-makers cannot purchase individual units of QALYs. Each program is supposed to produce a package of QALYs and the average price per QALY may differ by program size. Consequently, a threshold incremental cost-effectiveness decision rule is unable to determine whether a program represents an efficient use of resources.

Another limitation of economic evaluation has to do with the assumption that "a QALY is a QALY," meaning that QALY gains are implicitly valued equally irrespective of the beneficiary or the disease. Such practice has been an issue of debate because evidence tends to show that the public may prefer some QALY gains to others (Dolan *et al.*, 2008). In practice, although explicit QALY weighting is still uncommon, it seems it does implicitly exist. Recent developments in the UK illustrate such need to weight QALYs, for example, for those cases addressing end-of-life-prolonging drugs (NICE, 2009). The Netherlands has also responded to equity concerns by developing a framework that is primarily concerned with some idea of need, in particular, based on the controversial "proportional shortfall" (Van de Wetering *et al.*, 2013). Dealing with equity is not a straightforward task. Finding a systematic approach raises 2 important questions: (i) Which equity principle(s) are used to determine QALY weights? (ii) How can we derive practically applicable QALY weights that are in line with the chosen principles? These difficult and inherently normative questions complicate the formalization of methods to deal with equity concerns (Culyer, 2014; Musgrove, 1999; Shah *et al.*, 2013;).

Maximizing social benefits should imply, from a welfarist viewpoint, maximizing utility, not only as far as health is concerned but also accounting for other trade-offs. The utilitarian approach, consisting of the allocation of resources in order to maximize the health of the community as a whole versus some restrictive notion of egalitarian goals remains an open question. For example, "fair innings" is one of the many equity principles one may need to trade off against efficiency

(Williams, 1997). It captures the feeling that everyone is entitled to some "normal" span of health (usually expressed in life years) and anyone failing to achieve this has been cheated, while anyone getting more than this is "living on borrowed time." Productivity gains from health care spending are likely bounded by *fair innings* types of arguments from individual entitlements to health care access.

In spite of the limitations of economic evaluation, economic thinking has much to offer in the context of making decisions between competing claims on scarce health care resources. On the one hand, equity concerns are increasingly taken into explicit consideration in most priority setting processes (Culyer, 2012). On the other hand, although much is still to be accomplished, efforts are being made to provide frameworks for easier application of economic evaluation tools, like the controversial PBMA or Program Budgeting and Marginal Analysis (Donaldson and Mitton, 2009); or the Generalized Cost-Effectiveness Analysis, designed to allow policymakers to evaluate the efficiency of the mix of health interventions currently available and to maximize the capability to generalize results across settings (Torrance and Drummond, 2005); or the use of integer programming when data requirements are accomplished (Birch and Gafni, 2003) for constraint maximization problems.

Moreover, economic evaluation is receiving increasing attention as a means of setting regulated prices of goods and services provided within the benefits package boundary in most of the countries reviewed: *Value Based Prices* in **France** with higher therapeutic value (*SMR*), advocating greater coverage and higher prices. In **Germany**, reference pricing strategies have to follow the indication of the value as identified in cost effectiveness analysis. In **Sweden**, a new commitment for better therapeutic value is to be reflected in prices. In general, the idea that more risk-sharing contracts should be agreed upon for drug approvals with larger budget impacts is increasingly being accepted. Finally, the **UK**, in 2014, has tried to implement Value-Based Pricing and recommendations for treatment removal and delisting. Hence, the complex objectives faced by decision-makers, far from limiting the role of economic analysis, represent the challenges that economic models intend to accommodate.

References

Anel A, Glenngard AH, Merkur SM. 2012. *Health Care Systems in Transition: Sweden.* World Health Organization (ed.), Available at: http://www.euro.who.int/_data/assets/pdf_file/0008/164096/e96455.pdf?ua=1.

Anon. 2010. *Equality Act.* Available at: http://www.legislation.gov.uk/ukpga/2010/15/contents.

Anon. 2014. *NICE.* Available at: http://www.nice.org.uk/aboutnice/whoweare/who_we_are.jsp.

Birch S, Gafni A. 2003. Economics and the evaluation of health care programmes: Generalisability of methods and implications for generalisability of results. *Health Policy* 64(2): 207–219.

Brouwer W, Rutten FFH. 2010. Comment the efficiency frontier approach to economic evaluation: Will it help german policy making? *Health Economics* 19: 1128–1131.

Caro JJ, *et al.* 2010. The efficiency frontier approach to economic evaluation of health-care interventions. *Health Economics* 19: 1117–1127.

Clinical Evidence, B, BMJ Clinical Evidence Efficacy Cathegorizations. Available at: http://clinicalevidence.bmj.com/x/set/static/cms/efficacy-categorisations.html [Accessed 7 July 2014].

Culyer AJ. 2010a. *Evidence, Uncertainty and The Policy Pursuit of Fairness*. Rimini (Italy).

Culyer AJ. 2010b. Perspective and desire in comparative effectiveness research the central importance of context. *PharmacoEconomics* 28(10): 889–897.

Culyer T. 2012. *The Humble Economist.* In Cookson R, Claxton K (eds.). York: York Publishing Services.

Culyer AJ. 2014. *Social Values in Health and Social Care*. Available at: http://www.kingsfund.org.uk/sites/files/kf/media/commission-background-paper-social-values-health-social-care.pdf.

Culyer AJ, Wagstaff, A. 1993. Equity and equality in health and health care. *Journal of Health Economics* 12(4): 431–457.

Cutler DM, McClellan M. 2001. Is technological change in medicine worth it? *Health Affairs* 20(5): 11–29.

Dakin H, *et al.* 2013. The influence of cost-effectiveness and other factors on NICE decisions. *HERC Research Paper* (093).

Dickinson H, *et al.* 2011. Resource scarcity and priority-setting: from management to leadership in the rationing of health care? *Public Money & Management* 31(5): 363–370. Available at: http://www.tandfonline.com/doi/abs/10.1080/09540962.2011.598352 [Accessed 27 May 2014].

Dolan P. 1997. Valuations for EuroQol health states. *Medical Care* 35(11): 1095–1108.

Dolan P, *et al.* 2008. QALY maximisation and people's preferences: A methodological review of the literature. *Health Economics* 14(May): 197–208.

Donaldson C, Mitton C. 2009. *Priority Setting Toolkit: A Guide to the Use of Economics in Healthcare Decision Making*. BMJ Books, John Wiley & Sons.

Drummond M, Rutten F, 2008. The IQWiG Methodology Paper Version 1.0. *German Association of Research-Based Pharmaceutical Companies (VFA)*. Berlin, Germany.

Drummond M, Tarricone R, Torbica A. 2013. Assessing the added value of health technologies: Reconciling different perspectives. *Value in Health: The Journal of the International Society for Pharmacoeconomics and Outcomes Research* 16(1 Suppl): S7–S13. Available at: http://www.ncbi.nlm.nih.gov/pubmed/23317646 [Accessed 28 May 2014].

Field MJ, Gold MR. 1998. Summarizing Population Health. Institute of Medicine, Washington DC.

Ham C. 1998. Retracing the Oregon trail: The experience of rationing and the Oregon health plan. *BMJ: British Medical Journal* 316(7149): 1965.

Honoré PA *et al.* 2011. Creating a framework for getting quality into the public health system. *Health Affairs* (*Project Hope*) 30(4): 737–745. Available at: http://www.ncbi.nlm.nih.gov/pubmed/21471496 [Accessed 2 June 2014].

Husereau D, *et al.* 2013. Consolidated health economic evaluation reporting standards (CHEERS) statement. *BMC Medicine* 11(1): 80. Available at: http://www.biomedcentral.com/1741-7015/11/80 [Accessed 1 June 2014].

IOM. 2009. Initial National Priorities for Comparative Effectiveness Research. *The National Academies Press*. Available at: http://www.nap.edu/catalog/12648/initial-national-priorities-for-comparative-effectiveness-research.

IOM. 2011. Learning What Works: Infrastructure Required for Comparative Effectiveness Research: Workshop Summary.

IOM. 2012. Essential Health Benefits: Balancing Coverage and Cost. *The National Academies Press*. Available at: http://www.nap.edu/catalog.php?record_id=13234#toc.

IQWIG. 2009. *Institute for Quality and Efficiency in Health Care (IQWiG). Documentation of Comments on "Draft Method for Evaluating the Relation between Cost and Benefit in the German Statutory Health Insurance System, Version 2.0"* (*German Version*). Available at: http://www.iqwig.de/download/Dokumentation_der_Stellungnahmen_KNB-Methodenentwurf_2.0.pdf.

IQWIG. 2014. *IQWIG Introductory Brochure*. Available at: https://www.iqwig.de/download/IQWiG_informationflyer.pdf.

Jonsson E. 2009. History of health technology assessment in Sweden. *International Journal of Technology Assessment in Health Care* 25(Suppl 1(S1)): 42–52. Available at: http://journals.cambridge.org/abstract_S0266462309090412 [Accessed 12 December 2014].

Linander A. 2011. *Explicit Health Care Priority Setting in Practice — Clinical Managers "Views of Performing Vertical Prioritization in Västerbotten County Council"*. Available at: https://www.imh.liu.se/halso-och-sjukvardsanalys/prioriteringscentrum/publikationer/avhandlingar-forskningsrapporter/1.276990/EMasterthesis-Andrea Linander.pdf.

Lise Rochaix L, Xerri B. 2009. National Authority for Health: France. *Commonwealth Fund*.

Longson C, Littlejohns P. 2009. Update report on the application of the "end-of-life" supplementary advice in health technology appraisals. *National Institute for Health and Clinical Excellence*.

Lopez AD, Murray CC. 1998. The global burden of disease. *Natural Medicine* 4(11): 1241–1243.

Luce B, *et al.* 2010. EBM, HTA, and CER: Clearing the confussion. *The Milbank Quarterly* 88(2): 256–276. Available at: http://www.ncbi.nlm.nih.gov/pubmed/24597552.

McKie J, Richardson J. 2003. The rule of rescue. *Social Science & Medicine* 56(12): 2407–2419.

Mooney G, Wiseman V. 2000. Burden of disease and priority setting. *Health Economics* 9: 369–372.

Musgrove P. 1999. Public spending on health care: How are different criteria related? *Health Policy (Amsterdam, Netherlands)* 47(3): 207–23. Available at: http://www.ncbi.nlm.nih.gov/pubmed/10538919.

NICE. 2008. *Guide to the Methods of Technology Appraisal* NICE (ed.). London. Available at: http://www.nice.org.uk/media/B52/A7/TAMethodsGuideUpdatedJune2008.pdf.

NICE. 2005. Directions and Consolidating Directions to the National Institute for Health and Clinical Excellence 2005, 2(4): 1–6. Available at: http://www.nice.org.uk/niceMedia/pdf/DirectionFromSecretaryOfState2005.pdf.

NICE. 2009. Appraising life-extendeing, end of life treatments.

Poonacha TK, Go RS. 2011. Level of scientific evidence underlying recommendations arising from the National Comprehensive Cancer Network clinical practice guidelines. *Journal of Clinical Oncology: Official Journal of the American Society of Clinical Oncology* 29(2): 186–191. Available at: http://www.ncbi.nlm.nih.gov/pubmed/21149653 [Accessed 31 May 2014].

Sabik LM, Lie RK. 2008. Priority setting in health care: Lessons from the experiences of eight countries. *International Journal for Equity in Health* 7(Table 1), p. 4. Available at: http://www.pubmedcentral.nih.gov/articlerender.fcgi?artid=2248188&tool=pmcentrez&rendertype=abstract [Accessed 25 May 2014].

Schäfer W, *et al.* 2010. *The Netherlands: Health System Review.* Health System Transition 12(1): v–xxvii, 1–228.

Shah KK, *et al.* 2013. NICE's social value judgements about equity in health and health care. *Health Economics, Policy, and Law* 8(2): 145–165. Available at: http://www.ncbi.nlm.nih.gov/pubmed/22717361 [Accessed 27 May 2014].

Swedish Parliamentary Priorities Commission. Swedish Government, 1995. *Priorities in Health Care: Ethics, Economy, Implementation: Final Report from the Swedish Parliamentary Priorities Commission.* Swedish Government Official Reports 1995:5. Swedish Parliamentary Priorities Commission. (pp. 180) (ed.). Stockholm: Regeringskansliets Offsetcentral.

The Health Service in England. 2012. *Health and Social Care Act 2012.* Available at: file:///C:/Users/Upf/Documents/Laura/cres/scheffler/biblio/nice 2007n.pdf.

Torrance GW, Drummond MF. 2005. *Methods for the Economic Evaluation of Health Care Programmes.* Oxford University Press.

Towse A, Pritchard C. 2002. Does NICE have a threshold? An external view. In Office of Health Economics (ed.). *Cost-Effectiveness Thresholds: Economic and Ethical Issues.* London: Office of Health Economics: London, p. V37.

Tso P, *et al.* 2011. Developing a decision aid to guide public sector health policy decisions: A study protocol. *Implementation Science: IS* 6(1): 46. Available at: http://www.pubmedcentral.nih.gov/articlerender.fcgi?artid=3108337&tool=pmcentrez&rendertype=abstract [Accessed 23 May 2014].

Waldau S. 2010. *Waldau, Susanne. "Creating Organisational Capacity for Priority Setting in Health Care: Using a Bottom–Up Approach to Implement a Top-Down Policy Decision."*. Umeå University.

Van de Wetering EJ, *et al.* 2013. Balancing equity and efficiency in the Dutch basic benefits package using the principle of proportional shortfall. *The European Journal of Health Economics* 14(1): 107–115.

Williams B. 1962. The idea of equality. In Laslett P, Runciman W (eds.). *Philosophy, Politics and Society*. Oxford: Basil Blackwell, pp. 110–131.

Williams A. 1995. *The Measurement and Valuation of Health: A Chronicle*. University of York.

Williams A. 1997. Intergenerational equity: An exploration of the 'fair innings' argument. *Health Economics* 6(2): 117–132.

Estimating Health Care Treatment Costs

Alistair McGuire and Maria Raikou
LSE and University of Piraeus, Athens

This chapter considers the conceptual and many empirical problems associated with estimating health care costs. It does so by considering the estimation of such costs at different levels of aggregation — initially considering health costs incurred at the individual level, including those arising from treatments undergoing clinical trials, and then at the hospital level, the latter being the sector with the largest level of expenditure in most health care systems. The topics covered include the representativeness of sample populations, the importance of skew in the health care cost distribution, issues of censoring, and missing data and their relevance to the estimation process. The consistency of relevant estimators is assessed through discussion of transformation, linkage and general linear methods. Attention then turns to the hospital sector, where lack of knowledge of the underlying production process is a considerable drawback in specifying appropriate cost functions. The amendment of hospital cost functions to particular concerns, including the hospital's control of demand and reactions to demand uncertainty, are outlined. Given the importance of health care cost estimation in helping to risk adjust and predict future health care expenditure levels, as well as help determine reimbursement levels within the hospital sector, more attention needs to be given to this area of research.

Introduction

Traditionally, to analyze cost data in any sector, an understanding of the underlying production process must be understood. This is difficult in the health care sector, as the production process does not consist of a one-to-one relationship between inputs and outcomes. The health care production process, that is the conversion of treatment inputs into defined outputs, is more fungible. As health care becomes more complex, it becomes increasingly important to deliver in a timely fashion, increasingly poorly substitutable across patients, and different combinations of inputs may give rise to similar outcomes. Moreover, even the outcomes are difficult to monitor. Monitoring changes in health status are difficult, and outcomes can be measured in a number of ways. Individuals may experience changes in their life expectancy because of an intervention. These changes may be associated with changes in their quality of life. Perhaps only intermediate outcomes, such as cases treated, are monitored. In other words, various aspects of production are subject to more variability than standard textbook examples.

Normally, a cost framework is developed by attaching unit costs to input volumes as they relate to outcomes. Unit costs being the individual cost levels of specific treatment (resource) volumes. Given the difficulties in defining production relationships at the individual level in the health care sector, there are additional complications in attaching costs. Thus, the modeling of health care costs is challenging. This chapter will outline these challenges, given that costs may be defined at different levels of aggregation, e.g., at the individual patient level, the treatment population level or the system-wide level. First, we will review some of the difficulties that arise in modeling health care costs, even with access to well-defined experimental data, as gained through individual patient costs associated with randomized controlled trials. Second, we will consider the issue of analyzing individual health care costs more generally, when the patient population is more heterogeneously defined. Finally, we will review the literature on hospital costs to illustrate the difficulties associated with analysis at a higher-level of aggregation. In all cases, the general difficultics noted apply.

Health Care Costs in Clinical Trials

The analysis of cost data in clinical trials is of interest because the outcomes to be examined are pre-specified, there are normally pre-defined notions of treatment to which costs are applied and there is a fixed timescale over which the data are to be collected. This differs from estimating costs in normal treatment settings where populations are more heterogeneous and the treatment time is not delimited. The main interest in estimating treatment costs within clinical trials lies in deriving estimates of the mean cost of treatment over the duration of the study. Cost data applied to clinical trials has received limited attention compared to effectiveness data, even though the estimation of treatment costs is a fundamental element in the calculation of the incremental cost-effectiveness ratio. A number of reviews cover specific aspects relating to how cost is actually measured and cost collection as proxies, such as charges or reimbursement levels, are commonly used (Brouwer *et al.*, 2001; Dranove, 1995; Gold *et al.*, 1996; Sculpher, 2001).

In the majority of clinical trial analyses, the cost elements are confined to those directly related to the treatment. However, for a societal-based analysis, all cost elements — even beyond those directly related to treatment — must be identified. Olsen (1994) highlights the importance of the inclusion of productivity losses as related to sick time, as a cost, even when a social welfare function is constrained to the consideration of health maximization alone.

The direct treatment costs are usually estimated by quantifying the resource use attributable to the intervention under study and attaching unit cost information on individual treatment items to these resources. Commonly, data restrictions lead to limited capture of economic variables alongside clinical studies. Unit costs are usually deemed of secondary importance and are normally obtained from alternative sources on the basis that any variation in total cost is due to variation in resource volumes across treatment centers, reflecting variation in clinical practice, while unit costs are not expected to vary substantially across centers (Spiegelhalter *et al.*, 1996). This appears to represent an extreme view as costs are known to vary across treatment centers thus providing evidence to the contrary.

Economic theory suggests that there should be some defined, predictable relationship between the mix of resources used in producing treatments and the relative costs of these resources, specifically that treatment centers should be operating on their minimum cost curves. If the treatment center were operating as a cost-minimizing firm, it would choose the least cost input combination to produce the desired level of output. A substitution away from the relatively more expensive inputs would result in a change in the mix of resources. Glick *et al.* (2001) and Raikou *et al.* (2000) illustrate the differences in cost estimates resulting from the use of averaging unit costs across treatment centers compared to use of individual center-specific unit costs and recommend using the latter approach because the former ignores the relationship between resource volumes and unit costs at each center and will result in biased estimates. Within related research addressing similar concerns in the context of multi-center clinical trials opinions on the appropriate methodology to be adopted diverge. Typically individual center costs are associated with aggregate treatment effect findings (cf Drummond and Pang, 2001).

In theory, cost ought to represent the true opportunity cost of the resource, reflecting the minimum cost required to keep the resource in its current use rather than some alternative use. Such costs are not available in the health care sector, so a number of proxies are used. In identifying which costs ought to be included in an economic evaluation, Johnston *et al.* (1999) suggest that it is enough to identify the major components of total cost by studying the expected frequency of occurrence of different cost-generating events and identifying resources associated with high unit costs. Therefore, if health care costs are dominated by hospital visits and these are the highest valued costs, hospital costs should be emphasized. Whynes and Walker (1995) and Knapp and Beecham (1993) suggest that it would be difficult to identify the important cost categories at the outset of a study, due to the variation in the distribution of costs across individual patients and the variation in the distribution of costs across disease areas. Gold *et al.* (1996) argue that ease of measurement is not a justifiable criterion for deciding which cost elements should be included in practice, while Glick *et al.* (2001, p. 121) note that there is no agreed upon manner for making these decisions.

Cost analysis raises a number of statistical problems, some of which are discussed in more detail when we turn to consider individual treatment cost analysis below. An important issue relates to the representativeness of a typical study population and whether results are generalizable to other populations, as well as the bias that could be present in the estimates due to omitted variables and potential confounders. Viewed within a linear regression setting, Mullahy and Manning (1995) argue that in clinical trials, the randomization process ought to appropriately account for confounding variables. In other words, randomization ought to ensure orthogonality between the covariates measured in the study and the unobservables in order to avoid the bias due to omitted variables.

Statistical estimation of treatment costs associated with clinical trials can be undertaken using a number of alternative approaches: Both parametric and non-parametric. A parametric approach may be preferred when there is interest in assessing covariate effects on cost or in the extrapolation of costs beyond the end of the study period or to different patient populations. On the other hand, a parametric approach imposes a particular distributional form on costs, which may not be justified. Additional concerns which influence the choice of the analytical methodology relate to patterns in the observed cost data and include positive skewness in the cost observations, a substantial proportion of zero costs, missing data, censoring and lack of independence in the cost observations in situations where each individual in the sample contributes multiple data points over time. These problems are considered further below. Similar topics are discussed in Heyse *et al.* (2001) and Lipscomb *et al.* (1998).

A major concern with clinical trial cost analysis is that of missing data, as generally less emphasis is given to this data. Rubin (1976) identifies various mechanisms that may cause missing data and identifies the weakest conditions under which it is appropriate to ignore the process that causes missing data. In situations where the process cannot be ignored, imputation of the missing cost data may be undertaken. If missing data are missing at random and the observed data are observed at random, the problem is trivial, but still needs addressed (Rubin, 1976, p. 582). If data are not missing at random, then the methods that should be used to handle missing data depend on the mechanism that causes the missing values.

Assuming the classic linear regression model given by

$$E(Y|X) = \beta_0 + \beta' X,$$

where var $(Y|X) = \sigma^2$ the problem is to derive estimates of the parameters and associated variances when some of the data are missing. We discussed the issue with regards to missing X's, but this does not restrict the outcome variable, which could have some missing values as well.

Complete case analysis discards the cases with missing values and leads to loss of information which could be a substantial problem if the proportion of cases with missing values is high. This approach is normally used only for providing a baseline method for comparisons. Another method is first to impute the missing X values and then to perform the regression of Y on X using the imputed X values, either by ordinary least squares or by a weighted least squares regression that attaches lower weights to the incomplete cases. A simple approach for imputing the missing X values is to replace the missing X's by their unconditional sample means. This method will result in inefficient and inconsistent estimates if there is substantial correlation in the data, especially if the other covariates are correlated with the variable that has missing values. An improvement is to use information on the observed X's in a case to impute the missing X's. Another method is to impute the missing X by using both Y and the observed X's for imputation. A further approach is to assume a joint distribution for Y and X, a typical choice being a multivariate normal distribution, and to estimate the parameters of this distribution by maximum likelihood (Little, 1992). The estimates of the parameters are then substituted into the regression model yielding maximum likelihood estimates of the regression parameters.

Such imputation methods can result in low standard error estimates because errors in the imputations are not taken into account. A solution was proposed by Rubin (1978) and is referred to as multiple imputation. According to this approach, instead of imputing a single mean for each missing value, $N \geq 2$ values are drawn from the predictive distribution of the missing values given the remaining covariates and Y, and then complete data analysis is repeated N times, once with each imputation substituted. The final estimate of the parameter is the sum of the parameter values obtained for each imputation divided by the number of imputations. Multiple imputations has the advantage that once the imputations are constructed, analysis proceeds by complete-data methods. Multiple imputations could be predictions based on an explicit model or they could be based on an implicit model for the missing values. An example of the latter is hot-deck imputation, which matches incomplete cases to complete cases using information on covariates and then imputes values from the complete cases.

Robins *et al.* (1994) proposed a class of estimators to account for a subset of regressors having missing values, either by design or happenstance. Their approach derives weights using the inverse of the probability of non-missingness to estimate costs. The resultant estimators of the conditional mean cost are consistent under the following conditions: The data are missing at random, in the sense of Rubin (1976), the probabilities of missingness are bounded away from zero and the probabilities of missingness are known or can be estimated parametrically.

Related to missing data is the problem of censoring, which occurs whenever some individuals' behavior with respect to the variable under study is not observed for the full time to the event of interest, with information being incomplete for these patients. This is a common problem in trial settings, but also an issue with observational data. Patients who are lost to follow-up, drop out of the study, or are observed until the end of the study period without having reached the event of interest are right censored. Estimators of interest are biased if no account is taken of censoring, with the bias increasing as the degree of censoring increases. Given that censoring is a missing data process, the statistical theory for analyzing missing data can also be applied to the problem of censoring. There are obviously circumstances in which the problem of missing data on some of the covariates can arise alongside the problem of censoring of the dependent variable. For example, Lin and Ying (1993b) have considered this issue within the context of the Cox proportional hazards regression model, where time to failure is subject to censoring. Under conditions where some of the regressors have missing values, and although the model adjusts for censoring of the dependent variable, the authors state that not accounting for the missing covariate values appropriately will result in biased and inefficient parameter estimates.

Initial attempts to adjust estimates of cost statistics for censoring were based on application of traditional survival analysis techniques to cost data (e.g., Fenn *et al.*, 1995; 1996). The assumption underlying the validity of these approaches is the assumption of independence between the variable of interest and its censoring variable. This implies independence between time to event and time to censoring when failure time data are considered and independence between cost at event and cost at censoring when cost data are analyzed. This assumption is normally violated with respect to cost to event data, due to the lack of a common rate of cost accrual over time among individuals, as patients who are in poorer health states generate higher costs per unit of time and consequently, are expected to generate higher cumulative costs at both the failure time and the censoring time (Lin *et al.*,

1997; Etzioni *et al.*, 1999). This positive correlation implies that removal of certain observations from the sample due to censoring affects the joint distribution of cost for the remaining observations in the sense that, at any point in time, future cost expectation is statistically altered by censoring. As a result, any analysis that does not model this dependency will lead to erroneous inferences. Consequently, cost estimators based on traditional survival analysis approaches are normally inappropriate in the analysis of censored cost data.

Lin *et al.* (1997) proposed two non-parametric estimators of average cost under conditions of censoring. Under both methods, the study period is partitioned into a number of sub-intervals, an estimate of average cost in the interval is derived and the estimator of cost for the whole duration of analysis is obtained by summing over the sub-intervals the interval cost estimates weighted by interval-specific Kaplan–Meier probability estimates of time to event (Kaplan and Meier, 1958). The difference between the two alternatives is that, the first only uses information on the total costs of uncensored individuals incurred up to the point of the individual's event in the estimating process, while the second uses information on intermediate individual cost history from all individuals. Both estimators are shown to be consistent under the assumption of independent censoring. An extension of this assumption is to require that the censoring mechanism is unrelated to cost levels, continuous distribution of failure time and a discrete pattern for the censoring distribution.

An alternative approach, proposed by Bang and Tsiatis (2000), allows arbitrary censoring distribution patterns and attempts to improve the efficiency of the proposed estimators by recovering information lost due to censoring by adding functionals of the cost history process in the estimating equations. The idea underlying all estimators in this class is the use of the inverse of the probability of an individual not being censored in the estimating equations. The first estimator uses cost information from the uncensored individuals alone, while the second estimator also incorporates information on intermediate cost history from censored individuals. Under the first approach, the estimate of mean cost is derived as the average of the complete individual costs weighted by the inverse of the Kaplan–Meier probability of an individual not being censored, evaluated at the point of the individual's death. Under the second approach, the duration of analysis is partitioned into a number of sub-intervals; the first estimator is used to derive the estimated cost incurred in each of these sub-intervals; and the final estimate of mean cost is derived by summing over these intervals. The advantage of the latter estimator is an increase in efficiency, by allowing use of additional cost information. Each of these estimators is accompanied by an improved variant that attempts to increase efficiency in the estimates through use of some functional of the cost history process that allows recovery of information lost due to censoring. Under independent censoring, all four estimators are shown to be consistent. A theoretical discussion of the non-parametric estimators described above has also been provided by O'Hagan and Stevens (2004).

Turning to the parametric approaches, Lin (2000) suggests a linear regression model approach in which cost is related to a set of individual covariates. The method derives estimates of the regression parameters accounting for the presence of censoring and is not restricted by the censoring pattern. Two estimators result from this approach. The first uses the individual total accumulated costs at the individual's point of death or censoring while the second makes use of multiple cost observations on each subject obtained at various points in time over the study period. The advantage of the latter estimator is an increase in efficiency by allowing use of cost information that is not used by the preceding estimator. In both cases, the estimates of the regression parameters are adjusted for censoring by incorporating the inverse of the probability of an individual not being censored evaluated at the point of the individual observed cost in the estimating equations. Both approaches derive consistent estimates for the regression parameters.

Raikou and McGuire (2004) attempted to assess the non-parametric estimators' performance empirically under heavy censoring. They identify two estimators that perform well under all conditions considered — namely, the estimator by Lin *et al.* (1997), using intermediate individual cost history information, and the estimator by Bang and Tsiatis (2000), also uses intermediate individual cost history information. A similar study by Raikou and McGuire (2009) of the parametric estimators' performance, under the same censoring conditions and using the same data, found that the regression methodology proposed by Lin (2000) that uses intermediate cost history information performs well under heavy censoring, resulting in cost estimates that are very close to the ones derived from application of the best performing non-parametric estimators mentioned above. Use of the inverse of the probability of an individual not being censored in the estimating equations is instrumental in deriving unbiased estimates of medical care costs under conditions of censoring. Nevertheless, the success of the approach is also dependent on the amount of available information on the cost history process, with the value of this information increasing as the degree of censoring increases.

A further study by Baser *et al.* (2006) applied the inverse probability-weighted least-squares method to estimate the effects of treatment on total medical cost, subject to censoring, in a panel-data setting. The authors assessed the performance of both inverse probability-weighted pooled ordinary-least squares (POLS) and inverse probability-weighted random effects (RE) models, and they found them to be consistent under conditions of dependent censoring. Moreover, given that unweighted POLS and RE estimators are consistent under independent censoring and more efficient under the homoscedasticity assumption, the authors suggest using the Hausman test to determine whether the independent censoring assumption is violated and whether the censoring bias creates statistically meaningful differences in the estimated coefficients.

Liu *et al.* (2007) proposed a joint RE model to account for the correlation between medical costs and survival through a pre-specified random effect allocated to individuals. The contribution of their model is, first, it accounts for the correlation between cost and survival and, second, it allows modeling the pattern of cost prior to death in order to capture the typically increasing costs of patients in the period prior to death. The method for estimating this pattern of cost accumulation is applicable if cost accumulation is considered as an additive effect that is limited at some fixed point in time before death. As such, the model allows estimation of the pattern of cost accumulation both after the time of entry and before death.

Another estimator for estimating treatment costs under conditions of censoring has been introduced recently by Basu and Manning (2010). Their method extends the class of two-part models to account for the presence of random censoring in the data while an attempt is being made to use the cost information from the intervals where censoring occurs. The main contribution is through differentiating between the effect of covariates on survival and the intensity of utilization without assuming discreteness in censoring of death times. This appears to be an improvement on the Lin *et al.* (1997) estimator.

A further issue inherent in data consisting of repeated measurements of the variables of interest is the dependency among the repeated measurements for any subject. In such circumstances, ordinary least squares regression is not an appropriate estimation procedure, as the assumptions concerning the error terms are no longer valid. The general procedure to analyzing such data in the econometric and statistical literature is to adopt a generalized linear regression model which accommodates more general patterns for the distribution of the disturbances. A class of generalized estimating equations for the regression parameters has been proposed by Liang and Zeger (1986), which result in consistent estimates of the regression parameters and their variances without requiring specification of the joint distribution of a subject's observations.

Partly in an attempt to resolve the problem of dependency among the multiple observations for each subject, Lipscomb *et al.* (1998) used the stratified variant of the Cox proportional hazards model, with time being the stratification variable in deriving estimates of patient cost within each stratum. They argue that a great advantage of this model is that it does not make any assumptions about the distributional form of the error terms, and as such, it is likely to be among the best alternatives when interest lies in modeling complex distributions, such as distributions of cost. In addition, they suggest that this model overcomes the problem of dependency between multiple observations on the same individual, as it assumes different baseline hazards for cost across different strata. Given, however, the criticism of this approach (e.g., Etzioni *et al.*, 1999), it seems unlikely that such a methodology would be useful.

In addition, this approach can also be adopted in the event of some observations being missing, in which case the same results hold, provided that data are missing completely at random in the sense of Rubin (1976). Within this framework of generalized linear regression, Lin (2000) derived estimators for the regression parameters when repeated measurements on the outcome variable were obtained within the context of censored cost analysis.

Health Care Cost Estimation in General

When moving from clinical trial settings to health care costs generally Jones (2011) and Jones *et al.* (2014) give good overviews. He distinguishes between the use of cost estimation for cost-effectiveness, which has been largely covered in the previous section, and for risk-adjustment. In the more general setting, risk-adjustment and prediction are the more important concerns. It is important in a number of environments where reimbursement agencies or insurance companies are interested in predicting health care costs in their own right, or for reimbursement purposes themselves. Here, econometric models of health care cost estimation at the individual patient level also face a number of issues. Some, such as missing data and censoring, have been covered above.

Relating the issue back to equation above, the issue is to risk-adjust and predict the conditional mean of the costs:

$$\hat{E}(y_i|x_i) = \hat{\mu}(x_i) = x_i\hat{\beta}$$

A number of initial issues present themselves. If the population over which the estimated expected health care costs relates to the whole population, there may be a high level of zeros returned, as some individuals will not incur costs. A two-part model is estimated, where the first part models the probability of incurring health care costs, and the second part models expected health care costs among the subset of the sample population who do incur costs. The expected level of health care cost is then a probability-weighted expected cost, with the weighting related to the expectation of actually incurring costs.

A second issue is that the distribution of treatment costs for individuals is liable to be heavily skewed. The raw data must therefore be transformed to meet the requirements of the linear estimation process, where the error terms are assumed to have a mean of zero, and the variance around the estimated mean cost is assumed constant. In empirical work, this has led to various transformations being applied to raw cost data. Logarithmic transformations were typically used to reduce skewness and return error distribution toward a normal distribution. Such transformations become *ad hoc*, at least for the first part of any two-part model, to incorporate the zero occurrences of health care costs. Even ignoring this issue, as Mullahy (2009) noted that the predicted mean after transformation, is on a log scale. To retransform into actual costs a smearing factor has to be applied, as simple exponential transformation does not return the true retransformed value. This smearing factor is relatively straightforward, unless heteroskedasticity is present; which, of course, given that we are dealing with individual treatment costs, it often is. Duan *et al.* (1983) suggested a general smearing estimator be applied, yet even here the form of the heteroskedascticity has to be known. In general, this need not be the case.

This has in turn, led to a number of other transformations being applied. These range from simple square root transformations to more general Box–Cox transformation. The latter are a class of essentially power-based transformations, where the transformation and therefore, the explicit functional form applied is based on *ad hoc* data fitting. In other words, the functional form fitted by the Box–Cox transformation is dictated by the sample data at hand. Different samples may therefore return different functional forms. Semiparametric models of individual treatment costs take this *ad hoc* specification further by extending the data fitting in such a way that iteration provides estimates of the cost parameters, which are then coupled with transformations of the error term imposed to ensure zero mean and constant variance. Heteroskedasticity can be imposed by imposing weights on the variance–covariance matrix. Again, the semiparametric estimates have to be retransformed, using a Duan *et al.* (1983) type-smearing process, to return expected cost estimates to the original scale. Although, again, the form of heteroskedascticity has to be known.

These transformation approaches are all agnostic with respect to the underlying production processes and treatment processes at work. The approaches are essentially data fitting, usually with some transformation to ensure a tractable functional form given the population sample of cost to hand. Clearly, this means the functional forms are not derived explicitly from any knowledge of the treatment process itself. Thus, while considerable progress has been made in estimating treatment costs from data, little improvement has been made in our knowledge of how these costs are generated. Maybe, given the wide variation in medical practice, this should not be considered a worrisome issue. However, it does mean that we cannot be certain, even if the statistical issues are resolved, that the returned expected treatment costs are representative of efficient practice. Not surprisingly, given the issues of skewness, transformation, and retransformation, a number of these approaches do not perform well empirically either, leaving a large amount of unexplained variance in treatment costs across individuals.

Considerable effort has therefore subsequently been made on the issue of functional form and estimation techniques, in particular, in the application of non-linear regression models to estimate mean treatment costs across individuals. Once again, for a thorough review see Jones (2011). A major benefit of this class of model is that it returns estimates of the mean cost to the original scale; therefore, there is no need to transform and retransform. An obvious extension to the earlier models was estimation through the generalized linear model (GLM). In the GLM approach, which encompasses a wide range of specifications, explicit assumptions have to be made about the functional form of the mean and the variance being analyzed. Essentially, a link function is used to make explicit the relationship between the expected mean and the variance. A wide choice of linkage functions is available, although the log link is commonly applied. Recently, Basu and Rathouz (2005) has suggested the use of a Box–Cox link function, to generalize the fit. The GLM approach has the additional advantage of explicit modeling of underlying heteroskedasticity if present. However, as Mullahy (2009) has noted, GLM approaches tend to perform badly under conditions of skewness.

These GLM approaches are related to the general nonlinear approach associated with exponential conditional mean (ECM) models. These are commonly considered for count and duration data, but have been extended to apply to treatment cost data also. As would be expected, the ECM approach makes different assumptions about the distribution of the expected treatment cost. While GLM makes assumptions concerning the expected mean and the relationship between the expected mean and variance, the ECM approach imposes a parametric distributional assumption on the entire distribution. These distributional assumptions allow for explicit modeling of skewness. Manning *et al.* (2005), Deb and Burgess (2003), and Jones *et al.* (2014) are examples of different distributional forms imposed on the data. In this approach, attention is increasingly being given to nested approaches and flexible distributions to allow as general an application to treatment costs as possible.

There has been evolution in terms of estimation technique. However, this has been gained through ever more sophisticated investigation of data fit. All these models remain theoretical agnostic with respect to underlying treatment processes. Whether these approaches are supportable then depends on the empirical evidence. There are a number of papers which compare model performance (Basu *et al.*, 2006; Hill and Miller, 2010; Manning *et al.*, 2005; Jones, 2011). Most use out-of-sample prediction or Monte Carlo techniques to validate these models. There is no overall winner in terms of performance. Different approaches, functional forms and distributional assumptions are assessed across a range of sample populations, mainly but not exclusively drawn from the US. The specification and functional forms differ markedly. Different models appear to perform differently across different sample populations and across different sub-samples drawn from within these samples. If there is any message to be drawn, it is that the earlier, simpler specifications (such as logarithmic transformations) tend to perform less well, but this is not always the case, than the more sophisticated recent approaches. However, there is no general claim to be made. If anything, a conclusion should perhaps be drawn that different specifications should be used within any given sample population to examine the robustness of expected cost estimates.

Hospital Cost Modeling

If we move to the next level of cost estimation, and consider aggregations of treated individuals within the hospital sector, similar observations can be made. There has, at this level of aggregation, been widespread disagreement in the findings of a large body of empirical work on hospital cost functions. All studies agree costs must be related to outcome; but that is as far as the agreement goes. In terms of the functional form used to specify this relationship, a large number of studies have used flexible functional forms; in particular translog cost models. These models use approximations, based on a Taylor expansion around points on the estimated cost function, to derive expected cost estimates of hospital activity (Breyer, 1987). The translog function is specified in logarithmic form, therefore while translog functions can be useful in dealing with multi-output conditions (as arise in hospitals) they tend not to be able to specify full output levels across a sample of hospitals if some display zero levels of output in some dimension. One example of this is if some hospitals include and others do not include maternity services as a dimension of their output. For comparative purposes across the sample, maternity services would have to be excluded. Moreover, it is a mistaken interpretation of flexible form functional forms to assume that they are approximating the underlying technological structure. The advantage of using a fully flexible form is that they place few restrictions on the underlying technological structure, but at the cost of not necessarily providing truly global approximations, and imposing strong assumptions with regards to separability.

The question remains how does hospital cost relate to output? Different studies have considered different exact relationships — few have considered the endogenous nature of demand and/or the production function reactions to stochastic demand (Gaynor and Anderson, 1995). Moreover, most have used the volume of beds, an input in the production process, as a measure of (output) scale, implying misspecification. This measure is, however, used as an output measure, and associated with short-term utilization rates leading to poor information on hospital scale or size (Granneman *et al.*, 1986).

Those who have reviewed this literature find that there are conflicting conclusions drawn across the large number of studies (Granneman *et al.*, 1986; Breyer, 1987; Vita, 1990). Cowing *et al.* (1983) in a review of the early literature, which is acknowledged to be based on *ad hoc* specifications, suggests that economies of scale, e.g., do hold for smaller scale hospitals but not for larger-sized hospitals (those over 200 beds). The latter, and possibly more theoretically-based literature is equivocal. To the extent that larger hospitals treat more complex cases and have greater depth or scope of production, which tends to include more specialized services, and noting that such characteristics tend to increase unit costs, this will bias economies of scale downwards. Indeed, there seems to be no general conclusion to be drawn on functional form or empirical findings on the relationship between hospital costs and output. As Gaynor and Vogt (2000) note there are large discrepancies in the empirical literature, even on the definition of hospital output. The latter literature has used specifications incorporating endogenous demand in flexible functional forms, or specifications which have been determined empirically through Box–Cox fitting of the sample data (Hughes and McGuire, 2003; Gaynor and Anderson, 1995). This latter literature finds limited evidence of (weak) economies of scale.

Concluding Remarks

The emphasis in this overview of the literature has been on the concepts underlying the empirical determination of treatment cost, either at the individual level or at the aggregate hospital level. As was noted, there are fundamental statistical issues to be resolved, even when individual treatment costs are well defined and proscribed as in sample data drawn from clinical trials. When investigation is moved to the analysis of individual treatment costs more generally, these issues multiply. When we move to higher levels of aggregation, the problems are not resolved. In part, this is because there is little understanding of the treatment processes that underlie these costs. In part, it reflects the real difficulties in trying to adequately capture expected treatment costs when the treated populations display heterogeneity and sample selection. The lack of understanding of medical practice variation means that estimating expected (average) treatment cost in any population is difficult. It remains of fundamental importance.

Given the high, and in most cases, growing health care expenditures it seems unacceptable that more is not known about costs at various levels of aggregation. Individual health care costs need to be better understood for a number of purposes.

Certainly as more attention is given to risk adjustment in setting insurance premiums, there needs to be more attention given to the forecasting of individual health care utilization and cost structures. At a more aggregate, hospital level, as payment structures increasingly move towards DRG reimbursement, the underlying cost structures faced by hospitals become more important.

This overview highlights the lack of understanding of cost behavior at any level within the health care sector. Few studies have attempted to follow individuals with respect to their incurred health care costs over time. Those that have, in particular clinical trial based cost studies, are biased in their choice of treatment population through their entry criteria and tend not to follow-up all observations to the pre-specified end point. The hospital cost estimates suffer from misspecification problems, do not make explicit the relationship between the production levels and costs, and therefore give a wide range of estimates depending on the adopted assumptions and specifications.

References

Bang H, Tsiatis AA. 2000. Estimating medical costs with censored data. *Biometrika* 87: 329–343.

Baser O, Gardiner J, Bradley C, Yuce H, Given C. 2006. Longitudinal analysis of censored medical cost data. *Health Economics* 15: 513–525.

Basu A, Rathouz P. 2005. Estimating marginal and incremental effects on health outcomes using flexible link and variance function models. *Biostatistics* 6(1): 93–109.

Basu A, Arondekar BV, Rathouz PJ. 2006. Scale of interest versus scale of estimation: Comparing alternative estimators for the incremental costs of a comorbidity. *Health Economics* 15: 1091–1107.

Basu A, Manning W. 2010. Estimating lifetime or episode-of-illness costs under censoring. *Health Economics* 19: 1010–1028.

Breyer, F. 1987. The specification of a hospital cost function. *Journal of Health Economics* 6: 147–157.

Brouwer W, Rutten F, Koopmanschap M. 2001. Costing in economic evaluation. In Drummond M, McGuire A. (eds.). *Economic Evaluation in Health Care: Merging Theory with Practice* Oxford University Press, pp. 68–93.

Cowing TG, Holtmann AG, Powers S. 1983. Hospital cost analysis: A survey and evaluation of recent studies. In *Advances in Health Economics and Health Services Research*, Vol. 1, pp. 257–303, JAI Press, Greenwich, CN.

Deb P, Burgess J. 2003. A Quasi-experimental Comparison of Econometric Models for Health Care Expenditures. *Economics Working Paper Archive at Hunter College 212*, Hunter College Department of Economics.

Dranove D. 1995. Measuring costs. *In*: *Valuing Health Care*, Sloan, FA (ed.). Cambridge University Press. pp. 61–75.

Drummond M, Pang F. 2001. Transferability of economic evaluation results. *In*: Drummond M, McGuire A. (eds.). *Economic Evaluation in Health Care: Merging Theory with Practice*, Oxford University Press, pp. 256–276.

Duan N, Manning WG, Morris CN. 1983. A comparison of alternative models for the demand for medical care. *Journal of Business and Economic Statistics* 1: 115–126.

Etzioni R, Feuer E, Sullivan S, Lin D, Hu C, Ramsey SD. 1999. On the use of survival analysis techniques to estimate medical care costs. *Journal of Health Economics* 18: 365–380.

Fenn P, McGuire A, Phillips V, Backhouse M, Jones D. 1995. The analysis of censored treatment cost data in economic evaluation. *Medical Care* 33: 851–863.

Fenn P, McGuire A, Backhouse M, Jones D. 1996. Modelling programme costs in economic evaluation. *Journal of Health Economics* 15: 115–125.

Gaynor, M, Anderson G. 1995. Uncertain demand, the structure of hospital costs, and the cost of empty hospital beds. *Journal of Health Economics* 14: 291–317.

Gaynor M, Vogt W. 2000. Antitrust and competition in health care markets. In Culyer A, Newhouse J. (eds.). *Handbook of Health Economics*, Vol. 1B, Elsevier Science, North-Holland.

Grannemann TW, Brown RS, Pauly MV. 1986. Estimating hospital costs: A multiple output analysis. *Journal of Health Economics* 5(2): 107–127.

Glick H, Polsky D, Sculman K. 2001. Trial-based economic evaluations: An overview of design and analysis. In: Drummond M, McGuire A. (eds.). *Economic Evaluation in Health Care: Merging Theory with Practice,* Oxford University Press, pp. 113–140.

Gold M, Seigal JE, Russell LB, Weinstein MC. (eds.). 1996. *Cost-Effectiveness in Health and Medicine.* Oxford University Press, New York.

Heyse JF, Cook JR, Carides GW. 2001. In: Drummond M, McGuire A. (eds.). *Economic Evaluation in Health Care: Merging Theory with Practice,* Oxford University Press, pp. 215–235.

Hill SC, Miller GE. 2010. Health expenditure estimation and functional form: Applications of the generalized gamma and extended estimating equations models. *Health Economics* 19: 608–627.

Hughes D, McGuire A. 2003. Stochastic demand, production responses and hospital costs. *Journal of Health Economics* 22: 999–1010.

Johnston K, Buxton M, Jones DR, Fitzpatrick R. 1999. Assessing the costs of healthcare technologies in clinical trials. *Health Technology Assessment Review* 6: 3.

Jones AM. 2011. Models for health care. In: Clements M, Hendry D. (eds.). *The Oxford Handbook of Economic Forecasting*. pp. 625–654. (OUP, Oxford).

Jones AM, Lomas J, Rice N. 2014. Applying Beta-type size distributions to healthcare cost regressions. *Journal of Applied Econometrics* 29: 649–670.

Kaplan EL, Meier P. 1958. Nonparametric estimation from incomplete observations. *Journal of the American Statistical Association* 53: 457–481.

Knapp M, Beecham J. 1993. Costing mental health services. *Psychological Medicine* 20: 892–908.
Liang KY, Zeger SL. 1986. Longitudinal data analysis using generalised linear models. *Biometrika* 73: 13–22.
Lin DY. 2000. Linear regression analysis of censored medical costs. *Biostatistics* 1: 35–47.
Lin DY, Ying Z. 1993. Cox regression with incomplete covariate measurements. *Journal of the American Statistical Association* 88: 1341–1349.
Lin DY, Feuer EJ, Etzioni R, Wax Y. 1997. Estimating medical costs from incomplete follow-up data. *Biometrics* 53: 113–128.
Lipscomb J, Ancukiewicz M, Parmigiani G, Hasselblad V, Samsa G, Matchar D. 1998. Predicting the cost of illness: A comparison of alternative models applied to stroke. *Medical Decision Making* 18 Supplement: S39–S56.
Little, RJA. 1992. Regression with missing *X*'s: A review. *Journal of the American Statistical Association* 87: 1227–1237.
Liu L, Wolfe R, Kalbfleisch J. 2007. A shared random effects model for censored medical costs and mortality. *Statistics in Medicine* 26: 139–155.
Manning W, Basu A, Mullahy J. 2005. Generalized modeling approaches to risk adjustment of skewed outcomes data. *Journal of Health Economics* 24: 465–488.
Mullahy J, Manning WG. 1995. Statistical issues in cost effectiveness analysis. In: Sloan, FA (ed.) *Valuing Health Care*, Cambridge University Press, Cambridge.
Mullahy J. 2009. Econometric modeling of health care costs and expenditures: A survey of analytical issues and related policy considerations. *Medical Care* 47: S104–108.
O'Hagan A, Stevens J. 2004. On estimators of medical costs with censored data. *Journal of Health Economics* 23: 615–625.
Olsen J. 1994. Production gains should they count in health care evaluations? *Scottish Journal of Political Economy* 79: 687–705.
Raikou M, McGuire A. 2004. Estimating medical care costs under conditions of censoring. *Journal of Health Economics* 23: 443–470.
Raikou M, McGuire A. 2009. Parametric estimation of medical care costs under conditions of censoring. *LSE Health Discussion Paper Series, Working Paper No*: 13. LSE Health.
Raikou M, Briggs A, Gray A, McGuire A. 2000. Centre-specific or average unit costs in multi-centre studies? Some theory and simulation. *Health Economics* 9: 191–198.
Robins JM, Rotnitzky A, Zhao LP. 1994. Estimation of regression coefficients when some regressors are not always observed. *Journal of the American Statistical Association* 89: 846–866.
Rubin DB. 1976. Inference and missing data. *Biometrika* 63: 581–592.
Rubin DB. 1978. *Multiple Imputation for Nonresponse in Surveys*. John Wiley, New York.
Sculpher M. 2001. The role and estimation of productivity costs in economic evaluation. In: Drummond, M, McGuire, A. (eds.). *Economic Evaluation in Health Care: Merging Theory with Practice*. Oxford University Press, pp. 94–112.

Spiegelhalter FA, Jones DR, Parmar MKB, *et al.* 1996. *Being Economical with the Costs.* Department of Epidemiology and Public Health Technical Paper 96-06. University of Leicester, Leicester.

Vita M. 1990. Exploring hospital production relationships with flexible functional forms. *Journal of Health Economics* 9: 1–21.

Whynes D, Walker AR. 1995. On approximations in treatment costing. *Health Economics* 4: 31–40.

Incentivizing Health Care Utilization and Health Outcomes*

William H. Dow
UC-Berkeley
wdow@berkeley.edu
Justin S. White
Stanford University
justinswhite@stanford.edu
Stefano Bertozzi
UC-Berkeley
sbertozzi@berkeley.edu

This chapter discusses arguments and evidence on the promise of incentives as a development tool for increasing the use of health care services and improving health outcomes. Incentives have been a controversial tool, but prominent initiatives in recent years have increased interest in understanding the circumstances under which they may be efficacious, as well as how they may best be employed in an ethical and cost-effective manner. The chapter examines both small, time-delimited incentives and larger repeated incentives embedded in social protection programmes such as Mexico's Oportunidades program. It summarizes evidence on the way incentive efforts have been used in various health care domains, including family planning, prenatal care, facility-based delivery, immunization, HIV testing, and medication adherence; in promoting non-medical health behaviors such as smoking cessation; and for health outcomes such as weight loss or avoidance of sexually transmitted infections. Finally, the chapter considers the most promising areas for future development policy exploration.

Keywords: Financial Incentives; Conditional Cash Transfer; Behavioral Economics.

---

*An earlier version of this paper was prepared for the United Nations Population Division expert paper series. We are grateful for helpful comments on that version from the population division staff as well as participants at the United Nations Expert Group Meeting on Priorities for Improved Survival: ICPD Beyond 2014. http://www.un.org/en/development/desa/population/publications/pdf/expert/2013-13_Dow-and-White_Expert-paper.pdf.

Introduction

This chapter discusses arguments and evidence on the promise of incentives as a development tool for increasing the use of health care services and healthy behaviors so as to improve health outcomes. Incentives have been a controversial tool, but prominent initiatives in recent years have increased interest in understanding the circumstances under which they may be efficacious, as well as how they may best be employed in a cost-effective manner. The accumulated knowledge base is larger in high-income countries than in less developed settings, with much that is still poorly understood, but it is a highly active area of current research.

The following section discusses central arguments underlying incentive-based policies, as well as general concerns about the use of incentives. It elaborates on the various pathways through which incentives operate and informs appropriate incentive design. A distinction is made between smaller time-delimited incentives versus larger repeated incentives embedded in social protection programs such as Mexico's well-known Oportunidades conditional cash transfer (CCT) program. Smaller, more frequent incentives may better capitalize on benefits from the psychological pathways described, whereas longer repeated incentives may yield health benefits, not only through the usual incentive channels, but also through poverty alleviation.

The chapter then summarizes evidence on the ways incentive efforts have been used in various domains. Examples of efforts to incentivize healthcare utilization have included maternal and child health care such as family planning, prenatal care, facility-based childbirth, and good childcare, including vaccination. Other domains for adult health care incentives have been screenings such as HIV testing and medication adherence such as for tuberculosis. The increasing burden of chronic disease also raises the prospect of using incentives for chronic disease prevention by rewarding non-medical health behaviors such as smoking cessation. Finally, in domains for which risky behaviors cannot be directly observed, there have been efforts to reward specific health outcomes, such as avoidance of sexually transmitted infections. The final section of the paper considers the most promising areas for future development policy exploration.

Why Incentives? Arguments Pros and Con

Incentives as a version of price subsidies

Subsidies have been a staple of efforts to increase the use of effective health services in countries worldwide (World Health Organization, 2010). Traditionally, these have taken the form of supply-side price subsidies that reduce user fees below cost, or infrastructure subsidies that expand the geographic availability of services, thereby improving access and lowering the "time price" to users. Yet supply-side subsidies have often proven difficult to administer. Subsidized health care services are frequently unavailable to the most vulnerable populations, and the quality of subsidized health care where available is often sub-standard. Promising efforts are now being made to target subsidies through free voucher schemes and to improve provider incentives for quality care through performance-based financing that rewards providers for targeted activities such as vaccinations, both of which are beyond the scope of this chapter (see Volume 1, Chapter 10, *Pay for Performance in Health Systems Around the Globe*).

Even where official prices for quality care are reduced to zero, substantial economic barriers to utilization still remain for patients, including the informal payments sometimes demanded by providers, out-of-pocket travel costs to health care facilities, and the "opportunity cost" of time spent travelling and waiting in long queues. These barriers are compounded by credit constraints and a lack of future-orientation that is frequently observed in settings characterized by poverty and daily uncertainty, which leads people to put off seeking health care. To combat these barriers, there has been increasing research and policy experimentation around using positive incentives to reduce user prices below zero: in other words, paying people to utilize targeted health services or to engage in health-enhancing behaviors more generally. This chapter reviews several different forms of positive incentives, including CCTs that make payments contingent on pre-specified activities such as receiving a certain number of antenatal visits (in contrast to unconditional cash transfers (UCTs) that make no requirements of cash recipients) and non-monetary incentives that include in-kind gifts such as food handouts during immunization campaigns.

Viewed relative to supply-side investments, positive incentives (hereafter, referred to simply as incentives) can be understood as an extreme along a continuum of price subsidies. Given their cost, incentives may be viewed as unaffordable in already over-stretched health care systems, but when designed and administered well for a given setting, incentive policies may lower costs and be more cost-effective overall relative to traditional supply-side subsidies. Whether incentives are more cost-effective than supply-side subsidies is a setting-specific empirical question that requires careful assessment of both costs and relative effectiveness. Examples of such an analysis are too few. The costs and effectiveness of incentives are especially difficult to assess when the incentives are embedded within CCT programs because the additional administrative costs needed to verify conditionality must be considered. The challenge of verification is related to the potential for incentive-based programs to exacerbate corruption temptations, which is a concern for any subsidy delivery mechanism, and depends on the nature of systems for monitoring program employees and middlemen who disburse the payments.

Ethical considerations

All interventions aimed at changing behavior raise concern about the potential for coercion, i.e., the potential to undermine personal freedom of choice by leading individuals to feel compelled to participate or to ignore risks. Positive incentives have been a particular target of concern, in part because poor, credit-constrained individuals may be especially susceptible to the "income effect" from the incentives. While the ethical considerations involved are highly nuanced and a full discussion is beyond the scope of this chapter, the general concerns are described briefly. A recent ethics working group (London *et al.*, 2012) stated that, "We propose that concerns around the potential for incentives to undermine recipient autonomy are misplaced when incentives are used to overcome economic obstacles or a lack of effective motivation, and when recipients are incentivized to engage in health-related behaviors or practices with which they are already familiar and which they regard as beneficial or worthwhile." It is a significant challenge to ensure that incentivized individuals have the autonomy to choose whether to engage in the targeted behavior (for example, without a family member preventing them), and that they also have access to the necessary tools, including sufficient availability of the relevant health care services. Gopichandran and Chetlapalli (2012), for example, argued that one high-profile program incentivizing facility-based childbirth may have been unethical due to uneven access to services, among other considerations. Similar ethical debates surround many other applications of incentives. Supporters of incentive programs often respond that it would be unethical to ignore the potential for incentives as a tool to decrease mortality and increase well-being, if incentives are substantially more effective than alternatives.

Psychological considerations

While traditional economic frameworks suggest that people respond similarly to subsidies and incentives, psychological frameworks suggest that people may well perceive and respond to them differently. The recent surge in research in "behavioral economics," which lies at the intersection of psychology and economics, has fostered a better understanding of the various pathways through which incentives may operate (see Volume 2, Chapter 11 in this Handbook, *Behavioral Economics*: *Health Applications in the US* and Volume 2, Chapter 12, *Behavioral Economics*: *Health Applications in the UK*). Several such pathways are discussed below, including small incentive nudges, along with discussion of how understanding these pathways may inform better incentive design. We do not discuss in depth the interaction of monetary incentives and social preferences such as trust, altruism, and reciprocity; for a review, see Fehr and Falk (2002) and Bowles and Polania-Reyes (2012).

The first pathway through which incentives are understood to operate is by increasing the individual's "extrinsic" motivation — that is, one's motivation to engage in an activity in order to earn a reward or avoid a punishment. Perhaps the most widely discussed concern about the efficacy and sustainability of incentives has been that "extrinsic" motivations (such as monetary incentives) may crowd out "intrinsic" motivation (Deci *et al.*, 1999). In other words, individuals might lose interest in a task if they had previously been paid to complete the same or a similar task. This crowd-out of intrinsic motivation could lead incentive-based approaches to be not only ineffectual, as the desired behaviors are not maintained after the incentives are removed, but even counterproductive. For example, it has been hypothesized that short-term incentives could lead to a form of reference dependence in which people come to expect continued incentives and could become unwilling to engage in a desired behavior or pay for a health service once the incentives end (Simonson and Tversky, 1992). While there have been examples of crowd-out in laboratory experiments and of reference dependence in certain settings (Simonsohn and Loewenstein, 2006), the field evidence is lacking (Cameron *et al.*, 2001), and some, such as Fehr and Falk (2002), have questioned the relevance and strength of the evidence base for real-world economic applications. Indeed, the research community has been developing a more nuanced picture beyond this simplistic intrinsic–extrinsic dichotomy. If people engage in some healthy behaviors out of fear for negative health outcomes, then this fear motivation is less likely to be affected by extrinsic incentives. More generally, in many situations intrinsic and extrinsic motivations are not zero-sum: extrinsic motivations may even help activate intrinsic motivation, and can lead to the formation of good health habits. For example, Charness and Gneezy (2012) find that payments for gym attendance led participants to continue going to the gym even after the payments were removed. Incentives also may help individuals to learn about and experiment with a task, which can boost long-run adoption of the task. Dupas (2014) finds that short-term subsidies for antimalarial bednets make recipients more willing to pay for unsubsidized bednets in the future, in contrast to what would be expected if recipients had experienced reference dependence.

A second pathway through which incentives are understood to operate is by overcoming individuals' tendencies to favor the present over future benefits. Substantial evidence suggests that individuals have a bias for the present, in effect overweighting the value of immediate costs and benefits relative to future costs and benefits (White and Dow, 2015). Economic incentives may be able to counter this urge toward immediate gratification. For example, incentivizing smoking cessation may help to offset the potential immediate pleasure that a person derives from smoking. Many of the benefits of smoking cessation are not realized until far in the future, and the incentives are designed to bring forward those benefits into the present. Some researchers have designed incentive packages explicitly to make incentives felt in the present, such as efforts to deliver small, frequent payments for salutary behaviors. For example, Volpp *et al.* (2008a) offered daily incentives to participants who met a daily weight loss goal.

A third set of pathways involve countering feelings of regret, loss aversion, and the tendency for individuals to overestimate small probabilities, per prospect theory (Kahneman and Tversky, 1979). Some researchers have implemented so-called combination lotteries that use two independent lotteries, one with a low probability of a large reward and the other with a high probability of a small reward (Volpp *et al.*, 2008a; 2008b). The systematic overweighting of small probabilities may make a combination lottery more effective than a more conventional lottery with the same expected value. Prospect theory also specifies that individuals tend to avoid potential losses more than they tend to be attracted to potential gains, a concept known as loss aversion. Volpp *et al.* (2008b) entered participants into a daily lottery but only paid out if the winner remained adherent to warfarin, an anticoagulant drug that prevents blood clots. In an effort to mobilize regret from a missed payoff, the investigators notified all non-adherent winners of the amount that they would have won had they been adherent, and non-adherence decreased substantially. Subsequent work showed that the effect is concentrated among patients outside of the therapeutic range at enrollment (Kimmel *et al.*, 2012); overall, the empirical literature on activating regret in this way is still limited.

Fourth, there is evidence that even small incentive nudges may be effective by signaling to individuals the importance of the task in the eyes of the designer of the incentives and thus encouraging them to modify their behavior. A physician who recommends a certain course of treatment makes her preferences known to the patient, and likewise, a government that subsidizes the same treatment sends a signal. However, such contextual inference may also lead a person to surmise from the presence of a reward that an unfamiliar task is not enjoyable, and thus to forgo the task; this represents another potential pathway for crowd-out of intrinsic motivation (Bénabou and Tirole, 2003). Thus, the process of extracting signals from incentives in the environment may have difficult-to-predict outcomes that depend on each person's beliefs and interpretation of the signals; again, the empirical evidence on such pathways is not well developed.

With all of the above pathways, a prerequisite for a nudge to take hold is that the signal — the incentive — needs to be visible to the individual. In such cases, the incentivized task gains a temporary outsized salience as the person contemplates how to earn the incentives. The chance to receive a reward for immunization, for example, may draw a person's attention to planning for the event, which is important given the many demands for the person's daily attention and commonly observed procrastination. Relatedly, even small incentives may be effective if they provide an alternative frame for justifying healthy behaviors to oneself or friends, such as an alternative reason for taking an HIV test rather than admitting potential risk. These types of small nudges may lose their salience over time, however, and may be best suited to one-time or short-term behavioral changes.

A further contribution from psychology derives from better understanding physiological pathways underlying behavior. Critical and sensitive periods may exist in which behavior changes can have more lasting effects, and brain research suggests that adolescents may be especially vulnerable to the adoption of risky health behaviors as well as to longer-run shaping of healthy behavior patterns. Slow brain development, especially in the limbic and prefrontal regions, leads to reduced cognitive control and increased sensitivity to rewards (Richards *et al.*, 2012). Incentives activate those same systems and thus can be used effectively to leverage these enhanced sensitivities for health promotion purposes. This line of research promises further insights in the coming years.

Design Features to Enhance Incentive Effectiveness

The details of how an incentive is designed and delivered may have substantial impacts on incentive effectiveness. Different designs can activate different psychological pathways that moderate or intensify the effects of the incentives. The below discussion focuses on several dimensions of potential importance: the size of the incentives, the delivery schedule, the certainty of reward, the unit incentivized (person, family member, or group), and the targeted population. The research literature on these design features is in a nascent phase, and much is drawn from high-income countries; there is relatively little generalizable knowledge to date about the circumstances in which certain features are preferred. Often, theoretical arguments are offered *in lieu* of empirical evidence. Due to the scarcity of research, this discussion is limited to a brief introduction of the issues that relate to each dimension.

All else equal, bigger incentives tend to be more powerful motivators. However, empirical research from behavioral economics concludes that people often discount future payoffs too heavily, ignore decisions that do not rise to the top of the mind, and use heuristics instead of decision rules, among other cognitive shortcuts (DellaVigna, 2009). Thus, factors such as the timing and salience of incentives may sometimes overwhelm the importance of the size of the incentive. Nevertheless, a larger incentive will always be at least as salient as a smaller incentive and often more so *ceteris paribus*, though doubling the incentives will not always double the impact.

Individuals may be highly sensitive to small, immediate rewards. If a person is indifferent between completing and not completing a health-related task, even a small incentive may be sufficient to motivate a person. For example, Thornton (2008) demonstrated that monetary rewards as small as $0.10 to $0.20 increased the willingness of individuals in rural Malawi to accept HIV testing by 43 percentage points. Higgins *et al.* (1991) were the first to test an escalating reward schedule that paid in increasing increments over time to ward off participant fatigue from setting in. This approach has been repeated in a number of studies that reward abstinence from substance use, similar to Higgins *et al.*'s (1991) original application of the design to cocaine use.

Another relevant dimension for any incentive-based program is the schedule of delivery. Behavioral economists, such as Loewenstein *et al.* (2013), have argued that small and frequent payments for good health behavior can be more effective than programs with large, lump-sum incentives that are less visible. For example, less salient benefits would include those added to an existing payment, as opposed to a separate additional payment, even if the total amount is held constant. Frequent incentives take advantage of individuals' psychological bias toward immediate rewards while at the same time serving as a counterweight for the lure of immediate gratification from unhealthy behaviors.

Some researchers have experimented with lottery-based incentives. For example, Volpp *et al.* (2008b) tested an intervention in which participants were eligible for a daily lottery if they met a weight loss goal. A key advantage of lotteries as contingent incentives is their potential cost-effectiveness. The lotteries also make use of people's tendency to over-estimate the probability of rare outcomes and desire to avoid regret (loss aversion) (Kahneman and Tversky, 1979). Head-to-head research on lottery versus other designs is rare though, with apparently conflicting results. Halpern *et al.* (2011) found that unconditional fixed incentives for clinicians' response to surveys were superior to low-probability and high-probability lotteries. However, Haisley *et al.* (2012) found that a lottery, the entry to which was conditional on 4 to 8 team members completing a task, was about one-third more effective at promoting personal health risk assessments than were grocery gift certificates and no additional incentives. Petry *et al.* (2007) found that lotteries were more effective than a fixed-value reward of equal expected value. More research is needed to understand the conditions under which these different incentive schemes are effective.

Another important design feature is the unit targeted by the incentives. The majority of incentives aim to influence individual behavior. However, others explicitly recognize the social context in which individuals operate by simultaneously targeting the behavior of multiple household members. CCT programs are the most common of this variety, often making incentives contingent on the behavior of all children within a household and sometimes of the parents as well. A newer, less tested approach awards incentives to groups or teams of individuals in an effort to marshal social support and social pressure. The evidence to date indicates that group incentive schemes are a promising approach for promoting smoking cessation (White *et al.*, 2013), physical activity (Babcock *et al.*, 2015), and weight loss (Jeffery *et al.*, 1983), and may be applicable to other health behaviors. A similar unit-level decision is who receives the incentive payment: in some cases, providing the payment to mothers or teens may have different effects from payments to fathers (Thomas, 1991; 1994).

A further consideration is the population that an incentive-based program targets. The expansion of CCT programs in Latin America was motivated by a desire to reduce health inequities through the redistribution of resources. The programs tended to target lower-income households as a way to maximize impact. As similar programs have spread to countries in Asia and Africa, they have tended to be available to the general population. In part, governments wish to avoid the potentially large costs of developing and maintaining a targeting mechanism (Ranganathan and Lagarde, 2012). This shift in emphasis toward stimulating population demand for health interventions and away from reducing health inequities gives second-generation programs a distinctly different flavor from their progenitors.

Prominent Health and Health Care Domains in Which Incentives Have Been Used

This section reviews the use of incentives across a variety of health and health care domains. As a whole, incentives have been used in a wide variety of contexts. In many of these domains there have been only a few studies, and most of these have been observational with imperfect statistical controls and failed to fully distinguish incentive effects from other aspects of the interventions. In some domains, the accumulated evidence is drawn primarily from high-income countries, with unknown generalizability to developing countries. In other domains, the discussion highlights a single major efficacy study but without confirmatory studies or longer-term effectiveness evaluations from scaled-up implementations.

The discussion divides programs into three categories based on the target of the incentives: health care-seeking behavior, non-medical health behaviors, and health outcomes. The first two targets are directed toward the behavioral processes that contribute to a person's health status. The latter target is directed toward aspects of a person's health status itself. Incentives for medical and non-medical behaviors differ in certain important ways from incentives for health outcomes. First, whereas the former categories of incentives seek to directly modify targeted health behaviors, incentives for health outcomes operate more indirectly, leaving it to the discretion of the potential recipient to decide which behaviors to change and how. Second, a major distinction lies in the extent to which the target is under the individual's control. Health care utilization and non-medical health behaviors are more plausibly under an individual's control (assuming supply-side service availability, and reasonable prices relative to income) whereas health outcomes are far less so. A person's genetic make-up, environmental conditions, culture, and economic constraints interact with a person's behaviors to produce a relationship in which a person's health-related behaviors only imperfectly shape subsequent health outcomes. The trade-offs among these types of incentives are further discussed below.

There is also a distinction between incentives employed in stand-alone programs versus larger incentives embedded in CCT programs. The first part of this section addresses primarily the former, while the last part addresses findings specifically from CCT incentives.

Incentivizing health care utilization

Due to the major policy focus on maternal and child health services in developing countries, it is not surprising that incentives have been explored in a wide range of related health care areas including family planning, prenatal care, facility-based childbirth, and good childcare such as vaccinations, among others. In addition to incentives directed at increasing utilization of those services, this review discusses incentives for health screening such as HIV testing, as well as for the growing emphasis on chronic disease maintenance efforts such as medication adherence.

- *Family planning*

There is a long history of governments using incentives related to family planning. Heil *et al.* (2012) recently reviewed the published literature evaluating such efforts, and found that while it is suggestive of substantial impacts, the available studies are primarily observational rather than randomized, generally lack strong statistical analysis, and suffer from possible self-reporting bias concerns. Furthermore, one set of efforts involved incentives for sterilization, which is fraught with ethical problems, and these controversial efforts may have contributed to widespread aversion to the idea of incentives. Somewhat less controversial efforts have included incentives for attending family planning education sessions, continuation of reversible contraceptives, and incentives for altered family size. The last of these has been employed as well by countries attempting to increase low fertility rates, but such efforts have not been systematically evaluated.

- *Facility-based childbirth*

A persistent maternal-infant health concern has been the low share of pregnant women in many poor settings who give birth in health facilities. Lim *et al.* (2010) reported on a large, national program in India (Janani Suraksha Yojana, or JSY) offering women \$15–\$30 cash incentives for facility-based deliveries. They found that the program increased the proportion of in-facility births by over 40 percentage points, with significant accompanying reductions in perinatal and neonatal mortality (the study lacked power to assess maternal mortality). Nevertheless, the program has been controversial. In many areas of the country, the health facilities were unprepared to provide increased capacity or quality of care was low, thus undermining the program, and uneven implementation resulted in lower take-up among the least educated women. Gopichandran and Chetlapalli (2012) argued that these and other problems combined to make the intervention unethical. Amudhan *et al.* (2013) found in a separate analysis that supply-side service expansions were of limited effect on their own, and that combining supply-side expansions with demand-side incentives yielded the largest increases in facility-based deliveries. The overall determination of whether the JSY program was cost-effective and a better use of resources than alternatives will be quite complex, but evidence does suggest that this type of incentive is effective. A related study by Powell-Jackson and Hanson (2010) observed a somewhat smaller increase in facility deliveries from a similar program in Nepal; the authors attributed the relatively smaller magnitude of the treatment effects to challenges in implementing the program (Powell-Jackson *et al.*, 2009), which is a common and often formidable challenge to such programs. Nguyen *et al.* (2012) found that institutional deliveries in affected areas of Bangladesh increased 10–20 percentage points after the introduction of free delivery and transportation vouchers for women and provider incentives.

- *Prenatal care*

The above-mentioned JSY program incentivizing institutional delivery in India was also found to increase prenatal care, but by a much smaller amount — and it is unclear whether this was due to the delivery incentive or separate provider incentives that were part of the program. Some have proposed amending the JSY program to explicitly incentivize prenatal care attendance — but the evidence in support of the proposal is difficult to extrapolate. Again, there are scattered studies that provide mixed evidence. Morris *et al.* (2004) estimated that a CCT incentive in Honduras significantly increased prenatal care; in contrast, Barber and Gertler (2008) found no impact of Mexico's Oportunidades conditional cash transfer program on prenatal care, but this was largely because of very high baseline rates.

In another intriguing study, Dupas (2005) found that distributing free bed nets at prenatal clinics in Kenya substantially increased take-up of prenatal services. Thus, the evidence reinforces that services such as prenatal care can be responsive to incentives, but the nature of recommended interventions will depend crucially on local circumstances.

- *Vaccination*

Much of the recent evidence on incentives for vaccination comes from CCT programs, discussed further below. But another common tactic has been stand-alone incentives in vaccination programs, such as free food to parents who bring their children for vaccination. These incentives are particularly attractive for hard-to-reach populations, such as in hotspots in the polio eradication effort. But as with many other uses of incentives, they have rarely been systematically evaluated, much less using randomized methods. One exception is the recent Banerjee *et al.* (2010) study of a randomized controlled trial in India, in which villages were randomized to receive either an immunization camp, a camp combined with small food incentives, or neither. After 18 months, child immunization rates were 18% with camps versus 6% in controls, but 39% when food incentives were added, as compared to less than 2% pre-intervention. The value of the incentive was designed to be roughly equivalent to the opportunity cost of the mother's time. Relatively unique among such studies, the authors also conducted a cost-effectiveness analysis and argued that the camps with food incentives had lower costs per immunized child than the camps alone, and that the intervention was cost-effective overall.

- *Disease screening*

One-time screening behaviors are a potentially promising target for incentives, as procrastination is a common barrier to such screenings. An example of this is HIV screening. Thornton (2008) found that in a Malawi HIV screening intervention only 34% of those without an incentive picked up their HIV test result, but even small incentives on the order of an hour's wages resulted in roughly doubling the percentage picking up their test results. This example is not directly generalizable to many HIV screening interventions that currently use rapid tests, but the result is nevertheless striking and suggestive of results that could be obtained for other related types of services. For example, Montoy *et al.* (2013) show in an unpublished working paper that incentives as small as $10 increased HIV screening rates at a US hospital by 15 percentage points from a 52% base.

• *Medication adherence*

Medication adherence has been frequently suggested as a promising target for incentive use, and there are many examples of medication adherence programs harnessing incentives. Most of the published studies evaluating such efforts have been conducted in high-income countries, with much less systematic evidence gathered from developing countries. Furthermore, much of the literature is based on observational designs, is frequently unable to distinguish the effects of patient incentives from accompanying supply-side efforts, and many studies were conducted among high-risk subpopulations that make generalization difficult. Galárraga *et al.* (2014) reviews HIV treatment adherence; Lutge *et al.* (2012) and Beith *et al.* (2009) both review tuberculosis treatment adherence; and DeFulio and Silverman (2012) and Petry *et al.* (2012) review the literature across multiple types of medications, with the latter providing a formal meta-analysis. Overall, the evidence indicates that indeed such incentives can be effective, but there is a fade-out of the effects after removal of the incentives.

Incentivizing non-medical health behaviors

Monetary incentives have been used extensively to modify non-medical health behaviors. Researchers began to adopt the approach, in one of the first applications of incentives in the health domain, as early as the 1960s. Many behavioral researchers call these incentives contingency management, which is the term used for substance abuse treatment that employs cash incentives to promote drug abstinence. Since the development of contingency management, the thrust of the literature has been on rewarding abstinence from use of addictive substances, including tobacco, although the techniques have been applied to a range of other behaviors. This section discusses the use of incentives for deterring substance use, abstaining from smoking, and promoting physical activity. Although this research is drawn largely from the United States, it is relevant to global health considerations as increasing chronic disease burdens in developing countries will make similar approaches important to consider in coming decades.

A meta-analysis of contingency management programs for substance use disorders found that they raised compliance 32% on average (Lussier *et al.*, 2006). Studies have also shown a positive effect of incentives on attendance of treatment sessions at a clinic. Most of the included studies focused on patients who were dependent on cocaine or opiates. Whereas pharmacological and psychosocial interventions have often failed to alter the cocaine consumption of users, financial incentives have proven a viable promoter of abstinence. The positive effects have also been found in the handful of studies that have looked at carryover effects after discontinuation of the incentives (Higgins *et al*., 1993, 2000; Silverman *et al*., 1996). The effect sizes were larger for studies that offered vouchers of greater monetary value.

Smokers' responsiveness to personal cash incentives for quitting has yielded mixed results. A meta-analysis indicates that contingency management has been more effective for treating opiate and cocaine use than tobacco use (Prendergast *et al*., 2006) (See also Volume 2, Chapter 6 in this Handbook on *Smoking*). A systematic review of cash incentives for smoking cessation concludes that, although incentives raise quit rates in the short term, they do not tend to translate into long-run abstinence (Cahill and Perera, 2011). Troxel and Volpp (2012), however, reanalyze the data from Cahill and Perera's (2011) systematic review. Their main finding is that most studies are under-powered to detect small to moderate treatment effects. Many studies included in the systematic review also suffer from high attrition rates, as high as 40–50% in some cases. These limitations imply that the weak empirical designs of published studies do not *yet* allow researchers to reliably infer the impact of monetary incentives on smoking cessation — a sobering conclusion given the substantial research effort in this area.

Some studies from the cash-for-quitting literature have shown positive results. Volpp *et al*. (2006) found that modest financial bonuses did not lead to lasting quits, whereas Volpp *et al*. (2009) found that larger financial bonuses ($250 for 6-month test passage, $400 for 12-month test passage) offered through a workplace program in the United States increased both short-term cessation and lasting quits. Another area of success has been incentive-based programs for pregnant and newly postpartum women who smoke. Higgins *et al*. (2012) conducted a review that indicated the intervention increased fetal growth, birth weight, and breastfeeding duration.

Physical activity is another domain in which monetary incentives have been tested in high-income countries. Mitchell *et al*. (2013) conducted a systematic review and meta-analysis of the effect of monetary incentives on exercise adherence. In the 11 randomized controlled trials identified by the authors, 8 found a significant increase in exercise associated with the incentive and the pooled results were also positive. However, only one of the studies lasted for more than 1 year (Jeffery *et al*., 1998). Larger incentives yielded larger effects. The largest gap in the literature is the post-intervention effect of the incentives. Charness and Gneezy (2012) produced the only available evidence on physical activity after the incentives ended; they found that an increase in gym attendance persisted for 5 weeks in one trial and 16 weeks in another. However, Acland and Levy (2015) replicated the study by Charness and Gneezy (2012) and found that the post-intervention effect tapered over time.

Incentivizing health outcomes

Health outcomes represent a relatively unexplored frontier in the incentivizing health landscape. Some of the earliest studies dating back to the 1970s used incentives for weight loss, although very little research on incentives for health outcomes was conducted in the subsequent two decades. Recently, there has been a renewal of interest, although the inherent multi-factorial nature of health outcome determination makes it more challenging than providing incentives for discrete, modifiable behaviors that are more plausibly under the control of the incentivized individuals. Below is an overview of research on outcome incentives for weight loss, other chronic disease biomarkers, and sexually transmitted infections.

As obesity rates have climbed in recent decades, some researchers have turned to incentives for promoting weight loss. A series of early studies by Jeffery *et al.* (1978; 1984) tested various types of deposit contracts or commitment contracts, in which individuals made a deposit that they kept only if they met a pre-specified weight loss target. Jeffery *et al.* (1993) provided $25 per week for cumulative weight loss along with behavioral therapy. The incentives had no impact on short-term or long-term weight loss relative to therapy alone. A resurgence of research began with Finkelstein *et al.* (2007). The authors presented evidence of modest weight loss at three months but no difference at 6 months for financial rewards ranging from $7 to $14 per percentage point of weight reduction. Volpp *et al.* (2008a) tested an intervention in which participants were eligible for a daily lottery if they met a weight loss goal. The lottery group lost 13 more pounds than the control group at the end of the 16-week intervention, which persisted to 9 pounds at 7 months. However, the advantage disappeared by 32 weeks (John *et al.*, 2011). Cawley and Price (2013) compared a cash bonus to commitment contracts for weight loss in 24 worksites and found that the bonus led to high attrition, whereas the contracts limited take-up but promoted greater weight loss. However, the complicated reward structure, which varied by worksite and was not randomly assigned, did not allow for a clean comparison.

Several employers have experimented with workplace wellness programs that provide rewards to employees who show improvements on health outcome measures. For example, the Safeway grocery store chain in the United States offers up to $800 in rebates on an individual's health insurance premiums (up to $1,600 for families) in exchange for improvements in biomarkers such as blood pressure, fasting glucose, cholesterol, body mass index, and tobacco use. A growing number of employers have implemented such programs on the promise that they can slow medical cost inflation for the firm and increase worker productivity. Despite some hints that wellness programs can save money for employers (Baicker *et al.*, 2010), little rigorous research has tested the proposition.

A very different domain in which incentives for health outcomes have been recently tested is the controversial area of sexually transmitted infections, a domain in which the inability to verify risky behaviors makes it impossible to incentivize reducing those behaviors. In settings of high HIV risk, progress has been made in slowing the AIDS epidemic, but many such as Padian *et al.* (2011) are calling for new and expanded prevention efforts. In this context, several recent studies have tested the potential for incentives that reward negative tests for sexually transmitted infections as a marker for risky sexual behavior. de Walque *et al.* (2012b) discussed this approach in more detail, but to date only a handful of early studies are available. Kohler and Thornton (2012) tested incentives for HIV-negative individuals in Malawi to stay negative for a 1-year period, finding no significant effect, but the study was not well-powered to examine HIV incidence. de Walque *et al.* (2012a) reported on a randomized trial in rural Tanzania that followed up every 4 months with incentive rewards for individuals who remained negative on tests for a range of curable sexually transmitted infections. That study found that after 1 year, $20 incentives every 4 months led to a 27% reduction in infections relative to a control group that received all aspects of the intervention (such as counselling, free testing and free treatment) other than the incentive payments. Galárraga *et al.* (2013) found that at-risk populations in Mexico City such as men who have sex with men, including male sex workers, stated that they were willing to accept money to reduce risks for HIV and other sexually transmitted infections. Similar ongoing trials in other settings are expected to publish further results soon. This area of investigation is quite early still though, as these are largely efficacy trials designed to test whether sexual health outcomes respond to incentives, and no study has yet tested a variant designed to be sustainable for scale-up in low-income settings. As with related CCT programs discussed below, however, even if found to be effective, the sustainability of programs to incentivize better sexual health may depend critically on the extent to which program funders consider the incentive payments to be stand-alone efforts to improve health in targeted high-risk populations, or instead as part of larger social welfare cash assistance programs.

Conditional Cash Transfer Programs

Since the implementation of Mexico's Progresa/Oportunidades/Prospera program beginning in 1997 (see Case Study), a number of governments — most prominently in Latin America — have adopted CCT programs that have multiple objectives, including both poverty alleviation and building human capital in key areas such as health. Often multi-sectoral in nature, these programs have commonly included health care conditionality incentives, so that in order to receive recurring cash payments, the individuals must have documentation of targeted health care use such as prenatal care, vaccination, and other well child care. Much has been written on the success of these programs, including reviews by Lagarde *et al.* (2007), Parker *et al.* (2008), and Fiszbein and Schady (2009). One of the most recent is a systematic review by Ranganathan and Lagarde (2012), who reviewed the findings from quasi-experimental or experimental evaluations of 13 different CCT programs; key findings from this review are summarized below. Despite large contextual differences across program designs and study settings, CCT programs have generally been found to be acceptable, scalable, and effective in significantly improving several health-related behaviors and outcomes.

Case Study: *Progresa — Oportunidades:* Mexico's Conditional Cash Transfer Program

Oportunidades, formerly known as *Progresa*, is a conditional cash transfer (CCT) program launched in Mexico in 1997. The program was initially motivated by the idea that poverty alleviation could be best accomplished through human capital investments in the poor, with the goal of increasing the income potential of future generations (Levy 2006).[1]

Progresa/Oportunidades aimed to accomplish this goal by conditioning the cash transfers on households' compliance with required health visits and school attendance. Not only did the cash transfers provided the households with additional income, but also by conditioning on health and education, the next generation may be better prepared for better paying jobs in the future. Cash was transferred to the female head of household, unless no female head was available. The justification for this targeting was that women were hypothesized to be more likely than men to invest the money in the household (e.g., food) rather than their own personal benefit. On the supply side, the government was supposed to provide schools and health centers if the households were expected to attend them (Levy and Rodríguez, 2005). Thus, *Progresa/Oportunidades* excluded communities without access to basic education and primary health facilities. These populations were served by other programs.

Enrolled households received a basic grant that was conditional on meeting minimum attendance requirements at a health clinic. A complementary education

[1]As of September 1, 2014, the program is called *Prospera.*

component provided additional cash to the household for students in grades 3–12, conditional on their enrollment and school attendance (at least 85%) (García-Ramírez 2013). The amount of the cash transfer increased annually, roughly in proportion to the increasing opportunity cost of the child's labor. Girls received a higher transfer than boys (except during primary school), because girls were less likely than boys to attend secondary school when the program started. Cash transfers were not provided for children below grade 3, partly to avoid paying for attendance that was already almost universal at grades 1 and 2, and because lengthening the time from birth to transfer onset could reduce any possible pronatalist effect of the program. Unlike the federally supported Aid to Families with Dependent Children (AFDC) program in the US, Mexican household eligibility depended on poverty but not fertility; households did not need to have children to be eligible, further decreasing the likelihood of an unintended pronatalist effect of the program (Gueron, 1987).

The health and nutrition services provided through the health clinics included: family planning, prenatal and postpartum care, nutrition and growth monitoring, vaccinations, and screening and treatment for infectious and chronic diseases. The required visits depended on age and sex, with the highest frequency for pregnant women and young children (Van de Gaer *et al.*, 2014). Households received supplemental nutrition for pregnant mothers and young children, although compliance with nutritional recommendations was not a condition for receiving funds.

The program provided cash to the families rather than goods in-kind, under the assumption that households were best informed about their needs. *Progresa/Oportunidades* gradually replaced a number of programs that subsidized specific commodities for the general population. Later modifications of *Progresa/Oportunidades* included increasing cash transfers to seniors older than 70 living in urban areas, compensation for increased energy costs, and supplemental transfers for households whose food expenditure was greater than half of their monetary income (García-Ramírez, 2013).

How was it rolled out?

In 1997, when the CCT program started, there were approximately 4.8 million households living in extreme poverty, totaling 27.5 million people and representing 29.3% of the total population. About 56% (15.4 million) lived in rural areas. Therefore, the program first prioritized the most impoverished populations living in rural areas.

Targeting became a challenge when the program was expanded to cover people in urban areas with more heterogeneous socio-economic status and a lower prevalence of poverty. The program grew rapidly: 140 thousand households were covered in 1997, 4.2 million in 2003, and 5.8 million in 2010. By the end of April 2014, the program covered 95.8% (5.8 million) of its target household universe (6.1 million). Women heads-of-household received the cash transfers in 96% of households (Levy and Rodríguez, 2005; Coordinación Nacional, 2010).

How was it evaluated?

The CCT program worked with researchers to carry out a rigorous prospective, randomized evaluation of the program's impact on health, nutrition and education. Subsequent phases were accompanied by modified evaluation protocols, including differential promotion, regression discontinuity, and propensity score matching, among others. The first phase of the program, the rural village implementation in 1997, incorporated 140,544 households in 3,369 randomly assigned localities. In early 2000, the CCT program included around 2.6 million families distributed in 72,345 localities (Adato and Hoddinott, 2010). This initial community randomization and subsequent phased roll-out enabled a strong suite of research designs that helped to set a new standard for rigorous evaluation of large social programs.

What were the key findings?

The key findings of several external studies include (García-Ramírez, 2013):

Educational Outcomes

- Reduction of child labor (40%) and boys' school dropout (17.4%) in rural areas.
- Increase in secondary school enrollment in rural areas, both for girls (28.7%) and boys (15.7%).
- Increase in high school enrollment, both in urban (10.1%) and rural (85%) areas.
- Increase in the proportion of women in secondary education, both in rural (from 83 girls for every 100 boys to 96) and urban areas (from 92 girls per 100 boys in seventh grade to 95, from 95 girls per 100 boys in seventh grade to 99, with girls already in the majority in the ninth grade).
- Increase in the probability of successfully transitioning from primary to secondary school in rural areas, both for girls (25.7%–32.5% depending on the age of the girl at the time of transition) and for boys (32.9%–41.5%).
- One additional year of school among 15–19 year old students in the program versus a control population in rural areas.

Health Care Utilization and Health Outcomes

- Reduction in hospital visits in children under two years old in rural areas (58%).
- Increase in effective demand for health services, both in rural areas (between 30% and 50% increase depending on age) and urban areas (between 25% and 30% increase).
- Increased demand for prenatal (3.5% higher than women not enrolled in the program) and well-baby visits.
- Reduction in maternal (11%) and infant (2%) mortality rates.
- Reduction in sick days per family in rural areas (20% for reduction for children 0–5 years old, and 11% for those 6–49 years old) and urban areas (24% for children 6–15 years old, 50% for those 16–40 years old).
- Increased food expenditure (10.4%).
- Increased average child height (1 cm) and weight (0.5 kg).
- Reduction in emaciation.
- Reduction in anemia (25.2%).
- Small reduction in pregnancy and genital herpes in adolescents.
- Reduction in respiratory infections (4.5%), fever (4%) and diarrheal episodes (2.6%) in children under two.

It is more difficult to discern the impact of the program on macro-level poverty indicators at the national level. Poverty measurements were first estimated in 1992, and include a variety of measures: alimentary poverty line (households are unable to purchase the basic food basket even if they expend their entire disposable income), capacities poverty line (disposable household income is insufficient to purchase the basic food basket and cover expenses related to health and education), and patrimonial poverty line (the disposable income of the household does not cover the expenses for the basic food basket, health, education, clothing, transportation and housing) (CONEVAL, 2012).

As seen in Figure 1, implementation of the program was associated with a relative reduction in every poverty measure, but absolute poverty increased from 1990 to 2010 in every measure except the number of households living in sub-standard housing. This may not be the best way to measure the impact of the program, especially since the 1995 financial crisis had a major impact (see Figure 2) and the program took a decade to scale up after its 1997 inception. The financial crisis of 2008 was an additional blow (CONEVAL, 2012). Thus, despite its successes, *Progresa/Oportunidades* has not yet solved the problems of Mexico's poor. Much remains to be done.

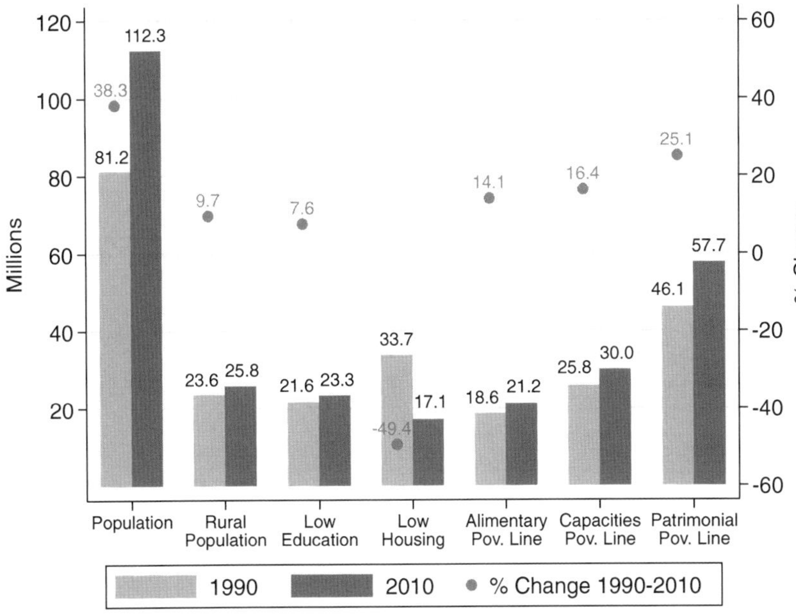

Figure 1. Demographic and SES changes in Mexico, 1990–2010

Note: The baseline poverty line is from 1992.
Source: INEGI (1990) and INEGI (2010).

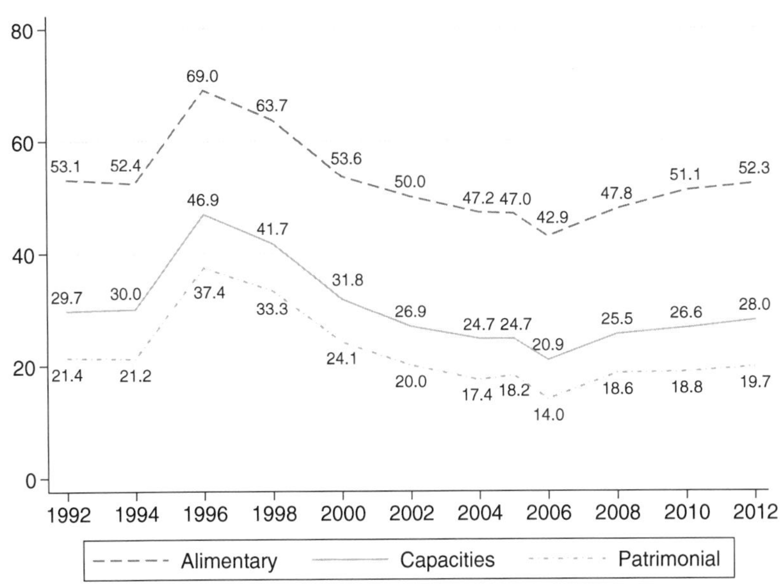

Figure 2. Percentage of the population of Mexico by poverty lines, 1992–2010

Source: CONEVAL (2012).

Ten studies have documented the impact of CCTs on the utilization of health services, such as the number of prenatal visits by pregnant women, well-child visits, and use of preventive health services. Uptake of prenatal visits was found to increase significantly in Honduras (Morris *et al.*, 2004) and in India where the incentives were not conditioned on clinic visits (Lim *et al.*, 2010). In Chile, where participating households received an UCT and advice from a social worker, Galasso (2011) reported no change in the share that received regular prenatal visits.

The evidence for preventive health visits among children in participating families is somewhat conflicting. There were no program effects on well-child visits in Mexico and Honduras but positive effects in Colombia, in Chile (among infants but not other ages), and in Nicaragua. A mixed picture emerged for a program-related bump in immunization coverage in Colombia, Honduras, Mexico, and Nicaragua. Certain populations of children benefited from increased coverage of certain vaccine types in each country.

One of the biggest successes of the CCT programs was the observed increase in height-for-age and decrease in stunting of children in participating households. Height-for-age is one of the best physiological measures of a child's health, nutrition, and development and highly predictive of later-life health. A positive impact on height occurred in Brazil, Colombia, Mexico, and Nicaragua (Lagarde *et al.*, 2007).

A key factor underlying the growth of CCT programs is their potential as a means for poverty alleviation. This could then potentially lead to even larger health and human development benefits in the future generation, i.e., the future children of better educated mothers, but it is too soon for systematic empirical evidence to evaluate such outcomes. Another attraction of CCT programs has been the potential for reduction of health inequities. Gopalan *et al.* (2013) review the literature and find that the programs often reach vulnerable populations, although in some cases the programs fail to reach the neediest households. Identifying poor households and targeting incentives to them is essential for maximizing social impact, but it is an enduring challenge for many CCT programs.

Recently, a small literature evaluating UCT programs has developed. UCTs differ from CCTs in that the former operate only via income increases, with no use of incentives — the targeted units receive the cash support with no monitoring of health care utilization, etc. Thus, comparing UCT to CCT programs provides a way to test the effects of specific incentives separate from income effects. UCTs are also administratively cheaper, but in the absence of incentives, they may have lower effectiveness in increasing health and health care. Baird *et al.* (2010; 2012) found that a CCT program for schooling in Malawi, with only schooling but not health-related incentive conditionality, nevertheless had important spillover effects on health, reducing the prevalence of teen pregnancy, HIV and herpes simplex infections in adolescent female recipients. The authors further compared the schooling effects to a UCT and found that the reduction in teenage pregnancy was due entirely to the impact of the UCT (Baird *et al.*, 2011). In a different setting, Akresh *et al.* (2012) implemented a 2-year program that randomly distributed transfers to parents that were either unconditional or conditional on routine health visits for infants. The CCT significantly increased the number of visits compared to the control group, whereas the UCT had no effect. Robertson *et al.* (2013) followed a similar design in Zimbabwe, with the CCT conditioned on several child wellbeing measures, including vaccination, but found no significant effect on vaccinations in either the UCT or CCT group, though the share of children who received birth certificates was highest in the UCT group. Despite the mixed evidence that shows no CCT advantage over UCTs in some cases, theory suggests that UCT effects on health behaviors may fade-out, as the novelty of the additional UCT income wears off and gets redirected to other less salutary household expenditures more quickly than with CCTs. Nevertheless, these disparate findings on UCT versus CCT programs reinforce the fact that much is still to be learned about the effects of incentives.

Discussion

Incentive approaches to health promotion have been eschewed by many stakeholders in debates over promising directions for population and development policies to improve health care utilization and health outcomes. This is often for good reason: incentives will rarely be the first-line policy approach, particularly in settings in which health knowledge is low and the supply of health services is inadequate. Yet some commentators appear to categorically reject the notion of incentives without careful comparison to traditional supply-side subsidies, without deep consideration of the competing ethical imperatives, and without knowledge of the accumulating economic and psychological evidence on their effectiveness. To be sure, some thoughtful and well-informed participants in such debates will continue to reject incentives for a variety of reasons. Yet the overall body of evidence reviewed above, despite its many limitations, conveys sufficient promise so as to suggest an obligation to continue formative research, policy experimentation, and rigorous evaluation of potentially cost-effective incentive-based approaches.

Among incentive approaches, CCT programs have been embraced most widely to date. It is perhaps not a coincidence that the first prominent such program, Mexico's *Progresa*, was developed by Mexican policy innovators rather than imposed from outside. The development community has a critical role in conducting evaluations of such programs, objectively assessing the promise and limitations, and working with local policymakers to refine their ideas for local adaptation of incentive programs. The wisdom of incentivizing specific domains in any given population and the detailed design decisions will depend critically on local considerations. Effectiveness of incentives will depend on many parameters including current prices (fees, time, and travel costs), incomes, disease prevalence, health service utilization, knowledge, attitudes, acceptability, administrative capacity, and so on. Also crucial for the design of CCT programs is the decision of which health domains to incentivize: Limited administrative capacity as well as incentivized individuals' limited attention both suggest the importance of focusing incentives on a narrow set of highly salient behaviors that reflect major national health priorities. Although none of the potential domains for incentives that were reviewed above are supported by a large body of unequivocally positive results, for many of them there is at least one setting in which a design has been adapted and found to be efficacious or effective.

When considering types of incentive domains, those that incentivize health outcomes have the smallest accumulated evidence base, and policy experimentation is likely to proceed slowly while awaiting a more robust body of knowledge from formative and efficacy studies.

Those domains that reward non-medical health behaviors have been studied in more detail in high-income settings, with few studies in developing countries. Yet growing chronic disease prevalence in developing countries will lead to increased attention to chronic disease prevention strategies in developing countries. Incentivizing health behaviors related to obesity, however, has not yet shown great promise. Substance abuse interventions such as contingency management may have generalizable promise for middle-income countries, and potentially low-income settings as well, though further work on potential cost-effectiveness will be needed. The demand for smoking cessation interventions in developing countries is likely to increase substantially in coming decades as well, and innovative approaches to harnessing incentives to increase their effectiveness holds great promise. As female smoking rates increase, incentives targeted at smoking cessation among pregnant women may become increasingly attractive to explore.

Finally, all of the discussed examples of incentivizing health care utilization hold promise for policy exploration in relevant settings. Maternal and child morbidity and mortality have improved dramatically in many developing countries in recent decades, but there is great scope for further increasing uptake of known effective interventions. Combining health education and health service supply expansions along with demand-side incentives creates potentially powerful synergies. These will require considerable administrative capacity, but mobile and digital technologies that are rapidly diffusing to even the lowest income settings may help reduce some of the administrative barriers. The increasing trend toward rigorous impact evaluation of policy experimentation will also help accelerate the ability to learn from successes and failures, so as to generate a much stronger evidence base to inform increasing development policy experimentation with incentives for health care utilization over the coming decades.

References

Acland D, Levy M. 2015. Naiveté, projection bias, and habit formation in gym attendance. *Management Science* 61(1): 146–160.

Adato M, Hoddinott J. (eds.). 2010. *Conditional Cash Transfers in Latin America*, International Food Policy Research Institute — The John Hopkins University Press, Baltimore.

Akresh R, Damien de Walque, Harounan Kazianga. 2012. Alternative cash transfer delivery mechanisms: Impacts on routine preventative health clinic visits in Burkina Faso. *National Bureau of Economic Research Working Paper No.* 17785.

Amudhan S, Kalaivani Mani, Sanjay K Rai, Chandrakant S Pandav, Anand Krishnan. 2013. Effectiveness of demand and supply side interventions in promoting institutional deliveries — a quasi-experimental trial from rural north India. *International Journal of Epidemiology* 42:769–780.

Babcock, P, Kelly B, Gary C, John H, Heather R. 2015. Letting down the team? Evidence of social effects of team incentives. *Journal of the European Economic Association*. In press.

Baicker K, David Cutler, Zirui Song. 2010. Workplace wellness programs can generate savings. *Health Affairs* 29(2): 1–8.

Baird, Sarah, Ephraim Chirwa, Craig McIntosh, Berk Özler. 2010. The short-term impacts of a schooling conditional cash transfer program on the sexual behavior of young women. *Health Economics* 19(S1): 55–68.

Baird Sarah J, Richard S. Garfein, Craig T. McIntosh, Berk Özler. 2012. Effect of a cash transfer programme for schooling on prevalence of HIV and herpes simplex type 2 in Malawi: A cluster randomised trial. *The Lancet* 379: 1320–29.

Baird Sarah, Craig McIntosh, Berk Özler. 2011. Cash, or condition: Evidence from a cash transfer experiment. *The Quarterly Journal of Economics* 126: 1709–1753.

Banerjee A, Duflo E, Glennerster R, D Kothari. 2010. Improving immunization coverage in rural India: a clustered randomized controlled evaluation of immunization campaigns with and without incentives. *British Medical Journal* 340: c2220.

Barber S, Gertler P. 2008. The impact of Mexico's conditional cash transfer program, Oportunidades, on birth weight. *Tropical Medicine and International Health* 2008a: 13.

Bénabou R, Tirole J. 2003. Intrinsic and extrinsic motivation. *The Review of Economic Studies* 70: 489–520.

Beith A, Rena Eichler, Diana Weil. 2009. Worldwide: incentives for tuberculosis diagnosis and treatment. In *Performance Incentives for Global Health-Potentials and Pitfalls*,

Rena Eichler, Ruth Levine, and the Performance-Based Incentives Working Group, ed. Washington, DC: Center for Global Development.

Bowles S, Polania-Reyes S. 2012. Economic incentives and social preferences: Substitutes or complements? *Journal of Economic Literature* 50(20): 368–425.

Cahill K, Rafael P. 2011. Competitions and incentives for smoking cessation. *The Cochrane Database of Systematic Reviews* 4: CD004307.

Cameron J, Banko KM, Pierce WD. 2001. Pervasive negative effects of rewards on intrinsic motivation: The myth continues. *Behavioral Analyst* 24(1): 1–44.

Cawley J, Price JA. 2013. A case study of a workplace wellness program that offers financial incentives for weight loss. *Journal of Health Economics* 32(5): 794–803.

Charness G, Gneezy U. 2012. Incentives to exercise. *Econometrica* 77(3): 909–931.

CONEVAL 2012. *Medición de La Pobreza. Evolución de Las Dimensiones de La Pobreza 1990–2012.* Available from: http://www.coneval.gob.mx/Medicion/Paginas/Evolucion-de-las-dimensiones-de-la-pobreza-1990-2010-.aspx>. [29 January 2015].

Coordinación Nacional del Programa de Desarrollo Humano Oportunidades 2010. *Matriz de Indicadores de Resultados Del Programa Oportunidades (por Entidad Federativa).* Available from: <http://www.oportunidades.gob.mx/Portal/work/sites/Web/resources/ArchivoContent/1182/IND_MIR_2010_06_SEP-OCT_RO_.xls>. [29 January 2015].

Deci, E L., Richard Koestner, Richard M. Ryan 1999. A meta-analytic review of experiments examining the effects of extrinsic rewards on intrinsic motivation. *Psychological Bulletin* 125(6): 627–668.

DellaVigna S. 2009. Psychology and economics: Evidence from the field. *Journal of Economic Literature* 47(2): 315–372.

DeFulio A, Silverman K. 2012. The use of incentives to reinforce medication adherence. *Preventive Medicine*, 55, Supplement: S86–S94.

de Walque, D, William H. Dow, Rose Nathan, *et al.* 2012a. Incentivising safe sex: a randomised trial of conditional cash transfers for HIV and sexually transmitted infection prevention in rural Tanzania. *BMJ Open*, 2: e000747.

de Walque, D, William H. Dow, Carol Medlin, Rose Nathan. 2012b. Stimulating demand for AIDS prevention: Lessons from the RESPECT trial. *National Bureau of Economic Research Working Paper No.* 17865.

Dupas P. 2005. The impact of conditional in-kind subsidies on preventative health behaviors: evidence from Kenya. Unpublished manuscript, EHESS-PSE, Paris; http://www.econ.ucla.edu/pdupas/TAMTAMpaper07.11.05.pdf.

Dupas P. 2013. Short-run subsidies and long-run adoption of new health products: Evidence from a field experiment. *Econometrica* 82(1): 197–228.

Fehr E, Falk A. 2002. Psychological foundations of incentives. *European Economic Review* 46: 687–724.

Finkelstein EA, Laura A. Linnan, Deborah F. Tate, Ben E. Birken. 2007. A pilot study testing the effect of different levels of financial incentives on weight loss among overweight employees. *Journal of Occupational and Environmental Medicine* 49(9): 981–989.

Fiszbein A, Schady N. 2009. Conditional Cash Transfers: Reducing Present and Future Poverty. World Bank, Washington, DC.

Galárraga O, Sandra G. Sosa-Rubí, César Infante, Paul J. Gertler and Stefano M. Bertozzi 2013. Willingness-to-accept reductions in HIV risks: conditional economic incentives in Mexico. *European Journal of Health Economics* 15(1): 41–55.

Galasso E. 2011. Alleviating extreme poverty in Chile: the short term effects of Chile Solidario. *Estudios de Economía* 38(1): 101–127.

García-Ramírez JS. 2013. *Progresa-Oportunidades y su contribución en la ruptura intergeneracional de la pobreza 1997–2010*. MA thesis. Universidad Complutense de Madrid.

Gopalan SS, Ronald Mutasa, Jed Friedman, Ashis Das. 2013. Health sector demand-side financial incentives in low- and middle-income countries: A systematic review on demand- and supply-side effects. *Social Science & Medicine* 100: 72–83.

Gopichandran V, Chetlapalli SK. 2012. Conditional cash transfer to promote institutional deliveries in India: Toward a sustainable ethical model to achieve MDG 5A. *Public Health Ethics* 5(2): 173–180.

Gueron JM. 1987. *Reforming Welfare with Work. Occasional Paper 2*, Ford Foundation, New York.

Haisley E, Volpp K, Pellathy T, Loewenstein G. 2012. The impact of alternative incentive schemes on completion of health risk assessments. *Am. J. Health Promot*, 26: 184–188.

Halpern SD, Kohn, A Dornbrand-Lo R, Metkus T, Asch DA, Volpp KG. 2011. Lottery-based versus fixed incentives to increase clinicians' response to surveys. *Health Serv Res.*, 46(5): 1663–1674.

Heil SH, Diann E. Gaalema, Evan S. Herrmann. 2012. Incentives to promote family planning. *Preventive Medicine* 55(S1): S106–S112.

Higgins ST, Alan J. Budney, Warren K. Bickel, John R. Hughes, Florian Foerg, Gary Badger. 1993. Achieving cocaine abstinence with a behavioral approach. *American Journal of Psychiatry* 150: 763–769.

Higgins ST, Dawn D. Delaney, Alan J. Budney, Warren K. Bickel, John R. Hughes, Florian Foerg, James W. Fenwick. 1991. A behavioral approach to achieving initial cocaine abstinence. *American Journal of Psychiatry* 148(9): 1218–1224.

Higgins ST, Conrad J. Wong, Gary J. Badger, Doris E. Haug Ogden, Robert L. Dantona. 2000. Contingent reinforcement increases cocaine abstinence during outpatient treatment and 1 year of follow-up. *Journal of Consulting and Clinical Psychology* 68(1): 64–72.

Higgins ST, Yukiko Washio, Sarah H. Heil, Laura J. Solomon, Diann E. Gaalema, Tara M. Higgins, Ira M. Bernstein 2012. Financial incentives for smoking cessation among pregnant and newly postpartum women. Preventive Medicine, 55, Supplement: S33–S40.

INEGI. 1990. *Censo General de Población y Vivienda 1990*. Available from: <http://www.inegi.org.mx/est/contenidos/proyectos/ccpv/cpv1990/default.aspx>. [29 January 2015].

INEGI. 2010. *Censo de Población y Vivienda 2010*. Available from: <http://www.inegi.org.mx/est/contenidos/proyectos/ccpv/cpv2010/Default.aspx>. [29 January 2015].

Jeffery RW, Wendy M. Bjornson-Benson, Barbara S. Rosenthal, Ruth A. Lindquist, Sharon L. Johnson. 1984. Behavioral treatment of obesity with monetary contracting: Two-year follow-up. *Addictive Behaviors* 9(3): 311–313.

Jeffery RW, Wendy M Gerber, Barbara S Rosenthal, Ruth A Lindquist. 1983. Monetary contracts in weight control: Effectiveness of group and individual contracts of varying size. *Journal of Consulting and Clinical Psychology* 51(2): 242–248.

Jeffery RW, Paul D. Thompson, Rena R. Wing. 1978. Effects on weight reduction of strong monetary contracts for calorie restriction or weight loss. *Behaviour Research and Therapy* 16(5): 363–369.

Jeffery R, Carolyn Thorson, Rena Wing, Lisa Burton. 1998. Use of personal trainers and financial incentives to increase exercise in a behavioral weight-loss program. *Journal of Consulting and Clinical Psychology* 66(5): 777–783.

Jeffery RW, Rena R. Wing, Carolyn Thorson, Lisa R. Burton, Cheryl Raether, Jean Harvey, Monica Mullen. 1993. Strengthening behavioral interventions for weight loss: A randomized trial of food provision and monetary incentives. *Journal of Consulting and Clinical Psychology* 61(6): 1038–1045.

John L, George Loewenstein, Andrea Troxel, Laurie Norton, Jennifer Fassbender, Kevin Volpp. 2011. Financial incentives for extended weight loss: A randomized, controlled trial. *Journal of General Internal Medicine* 26: 621–626.

Kahneman D, Tversky A. 1979. Prospect theory: An analysis of decision under risk. *Econometrica* XLVII: 263–291.

Kimmel, Stephen E., Andrea B. Troxel, George Loewenstein, Colleen M. Brensinger, Jane Jaskowiak, Jalpa A. Doshi, Mitchell Laskin, Kevin Volpp. 2012. Randomized trial of lottery-based incentives to improve warfarin adherence. *American Heart Journal* 164: 268 274.

Kohler HP, Thornton R. 2012. Conditional cash transfers and HIV/AIDS prevention: Unconditionally promising? *World Bank Economic Review* 26: 165–190.

Lagarde M, Andy Haines, Natasha Palmer. 2007. Conditional cash transfers for improving uptake of health interventions in low- and middle-income countries — a systematic review. *Journal of the American Medical Association* 298: 1900–1910.

Levy, S and Banco M. 1991 Poverty alleviation in Mexico. Vol. 679. Country Department II, Latin America and the Caribbean Regional Office, World Bank.

Levy S, Rodríguez E. 2005. *Sin herencia de pobreza: El Programa Progresa. Oportunidades de México*, IADB — Planeta, Mexico.

Levy, S. 2006. Progress Against Poverty: Sustaining Mexico's Progresa-Oportunidades Program. Washington, DC: The Brookings Institution.

Lim SS, Lalit Dandona, Joseph A Hoisington, *et al*. 2010. India's Janani Suraksha Yojana, a conditional cash transfer programme to increase births in health facilities: An impact evaluation. *The Lancet* 375(9730): 2009–2023.

Loewenstein G, David A. Asch, Kevin G. Volpp. 2013. Behavioral economics holds potential to deliver better results for patients, insurers, and employers. *Health Affairs* 32(7): 1244–1250.

London AJ, Borasky DA Jr, Bhan A, for the Ethics Working Group of the HIV Prevention Trials Network. 2012. Improving ethical review of research involving incentives for health promotion. *PLoS Med* 9(3): e1001193.

Lussier JP, Sarah H. Heil, Joan A. Mongeon, Gary J. Badger, Stephen T. Higgins. 2006. A meta-analysis of voucher-based reinforcement therapy for substance use disorders. *Addiction* 101(2): 192–203.

Lutge EE, Charles Shey Wiysonge, Stephen E Knight, Jimmy Volmink. 2012. Material incentives and enablers in the management of tuberculosis. *The Cochrane Database of Systematic Reviews* 1: CD007952.

Mitchell MS, Jack M. Goodman, David A. Alter, Leslie K. John, Paul I. Oh, Maureen T. Pakosh, Guy E. Faulkner. 2013. Financial incentives for exercise adherence in adults. *American Journal of Preventive Medicine* 45(5):658–667.

Montoy JC, William H. Dow, Beth Kaplan. 2013. Small incentives and nudges for HIV testing. *Working paper*.

Morris S, Flores R, Olinto P, Medina JM. 2004. Monetary incentives in primary health care and effects on use and coverage of preventive health care interventions in rural Honduras: cluster randomised trial. *Lancet* 364: 2030–2037.

Nguyen Ha TH, Laurel Hatt, Islam, Mursaleena Islam, Nancy L. Sloan, Jamil Chowdhury, Jean-Olivier Schmidt, Atia Hossain, Hong Wang. 2012. Encouraging maternal health service utilization: an evaluation of the Bangladesh voucher program. *Social Science & Medicine* 74: 989–996.

Padian NS, McCoy SI, Karim SS, Hasen, N Kim J, Bartos M, Katabira K, Bertozzi SM, Schwartländer B, Cohen MS. 2011. HIV prevention transformed: The new prevention research agenda. *Lancet* 378(9787): 269–78.

Parker, Susan W., Luis Rubalcava, Graciela Teruel. 2008. Evaluating conditional schooling and health programs. Chapter 62 in: *Handbook of Development Economics*, Volume 4, ed. T. Paul Schultz and John A. Strauss. pp. 3963–4035.

Petry NM, Alessi SM, Hanson T, Sierra S. 2007. Randomized trial of contingent prizes versus vouchers in cocaine-using methadone patients. *Journal of Consulting and Clinical Psychology*. 75: 983–991.

Petry NM, Rash CJ, Byrne S, Ashraf S, White WB. 2012. Financial reinforcers for improving medication adherence: findings from a meta-analysis. *American Journal of Medicine* 125(9): 888–896.

Powell-Jackson T, Kara Hanson. 2010. Financial incentives for maternal health: Impact of a national programme in Nepal. *Journal of Health Economics* 31(1): 271–284.

Powell-Jackson T, Joanna Morrison, Suresh Tiwari, Basu Neupane, Anthony Costello. 2009. The experiences of districts in implementing a national incentive programme to promote safe delivery in Nepal. *BMC Health Services Research* 9: 97.

Prendergast M, Deborah Podus, John Finney, Lisa Greenwell, John Roll. 2006. Contingency management for treatment of substance use disorders: A meta-analysis. *Addiction* 101(11): 1546–1560.

Ranganathan M, Lagarde M. 2012. Promoting healthy behaviours and improving health outcomes in low and middle income countries: A review of the impact of conditional cash transfer programmes. *Preventive Medicine* 55, Supplement: S95–S105.

Richards JM, Rista C. Plate, Monique Ernst. 2012. Neural systems underlying motivated behavior in adolescence: Implications for preventive medicine. *Preventive Medicine* 55, Supplement: S7–S16.

Robertson L, Phyllis Mushati, Jeffrey W Eaton, *et al.* 2013. Effects of unconditional and conditional cash transfers on child health and development in Zimbabwe: A cluster-randomised trial. *The Lancet* 381: 1283–1292.

Silverman K, Higgins, Stephen T, Brooner, Robert K., *et al.* 1996. Sustained cocaine abstinence in methadone maintenance patients through voucher-based reinforcement therapy. *Archives of General Psychiatry* 53: 409–415.

Simonson I, Tversky A. 1992. Choice in context — tradeoff contrast and extremeness aversion. *Journal of Marketing Research* 29(3): 281–95.

Simonsohn U, Loewenstein G. 2006. Mistake #37: The effect of previously encountered prices on current housing demand. *Economic Journal* 116(508): 175–199.

Thomas D. 1991. Intra-household resource allocation: An inferential approach. *Journal of Human Resources* 25(4): 635–664.

Thomas D. 1994. Like father, like son; like mother, like daughter: Parental resources and child height. *Journal of Human Resources* 29(4): 950–988.

Thornton RL. 2008. The demand for, and impact of, learning HIV status. *American Economic Review* 98(5): 1829–1863.

Troxel AB, Volpp KG. 2012. Effectiveness of financial incentives for longer-term smoking cessation: Evidence of absence or absence of evidence?" *American Journal of Health Promotion* 26(4): 204–207.

Van de Gaer D, Vandenbossche J, Figueroa JL. 2014. 'Children's Health Opportunities and Project Evaluation: Mexico's Oportunidades Program'. *The World Bank Economic Review* 28(2): 282–310.

Volpp KG, Andrea Gurmankin Levy, David A. Asch, *et al.* 2006. A randomized controlled trial of financial incentives for smoking cessation. *Cancer Epidemiology and Biomarkers Prevention* 15(1): 12–18.

Volpp KG, Leslie K. John, Andrea B. Troxel, Laurie Norton, Jennifer Fassbender, George Loewenstein. 2008a. Financial incentive-based approaches for weight loss: A randomized trial. *Journal of the American Medical Association* 300(22): 2631–2637.

Volpp K, George Loewenstein, Andrea Troxel, Jalpa Doshi, Maureen Price, Mitchell Laskin, Stephen Kimmel. 2008b. A test of financial incentives to improve warfarin adherence. *BMC Health Services Research* 8(1): 272.

Volpp KG, Andrea B. Troxel, Mark V. Pauly, *et al.* 2009. A randomized, controlled trial of financial incentives for smoking cessation. *New England Journal of Medicine* 360(7): 699–709.

White JS, Dow WH. 2015. Intertemporal Choices for Health. Roberto CA, Kawachi I (eds.). Behavioral Economics and Public Health, Oxford University Press.

White JS, William H. Dow, Suthat Rungruanghiranya. 2013. Commitment contracts and team incentives: A randomized controlled trial for smoking cessation in Thailand. *American Journal of Preventive Medicine* 45(5): 533–542.

World Health Organization 2010. World Health Report 2010: Health systems financing: the path to universal coverage.

Economic Evaluation of Health Care Programmes and Interventions: Applications to Low- and Middle-Income Countries

Paul Revill*, **Beth Woods, and Mark J. Sculpher**
Centre for Health Economics, University of York, United Kingdom

In countries across the globe, difficult decisions have to be made as to how health care is financed, organized, and provided to meet the needs of populations. The tools of economic evaluation (e.g., cost-effectiveness analysis) offer means to inform the allocation of scarce health system resources. Recent years have seen a number of notable developments in the methods of economic evaluation, often driven by the demands of policymakers. These developments have usually arisen to address policy needs expressed in some higher income countries (e.g., the UK, Australia, and Canada). In contrast, the field of economic evaluation as applied to inform decisions in low- and middle-income countries (LMICs) has generally evolved along quite distinct lines. This chapter explores the policy challenges faced within LMICs, the possible contributions of recent methods developments to addressing these challenges and areas in which further methods research would be of value. These include estimating cost-effectiveness thresholds, characterizing and exploring the implications of uncertainty, reflecting non-budgetary (demand- and supply-sides) constraints and incorporating non-health effects and equity concerns. In addition to the development of suitable methods, the use of economic evaluation to improve population health in LMICs will also require political commitment and local ownership of decision processes.

Keywords: Economic Evaluation; Methods; Low and Middle Income Countries (LMICs).

* Centre for Health Economics, University of York, Heslington, York, YO10 5DD, United Kingdom. Tel: (+44) 1904 321488, E-mail: paul.revill@york.ac.uk.

Introduction

In countries across the globe, difficult decisions have to be made (whether implicitly or explicitly) as to how health care is financed, organized and provided to meet the needs of populations. The range of interventions that could generate health gains for patients invariably exceeds what can be provided from available budgets. The decisions made affect the kinds of interventions provided, who receives health care, who goes without, and ultimately aggregate population health attainment. These decisions have to be made in all countries — from Switzerland to Swaziland — but the levels of available resources and health care needs differ widely across settings. It is estimated that, somewhat incongruously, only 15% of global health care expenditure is in low- and middle-income countries, where 85% of people live and which contain 92% of the world's disease burden (World Health Organization, 2012). Resource availability affects the types of interventions that can be provided and also the kinds of assessments of the costs and benefits of interventions that are feasible and required in different contexts exhibiting different features.

In this chapter, we explore the tools and approaches available to inform health care resource allocation decisions in different kinds of health care systems. We use World Bank definitions to make a broad distinction between high-income and low- and middle-income countries (LMICs) (World Bank, 2015). This separation is made for convenience and does not deny the wide range of experiences within these two categories. The chapter focuses on identifying opportunities to improve the methods of economic evaluation in LMICs. Other barriers to the useful application of economic evaluation such as local research capacity and decision-context barriers (e.g., understanding of methods by policymakers, as well as social, political, institutional and ethical factors (Yothasamut *et al.*, 2009)) are acknowledged but are beyond the scope of this chapter.

The field of economic evaluation

Health economic evaluation comprises the set of tools and approaches to inform a wide range of resource allocation decisions related to individual health technologies (e.g., drugs, diagnostics, medical devises) and/or health care programs (e.g., commissioning structures, performance management systems, service organization, service delivery, public health interventions, communication programmes, individual loans or subsidies). A key principle for the application of economic evaluation methods is that alternatives should be recommended if the commitment of resources to their provision results in health gains and other benefits that exceed what would have been generated from the other alternative priorities that must be forgone (i.e., if gains exceed opportunity costs; where opportunity costs reflect the gains forgone through resources being unavailable for other purposes) (Drummond *et al.*, 2005).

Decision-makers charged with making difficult resource allocation decisions require appropriate economic analyses supported by reliable evidence. Economic methods therefore tend to dominate and a wide range of economics sub-disciplines have effectively contributed to informing choices in health care. Most notably, the toolkits of cost–benefit analysis (CBA) and cost-effectiveness analysis (CEA) have been used to compare competing alternatives, particularly relating to drugs and other clinical interventions (Drummond *et al.*, 2005). However, other economics sub-disciplines have also contributed in various ways. Behavioral economics studies, for instance, have shown how demand for, and adherence to, health-improving interventions can be effectively generated (Gaarder *et al.*, 2010; Volpp *et al.*, 2008), and how paying health care providers differently affects the type and level of care delivered (Basinga *et al.*, 2011; Chalkley and Malcomson, 2000). Tools of inequality analyses have examined the extent to which different health care arrangements affect the distribution of health, health care and health care costs and whether or not this can be judged equitable (Kakwani *et al.*, 1997; Wagstaff and Vandoorslaer, 1992).

In addition to economics, other disciplines also have had key roles in informing choices. Within the field of quantitative analysis, for instance, operations research techniques have been applied to issues as diverse as informing health care facility location (Ndiaye and Alfares, 2008; Rais and Viana, 2011), capacity planning in hospitals (Green and Savin, 2008; Rais and Viana, 2011), and designing systems to manage patient flows (Jiang and Giachetti, 2008; Rais and Viana, 2011). Non-quantitative approaches such as qualitative social science, political science, legal disciplines and ethics have also had a role in shaping, weighting and interpreting available evidence to determine health care policy.

Economic evaluation as a field is, therefore, not restrictive in the types of techniques employed but instead draws upon and utilizes available evidence and analyses as deemed useful according to the requirements of the policy questions at hand.

Principles and methods

An important distinction needs to be made between the principles required to coherently inform resource allocation and the methods of analyses adopted. Whereas principles will generally hold across contexts, for different kinds of decisions, methods will justifiably differ; not least in relation to the resourcing and capacity for evidence generation and analyses.

The Bill and Melinda Gates Foundation (BMGF) has recently launched guidelines and a ‘reference case’ for the economic evaluation studies it funds that outlines principles of best practice (see Table 1) (Bill and Melinda Gates Foundation, 2014). The principles were agreed upon by a large group of specialists. They are motivated by two key underlying concerns. Firstly, decisions about the allocation

Table 1. Principles of economic evaluation

Statement of principles
1. An economic evaluation should be **communicated clearly and transparently** to allow the decision maker(s) to **interpret** the methods and results.
2. The **comparators** against which costs and effects are measured should accurately **reflect the decision problem**.
3. An economic evaluation should **consider all available evidence relevant** to the decision problem.
4 The **measure of health outcome** should be appropriate to the decision problem, should capture measurements of both length of life and quality of life, and should be generalizable across disease states.
5. All differences in expected **costs and resources used** in delivering interventions to the target population(s) should be incorporated into the evaluation.
6. The **time horizon** used in an economic evaluation should be of sufficient length to capture all costs and effects **relevant to the decision problem**; an appropriate **discount rate** should be used to **discount cost and effects to present values**.
7. **Non-health effects** and **costs that do not fall on the health budget** that are associated with gaining or providing access to health interventions should be identified where relevant to the decision problem. All **costs and effects should be disaggregated**, either by sector of the economy or by who incurs them.
8. The **effects** of the intervention **on sub-populations** within the decision problem **should be explored** and the **implications** appropriately **characterized**.
9. The **uncertainty** associated with an economic evaluation should be appropriately **characterized**.
10. The impact of implementing the intervention on **health budget and on other constraints** should be clearly and separately **identified**.
11. An economic evaluation should explore the **equity implications** of implementing the intervention.

Sources: Bill and Melinda Gates Foundation (2014). Methods for Economic Evaluation Project (MEEP) — Final Report.

of health care resources only make sense if they create 'value' at a local level (i.e., recommendations made at higher levels that are at odds with the health care contexts in particular jurisdictions are unlikely to improve population health and welfare). Secondly, to determine value at a local level requires ensuring benefits exceed opportunity costs.

The principles defined in the BMGF guidelines are outlined in Table 1. They cover features such as: the choice of comparators in a study (stating: '*all comparators reflecting a decision problem should be included*'); what evidence should be considered ('*all available relevant evidence*'); how health outcomes should be measured ('*in a way that is generalizable across diseases*'); which health care costs should be included ('*all those differing across evaluated alternatives*'); how non-health effects and non-health care costs should be reported ('*disaggregated across economic sectors or by who incurs them*'); and the manner in which results should be presented to policymakers (‘*uncertainty should be appropriately characterized*’); as well as other features.

The BMGF Guidelines are primarily intended for studies informing decisions in low- and middle-income country settings but could equally be applied to high-income contexts. However, what these key principles mean in different contexts, for different kinds of decision problems, in studies undertaken by groups with different skill mixes, backed by differing levels of resources, is justifiably non-prescriptive. The principles are intended to support rather than to dictate the choice of analytical methods and may suggest further methods development to meet policy needs.

It is useful to explore how specific methods have been developed within different contexts. We do this, first, for higher-income settings and then for low- and middle-income settings. Important unresolved methods concerns for lower-income country are then outlined, motivated by recognition of the key principles, and assessment made of how these methods concerns may appropriately be addressed.

Use of economic evaluation in high-income countries

- *Foundations of approach*

The role of economic analysis in informing social choice in high-income settings has its roots in welfare economics. Policy choices are assessed by their impact on a social welfare function which focuses on individuals’ utilities. Theoretically, this allows us to rank all possible policy choices. This includes policies which differ in terms of the sets of health care activity delivered, and those which differ in terms of the budget allocated to health care vis-à-vis non-health care activity.

The notion that a maximand determined by individual utilities may not be an appropriate basis for health care policy choices has been discussed extensively. At the core of this debate is the concern that welfarism ignores all non-utility information about people (Culyer, 2012). In particular, that it ignores what commodities may enable us to do (our capabilities) and other characteristics that determine wellbeing. It also goes against widely stated preferences from politically legitimate sources — such as national governments — that improving population health is a primary objective of health care systems.

An alternative paradigm, extra-welfarism, broadens the evaluative space from individual utilities to place direct value on other relevant outcomes (Brouwer *et al.*, 2008; Culyer, 2012). This normative foundation also allows interpersonal comparisons of these outcomes. In health economics, health has been used extensively as the single maximand (and wider constituents of well-being are ignored). This is consistent with the typical policy context whereby health care agencies are assigned health objectives and constrained by a fixed budget. Perhaps the most well-known agency that has used this approach is the National Institute for Health and Care Excellence

(NICE), which makes recommendations regarding health care interventions for the National Health Service in England and Wales. Similar agencies have roles in other countries such as the Pharmaceutical Benefits Advisory Committee (PBAC) in Australia, the Canadian Agency for Drugs and Technologies in Health (CADTH), and the Pharmaceutical Management Agency (PHARMAC) in New Zealand.

The incremental cost-effectiveness ratio (ICER) has been used to operationalize this framework in economic evaluation. Where an intervention results in more health and higher costs (or less health and lower costs) than the available alternative, an ICER is calculated as the ratio of incremental costs and incremental health. Alternatively, an intervention may result in lower costs and more health (or higher costs and less health). In these cases the implications for decision-making are straightforward and an ICER is not calculated. To interpret whether an ICER is acceptable, a cost-effectiveness threshold is required. In the context of health care systems with fixed budgets or limits on increased expenditure this threshold should reflect the opportunity costs (health forgone) that would result from the costs imposed with the new intervention (Culyer *et al.*, 2007).

The economic evaluation approach outlined here — founded on extra-welfarism — has been applied extensively in high-income countries. The degree to which economic evaluation as opposed to clinical criteria or other considerations are used to make funding decisions, however, varies widely across countries (Sculpher and Drummond, 2006).

- *Development of methods*

The demands of policymakers have driven a number of significant methods developments in high-income countries. Two prominent examples of these are mixed treatment comparisons and methods for incorporating uncertainty appropriately into decision-making.

Mixed treatment comparisons represent a set of statistical tools that allow interventions not directly compared in randomized controlled trials (RCTs) to be compared using the available RCT evidence. These methods were developed to meet the clear need of decision-makers to compare all relevant interventions and a scientific preference for using RCT evidence to inform measures of relative effect. Mixed treatment comparisons are now considered important evidence by a range of reimbursement agencies in high-income countries (Jansen *et al.*, 2011; Salanti, 2012).

For typical health care investments, governments should be risk neutral and, therefore, make decisions on the basis of expected values (Claxton, 1999). However, uncertainty should not be ignored in decision-making. A framework for incorporating the consequences of uncertainty into decision-making has been developed (Claxton *et al.*, 2012). This evaluates the cost of the uncertainty (or potential value of further information), the possibility and cost of research to reduce the uncertainty and any irreversible costs associated with making a decision. Quantification of these elements can then be used to determine whether an intervention should be approved, rejected, approved alongside further research or used only in research.

Both of these methods examples also highlight the important contributions made by researchers outside the field of economics to economic evaluation methods. The work on mixed treatment comparisons has been led by biostatisticians, and statistical decision theory provided the foundation for methods to incorporate uncertainty into decision-making processes.

Use of economic evaluation in low- and middle-income countries

There is a wide and diverse spectrum of health care systems in low- and middle-income countries (LMICs). However, in comparison to higher-income settings, some distinct features are often evident. Most noticeably, systems overall operate under more severe resource constraints — this includes not only financial, but also human, capital and infrastructural resources — which limit the scope of interventions that can be fully provided to populations.

Limited resources also result in managerial and stewardship challenges. Health care systems in LMICs, particularly in the lowest income countries, can in general be characterized as being more fragmented than in richer countries. They have less prepayment of health care, often multiple fund pools (e.g., from taxation, social/community health insurance schemes, direct donor/non-governmental organization contributions as well as from vertical disease funding that focuses on a particular disease or group of diseases), generally greater reliance on out-of-pocket (OOP) contributions, and a mix of provider types (public, faith-based, private and sometimes informal providers and traditional practitioners).

The kinds of policy problems addressed by economic evaluation studies can differ due to these and other features. Infectious diseases still tend to predominate, although the burden of non-communicable disease is rising (Lozano *et al.*, 2012). Furthermore, evidence on relative effectiveness and even costs is frequently derived from outside the jurisdiction in which an assessment is made. As a result of diverse funding pools, high reliance on OOP payments and high background levels of poverty, the consequences associated with the receipt or non-receipt of interventions can extend well beyond measures of health alone.

The development of economic evaluation methods for LMICs has been motivated by these and other features of health care systems but has evolved along somewhat distinct lines from higher-income settings. The principles behind economic evaluation are universal. However, there are certain methods features applied within LMICs (most particularly in the more donor dependent low-income countries) that are not generally adopted elsewhere, and some methods developed within higher-income settings are not widely applied in LMICs.

The World Health Organization (WHO), through the CHOosing Interventions that are Cost-Effective (CHOICE) team, has played a central role in the application of cost-effectiveness analysis (CEA) in LMICs with the development of generalized cost-effectiveness analysis (G-CEA) (Acharya *et al.*, 2004). This approach is intended to identify "best buys" from amongst large numbers of interventions, sometimes modeled at the level of whole regions (e.g., Sub-Saharan Africa or South-East Asia). Analyses begin from a 'null' position whereby it is assumed that no interventions are provided within a health care system and those providing health gains at lowest cost are then identified for prioritization. The approach has been described as providing 'broad brush' guidance to resource allocation. Data requirements to model large numbers of interventions across many countries are substantial, and analyses often draw upon evidence on relative effectiveness from diverse settings, even from high-income contexts. However, by starting from a null situation, this approach does not reflect how existing health care infrastructures need to be adjusted to deliver interventions and how this is likely to affect the costs (and cost-effectiveness) of alternatives.

The Disease Control Priorities Project (DCPP) is another major initiative informing resource allocation decisions in LMICs (www.dcpp.org). The DCPP is a joint enterprise funded primarily by BMGF and contributed to by staff of the World Bank, the World Health Organization, the Fogarty International Center of the National Institutes of Health and the National Library of Medicine. Two DCPP reports have been produced (Jamison *et al.*, 1994; Jamison, 2006), with a third report currently under development. The reports are compendiums on the state of knowledge on health care delivery and "best buys" within disease areas. For the third report, an approach of extended cost-effectiveness analysis (E-CEA) is being adopted that combines concern for health maximization, the distribution of health in a population and protection against financial risk (Verguet *et al.*, 2013; 2014) (see Sections "Non-Health Costs and Effects" and "Equity Considerations" for further details). The DCPP analyses also tend to be undertaken by international teams predominantly resident in high-income settings.

In addition to the WHO G-CEA and DCPP approaches, other academic and consultancy groups also undertake analyses to inform decisions in LMICs. A recent review reveals that these draw to some extent on methods developed by the WHO and DCPP teams (Bill and Melinda Gates Foundation, 2014). However, there is wide heterogeneity of methods applied, the quality of studies is variable and comparability between different study results is limited (Bill and Melinda Gates Foundation, 2014). This variation in itself highlights lack of consensus over key methods features.

In the following section, we outline a non-exhaustive list of methods issues for the conduct of economic evaluations in LMICs; highlighting the importance of each consideration, critiquing existing approaches developed for LMICs and assessing how methods could potentially be improved to meet policy needs more appropriately.

Methods Issues in the Application of Economic Evaluation in LMICs

Locally relevant decision-making parameters

The BMGF Guidelines (Bill and Melinda Gates Foundation, 2014) provide a fundamental insight that economic evaluations only add value if they make sense at a local level leading to configurations of health care services likely to improve population health. It is, therefore, crucial that evaluations use locally-relevant decision-making parameters. Two in particular can be highlighted: The cost-effectiveness threshold, used to assess value; and the discount rates applied to future costs and benefits.

- *Cost-effectiveness thresholds*

The cost-effectiveness threshold represents the cost per unit of health gain — measured in quality-adjusted life years (QALYs), or disability-adjusted life years (DALYs) averted — the health care system is willing to incur to fund an intervention offering health gains. It is, therefore, central to determining cost-effectiveness.

The use of thresholds to improve population health relies upon their reflecting opportunity costs, defined in terms of the benefits forgone as a result of the commitment of resources to a particular intervention due to their being unavailable for other purposes. In practical terms this means that the ICER (additional costs per health gain) associated with an intervention should be less than ICERs of other interventions displaced or forgone (sometimes termed the 'shadow price of the budget constraint').

If policymakers had full information about the costs and effects of all possible interventions they could, in principle, determine an optimal allocation of resources by only funding those that maximize health from within available budget constraints. This, in principle, could be achieved through mathematical programming (McKenna *et al.*, 2010). In practice, such full information is generally not available, so thresholds inform decisions at the margin: That is, what new interventions are targets for investment and what existing interventions would be used to release resources through disinvestment.

Most interventions result in only marginal budgetary changes so it is unlikely they will affect the shadow price of the budget constraint. However, some interventions, and programmes in particular, constitute such large calls on budgets that they are non-marginal and can affect cost-effectiveness thresholds. For instance, in many areas of Sub-Saharan Africa, provision of antiretroviral therapy (ART) for HIV/AIDS represents such a large proportion of overall health care expenditure that opportunity costs are likely to be greater (and the appropriate threshold less) than if ART was not provided and the same overall level of resources was still available. For applied economic evaluation, it is necessary to consider whether budgetary changes are marginal or non-marginal and how this affects measures of opportunity costs (Claxton *et al.*, 2010).

The cost-effectiveness literature for LMICs is notable for the lack of critical reflection on what thresholds represent and how they can be informed. The WHO in 1996 judged interventions with ICERs below a threshold of $150 as having 'attractive' cost-effectiveness and below $50 as having 'very attractive' cost-effectiveness (WHO, 1996). Currently, the WHO G-CEA Guidelines use gross domestic product (GDP) per capita to judge any intervention with an ICER below three times GDP per capita as 'cost-effective' and those below one times GDP per capita as 'very cost-effective' (Acharya *et al.*, 2004; WHO, 2012). However, a number of countries have large coverage gaps for interventions well below these thresholds (Bowie and Mwase, 2011) suggesting the thresholds are far too high to reflect opportunity costs (Revill *et al.*, 2014).

A review of decision rules for LMICs (Shillcutt *et al.*, 2009) identified another basis for informing thresholds. This is the notion they could reflect what the public is "willing to pay" (WTP) to achieve health gains or "willing to accept" (WTA), in terms of financial compensation, to take on health-threatening risks. Estimates of WTP/WTA for a QALY have been generated by studies conducted in LMICs including in Thailand and Malaysia (Lim *et al.*, 2013; Thavorncharoensap *et al.*, 2013). It is important, however, to distinguish issues of *value* and issues of *fact*. If budgets are not aligned to a level at which public willingness to pay/accept matches opportunity costs, basing reimbursement decisions on WTP/WTA will result in suboptimal health outcomes in the population. If current budgets are not believed to reflect societal preferences (and may, for example, reflect vested interests or historical budget allocation patterns) WTP/WTA valuations may provide a basis for establishing the appropriate health care budget. However, it is not certain that setting budgets at such levels would be normatively correct insofar as authorities (e.g., ministries of finance) that generate and allocate resources across government departments have claims to legitimacy.

Methods for determining thresholds in LMICs

There is still a high degree of uncertainty over threshold values even in settings in which the methods of economic evaluation are most established (e.g., in European countries), and few authorities state explicitly what their thresholds are. It has been recommended that policymakers should avoid setting specific thresholds and instead undergo processes of "threshold searching" by identifying the least cost-effective intervention currently provided and the most cost-effective intervention not yet routinely available (Culyer *et al.*, 2007).

This approach could also be undertaken in some LMICs, especially those in which a greater number of economic evaluations take place. Although attempts have been made to investigate the cost-effectiveness of interventions falling inside and outside the budget envelope in particular jurisdictions (Bowie and Mwase, 2011), this approach has not been widely used. Most countries remain far from being able to reasonably determine their local thresholds.

An alternative approach is to estimate the marginal productivity of health care expenditure *across* countries. There is now good evidence, using multi-country panel data, that health outcomes improve as countries increase spending on health care, although at a diminishing rate (Moreno-Serra and Smith, 2014). Understanding this relationship could indicate whether certain interventions/programmes are likely to increase or reduce productivity in the health sectors of different countries with particular levels of resources and health care needs.

Clearly, some countries will be more efficient than average in converting health care expenditure into health outcomes (for example, due to how they finance and organize health care or due to non-health care factors including absence of war, geography and climate); whereas others will be less efficient. In countries with greater efficiency, the local thresholds will be lower than that estimated using cross-country variations. In those with lower productivity, the thresholds will be higher. This may indicate that substantial health gains can be achieved more through internal reorganization of the health care system (e.g., through disinvesting in cost-ineffective interventions and continuing to scale-up of highest value interventions) rather than spending on the adoption of new interventions and programmes.

The financing of LMIC health care systems is often very fragmented with an array of fund pools. For instance, in addition to public financing, non-governmental organizations (NGOs), bilateral and multilateral donors, private financing and others may contribute certain inputs to health care delivery. Sometimes funding and purchasing is coordinated (this may even include the pooling of funds into one overall budget (Peters and Chao, 1998)), but often this is not the case. Where there are multiple budgets, there could be multiple thresholds (e.g., the threshold for HIV interventions could differ from the threshold for malaria interventions when these are subject to different budgets). Where multiple thresholds do exist (e.g., for disease funding silos) this gives an indication of how funding can be reallocated to improve overall efficiency (i.e., to where thresholds are lowest/opportunity costs highest).

Interventions considered for investment in LMICs are more likely to represent a large proportion of health care spending. Methods to assess opportunity cost in the face of non-marginal resource allocation changes, as well as reflecting sometimes rapidly changing health care budgets, are therefore likely to be important. Non-threshold methods for appraising the value of alternative resource allocation options could also be considered. For example program-budgeting and marginal analysis (PBMA) (Mitton and Donaldson, 2003) establishes value by determining the health generated by shifting finance between health care budgets, with a focus on specific types of investment and disinvestment. This could even be used as a method of "threshold searching" by forcing decision makers to reveal the programmes where they believe low value is being achieved at the margin.

Suitable measures of opportunity cost are also required to guide research decisions (see Section "Uncertainity") as well as possible health system investments on both the supply-side (Section "Other Constraints in the Delivery of Health Care") and demand-side (Section "Demand-Side Factors Affecting Receipt of Health Care").

- *Discount rates*

When the costs and effects of alternatives have different time profiles it is necessary to express them in present value terms so these can be compared. This requires discounting.

A recent literature review showed that most studies in LMICs follow the WHO-CHOICE Guidelines recommendation of a 3% discount rate on both costs and health outcomes (Bill and Melinda Gates Foundation, 2014). It is unclear, however, how this recommendation was determined and, therefore, uncertainty remains over what the correct discount rate should be in different contexts, and even whether the same discount rate should be used for costs and health outcomes. A higher discount rate for costs (benefits) would balance analyses more in favor of alternatives with costs (benefits) realized in later (earlier) periods, with the opposite being true for lower discount rates. Discounting can, therefore, affect which interventions/programmes are recommended for investment.

Methods for determining discount rates

The discount rates adopted for most social investment programmes depend in part on three core underlying reasons for discounting. All else being equal, discount rates should be higher (lower) (1) the higher (lower) individuals' time preferences are to bring forward benefits and delay costs; (2) the higher (lower) the risk of future catastrophic events such that future projections are not realized; and (3) the higher (lower) the economic growth in a country. These are the three components that make up the Ramsey discount formula (Ramsey, 1928), used by many Treasuries/

ministries of finance (Treasury, 2003). The social rates of discount chosen by countries to evaluate public works programmes tend to be higher in low income countries (8–15%) than in higher-income settings (3–7%), most likely as a result of differences in perceived social opportunity costs of public funds across countries (Zhuang *et al.*, 2007).

The 'correct' discount rates, however, depend upon what objective is being maximized (e.g., within health care, whether the objective is to maximize health or a wider measure of social welfare, which could be defined as the consumption value of health — the rate at which individuals are willing to forego other forms of consumption to achieve health improvement), whether there is a fixed budget constraint and on the decision rule. Recent methods research has highlighted how discount rates can be informed within jurisdictions (Claxton *et al.*, 2011). Research to determine discount rates within LMICs would be valuable and could determine whether evaluations should balance relatively in favor of interventions with more immediate or delayed health gains (e.g., this may affect choices of treatment vs. preventative strategies).

Outcomes and local preferences

Economic evaluation requires a measure of health outcomes, capturing both changes in mortality and morbidity that can reasonably be compared across disease areas. There has long been debate in the literature over what constitutes the most appropriate measure of health (Drummond *et al.*, 2005; Gafni and Birch, 1997; Gold *et al.*, 2002; Williams, 1999). The measure that has come to be used most frequently in high-income (and also a number of middle-income) countries is the quality-adjusted life year (QALY) (Drummond *et al.*, 2005). This has a number of advantages — it is easily comprehendible, and it is a generic measure of health gain that can be compared across diverse interventions. Importantly, it provides a means of comparing the gains from new investments to the health forgone as a result of opportunity costs. However, the QALY is not the only outcome measure that exhibits these qualities, and alternatives have been proposed.

The Healthy Year Equivalent (HYE) is an attempt to overcome some of the restrictive assumptions of QALYs (Mehrez and Gafni, 1989). These include that individuals are willing to sacrifice a constant proportion of remaining life years in order to achieve a given improvement in health regardless of the time spent at different levels of health and individuals preferences for health states are unaffected by the sequence in which health states occur. However, the sheer number of possible lifetime health profiles limits its applicability, and thus it has rarely been used in applied work.

Both the WHO-CHOICE and DCPP approaches measure health on the basis of reductions in mortality and morbidity, as measured in the number of disability-adjusted life years (DALYs) averted which has become the most used measure in LMICs (Bill and Melinda Gates Foundation, 2014). DALYs were originally developed in the early 1990s and attempted to focus attention on those diseases that resulted in the greatest worldwide mortality and morbidity (World Bank, 1993). Premature death, which forms the basis for DALY measurement, is defined relative to the country in the world with the highest life expectancy, Japan, which is unlikely to be a realistic achievement for many countries.

Whatever the measure used, it is important that valuations reasonably reflect patients' health-related quality of life (HRQoL). Valuations of HRQoL for QALY calculations are typically derived using general population preferences elicited via large-scale jurisdiction-specific surveys. DALYs also combine mortality and morbidity, but disability is a much more restricted concept than HRQoL, relating only to functional status. Initial DALY weights were obtained from a panel of health care professionals although the latest weights are now based upon representative surveys in five countries (Bangladesh, Indonesia, Peru, Tanzania, and the USA), as well as a web survey, and broadly similar valuations are reported across settings (Salomon *et al.*, 2012). This contradicts findings from some other studies that have reported cultural differences have notable effects on health state valuation (Jelsma *et al.*, 2003; Swinburn *et al.*, 2012).

Methods for reflecting local preferences

Any outcome measure used for economic evaluation needs to offer some means of trading off between the different dimensions of HRQoL, and between HRQoL and survival duration. These trade-offs are inherently value-based and, for QALYs and DALYs, have been based on individuals' preferences. Ideally, the chosen measures of health outcomes should reasonably reflect local preferences (which may vary according to culture, health care availability and support from social institutions (Kularatna *et al.*, 2013)) for economic evaluation to deliver value at the local level. As for all other sources of evidence in an economic evaluation seeking to inform local decisions, however, whether the cost of collecting local preference data is justified needs to be considered in the context of the value of this additional information (see Section "Uncertainity"). For evidence such as prevalence, baseline risks, treatment effects and risks of side effects, there may be cases where data exist from other jurisdictions with similarities to the location of the decision and/or where the cost-effectiveness of a given programme or intervention are not sensitive to uncertainty in those parameters. In these situations, there may be little value in collecting additional local data. This principle also applies to preference data, although these are generally collected once for a given jurisdiction rather than on a study-by-study basis, so the research cost is effectively spread over many decisions.

The use of DALYs in LMICs, instead of QALYs as used in other settings, has undoubtedly created a separation in the field of research that appears to have offered little or no benefit. Instead, it may have frustrated the translation of novel methods to inform decision-making also in lower-income contexts. The economic evaluation community working within LMICs needs to consider whether this separation is justifiable. Perhaps the more widespread use of QALYs, based upon local valuation sets, would assist in the faster diffusion of leading methods across settings.

Uncertainty

Any economic evaluation will provide results that are uncertain. The underlying evidence base will comprise of studies with finite sample size. This evidence will, therefore, be associated with a level of uncertainty; this is generally labelled "parameter uncertainty." Parameter uncertainty also reflects the fact that studies informing parameters may suffer from limitations in terms of internal or external validity and relevance to the setting of interest. In LMICs, future prices of pharmaceuticals may also represent a key source of uncertainty. As well as uncertainties in the evidence base, any analysis of cost-effectiveness involves a series of assumptions and analytic decisions. As different decisions could almost certainly have been made, structural uncertainty will also be present. Both types of uncertainty contribute to decision uncertainty, i.e., uncertainty regarding which intervention should be adopted. The BMGF Guidelines emphasize the importance of characterizing uncertainty (Bill and Melinda Gates Foundation, 2014). This section explores ways in which a greater understanding of the implications of uncertainty could usefully inform decision-making.

Uncertainty is costly due to both the possibility that a wrong decision may be made and the implications of making the wrong decision (i.e., the health lost). Obtaining further information is valuable to the extent that it reduces these costs. This can be assessed using formal value of information methods (Claxton, 1999) that compare the value of reducing uncertainty to the cost of further research. If further research can be conducted concurrently with implementation and the intervention has no significant irreversible costs, then the decision of whether to adopt the intervention now (the adoption decision) and the decision of whether to conduct research to improve decision-making in the future can be separated. Current decision-making should be based on expected costs and effects and research commissioned if it is expected to generate value (Claxton, 1999).

In reality, irreversible costs are likely to be important in LMICs where introduction of basic health provisions may involve large capital or other set-up expenditures. Research may not be feasible following implementation of an intervention, for example due to the ethical and practical challenges of randomization; or, for example, in the case of infectious diseases, because the dynamics of infectious disease transmission may have been irreversibly altered by the intervention.

Where irreversible costs exist or implementation of a program removes opportunities for research, the interplay between the adoption decision and the research decision needs to be considered. In these situations, delaying a decision may generate more health than making a decision based on current expected cost-effectiveness. Delaying a decision may generate more health either because it avoids costly start-up expenditure (e.g., recruitment of additional staff, training or capital investments) for an intervention that may be discontinued due to not being cost-effective once new evidence emerges; or because it allows research to be conducted that allows a better decision to be made (Claxton *et al.*, 2012).

In practice, decision-makers do not appear to be adequately considering the interplay between adoption decisions and research efforts. For example, the WHO 2013 Consolidated HIV Treatment Guidelines (WHO, 2013) recommended earlier HIV treatment (i.e., treatment of adults with CD4 counts in the arrange 350–500 per μL). These recommendations were made on the basis of limited evidence and in a period when a trial designed to directly assess the benefits of early ART-initiation was ongoing (the Strategic Timing of AntiRetroviral Treatment (START) trial (Babiker *et al.*, 2013)). The benefits of delaying the adoption decision in light of ongoing research should have been examined in this case. If the trial and associated decision analysis show earlier initiation either leads to worse health outcomes for patients or is cost ineffective it is likely to be difficult and costly to reverse the Guidelines recommendations.

In the context of priority setting for LMICs, the WHO G-CEA includes stochastic league tables as a potential representation of uncertainty in adoption decisions. Stochastic league tables present probabilities that each intervention will be included in the optimal set of interventions conditional upon the available health care budget (Acharya *et al.*, 2004). This approach extends the information requirements beyond the considerable requirements of deterministic G-CEA (which requires cost and effect estimates for all interventions) to a requirement for estimates of the distribution of cost and effect estimates for all interventions and their correlation within and across interventions. The Stochastic League Table presentation provides no information on the likelihood that a given *combination* of interventions is optimal (Koffijberg *et al.*, 2012). The informational requirements and the unclear implications of the results of Stochastic League Table results make it unlikely that they will represent a useful tool for decision-making in most cases.

Methods for accounting for uncertainty

The decision of whether to adopt a technology, adopt a technology and commission more research, commission more research and delay adoption, or simply delay adoption while uncertainties resolve will depend on the size of the population, cost of uncertainty, cost of research, availability of ongoing research, feasibility of simultaneous adoption, and research and irreversible costs.

Robust quantification of all of these attributes in the form of a full value of information analysis is unlikely to be feasible or necessary for all cost-effectiveness analyses. However, the principles of decision-making under uncertainty should be followed, regardless of the analyses available. Where probabilistic models are available, the potential benefits of research can be quantified using existing analyses (Claxton, 1999). If concurrent research and adoption is feasible, these benefits can be compared to research costs. Where adoption would prohibit research, the benefits of research can be compared to the costs of research and the costs of delaying adoption. Cases where research is expected to be valuable could then be triaged to more formal and advanced value of information analyses to determine the benefits of alternative types of research (e.g., trials, observational studies, costing studies). An assessment of the potential importance of irreversible costs could be made by comparing the time profile of irreversible costs to the time profile of expected net benefits. This would allow for an informed appraisal of the benefits of delaying access in order to allow uncertainties to resolve (via commissioned research or otherwise).

The Stochastic League Tables Approach highlights the fact that both the adoption decision and decisions to commission further research may differ when a hard budget constraint is imposed (McKenna *et al.*, 2010). A hard budget may be a more relevant concept in the context of LMICs where separate funding silos exist and individual intervention costs may represent more significant proportions of the available budget. The exact impact of a hard budget constraint will depend on the extent to which decision makers are expected to be able to respond to realizations of uncertainty. Further research is required to develop methods for decision-making in the face of uncertainty and a hard budget constraint.

Finally, as discussed in the context of preference data in Section "Outcomes and Local Preferences", relevance of the available data is likely to represent a fundamental source of uncertainty in the context of LMICs where information on key parameters is frequently generalized across jurisdictions. Formal quantification of the impact of (ir)relevance on expected cost-effectiveness and uncertainty via expert elicitation may be appropriate in some instances (Turner *et al.*, 2009). This could allow both an assessment of whether uncertainties around relevance should impact the adoption decision or necessitate further (for example, local) research efforts.

Other constraints in the delivery of health care

The challenges to the delivery of health care in many LMICs extend well beyond limited finances alone, and how these finances are provided. They also include other constraints in key health sector inputs such as human, capital and infrastructural resources; as well as the general environment in which health care is delivered and received.

In recent years, recognition has grown of the importance of health systems in affecting health care delivery and health attainment (Alliance for Health Policy and Systems Research/World Health Organization, 2009; Mills, 2014; World Health Organization, 2000). Although health care systems are more than the sum of their constituent parts, there are core inputs required if health care is to be provided widely and effectively: These include health care facilities, human resources and other supporting infrastructures (e.g., laboratories). Importantly, the way in which these are organized and managed is also likely to affect health outcomes.

A number of frameworks have been put forward to characterize the delivery constraints that may impede effective health care (Alliance for Health Policy and Systems Research/World Health Organization, 2009; Ensor and Cooper, 2004; Hanson *et al.*, 2003; Mills, 2014). A framework from the WHO Commission on Macroeconomics and Health, in particular, highlights how constraints can take affect around different functions of health care systems (e.g., in financing, governance, service delivery) but also at different levels (e.g., households and communities, national governments and even globally) (Hanson *et al.*, 2003; Mills, 2014). This implies a huge breadth of potential policies that could improve health system performance.

The importance of different constraints for the delivery of particular interventions or programmes depends upon context and the degree to which the constraint limits delivery. In some cases, it may be possible through quite simple measures to relax a constraint (e.g., if certain facility infrastructures are required but not currently available, investment could rectify this). However, often constraints cut across the health sector, and even beyond, and can only be addressed through more fundamental changes in the health care environment (e.g., if health system managerial and stewardship capacity is limiting health care delivery, it is difficult to envisage how this can immediately be overcome with investment alone).

Methods for incorporating other constraints

To inform policy effectively, economic evaluations need to reflect the existing configurations and constraints in health care delivery; whether these be in terms of financing and/or other key inputs to services. The WHO G-CEA assumption of a 'null' situation (Acharya *et al.*, 2004), in which policy alternatives are evaluated assuming nothing is currently provided, pays too little attention to the difficulties and costs of implementing interventions and programmes. Implementation costs also have opportunity costs, and ignoring them risks generating misleading conclusions. Moreover, in the face of uncertainty and irreversibility, such costs may affect the range and feasibility of future options.

Evaluations may seek, as a first take, to inform policies that maximize health within prevailing constraints. In this case, where health system inputs are limited, analysts need to consider the opportunity costs associated with inputs upon which interventions/programmes draw. For instance, if the introduction of a new screening programme were to divert limited human resources from an immunization programme, the health consequences of this should be reflected. This implies that, as well as a cost-effectiveness thresholds associated with financing requirements, there may also be separate and different thresholds depending upon the particular resource inputs used.

In some cases — for example where the supply of interventions is limited by production constraints — incorporating a nonlinear cost function may be appropriate. For example, a certain level of provision may be achievable at current unit costs, whereas beyond this point, additional production facilities may have to be set up, increasing unit costs. This may require more detailed analyses than typically conducted in high-income countries where unit costs are generally assumed to be constant.

Analysts could also investigate, however, whether supply-side constraints (e.g., limited numbers of health care workers or laboratory infrastructures) can be effectively overcome through investments enabling better delivery. Software such as the One Health Tool (Health Systems Financing and Governance Department, WHO, 2013) and the Marginal Budgeting for Bottlenecks tool provide a means for estimating the costs and health outcome consequences of removing supply side constraints. These tools have generally been considered as a means for assessing the cost implications of reaching specific goals (for example, Millennium Development Goals) rather than as a basis for assessing the value for money of alternative uses of the health budget. Value of implementation analysis (Fenwick *et al.*, 2008; Walker *et al.*, 2013) offers a framework for assessing the value for money of policies (which could include the removal of supply side constraints) that increase the coverage of cost-effective interventions. Combining the information currently being collated in tools such as the One Health Tool with a value of implementation approach could provide an efficient way to establish priorities for supply-side interventions. Improvements in routine data collection could increase the robustness and value of these analyses. Further work could explore the value of increasing the type and quality of routine data collection to inform these and other analyses used in health care decision-making.

Demand-side factors affecting receipt of health care

The availability of health care is only one factor that affects health attainment. Health outcomes also rely, importantly, on other environmental factors (including those in the realm of public health) and on individuals' demand for health and health care.

The Grossman Model of health production highlights that demand for health care is derived from the demand for health itself (Grossman, 1972). Health has value for its own sake and also instrumental value, improving work and leisure. Individuals are both producers and consumers of health. They decide how much to invest in health from their limited time and resources (e.g., on health improving efforts and avoiding unhealthy behaviors), based upon the benefits health provides compared to other forms of consumption. Their consumption of health care depends upon its direct (e.g., prices), indirect (e.g., travel times/costs) and opportunity costs (what else they could do with their time and money), as well as expected health improvements.

Until relatively recently, the literature in LMICs focused overwhelmingly on the supply of health care. There is now growing recognition of the role individual behaviors play in determining demand for health care and health attainment (Ensor and Cooper, 2004; Mills, 2014). Effective health care ultimately requires some interaction between provider and recipient. Demand-side constraints can prohibit this or impact the effectiveness of this interaction. These can operate at the individual level (e.g., due to limited knowledge of effective health care), within households (e.g., household wealth and relationships) or at community levels (e.g., certain communities, particularly those in more rural locations, often have more limited access to health care).

Potential responses to ineffective demand depend upon the kinds of constraints that operate. For instance, if the issue is lack of knowledge on health care choices, information campaigns may have a role. If constraints relate more to the time and costs patients face in accessing health care, particularly for 'harder-to-reach' communities, configuring health care so services are provided closer to where patients live may be beneficial. Increasingly, there is interest in the use of financial and in-kind incentives to encourage patients to act in ways likely to improve their health — whether this be taking preventive actions (Banerjee *et al.*, 2010), accessing services (Glassman *et al.*, 2013), or adhering to treatments (Volpp *et al.*, 2008).

Methods for incorporating demand-side factors

In many cases, the demand for health care is not exogenously set and policy choices, including those related to how interventions are provided, can affect patient demand.

Economic evaluation needs to reflect how different alternatives may affect patient demand and what this means for the total costs and health gains associated with policy choices whenever this differs across alternatives. Recognizing demand constraints also raises the question of how these can effectively be overcome. Value of implementation analysis (Fenwick *et al.*, 2008; Walker *et al.*, 2013) holds potential in evaluating demand-side measures in light of other calls on resources and their opportunity costs.

There is somewhat of a separation in expertise, even within the discipline of economics, between researchers working on demand-side issues and those undertaking economic evaluation. All health care requires some interaction between provider and recipient, so engagement between different specialists and methods research to reconcile the supply and demand sides of provision holds potential to inform policy more fully.

Non-health costs and effects

In addition to health outcomes and direct costs falling on the health budget, other costs and consequences of interventions may also be important. Non-health effects and costs that fall outside the health budget may be important because alternative interventions can result in different non-health effects that have social value (or cost). These costs and benefits may be borne by non-health public sector organizations, donors or individuals. In health systems in which a significant proportion of interventions are funded through OOP payments, financial consequences for individuals may be particularly important. In this context, financial risk protection as a potentially important non-health consequence of health care provision has recently been explored (Verguet *et al.*, 2014). Non-health costs and effects may also be particularly important in LMICs due to the absence of the welfare state and other "safety nets" generally more widely available in higher income countries. This may result in the ill-health of individual family members having profound health and non-health household level impacts.

Methods for incorporating non-health costs and effects

The BMGF Guidelines recognize the potential importance of non-health effects and costs and require that these are reported separately from direct health costs and effects (Bill and Melinda Gates Foundation, 2014). This requirement for separate reporting reflects the challenges of including non-health costs and effects within a single policy evaluation. Most fundamentally, including the effects would require a social welfare function to be specified (Claxton *et al.*, 2010). This is generally considered an impossible task, requiring consensus on the arguments of the social welfare function, as well as the weight each should be given and how the weights interact. The alternative to such aggregation — a deliberative approach considering the full set of health and non-health costs and benefits — does still, however, require information about non-health costs and benefits as well as some basis for understanding how these might be traded off against health. This may be considered within a multiple criteria decision analysis framework (see Section "Equity Considerations").

To operationalize a decision-making approach where non-health costs and effects are sensibly accounted for, further empirical research is warranted. This would consider a range of aspects including the need to understand the consumption value of health in relation to the cost-effectiveness threshold in LMICs. As discussed in Section "Cost-Effectiveness Thresholds", some empirical work has already been conducted to determine the consumption value of health (Lim *et al.*, 2013; Thavorncharoensap *et al.*, 2013). However, very little empirical work has been conducted to estimate cost-effectiveness thresholds. This information could be used to establish the desirability of alternative policy options intended to account for non-health costs and benefits — including policies which have been applied in high-income countries (Claxton *et al.*, 2010). In the context of donor-funded programmes, further work would be required to understand donors' implicit value function. If the preferred policy option requires non-health costs and effects to be incorporated formally or informally into decision-making, identification of the most important types of non-health costs and effects to include and of robust methods to measure and value these effects will be required. An understanding of the non-health costs and effects of activity displaced by new programmes would also be required — a formidable task.

Equity considerations

Equity in health has long been recognized alongside efficiency as a dual and sometimes competing priority for health care decision-makers. Equity is likely to be a fundamental policy objective in LMICs given the potential for individuals to experience very poor but avoidable states of health and for under-provision of basic health interventions.

Three broad approaches to equity have been applied in the economic evaluation field. The first — and probably most commonly applied — is a deliberative approach. Here, the equity implications of decisions are considered in the context of a set of broad social value judgments on whether the valuation of health should depend upon certain patient characteristics (e.g., socio-economic status or burden of disease) (see Shah *et al.*, 2013). Although these social value judgments may contain commitments to reduce health inequalities, in practice decision-makers have rarely departed from the judgment that 'a QALY is a QALY is a QALY' (Shah *et al.*, 2013). This may reflect a lack of information regarding the equity implications of policy alternatives, a lack of understanding of relevant preferences with respect to efficiency-equity trade-offs and the politically controversial nature of equity concerns.

Multi-criteria decision analysis (MCDA) has been proposed as an alternative to the deliberative process (Johri and Norheim, 2012). MCDA formalizes the decision-making approach outlined above by aggregating attribute values (e.g., efficiency, equity) for each intervention in a way that reflects their importance to the decision-maker (Thokala and Duenas, 2012). MCDA suffers from the same challenges as deliberative decision-making, but can encourage explicit consideration of all included attributes and could improve the consistency and transparency of decisions.

A third approach involves quantifying the health loss (gain) considered equivalent to a given increase (reduction) in inequality. The Distributional Cost-Effectiveness Analysis (DCEA) framework has recently been developed to evaluate interventions in this way (Asaria *et al.*, 2014). DCEA compares health distributions associated with alternative interventions, including the distributional consequences of opportunity cost, and involves specifying a social welfare function to trade off efficiency and equity objectives.

In the LMIC setting, an Extended Cost-Effectiveness Analysis (E-CEA) framework has been developed and applied in a number of case studies (Verguet *et al.*, 2013; Verguet *et al.*, 2014). ECEA extends standard economic evaluation by presenting three additional dimensions on which health care provision may impact: reduced OOP payments, protection against financial risk and the distribution of health. ECEA results are presented in a disaggregated format similar to a cost-consequence analysis (i.e., results are presented for each dimension). ECEA can, therefore, be thought of as a potentially important tool to inform a deliberative approach to equity considerations.

The case studies developed to date illustrate the importance of adequately capturing, for each dimension, both the benefits of interventions and their opportunity cost. In the tuberculosis (TB) and rotavirus case studies (Verguet *et al.*, 2013; 2014), benefits of treatment are quantified in terms of deaths avoided. No adjustment is made for differences across income levels in life expectancy following disease survival. This may have significant impacts in terms of total health gains and the distribution of health gains. The benefits of reduced private expenditure are presented in cash terms. These cash gains are not adjusted in any way to reflect the marginal value of income — this may make it difficult for decision-makers to weigh-up gains made on this dimension by individuals at different income levels. The case studies to date have included limited quantification of opportunity cost. The rotavirus case study simply presents the impact on government spending. Secondary analyses in the TB case study incorporate the opportunity cost of the intervention by including the private expenditure implications of a tax. This ignores the opportunity cost of diverting whatever that tax could otherwise be used for to fund the TB programme. These alternative uses of funds could have important benefits on each dimension evaluated, which could potentially exceed those of the TB programme. The approach also assumes that individual programmes could be funded by tax increases rather than by the existing tax base which may not be realistic.

Methods for incorporating equity considerations

Any attempt to incorporate equity considerations into policy choices requires information about the distribution of consequences (health, monetary, other) associated with each alternative course of action. This should include the distributional consequences of displaced activities (opportunity costs) as well as the distributional consequences of different interventions in the target population. An assessment of whether this information is likely to change decision-making may represent a practical way of triaging cases for more detailed equity analysis. This could be made on the basis of the cost-effectiveness results observed in the absence of equity considerations and the extent to which distributions of health are expected to differ between interventions.

Decision-makers choosing between interventions which offer efficiency–equity trade-offs are likely to require more information on the preferences of those they represent than are currently available. Depending on the nature of health care financing, these preferences may most appropriately represent those of donors, health care recipients or the general public. Further work is required to identify the value of understanding different groups' preferences and to develop methods for eliciting these preferences.

Further work is also required to establish whether the information required to model the distribution of consequences of alternative policies is available in LMICs, and the value of increasing access to such data if it is not. Previous work, for example, has required estimates of treatment coverage, out of pocket expenditure, disease incidence and disease-specific mortality by income level to allow the effects of interventions to be presented by income quintile (Verguet *et al.*, 2013; 2014).

Discussion

The application of economic evaluation methods to the resource allocation problems facing health sectors in low-income countries following the principles outlined in the BMGF reference case holds potential to bring a number of benefits. Most importantly, it would lead to decision-making by national authorities more likely consistent with the maximization of health and other benefits from limited available resources. Although other disciplines have important roles to play, the key decisions are ultimately questions of economics and rely heavily on economic methods.

This chapter has outlined a non-exhaustive list of key unanswered methods concerns for the fuller application of economic evaluation to LMICs. These are summarized in Table 2. We have suggested in the chapter some ways in which

Table 2. Questions for future methods research

Topics	Research questions
1. Quantifying opportunity cost	• How can jurisdiction-specific estimates of a cost-effectiveness threshold be generated efficiently and with reasonable precision in LMICs? o How can decision-making reflect the implications of non-marginal changes and rapid budget changes for opportunity cost? o Is there a need to reflect the plurality of funding sources when estimating opportunity cost and how should this be done?
2. Understanding the relative importance of costs and benefits now and in the future	• How can jurisdiction-specific estimates of a discount rate be generated efficiently and with reasonable precision in LMICs?
3. Local preferences	• How can local preferences be realistically reflected in economic evaluations in LMICs?
4. Decision making in the face of uncertainty	• Methods are already available to determine the impact uncertainty should have on implementation and research decisions. How can these methods usefully be applied in LMICs? • When and how should a lack of locally relevant data impact upon implementation and research decisions?
5. Constraints and "bottle-necks" in health care delivery	• How can interventions which target supply-side constraints be evaluated appropriately?
6. Demand for health care	• How can interventions which target demand for health care be evaluated appropriately?
7. Non-health implications of health care spending	• Which non-health effects of health care are most important in LMICs and how and when should these be quantified? • How should policymakers' trade-off health and non-health implications of different policy choices? • Can the non-health consequences of displaced activities be quantified and what implications does this have for incorporating non-health effects in economic evaluation?
8. Equity implications of resource allocation	• Which dimensions of inequity are of most to concern to decision-makers? • How and when should the equity implications of interventions be considered? • How should policymakers evaluate efficiency–equity trade-offs? • Can the equity implications of displaced activities be quantified and what implications does this have for incorporating distributional considerations in economic evaluation?

(*Continued*)

Table 2. (*Continued*)

Topics	Research questions
9. Routine data	• How does the availability of routine data impact on our ability to evaluate different types of health care interventions? • How does the availability of routine data impact on our ability to incorporate non-health and equity implications of resource allocation decisions? • What value could increasing the collection and quality of routine data have in improving resource allocation decisions?
10. Topic selection and scoping	• How should topics for economic evaluation be prioritized in LMICs? • How can scoping be used to identify evaluations where more extensive analyses (e.g., of non-health effects or equity) are required?

these could be addressed using existing methods, and example to demonstrate how these approaches would provide valuable areas of future research. In other cases, *de novo* methods will be required. The common theme running through each methods issue is the centrality of determining value — through recognizing the opportunity costs of spending limited resources in terms of what is forgone elsewhere in a health care system. Economic evaluations only really make sense if they support decisions which can create value at a local level, and this requires reflecting the realities of localized constraints. Decisions made at higher levels (e.g., regionally, internationally) also have to ultimately contribute to health improvement at local levels.

The tools of economic evaluation have been applied now in global health, at least to some degree, for the best part of two decades. The two major initiatives to date — WHO-CHOICE and the Disease Control Priorities Project (DCPP) — can be characterized, however, as being predominantly top–down approaches: Based upon the collation of evidence and provision of guidance at an international level. Whilst they have had important roles informing policymakers, especially at international levels, it is not clear that their recommendations have been consistent with local, within-country priorities based upon the constraints faced.

A major danger, if evaluations are not grounded within local realities, is that analysts may become more affected by international influences — including specialist clinicians, industry representatives, or other groups with specific interest in promotion of particular diseases and/or interventions/programmes — than by policy needs within lower-income countries. Whilst it is not clear the extent to which this has occurred, many working in this area feel that a large proportion of analyses do not adequately reflect the difficult decisions and trade-offs faced by within-country policymakers.

A new initiative — the International Decision Support Initiative (www.idsi-health.org) — has recently been established to inform health priorities at a local level. The idea behind iDSI is to support countries, on a demand-led basis, in setting up the evaluation processes and institutions, and informing countries on suitable methods required to make difficult decisions on resource allocation. The initiative holds promise that value for money criteria becomes central in the design of health care systems and in the provision of services, based upon the recognition of localized constraints. However, this is clearly no trivial task — it requires political commitment to establish such institutions and processes, capacity for these to be managed and also, crucially, guidance on the methods that can be used to inform such decisions.

Considering resource allocation across a country's health care system gives rise to the vast universe of possibilities regarding what policies can be pursued and what kinds of analyses, based upon limited resources and capacities available, can inform areas of focus and the choice of policies. Such choices can be guided by calls for universality in access to health care (Frenk and de Ferranti, 2012). This chapter has highlighted that policymakers need to think beyond the delivery of specific health care interventions or programmes to consider also prospects for improved implementation and generating demand. Potential policies can relate to all functions of the health care system. The importance of appropriate topic selection upon which analyses should focus is evident in this light. Analyses need to be geared towards areas of greatest importance and not just relate to the latest 'new' interventions. Routine data as a means for understanding current disease and treatment patterns is likely to be an important input in informing topic selection. Further research is required to determine routine data that would be most valuable in informing both topic selection and economic evaluations and to determine better means for prioritizing topics for evaluation.

The centrality of determining value based upon local contexts and constraints implies that a key area of work for the more thorough application of economic evaluation methods in LMICs, regardless of the particular policy question at hand, is to assess the benefits forgone whenever interventions or programmes are implemented. Cost-effectiveness analyses, as routinely applied within higher-income settings, assumes the allocation of a fixed overall health care budget with the sole purpose of generating 'health' amongst the population. In many lower-income settings, reliant on pluralistic sources of financing, the notion of one overall health budget is less plausible. Interventions with non-marginal budget impacts and rapid changes to the health care budget are also more likely in the context of LMICs. Further work is required to determine how these factors can be reflected in estimates of opportunity cost.

Priority lists of cost-effective care in the form of "health benefits plans" have been used as a basis for priority setting in LMICs (Glassman and Chalkidou, 2012). To align with the principles of economic evaluation, benefit plans should only include interventions which would generate value at the local level. They should be based as much as possible on evaluations conducted using locally relevant data and should use local estimates of opportunity cost. Design of benefits plans should consider the potential for any large proposals for expenditure to displace activity that is more valuable than suggested by a threshold value which reflects opportunity cost at the margin.

To ensure that policy decisions deliver value locally, more focus could be given to ensuring that key parameters that determine the relative value of different interventions reflect local preferences. This should include use of locally relevant discount rates and health state preferences.

The delivery and receipt of interventions often draws upon a number of sources of funding, as well as additional resources (human, capital and infrastructural, as well as financial), and is more likely to result in consequences beyond those captured in measures of health alone. The incorporation of these considerations, when this is deemed to be necessary, also still requires further methods research as highlighted in this chapter. For a number of the methods issues highlighted — in particular the inclusion of non-health effects (see Section "Non-Health Costs and Effects") and concerns for equity (see Section "Equity Considerations") — the literature is still far from a consensus on how these can best be reflected within any (high- or low-income) setting. It remains unclear whether formal incorporation of these concerns, perhaps distilled into a single number in evaluations, is even desirable. The alternative is for multiple sources of evidence (e.g., on costs, health gained, equity, non-health effects) be instead presented independently to decision-making authorities which can then weigh the merits of the evidence which they have been provided. Crucially, any wider effects of health care interventions need to be reflected in opportunity costs.

However, the aggregation of multiple criteria — whether done formally in analyses or informally through a deliberative process — relies upon some social value judgment. What these value judgments are, and the ethical bases upon which they can be made, requires careful consideration. There is inevitable danger that decisions turn on the preferences, idiosyncrasies and even biases of the individual decision-makers in place at any one time. Therefore, research to highlight the range of trade-offs between competing concerns, how these can be reasonably weighed, and who should undertake the weighting, is always likely to remain valuable. A key issue then is when are extensions to the more routine application of cost-effectiveness analysis (e.g., to reflect equity concerns, to assess whether to implement a policy now or postpone implementation until further research is conducted) required and how can this be determined.

The principles of decision-making under uncertainty are not generally embedded in high-income country resource allocation decision-making (Kent *et al.*, 2013). "Lessons learned" from the experiences of educating decision-makers in relevant concepts and simplifying the required analyses should be used to inform development of these methods for LMICs.

In countries where economic evaluation is most routinely used to inform policy decisions (e.g., in Europe, Canada, and Australia) substantial research capacity has been built up over the years to produce, review and critique analyses. This critical mass is sustained through demand for such expertize from institutions charged with informing policy within jurisdictions (e.g., NICE in the UK, CADTH in Canada), and methods development has been motivated by and responded to policy needs.

In contrast and by comparison, the economic evaluation field as applied within lower-income settings remains underdeveloped, with only limited research on the development of suitable methods. Many current studies are funded alongside clinical research studies and often through the same funding channel. This risks compromising the impartiality of economics research in informing overall resource allocation but also provides limited scope for transformative methods research and the building of long-term technical capacity. The development of local institutions with responsibility for translating evidence to inform resource allocation decisions will hopefully encourage development of more contextually appropriate methods and data.

Building capacity for research in LMICs is likely to be a slow process and, in some countries, only very limited research resources may be available even in the longer term. It is, therefore, imperative that, in addition to efforts taken to improve economic evaluation methods in LMICs, efforts are also made to disseminate the methods in way that is accessible to researchers working across LMICs.

Capacity for economic evaluation is limited not only in lower-income settings but also amongst researchers working in this area in high-income countries — many of whom are expected to take supervisory roles when working in these contexts. The substantive body of research capacity built up around health technology assessment (HTA) institutions in higher-income settings rarely if ever applies its expertize to health problems facing lower-income countries. This is partly the result of a largely unnecessary separation in this field of study (DALYs in global health, as opposed to QALYs used in all other settings, is just one example), but it is also due to inadequate financing of research for LMICs. To address this situation would require large up-front investment and long-term commitment in the economic evaluation field from funders in global health.

Increasing capacity in economic evaluation for low-income contexts is itself, however, not sufficient. The transition from suboptimal allocations to achieving greatest gains from available health sector resources requires substantial political commitment and relies upon country ownership of decisions. This task will be challenging and involve difficult choices — such as closing some services and redirecting health workforces — with substantial associated transaction costs of change. Even discussing opportunity cost, for example when setting a cost-effectiveness threshold, can be politically controversial. It is only through commitment to these at the level of jurisdictions, which requires the establishment of mandated institutions and processes (such as those being supported by iDSI), that these difficult decisions can and will be made. In turn, within-country institutions can provide the foundation for research suitable to the needs policymakers in LMICs.

Acknowledgments

Centre for Health Economics received funding from the International Decision-Support Initiative (www.idsihealth.org) for this work. IDSI is multi-institution initiative coordinated by NICE International that has received funding from the Bill and Melinda Gates Foundation and the Department for International Development, United Kingdom Government.

The authors wish to thank the following individuals for their helpful comments and suggestions: Yot Teerawattananon, Nattha Tritasavit, Peter Smith, Ranjeeta Thomas, Amanda Glassman, Francis Ruiz, and Kalipso Chalkidou. Any remaining errors or omissions are those of the authors.

References

Acharya A, Adam T, Baltussen R, Evans D, Hutubessy R, Murray CJL, Tan Torres, T. 2004. *Making Choices in Health. WHO Guide to Cost-Effectiveness Analysis*, World Health Organization.

De Savigny D, Taghreed A. 2009. Systems thinking for health systems strengthening. Geneva, Switzerland: Alliance for Health Policy and Systems Research, World Health Organization.

Asaria M, Cookson R, Griffin S. 2014. Incorporating Health Inequality Impacts into Cost-Effectiveness Analysis. In: Culyer AJ. (ed.). Elsevier.

Babiker AG, Emery S, Fatkenheuer G, Gordin FM, Grund B, Lundgren JD, Neaton JD, Pett SL, Phillips A, Touloumi G, Vjechaj MJ, Group ISS. 2013. Considerations in the rationale, design and methods of the strategic timing of antiretroviral treatment (start) study. *Clinical Trials* 10: S5–S36.

Banerjee AV, Duflo E, Glennerster R, Kothari D. 2010. Improving immunisation coverage in rural India: Clustered randomised controlled evaluation of immunisation campaigns with and without incentives. *British Medical Journal* 340: c2220.

Basinga P, Gertler PJ, Binagwaho A, Soucat ALB, Sturdy J, Vermeersch CMJ. 2011. Effect on maternal and child health services in Rwanda of payment to primary health-care providers for performance: An impact evaluation. *Lancet* 377: 1421–1428.

Bill and Melinda Gates Foundation 2014. Methods for Economic Evaluation Project (MEEP) — Final Report. A partnership between Bill and Melinda Gates Foundation, NICE International, the Health Intervention and Technology Assessment Program (Thailand), and the University of York, Centre for Health Economics.

Bowie C, Mwase T. 2011. Assessing the use of an essential health package in a sector wide approach in Malawi. *Health Research Policy and Systems* 9: 4.

Brouwer WB, Culyer AJ, Van Exel NJ, Rutten FF. 2008. Welfarism vs. extra-welfarism. *Journal of Health Economics* 27: 325–338.

Chalkley M, Malcomson JM. 2000. Government purchasing of health services. *Handbook of Health Economics* 1: 847–890.

Claxton K. 1999. The irrelevance of inference: A decision-making approach to the stochastic evaluation of health care technologies. *Journal of Health Economics* 18: 341–364.

Claxton K, Palmer S, Longworth L, Bojke L, Griffin S, Mckenna C, Soares M, Spackman E, Youn J. 2012. Informing a decision framework for when NICE should recommend the use of health technologies only in the context of an appropriately designed programme of evidence development. *Health Technology Assessment* (*Winchester, England*) 16: 1–323.

Claxton K, Paulden M, Gravelle H, Brouwer W, Culyer AJ. 2011. Discounting and decision making in the economic evaluation of health-care technologies. *Health Economics* 20: 2–15.

Claxton K, Walker S, Palmer S, Sculpher M. 2010. Appropriate Perspectives for Health Care Decisions. *CHE Research Paper 54.*

Culyer A, Mccabe C, Briggs A, Claxton K, Buxton M, Akehurst R, Sculpher M, Brazier J. 2007. Searching for a threshold, not setting one: The role of the National Institute for Health and Clinical Excellence. *Journal of Health Services Research & Policy* 12: 56–58.

Culyer T. 2012. *The Humble Economist.* York, York Publishing Services Ltd.

Drummond M, Sculpher M, Torrance G, O'Brien B, Stoddart G. 2005. *Methods for the Economic Evaluation of Health Care Programmes. 3rd Edition*, Oxford Medical Publications.

Ensor T, Cooper S. 2004. Overcoming barriers to health service access: Influencing the demand side. *Health Policy Plan* 19: 69–79.

Fenwick EF, Claxton K, Sculpher MJ. 2008. The value of implementation and the value of information: Combined and uneven development. *Medical Decision Making* 28: 21–32.

Frenk J, De Ferranti D. 2012. Universal health coverage: Good health, good economics. *Lancet* 380: 862–864.

Gaarder MM, Glassman A, Todd JE. 2010. Conditional cash transfers and health: Unpacking the causal chain. *Journal of Development Effectiveness* 2: 6–50.

Gafni A, Birch S. 1997. QALYs and HYEs (healthy years equivalent). Spotting the differences. *Journal of Health Economics* 16: 601–608.

Glassman A, Chalkidou K. 2012. Priority Setting in Health: Building Institutions for Smarter Public Spending. A Report of the Centre for Global Development's Priority-Setting Institutions for Global Health Working Group.

Glassman A, Duran D, Fleisher L, Singer D, Sturke R, Ageles G, Charles J, Emrey B, Gleason J, Mwebsa W, Saldana K, Yarrow K, Koblinsky. 2013. Impact of conditional cash transfers on maternal and newborn health. *Journal of Health, Population and Nutrition (JHPN)* 31.

Gold MR, Stevenson D, Fryback DG. 2002. HALYs and QALYs and DALYs, Oh My: Similarities and differences in summary measures of population health. *Annual Review of Public Health* 23: 115–134.

Green LV, Savin S. 2008. Reducing delays for medical appointments: A queueing approach. *Operations Research* 56: 1526–1538.

Grossman M. 1972. Concept of health capital and demand for health. *Journal of Political Economy* 80: 223–225.

Hanson K, Ranson MK, Oliveira-Cruz V, Mills A. 2003. Expanding access to priority health interventions: A framework for understanding the constraints to scaling-up. *Journal of International Development* 15: 1–14.

Health Systems Financing And Governance Department, WHO. 2013. OneHealth tool: Supporting intergrated strategic health planning, costing and health impact analysis.

Jamison DT. 2006. Investing in Health. In Jamison DT, Breman JG, Measham AR, Alleyne G, Claeson M, Evans DB, Jha P, Mills A, Musgrove P. (eds.). *Disease Control Priorities in Developing Countries.* 2nd Edition. Washington (DC).

Jamison DT, Bobadilla JL, Mosley WH, Measham AR. 1994. *Disease Control Priorities in Developing Countries*. Oxford University Press.

Jansen JP, Fleurence R, Devine B, Itzler R, Barrett A, Hawkins N, Lee K, Boersma C, Annemans L, Cappelleri JC. 2011. Interpreting indirect treatment comparisons and network meta-analysis for health-care decision making: Report of the ISPOR Task Force on Indirect Treatment Comparisons Good Research Practices: Part 1. *Value in Health: The Journal of the International Society for Pharmacoeconomics and Outcomes Research* 14: 417–428.

Jelsma J, Hansen K, De Weerdt W, De Cock P, Kind P. 2003. How do Zimbabweans value health states? *Population Health Metrics* 1: 11.

Jiang LX, Giachetti RE. 2008. A queueing network model to analyze the impact of parallelization of care on patient cycle time. *Health Care Management Science* 11: 248–261.

Johri M, Norheim OF. 2012. Can cost-effectiveness analysis integrate concerns for equity? Systematic review. *International Journal of Technology Assessment in Health Care* 28: 125–132.

Kakwani N, Wagstaff A, Vandoorslaer E 1997. Socioeconomic inequalities in health: Measurement, computation, and statistical inference. *Journal of Econometrics* 77: 87–103.

Kent S, Briggs A, Eckermann S, Berry C. 2013. Are value of information methods ready for prime time? An application to alternative treatment strategies for NSTEMI patients. *International Journal of Technology Assessment in Health Care* 29: 435–442.

Koffijberg H, De Wit GA, Feenstra TL. 2012. Communicating uncertainty in economic evaluations: Verifying optimal strategies. *Medical Decision Making: An International Journal of the Society for Medical Decision Making* 32: 477–487.

Kularatna S, Whitty JA, Johnson NW, Scuffham PA. 2013. Health state valuation in low- and middle-income countries: A systematic review of the literature. *Value Health* 16: 1091–1099.

Lim YW, Shafie AA, Hassali MAA, Chua GN. 2013. Exploring the feasibility of the instrument used in determination of willingness-to-pay per quality-adjusted life-year in Malaysia. *Value in Health* 16: A596–A597.

Lozano R, Naghavi M, Foreman K, Lim S, Shibuya K, Aboyans V, Abraham J, Adair T, Aggarwal R, Ahn SY, Alvarado M, Anderson HR, Anderson LM, Andrews KG, Atkinson C, Baddour LM, Barker-Collo S, Bartels DH, Bell ML, Benjamin EJ, Bennett D, Bhalla K, Bikbov B, Bin Abdulhak A, Birbeck G, Blyth F, Bolliger I, Boufous S, Bucello C, Burch M, Burney P, Carapetis J, Chen H, Chou D, Chugh SS, Coffeng LE, Colan SD, Colquhoun S, Colson KE, Condon J, Connor MD, Cooper LT, Corriere M, Cortinovis M, De Vaccaro KC, Couser W, Cowie BC, Criqui MH, Cross M, Dabhadkar KC, Dahodwala N, De Leo D, Degenhardt L, Delossantos A, Denenberg J, Des Jarlais DC, Dharmaratne SD, Dorsey ER, Driscoll T, Duber H, Ebel B, Erwin PJ, Espindola P, Ezzati M, Feigin V, Flaxman AD, Forouzanfar MH, Fowkes FG, Franklin R, Fransen M, Freeman MK, Gabriel SE, Gakidou E, Gaspari F, Gillum RF, Gonzalez-Medina D, Halasa YA, Haring D, Harrison JE, Havmoeller R, Hay RJ, Hoen B, Hotez PJ, Hoy D, Jacobsen KH, James SL, Jasrasaria R, Jayaraman S, Johns N, Karthikeyan G, Kassebaum N, Keren A, Khoo JP, Knowlton LM, Kobusingye O, Koranteng A, Krishnamurthi R, Lipnick M, Lipshultz SE, Ohno SL, *et al.* 2012. Global and regional mortality from 235 causes of death for 20 age groups in 1990 and 2010: A systematic analysis for the Global Burden of Disease Study 2010. *Lancet* 380: 2095–2128.

Mckenna C, Chalabi Z, Epstein D, Claxton K. 2010. Budgetary policies and available actions: A generalisation of decision rules for allocation and research decisions. *Journal of Health Economics* 29: 170–181.

Mehrez A, Gafni A. 1989. Quality-adjusted life years, utility theory, and healthy-years equivalents. *Medical Decision Making* 9: 142–149.

Mills A. 2014. Health care systems in low- and middle-income countries. *New England Journal of Medicine* 370: 552–557.

Mitton CR, Donaldson C. 2003. Setting priorities and allocating resources in health regions: Lessons from a project evaluating program budgeting and marginal analysis (PBMA). *Health Policy* 64: 335–348.

Moreno-Serra R, Smith PC. 2014. Broader health coverage is good for the nation's health: Evidence from country level panel data. *Journal of the Royal Statistical Society: Series A* (*Statistics in Society*) 178(1): 101–124.

Ndiaye M, Alfares H. 2008. Modeling health care facility location for moving population groups. *Computers & Operations Research* 35: 2154–2161.

Peters D, Chao S. Y. 1998. The sector-wide approach in health: What is it? Where is it leading? *International Journal of Health Planning and Management* 13: 177–190.

Rais A, Viana A. 2011. Operations research in healthcare: A survey. *International Transactions in Operational Research* 18: 1–31.

Ramsey FP. 1928. A mathematical theory of saving. *The Economic Journal* 38: 543–559.

Revill P, Walker S, Madan J, Ciaranello A, Mwase T, Gibb D.M, Claxton K, Sculpher MJ. 2014. Using cost-effectiveness thresholds to determine value for money in low- and middle-income country healthcare systems: Are current international norms fit for purpose? *Centre for Health Economics Research Paper 98.* The University of York.

Salanti G. 2012. Indirect and mixed-treatment comparison, network, or multiple-treatments meta-analysis: Many names, many benefits, many concerns for the next generation evidence synthesis tool. *Research Synthesis Methods* 3: 80–97.

Salomon JA, Vos T, Hogan DR, Gagnon M, Naghavi M, Mokdad A, Begum N, Shah R, Karyana M, Kosen S, Farje MR, Moncada G, Dutta A, Sazawal S, Dyer A, Seiler J, Aboyans V, Baker L, Baxter A, Benjamin EJ, Bhalla K, Bin Abdulhak A, Blyth F, Bourne R, Braithwaite T, Brooks P, Brugha TS, Bryan-Hancock C, Buchbinder R, Burney P, Calabria B, Chen H, Chugh SS, Cooley R, Criqui MH, Cross M, Dabhadkar KC, Dahodwala N, Davis A, Degenhardt L, Diaz-Torne C, Dorsey ER, Driscoll T, Edmond K, Elbaz A, Ezzati M, Feigin V, Ferri CP, Flaxman AD, Flood L, Fransen M, Fuse K, Gabbe BJ, Gillum RF, Haagsma J, Harrison JE, Havmoeller R, Hay RJ, Hel-Baqui A, Hoek HW, Hoffman H, Hogeland E, Hoy D, Jarvis D, Karthikeyan G, Knowlton LM, Lathlean T, Leasher JL, Lim SS, Lipshultz SE, Lopez AD, Lozano R, Lyons R, Malekzadeh R, Marcenes W, March L, Margolis DJ, Mcgill N, Mcgrath J, Mensah GA, Meyer AC, Michaud C, Moran A, Mori R, Murdoch ME, Naldi L, Newton CR, Norman R, Omer SB, Osborne R, Pearce N, Perez-Ruiz F, Perico N, Pesudovs K, Phillips D, Pourmalek F, Prince M, Rehm JT, Remuzzi G, Richardson K, *et al.* 2012. Common values in assessing health outcomes from disease and injury: Disability weights measurement study for the Global Burden of Disease Study 2010. *Lancet* 380: 21292143.

Sculpher MJ, Drummond MF. 2006. Analysis sans frontieres: Can we ever make economic evaluations generalisable across jurisdictions? *Pharmacoeconomics* 24: 1087–1099.

Shah KK, Cookson R, Culyer AJ, Littlejohns P. 2013. NICE's social value judgements about equity in health and health care. *Health Economics, Policy, and Law* 8: 145–165.

Shillcutt SD, Walker DG, Goodman CA, Mills AJ. 2009. Cost effectiveness in low- and middle-income countries: A review of the debates surrounding decision rules *Pharmacoeconomics* 27: 903–917.

Swinburn P, Shingler SL, Kim WS, Chao TY, Huang H, Liu Y, Acaster S. 2012. Health State utilities for Relapsed/Refractory (Rel/Ref) Hodgkin's Lymphoma (HL) and Systemic Anaplastic Large-Cell Lymphoma (SALCL): Asian Pacific Country Data. *Value in Health* 15: A657–A657.

Thavorncharoensap M, Teerawattananon Y, Natanant S, Kulpeng W, Yothasamut J, Werayingyong P. 2013. Estimating the willingness to pay for a quality adjusted life year in Thailand: Does the context of health gain matter. *ClinicoEconomics and Outcomes Research* 5: 29–36.

Thokala P, Duenas A. 2012. Multiple criteria decision analysis for health technology assessment. *Value in Health: The Journal of the International Society for Pharmacoeconomics and Outcomes Research* 15: 1172–1181.

Treasury HMS. 2003. *The Green Book: Appraisal and Evaluation in Central Government: Treasury Guidance*. Stationery Office.

Turner RM, Spiegelhalter DJ, Smith GCS, Thompson SG. 2009. Bias modelling in evidence synthesis. *Journal of the Royal Statistical Society. Series A* (*Statistics in Society*) 172: 21–47.

Verguet S, Laxminarayan R, Jamison DT. 2014. Universal public finance of tuberculosis treatment in India: An extended cost-effectiveness analysis. *Health Economics* 24(3): 318–332.

Verguet S, Murphy S, Anderson B, Johansson KA, Glass R, Rheingans R. 2013. Public finance of rotavirus vaccination in India and Ethiopia: An extended cost-effectiveness analysis. *Vaccine* 31: 4902–4910.

Volpp KG, Loewenstein G, Troxel AB, Doshi J, Price M, Laskin M, Kimmel SE. 2008. A test of financial incentives to improve warfarin adherence. *BMC Health Services Research* 8: 272.

Wagstaff A, Vandoorslaer E. 1992. Equity in the finance of health-care — Some international comparisons. *Journal of Health Economics* 11: 361–387.

Walker S, Faria R, Dixon S, Palmer S, Sculpher M. 2013. Getting Cost-Effective Technologies into Practice: The value of implementation. Policy Research Unit in Economic Evaluation in Health and Care Interventions: School of Health and Related Studies (SHARR), University of Sheffield & Centre for Health Economics (CHE), University of York.

WHO. 2012. *World Health Organization, Cost-Effectiveness Thresholds. http://www.who.int/choice/costs/CER_thresholds/en/index.html* [Online]. [Accessed 30 April 2012].

WHO. 2013. Consolidated Guidelines on the Use of Antiretroviral Drugs for Treating and Preventing HIV Infection: Recommendations for a public health approach.

Williams A. 1999. Calculating the global burden of disease: Time for a strategic reappraisal? *Health Economics* 8: 1–8.

World Bank. 2015. Data: Country and Lending Groups. [ONLINE] Available at: http://data.worldbank.org/about/country-and-lending-groups [Accessed 14 September 15].

World Bank. 1993. *World Development Report: Investing in Health*. World Bank and Oxford University Press.

World Health Organization. 1996. *Investing in Health Research and Development. Report of the Ad Hoc Committee on Health Research Relating to Future Intervention Options. Geneva: World Health Organization.*

World Health Organization. 2000. *The World Health Report 2000: Health Systems: Improving Performance.*

World Health Organization. 2012. *Spending on Health: A Global Overview* [Online]. Available: http://who.int/mediacentre/factsheets/fs319/en/index.html [Accessed 17 February 2014].

Yothasamut J, Tantivess S, Teerawattananon Y. 2009. Using economic evaluation in policy decision-making in asian countries: Mission impossible or mission probable? *Value in Health* 12: S26–S30.

Zhuang J, Liang Z, Lin T, De Guzman F. 2007. *Theory and Practice in the Choice of Social Discount Rate for Cost–Benefit Analysis: A Survey*. Asian Development Bank.

Inequalities and Inequities in Health and Health Care*

Marisol Rodríguez
University of Barcelona

Rosa Urbanos-Garrido
Complutense University of Madrid

Inequalities in health and health care in the form of a social gradient are a long persisting phenomenon across and within countries, and in many cases gaps have widened over time. Nevertheless, inequities only arise when inequalities are unfair and avoidable by reasonable action. The magnitude and the direction of the gradient largely vary across time, regions, diseases, genders and socioeconomic indicators. Unfortunately, the exact mechanisms by which socioeconomic status (SES) drives better or worse health are not well known or understood as yet. Socioeconomic and geographical disparities are also present in the access to and the use of health care services, even despite worldwide progress on the road to universal health care coverage. There are no universal prescriptions for effectively reducing inequities. Moreover, at the level of action, not all the recommendations by experts are possible or desirable aims for intervention for those in charge of designing policies. Although health Millenium Development Goals (MDGs) have shown significant progress during the 21st century, major efforts are still needed to combat illnesses that particularly affect the worse off, and to provide better access to health care. The fight against inequities in health and health care should remain relevant targets in the global agenda.

Keywords: Inequalities; Inequities; Social Gradient.

---

*Parts of Sections "Chief Measures", "Are Health Care Systems Inequitable? By How Much?" and "Some Considerations about Future Actions" draw from a teaching unit written by Marisol Rodríguez for the online International Master in Health Economics and Pharmacoeconomics at UPF Barcelona School of Management.

Introduction

Although during the last century average life expectancy has doubled and the global amount of health care resources has largely been increased, inequalities in health and health care persist across and within countries, and in many cases gaps have widened over time. Undoubtedly, not all the differences in health status or in the distribution of health care between different population groups are of concern, but only those which may be considered unfair and avoidable by reasonable action (Whitehead, 1992; CSDH, 2008) or, to put it another way, those that can be labelled as inequitable. The existence and growth of these inequalities may be judged as one of the urgent global health problems which should be addressed not only at a national level, but also by the international community.

As unfair inequalities in health may be seen as a global phenomenon, the text will focus on low- and middle-income countries, as well as on high-income countries. Every section of the chapter will include references to both geographical contexts.

Several dimensions of inequity can be analyzed, as population groups may be distinguished by their socioeconomic status (SES), their geographical location, their gender or their race, among other relevant characteristics. All these dimensions should be taken into account when inequity is analyzed and addressed. Therefore, in this chapter, we will try to illustrate most of them with recent data.

Section "Conceptual Framework" addresses the conceptual framework for both equity in health and health care. Section "Health Inequalities: Measurement and Empirical Evidence" presents the worldwide empirical evidence of socioeconomic inequalities in health and highlights issues about their measurement and the suitability of existing indicators to guide policy. Equity in health care is analyzed in Sections "Inequalities in the Access to Health Care" and "Inequity in the Utilization of Health Care" from two complementary perspectives: The access to and the utilization of health services, respectively. The chapter ends with Section "From Theory to Practice: Addressing Health & Health Care Disparities," where courses of action are suggested to reduce health and health care disparities.

Conceptual Framework

Although the phenomenon of socioeconomic inequalities in health is not new, its rediscovery at the end of the 20th century contributed to a radical change in the analysis of the determinants of health itself. In effect, health and sickness are no longer understood as being caused only by biological and medical care factors, but increasingly as a function of social, psychological and behavioral factors that are far from alien to the socioeconomic context. It is a change that has brought about the full and generalized integration of social factors into the determinants of health. This, in turn, is affecting the traditional scope of public health. Social factors and health inequalities are now current topics involved under the standard trilogy of prevention, protection and promotion that enter the definition of public health.

Inequalities in health and health care may be due to different factors. If, as it was mentioned in the introduction, they are unavoidable (for instance, health disparities due to age) or acceptable (more health care resources allocated to the needy), they cannot be labelled as unfair. Therefore, it is necessary to determine when inequalities in health and health care are due to factors than can (or cannot) be ethically justified (Fleurbaey and Schockkaert, 2012).

Equity in health care

Clinical needs and preferences (as well as appropriateness of intervention) are seen as legitimate reasons for health care differences across population groups (Fleurbaey and Schockkaert, 2012). Hence, if two groups have different needs, they should be treated differently by the health system (generally it is assumed that needy groups should receive more care). Furthermore, if those groups are equally needy but they have different preferences about health care (e.g., one of them prefers not to be treated), differences in treatment may also be considered legitimate. Julian Le Grand, in a classical work (Le Grand, 1991), proposed that in a context where choice sets are equal and choices are freely made, any resulting distribution should be considered equitable. Then, the question about how to define a free choice arises. According to Roemer, real freedom of choice can only be guaranteed when all the individuals are equally aware of the costs and benefits linked to an action. Therefore, equality of opportunity is only possible provided that the impact of exogenous circumstances on personal choices has been counteracted (Roemer, 1998). That is to say, even preferences may be considered an illegitimate factor in some cases, since the choices we make are highly influenced by a complex set of — at least partially exogenous — social and economic factors that include our income, education, labor status and the place we live.

Difficulties, both conceptual and operational, to delimit when a situation derives from personal and free choices, may lead to advocating that basic needs should be guaranteed for all, irrespective of their responsibility (Cappelen and Norheim, 2005; Segall, 2010). They also may justify defining equity as not only equal access to available care for equal need, but also as equal use for equal need (Whitehead, 1992), then ignoring the role played by patients' preferences in the utilization of health care resources — which, although limited by asymmetric information, may not be negligible. Furthermore, disparities in the use of health care are important in the assessment of equity as utilization is basically determined by health care providers, and also may be strongly influenced by patients' socio-economic characteristics. Even in quite egalitarian countries, such as Norway, there is evidence showing that highly educated cancer patients are more likely than other patients to be transferred to the two specialized hospitals in the capital, where more advanced treatment may be provided by a highly skilled staff (Fiva *et al.*, 2014). This study also suggested that a substantial part of the educational difference in cancer survival in the analyzed regions was due to differences in access to and utilization of specialized treatment. As treatments in Norway did not depend on the ability to pay, it was suggested that highly educated people gained access to specialized treatments possibly using an information or competency advantage. Moreover, doctors' preferences, skills, abilities, and access to information and resources are also a relevant factor of inequalities in utilization of health care (in terms of quantity and quality of services).

However, equity goals in national health legislation across countries are usually defined in terms of equality of access — relative to equal need (Olsen, 2013). Both aspects, access to and use of health care, although closely related, will deserve separate attention.

Some clarifications about equity in health care should be made at this point. Usually, it is implicitly assumed that more access to health care and more use of medical services are better than less (particularly when literature refers to pro-rich or pro-poor inequity, meaning inequities that favor one or the other socioeconomic group). However, this must be carefully discussed, since higher use of health care resources may be associated either with a better opportunity to be healthy or with a higher risk of losing health. Some evidence points to iatrogenic damage as the third leading cause of death in the US (Starfield, 2000). Moreover, when for-profit organizations are in charge of health care provision, particularly when working on a fee-for-service basis, it is quite common to see how medical care received by patients exceeds the appropriate amount, even in less developed countries (LDC), as Kremer and Glennerster (2012) pointed out.

Therefore, inequity in the use of health services only may be considered as "favoring" a certain group if it leads this group to better health (or, at least, to a better opportunity to be healthy). When unfair and avoidable inequalities are related to overuse of health care services, both equity and efficiency issues arise. Firstly, equity is concerned if a systematic discrimination against one group is identified, although it is necessary to know what the effects on health of such discrimination are before taking a course of action. Secondly, as better use of health resources is possible, efficiency may be improved. And insofar as resources newly available from efficiency improvements are used to alleviate the situation of needy groups, equity may be doubly fostered.

Thus, although inequalities in access to and use of health care for those with equal need are usually labelled as "inequities", we should keep in mind that this assessment is not straightforward. Unfortunately, this issue is difficult to investigate in a proper way when big areas of medical attention are considered (primary care or specialized outpatient or inpatient care, for instance). That is why it is increasingly important to narrow the scope of studies focusing on disparities and inequalities in health care by analyzing specific medical processes or medical conditions. However, until data about the quality and adequacy of health care is made more frequently available, it will be difficult to advance on the assessment of inequity.

Equity in health

Whitehead (1992) defined as unfair all those health inequalities due to health-damaging behavior (in instances where the degree of lifestyle choice is severely restricted); to exposure to unhealthy, stressful living and working conditions; and to inadequate access to essential health care and other public services. Some years later, the Commission on Social Determinants of Health developed a conceptual framework showing the variables influencing equity in health and well being and the channels that transmit their effects, which is broadly accepted (Figure 1). It distinguishes between structural or social determinants of *health inequities*

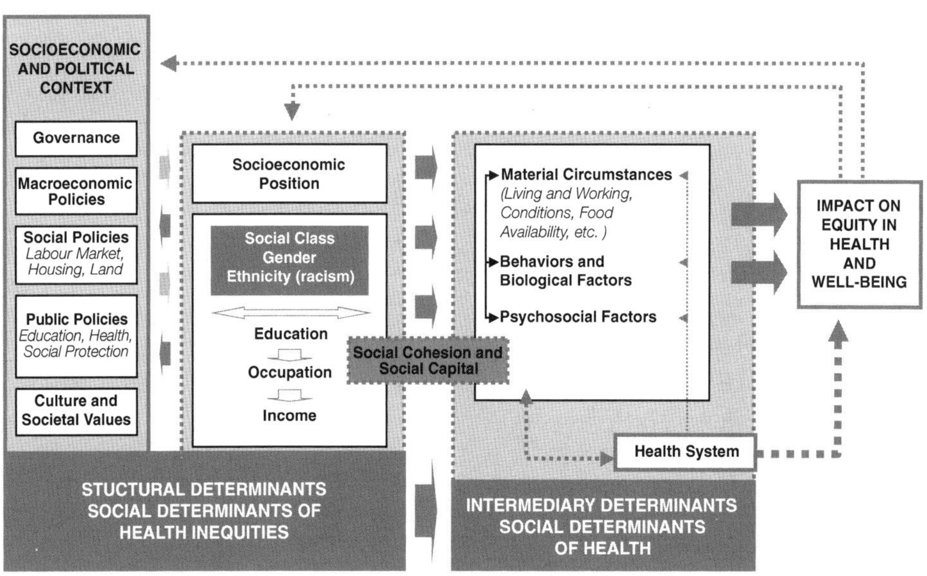

Figure 1. CSDH conceptual framework

Source: WHO (2010a).

(caused by the social, economic and political context resulting in an individual's social position) and intermediary or social determinants of *health* (caused by structural factors), which include material circumstances, behavioral, biological and psychosocial factors, and also the health system itself (WHO, 2010a). The former may be considered as "the causes of the causes," which are responsible for social disadvantage and also for health gradient. The intermediary determinants of health are therefore a consequence of these structural factors, and have a direct influence on health outcomes.

Two main features should be highlighted in this conceptual framework. Firstly, the "lifestyle" approach, where individuals are the main parties responsible of their own health, seems to be definitely dismissed and substituted by the "living conditions" approach, where most of circumstances affecting health are not chosen by the person. Therefore, this framework suggests that since responsibility for health outcomes and distribution is largely collective, social intervention should be called for. Secondly, the reduction of inequities requires the design of global and intersectoral strategies, not merely focused on the health care system. We will return to these points in Section "Inequity in the Utilization of Health Care".

Since by our definition health inequalities must be not only unfair but also avoidable to be labelled as inequities, it may be discussed the extent to which the above-mentioned determinants may be avoided through what the World Health Organization (WHO) calls 'plausible' interventions (WHO, 2010b). It is not clear if this means that the interventions have to just be feasible or also not too costly (Olsen, 2013). But as huge differences in health between and within countries are mainly considered "a matter of social justice", and fighting against them is seen as an "ethical imperative" (CSDH, 2008), for our purposes we will deem that any action trying to impact health determinants — whether structural or intermediary — is plausible, although not always may be regarded as unambitious.

The conceptual framework shown in Figure 1 is valid for all countries, irrespective of their level of income and development. However, interventions designed to reduce health inequities should be regionally adapted, since main causes of illness and death substantially differ across countries. In low-income countries, childhood underweight, unsafe water and hygiene, unsafe sex, suboptimal breastfeeding and indoor smoke from solid fuels are the five leading risk factors causing losses of Disability-Adjusted Life Years (DALYs), whilst for middle- and high-income countries, major causes of DALY losses are related to alcohol and tobacco use, overweight and obesity, high blood pressure and hyperglycemia (WHO, 2009). These differences suggest that, although health inequalities are generated and transmitted through common channels all around the world, the relative weight of health determinants — and determinants of health inequities — may be quite different across world regions.

Poverty and lack of access to basic goods and services (food, clean water, sanitation and health services, among others) are the main sources of health inequalities in low-income countries. New analysis also shows that power imbalances between social groups and even gender inequalities in low-income countries are linked to reduced access to clean water and to fewer sanitation improvements, land degradation, and deaths due to indoor and outdoor air pollution, amplifying the effects associated with income disparities (UNDP, 2011). Environmental degradation (greenhouse gas emissions, deforestation, desertification) also has wider effects on LDC, where fewer coping tools (fragile public institutions, poor funding, etc.) are available (UNDP, 2011).

Furthermore, some health threats linked to climate change, such as floods, hurricanes and rising temperature and humidity, are of particular concern in least developed countries (LDC). Siegel (2012) pointed out that climate change will expand the areas where certain infectious diseases — for instance, malaria — are endemic, and highlighted how health impacts will be particularly felt in the LDC because of the limited ability of their public health systems to respond, the great poverty of the population, and their poor stock of initial health capital, while more developed countries will be better able to cope with the effects of extreme temperatures or other climatic shocks. The impact of these weather events may also result in periodic crop failures associated with chronic hunger and famine, which have been characteristic of the Sub-Saharan area.

The recent Ebola outbreak in Africa is another example of how health impacts of epidemics are singularly severe in those countries with very weak health systems, lacking human and infrastructural resources, which also have suffered from long periods of war and conflict. In summary, many health problems are intensified in LDC due to several factors, such as rapid population growth, high rates of poverty and illiteracy, lack of social protection structures, inadequate access to health care and health facilities, unstable political environments, the fragility of public institutions and corruption (Siegel, 2012).

Health Inequalities: Measurement and Empirical Evidence

Measurement methods and concerns

At first glance, measuring inequality should not be a difficult or controversial issue. Inequality is a statistical concept that expresses the greater or lesser concentration or dispersion in the distribution of a characteristic or resource in a particular population. Following certain rules, it should be relatively simple to construct indicators to summarize the degree of inequality that comes out of such a distribution. However, different indicators have different properties, with pros and cons, so that in fact no perfect measure exists. Moreover, inequalities in health carry an implicit moral judgement that makes the topic much more complex and contentious. Not least so because the way we measure and present the facts about inequalities is going to shape, in part, how we understand them and how we will go about tackling them (Braveman, 2006).

An initial issue is whether it is relevant or, indeed, useful to calculate inequalities by themselves (univariate measure) or whether it is better to calculate inequalities in health associated to some socioeconomic variable (bivariate measure). In the first case, the distribution of a certain health measure would be appraised without taking into consideration any other characteristic of the individual or the group. In the second case, we would be estimating socioeconomic inequalities in health, that is to say, evaluating the degree of inequality of the health measure in relation to certain socioeconomic attributes pertaining to each individual or group. For example, we could look at differences in life expectancy by educational level or variations in child mortality between poor and rich regions. To do so, first of all we need to define the socioeconomic variable against which health is going to be compared and then cut it into categories or sets of values. These categories or sets of values constitute a common measurable feature shared by individuals, regions or areas grouped in this manner.

The univariate approach was advocated by several officials at WHO on the occasion of the publication of its World Health Report 2000 (Gakidou *et al.*, 2000; Murray, 2001). They contended that it was more objective to calculate inequalities in "health expectancy" between individuals in the strict sense, without grouping them together socioeconomically, i.e., simply comparing "healthy" and "unhealthy" without examining who the healthy and unhealthy are. This attempted asepsis was charged with being very ideological, and the WHO was severely criticized for it (Navarro, 2000; Braveman *et al.*, 2001). Braveman *et al.* forcefully argued that a comparison of health indicators between individuals or groups (neighborhoods, regions, countries, etc.), without taking into account socioeconomic characteristics, would remove the moral weight attached to inequalities in health and would fail to serve as a useful tool for guiding resource allocation or target policies.

The standard approach is, however, to use a bivariate measure in order to highlight *socioeconomic* inequalities in health. The socioeconomic indicators used most often as reference variables are income, education, occupation, social class (which usually is a composite of the other three), gender, race and urban/rural location. Given that, in most societies, aversion to health inequalities is indeed aversion to socioeconomic inequalities in health, we do not doubt of the necessity of using such socioeconomic indicators in order to present the data and foster concern for health inequalities. However, for inequalities presented in this matter to really inform effective policies, it is crucial that we fully understand the causation mechanisms linking one to the other (Deaton, 2013). Too broad a concept of SES may not be helpful in unravelling causation and thinking about policies.

In spite of great efforts by many authors and institutions (notably, those of the WHO's Commission on Social Determinants of Health already mentioned), the exact mechanisms by which socioeconomic advantage or disadvantage drives better or worse health are not well known or understood as yet. That lessens the suitability of these indicators to guide policy. Take, for instance, the case of stunting in India, a very serious problem that affects 65 million Indian children under the age of 5, including a third of children from the country's richest families. Efforts by families and communities to feed their children are often failing; the reason, now becoming apparent, is poor sanitation. The nutrients that children consume are being diverted away from growth and brain development to fighting infections, thus sanitation and not lack of food is emerging as a principal explanation for stunting and other health problems (Harris, 2014). Poor sanitation has to do with the lack of community infrastructure, but also with a rooted habit of defecating outdoors (it is estimated that half of India's population defecates in the open; more than in any other country of the world).

Interestingly, a well-documented and puzzling phenomenon is that child mortality is much higher among Hindu children than among Muslim children in India, even though Muslims generally have lower SES: They belong to lower castes, and they are poorer and less educated (Bhalotra *et al.*, 2010). Multiple socioeconomic variables, as well as possible differences in childcare practices, have been tested to explain this gap without much success (Guillot and Allendorf, 2010). However, according to the latest research by Geruso and Spears (2014) the 18% difference in infant mortality can be fully explained by the fact that Muslims are far more likely than Hindus to use latrines and, more importantly, to live next to others also using latrines, thus avoiding negative externalities from neighbors. The implication of this finding for our purposes is clear. Inequalities in health measured using SES or ethnicity as grouping variables may sometimes miss or overlook the true causes at work, directing resources, unintentionally, toward the wrong programs (in this case, more money for food or income programs instead of for sanitation or public health education to change population habits). Of course, this is not to imply that everywhere stunting should be fought with sanitation or changing defecation habits. In Afghanistan, the prevalence of stunting among children under 5 is even higher, but defecating in the open a much less frequent practice.

Although some authors see the link between education and health as more sound and stable, there is evidence that shows that their relationship can be quite variable between countries and between sexes, making it difficult to identify a definite pattern. This variability is demonstrated, for example, by Von dem Knesebeck *et al.* (2006), who calculated the odds ratio (OR) of self-rating health as poor, comparing individuals with a low educational level to those with an educational level other than low among a sample of 42,359 individuals from 22 European countries. The OR was not significant for Ireland, Italy and the UK. However, it was significant for women but not men in Austria, Denmark, Germany, the Czech Republic, Norway, Sweden, and Switzerland and, on the contrary, significant for men but not women in Belgium, the Netherlands, and Spain. Finally, it proved significant for both sexes in the remaining countries: France, Finland, Greece, Hungary, Poland, Portugal, and Slovenia.

Moreover, access to education improved greatly in most of these countries in the second half of the 20th century. In Spain, the proportion of people with no education (unable to read or write or only some primary education) diminished dramatically and the average level of education increased extraordinarily, and yet socioeconomic inequalities in health augmented (Regidor *et al.*, 2006). One possible hypothesis is that the meaning of education and other measures of SES has changed over the past 50 years (Regidor, 2008), thus changing the stance of these indicators on the causal pathway to health. Lack of years of formal education in a contemporary young adult could reflect very adverse events in his or her infancy that serve as a predictor of today's not so healthy habits, while illiteracy among our parents and grandparents, which was much more common, would be less predictive of unhealthy lifestyles or reduced ability to cope with life.

The same goes for occupation. In high-income countries, the decline in manufacturing and manual jobs and the growth of service-oriented work imply a reduction in some of the traditional physical and environmental health risks. However, the standard division between manual and non-manual occupations has probably lost its predicting power with regards to health. It may now be more important to distinguish between "standard" full-time permanent contracts and the plethora of atypical working arrangements (freelance, part-time with variable hours, temporary jobs, etc.) that sum up to job insecurity and its toll of bad health (Robone *et al.*, 2010; Solé *et al.*, 2013).

To summarize, the path leading from income (or the other indicators of SES) to health may be a long and erratic one (O'Donnell, 2015). Improving the distribution of income and the general level of education and working conditions may be good things in themselves and would enhance population well-being. But socioeconomic inequalities in health may still persist despite these improvements, and tackling them might require a more specific approach that is most likely different from one country to the next. To be sure, this is not to deny that there is overwhelming evidence that, generally, individuals with a higher socioeconomic position have better health status than those who are worse off. Nor to advocate for measures that do not take into account SES, because that would imply changing altogether the focus of attention and failing to capture the socioeconomic dimension of inequalities in health. We are only saying that evidence of association is not the same as causation. Since policymakers need more evidence of the latter, research on this topic should be moving on to deliver it.

Chief measures

In order to know the magnitude, characteristics and time trends of health inequalities, various measurement tools can be used. Most of them have primarily been developed in the framework of social epidemiology, with some interesting contributions from economics. Depending on what we are interested in measuring, we will choose different methods; and depending on what tool we choose, we will get different results. Regidor (2004a; 2004b) offers a good classification and overview of measures, remarking that it is recommendable to use and compare more than one in order to obtain a more complete vision of health inequalities (Regidor, 2004a).

Some characteristics should be taken into account in determining the appropriate measurement tool. First of all, the type of data available, and whether the data is of aggregate or individual nature, is important to consider. The use of aggregate data tends to weaken the ability to identify associations between variables and makes it more difficult to analyze and control for confounding factors. However, ecological studies have the advantage that they take into account the contextual effect of the area of residence. Second, in comparing different measurement tools, there are pros and cons to each. Some measures, such as the quotient or the difference between socioeconomic groups, analyze information solely on the basis of two groups (e.g., the richest 20% of the population vs. the poorest 20%) and ignore the information on intermediate groups. In contrast, other measures such as the concentration index (CI) or the slope and relative indices of inequality consider all groups included in the study. Effect measures do not take into account the size of the groups whereas total impact measures do. Finally, it is important to distinguish between absolute and relative measures. With absolute measures, we are answering the question, "What is the additional risk of one group with respect to the other?" in absolute terms. Whereas with relative measures, we are answering the question, "How many times more risk does one group have than the other?" Most of the times, we can convert absolute measures to relative ones and vice versa.

Measures that do not take into account the whole population

- *Differences and quotients*

Differences and quotients are the simplest and most intuitive measures of health inequalities. The former are absolute measures and are calculated as the simple difference between the indicators or rates of two groups. The latter are relative measures that are calculated as a quotient or ratio between these rates. For example, given that the mortality rate of white children in the US in 2007 was 5.6 (per 1,000 live births) and the mortality rate of black children was 13.3, the difference stands at 7.7 more deaths per 1,000 live births among black children. Expressed as a ratio (or quotient), it tells us that the relative risk of mortality of black children is almost 2.4 times that of white children.

One limitation of these measures is that, when choosing the two groups, we need to avoid groups that are so broad that the differences are blurred, or groups that are so extreme that they conceal the experiences of the intermediate groups. Another important limitation of these measures is that they do not take into account how individuals are distributed in each category, that is, the group's size and variations that may be present. This can distort comparisons between populations and between time periods within a single population. For example, surely the size and characteristics of the educational group that has received "only primary studies" vary widely among countries that are at very different stages of development and have changed much over time. It is important to be aware of these limitations in both the selection of groups for comparison and in the interpretation of results.

Finally, as we have said, the two measures reflect different concepts, and we cannot say that one is better than the other. Epidemiologists tend to attach greater importance to relative measures, even though a health problem may show large relative differences yet be of little numerical importance (take, for example, a rare disease with a prevalence rate of 8 people per 100,000 in one group and 2 people per 100,000 in another group. The relative risk is 4 — very high — but the absolute difference is 6 people per 100,000). Absolute measures are perhaps a better expression of the magnitude and the social relevance of a health problem since, when we calculate ratios, the units disappear and we lose sight of the magnitude of the problem. Although absolute differences can be converted into relative differences and the other way around it is important to remark that they offer different — sometimes even opposite — perspectives of the evolution of inequalities over time. As an example, let us suppose that the infant mortality rate (IMR) of poor children in a country was 13.3 per 1,000 live births in 2007 and it dropped to 5.5 in 2014, while the evolution of the IMR of rich children changed from 5.6 to 2.0 over the same period. We would say that the absolute difference in IMR between poor and rich children had diminished from 7.7 per 1,000 live births in 2007 to 3.5 in 2010, i.e., less than half the difference in 2007. However, the relative difference (ratio between the IMR of poor children and the IMR of rich children) would have gone from 2.37 to 2.75, that is, it would have increased. The reason is that, proportionally, the drop in the IMR was smaller among poor children than among rich children. In this sense, relative differences are more useful in observing which group has had a more favorable trend. Altogether then, when it comes to looking into the evolution of inequality, it is wise to compare different measures.

- *OR and population attributable risk*

The term "odds" refers to the probability or likelihood of something happening as opposed to it not happening. For example, developing influenza over the year compared to not developing it. The odds of an event happening to one group of people may differ from the odds of that same event happening to another group of people. The comparison of the odds between the two groups is the OR, that is, the ratio of two odds.

If the event we are measuring is a health or health care utilization variable and those two groups are defined by some SES characteristic (e.g., poor and rich, black and white, qualified and unqualified workers), then the OR can be interpreted as a measure of socioeconomic health inequality. For example, if we are comparing disability events between blue-collar and white-collar workers and we find an OR of, say, 1.5, it means that the odds of blue-collar workers suffering a disability event is 1.5 times as high as the odds of white-collar workers suffering a disability event, or an increase of 50% in the odds of blue-collar workers experiencing a disability event. One interesting characteristic is that OR are related to logistic regression, so that most statistical software already directly provides the OR of the variable of interest, taking into account the effect of the other variables present in the equation. It is quite common to find inequalities expressed in terms of OR in the literature.

Population attributable risk (PAR) is a measure of total impact which, by definition, takes into account the size of the groups. In keeping with the SES example, the PAR would be calculated as the difference between the general (average) rate of some outcome in the population and the rate among the highest socioeconomic group, expressed as a percentage of the general rate. Values far from zero indicate greater inequality. The PAR measure enables us to answer questions such as: How many child deaths could be avoided if all groups had the same IMR as the most advantaged group? Nevertheless, its reliance on the population average may mask big differences between the best-placed group or area and the worst-placed. If the majority of the population is fairly well off and has favorable health indicators, the gap between the best-placed group and the population average may not be large. However, the spread between the worst-placed and the best-placed could still be large, and the PAR would not reflect this. For this reason, although the PAR is widely used in epidemiology, it is less widespread in the context of inequalities.

Measures that take into account the whole population

- *The concentration curve and concentration index*

The CI was originally proposed under the framework of a multinational research project on equity issues financed by the European Community and led by Wagstaff and Van Doorslaer. It is based on the concentration curve, a particular case of the Lorenz Curve where the cumulative proportions of the population, beginning with the most disadvantaged socioeconomic individuals or groups and ending with the least disadvantaged, are plotted against the cumulative proportions of health, represented in the y-axis (Wagstaff, *et al.*, 1991). Groups are usually formed by dividing the population into "ten percents" (deciles) or "twenty percents" (quintiles). In this way, by looking at the inequality area between the concentration curve and the 45-degree line, we can visualize the degree of socioeconomic inequality in a chosen health indicator.

The concentration curve can lie below or above the 45-degree line. Taking into account that health tends to show a positive gradient with respect to SES, if the indicator chosen constitutes a measure of "good" health (for instance, life expectancy) the concentration curve will lie below the diagonal, because the least advantaged groups will usually accumulate a less than proportional share of "good" health. However, if the y-axis represents some measure, of ill health (for example, the proportion of people in each socioeconomic group who rates their health as poor or very poor), the concentration curve will lie above the diagonal, because the least advantaged groups will tend to accumulate a higher percentage of ill health compared to their share in the population.

The health CI derives from this concentration curve. The CI corresponding to a concentration curve is equal to twice the area between the concentration curve and the 45-degree line. By convention, a positive sign is given to the areas below the diagonal, and a negative sign to areas of inequality above the diagonal. Thus, the CI varies between −1 (meaning that health — typically "bad" health — is particularly concentrated in the most disadvantaged members of the population) and +1 (meaning that health — typically some measure of "good health" — is disproportionally concentrated in the hands of the most advantaged).

Figure 2 illustrates the construction of concentration curves using the data provided in Table 1, showing health limitations experienced by individuals in 2007 in Cyprus. As the poorest 20% of the population accounts for a disproportionately high percentage of health limitations (39%), the curve lies above the diagonal and the CI will have a negative sign. If the proportion of the population in each income quintile exactly corresponded to the proportion of the population who report health limitations, then the concentration curve would be a straight line coinciding with the 45-degree line. There would be no inequalities and the CI would be equal to zero.

The CI has numerous advantages: Its calculation includes all individuals in the population, it is possible to work with individual or grouped data, it is sensitive to changes in the distribution of the population across different socioeconomic

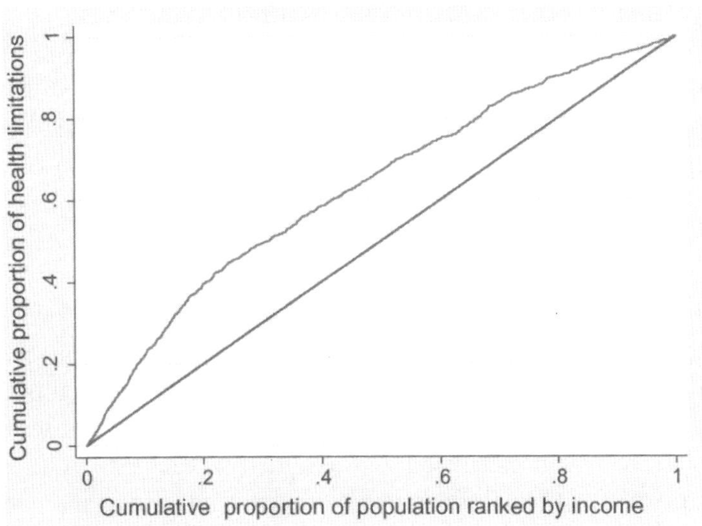

Figure 2. Concentration curve of health limitations in Cyprus

Source: Costa-Font and Hernández-Quevedo (2012).

Table 1. Health limitations reported by individuals in Cyprus, by income quintile.

Quintile	Proportion of all health limitations reported	Cumulative proportion
1 (poorest 20%)	0.390	0.390
2	0.196	0.586
3	0.171	0.757
4	0.154	0.911
5	0.089	1.000
Total	1.000	

Source: Costa-Font and Hernández-Quevedo (2012).

categories, it can be used to compare inequalities in health over time and among different places, and it can be decomposed into the contributions of individual variables so that we can know which factors are most responsible for any inequalities observed. The only requirement is that one must be able to order the various SES categories in accordance to a strict hierarchical ranking (Regidor, 2004b). Continuous variables, such as income or years of schooling are most suitable for this purpose whereas variables such as gender and race/ethnicity would not be suitable. Nevertheless, in recent years, some shortcomings have been pointed out and suggestions to correct those problems have been made (Wagstaff, 2005; Erreygers, 2009).[1]

[1]See Fleurbaey and Schokkaert (2012) for a more thorough and mathematical explanation of the index, its limitations and corrections, and the normative assumptions underlying it.

- *The slope and relative indices of inequality*

Both the slope and relative indices of inequality are regression based, and therefore include all individuals or groups in a population. The slope index of inequality (SII) represents the coefficient in the regression of a health variable on a hierarchical ranking of each socioeconomic category defined on certain social scale. The SII can be interpreted as the absolute change in health level or in the frequency of a health problem when one goes from the highest level in the social hierarchy to the lowest level.

An example is provided in Figure 3, showing the SII in the London borough of Tower Hamlets (Murage *et al.*, 2012). The socioeconomic indicator represented in the x-axis is the Index of Multiple Deprivation, or IMD (based on 7 metrics, including income, employment, education, barriers to housing and services, etc.). An IMD score has been calculated and assigned to each LSOA (Lower Super Output Area, which are small geographical units with an average population of about 1,500) within the borough. LSOAs are then ranked and aggregated into socioeconomic categories (in this case, deciles, that is, 10 equal groups of LSOAs) starting with the most deprived and ending with the best-off (least deprived). Health (indicated by life expectancy) is represented in the y-axis.

The life expectancy of each IMD decile is marked with a dot positioned at the mid-point of the decile range, with the segments representing confidence

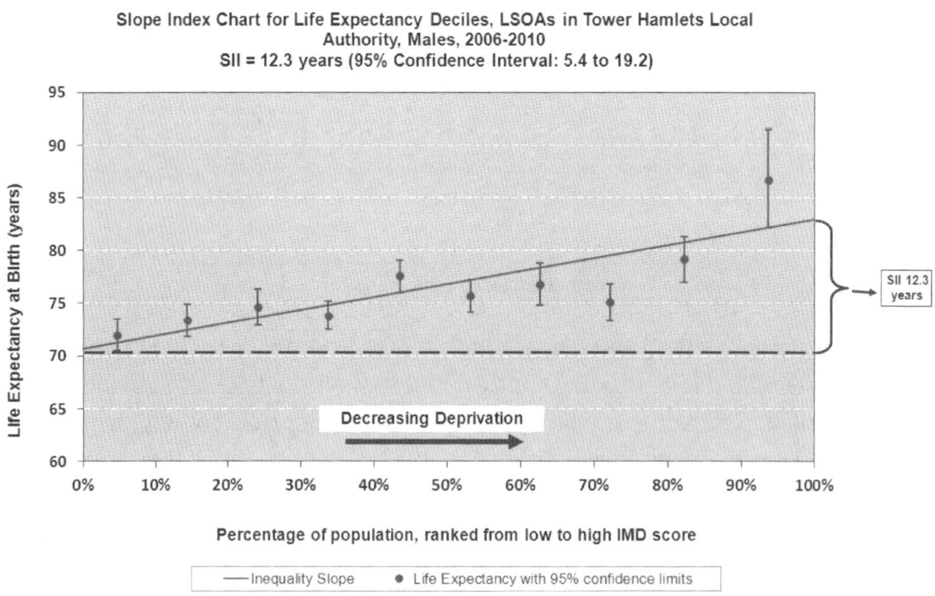

Figure 3. Slope Index of Inequality for male life expectancy by IMD in Tower Hamlets borough (London), 5-year average, 2006–2010

Source: Murage *et al.* (2012).

intervals. The solid line on the graph is a linear regression line of best fit for the data, calculated by the usual least squares method. Now, the SII is simply the gradient of that line. Therefore, it is a single score which represents the gap in years of life expectancy between the best-off LSOAs (at 100% on the x-axis) and worst-off LSOAs within the local authority. In this case, the SII is 12.3 years.

Since the absolute gap between hierarchical categories may change over time while relative differences remain constant (this would happen if, for example, everyone's health doubled, widening absolute differences), the SII is not well suited for establishing comparisons of inequality in health over time. One alternative that has been proposed is the relative index of inequality (RII), which can be estimated by dividing the SII by the mean level of health. A larger RII in one population than in another may be attributable to a larger socioeconomic gradient in health and/or to a larger inequality in the way individuals are distributed across the different socioeconomic categories.

- *The Gini index*

The Gini index, which is based on the Lorenz curve, is calculated from a plot of the cumulative proportion of the population ranked by health — beginning with the sickest person, group or country and ending with the healthiest one — on the x-axis against the cumulative share of health in the population on the y-axis. So, it measures inequalities in the strict sense (Regidor, 2004a), without taking into account any socioeconomic attribute of those persons/groups/countries. Therefore, as argued at the beginning of Section "Measurement Methods and Concerns," it cannot really be considered a measure of *socioeconomic* inequalities in health. In the next section, we will see an example of use of this index in the European Commission Report "Health inequalities in the EU."

Evidence of health inequalities

The evidence that health inequalities exist in all countries and in the form of a social gradient is overwhelming. Socioeconomic health inequality exists even in the countries with the most egalitarian income distributions (e.g., the Nordic European countries), and is not exclusive to comparisons between rich and poor countries. However, the magnitude and the direction of the gradient show variations from one disease to another, from one time period to another, from one place to another, between genders, and between SES indicators used.

The issue of social inequalities in health has been on the political and research agenda of almost all countries since the appearance of the Black

Report[2] in 1980 in the UK, a true milestone in this field, which confirmed the persistence of widespread health inequalities among the population despite 30 years of free and universal health care through the National Health Service (Townsend and Davidson, 1992). The diagnosis was clear: Although health in general had improved in the decades prior, the advances of the poor had not been parallel to those of the rich, who had improved much more, thus widening the gap between the two social classes. A total of 37 recommendations, some of them very specific, were issued, directed in part to the health services sector but basically aimed at eradicating poverty and improving living conditions for the lower classes. Its publication caused uproar in British society, and its impact was and continues to be huge. Yet the reception given to the report by the British Government was icy. The Conservative Secretary of State for Social Services wrote clearly and bluntly in the foreword that the additional expenditure that would be required to follow the report's recommendations was quite unrealistic, and that the government would not, therefore, endorse them.

Turning to a global view of health inequalities, Figure 4 (freely available from the Gapminder Foundation at http://www.gapminder.org/GapminderMedia/wp-uploads/Gapminder-World-2012.pdf) shows that there are more than 30 years' difference between life expectancies in countries with the highest levels and those with the lowest. The former are all rich countries (in terms of income per person) and the latter are all poor countries. But at the intermediate positions we have a great variety of countries with similar life expectancies but very different income levels (compare, for example, Kuwait and Nicaragua, or the US and Costa Rica) or the same income levels but quite different life expectancies (for instance, South Africa and Cuba). The implication is obvious: Money matters, but it is not the only factor explaining inequalities in health at the international (between countries) level. Public policy and the social organization of the country also tend to be decisive.

Figure 5 shows differences in the under-five mortality rate (probability of dying between birth and exactly 5 years of age per 1,000 live births) by quintiles[3] of household wealth in 5 countries. We can observe differences in the average

---

[2] Also known as the Report of the Working Group on Inequalities in Health, the Black Report was published by the UK Department of Health and Social Security and named after the chairman of the expert committee Sir Douglas Black. The report, which had been commissioned in 1977 by David Ennals, Labor Secretary of State, appeared when the conservative party of Margaret Thatcher had gained power.

[3] Quintiles are obtained by dividing the population in 5 equal groups, so that each one contains 20% of the population.

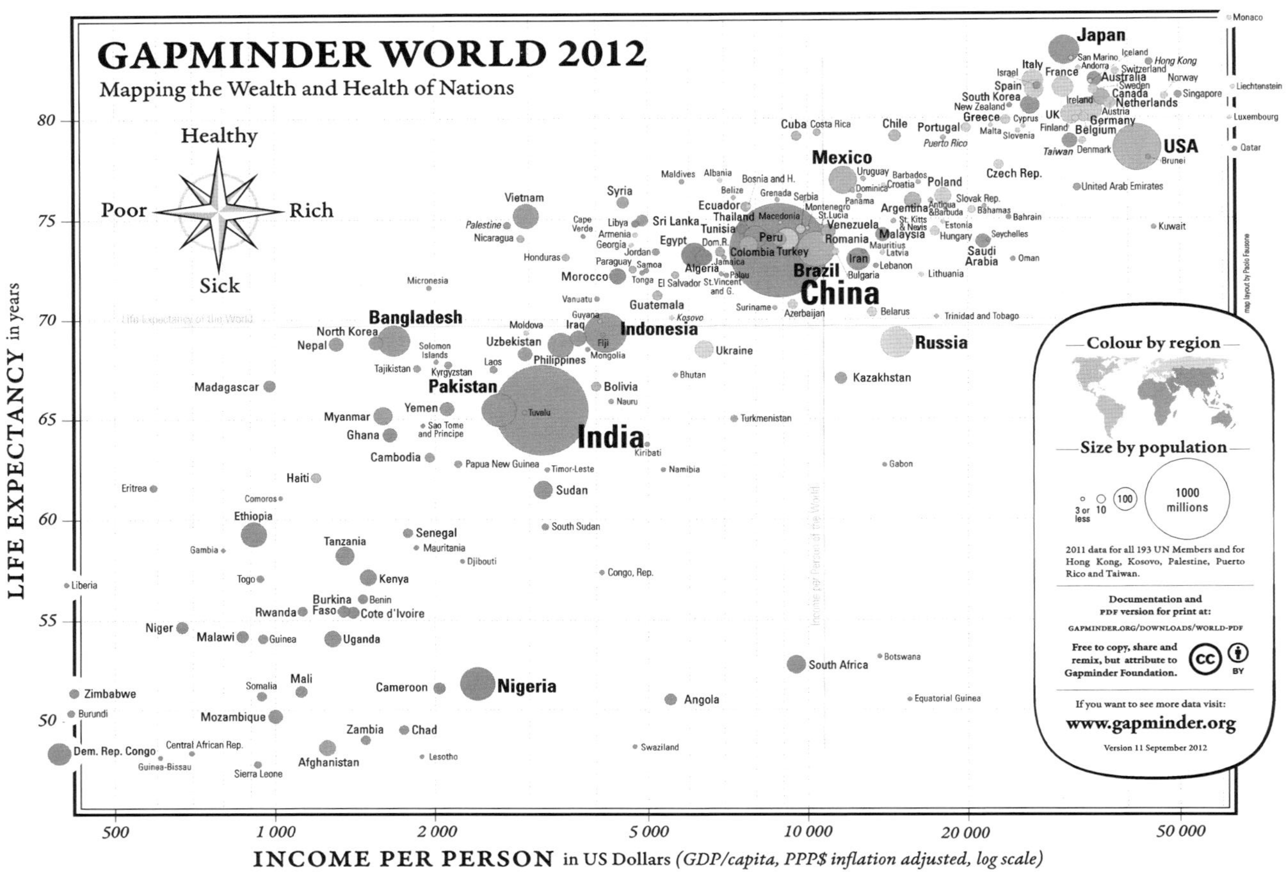

Figure 4. Life expectancy at birth (years) and income per person in the world, both sexes, 2011

Source: Gapminder Foundation 2012.

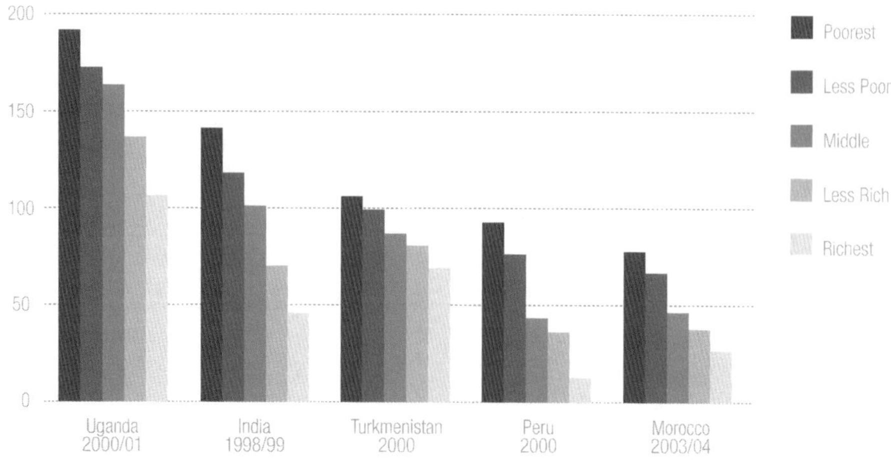

Figure 5. Under-five mortality rate (per 1,000 live births) by quintile of household wealth in five countries

Source: Commission on Social Determinants of Health (2008). World Health Organization (2008), p. 30.

mortality level, but also and most importantly, a substantial wealth gradient in all the countries except Turkmenistan. So, within each country, again money matters, but its influence does not seem to be the same everywhere, the gradient being much steeper in Peru or India. Interestingly, mortality in children under five coming from the poorest wealth quintile in Morocco is lower than that in children from the richest quintile in Uganda, which once more hints at money not being enough to counteract all the hardships that come with other contextual factors (macroeconomic, infrastructural, environmental, social, access to health care, etc.). In that sense, being the "richest" in one country may be more comparable to being "less rich" or "middle" in another country.

Focusing on health inequalities within developing countries is of high interest, since they may account for nearly half of the global health gap between developed and developing world regions, such as Amouzou *et al.* (2014) prove for under-five mortality. These authors use data from Demographic and Health Surveys conducted between 1995 and 2010 in 67 developing countries and calculate, using a PAR approach, that about half of the under-five mortality gap between developed and developing countries can be reduced by lowering the under-five mortality rate in each developing country to the level enjoyed by the top economic stratum (the top wealth decile) of these countries. The authors warn that the choice of reference group (top 5% or 20% instead of the top 10%) delivers quantitatively different results, but what is important is the sense of magnitude conveyed in this case.

Between-country variability in the magnitude of inequalities in health is also very large, as demonstrated for example in Western Europe (Mackenbach *et al.*, 2008; WHO Regional Office for Europe, 2013a). Mackenbach *et al.* analyzed mortality rates (based on 3.5 million deaths) and prevalence of poor self-assessed health (based on national health or multipurpose surveys) related to education and income in 22 European countries. They used the slope index of inequality and a regression-based relative index of inequality so that both measures, then, take into account the whole population and remove variability in the size of socioeconomic groups as a source of variation in the comparison of inequalities. Through this approach, they found that education-related inequalities in mortality are highly variable, smaller in the Southern European populations and biggest in the Eastern and Baltic regions. The between-country variations in self-assessed health were not as great, but their geographic pattern differed. In addition to demonstrating the inequalities between countries, an implication worth noting of this result is that it would be ill-advised to generalize from inequalities in mortality to inequalities in other indicators of health, especially self-reported indicators since cultural and social factors, as well as the idiosyncrasy of each country may highly influence the perception of illness. Sen (2002a) nicely illustrated this issue by comparing life expectancy and self-reported morbidity in the US and India (the country as a whole and two states): The countries and territories that enjoyed higher life expectancy were also the countries and territories with higher reported morbidity.

Based precisely on the unexpectedly smaller magnitude of inequalities among the Southern European countries, compared to those among the Northern ones, Mackenbach *et al.* concluded that inequalities seem unrelated to political factors, specifically, to the extent and generosity of welfare policies. Still, they affirmed that the wide variability among European countries overall in mortality inequalities implies that there is room for reducing them through interventions that address the structural and intermediary determinants of inequalities in health. This being obvious, we would add that this variability hints, once more, at our ignorance of the true mechanisms that originate and sustain inequalities in health.

A different example of evidence of a socioeconomic gradient within a high-income country is provided in Figure 6, which displays several indicators of health by income levels in the US in 2009. Figures are based on data from the Centers for Disease Control and Prevention, the National Center for Health Statistics and the National Health Interview Survey. As income level rises, a pattern of decreasing frequency is shown for all of the health problems reported, differences being steeper in the case of psychological distress and self-reported poor/fair health.

In several countries, and especially in the US where such data is routinely collected, there is also compelling evidence of the association between race/ethnicity and health outcomes. For instance, in 2006, the IMR in the US of babies born to non-Hispanic black women was 13.35 per 1,000 live births, compared with a rate of 5.58 for non-Hispanic white women (reference category). That means an absolute difference of 7.77 percentage points or a 139.2% higher rate in the case of non-Hispanic black women. In contrast, IMRs were 4%, 18%, and 19% lower than the reference group for Mexican (5.34) Asian/Pacific Islander (4.55) and Central

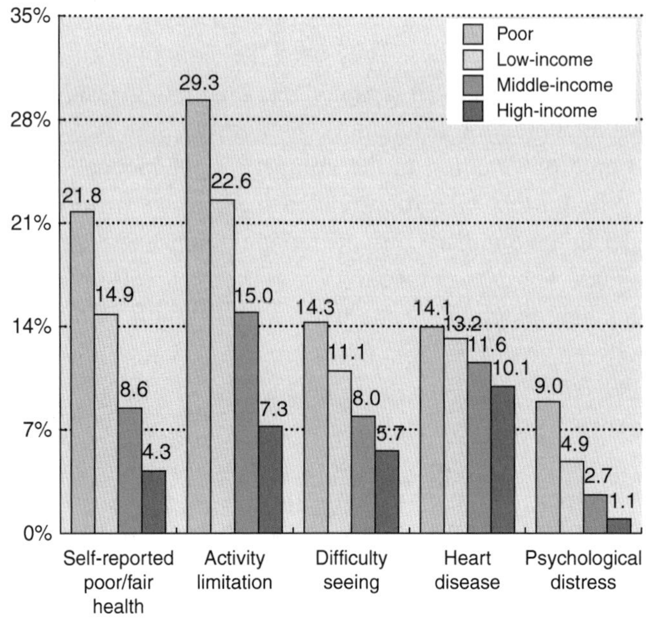

Figure 6. Frequency of several health problems by income level, US 2009

Notes: Income groups based on family income, size and composition, relative to the federal poverty line (FPL). In 2009, the FPL for a two-adult, two-child family was $21,756. Poor defined as less than 100% FPL; low-income as 100% to less than 200% FPL; middle-income as 200% to less than 400% FPL; high-income as equal to or greater than 400% FPL. Estimates for adults 18 and over except for self-reported health, shown for all persons. Activity limitations include difficulty bathing or preparing meals, for example.

Source: Jank and Owens (2015).

or South American (4.52) women, respectively (MacDorman, 2011). Percentage changes from 2000 to 2006 in IMRs for each racial/ethnic group were not statistically significant, although the country average IMR did fall a meagre 3%, or 0.21 percentage points (from 6.89 in 2000 to 6.68 in 2006). Percentage changes for each racial/ethnic group were not statistically significant. As the author noted, the US seems unable to drill through an apparent infant mortality plateau and to narrow black–white disparities. As a point of comparison, the IMR in the 27 country-members of the European Union decreased by 17% between 2000 and 2005, from 5.9 to 4.9 per 1,000 live births (European Commission, 2013).

Racial disparities have also been reported for many other health measures and risk factors. For example, during the period between 1980 and 2007, the age-adjusted maternal mortality rate of black women was always much higher (2- or 3-fold) than that of white women (PAHO, 2012). Grouping individuals by race or ethnic group is undoubtedly useful to raise awareness about these disparities; however, a question often posed is whether it is race by itself (discrimination) that matters or rather SES (blacks being probably overrepresented in the lower income, educational, occupational or social class groups). Fleurbaey and Schokkaert (2012) discussed this issue in some depth, showing how it is possible to apply an Oaxaca–Blinder decomposition to estimate each effect separately and the interaction between both of them, so that racial disparities would be the sum of the "direct" effect of race and the indirect effect that works through the effect of SES on health. Kawachi *et al.* (2005) contended that class and race should be recognized as distinct but intertwined determinants of disparities in health and that excessive emphasis on race is actually a way of downplaying the importance of class or SES.

We turn now to the crucial issue of whether inequalities in health are narrowing or enlarging. The conventional wisdom in the past decade has been that inequalities widened at the end of the 20th century, at least in Europe. Several studies, with very explicit titles, pointed in that direction: Mackenbach *et al.*, 2003; Regidor *et al.*, 2006; Murphy *et al.*, 2006; Department of Health 2009; Palosuo *et al.*, 2009. In the first of these studies, which has been extensively cited, Mackenbach *et al.*, analyzed data on mortality by educational level and occupational class in six European countries: Finland, Sweden, Norway, Denmark, England/Wales and Italy (Turin), in two periods: 1981–1985 and 1991–1995. Their conclusion was that absolute differences in total mortality were fairly stable (except in Finland) but relative inequalities had increased.[4] The main reason was that mortality from cardiovascular diseases had declined proportionally more in the upper socioeconomic groups. Other causes of death (lung cancer, breast cancer, etc.) also contributed to the widening gap due to increasing mortality rates in lower socioeconomic groups in several countries.

Regidor *et al.* (2006) also found that, in Spain, income-related inequalities in mortality and disability were greater in 2000 than in 1985. Since this happened in a period in which income inequality had diminished, the authors call attention to the fact that a reduction in health inequalities does not necessarily parallel a reduction in socioeconomic inequality. In the case of Russia, Murphy *et al.* (2006) studied the period of a sharp rise in mortality after 1990 and concluded that it had predominantly affected less educated men and women. Since mortality among the better educated (university level) had improved, the divergence had become greater. In an extensive report for Finland, Palosuo *et al.* (2009) concluded that the evolution of average population health between 1980 and 2005 was positive (life expectancy of men and women at age 35 had increased 4.6 and 3.4 years, respectively), but socioeconomic inequalities in health had generally stayed or widened

[4]For example, as can be seen in their Table 1, the age-standardized mortality rate of manual male workers in Norway went from 5.2 per 1,000 persons in 1983 to 4.3 in 1993; while that rate dropped from 3.7 to 2.8 in the case of non-manual workers. The decline (absolute difference) was 0.9 in both occupational groups, but the relative difference increased from 1.4 (5.2/3.7) to 1.53 (4.3/2.8). What happened is that the mortality rate of manual workers decreased by 17% whereas the decline was higher (24%) in the case of non-manual workers.

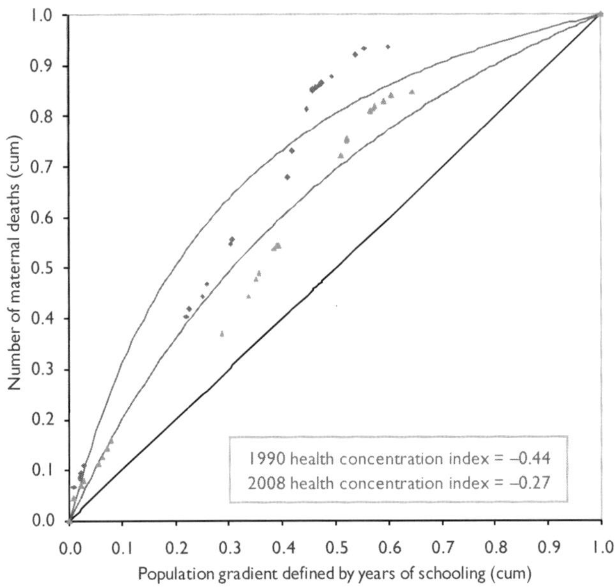

Figure 7. Inequality in maternal mortality according to years of schooling, Region of the Americas, 1990 and 2008

Source: PAHO (2012).

(the difference between upper white-collar and blue-collar workers augmented 1.1 years for men and 1.0 years for women). Finally, to illustrate the case of the UK (England), a country with a long tradition of studies in health inequalities, we cite here a report reviewing the developments over the 10 years since the Acheson Report — a follow-up to the Black Report — that had been published in 1998 and had showed a widening health gap between different social groups. Almost 10 years after the Acheson Report, in 2005–2007, IMR and average life expectancy had improved notably, but inequalities persisted or had increased slightly. In particular, the absolute difference in life expectancy between males in the general population and those living in disadvantaged areas (70 local authority areas with the worst health and deprivation indicators, accounting for 28% of the general population) had augmented from 1.9 to 2.1 years. Similarly for females, the gap had gone from 1.4 to 1.6 years (Department of Health, 2009).

Notwithstanding these results, we cannot say that the evidence on this issue of the growing or narrowing of health inequalities is conclusive. For example, Figure 7 plots the number of the maternal deaths against the mother's number of years of schooling for 1990 and 2008 in the WHO Region of the Americas. Both concentration curves show that maternal deaths are disproportionally concentrated among mothers with the lowest years of schooling. Nevertheless, while the degree of inequality is still large, it has diminished significantly in the period between 1990

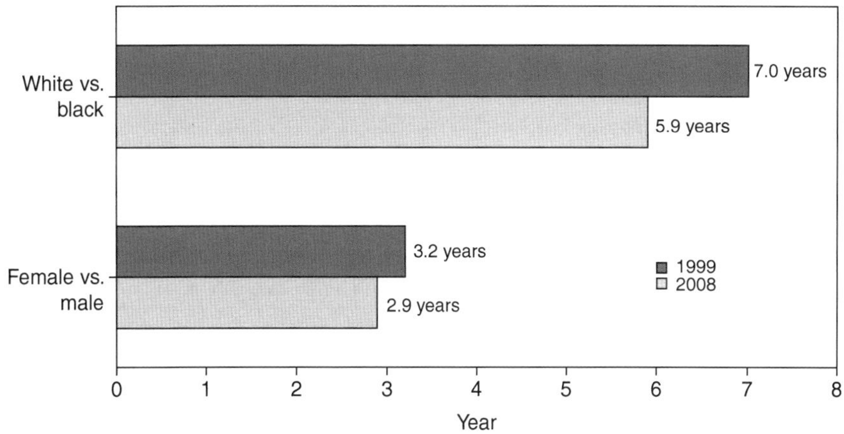

Figure 8. Disparities in expected (at birth) years free of activity limitation caused by chronic conditions, by race and sex, US, 1999–2008

Source: Molla (2013).

and 2008. The concentration curve for 2008 is closer to the 45-degree line and the CI has dropped from –0.44 to –0.27.

Similarly, for indicators of health such as the expected (at birth) years free of activity limitation caused by chronic conditions, Figure 8 shows that racial disparities and the gender gap in the US also appear to have narrowed.

In its report on "Health inequalities in the EU", released in December 2013, the European Commission also claimed contemporary reductions in health inequalities for some indicators between the EU-27 member states (prior to the incorporation of Croatia in July 2013) (European Commission, 2013). This report, which was the result of a consortium led by Sir Michael Marmot, exhibited data that demonstrated: (i) Improvements in life expectancy and the IMR in almost all countries between 2001 and 2010, (ii) improvements in the degree of inequality for a small number of indicators, while for others there had been no change and, for a few, a deterioration, and (iii) that anyhow sizeable gaps in health still existed between member states of the EU.

With respect infant mortality, Figure 9, taken from the above-referenced report, shows that in 2000, there was a gap of 15.2 deaths per 1,000 live births between the countries with the highest and lowest rates (Romania 18.6 and Sweden 3.4). In 2010, the gap had declined to 7.5 (Romania 9.8 vs. Finland 2.3). Taking into account all 27 countries and not just the extremes, the Gini Coefficient of inequality (which weighs for the number of births in each country) shows a year-on-year reduction in inequality, with a 26% drop over the whole period. However, there was still more than a 4-fold difference in the chance of a baby under 1 year old dying between the highest and lowest ranking member states. As

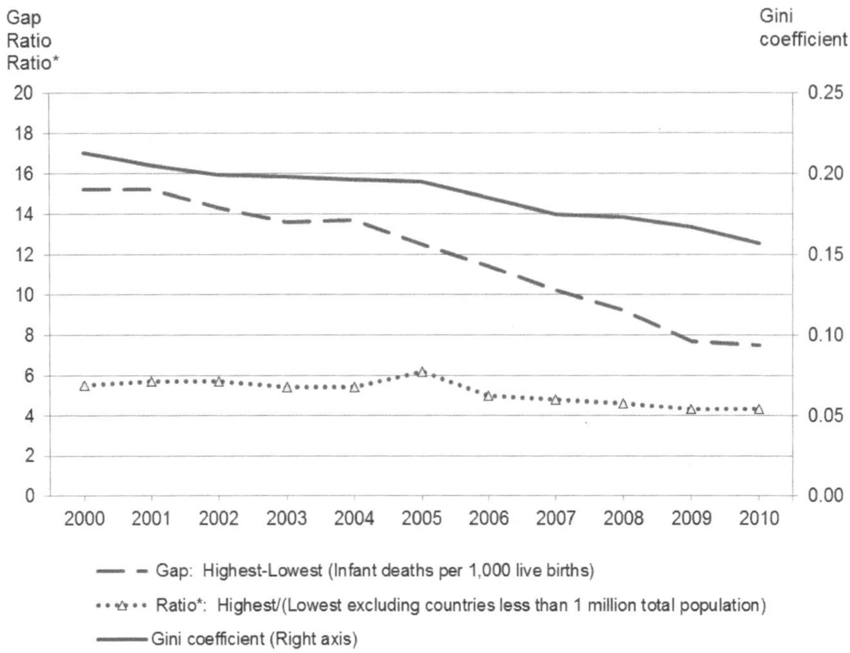

Figure 9. Selected measures of inequality in infant mortality between EU-27 Member States, 2000–2010

Notes: The countries with less than 1 million total population are Cyprus, Luxembourg and Malta.
Source: European Commission (2013).

far as differences in life expectancy at birth, (not shown in the figure) the Gini Coefficient between EU member states decreased by 3.5% for males and by 10.4% for females over the period 2000 to 2010.

Now, we should stress that, as we saw at the end of Section "Chief Measures", the Gini index is not really a measure of socioeconomic inequality in health. Here, countries are ranked according to the level of health (from the country with the worst indicator to the best) and not according to any socioeconomic variable. Although the two go often together, the correlation is not perfect. For example, Luxembourg has the highest income per capita in Europe, but its IMR in 2010 was higher than that of Portugal or Slovenia, much poorer countries. Other variables aside from income may be at work, for instance, health care coverage of immigrant population.

The "Health inequalities in the EU" report did have a section on the relationship between social and health inequalities. In this section, it analyzed the relationship between individual socioeconomic characteristics and self-reported health and mortality, revealing the existence of important socioeconomic gradients, measured by the slope index of inequality (SII), for three SES indicators: Education, income and material deprivation. In the case of income, the SIIs for life expectancy at birth and life expectancy at age 50 for women were 5.4 and 4.5, respectively, indicating that across the whole of the EU, females in the richest regions could expect to live about 5.4 years longer than females in the least affluent regions, and the corresponding difference in life expectancy at 50 was 4.5 years. The variation in female life expectancy between member states was smaller than for males. Similarly, educational gradients for women were less steep. In fact, the steepest social gradients were observed between material deprivation as SES indicator and most measures of health.

Trend data on self-reported health for 2007–2010 (which more or less coincides with the Great Recession) do not provide robust evidence of either a reduction or an increase in socioeconomic inequalities in self-perceived health status, the period being too short. Since monitoring of socioeconomic inequalities in health at the EU level is still at an early stage, it will be some years before trends can be measured reliably (European Commission, 2013).

Inequalities in the Access to Health Care

As is the case with inequalities in *health*, we face now a global problem visible across and within countries: Access to *health care* is generally better in high-income and more developed countries, and rich people have more access than poor people to health care within each country. Although in most high-income world regions inequality in access to health care is a secondary factor explaining health inequities,[5] in poor countries, unequal access and quality of health care is considered a major determinant of inequality in health (Gwatkin, 2002).

Following Whitehead (1992), equal access to available care for equal need implies "equal entitlement to the available services for everyone, a fair distribution throughout the country based on health care needs and ease of access in each geographical area, and the removal of other barriers to access".

Equal entitlement to available services for everyone: The road to Universal health care coverage

Universal health coverage (UHC) ranks high on the policy agenda, particularly since it was endorsed by the World Health Assembly in 2005 and further supported by the World Health Report 2010 (WHO, 2010c). Health policy reforms have been oriented to this goal in high-income countries (e.g., the US, with the approval of the Patient Protection and Affordable Care Act in 2010) and also in medium- and low-income countries, such as Mexico, Colombia, Peru, Ghana, Tanzania, Thailand, and Vietnam, among others (WHO, 2014a). While during the recent economic

[5] An exception has to be made for the US, where lack of access to health care has been the most significant contributing factor to poor quality of care for the uninsured groups of population (US Department of Health and Human Services Agency for Healthcare Research and Quality, 2014).

recession, public health spending has fallen in many European countries, particularly in those most affected by the economic crisis (such as Greece, Ireland and Spain), some countries outside Europe have registered significant public health spending growth rates, mainly due to efforts toward universal health care coverage, such as Chile (7.2% growth in 2011–2012) and Mexico (10.7% growth) (OECD Health Data, 2014). However, although countries in the American Region have reinforced their commitment to UHC during the period 2006–2010, the goal of guaranteeing basic health care access to everybody is far from being accomplished. A high proportion of population still does not have access to basic services and depends on fragmented and segmented health systems, and about 30% of people living in this region cannot afford health care (PAHO, 2012).

The group of BRICS countries (Brazil, the Russian Federation, India, China and South Africa) has also undertaken health-system reforms to make progress towards UHC over the past two decades, but these countries still face important challenges. Brazil, for instance, has difficulty attracting qualified health workers to remote areas, and formal and informal out-of-pocket (OOP) payments for health care act as significant barriers to access in India, China and the Russian Federation (Rao *et al.*, 2014).

Measures of service coverage for prevention and treatment interventions by region, in the aggregate and stratified by income, are shown in Figure 10. Shortfalls

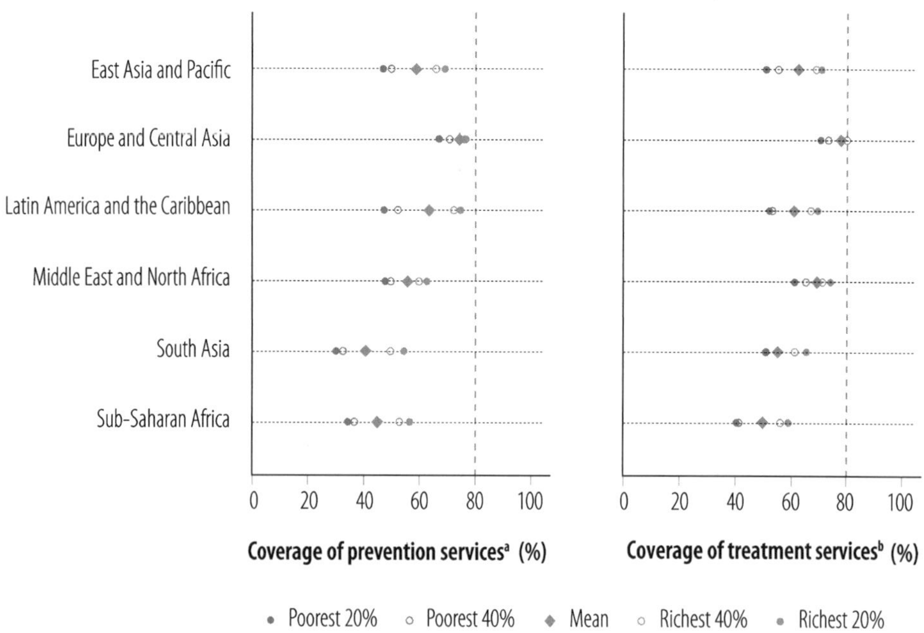

Figure 10. Coverage of prevention and treatment services, by region

Source: World Health Organization and International Bank for Reconstruction and Development/The World Bank (2014).

in coverage relative to the 80% coverage target (the vertical dotted line), jointly set by the WHO and The World Bank Group on the basis of consultations and discussions with country representatives, technical experts and global health and development partners as a way for monitoring progress towards UHC, can be seen for all regions. Social gradient is significant for both prevention and treatment measures, since coverage is lower among the poorest 20% and 40% of the population than the richest 60% and 80% in all regions (WHO and IBRD/World Bank, 2014).

UHC comprises not only access for all to the quality health services needed, but also the absence of financial hardship. Two commonly used indicators to measure the level of financial protection in health are the incidence of "catastrophic" health expenditures and the incidence of impoverishment due to OOP health payments (The World Bank, 2014).[6]

Although relevant information for many low-income countries is missing, particularly for the African Region, available data show that the average incidence of catastrophic health expenditure in this region is around 3%, with a range from almost 0% to around 8%.

This figure still hides important socioeconomic disparities, since the average incidence among the poorest quintiles in these countries was over 4.5%, while it hardly reached 2% in the richest quintiles. It is also known that over 8 million of Africans are impoverished due to OOP health expenditures (Musango *et al.*, 2013). It has to be considered that financing schemes in most LDC still require direct payments at the point of delivery. Although the poor are often exempt from user fees levied at public health facilities in low-income countries, these exemptions are not always respected since providers are not compensated for lost revenues (Flores *et al.*, 2013).

Rates of financial protection against catastrophic health payments are much lower than those of financial protection against impoverishing in all world regions, as Figure 11 shows. It may also be seen that the poorest 20% and 40% have the lowest protection against impoverishing expenditure, whereas for catastrophic spending, the poor appear to be worse off only in South Asia (WHO and IBRD/World Bank, 2014).

A recent work about the prevalence of catastrophic payments among population groups in some Latin-American countries found a high dispersion in the proportion of households showing this problem (from 1% to 25%), which was related to coverage and protection provided by the health systems. Main explanatory factors of catastrophic spending were found to be rurality, low levels of

---

[6]The incidence of "catastrophic" health expenditures indicates the proportion of households that incur health payments that are higher than their resources. Meanwhile, the incidence of impoverishment due to OOP health payments indicates the percentage of households that is pushed into poverty, or deeper into poverty, because of health spending (WHO and IBRD/World Bank, 2014).

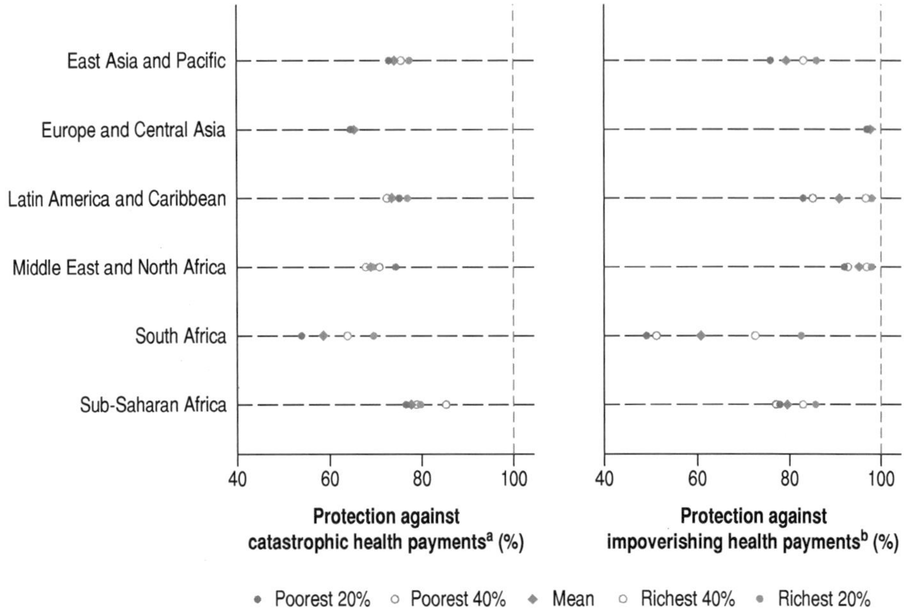

[a] Percentage of the population not spending more than 25% of non-food expenditure on health care.

[b] Percentage of the population neither impoverished by out-of-pocket payments nor pushed further into proverty by them.

Figure 11. Financial protection measures against catastrophic and impoverishing health payments, by region

Source: World Health Organization and International Bank for Reconstruction and Development/The World Bank (2014).

earnings, the presence of elderly people in households and the absence of health insurance (Knaul *et al.*, 2011).

OOP payments as a percentage of private expenditure on health are significantly higher in low- and middle-income countries compared to high-income countries, although its proportion fell during the latest years, particularly for the first group. According to the WHO (2014b), this indicator decreased from 84.1% in 2000 to 76.2% in 2011 for low-income countries, while percentages decreased from 89.6% to 87.1% in lower-middle-income countries, from 80.2% to 74.2% in upper-middle-income countries and from 38.5% to 37.6% in high-income countries.

In Europe, financial barriers to access to basic health care services is not an issue, since in most countries there is free or almost free access for children, poorer adults, and high users of health care (Masseria *et al.*, 2009). However, as Figure 12 shows, the report of unmet needs due to access barriers may not be negligible for some European countries, such as Greece or Bulgaria.

Social gradient in access to health care is also present within European countries. The proportion of people reporting unmet needs is always higher in the lowest

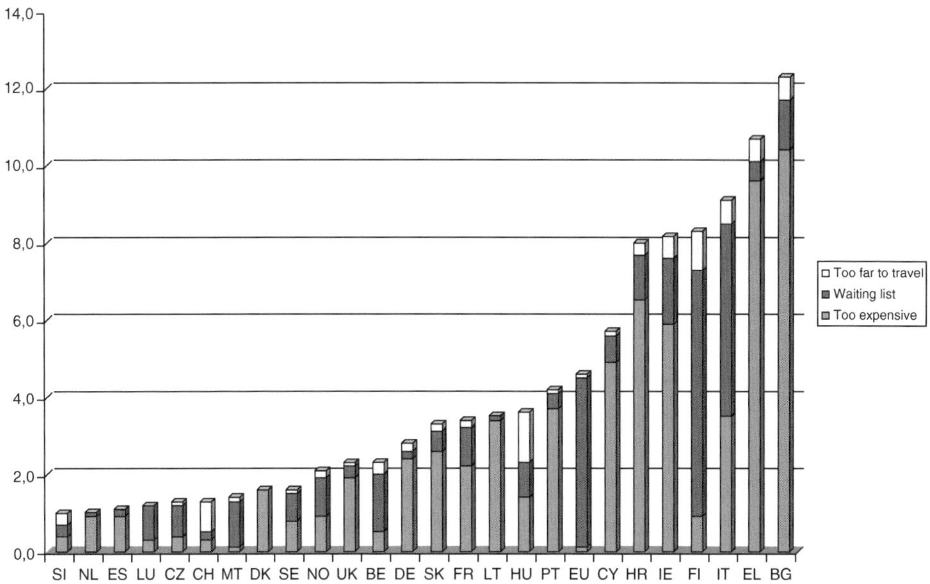

Figure 12. Proportion of the population reporting unmet needs due to access barriers in Europe, 2012

Note: Data for Austria, Ireland and Turkey are not available.

Source: Eurostat (2014).

income quintiles, with inequalities particularly pronounced in Belgium, far followed by Spain, Italy, France and Malta. Moreover, waiting times to be diagnosed and treated tend to favor the most socioeconomically advantaged patients even in universal health care systems such as the UK or Spain (Pell *et al.*, 2000; Laudicella *et al.*, 2012; Abásolo *et al.*, 2014). Even the general practitioner (GP) may act as a barrier leading to social inequalities in the access to some medical services. Kelly-Irving *et al.* analyzed, for a sample of French patients, agreement/disagreement between GP and patient on the patient's health status. They showed how those patients with low and medium educational levels were at higher risk of being overestimated by GP's with respect to self-reported health, compared to highly educated patients (Kelly-Irving *et al.*, 2011). Their findings suggested that, perhaps as a consequence of not being able to reliably transmit information about their health status, people with a lower education could suffer from lack of advice and treatment and, ultimately, this could lead to the persistence of health inequalities.

Allocation of health care resources

From a global perspective, it is well known that health care resources are allocated in inverse relation to health needs. Poor countries, which concentrate higher rates

Table 2. Availability of health care resources by groups of countries. Selected indicators

	Physicians (per 10,000 population)[a]	Nursing and midwifery personnel (per 10,000 population)[a]	Hospital beds (per 10,000 population)[b]	Radiotherapy units (per million population)[c]
Low-income	2.4	5.4	21	0.2
Lower-middle-income	7.8	17.8	10	0.6
Upper-middle-income	15.5	25.3	32	2.2
High-income	29.4	86.9	54	8.3
Global	14.1	29.2	27	2.5

Notes: [a]2006–2013; [b]2006–2012; [c]2013.

Source: World Health Statistics (2014).

of mortality and morbidity, have significant less health workers and hospital beds than middle- and high-income countries. LDC suffer from a chronic shortage of human resources, low availability and affordability of essential medicines, and inadequate infrastructure of health facilities. Additionally, at a time when physicians and nurses are most needed in the LDC, they have been recruited away to the West (Siegel, 2012), and absence rates within countries are quite high. Even when the staff is present, sometimes they do not have knowledge of basic procedures, or there may also be a gap between what health care providers know they should do and what they do in practice (Kremer and Glennerster, 2012). Table 2 shows world disparities in some indicators of the availability of health resources, such as health workforce, infrastructure and technologies.

Marked geographic inequalities are also frequent within many countries across regions and between urban and rural contexts, again as a consequence of disparities in the availability of health care resources. For instance, in Ethiopia, 50.8% of all births in the urban population are attended by a skilled provider, while in the rural population the proportion is merely 4.0% (WHO, 2014b). Although physicians practicing in the LDC work mostly in the large cities, a large share of the population inhabiting these countries lives in rural areas, particularly in Sub-Saharan Africa, where the rural population exceeds 60% of the total population of many countries (Siegel, 2012). Furthermore, health workers in African countries usually earn less in rural areas than their urban counterparts, which is a perverse incentive to place resources where they are more needed (Soucat and Scheffler, 2013).

Evidence suggests that free access to health care does not guarantee equity in distribution, particularly when resources are allocated to health care institutions and populations without taking into account equity criteria. Diderichsen (2004) explained how need-based resource allocation formulae might serve as useful tools to promote equity, and summarized the formulae used by some high-income countries (such as the UK and Sweden), and low- and middle-income countries (such as Uganda and South Africa), where different types of need variables (such as age, mortality or morbidity rates, rates of unemployment or deprivation indices) were employed to allocate more health resources to those areas where needy and deprived groups are concentrated. Resource allocation formulae may also be adapted to reduce disparities across ethnic groups, as in New Zealand, where more resources are allocated to those areas where Maoris live, in order to balance the underutilization of health care facilities by this minority group.

Other barriers to access

Geographic or cultural barriers may also hinder access to health care. Many LDC countries suffer from geographic difficulties related to distance and lack of transportation, particularly in mountainous countries, such as Bolivia and Nepal, but also in other countries such as Namibia and Zimbabwe (Kremer and Glennerster, 2012). Cultural concerns arising from women's roles and status are common in Armenia, Bolivia, Cambodia, Nicaragua, Nepal, and Peru (Kremer and Glennerster, 2012). Women also face huge barriers in accessing health services in some countries due to restricted decision-making and mobility, and to norms that restrict interaction with males outside the family, as in Afghanistan and other Muslim countries (WHO, 2013).

Inequity in the Utilization of Health Care

Are health care systems (in)equitable? by how much?

It is now beyond question that universal free access to health services is not enough to reduce disparities in health. However, this does not mean that we should ignore or disregard its contribution to differences in health levels, which can be significant, above all in lower-income countries. Nor does it mean that equity in the utilization of health services is not a desirable goal in itself (Sen, 2002b).

The evidence on socioeconomic inequality in the utilization of health care services is overwhelming. An example is provided in Figure 13, which displays poor–rich inequalities in five indicators of maternity and child health care use in 45 developing countries (Houweling *et al.*, 2007). Apart from differences between rich and poor (household wealth was measured through a composite index taking into account ownership of durable goods, housing quality and water and sanitation facilities), the graph also shows the median level for each indicator in the total population. Interestingly, although the median for professional delivery care and the treatment of acute respiratory infections are very similar, disparities are much larger for the former (measured as the percentage of births attended by a medically trained person).

However, as explained in Section "Conceptual Framework," in a strict sense, differences in utilization do not themselves imply inequity. An assessment of

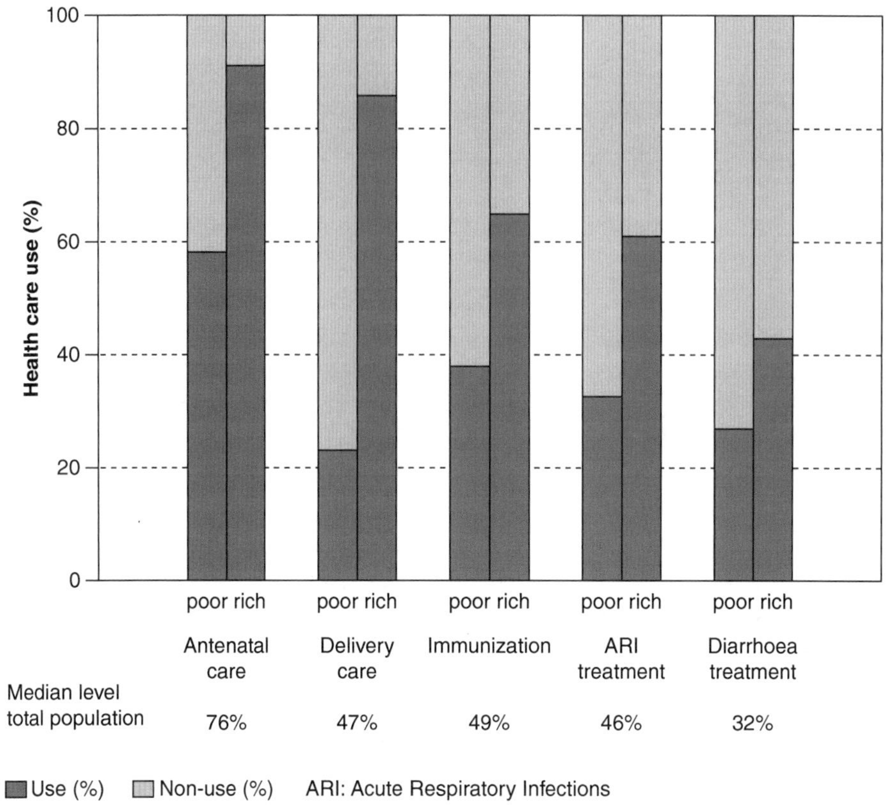

Figure 13. Maternity and child health care use among the poorest and the richest 20% wealth group across 45 developing countries

Source: Houweling *et al.* (2007).

whether inequalities in utilization are related to need is required before inequalities can be labelled as inequities. Panels A and B in Figure 14 bring to the fore a comparison between utilization and need. It shows that use of the human papillomavirus (HPV) vaccine in the 50 states of the US is positively correlated with state income and inversely correlated with the cervical mortality rate, which can be interpreted as an indicator of need (Bach, 2010).

Being able to state whether the provision of health care services follows or does not follow need is useful, but if we want to make comparisons between services, between regions/countries, or within countries or services over time it is necessary to be able to say by how much, that is, to arrive at a number informing about the scale of inequity. Wagstaff *et al.* (1989) first developed a methodology based on the concentration curve and the CI to quantify the degree of (in)equity in the delivery of health care services that, with some improvements, has been profusely used in the literature ever since.[7] Following the public economics principle of "horizontal

[7] The step-by-step methodology can be consulted in O'Donnell *et al.* (2008).

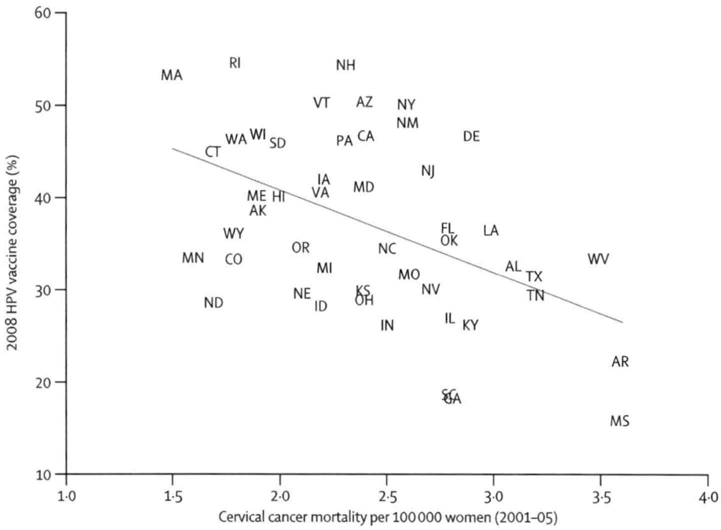

(a)

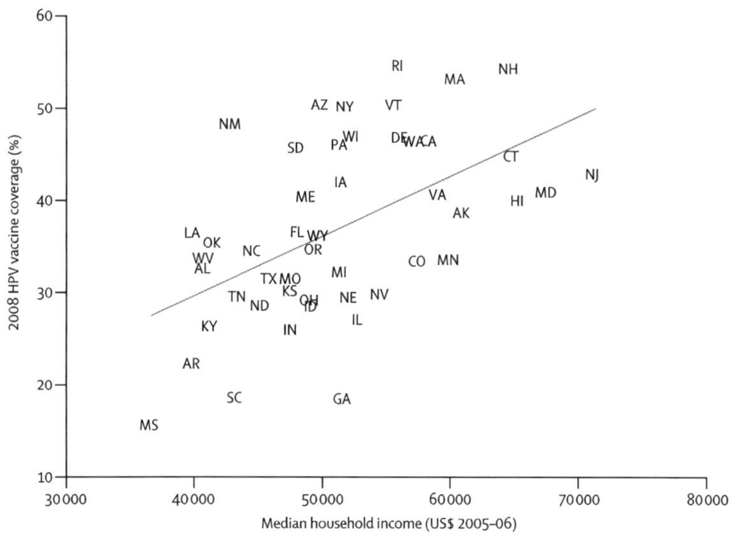

(b)

Figure 14. Correlation between HPV vaccine coverage rate in girls aged 13–17 and cervical cancer mortality rate (Panel A) and median income (Panel B) in US states

Source: Bach (2010).

equity" (giving the same treatment to people in an identical situation), the equity criterion in the health field is phrased as: *Equal treatment for equal need, irrespective of level of income or any other socioeconomic characteristic.*

The assessment of the equity criterion thus entails taking into account legitimate or need-determined differences in utilization. Standardizing for differences

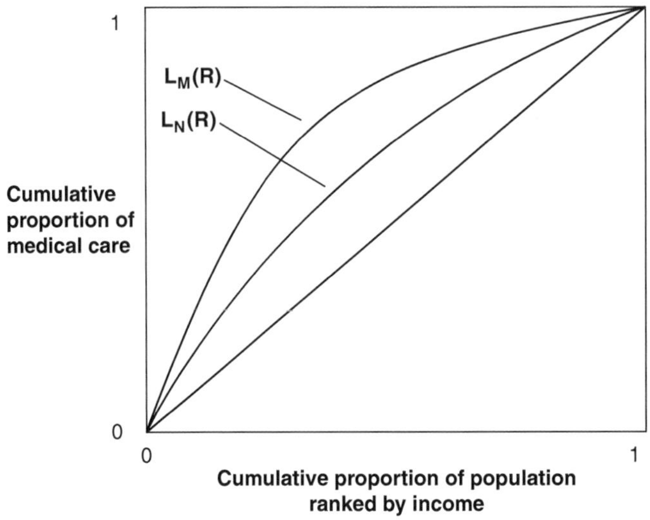

Figure 15. Concentration curves of utilization and need of health care
Source: van Doorslaer *et al.* (2000).

in need can be done either through a direct or indirect method. Indirect standardization involves comparing the actual distribution of care by income level (or any other similar ranking indicator such as wealth or household expenditures) with the distribution of need-expected (or need-predicted) utilization by the same income groups. Need-expected use, obtained for each individual as the predicted utilization of a regression on need indicators, is the amount of health care an individual ought to receive if he/she was treated as others with the same need characteristics are, on average, treated by the system. As van Doorslaer *et al.* (2000) remarked, this interpretation implies that the average relationship between need indicators and utilization is the implicit norm for assessing equity in a particular health system or country. Or, in other words, that "on average, the system gets it right." In empirical studies, need characteristics are represented by demographic factors (age and sex) plus several types of health status and morbidity indicators such as self-rated health, presence of chronic conditions, days of restricted activity, etc. The three most common types of services analyzed to measure utilization are GP visits, specialist visits and hospitalizations, with the first two being sometimes aggregated as "doctor's visits." But other indicators can also be used; for example, emergency room visits or screening procedures. When the average price of each type of service is available one can multiply these prices by the quantity of services utilized thus obtaining and indicator of health expenditure absorbed or received.

Figure 15 illustrates this method. The degree of socioeconomic inequality in the utilization of health care services is represented by the concentration curve $L_M(R)$. This curve is defined as in Section "Health Inequalities: Measurement and

Empirical Evidence" and it represents the cumulative proportion of medical care actually used by each successive income group, given its utilization of the type of service (or bundle of services) considered. On the other hand, the curve $L_N(R)$ represents the cumulative distribution of need (or need-expected use) for the successive income levels. Note that concentration curves $L_M(R)$ and $L_N(R)$ are both drawn above the diagonal. This is presupposing that need and utilization of medical care are concentrated amongst the poor.

From these curves one can derive the concentration indices CI_M and CI_N, where CI_M is the CI or degree of inequality in the utilization of medical care and it is determined by the area between curve L_M and the 45-degree line. Similarly, CI_N is the CI or degree of inequality in the distribution of need-expected or need-predicted use and it is determined by the area between curve L_N and the 45-degree line. Need-predicted utilization is usually calculated by a linear regression of utilization on need characteristics as regressors. In the graph, since the $L_M(R)$ curve lies further away from the 45-degree line than the $L_N(R)$ curve, the area enclosed is greater implying a higher CI, that is, larger inequality in the distribution of health care utilization than in the distribution of need or need-expected use.

By comparing these two concentration curves and their corresponding indices, we conveniently arrive at a single number able to describe the amount or degree of horizontal (in)equity in the health system or health service considered. The horizontal inequity (HI) index is defined as the difference between the two CIs: $HI = CI_M - CI_N$. Given that, by convention, the CI receives a negative sign when the concentration curve lies above the diagonal and a positive sign when the concentration curve lies below the diagonal, the HI index can be either positive or negative. A positive value of the HI index indicates that there is inequity favoring the rich.[8] This happens, for example, when CI_M and CI_N are both negative and $CI_N > CI_M$ (curve L_N would lie above curve L_M). This would indicate that the greater need of the poor is not met with a proportionally equal quantity of care. In contrast, the rich receive more care than they ought to, given their need. Clearly, the HI index is also positive and inequity is pro-rich when ill health (need) is proportionally higher among the poor (CI_N is negative) but health care utilization is more concentrated among the rich (CI_M is positive). We will see examples of this happening below. An HI equal to zero indicates absence of inequity, i.e., that medical care and need are proportionally distributed across income groups.

When HI is negative, the inequity (meaning violation of the principle of equal treatment for equal need) favors the poor. Most commonly, this occurs when the

[8] All throughout this section, the expressions "favoring the rich" or "favoring the poor" are used in the sense of bias or non-need proportionality in the utilization of medical care by one or another socioeconomic group. As it was remarked in Section "Equity in Health Care," the expression does not necessarily imply that better health is derived from that disproportional consumption.

curve L_M lies outside curve L_N (Figure 15) and the poor receive proportionally more care than they ought to. That is, CI_M and CI_N are both negative and $CI_M > CI_N$. These calculations can be done for the entirety of the health services, or can be broken down for each type of service separately, as it is often the case.

Direct standardization for differences in need implies calculating the health care utilization that each individual (or income group) would have with the income and other non-need attributes he/she has, if he/she had the same need characteristics as the population as a whole. It is based on a linear regression that includes both need and non-need factors as explanatory variables. Once observable need indicators have been controlled for, any residual variation in utilization is imputable to the non-need factors and, therefore, deemed inequitable. The degree of inequity is given by the size of the CI of the resulting need-standardized distribution of health care utilization, that is, the comparison of the need-standardized concentration curve with the 45-degree line (equal distribution).

Finally, for policy purposes, being able to unfold the causes of inequalities and inequities in health can be very useful. Wagstaff *et al.* (2003) proposed a method to decompose the CI of any variable (health or health care utilization) into its contributing explanatory factors and their relative importance. The authors also showed how changes over time in the inequality of the variable of interest can be decomposed into changes in the degree of inequality in its determinants, plus changes in the means of those determinants, plus changes in the extent of their impact on the variable of interest. Among other nice features, this decomposition allows for apprising possible trade-offs between policies directed at improving the means of the explanatory factors (e.g., the mean level of education) and policies directed at reducing the inequality in those factors (e.g., reducing the gap in years of schooling).

International evidence of (in)equity in health care utilization

We now present several works describing the situation in developed and developing countries. In industrialized countries, most of them with universal or quasi-universal health care systems (the greatest exception being the US) a recurrent finding is that individuals in lower-income groups are intensive users of health services. But since need is likewise concentrated in lower-income groups we cannot know for certain whether there is inequity or not. What really matters is the inequality left after accounting (or standardizing) for need, i.e., the horizontal inequity.

Table 3, adapted from Lu *et al.* (2007) depicts both, the income-related inequality and the horizontal inequity in the utilization of several types of health care

Table 3. Income-related inequality (C index) and inequity (HI index) in annual per capita probability of use and volume of utilization of several types of health care services in Hong Kong, South Korea and Taiwan

	Hong Kong						**South Korea**						**Taiwan**					
	Prob*	*C*	**HI**	Total no.	*C*	**HI**	Prob*	*C*	**HI**	Total no.	*C*	**HI**	Prob*	*C*	**HI**	Total no.	*C*	**HI**
Outpatient visits																		
Western doctor	0.18	**0.0185**	**0.0927**	8.27	**0.0241**	**0.1037**	0.16	**–0.0921**	–0.0090	9.76	**–0.0975**	–0.0234	0.35	**–0.0180**	**0.0209**	8.39	**–0.0581**	0.0014
LTM practitioner	0.03	**0.0574**	**0.1195**	2.55	0.0237	**0.1237**	0.02	–0.0178	0.0862	1.38	–0.0321	–0.0726	0.08	**0.0426**	**0.0675**	2.19	0.0232	**0.0507**
Dentist	0.31	**0.2612**	**0.2698**	1.14	**0.2266**	**0.2386**	0.02	0.0283	0.0333	1.12	–0.0155	–0.0262	0.09	**0.0738**	**0.0830**	2.58	0.0171	0.0272
Hospital services																		
Emergency Room	0.01	**–0.2226**	**–0.1751**	0.22	**–0.2518**	**–0.2013**	NA	NA	NA	NA	NA	NA	0.10	–0.0198	0.0218	0.14	–0.0202	**0.0403**
Inpatient admission	0.07	**–0.0502**	**0.0638**	0.14	**–0.0954**	**0.0468**	0.10	**–0.0744**	**–0.0627**	0.07	**–0.0734**	–0.0506	0.07	**–0.1165**	**–0.0381**	0.09	**–0.1309**	–0.0236

Notes: LTM: licensed traditional medicine, Prob*: Probability of use of outpatient visits/inpatient admissions in the previous year. Total no.: Total number of visits/admissions/hospital days per person per year (including those with zero consumption). Statistically significant ($p<0.05$) C and HI indices are in bold type.

Source: Adapted from Lu *et al*. (2007).

services in three high-income Asian economies: Hong Kong, South Korea, and Taiwan.[9] All three economies enjoy health systems inline with the egalitarian tradition, meaning universal coverage and access to a fairly comprehensive range of services. Income-related inequity in utilization is calculated after standardizing for differences in need, proxied by age, gender and health indicators: Self-assessed health and activity limitations. Looking at the first line we observe that there is pro-poor inequality in the probability of visiting a western doctor in South Korea and Taiwan (negative sign of the C indices), but pro-rich inequality in Hong Kong (C index exhibits a positive sign). After controlling for need, inequity (HI) is not significantly different from zero in South Korea but it becomes pro-rich in Taiwan. Both the probability of a visit and the total number of visits to a licensed traditional medicine practitioner show pro-rich inequity in Hong Kong and Taiwan whereas we cannot reject the hypothesis that they are evenly distributed in South Korea. Finally, all three territories show pro-poor bias for inpatient care. However, after adjusting for income-related differences in need, the bias becomes slightly pro-rich in Hong Kong.

Regarding evidence for the OECD countries, after two decades of studies (van Doorslaer and Wagstaff, 1992; van Doorslaer *et al.*, 2000; 2002; 2006; Devaux and Looper, 2012; just to mention some of those covering a wide number of countries) the main conclusions can be summarized by saying that: (i) Substantial cross-country differences in mean levels of use are observed for most types of services, (ii) in general, GP visits show pro-poor inequality but given that the poor also have more need, there is little or no significant inequity, (iii) on the contrary, specialist care tends to be unequally distributed across income groups, with significant inequity favoring the rich remaining in most countries after adjusting for need, (iv) the evidence with respect hospital care is mixed, with a tendency to be equitably distributed, (v) quite pro-rich inequality and inequity in dental care emerges, and (vi) inequalities (comparing the two more recent among those studies) have remained quite stable and country rankings have hardly changed.

Since the main bleak area lies in the unequal distribution of specialist visits, it is worth going into some detail and to comment a bit more on the last of those studies, that by Devaux and Looper (2012). Figures 16 and 17 make ostensibly clear the divergence in the pattern of use of GP's and specialists in the OECD countries included. The value of the index for each country is represented with a dot; the height of the bar represents the confidence interval of the HI. Whenever the confidence interval crosses the zero line it means that the HI is not statistically significantly different from 0; that is, given the same need, the likelihood of seeing a doctor for people with a lower income is the same as for people with higher income. We observe that while consultations with a GP tend to be equitable or to display very low inequity (favoring the rich in the case of the probability; biased

[9]Note that here the acronym for the concentration index of inequality in utilization is shortened to C.

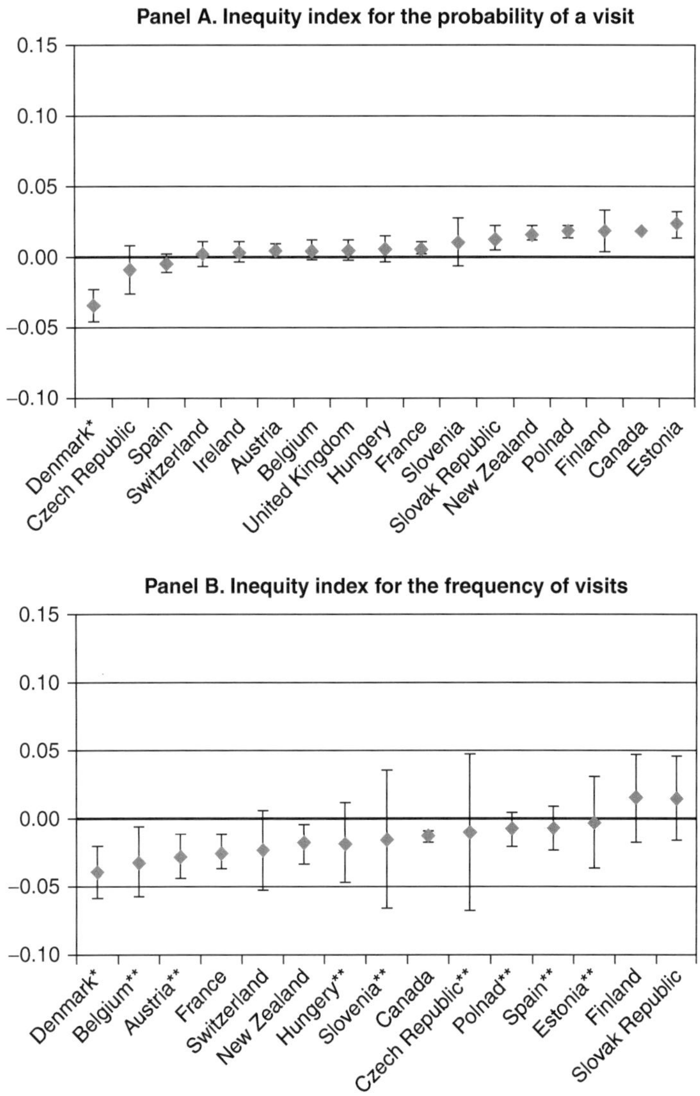

Figure 16. Horizontal inequity index for GP visits in the past 12 months in several OECD countries, 2009 (or latest year)

Notes: (*) visits in the past 3 months in Denmark. (**) counts in the past 4 weeks.

Source: Devaux and Looper (2012).

towards the poor in the case of the frequency of visits), the probability and frequency of specialist visits shows pro-rich inequity in many of the countries, especially large in Switzerland, Estonia, Finland, France, and Spain.[10] The significant

[10]The United States does not appear in these graphs because there was no information available on the breakdown between GP and specialist visits. When the aggregate "doctor visits" is used, Devaux and Looper (2012) find that both the probability and the frequency of visits to a doctor exhibit high

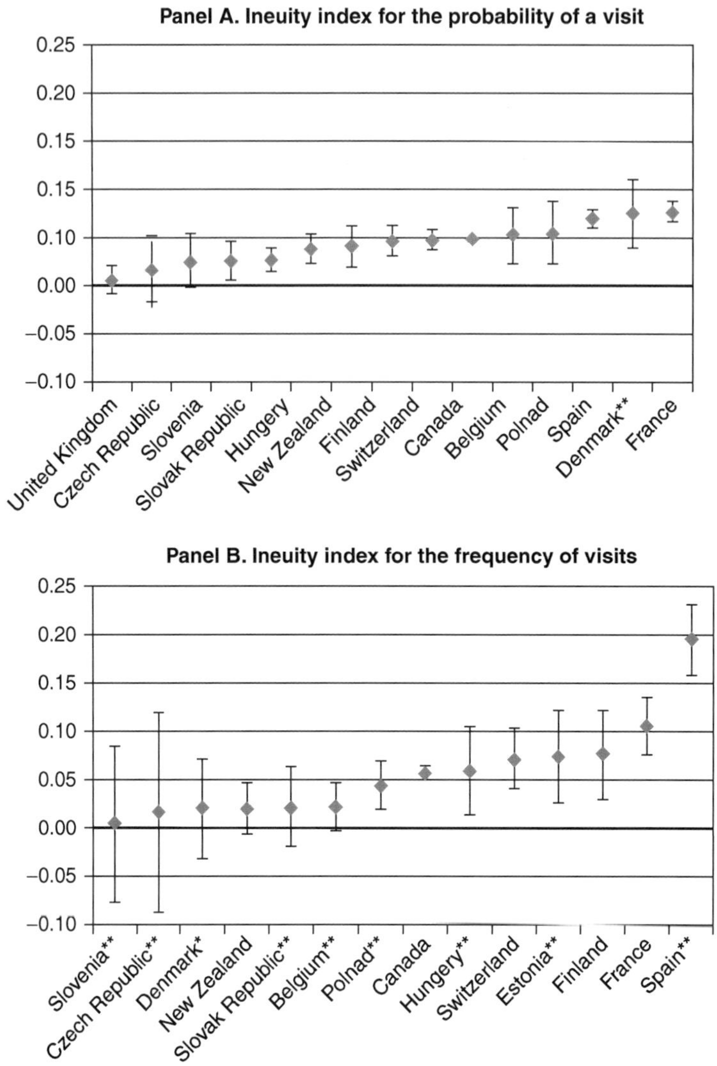

Figure 17. Horizontal inequity index for specialist visits in the past 12 months in several OECD countries, 2009 (or latest year)

Notes: (*) visits in the past 3 months in Denmark. (**) counts in the past 4 weeks.

Source: Devaux and Looper (2012).

inequities in GP visits in Denmark could perhaps be explained by the shorter recall period in the survey used. The outlier position of Spain in the frequency of specialist visits is probably related to the gate-keeper role of GPs in the public sector and

---

and significant pro-rich inequity (HI for the probability of a visit equal to 0.060 and HI for the total number of visits equal to 0.084).

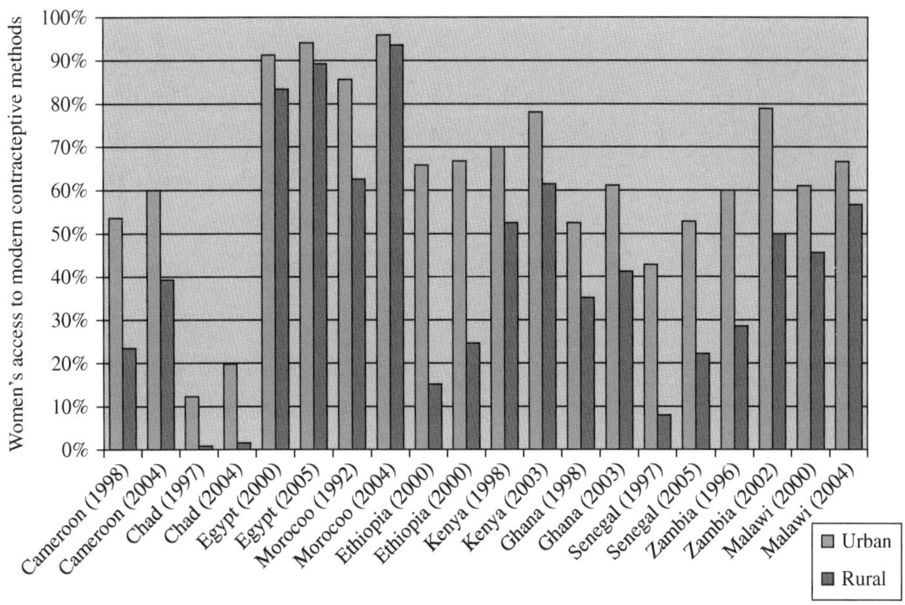

Figure 18. Women's access to modern contraceptive methods in 10 African countries stratified by urban and rural residence

Source: Mutangadura *et al.* (2007).

to private sector visits paid out of pocket or through private insurance, which is concentrated among the richer and more educated groups of the population.

In certain places, like the African continent, an urban/rural stratification is essential when unveiling inequalities in health care utilization. With data from Demographic Health Surveys (DHS) in 10 African countries, Mutangadura *et al.* (2007) showed that there are large disparities both by level of wealth and urban/rural location in the utilization of several types of maternal and child health services: Women's access to modern contraceptive methods, access to prenatal care services, access to delivery assistance, child immunization and children's attendance to health facilities. In fact, inequalities between urban/rural settings are sometimes greater than among wealth quintiles. Just as an example, Figure 18 portrays a deep urban/rural divide in access to modern contraceptive methods, which include oral contraceptives, intrauterine devices, voluntary sterilization, condoms and injectables.

The chart reveals that in this, like in many other domains, to talk about "Africa" is an overgeneralization, since there are enormous differences in levels of contraceptive use between some of the countries selected. Urban/rural disparities are very big in some countries (mainly Chad, Ethiopia and Senegal) but rather small in other countries (particularly, Egypt and Morocco). Finally, by looking at the dates one can conclude that the gap has tended to narrow over time, although not everywhere and not at the same pace. On the positive side, the authors mention that the overall pattern of utilization by sex of the child shows hardly any differences. Male and female children with acute respiratory infections or diarrhea are taken to a health care facility in very similar percentages in practically all the countries studied.

DHS are a very good source of data because they are updated regularly and they are available for many countries. However, they have a limitation: They focus on maternal and childcare so that generally they only contain information on health care use and health status of women at childbearing age and their children. Therefore, they leave an empty gap with regards to other adults' health and health care utilization, especially taking into account the expected rise in the prevalence of chronic diseases in Africa and other developing areas of the world (Ng *et al.*, 2010). Over the next 10 years, the African continent is projected to experience the largest increase in death rates from cardiovascular disease, cancer, respiratory disease and diabetes, which will entail a tremendous challenge for African health care systems at the financial, organizational and policy level (de-Graft *et al.*, 2010).

This information gap can be partly filled by using the World Health Surveys (WHS) conducted by the WHO in 2003 across a large set of countries. Bonfrer *et al.* (2012) employ such WHS (supplemented with DHS data for several years) for 18 sub-Saharan countries in order to estimate and compare inequalities and inequities in health care delivery in those countries. Another advantage of the WHS is that they encompass detailed data on, mostly self-reported, adult health indicators, thus allowing for more extensive measurement of need, although the information on health care utilization is somewhat more limited.

Table 4 reproduces the main results from Bonfrer's *et al.* (2012) study. First, we observe that for all countries for which data are available, the utilization of maternal care demonstrates considerable inequalities favoring the better-off (the concentration indices are all positive and in general quite high). Secondly, although inequalities in the use of *any* health care are smaller, they also favor the better-off, except in Mauritius, Zambia and Zimbabwe which exhibit negative, pro-poor, CIs (although that of Zimbabwe is not significant). Thirdly, the rich also concentrate a larger share of inpatient care (the concentration indices are all positive, except for Mauritius) but inequalities for this type of care seem even smaller in 13 of the 18 countries. *Inpatient care* means inpatient care use in the last 5 years and, given survey limitations, *any care* means inpatient care or outpatient care *only* if the individual respondent has used no inpatient care. After adjusting for need, all the countries (except, again, Mauritius) show positive horizontal inequity indices (here represented by I). They are highest for Côte d'Ivoire, Ghana and Mauritania and smallest for Mali (*inpatient care*), and Zambia and Zimbabwe (*any care*).

Table 4. Concentration indices (CI) for maternal and general health care and inequity indices (I) for general health care

Maternal care	**BFA**	**TCD**	**COM**	**COG**	**CN**	**ETH**	**GHA**	**KEN**	**MWI**	**MLI**	**MRT**	**MUS**	**NAM**	**SEN**	**SAF**	**SWZ**	**ZNB**	**ZWE**
Sufficient antenatal care (CI)	0.15	0.27	0.39	0.23	0.37	0.21	0.25	0.25	0.15	0.30	n/a	n/a	0.11	0.28	n/a	0.10	0.07	0.13
Skilled birth attendance (CI)	0.35*	0.33*	0.47*	0.26	0.49*	0.17	0.44**	0.46*	0.29*	0.36*	n/a	n/a	0.34*	0.66*	n/a	0.34*	0.54*	0.30*
General health care																		
Any care (CI)	0.11	0.09	0.11	0.08	0.16	0.05	0.11	0.07	0.07	0.05	0.12	–0.06	0.03	0.10	0.08	0.07	–0.04	*–0.05*
Any care (I)	0.12	0.10	0.10	0.06	0.15	0.07	0.13	0.12	0.09	0.05	0.13	0.00	0.05	0.08	0.06	0.03	0.01	0.01
Inpatient care (CI)	0.08**	0.06**	0.05**	0.03**	0.08**	0.04	0.07**	0.04	0.06	*0.01***	0.09	–0.10	0.06	0.04**	0.11	0.07	0.03**	0.05**
Inpatient care (I)	0.08	0.06	0.04	0.02	0.08	0.04	0.08	0.06	0.06	0.00	0.10	–0.04	0.06	0.03	0.10	0.04	0.06	0.05

Notes: *All the CIs are significantly different from 0 at $\alpha = 0.05$ apart from the two in italics. **CI Skilled birth attendance differs significantly from CI sufficient antenatal care. ***CI Inpatient care differes significantly from CI any care. The abbreviations of the countries represent respectively Burkina Faso, Chad, Comoros, Congo, Côte d'Ivoire, Ethiopia, Ghana, Kenya, Malawi, Mali, Mauritania, Mauritius, Namibia, Senegal, South Africa, Swaziland, Zambia and Zimbabwe.

Source: Bonfrer *et al.* (2012).

Thus, the authors conclude, health care utilization in sub-Saharan countries does not match needs. After performing a decomposition analysis, their conclusion is that health care utilization is largely determined by wealth and education. Nonetheless, they call attention to two important methodological problems encountered in identifying the extent of inequity in these resource-frail settings. First, as we have already mentioned, conventional methods to investigate horizontal equity assume implicitly that the observed average relationship between need and utilization in a given country can be taken as the norm against which to evaluate need-expected use and deviations from it. While that assumption may be reasonable in high-income countries with well-developed health care systems, it does not seem very likely to hold in countries with very weak health systems where (lack of) ability to pay usually is the main factor determining effective access to care. In such settings, it is awkward to assume that, on average, the health systems "gets it right".

Another important problem is heterogeneity reporting, that is, the tendency of people with the same objective health but different socioeconomic background to respond to questions about their health differently. Specifically, they argue, the poor tend to understate their need because they have less information, lower health expectations and probably different frames of reference. A phenomenon that is not exclusive to African countries (see Bago d'Uva *et al.*, 2008 for India, Indonesia and China) and to which we have already made reference citing Sen (2002a).

Bonfrer *et al.* checked and confirmed the existence of this under-reporting bias by comparing self-reported problems in DHSs (e.g., children diarrhea) with more objective measures (e.g., underweight) included in the same surveys. Because the poor underestimate their needs, the concentration indices for need found are positive for some countries, thus appearing as if health problems and need for health care were higher among the rich. The implication is that the horizontal inequity calculated is biased downwards. See that for several countries (notably South Africa, Senegal, Swaziland and Congo) the inequity index (I) is smaller than the utilization concentration index (CI), a clear hint that the CI for need is positive (remember that, in our terminology, $HI = CI_M - CI_N$). If the true CI for need was negative, the inequity index would be higher than it appears to be. In sum, Bonfrer *et al.* conclude that relying on self-reported measures of health may lead to an underestimation of the degree of inequity if the poor understate their needs.

The case of Latin America and the Caribbean is particularly interesting because of the rapid economic and social changes experienced in the region in the last two decades. The region has long been characterized by high levels of income inequality — as measured by the Gini index — and low level of public expenditures over GDP. For example, in 1990 the wealthiest 20% of the population earned 52.4% of the area's income, while the poorest 20% earned only 4.5%, for a ratio of 11.6:1 (Alleyne *et al.*, 2002). This resulted in huge differences in health and health care utilization. However, the situation both in terms of economic growth and health outcomes has improved notoriously in the last 10–15 years, so that some of the countries in the region now enjoy a relatively good position in the developing world context (Etienne, 2013). In addition, several of the countries have undertaken profound reforms in their health care systems directed at expanding health care coverage, above all of the poor and uninsured. Still, the pattern in the region is one of highly segmented health care systems where social insurance for the employed coexists with other forms of public insurance for the poor and those working in the informal sector, plus several networks of private insurance providers and OOP payments still being very prevalent.

The extent to which these changes have had a reflection in inequality and inequity in the utilization of health care services can be tracked through two waves of studies conducted by the Pan American Health Organization (PAHO) within the EquiLAC Project. The first wave of studies, done between June 1998 and January 1999, included Brazil, Ecuador, Guatemala, Jamaica and Mexico. EquiLAC-II studies, whose results were published in 2013, comprised of Brazil, Chile, Colombia, Jamaica, Mexico and Peru. In both occasions, these countries accounted for more than two-thirds of the Latin America and Caribbean region's population. And in both occasions the different authors followed the conventional methodology firstly developed by Wagstaff and van Doorslaer that we have explained in this section.

Suárez-Berenguela (2001) summarized the results of the EquiLAC-I project. As he described, in all of the countries analyzed health care was pro-rich. After adjusting for need, the HI index was positive and elevated in all cases implying that the different health care services considered (labelled curative care, preventive care, chronic care, and hospitalizations) were not distributed according to need, with the rich receiving a higher than proportional share. Since, according to the same summary study, the financing of the public component of health care systems tended to be regressive (at least in Ecuador, Guatemala, Jamaica and Mexico), the conclusion was frankly disappointing: In some of these countries, the existence of a public health system was actually negative for the poor because the poor contributed to it proportionally more but used it proportionally less given their need. The main reason why the financing of the public component of health systems tended to be regressive was because government expenditure on health was basically financed with general tax revenues, which in these countries were overwhelmingly made up by indirect taxes, shown to be highly regressive (Inter-American Development Bank, 1998). From a benefits–incidence perspective (distribution of the benefits of government expenditures on health) a salient although not unusual result was that government expenditure on health followed an increasing gradient when going from the poorest to the richest quintiles in Ecuador and Guatemala. While it is generally accepted that government health expenditures should primarily benefit the poor, in practice, in most developing countries the

Table 5. Evolution of inequality and inequity in the utilization of several health care services in Latin America

Country	Date	Physician visits (probability)[a]		Physician visits (total number)[b]		Hospitalizations (prob.)	
		CI	HI	CI	HI	CI	HI
Brazil	2003	0.0518	0.0653	0.0581	0.1030	–0.0470	0.0128
	2008	0.0398	0.0518	0.0429	0.0868	–0.0411	0.0189
Difference[c]		*Down*	*Down*	*Down*	*Down*	*Down*	*Up*
Chile	2003	0.0820	0.1780	0.0840	0.0210	–0.0030	0.0690
	2009	0.0210	0.0790	0.0170	0.0970	–0.0410	0.0150
Difference		*Down*	*Down*	*Down*	*Up*	*Up*	*Down*
Colombia	2003	0.0529	0.0576	n.a.	n.a.	0.0460	0.0773
	2008	0.0381	0.0373	n.a.	n.a.	0.0012	0.0361
Difference		*Down*	*Down*			*Down*	*Down*
Jamaica	2004	–0.0100	0.0160	–0.0170	0.0219	n.a.	n.a.
	2007	0.0590	0.0800	0.0940	0.1210	n.a.	n.a.
Difference		*Up*	*Up*	*Up*	*Up*		
Mexico	2000	0.0081	0.0575	n.a.	n.a.	0.0092	0.0479
	2006	0.0041	0.0525	n.a.	n.a.	–0.0096	0.0269
Difference		*Down*	*Down*			*Down*	*Down*
Peru	2004	0.1830	0.2171	n.a.	n.a.	0.1445	0.1443
	2008	0.1000	0.1422	n.a.	n.a.	0.1528	0.1515
Difference		*Down*	*Down*			*Up*	*Up*

Notes:
[a]For Brazil and Chile, this is the probability of "any physician visit" (any visit to a physician for any reason — health problem or prevention — during the last 12 months). For Colombia, Jamaica, Mexico and Peru, it is the probability of "any curative visit" (any visit to a health care facility or professional due to illness or accident in the past 4 weeks).
[b]Total number of physician visits in Brazil and Chile. Total number of curative visits in Jamaica.
[c]"*Difference*" indicates the direction of the change in the inequality and inequity indices taking into account the absolute value of the numbers.
Sources: Own elaboration based on Almeida *et al.* (2013); Barraza-Llorens *et al.* (2013); Petrera *et al.* (2013); Ruiz *et al.* (2013); Scott and Theodore (2013); Vasquez *et al.* (2013).

opposite is the case (Castro-Leal *et al.*, 2000; O'Donnell *et al.*, 2007; Wagstaff, 2010). One possible reason is that the better endowed public health care facilities tend to be in the urban settings.

In Table 5, we summarize the main results of the EquiLAC-II project using the six country research studies that came out of it (Almeida *et al.*, 2013; Barraza-Llorens *et al.*, 2013; Petrera *et al.*, 2013; Ruiz *et al.*, 2013; Scott and Theodore, 2013; Vasquez *et al.*, 2013). All six analyzed changes over time using nationally representative household surveys for at least two points in time. In spite of great efforts to share a common methodology (Almeida and Sarti, 2013), neither the set of socioeconomic and health utilization variables nor their definition is exactly the same for every country. For example, the ranking variable is monthly household income per equivalent adult for all the countries except Peru, for which only monthly household expenditure per equivalent adult was available.[11] As for health care utilization, the breakdown between GP visits and specialist visits is only available for Chile and preventive dentist visits are only collected in Colombia. Therefore, the table only reflects the results for the most basic categories: Physician visits (probability and total number) and hospitalizations. But even these are not available for all of the countries, the definitions are not exactly the same and the recall period varies. Two countries, Brazil and Chile, report results for 3 years, but we have only included those corresponding to the two more recent surveys.

Several comments stem out of Table 5. First of all, most concentration indices exhibit a positive sign indicating that the better-off segments of the population use more medical care than their proportional share. The exceptions are hospitalizations in Brazil (both years) and Mexico (2006) and physician visits in Jamaica for 2004. However, over the time span covered by the surveys reported, the bias towards the rich decreases in all the countries (except Jamaica) as shown by the smaller CIs. On the other hand, all the HI indices without exception are positive showing that there is inequity favoring the rich; that is, in all these countries the share of health services consumed by the better-off is proportionally higher than it ought to be given their need. In many of the countries, the poor report worse self-assessed health and more limitations, but often it is the rich who declare more chronic illness. Possibly, the rich do have more chronic illness because they tend to live longer, but it could also be that they have a higher probability of being diagnosed with these diseases because of their greater consumption of (quality) doctor's visits.

The most positive finding is that, in general, the HI indices also fall, thus implying that there has been progress in the equity in the delivery of most of these services in the region. Remarkable examples are Chile and Peru for the probability of physician visits. The main exceptions to this general trend are hospitalizations in Brazil and Peru and above all physician visits — the only service for which

[11]Interestingly, the 2006 Mexican Survey contained three ranking living standard variables: Household income, household expenditures and household wealth. The table reflects the results for household income (because that is the variable employed in most of the other countries), but it is worth noting that the concentration indices and the horizontal inequity indices reported for the other two socioeconomic ranking variables are generally higher. This illustrates how sensitive the results are to the ranking variable used.

information is available — in Jamaica. It would seem that economic growth, lower income inequality, increased health expenditures and reforms of the health care system are paying off.[12] According to World Bank data, the GDP per capita in constant USD increased between 2001 and 2013 by an impressive 77% in Peru, 45% in Chile, 43% in Colombia, 32% in Brazil and 13% in Mexico (no data for Jamaica). More or less during the same period, the Gini index for income inequality went down by 7 points in Brazil, by around 5 points in Chile, Colombia, and Peru; in Mexico it fell by 3.8 points, while there was no improvement in Jamaica (World Bank, 2015). Public health care expenditures as a percentage of GDP increased between 2001 and 2013 by 51% in Brazil and Jamaica, 47% in Mexico, 40% in Chile and Colombia and 23% in Peru (World Bank, 2015). Five of the six countries have reached levels of health care coverage above 90% (Etienne, 2013); taking into account their population weight in the region, this means a lot of people have now some sort of health insurance coverage. Still, when the inequity in the utilization of health care services is decomposed into its main contributing factors, insurance coverage (in some cases, private insurance) comes up high as a reason explaining those inequities, together with income (or any similar measure of living standard) and education.

Geographic inequalities

Unwarranted geographical variations in medical practice is a well-known phenomenon which has been widely studied in high-income countries (HIC) (Skinner, 2012); indeed, it constitutes another way of looking at inequalities (not necessarily in favor of the rich) in health care utilization. According to evidence, a significant number of clinical procedures show a high variability rate which cannot be mostly explained by differences in population needs, thus breaking the horizontal equity principle. As Peiró and Maynard (2015) remarked, "*at least at the population level, geography, not morbidity, is the main determinant of health care utilization and health expenditure*". It is also well known that variation in medical practice is reduced to a minimum when the clinical value of a certain procedure is highly consensual. For example, appendectomy or hip replacement variation rates are, in general terms, quite low, and mainly depend on the need characteristics of the covered population (Meneu and Peiró, 2008). However, it is quite common to find high variation rates attached to those procedures with high doses of uncertainty,

[12] Of course, this is not to imply that these factors constitute a general solution to reduce health inequalities that is going to work forever and everywhere. As we pointed out at the beginning of Section "Health Inequalities: Measurement and Empirical Evidence", and we will discuss still further in the next section, tackling health inequalities is a much more complex issue. For instance, once a certain level is reached, increasing health expenditures or reducing broad socioeconomic inequalities may not work as the experience of some high-income countries demonstrates.

such as prostatectomy, inguinal hernia repair or knee arthroplasty, among others. Clinical practice may be, in those cases, very influenced by supply volume and/or by the financial incentives for providers.

Moreover, several studies show the presence of income-related inequality in medical practice for several procedures such as prostatectomy, the above mentioned, among many others, pointing at a higher use of medical services in those geographical areas with high income levels, once the population has been need-standardized. This situation, which in standard literature would be identified as pro-rich (areas) inequity, should not be recognized as favoring people living in rich areas, due to the fact that this inequity could be indicative of excess health care consumption and/or utilization of ineffective or damaging procedures by those living in rich areas. Actually, it seems to be the case that, at least in the European and the US contexts, higher spending regions do not achieve better outcomes (Fisher *et al.*, 2003; Peiró and Maynard, 2015). A similar argument was exposed in Section "Conceptual Framework" when equity issues were discussed from a socioeconomic (instead of geographical) perspective. Although there is profuse evidence about horizontal (pro-rich) inequity in the delivery of specialized outpatient health care, in some cases it might be related to an overconsumption of services. For instance, when analyzing socioeconomic inequalities in pregnancy control, it has been found that in the more privileged classes there was a higher proportion of women receiving excessive medical care (defined as more than 12 obstetric visits and more than three ultrasound scans, which may introduce unknown risks) (Cano-Serral *et al.*, 2006). Therefore, more research on specific procedures is needed in order to identify if those groups or areas showing a more intensive use of services are benefiting from inequity.

From Theory to Practice: Addressing Health and Health Care Disparities

How should health inequalities be addressed?

- *What is being done to reduce health inequities?*

As it has been stated previously, there is still a huge gap in the outcomes of various health indicators across world regions, which requires major efforts in order to reduce mortality in the poorest countries, particularly child mortality. Large reductions in child mortality in Africa have mainly been achieved through action on immunization, family planning, nutrition and treatment of childhood illnesses, but additional efforts are needed by providing essential care during childbirth and immediately afterwards (Save the Children, 2014). Amouzou *et al.* (2012) attributed the success of Niger, which is considered the best example in reducing child mortality, to public policies supporting universal access to health care, the provision of free health care for pregnant women and children, and decentralized nutrition programs. The promotion of education is also relevant in the design of strategies aimed at reducing illness and mortality in poor countries. For instance, recent evidence suggests that girls' secondary school enrollment, as it significantly increased the likelihood of abstaining from sex, could be strongly associated with the successful decline in HIV rates registered in Uganda in the early 1990s (Alsan and Cutler, 2013).

From the within-countries perspective, methodological developments in health economics mentioned in the previous section have allowed the identification and measurement of factors explaining income-related health (and health care) inequality, through the decomposition of the health (and health care) CI (Wagstaff *et al.*, 2003; O'Donnell *et al.*, 2008). A comparative study showed, by using these new health economics methods, how unemployment and economic deprivation were the main determinants of health inequalities within European countries (Hernández-Quevedo *et al.*, 2010), then pointing out which were the action lines to address this problem. The strategy the EU designed to address health inequalities is quite coherent with these results, since it tends to focus on people experiencing poverty, disadvantaged migrants and ethnic minority groups, people with disabilities, homeless people, children and the elderly (European Commission, 2013). Furthermore, the EU is developing different initiatives aimed at alleviating unemployment and its consequences, particularly for youth, and at fighting child poverty and social exclusion (e.g., the Youth Employment Initiative, the Europe 2020 Strategy, the Comenius Program, etc.). Since poor early life circumstances are associated with poor health in adulthood, these initiatives may result in a future reduction of health inequalities.

In many European countries, the level of access to basic services cannot be considered a main determinant of health inequities within the country, as broad coverage of basic services is provided. Although some access barriers are also present in Europe (cost sharing arrangements, geographical and organizational barriers, *etcetera*), high priority to universal access is given (Wörz *et al.*, 2006). But in countries in other geographic areas, the picture is quite different. For instance, Gwatkin *et al.* (2000) found that the differential reach of immunization programs across income groups is responsible for some of the social inequalities in health within low- and middle-income countries, with richer quintiles benefiting from much better coverage even though preventable infectious diseases predominate among the poor. Victora *et al.* (2012) associated the reduction of socioeconomic inequalities in health within countries with rapid changes in overall coverage of skilled birth attendants, measles vaccination and use of insecticide-treated bed nets. The role of social protection is also emphasized by some studies. For example, Baeten *et al.* (2013) found that health disparities in China were related to rising income inequality and, in particular, to the adverse health and income experiences of older people. They suggested that social protection at older ages via replacement incomes and pensions may be one of the most important policy levers for reducing social inequalities in health among Chinese.

Most available evidence about how to address health inequities is related to the socioeconomic dimension. Nevertheless, the ethnic perspective is also of interest in some contexts, such as in the US. A recent study, after showing a significant racial gap in survival rates among patients suffering from a chronic condition in an equal-access health care system, proves that beyond socioeconomic differences across racial groups (which account for 20% of the survival difference) and differences in quality of clinical care within health facilities (which account for 5%), most of racial gap is due to patients' adherence to recommended clinical therapy, thus suggesting that policies are needed that improve both physicians' awareness of clinically recommended therapies, as well as patients' response and adherence to therapy (Simeonova, 2013).

As the CSDH framework shown in Section "Conceptual Framework" pointed out, the reduction of health inequities requires the design of global and multisectoral strategies. In Europe, different strategies of intersectoral cooperation are being implemented in order to address health inequity. For instance, Norway and Slovenia have reduced some of the coverage gaps in the social security system for vulnerable groups (such as the elderly, children and mothers) and developed policies to reduce precarious employment, hence trying to modify structural determinants of health and living conditions. The 'national breakfast' initiative in Norwegian kindergartens, which guarantees access to a nutritious meal every school day, is another example of how cooperation across government departments may contribute to health equity goals by improving living conditions and health-related behaviors (WHO, 2012). Yet another example is the Sure Start Program in England, which provides free education, home health care and maternity cash benefits to young children and their families in disadvantaged areas, thus trying to reduce health inequities by focusing on least advantaged groups. The multisectoral perspective is based on involving in health programs the different sectors of the public administration levels. This is the core of the well-known strategy 'Health in All Policies', which was firstly proposed under the Finnish Presidency of the European Union in 2006. However, multisectoral action has also been developed in non-European contexts, such as in United States, Costa Rica, Canada, Ghana and Peru.

Despite efforts to reduce socioeconomic inequalities in health, all countries have faced challenges. Major barriers to addressing health inequities at the national level were identified at the World Conference on social determinants of health, held in Brazil in 2011. Among the barriers, a lack of trust between government ministries and other institutions and organizations was seen as a problem in implementing effective actions to address social determinants, particularly in Europe. In Ghana, funding gaps in government health budgets were identified as a crucial barrier, which may also extend to other countries in the region. In Peru, unemployment and corruption were identified as primary barriers for addressing national health inequities by the Peruvian Minister of Health himself (WHO, 2012a).

- *Some considerations about future action*

Policy decision-making is hindered by the complexity underlying the relationship between socioeconomic inequalities and health. In addition, conceptual ambiguity raises doubts about the objective pursued and how to pursue it. All too often, it is unclear whether governments aim at reducing socioeconomic inequalities in health even if it is at the cost of lowering the average level of health; at improving the health of the whole population, but to a greater extent the health of those in a worse socioeconomic position (e.g., central to the vision of the Public Health Outcomes Framework for England 2013–2016 (Department of Health, 2012) is "improving the health of the poorest fastest"); at improving the health of those with worse health, regardless of their socioeconomic position; at lowering socioeconomic inequalities with the understanding that this will cause a reduction in health inequalities; or at doing all these things at once (Regidor, 2008).

Even apart from the lack of a thorough grasp of the transmission mechanisms, we have to bear in mind that often it will be more feasible to act on the mediating factors than to alter the ultimate causes. At the level of action, of *realpolitik*, not all the links detected by experts are possible or desirable targets for intervention for those in charge of designing policies. If they were, from a purely analytical point of view, the recipe would be simple: Dilute socioeconomic inequalities, and their effect on health will disappear. However, it is important to expressly take into account the political and economic restrictions on measures for correcting inequalities, including budget constraints, opportunity costs, the redistributive impact of funding corrective measures, and so on.

As the reduction of socioeconomic inequalities is not an easy task, most governments opt for a mixed approach: Partially reducing socioeconomic inequalities, admitting that they will not disappear, and directly targeting the mediating factors, by improving health-related living or working conditions, encouraging healthy habits, or improving disadvantaged groups' access to basic services. This brings us back to the CSDH framework. The intermediary determinants (material circumstances and biological, behavioral and psychosocial factors) involve different exposures and different vulnerability to health risks for different groups within the population. Inline with this, in its more recent publications, the CSDH has proposed a framework for action to reduce health inequalities which focuses on three key elements that can be aimed at either the macro (macroeconomic policies), meso (community) or micro (individual) level:

(1) Policies for mitigating social stratification (economic, gender, etc.).
(2) Measures for reducing exposure to health risks for the least advantaged.
(3) Policies for lowering the vulnerability to risk (i.e., the susceptibility and magnitude of impact for a given exposure) of less favored individuals.

In fact, one of the most perennially occurring political dilemmas is the choice between universal measures and programs aimed at specific groups (Korpi and Palme, 1998; Marx *et al.*, 2013). For example, a program against smoking in schools in economically deprived neighborhoods is different from one that fights smoking through a campaign in the media. There is no consensus in the literature, and in real life, the most common approach is to combine these two types of action. Many countries apply measures that target specific groups, while others choose to act universally. Sweden offers an example of the latter type of policies. The Swedish Strategy is based on the belief that improvements in universal welfare are the best way to progress in the reduction of inequalities, and therefore takes great stock in social and environmental factors.

Along the same lines, Rose (2001) argued that the strategy targeting risk groups could be ineffective at altering behaviors. Given that the individuals in the same risk group share certain health-related habits (drinking, exercise, diet, etc.), altering their behavior to set them apart from their peers may prove to be too costly for the individual and ultimately have no effect. Therefore, a general strategy aimed at converting certain behaviors into "non-normal" from a peer-group perspective may be more effective. An example that is often cited is again that of smoking — although critics point out that the first to give up smoking as a result of these campaigns are the socioeconomically most advantaged. For this reason, Gwatkin, Victora and other authors contended that the reduction of inequalities will always be greater if action is first taken on the least advantaged groups. Without specific measures aimed at the most disadvantaged groups, policies may achieve their objectives in terms of averages but may maintain or widen gaps in mortality and morbidity rates. Universal measures ultimately amount to a "top–down" strategy, in which achievements are initially concentrated in the rich and gradually trickle down to lower-income groups. This is what Victora called the 'inverse equity hypothesis' and, at that time, would explain the increase in inequalities in infant mortality in countries like Brazil even when the general rate had fallen (Victora *et al.*, 2000).

Moreover, Deaton (2013) claimed that public interventions should distinguish between children and adults, according to the different mechanisms causing health outcomes for both groups. Whilst in the case of children the focus should be on "breaking or weakening the injustice of parental circumstances determining child outcomes", the reduction of health inequalities in adults should depend on what is seen as the primary cause of health. If income is the main determinant of health, health inequalities should be addressed through redistribution, but if ill health is not the consequence but the cause of low income, the main priority for adults should be "the prevention of the impoverishment that can come from ill-health, through loss of the ability to work, or through the costs of treatment".

There is no best strategy to fight against health inequities. Moreover, there is very little evaluation in this field on which the pros and cons of various approaches. A study published by the Health Development Agency showed that, in the United Kingdom at least, out of all the studies that specifically analyzed interventions, only 10% evaluated the outcomes (Milward *et al.*, 2001). And to the day, this percentage might not have substantially improved.

Furthermore, there is no consensus about the right evaluation methods. On the one hand, quasi-experimental studies and randomized trials, which include a control group, offer the most robust results. However, because of the ethical dilemmas raised by these types of studies, their application is rather scarce. On the other hand, if we adopt strict criteria to select evidence by focusing systematic review of health effects of interventions on randomized trials, we run the risk of ignoring some evaluation studies that could contribute to valuable experience and knowledge. Although there is no formula for success, some general recommendations can be drawn from the numerous publications on this topic. Firstly, the provision of education and information about health-related behaviors should be emphasized. Secondly, a multidisciplinary approach, involving several departments and ensuring proper coordination, should be adopted in the design of strategies aimed at reducing health inequities. Moreover, direct involvement of those individuals to whom the intervention is addressed should be ensured, in order to promote effectiveness. Also, attention to the cultural specificities of the group/s to which the policy is addressed should be given. Besides, the participation of members of the community in program planning and implementation should be promoted. The promotion of individual responsibility is recommendable as well: This is what is sought, for example, through conditional cash transfer programs such as *Oportunidades* (now named *Prospera*) in Mexico and *Bolsa Familia* in Brazil. Finally, interventions should be persistent in order to guarantee they have effects over time.

Reducing health care disparities

The reduction of health care disparities can be strengthened by addressing (singly or in combination) the different hurdles to health care, as defined by Wörz *et al.* (2006), which would include:

(1) Increasing the proportion of the population covered for health care.
(2) Defining basic and priority benefits covered by health care systems.
(3) Protecting vulnerable groups (low income families, children, pensioners, chronic patients, *etcetera*) against cost-sharing.
(4) Reducing geographical barriers to access, then guaranteeing geographical proximity to health care providers.
(5) Reducing organizational barriers to access, and
(6) Promoting equitable utilization of accessible services.

Some of these measures are inline with those recommended by the WHO Consultative Group on Equity and UHC, whose final report was published in 2014. This report suggested a strategy to those countries seeking fair and equitable progress toward UHC which comprises, firstly, the expansion of coverage for high-priority services to everyone. High-priority services should include those addressing communicable diseases, reproductive health, nutrition and other non-communicable diseases — including mental disorders — and injuries. Secondly, the WHO recommended the elimination of OOP payments while increasing mandatory, progressive prepayment with pooling of funds (WHO, 2014b).

Mexico has been one of the countries that successfully reduced catastrophic payments by introducing government-funded health insurance. The *Seguro Popular* was launched in 2003 and has achieved a reduction in the proportion of households spending more than 30% of their post-subsistence income on health from 8.4 to 6.5% (Azuara and Marinescu, 2013). Some other countries have tried to reduce the incidence of catastrophic health expenditure by removing user fees, but sometimes this needs to be accompanied by other mechanisms to reduce the burden of OOP costs and improve access to care, particularly among the poorest (Musango *et al.*, 2013). This is the case of Uganda, where incidence of catastrophic health expenditure increased — although only in the short term — after user fees abolition in 2001, as private providers remained the preferred choice for patients. Furthermore, the removal of fees had an unwanted effect: Health workers' morale declined as their salaries decreased because of the reduction of funds (Nabyonga *et al.*, 2013).

Flores *et al.* (2013) have shown how Cambodian Health Equity Funds could be a mechanism to make user fee exemptions more effective. These funds are mostly financed by international donors and give NGOs responsibility for assessing eligibility and compensating providers for lost revenue. They may reduce OOP payments by 35% on average, with a larger effect for poorer households. Moreover, in some rich countries the exemption of user fees for low-income people has effectively improved access to care and reduced social inequalities (van Doorslaer *et al.*, 2006).

With respect to geographical barriers to access, regulatory intervention may be useful to reduce inequalities within countries. In the Netherlands, the Ministry sets a standard for maximum travelling time to hospital and to a GP. This measure, along with the high population density, explains that the Netherlands is one of the countries with the highest proportion of people with uniform proximity to hospitals and GPs (Wörz *et al.*, 2006).

Most LDC will need to leverage more resources in order to widen coverage and promote better health care access for disadvantaged people. However, in addition to getting more funds, some other strategies should be followed to battle organizational obstacles to health care for the worse-off. For instance, cooperation between public and private sectors has to be studied to explore its potential for reducing disparities. A change from competition to collaboration among providers, and from marketization and privatization to governmental planning is taking place in many countries, since some of the previous reforms have proved to be misleading (Lister, 2008). A more effective regulation of the private sector is needed in order to ensure quality of care, rational health service provision and cost control (Nabyonga *et al.*, 2013). Nonetheless, there is still room to see how public and private actors may interact to provide more and better health care to all.

Also, the configuration of health services delivery and/or the attitude of health workers when treating health problems have to be highlighted as factors that may act as obstacles to accessing care, and therefore should be addressed in order to remove health care inequities. For instance, promoting training and increasing the capacity of health care workers and services in order to better respond to gender-sensitive health issues have been recommended in the reform of health systems (WHO, 2013). Developing the capacity to better treat the most vulnerable groups (such as ethnic minorities, migrants, and other socioeconomically disadvantaged people) should also be considered as a good strategy to combat health care inequities.

Lastly, regarding the equitable utilization of accessible services, it has been shown in Section "Inequity in the Utilization of Health Care" how socioeconomic inequalities in the use of medical services vary depending on the type of the care provided. Moreover, we have seen that there is a "pro-rich" bias in specialized services which cannot be explained by differences in clinical needs. This bias could be reduced if health systems were to give more attention to primary care, in terms of human resources (more professionals) and a higher access to technologies that increase the proportion of health problems that may be diagnosed and treated without the intervention of specialized care. Empirical evidence also suggests that public spending in primary health care is more equitable than spending in secondary care (Anselmi *et al.*, 2014), but primary care remains with a low proportion of health resources and nothing leads us to think that this picture will substantially change in the coming years.

Big policy issues: The role of international institutions in global equity

The number of multilateral institutions involved in global health has rapidly grown in recent years. Development assistance for health (DAH) almost tripled between 2000 and 2011, from $11 billion to $28 billion (Elovainio and Evans, 2013). However, it has not been enough to eliminate health and health care inequalities, as it has been shown in the previous sections. Besides, DAH fell for the first time in 2011 and then rose slightly in 2012, what has been suggested that could be signaling a new phase of no growth (Institute for Health Metrics and Evaluation, 2012). The priority health themes were HIV and AIDS (which received up to 30% of all DAH in 2010), followed by maternal, newborn and child health (23.3%). Tuberculosis and malaria received less than one-third of funds allocated to HIV and AIDS. Other health focus areas, such as health-sector support and noncommunicable diseases, represented about 5.0% and 0.8% of DAH in 2010, respectively (World Vision International, 2013).

The potential role played by DAH in the reduction of inequalities is quite large, as it gives a significant amount of resources to low-income countries to combat illnesses that particularly affect the worse-off, and to provide better access to health care. However, the adequacy of DAH in relation to global health challenges has been firmly questioned, as DAH is perceived as insufficient and inequitably distributed, it does not address income-related disparities within and between countries, and it is strongly biased to the priority areas highlighted by the United Nations MDGs framework rather than emphasizing a health care integration and universal health rights (Garay, 2012).

Health MDG (reducing child mortality, improving maternal health and combatting HIV/AIDS, malaria and other diseases) have shown significant progress during the 21st century, although the targets will not be fully attained by 2015. However, advances may be hiding important socioeconomic, ethnic and gender health disparities, as indicators used to measure progress are based on national average figures. Furthermore, it has been suggested that the focus on MDG in isolation should be substituted by an integrated social, ecological and economic approach to more effectively promote health and human development (Garay, 2012).

The strategies designed to stimulate both sustainability and human development also should foster stronger accountability and democratic processes at country level, partially through support for an active civil society and media (UNDP, 2011). Successful approaches involve inclusive institutions that pay more attention to disadvantaged groups and also reinforcing coordination of budgets and interventions across all the development partners (UNDP, 2011).

It has been suggested that the main national contributors to DAH should improve policy coherence for development, contribute to building up the capacity of national systems to monitor health equity by strengthening the national information systems, and support comprehensive social protection systems in low-income countries (Koller *et al.*, 2010). But the requests for strong reforms are also directed at WHO (Working Group on Health Financing, 2014). The WHO has been developing a reform process since 2010 in response to financial and governance problems, partially due to the emergence of new actors in the global health scene. This reform is aimed at enhancing a more strategic approach to priority setting in order to focus WHO's activities and improving its effectiveness, tightening collaboration with relevant stakeholders (NGO's, foundations, *etcetera*) to promote greater coherence in global health and strengthening technical and policy support to Member States (WHO, 2010d). However, some critical voices argue that this process does not ask fundamental questions about WHO's place in the present international system for health and that deeper changes should be implemented to allow the WHO to effectively overcome challenges of global health (Clift, 2013). A global coalition of civil socicty and academics — the Joint Action and Learning Initiative on National and Global Responsibilities for Health (JALI) — has asked WHO to adopt a Framework Convention on Global Health (FCGH), where equity issues are of major concern. This would require "*defining national responsibilities for the population's health; defining international responsibilities for reliable, sustainable funding; setting global health priorities; coordinating fragmented activities; reshaping global governance for health; and providing strong and global health leadership through the World Health Organization*" (Gostin, 2012).

Beyond the MDG, the post-2015 agenda of international development goals is now under discussion. The fight against health and health care inequities should remain as relevant targets in this global agenda.

References

Abásolo I, Negrín M, Pinilla J. 2014. Equity in specialist waiting times by socioeconomic groups: Evidence from Spain. *European Journal of Health Economics* 15: 323–334.

Alleyne GAO, Castillo-Salgado C, Schneider MC, Loyola E, Vidaurre M. 2002. Overview of social inequalities in health in the Region of the Americas, using various methodological approaches. *Revista Panamericana de Salud Pública/Pan American Journal of Public Health* 12: 388–397.

Almeida G, Sarti FM. 2013. Measuring evolution of income-related inequalities in health and health care utilization in selected Latin American and Caribbean countries. *Revista Panamericana de Salud Pública/Pan American Journal of Public Health* 33: 83–89.

Almeida G, Sarti FM, Ferreira FF, Diaz MD, Campino AC. 2013. Analysis of the evolution and determinants of income-related inequalities in the Brazilian health system, 1998–2008. *Revista Panamericana de Salud Pública/Pan American Journal of Public Health* 33: 90–97.

Alsan MM, Cutler DM. 2013. Girls' education and HIV risk: Evidence from Uganda. *Journal of Health Economics* 32: 863–872.

Amouzou A, Habi O, Bensaïd K, and the Niger Countdown Case Study Working Group. 2012. Reduction in child mortality in Niger: A Countdown to 2015 country case study. *The Lancet* 380: 1169–1178.

Amouzou A, Kozuki N, Gwatkin DR. 2014. Where is the gap?: The contribution of disparities within developing countries to global inequalities in under-five mortality. *BMC Public Health* 14: 216. doi: 10.1186/1471-2458-14-216.

Anselmi L, Lagarde M, Hanson K. 2014. Equity in the allocation of public sector financial resources in low- and middle-income countries: A systematic literature review. *Health Policy and Planning.* doi: 10.1093/heapol/czu034.

Azuara O, Marinescu I. 2013. Informality and the expansion of social protection programs: Evidence from Mexico. *Journal of Health Economics* 32: 938–950.

Bach P. 2010. Gardasil: From bench, to bedside, to blunder. *The Lancet* 375: 963–964.

Baeten S, Van Ourti T, van Doorslaer E. 2013. Rising inequalities in income and health in China: Who is left behind? *Journal of Health Economics* 32: 1214–1229.

Bago d'Uva T, van Doorslaer E, Lindeboom M, O'Donnell O. 2008. Does reporting heterogeneity bias the measurement of health disparities? *Health Economics* 17: 351–375.

Inter-American Development Bank. 1998. Facing Up to Inequality in Latin America. Economic and Social Progress in Latin America. 1998–1999 Report. Washington, DC: IDB.

Barraza-Llorens M, Panopoulou G, Diaz BY. 2013. Income-related inequalities and inequities in health and health care utilization in Mexico, 2000–2006. *Revista Panamericana de Salud Pública/Pan American Journal of Public Health* 33: 122–130.

Bhalotra S, Valente C, Van Soest A. 2010. The puzzle of Muslim advantage in child survival in India. *Journal of Health Economics* 29: 191–204.

Bonfrer I, Van de Poel E, Grimm M, van Doorslaer E. 2012. Does health care utilization match needs in Africa? Challenging conventional needs measurement. *iBMG Working Paper* W2012.02, Erasmus University, Rotterdam.

Braveman P. 2006. Health disparities and health equity: Concepts and measurement. *Annual Review of Public Health* 27: 167–194.

Braveman P, Starfield B, Geiger HJ. 2001. World Health Report 2000: How it removes equity from the agenda for public health monitoring and policy. *British Medical Journal* 323: 678–680.

Cano-Serral G, Rodríguez-Sanz M, Borrell C, Pérez MM, Salvador J. 2006. Desigualdades socioeconómicas relacionadas con el cuidado y el control del embarazo. *Gaceta Sanitaria* 20: 25–30.

Cappelen AW, Norheim OF. 2005. Responsibility in health care: A liberal egalitarian approach. *Journal of Medical Ethics* 31: 476–480.

Castro-Leal F, Dayton J, Emery L, Mehra K. 2000. Public spending on health care in Africa: Do the poor benefit? *Bulletin of the World Health Organization* 78: 66–74.

Clift C. 2013. The Role of the World Health Organization in the International System. *Centre on Global Health Security Working Group Papers*. Working Group on Governance, Paper 1. Chatham House, The Royal Institute of International Affairs.

Commission on Social Determinants of Health (CSDH). 2008. *Closing the Gap in a Generation: Health Equity Through Action on the Social Determinants of Health*. Geneva, World Health Organization.

Costa-Font J, Hernández-Quevedo C. 2012. Measuring inequalities in health: What do we know? What do we need to know? *Health Policy* 106: 195–206.

Deaton A. 2013. What does the empirical evidence tell us about the injustice of health inequalities? In Eyal N, Hurst SA, Norheim OF, Wikler D. (eds.). *Inequalities in Health: Concepts, Measures, and Ethics*. Oxford: Oxford University Press.

Department of Health 2009. *Tackling Health Inequalities: 10 Years On — A Review of Developments in Tackling Health Inequalities in England over the Last 10 years*. Department of Health, London.

Department of Health 2012. *The Public Health Outcomes Framework for England, 2013–2016*. Department of Health, London.

Devaux M, Looper M. 2012. Income-related inequalities in health service utilisation in 19 OECD countries, 2008–09. *OECD Health Working Paper* 58.

de-Graft AA, Unwin N, Agyemang C, Allotey P, Campbell C, Arhinful D. 2010. Tackling Africa's chronic disease burden: From local to the global. *Globalization and Health* 6: 5 doi: 10.1186/1744-8603-6-5.

Elovainio R, Evans DV. 2013. Raising and Spending Domestic Money for Health. *Centre on Global Health Security Working Group Papers*. Working Group on Financing, Paper 2.

Erreygers G. 2009. Correcting the concentration index. *Journal of Health Economics* 28: 504–515.

Etienne CF. 2013. Equity in health systems. *Revista Panamericana de Salud Pública/Pan American Journal of Public Health* 33: 79–80.

European Commission. 2013. *Health Inequalities in the EU — Final Report of a Consortium. Consortium Lead: Sir Michael Marmot*. European Union.

Eurostat. 2014. http://epp.eurostat.ec.europa.eu/portal/page/portal/employment_social_policy_equality/social_protection_social_inclusion/indicators/health_long_term_care [7 August 2014].

Fisher ES, Wennberg DE, Stukel TA, Gottlieb DJ, Lucas FL, Pinder EL. 2003. The implications of regional variations in Medicare spending. Part 2: Health outcomes and satisfaction with care. *Annals of Internal Medicine* 138: 288–298.

Fiva JH, Hægeland T, Rønning M, Syse A. 2014. Access to treatment and educational inequalities in cancer survival. *Journal of Health Economics* 36: 98–111.

Fleurbaey M, Schockkaert E. 2012. *Equity in Health and Health Care*. In Pauly M, McGuire TG, Pita-Barros P. (eds.). *Handbook of Health Economics*, Vol. 2: 1003–1092. Elsevier, North-Holland.

Flores G, Ir P, Men CR, O'Donnell, van Doorslaer E. 2013. Financial protection of patients through compensation of providers: The impact of health equity funds in Cambodia. *Journal of Health Economics* 32: 1180–1193.

Gakidou EE, Murray CJ, Frenk J. 2000. Defining and measuring health inequality: An approach based on the distribution of health expectancy. *Bulletin of the World Health Organization* 78: 42–54.

Garay, JE. 2012. *Global Health Equity. The Challenge for a New Global Health Framework. The US and EU Policies and Opportunities to Improve Global Health*. Unpublished document.

Geruso M, Spears D. 2014. Sanitation and health externalities: Resolving the Muslim mortality paradox. https://laits.utexas.edu/~mlg2296/images/MuslimSanitation.pdf [14 July 2014].

Gostin LO. 2012. A framework convention on global health: Health for all, justice for all. *Journal of the American Medical Association* 307: 2087–2092.

Guillot M, Allendorf K. 2010. Hindu–Muslim differential in child mortality in India. *Genus* 66: 43–68.

Gwatkin DR, Rutstein S, Johnsson K, Pande R, Wagstaff A. *Socioeconomic Differences in Health, Nutrition and Population*. Washington (DC). World Bank 2000. Health, Nutrition and Population Paper.

Gwatkin DR. 2002. Reducing health inequalities in developing countries, In Detels R, McEwen J, Beaglehole R, Tanaka H. (eds.). *Oxford Textbook of Public Health*. Oxford University Press.

Harris G. 2014. Poor Sanitation in India May Afflict Well-Fed Children With Malnutrition. *The New York Times*, July 13, Online Edition.

Houweling TAJ, Ronsmans C, Campbell OMR, Kunst AE. 2007. Huge poor–rich inequalities in maternity care: An international comparative study of maternity and child care in developing countries. *Bulletin of the World Health Organization* 85: 745–754.

Hernández-Quevedo C, Masseria C, Mossialos EA. 2010. Analysing the Socioeconomic Determinants of Health in Europe: New Evidence from EU-SILC. Luxembourg: Eurostat *Working Paper*.

Institute for Health Metrics and Evaluation. 2012. *Financing Global Health 2012: The End of the Golden Age?* Seattle, WA: IHME.

Inter-American Development Bank. 1998. Facing Up to Inequality in Latin America. Economic and Social Progress in Latin America. 1998–1999 Report. Washington, DC: IDB.

Inter-American Development Bank. 1999. *Progreso económico y social en América Latina: América Latina frente a la desigualdad. Informe 1998–99.* Washington, DC.

Jank S, Owens L. 2015. Inequality in the United States. Understanding Inequality with Data. The Stanford Center on Poverty and Inequality. http://web.stanford.edu/group/scspi/slides.html [26 February 2015].

Kawachi I, Daniels N, Robinson D. 2005. Health disparities by race and class: Why both matter. *Health Affairs* 24: 343–352.

Kelly-Irving M, Delpierre C, Schieber AC, Lepage B, Rolland C, Afrité A, Pascal J, Cases C, Lombrail P, Lang T. 2011. Do general practitioners overestimate the health of their patients with lower education? *Social Science & Medicine* 73: 1416–1421.

Knaul FM, Wong R, Arreola-Ornelas H, Mendez O. 2011. Household catastrophic health expenditures: A comparative analysis of twelve Latin American and Caribbean Countries. *Salud Pública de México* 53: 85–95.

Koller T, Villar E, Alonso PL, Robert M, Rasanathan K. 2010. Global health inequalities and social determinants of health: Opportunities for the EU to contribute to monitoring and action. In *Moving Forward Equity in Health: Monitoring Social Determinants of Health and the Reduction of Health Inequalities. An Independent Expert Report Commissioned through the Spanish Presidency of the EU.* Ministry of Health and Social Policy of Spain.

Korpi W, Palme J. 1998. The paradox of redistribution and strategies of equality: Welfare State Institutions, inequality, and poverty in the Western Countries. *American Sociological Review* 63: 661–687.

Kremer M, Glennerster R. 2012. Improving health in developing countries: Evidence from randomized evaluations. In Pauly M, McGuire TG, Pita-Barros P. (eds.). *Handbook of Health Economics,* Vol. 2, pp. 201–315. Elsevier, North-Holland.

Laudicella M, Siciliani L, Cookson R. 2012. Waiting times and socioeconomic status: Evidence from England. *Social Science & Medicine* 74: 1331–1341.

Le Grand J. 1991. *Equity and Choice: An Essay in Economics and Applied Philosophy.* Harper Collins Academic, London.

Lister J. 2008. *Globalization and Health Systems Change.* Globalization Knowledge Network, Research Papers.

Lu JR, Leung GM, Kwon S, Tin KYK, van Doorslaer E, O'Donnell O. 2007. Horizontal equity in health care utilization evidence from three high-income Asian countries. *Social Science & Medicine* 64: 199–212.

MacDorman MF. 2011. Infant deaths — United States, 2000–2007. Health Disparities and Inequalities Report — United States, 2011. *Centers for Disease Control and Prevention Morbidity and Mortality Weekly Report* 60: 49–51.

Mackenbach JP, Bos V, Andersen O, Gardano M, Costa G, Harding S, Reid A, Hemström Ö, Valkonen T, Kunst A. 2003. Widening socioeconomic inequalities in mortality in six Western European countries. *International Journal of Epidemiology* 32: 830–837.

Mackenbach JP, Stirbu I, Roskam A-JR, Schaap M, Menvielle G, Leinsalu M, Kunst AE, for the European Union Working Group on Socioeconomic Inequalities in Health. 2008. Socioeconomic inequalities in health in 22 European countries. *The New England Journal of Medicine* 358: 2468–2481.

Marx I, Salanauskaite L, Verbist G. 2013. The Paradox of Redistribution Revisited: And That It May Rest in Peace? *IZA Discussion Paper* No. 7414; May 2013. CSB, University of Antwerp.

Masseria C, Irwin R, Thomson S, Gemmill M, Mossialos E. 2009. *Primary Care in Europe. Policy Brief.* The London School of Economics and Political Science.

Meneu R, Peiró S. 2008. Desigualdades en la efectividad y utilización de los servicios sanitarios e implicaciones de equidad. In Rodríguez M, Urbanos R (eds.). *Desigualdades sociales en salud. Factores determinantes y elementos para la acción,* pp. 167–188. Elsevier Masson.

Milward L, Kelly M, Nutbeam D. 2001. *Public Health Intervention Research: The Evidence*. London: Health Development Agency.

Molla M. 2013. Expected Years of Life Free of Chronic Condition — Induced Activity Limitations — United States, 1999–2008. Health Disparities and Inequalities Report — United States, 2013. *Centers for Disease Control and Prevention Morbidity and Mortality Weekly Report* 62: 87–92.

Murage P, Hamm J, Brannan M (on behalf of the London Regional Public Health Group and the London Health Inequalities Network). 2012. The Slope Index of Inequality (SII) in Life expectancy: Interpreting It and Comparisons Across London. Regional Public Health Group-London (Department of Health). http://www.instituteofhealthequity.org/projects/the-slope-index-of-inequality-sii-in-life-expectancy-interpreting-it-and-comparisons-across-london [21 February 2015].

Murphy M, Bobak M, Nicholson A, Marmot M, Rose R. 2006. The widening gap in mortality by educational level in the Russian Federation, 1980–2001. *American Journal of Public Health* 96: 1293–1299.

Murray JL. 2001. Commentary: Comprehensive approaches are needed for full understanding. *British Medical Journal* 323: 680–681.

Musango L, Saksena P, Toure B. 2013. Financial risk protection in the African Region. *African Health Monitor* 17: 4–5.

Mutangadura G, Gauci A, Armah B, Woldemariam E, Ayalew A, Egu B. 2007. *Health Inequalities in Selected African Countries: Review of Evidence and Policy Implications.* United Nations Economic Commission for Africa, Addis Ababa, Ethiopia, http://www.uneca.org/sites/default/files/page_attachments/gladys_mutangadura_adrian_gauci_kasirim_nwuke_bartholomew_0.pdf [28 February 2014].

Navarro V. 2000. Assessment of the World Health Report 2000. *The Lancet* 356:1568–1601.

Nabyonga J, Mapunda M, Musango L, Mugisha F. 2013. Long-term effects of the abolition of user fees in Uganda. *African Health Monitor* 17: 30–35.

Ng N, Kowal P, Kahn K, Naidoo N, Abdullah S, Bawah A, Binka F, Chuc N, Debpuur C, Egondi T, Gómez-Olivé F, Hakimi M, Hirve S, Hodgson A, Juvekar S, Kyobutangi C, Minh H, Mwanyangala M, Nathan R, Razzaque A, Sankoh O, Streatfield P, Thorogood M, Wall S, Wilopo S, Byass P, Tollman S, Chatterji S. 2010. Health inequalities among older men and women in Africa and Asia: Evidence from eight Health and Demographic Surveillance System sites in the INDEPTH WHO-SAGE study. *Global Health Action Supplement* 2. doi: 10.3402/gha.v3i0.5420.

O'Donnell O, Rannan-Eliya RP, Somanathan A, Adhikari SR, Harbianto D, Garg CC, Hanvoravongchai P, Huq MN, Karan A, Leung GM, Ng CW, Pande BR, Tin K, Tisayaticom K, Trisnantoro L, Zhang Y, Zhao Y. 2007. The incidence of public spending on healthcare: Comparative evidence from Asia. *The World Bank Economic Review* 21: 93–123.

O'Donnell O, van Doorslaer E, Wagstaff A, Lindelow M. 2008. *Analyzing Health Equity Using Household Survey Data. A Guide to Techniques and their Implementation.* World Bank Institute.

O'Donnell O, Van Doorslaer E, Van Ourti T. 2015. Health and Inequality. In Atkinson AB and Bourguignon F (eds.). Handbook of Income Distribution. Vols. 2A and 2B, Chapter 17. North-Holland, Amsterdam.

Olsen JA. 2013. Concepts of Equity and Fairness in Health and Health Care. In Glied S, Smith PC (eds.). *The Oxford Handbook of Health Economics*, Chapter 34. Oxford University Press.

PAHO. 2012. *Health in the Americas. Regional Outlook and Country Profiles. 2012 Edition.* http://www.paho.org/saludenlasamericas/index.php?option=com_content&view=article&id=9&Itemid=14&lang=en [7 July 2014].

Palosuo H, Koskinen S, Lahelma E, Kostiainen E, Prättälä R, Martelin T, Ostamo A, Keskimäki I, Sihto M, Linnanmäki E (eds.). 2009. *Health Inequalities in Finland. Trends in Socioeconomic Health Differences 1980–2005*. Ministry of Social Affairs and Health Publications, Helsinki.

Peiró S, Maynard A. 2015. Variations in health care delivery within the European Union. *European Journal of Public Health* 25 (Suppl. 1): 1–2.

Pell JP, Hart JT, Pell AC, Norrie J, Ford I, Cobbe SM. 2000. Effect of socioeconomic deprivation on waiting time for cardiac surgery: Retrospective cohort study Commentary: Three decades of the inverse care law. *British Medical Journal* 320: 15–19.

Petrera M, Valdivia M, Jimenez E, Almeida G. 2013. Equity in health and health care in Peru, 2004–2008. *Revista Panamericana de Salud Pública/Pan American Journal of Public Health* 33: 131–136.

Rao KD, Petrosyan V, Araujo EC, McIntyre D. 2014. Progress towards universal health coverage in BRICS: Translating economic growth into better health. *Bulletin of the World Health Organization* 92: 429–435.

Regidor E. 2004a. Measures of health inequalities: Part 1. *Journal of Epidemiology and Community Health* 58: 858–861.

Regidor E. 2004b. Measures of health inequalities: Part 2. *Journal of Epidemiology and Community Health* 58: 900–903.

Regidor E, Martínez E, Astasio P, Ortega P, Calle MA, Dominguez V. 2006. Trends in socioeconomic inequalities and socioeconomic inequalities in self-perceived health in Spain. *Gaceta Sanitaria* 20: 178–183.

Regidor E. 2008. Desigualdades socioeconómicas en la exposición al riesgo y en salud. In Rodríguez M, Urbanos R (eds.). *Desigualdades sociales en salud. Factores determinantes y elementos para la acción,* pp. 11–40. Elsevier Masson.

Robone S, Jones A, Rice N. 2010. Contractual conditions, working conditions and their impact on health and well-being. *The European Journal of Health Economics* 12: 429–444.

Roemer JE. 1998. *Equality of Opportunity*. Harvard University Press.

Rose G. 2001. Sick individuals and sick populations. *International Journal of Epidemiology* 30(3): 427–432.

Ruiz F, Zapata T, Garavito L. 2013. Colombian health care system: Results on equity for five health dimensions, 2003–2008. *Revista Panamericana de Salud Pública/Pan American Journal of Public Health* 33: 107–115.

Save the Children. 2014. *Ending Newborn Deaths. Ensuring Every Baby Survives*. The Save the Children Fund.

Scott E, Theodore K. 2013. Measuring and explaining health and health care inequalities in Jamaica, 2004 and 2007. *Revista Panamericana de Salud Pública/Pan American Journal of Public Health* 33: 116–121.

Segall S. 2010. *Health, Luck and Justice*. Princeton: Princeton University Press.

Sen A. 2002a. Health: Perception versus observation. *British Medical Journal* 324: 860–861.

Sen A. 2002b. Why health equity? *Health Economics* 11: 659–666.

Siegel JS. 2012. *The Demography and Epidemiology of Human Health and Aging*. Springer Science+Business Media B.V.

Simeonova E. 2013. Doctors, patients and the racial mortality gap. *Journal of Health Economics* 32: 895–908.

Skinner J. 2012. Causes and consequences of regional variations in health care, In Pauly M, McGuire TG, Pita-Barros P (eds.). *Handbook of Health Economics*, Volume 2, pp. 45–94. Elsevier, North-Holland.

Solé M, Díaz-Serrano L, Rodríguez M. 2013. Disparities in work, risk and health between immigrants and native-born Spaniards. *Social Science & Medicine* 76: 179–187.

Soucat A, Scheffler R. 2013. Labour market analysis of human resources for health. In Soucat A, Scheffler R, Ghebreyesus A (eds.). *The Labour Market for Health Workers in Africa. A New Look at the Crisis*, pp. 1–12. The World Bank.

Starfield B. 2000. Is US health really the best in the World? Commentary. *Journal of the American Medical Association* 284: 483–485.

Suárez-Berenguela R. 2001. Health system inequalities and inequities in Latin America and the Caribbean: Findings and policy implications. In *Investing in Health: Social and Economic Returns*. Pan American Health Organization.

Townsend P, Davidson N (eds.). 1992. The Black Report. In Townsend P, Davidson N, Whitehead M. (eds.). *Inequalities in Health. The Black Report and the Health Divide*. Penguin Books, 2nd Edition, London.

United Nations Development Programme. 2011. *Human Development Report 2011. Sustainability and Equity: A Better Future for All*. Palgrave Macmillan; New York.

U.S. Department of Health and Human Services. Agency for Healthcare Research and Quality. 2014. National Healthcare Disparities Report. *AHRQ Publication* No. 14-0006.

van Doorslaer E, Wagstaff A. 1992. Equity in the delivery of health care: Some international comparisons. *Journal of Health Economics* 11: 389–411.

van Doorslaer E, Wagstaff A, van der Burg H, Christiansen T, De Graeve D, Duchesne I, Gerdtham UG, Gerfin M, Geurts J, Gross L, *et al.* 2000. Equity in the delivery of health care in Europe and the US. *Journal of Health Economics* 19: 553–583.

van Doorslaer E, Koolman X, Puffer F. 2002. Equity in the use of physician visits in OECD countries: Has equal treatment for equal need been achieved? In: *Measuring up: Improving Health Systems Performance in OECD Countries*, pp. 225–248. OECD, Paris.

van Doorslaer E, Masseria C, Koolman. 2006. Inequalities in access to medical care by income in developed Countries. *Canadian Medical Association Journal* 174: 177–183.

Vasquez F, Paraje G, Estay M. 2013. Income-related inequality in health and health care utilization in Chile, 2000–2009. *Revista Panamericana de Salud Pública/Pan American Journal of Public Health* 33: 98–106.

Victora CG, Vaughan JP, Barros FC, Silva AC, Tomasi E. 2000. Explaining trends in inequities: Evidence from Brazilian child health studies. *The Lancet* 356: 1093–1098.

Victora CG, Barros AJ, Axelson H, Bhutta ZA, Chopra M, França GV, Kerber K, Kirkwood BR, Newby H, Ronsmans C, Boerma JT. 2012. How changes in coverage affect equity in maternal and child health interventions in 35 Countdown to 2015 countries: An analysis of national surveys. *The Lancet* 380: 1149–1156.

Von dem Knesebeck O, Verde PE, Dragano N. 2006. Education and health in 22 European countries. *Social Science & Medicine* 63: 1344–1351.

Wagstaff A. 2005. The bounds of the Concentration Index when the variable of interest is binary, with an application to immunization inequality. *Health Economics* 14: 429–432.

Wagstaff A. 2010. Benefit incidence analysis. Are government health expenditures more pro-rich than we think? *Policy Research Working Paper* 5234. The World Bank.

Wagstaff A, Paci P, van Doorslaer E. 1991. On the measurement of inequalities in health. *Social Science & Medicine* 33: 545–557.

Wagstaff A, van Doorslaer E, Paci P. 1989. Equity in the finance and delivery of health care: Some tentative cross-country comparisons. *Oxford Review of Economic Policy* 5: 89–112.

Wagstaff A, van Doorslaer E, Watanabe N. 2003. On decomposing the causes of health sector inequalities, with an application to malnutrition inequalities in Vietnam. *Journal of Econometrics* 112: 219–227.

Whitehead M. 1992. The concepts and principles of equity in health. *International Journal of Health Services* 22: 429–445.

Working Group on Health Financing. 2014. *Shared Responsibilities for Health. A Coherent Global Framework for Health Financing*. Final Report of the Centre on Global Health Security. Chatham House Report; Chatham House, The Royal Institute of International Affairs.

World Bank. 2015. *World Development Indicators*, updated March 2015. http://databank.worldbank.org/data/views/variableselection/selectvariables.aspx?source=world-development-indicators [12 March 2015].

World Health Organization. 2009. *Global Health Risks. Mortality and Burden of Disease Attributable to Selected Major Risks*. WHO, Geneva.

World Health Organization. 2010a. A conceptual framework for action on the social determinants of health. Social determinants of Health. *WHO Discussion Paper 2*.

World Health Organization. 2010b. *Equity Social Determinants and Public health Programmes*. WHO, Geneva.

World Health Organization. 2010c. *The World Health Report 2010 — Health Systems Financing: The Path to Universal Health Coverage*. WHO, Geneva.

World Health Organization. 2010d. *The Future of Financing for WHO. Summary of a Consultation*. EB128/INF.DOC./2, 16 December 2010. WHO, Geneva.

World Health Organization. 2012a. *World Conference on Social Determinants of Health: Meeting Report, Rio de Janeiro, Brazil, 19–21 October 2011*. WHO, Geneva.

World Health Organization. 2013a. *Review of Social Determinants and the Health Divide in WHO European Region: Final Report*. WHO, Regional Office for Europe, updated reprint 2014.

World Health Organization. 2013b. *Increasing Access to Health Care Services in Afghanistan with Gender-Sensitive Health Service Delivery*. WHO, Regional Office for the Eastern Mediterranean.

World Health Organization. 2014b. World Health Statistics 2014.

World Health Organization. 2014b. *Making Fair Choices on the Path to Universal Health Coverage*. Final report of the WHO Consultative Group on Equity and Universal Health Coverage.

World Health Organization and International Bank for Reconstruction and Development/ The World Bank. 2014a. *Monitoring Progress Towards Universal Health Coverage at Country and Global Levels. Framework, Measures and Targets*. WHO and World Bank Group.

World Vision International. 2013. *Development Assistance for Health. Donor Landscape for Health Financing*. Global Health and WASH.

Wörz M, Foubister T, Busse R. 2006. Access to health care in the EU Member States. *EuroObserver* 8: 1–4.

Index

A
Ability to Pay (*see also* ATP), 191, 202, 235, 241, 244, 258, 260, 263, 492, 534
Absorptive Capacity, 56, 70
Abuja Declaration, 11, 22, 25,
Academic Medical Centers, 181, 210
Accountability, 7, 9, 11, 56–57, 72, 76–78, 133, 258, 271, 284, 296, 304
Accuracy, 177, 203–205
Actuarial Cells, 320–323, 340
Actuarial Risk Sharing Mechanism, 233
Actuarial Science, 220
Additional Borrowing, 67
Adjusted Clinical Groups (*see also* ACG), 320, 323–326, 332– 336
Administrative Barriers, 444
Administrative Costs, 39, 41, 235, 260, 296, 352, 396, 423
Administrative Expenditure, 261
Administrative Logjams, 77
Adult Height, 74
Adverse Selection, 227, 230, 255, 259, 263, 275–276, 298, 300, 317
Age and Gender, 49, 319–320, 333, 337, 351
Age/Sex/Disease Projections, 212
Aggregate Factors, 40–42
Aggregated Diagnostic Groups (*see also* ADGs), 332–333
Aggregation, 178, 190, 343, 403–404, 415–416, 473, 480
Aging, 19, 31, 38–39, 49, 64, 69, 115, 124, 130–131, 177–178, 180–202, 270, 341, 363
Agricultural Economies, 182
Agricultural Implications, 171
Agricultural Workers, 54
Ambulatory Clinics, 240
Amenity Beds in Hospitals, 276
Anemia, 74, 440
Antenatal Care, 522, 533
Antiretroviral Treatment, 160, 468
Archipelago, 342
Asian Financial Crisis, 95
Asymmetrical Information, 259
ATM Framework, 93, 107
Automatic Stabilizers, 108
Automobile Ownership, 206
Autoregressive Integrated Moving Average (*see also* ARIMA) Analysis, 196
Aversion Behavior, 104–105

B
Bacteriology, 209
Banking Crises, 86
Basing Payments, 354
Behavioral Change, 127, 166, 427
Behavioral Economics, 421, 424, 427, 455

Beneficiary Identification, 107, 295
Beneficiary Registration, 107
Benefit Expenditure, 261
Benefit–Cost Ratio, 6
Benefits Package, 259
Bidirectional Granger-Causality, 34
Bill and Melinda Gates Foundation (*see also* BMGF), 455
Box–Cox Link Function, 414
Breast Cancer, 368–369, 511
Budget Allocation, 57, 62, 98, 117–118, 280, 311, 323, 356, 462
Budget Constraint, 23, 65, 77, 124, 186, 365, 375, 396, 461, 465, 469
Budgeting Process, 1, 57, 124, 314
Bundled Payments, 314, 317, 354
Burial Insurance, 235
Business Cycle, 60, 86–91, 128–131, 178, 187, 192–194, 202
Business Index, 98

C

Cambodia's Health Equity Funds (*see also* HEFs), 295, 297, 545
Canadian Agency for Drugs and Technologies in Health (*see also* CADTH), 458, 481
Capital Expenditure on Investments, 221, 223
Cataracts, 368–369
Center for Global Development (*see also* CGD), 85
Central Government Funding of Health Care, 235
Cerebrovascular Disease, 168
Cervical Cancer Mortality Rate, 523
Cession Contract, 262
Changes in Financing Health care, 39
Charity, 209
Child Immunization, 432
Child Stunting, 74
Childbirth, 202, 422, 424, 430–431, 539
Childcare, 430
Childhood Diseases, 103
Chile
Fondo Nacional de Salud (*see also* FONASA), 343
Universal Access with Explicit Guarantees (*see also* AUGE), 296
Ministry of Health of Chile, 352
China's New Cooperative Medical Scheme (*see also* NCMS), 298–300
Chronic Conditions, 41, 107, 321, 326, 334, 513, 524
Chronic Disability Payment System (*see also* CDPS), 332, 335
Chronic Illnesses, 115, 352, 537
Civil Unrest, 206
Clinical Classification System (*see also* CCS), 335
Clinical Commissioning Groups (*see also* CCG), 382
Clinical Risk Group (*see also* CRG), 324, 332–334,
Clinics, 191, 211, 240, 252, 256–257, 311–312, 349, 351, 432, 438
Clothing, 440
CMS–HCC Model, 330
Commission on Social Determinants of Health (*see also* CSDH), 490, 493–494, 541–542
Committee on the Costs of Medical Care (*see also* CCMC), 198
Commodity Stabilization Funds, 88
Community Health Centers (*see also* CHCs), 346
Community Health Insurance, 235, 459
Community Rating, 259, 262–263, 339
Compulsion, 275–277, 288, 301
Computable General Equilibrium (*see also* CGE) Model, 155, 165–171
Concentration Curve, 42–43, 502–503, 512–513, 523–526
Concentration Index (*see also* CI), 42–44, 499, 502, 512, 522–534

Conditional Cash Transfer (*see also* CCT), 421–436, 442–444, 544
Consolidated Health Economic Evaluation Reporting Standards (*see also* CHEERS) Statement, 371
Contingency Management, 433–434, 444
Contributory-based Entitlement Options, 292
Co-payments, 188
Copenhagen Consensus, 74
Core Government Budgets, 231–232
Corporate Tax, 269
Correlation Coefficient, 129
Corruption, 24–25, 77, 79, 91, 231, 235
Cost Collection, 404
Cost Containment, 8, 20, 331, 334, 344, 353–354
Cost of Health Services Utilization, 315
Cost of Illness Approach, 155
Cost Sharing, 363
Cost–Benefit Analysis (*see also* CBA), 371–376, 455
Cost-consequences Analysis, 372
Cost-effective Interventions, 73, 471
Cost-effectiveness (*see also* C-E) Threshold, 384
Cost-effectiveness Analysis (*see also* CEA), 56, 371–375, 453, 455, 460, 475
Cost-effectiveness Ratio, 373–374, 404, 458
Cost-minimization Analysis (*see also* CMA), 371–372
Cost–Utility Analysis (*see also* CUA), 371–372
Countercyclical Policy, 55, 86–88, 126, 129
Countercyclical Response, 88
Counter-cyclicality, 83
Cream Skimming, 230, 259–260
Credit Constraints, 88
Crisis Literature, 87
Crisis Pathways, 128
Crisis Typology, 86
Crop Insurance, 235
Cross-Country Analysis, 71
Cross-Country Regressions, 54, 68
Cross-subsidies, 260
Cross-subsidization, 225
Crowd-out Effect, 16, 23, 26, 68, 102, 425
Currency Crises, 86
Cyclicality of Health Expenditures, 2
Cyclicality of Health Spending, 88

D

Deadweight Losses, 228
Debt Sustainability, 67
Decennial Employment and Expenditures, 198
Decision-making, 40, 367
Delivery Immunization, 421, 522
Diarrhoea, 522
Delphi Method, 260
Democracy, 24
Demographic Adjusters, 322
Demographic Dividend, 109
Demographic Drag, 130
Demographic Health Surveys (*see also* DHS), 531
Demographic Models, 320
Demographic Profile, 110
Demographic Trajectories, 113
Demographic Transition, 49, 109
Demographic Waves, 48–49, 55, 113
Demographic/disease Changes, 208
Demographics, 18, 168–170, 316
Dependency Ratio, 41
Depression, 168, 190, 196, 368–369, 392
Descriptive Analyses, 40
Deterioration, 91
Development Assistance for health (*see also* DAH), 25, 55, 68
Development Partners (*see also* DPs), 75
Diabetes, 168, 327, 342, 385, 392, 532
Diagnoses-based Models, 320

Diagnosis-related Groups (*see also* DRGs)
DRG payments, 319, 328, 347
DRG reimbursement, 417
Diagnostic Cost Group (*see also* DCG), 320, 345
Diagnostic Testing, 209
DICE Model, 169
Direct Link between Payments and Outcomes, 7
Direct Productivity Increases, 50
Direct Taxation, 290
Disability Adjusted Life Years (*see also* DALYs), 156, 366
Disease Control Priorities Project (*see also* DCPP), 460, 478
Disease Screening, 432
Distributional Cost-Effectiveness Analysis (*see also* DCEA), 475
DOHA Declaration, 160
DOHA Protocol, 161

E

East Asia and the Pacific (*see also* EAP), 36, 80
Ebola Epidemic, 1, 99
Ebola Outbreak, 98
Ebola Response, 102
Economic Burden of Disease, 50
Economic Committee for Health Care Products (*see also* CEPS), 389
Economic Cycles and Spending, 8
Economic Effects, 97, 157, 165, 169
Economic Evaluation in Health Care, 80
Economic Management, 115
Economic Sustainability, 65
Economics of Health Insurance, 224
Education, 2, 4, 11, 41, 48, 188, 194, 206, 218, 342, 365, 389, 430, 437, 440, 491, 541
Efficiency Analysis, 78
Efficiency Gains, 55
Elastic Demand, 260
Elasticity, 131
Eligibility Assessment, 107
Environmental Aspects, 42
Epidemiology, 17, 41
Episode Risk Groups (*see also* ERGs), 332–335
Episode Treatment Groups (*see also* ETGs), 333
Equitable Financing, 20
Equity Implications, 456
Equity in Health Care, 490–492, 525–526
Essential Health Benefits (*see also* EHB), 381
Ethical Confidentiality, 255
Ethical Dilemmas, 376
Ethnic Fractionalization, 73
Ethnicity, 342
Ethno-linguistic Heterogeneity, 24
Europe and Central Asia (*see also* ECA), 18, 63
European Union (*see also* EU), 107, 510, 541
Evidence of Health Inequalities, 505
Evidence-based Priority Setting, 64, 107
Evidence-based Responses, 64
Excess Cost Growth (*see also* ECG), 39, 178
Excess Growth (*see also* EG), 31
Panel Data Methods, 34
Excess Health Expenditure Growth, 131
Expansions and Contractions, 60
Experience Rating, 261
Exponential Conditional Mean (*see also* ECM) model, 414
External Cross-currents, 192
External Donor Funding, 223
Extrapolation, 190

F

Facility-based Delivery, 421
Failure Time and Censoring Time, 408
Family Planning, 421
Federal and State Regulatory Requirements, 39

Fee-for-Service (*see also* FFS)
FFS payment systems, 346
FFS reimbursement, 348
FFS-only mechanism, 348
Female Representation, 24
Financial Access, 74, 127, 291, 299
Financial Hardship, 75, 232, 268, 517
Financial Incentives, 421
Financial Resources, 340
Financial Risk in Health Care, 217
Financial Services, 206
Financial Sustainability, 16, 65
Fiscal Austerity, 63
Fiscal Burdens, 205
Fiscal Envelope, 124
Fiscal Expansion, 67
Fiscal Inertia, 184
Fiscal Policy, 131
Fiscal Position/space, 41
Fiscal Space Analysis (*see also* FSA), 14, 59
Fiscal Space Assessment, 71
Fiscal Space for Health, 84, 132
Fiscal Sustainability, 63, 132
FONASA Payment System, 344
Food Basket, 440
Food Expenditure, 440
Food Subsidies, 295
Forecasting, 178
Foreign Aid, 24
Fragmented Delivery and Financing, 41
Framework for Uncertainty, Negotiation and Distribution (*see also* FUND) Model, 169
Free-riding, 261
Front Page Treatments, 39
Fungibility, 67

G

Gender Inequality, 73
General Circulation Models (*see also* GCMs), 169
Generalized Cost-Effectiveness Analysis, 398
Generalized Linear Model (*see also* GLM), 414
Geographic Area, 342
Geographic Units, 182
Geographical Barriers, 545
Germany, 386
Gini Index, 505
Global Assessment Tool, 97
Global Disease Burden, 221
Global Economic Crisis (*see also* GEC), 15
Global Health Care Payment Systems, 311
Global Health Care, 217
Global Health Partnerships, 75
Global Health Protection Fund, 132
Global Health Spending Trends, 2
Global Patterns of Health Spending, 15
Global Trend, 27, 30
Global Vulnerability Assessment, 97
Globalization, 155, 157
Governance, 7, 9, 56, 71, 96, 118, 126
Government Agency, 315
Government Budget Constraints, 65
Government Budget, 25, 28, 69, 106, 117, 188, 279–281
Government Efficiency, 71, 77
Government Health Expenditures (*see also* GHE)
GHE cycles, 119
Growth rate in GHE, 29, 63
Income elasticity of GHE, 35–36
Government Interventions, 217, 224
Government Mandates, 39
Government Priorities and Policies, 7
Government Responsiveness, 100
Government Social Expenditure, 52
Government's Budgeting, 70
Government-subsidized Public Hospitals, 240
Greenhouse Gas Reductions, 167
Gross Domestic Product (*see also* GDP)
expenditures as a share of GDP, 177
GDP fluctuations, 187

GDP growth rate, 18
GDP-neutral impact, 167
real GDP growth, 204
Grossman Model, 472
Growth Elasticity of Poverty (*see also* GEP), 133
Growth elasticity of poverty (*see also* GEP), 42
Concentration Index, 42
Polity or International Country Risk Guidance (*see also* ICRG) Index, 43
Country Policy and Institutional Assessment (*see also* CPIA) Index, 43
Growth in Health Spending, 8
Growth in Real Health Expenditures, 195
Growth Models, 164
Growth Surges, 196
Growth Trends, 1
Guilds, 209

H

H1N1 (Swine Flu) Pandemic, 166
Hazards Regression Model, 408
Health and Economic Growth, 2
Health and Nutritional Expenditure
Health and Social Protection, 56
Health Care Coordination, 341
Health Care Cost Estimation, 412
Health Care Disparities, 545
Health Care Financing Policy, 2
Health Care Financing, 51, 363
Health Care Funding, 217
Health Care Payment, 217
Health Care Providers, 256
Health Care Resources, 74, 519
Health Care Sector, 405
Health Care Use, 522
Health Crises, 96
Health Economic Analysis, 164
Health Emergencies, 96
Health Financing Policy, 69, 271
Health Financing, 96, 217
Health Funding, 66
Health Gains, 5, 122, 167, 341, 383–384, 454, 46
Health in All Policies, 541
Health Inequalities, 513
Health Insurance Act of 2006, 248
Health Insurance Organizations, 254
Health Insurance Programs, 226, 246, 256, 298, 336
Health Outcomes, 6
Health Plan, 328
Health related Poverty, 55
Health Sector Investments, 1
Health Sector Reforms, 63
Health Spending and Economic Crisis, 2
Health Spending, 8,178
Health System Factors, 40
Health System Reform, 268
Health System Resilience, 103
Health System Vulnerability, 95
Health Systems' Complexity, 341
Health Technology assessment (*see also* HTA), 81
Health Workforce, 96, 138, 520
Healthcare Payments Systems, 311
Health-Growth Nexus, 11
Health-related Quality of Life (*see also* HRQoL), 466
Health-seeking Behavior, 93
Health-specific Knowledge, 120
Healthy Diet, 168
Heart Attack, 369
Hierarchical Condition Category (*see also* HCC) Model, 320, 330
High-Income Countries (*see also* HICs), 20, 35, 113
Hippocratic Oath, 178
HIV/AIDS
AIDS-related Mortality, 53
decline in HIV rates, 540
explosion of HIV/AIDS, 6
high prevalence of HIV/AIDS, 57

HIV screening, 432
HIV testing, 421
HIV/AIDS prevention and treatment, 47
medication for HIV, 161
scaled-up investments in HIV/AIDS programs, 75
Hospital Cost Functions, 415
Hospital Cost Modeling, 415
Household-level Factors, 127
Housing Characteristics, 120, 322
Housing, 440
HPV Vaccine Coverage Rate, 523
Human Capital Accumulation, 48
Human Capital Formation, 52
Human Capital Investment, 48
Human Capital Theory, 48
Human Capital, 4
Human Development Index, 98
Human Development, 4, 52
Human opportunity index (*see also* HOI), 122
Human Resources for Health, 101
Human Rights Perspectives, 62
Human Security, 272
Hypertension, 342

I

Illness-based Indicators, 354
Imitation Effect, 18
Immigration Status, 342
Impact Evaluation (*see also* IE), 41, 53, 123
Impact of Fiscal Capacity, 91
Impact of National Income, 91
Imperfect Monitoring, 283
Incentive Effectiveness, 427
Incentives for Sterilization, 430
Income Elasticity of Health Expenditures, 133
Income Elasticity of Total Health Expenditure, 35
Income Growth, 114
Income Tax, 269, 281, 298
Incremental Cost-effectiveness Ratio (*see also* ICER), 373
India's RSBY Program, 288
Indigence, 342
Individual Budgets, 188
Industrial Revolution, 210
Inelastic Demand, 260
Inequalities in Health and Health Care, 491
Inequities, 56, 120, 123, 222, 429, 442, 489–493, 526, 544–549
Infant Mortality, 206
Inflationary Financing, 67
Influenza Pandemics, 166
Information Asymmetry, 41, 230, 254
Institute of Medicine (*see also* IOM), 378
Institutional and Organizational Context, 56
Institutional and Knowledge Issues, 40
Institutions and Governance, 7, 88
Insurance Competition, 270
Insurance Coverage, 363
Insurance Death Spirals, 230
Insurance Effect, 41, 243
Insurance Premiums, 239
Insurance-based Funding, 232
Integrated Assessment Models (*see also* IAMs), 168
International Labor Organization (*see also* ILO), 196
Intrinsic–Extrinsic Dichotomy, 425
Ischemic Heart Disease (*see also* IHD), 168
Keynesian Theory, 85

L

Labor Market Effects, 229
Labor Market Participation, 61
Labor Market, 230
Labor Mobility, 73
Labor Productivity, 53
Lags, 177–178, 187, 194

Latin America and the Caribbean (LAC), 18, 36
Less Developed Countries (*see also* LDC), 492
Life Expectancy, 39, 156
Life-saving Interventions, 109
Linear Regression Model, 407
Literacy, 206
Literacy, 5, 41, 119, 206
Logarithmic Transformations, 413
Longevity, 207
Long-range Planning, 181
Long-run Growth Trends, 194
Long-Run Trends, 196
Long-term Cost, 41
Long-term Planning, 125
Loss Aversion, 426
Low-Birthweight Infants, 369
Lower-Middle Income Countries (*see also* LMICs), 35
Low-Income Countries (*see also* LICs), 35, 113

M

Macro Analysis, 47
Macro Effects, 230
Macro Evidence, 9, 48
Policy Sequencing, 9
Macroeconomic Growth, 54
Macroeconomic Stability, 67
Macroeconomics, 155
Macroeconomists, 48
Solow Economic Growth Model, 48
Macro-Fiscal Constraints, 3
Macro-Fiscal Environment, 60
Macro-Fiscal Objectives, 66
Mainstream Public Finance Theory, 11
Malaria, 13, 103
Male Sex Workers, 436
Malnutrition, 74
Malpractice Litigation, 42
Management Information Systems (*see also* MIS), 106
Mandates, 39, 188, 237–239
Marginal Payments, 314
Market Distortion, 231
Market Failure, 261
Marketplace Issues, 41
Maternal and Childhood Nutrition, 74
Maternal Mortality, 224
Maternal Nutrition and Health, 53
Mean Absolute Percentage Error (*see also* MAPE), 203
Medical Care System, 188
Medical Care, 38
Medical Costs, 177, 207–209, 411
Medical Nihilism, 209
Medical Products, 96
Medical Provision, 115
Medical Spending, 178
Medical Tourism, 162
Medical Underwriting, 261
Medication Adherence, 421, 433
Medium-term Expenditure Framework (*see also* MTEF), 16, 132
Methodological Barriers, 80
Mexico's Demographic and SES Changes, 441
Micro Analysis, 47
Micro Evidence, 9
Micro Loans and Savings, 235
Microeconometric Studies, 50
Middle East and North Africa (*see also* MENA), 36
Middle-income Countries (*see also* MICs), 94, 113
Millenium Development Goals (*see also* MDGs)
  MDG agenda, 58
  MDG health targets, 82
  MDG targets, 21
Ministries of Health and Finance, 1
Ministry of Civil Affairs, 299
Ministry of Health (*see also* MOH), 65
Ministry of Planning and Finance (*see also* MPF), 65

Mitigation of Crisis Effects, 107
Mitigation Policy Options, 127
Monetary Units, 371
Monitoring Changes in Health Status, 404
Monitoring Tools, 64
Monolithic Systems, 250
Moral Hazard, 230, 254
Moral Pricing Transparency, 41
Morbidity and Mortality, 42, 103, 165, 211, 355, 387, 444
Multi-criteria Decision Analysis (*see also* MCDA), 474
Multi-pillar System, 250
Multiple Technology Appraisal (*see also* MTA), 382
Multiplicitous Agency, 76
Multispectral Coordination, 124

N

National and Global Health Expenditure, 202
National Board of Health and Welfare (*see also* NBHW), 392
National Comprehensive Cancer Network (*see also* NCCN), 367
National Health Accounts (*see also* NHA), 125
National Health Expenditures (*see also* NHE), 188, 194
National Health Insurance Scheme, 283
National Health Insurance System (*see also* NHIS), 340
National Health Service (*see also* NHS), 81
National Institute for Clinical Excellence (*see also* NICE), 81
National Institute for Health and Care Excellence (*see also* NICE)
National Treatment, 164
Neoclassical Growth Model, 48
Neoclassical Theory, 85
Netherlands
    Dunning Report, 394
    Dutch policymakers, 248
Dutch's health insurance system, 248
New Rural Cooperative Medical Scheme (*see also* NRCMS), 352
Non-Communicable Diseases (*see also* NCDs)
    NCD burden, 7, 9, 38
    NCD-related health effects, 158
prevalence of NCDs, 41
Non-Contributory-based Entitlement Options, 292
Non-Demographic Factors, 17
Nongovernmental Organizations, 68
Non-Health Costs, 473
Non-Health Effects, 456
Non-Income Factors, 37
Non-Parametric Estimators, 409
Non-Profit Organization, 378
Nonrandom Cost Variation, 312
Non-Universal Social Insurance, 228
Non-Workers, 226
Norms and Standards, 41
North America (*see also* NAC), 22, 36–37, 91
Nudge, 427
Nutrition, 44, 158–159, 438

O

Odds Ratio (*see also* OR), 497
Official Development Assistance (*see also* ODA), 36
Ordinary Least Squares (see also OLS), 325, 407, 411
One Health Tool, 73, 471
Operations Research, 220
Optimal Risk Adjustment, 318
Oral Rehydration Therapy, 44
Oregon Alternative Payment Methodology (*see also* APM), 346
Organisation for Economic Co-Operation and Development (*see also* OECD)
    OECD countries, 15, 23, 33–39, 193, 208, 233, 329, 528–230

OECD dataset, 179
OECD health data, 179
OECD health expenditure, 201
OECD structure, 179
Organizational Barriers, 540
Organizational Subgroups, 186
Organized Delivery System (*see also* ODS), 340
Outbreak of NDM1 in the UK, 162
Out-of-pocket (*see also* OOP)
out-of-pocket expenditures, 21
out-of-pocket payments, 518
out-of-pocket spending, 36
Output Gap, 134
Over Insurance, 230

P

PAGE Model, 169
Palliative or Extended Care, 217
Panel Data Analyses, 38
Pathology, 209
Patient Advocacy, 255
Patient Protection and Affordable Care Act (*see also* ACA), 283
Patient Protection and Affordable Care Act (*see also* ACA), 380
Patient–Healer Relationship, 253
Pay-for-Performance (*see also* P4P)
P4P measures, 347
P4P payments, 347
P4P programs, 329
P4P schemes, 329
Payment for Results (*see also* PFR), 344
Performance-based Financing (*see also* PBF), 82, 286
Personal Income Growth, 39
Pharmaceutical Benefits Advisory Committee (*see also* PBAC), 458
Pharmaceutical Companies, 210
Pharmaceutical Management Agency (*see also* PHARMAC), 458
Pharmaceutical Prescription-based Models, 321
Pharmacy, 312
Pharmacy-based Cost Groups (*see also* PCGs), 321
Physical Capital, 4, 47–50
Physical Environment and Infrastructure, 42
Pilot Scale, 53
Plan Nacer, 351
Policy Formulation, 21
Policy Implications, 178
Policymakers, 1
Political Economy, 64
Political Promises, 241
Pooled Ordinary-Least Squares (*see also* POLS), 410
Pooled Sources of Funding, 231
Pooling, 20
Poor Cognitive Development, 74
Population Affiliation, 273, 298
Population Attributable Risk (*see also* PAR), 501
Population Dynamics, 109
Population Size, 47
Poverty and Inequality, 42
Poverty Headcount, 42
Poverty Reduction Strategy Paper (*see also* PRSP), 120
Poverty Reduction, 4, 8, 54, 115
Prediction Measure (*see also* CPM), 326
Premium-based Risk Adjustment Systems, 315
Prenatal Care, 353, 421–422, 531
Preston Curve, 44
Primary Care Activity Level (*see also* PCAL), 330
Primary Care Trusts (*see also* PCTs), 382
Primary Care Trusts, 322
Primary Deficit, 41
Principles of Economic Evaluation, 456
Prioritization and Consolidation, 23
Priority Setting in Health Care, 78
Private Insurance, 228
Private Voluntary Insurance, 237

Privatization, 4
Procyclical Policy, 84, 129
Procyclical/Countercyclical Policy, 86
Productivity, 47
Programme-Budgeting and Marginal Analysis (*see also* PBMA), 464
Pro-rich, 240
Prospective Payments, 314
Protocols Compliance, 345
Provider Density, 41
Provider Payment Methods (*see also* PPMs), 268, 285–286
Psychology, 220
Public and Private Financing, 180
Public Budget Allocations, 68
Public Expenditure Review (*see also* PER), 14, 55–56
Public Expenditure Tracking Survey (*see also* PETS), 57–58, 66–70, 78–80
Public Finance Management, 25, 56, 60, 126
Public Finance Theory, 62
Public Financial Management (*see also* PFM), 78, 301–302
Public Goods, 262
Public Health Impacts, 167
Public Health Insurance, 227
Public Health Risks, 156
Public Health Services, 44
Public Mandatory Insurance, 237
Public Sector Performance, 76
Purchasing Reforms, 76
Purse Strings, 254

Q

Qualified Health Plans (*see also* QHPs), 380
Quality Adjusted Life Expectancy (QALE), 365
Quality Adjusted Life-Year (*see also* QALY), 365
Quality of Care, 42, 71, 120, 241, 254, 288, 329, 341–346, 355
Quantitative Analyses, 40
Quantitative Assessment, 97
Quantitative Service Delivery Survey (*see also* QSDS), 58

R

Random Effects (*see also* RE) Models, 410
Random Noise, 192
Randomized Controlled Trials (*see also* RCTs), 458
Reduction in Emaciation, 440
Regression Models, 323
Regression Parameters, 410
Regulation, 41, 158, 160, 162, 230, 259, 377
Rehabilitation, 217–218, 263, 392
Reimbursable Drug, 389
Reimbursement Levels, 403
Reinsurance, 262
Relative Index of Inequality (*see also* RII), 505
Reprioritization, 55
Reproductive, Maternal, Newborn, and Child Health (*see also* RMNCH), 73
Resource Allocation Working Part (*see also* RAWP), 322
Resource Allocation, 2, 11, 60–76, 122, 217, 220, 279, 293, 322–323, 336–343, 363–369, 454–464, 476–481, 496, 520–521
Resource Tracking System, 70
Results-based Financing (*see also* RBF), 7, 270, 286, 297, 346
Retirees, 226
Revenue Raising, 275
Revenue–Expenditure Ratio, 19
Revised International Health Regulations, 156
RICE Model, 169
Risk Adjusters, 317
Risk Adjustment, 248, 311
Risk Equalization, 262

Risk Mitigation, 107
Risk Premium, 238
Risk Rating, 263
Risk Segregation, 263
Risk selection Incentives, 317
Risk Selection, 248, 263
Risk Sharing, 263
Role of Health in Economic Development, 4
Rotavirus, 475
Rwanda's Community Based Health Insurance (*see also* CBHI), 298

S
Scarce Households, 244
Scarce Public Resources, 80
Sea-level Rise (*see also* SLR), 169
Secretary of Health and Human Services (*see also* HHS), 380
Sector Rationalization, 20
Self Insurance, 263
Service Capacity, 41
Service Delivery Indicator Survey (*see also* SDI), 58
Service Delivery Network, 120
Severe Acute Respiratory Syndrome (*see also* SARS), 156
Singapore's Multi-Pillar Health Insurance, 251
Single Technology Appraisal (*see also* STA), 382
Single-Parent Households or Orphanage, 53
Skewness, 413
Skilled Birth Attendance, 103
Slope Index of Inequality (*see also* SII), 504
Smoking Cessation, 421
Social Accounting Matrix (*see also* SAM), 165
Social Cohesion, 272
Social Gradient, 489
Social Health Insurance (*see also* SHI), 263, 270, 277
Social Security Systems, 64
Social Status, 342
Social Value Judgments, 376
Socio-economic and Individual Determinants, 40–42
Socioeconomic Benefits, 40
Socioeconomic Status (*see also* SES), 489
Sociology, 220
Socio-political Risks, 24
Solvent Demand, 260
South Asia, 36
Sovereign Debt Crises, 86
Staff Absence Survey (*see also* SAS), 58
Streamlining Expenditures, 1
Suboptimal Development Path, 232, 234
Sub-Saharan Africa, 22
Subsidies and Risk-Pooling, 188
Subsidizing Basic Care, 244
Supplier-Induced Demand, 41
Supply-side Funding, 302
Survey-based Models, 321
Sustainable Development (*see also* SDGs), 5, 99
System Vulnerability,
Systematic Sector Diagnostics, 126
System-level Factors, 127

T
Taskforce on Innovative International Health Financing for Health Systems, 21
Tax Collection Capacity, 297
Tax Reduction, 61
Tax Revenue, 41
Technical and Allocative Efficiency, 230
Technological Advancements, 64
Technological Dynamism, 184
Technological Innovation, 363
Technology Development and Diffusion, 41
Technology Diffusion, 38

Temporal Units, 182
Thailand's National Health Security Office (*see also* NHSO), 288
Tobacco Control, 158
Total Fertility Ratio (*see also* TFR), 41
Tracking Service Utilization
Tracking Surveys, 79
Trade Agreements, 163
Trade in Services, 161
Trade Liberalization, 4
Transaction Costs, 206
Transitory Noise, 194
Transparency and Accountability, 271
Transportation, 191, 396, 521
Trends in Health Expenditure, 28
Trends in Health Status, 8
Triple Transition, 30
Truncated Demand, 261
Tuberculosis (*see also* TB), 103, 212, 342, 433, 475, 547
Two-way Causality, 52

U

Uncertainty of Outcomes, 254
Unconditional Cash Transfers (*see also* UCTs), 423
Under Insurance, 230
Underdevelopment, 4
Market-Oriented Reforms, 4
Underfunding, 231
Underwriting, 263
Unemployment, 87, 94, 158, 278, 322, 337, 521, 540
United Kingdom (*see also* UK)
  UK's National Health Service (*see also* NHS), 163
  UK's synthetic indices method, 322
  UK's Transport Sector Emissions, 167
United States (*see also* US)
American Recovery and Reinvestment Act (*see also* ARRA), 380
National Bureau of Economic Research's (*see also* NBER's), 86
  US centers for Medicare and Medicaid Services (*see also* CMS), 330
  US Congress and Senate, 230
  US Department of Health and Human Services (*see also* HHS) 340
  US health insurance marketplace system, 326
  US Medicare program, 211, 339
  US office of the actuary, 191
  US society of actuaries, 335
Universal Coverage Scheme (*see also* UCS), 293
Universal Declaration of Human Rights, 272
Universal Health Care, 217, 233, 506, 515, 519, 526
Universal Health Coverage (*see also* UHC)
  financing for UHC, 302
  ideology of UHC, 270
  UHC goals, 301
Universal Primary Health Care, 76
Upper-Middle-Income Countries (*see also* UMICs), 35
Urbanization, 170
User Fees, 238, 244, 271, 294–297, 422, 517, 545

V

Vaccination, 44, 432
Vaccines and Technology, 96
Valuation of life years (*see also* VLY), 6
Value for Money, 10
Value-added Tax, 269
Value-for-Money Dimension, 28
Variable Lags, 194
Virtual Revolution, 209
Voluntary Health Insurance (*see also* VHI), 275
Vulnerability Assessment Framework, 95

W
Wages, 57
Water and Sanitation, 48
Willingness to Pay (*see also* WTP), 263
World Bank Group
Development Impact Evaluation Initiative (*see also* DIME), 122
Independent Evaluation Group (*see also* IEG), 53
World Development Indicators (*see also* WDI), 125
World Development Report, 2
World Health Organization (*see also* WHO)
WHO Constitution, 272
WHO Global Health Observatory, 135
WHO's Commission on Macro Economics and Health, 2
WHO's emergency, 96
WHO's health system, 96
WHO's NHA, 134
WHO's toolkit, 96
World Trade Organization (*see also* WTO)
General Agreement on Trade in Health Services (*see also* GATS), 161
Trade Related Intellectual Property Rights (*see also* TRIPS), 160

Y
Youth Dependency, 114

Z
Zero-sum Effect, 68